www.harcourt-international.com

Bringing you products from all Harcourt Health Sciences companies including Baillière Tindall, Churchill Livingstone, Mosby and W.B. Saunders

- ▶ **Browse** for latest information on new books, journals and electronic products

- ▶ **Search** for information on over 20 000 published titles with full product information including tables of contents and sample chapters

- ▶ **Keep up to date** with our extensive publishing programme in your field by registering with eAlert or requesting postal updates

- ▶ **Secure online ordering** with prompt delivery, as well as full contact details to order by phone, fax or post

- ▶ **News** of special features and promotions

If you are based in the following countries, please visit the country-specific site to receive full details of product availability and local ordering information

USA: www.harcourthealth.com

Canada: www.harcourtcanada.com

Australia: www.harcourt.com.au

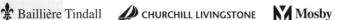 Baillière Tindall    CHURCHILL LIVINGSTONE   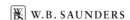 Mosby   W.B. SAUNDERS

The Treatment of Pain with Chinese Herbs and Acupuncture

痛證中醫藥治療

To my professor, Professor Shi Zhongan
To my wife and children

For Churchill Livingstone:

Publishing Manager, Health Professions: Inta Ozols
Project Development Manager: Dinah Thom
Project Manager: Jane Dingwall
Designer: George Ajayi

The Treatment of Pain with Chinese Herbs and Acupuncture

痛證中醫藥治療

EDITED BY

Sun Peilin MD

Professor of Medicine, Guangxi College of Traditional Chinese Medicine and Jiangxi College of Traditional Chinese Medicine, China; Professor in Traditional Chinese Medicine, Jing Ming College of Oriental Medicine, Belgium

FOREWORDS BY

Shi Zhongan MD

Formerly Professor of Medicine, Faculty of TCM Literature, Nanjing University of Traditional Chinese Medicine, Nanjing, China

Steven K. H. Aung MD FAAFP

Associate Clinical Professor, Departments of Medicine and Family Medicine, University of Alberta; Adjunct Professor of Extension, University of Alberta: Associate Clinical Professor, New York University College of Dentistry; President, Canadian Medical Acupuncture Society; President, World Natural Medicine Foundation; President College of Integrated Medicine

Peter Deadman BAc

Editor of the Journal of Chinese Medicine, Brighton, UK

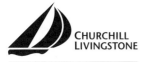

CHURCHILL LIVINGSTONE

EDINBURGH LONDON NEW YORK PHILADELPHIA ST LOUIS SYDNEY TORONTO 2002

CHURCHILL LIVINGSTONE
An imprint of Harcourt Publishers Limited

© Harcourt Publishers Limited 2002

✎ is a registered trademark of Harcourt Publishers
Limited

The right of Sun Peilin to be identified as editor of this work
has been asserted by him in accordance with the Copyright,
Designs and Patents Act 1988.

First published 2002

ISBN 0 443 07127 6

British Library Cataloguing in Publication Data
A catalogue record for this book is available from the British
Library

Library of Congress Cataloging in Publication Data
A catalog record for this book is available from the Library
of Congress

Note
Medical knowledge is constantly changing. As new
information becomes available, changes in treatment,
procedures, equipment and the use of drugs become
necessary. The editors, contributors and publishers have
taken care to ensure that the information given in this text is
accurate and up to date. However, readers are strongly
advised to confirm that the information, especially with
regard to drug usage, complies with the latest legislation and
standards of practice.

The
publisher's
policy is to use
**paper manufactured
from sustainable forests**

Printed in China

Contents

Contributors

Primary contributors

Shen Xiaoxiong MD PhD
Research Scientist, Department of Endocrinology,
University of California, Los Angeles, USA

Yao Fengli MD
Former Professor of Medicine, Beijing University of
TCM, Beijing, China

Yang Yifan MD MSc
Private Practitioner and Lecturer, The Netherlands;
Former Lecturer in Medicine, Beijing University of
TCM, Beijing, China

Jiang Hongbing MD
Professor and Director of the Institute for Basic
Education, Guangxi College of TCM, Guangxi, China

Secondary contributors

Yang Guohua MD
Professor of Medicine, Beijing University of TCM and
Wang Jing Hospital, Beijing, China

Sun Yijun MB
Lecturer in Medicine, The International Training
Centre, Beijing University of TCM, Beijing, China

Ma Liangxiao MB
Lecturer in Medicine, The International Training
Centre, Beijing University of TCM, Beijing, China

Forewords

Foreword by Shi Zhongan

Traditional Chinese Medicine (TCM), one of the most important components of Chinese culture, has a long-standing history and consists of a profound and extensive source of knowledge. It has made a great contribution to the well-being and prosperity of the Chinese people. At present, TCM is also becoming well known outside China, playing a unique role in the health of people of other nationalities.

The key point of TCM is treatment based on differentiation. Differentiation involves a search for the pathology of a condition by systematically examining the patient's signs and symptoms, as well as other clinical information. The treatment utilises either Chinese herbal medicine or acupuncture, or a combination of both, so as to eliminate the causative factors and alleviate the pain.

Pain is the primary syndrome, and it occurs during the everyday life of most people. Hence the search for effective treatments for pain control has been one of the main medical tasks for all practitioners of different modalities over the centuries. Some valuable experiences and excellent techniques are recorded in the voluminous literature, and yet no single TCM monograph that deals systematically with this topic has been published to date. From this point of view, the compilation of such a text is of great significance, which could prove valuable for TCM practice.

Sun Peilin, one of my students, is modest, full of curiosity and eager to learn. Whilst compiling his previously published book on Bi syndrome, he became aware of research findings on pain treatment by both TCM and Western medicine and began to collect this literature. Ten years ago, he emigrated to Europe but our correspondence and academic exchange have never ceased. He never felt ashamed to ask questions and always tried his best to increase his theoretical knowledge and improve his clinical practice. Four years ago, he started to compile this book on pain treatment in English, but as he was so busy with his lecturing and daily clinical practice he found it impossible to complete such a huge work alone. So he has invited some other professors and colleagues of TCM who share the same interests to collaborate in this book and add their considerable clinical experience on pain treatment.

The first part of this book describes in detail the aetiology and pathology of pain, the differentiation of pain and the therapeutic characteristics and principles. The following chapters deal with pain syndromes in 46 areas of the body. The discussion in each chapter covers the general characteristics, related disorders in Western medicine, aetiology, pathology, the general principle of treatment, Chinese herbal and acupuncture treatment and case histories. In particular, there are interesting and practical explanations and modifications given for the herbal and acupuncture treatments. This book should be a valuable reference for the practice, teaching and research of both TCM and Western medicine, and I congratulate the authors on its publication. It is my pleasure to write a foreword for this book.

Shi Zhongan

序

　　中医学源远流长，学科丰富，是中华民族优秀文化的重要组成部分，对中华民族的生息繁衍作出过卓越的贡献。目前，中医学正在走向世界，为世界人类的健康而发挥独特作用。

　　中医学之菁华，荟萃于辨证施治。所谓辨证就是系统分析，谨守病机；所谓施治就是或药或针，去除病因，减少痛苦。

　　痛证是人类在生存发展过程中所遇到的首要病证，而寻求对痛证的有效的治疗一直是历代特别是当代各科医生研究的主要内容之一，其研究结果也散落于浩瀚的文献之中，缺乏系统论述的专著。因此，编著中医药对痛证的治疗方面的书籍具有十分重大的理论意义和实践价值。

　　我的学生孙培林谦虚好学，善于钻研，他在出版有关痹证治疗专著期间，就已开始关注中西医对痛证治疗方面的研究成果和资料收集。十年之前，他虽移居海外，但与我在学术上仍然保持良好的联系，虚心请教，孜孜不忘提高自己的中医理论和实践水平。四年前他就开始此书的英文纂写，可是他的诊务和教学十分繁忙，无法个人完成此巨著。于是，他又联合组织了一批志同道合，有一定临床和教学经验的大学教授和医生共同参与编纂。经期年努力，初稿终于完成。随后，孙培林一人又数易其稿，统一体例，修订不足，芟除芜杂，完善施治，而成此书，其难度可想而知。

　　是书首章详尽论述痛证的病因病机，辨证以及治疗特点和原则，随后章节广罗各类常见痛证凡四十六例，一一详析。各证述以概述，现代医学相关疾病，病因病机，理法方药针贯珠一线，特别是随证加减，更是实用明了，实可为中医和中西医结合的医、教、研各方面所借镜。行将付梓问世，值得庆贺。欣喜之余，乐为之序。

沈仲宽　教授

南京中医药大学

2002 夏

Foreword by Steven K. H. Aung

Pain is a major subject in any medicine. According to the distinguished physician Albert Schweitzer: 'We all must die. But if I can save him from days of torture, that is what I feel is my great and ever new privilege. Pain is a more terrible lord of mankind than even death himself.' Therefore, it is extremely important that we thoroughly understand the subject of pain as well as the proper approach to it. In the early 1990s, the International Association for the Study of Pain was formed by physicians who were vitally interested in looking into the deeper understanding of medical pain control. The association, which currently has over 6000 members from over 100 countries, has annual conferences on pain management in various venues around the world.

Presently, total pain control remains a constant challenge for medical and primary health care providers, especially with respect to safe, natural and inexpensive pain management modalities for the benefit of patients everywhere.

Dr Sun Peilin, who presently resides in Belgium, graduated from the Suzhou Medical Academy in 1981. He has served in Yangzhong People's Hospital as a physician and in 1990 obtained a master's degree in medicine at Nanjing University of Traditional Chinese Medicine. He has served as a lecturer in the Nanjing Acupuncture Training Center as well as the WHO Nanjing Collaborative Center for Traditional

Medicine. At present, he is associated with the Jiangxi College of Traditional Chinese Medicine and Guangxi College of Traditional Chinese Medicine. He has written more than 30 articles on various aspects of TCM.

Dr Sun has carefully written this present book on pain, encompassing aetiology, pathogenesis and differentiation of syndromes. He takes a step-by-step approach to TCM pain management. This book is comprehensive, dealing with various types of physiological and pathological pain in detail, which is a valuable part of this book. I would say that his work is well done and will be a suitable reference for those who are interested in TCM pain control, especially in the areas of acupuncture and herbal medicine.

In my opinion, Dr Sun has done the best that he can to share his valuable knowledge and experience with all of us around the world to help in our quest to control pain. May we all learn the special techniques to help our patients be free from pain. Most of all, we must never forget about considering total pain, which encompasses the body, mind and spirit. The most important thing is to be compassionate to our dear, suffering patients. Dr Sun's book will no doubt help us in this worthwhile direction.

Steven K. H. Aung

Foreword by Peter Deadman

The last 25 years have witnessed a phenomenal growth in interest in Traditional Chinese Medicine. Although many factors have played a part in this, a single event may be seen to encapsulate the moment when acupuncture in particular was brought into the spotlight. The journalist, James Reston, accompanying President Nixon to China in 1972, wrote a front-page article in the *New York Times*, telling of his emergency appendectomy. Chinese doctors used acupuncture to control Reston's post-surgical pain, and his recovery was swift. Intrigued by Reston's report, doctors began visiting Chinese hospitals to observe Oriental medicine being practised. The hospitals responded with training programmes which soon drew professionals from other Western countries.

It is appropriate that this famous event demonstrated the ability of acupuncture to ease and control pain, as its role in the treatment of pain has probably aroused more interest within the orthodox medical community than any other aspect of Traditional Chinese Medicine. Even relatively untrained acupuncturists may observe significant results in the clinic, since at the most basic level the local insertion of a needle into a site of pain can offer relief. Furthermore, both the effects and the mechanism of acupuncture analgesia are exciting subjects for research. Perhaps unsurprisingly, these factors have contributed, within the orthodox medical community, to the idea that the treatment of pain is relatively simple and empirical, and that the basic practice of needling local and adjacent sites, whether chosen on the basis of traditional acupuncture points or modern trigger point theory, is all that Chinese medicine usefully has to offer. The rest, the centuries of traditional theory, can be dispensed with as irrelevant and out-dated.

Only those unaware of the true depth and richness of Traditional Chinese Medicine are likely to hold such ideas. The insertion of needles or the prescribing of a mixture of herbs is the final act in a refined process of analysis and discrimination, and the most effective treatment can only be determined by this process. Central to this process is the understanding of the theory of ben (root) and biao (branch or manifestation). The same manifestation (biao) may have different roots (ben), for example pain in the face may be due to heat or cold, excess or deficiency, external environmental factors or internal disharmony. If treatment only focuses on treating the symptom, the effect of treatment will be diminished, being less effective and more temporary. By using the traditional methods of diagnosis, differentiation and treatment selection, true Traditional Chinese Medicine seeks to combine treatment of the root cause or disorder with treatment of its symptoms (manifestations). By treating the root, any underlying disease may be helped or cured and treatment of the symptom will be supported and amplified. Wherever possible, the aim of Chinese medicine is to treat the disorder at all its levels and by doing so offer much more than palliative relief.

One aspect of root differentiation that has special significance in the treatment of pain is the role of mental and psychological states. Disharmony of the emotions is one of the traditional causes of disease, and certain emotional habits, for example emotional repression, can play an important role in the development of painful disorders. At the same time, prolonged pain can of itself injure a person at the psycho-emotional level. Addressing treatment at this level (for example by calming the mind) as well as by giving appropriate emotional support can play a vital role, especially in the treatment of chronic pain.

Given the prevalence of painful disorders, their frequent presentation at Chinese medicine clinics, and the considerable distress they cause, a comprehensive textbook on this subject is especially welcome. Dr Sun Peilin has long specialised in this subject and he brings to it a deep grounding in traditional Chinese medicine history and theory, combined with extensive clinical practice. True to the best tradition of Chinese medicine, this book emphasises that only with proper differentiation can effective treatment be given.

Peter Deadman

Preface

This book is aimed at students and practitioners of acupuncture and Chinese herbs, as well as practitioners of Western medicine. Both beginners in TCM and experienced practitioners can use this book for reference, practice, teaching and research.

My students have often asked me what the difference is between Bi syndrome and pain syndrome. It can be explained in this way: the main complaint of Bi syndrome in the early stages is pain in the joints and muscles, but it seldom involves the internal organs. The chief causative factor for Bi syndrome is invasion of a mixture of Wind, Cold and Damp. Because of the successes of Western medicine and good health care systems, it is unusual to see many patients with Bi syndrome in the second or later stages. As a consequence, treatment of Bi syndrome focuses on dispelling external pathogenic factors. However, pain syndrome can be caused by many other kinds of pathogenic factors as well as Wind, Cold and Damp. In this sense, it can be said that pain syndrome actually encompasses the contents of Bi syndrome.

The idea for writing this book came to me 8 years ago when I was busy writing a book on Bi syndrome. During the course of this, I found that many pain syndromes could not be clearly described or included in the book, so I began to collect together data on pain control in TCM and drew on my own experience as a clinician and teacher as well as that of my tutor, Professor Shi Zhongan, and my colleagues. Besides supplying me with knowledge, they also gave me a lot of encouragement. Slowly the book gradually took shape. However, because of my busy clinical practice and extensive teaching both at home and abroad, it took me about 2 years before one chapter of the book

was roughly completed. In 1996, I sent this text to the publishers and they expressed an interest in publishing it. However, my time was so limited that I could not finish the book by myself. I consequently invited a few other authors, who are qualified professors and medical doctors in both teaching and clinical practice, to join this writing team. Thanks to the efforts of all the authors, the draft manuscript was finished before the summer of 1998. Since then it has taken all my spare time to revise, edit and modify the contents and, since the only time available for me to work on it was after my practice in the evening, it was quite usual for me to work until the middle of the night! Luckily, I have continually received the support of my family over this period. It was an enormous pleasure for me to see the manuscript finally completed.

The first part of the book is an intensive inquiry into the general aspects of the aetiology of pain, its pathology, treatment principles, acupuncture point selection and steps in treatment. This part serves as a general guide for readers.

The other parts divide the discussion on pain into 46 chapters according to anatomical regions. These chapters provide descriptions of not only the aetiology and pathology for each type of pain, but also the different treatments with Chinese herbs and acupuncture. For each topic, key points are given about differentiation, explanations of herbs and acupoints selected for the treatment and individual modifications, in order to present readers with practical and easily accessible information.

Since it is difficult to find one standard classic herbal formula that fits all complaints, most of the prescriptions mentioned in the herbal treatments have been modified according to the individual situation. Moreover, since not all the readers will feel confident about their knowledge of individual Chinese herbs, useful patent remedies are also suggested. Nevertheless, it should be borne in mind that there is never one patent remedy that can alleviate a specific pain sufficiently without the addition of acupuncture treatment for individual complaints.

We sincerely hope that our colleagues, friends and readers will provide suggestions and comments after reading this book so that it can be modified for any future edition.

All the authors of this book would feel happy if this book serves its purpose in helping to alleviate pain and treat illness.

Belgium, 2002   Sun Peilin

Acknowledgements

This book would not have been published in its present state without the help of many friends and colleagues. In particular, I am deeply indebted to my tutor, Professor Shi Zhongan from Nanjing University of Traditional Chinese Medicine, China. He encouraged me so much in studying, practising and teaching TCM both in China and abroad. He taught me not only how to study at university, but also how to treat people. In particular, I would like to thank him at the age of 84 for writing a foreword and skilfully undertaking the ancient style of Chinese calligraphy for the title of this book.

I am grateful to Dr Robert Rinchart for his many good suggestions in writing this book and also to Mr Jan Schroen and Mrs Ineke van de Ham for their help in checking the English and correcting the writing style in some parts of the book. I am indebted to Mrs Zhou Wei for continually providing me with so much essential information for the book, and also to Professor Chen Zhiqiang for his contribution on acupuncture treatment in the section on back pain. I am very grateful to Mr Yao Zhiguo for spending so much of his spare time in producing the basic layout of the book, and also to the staff of Churchill Livingstone, in particular Inta Ozols, Dinah Thom and Martina Paul, for their expertise and efficiency.

Finally, I owe much to my wife, Yuqing, and my three children, for allowing me to devote a considerable part of my spare time to the book that we would otherwise have spent together.

Sun Peilin

General introduction 概论

Introduction 1
简
述

Discussion on pain

Traditional Chinese Medicine (TCM) is probably one of the oldest complementary therapies and continuously practised systems of medicine in the world. Developed through empirical observation by the Chinese over thousands of years, this unique medical system is used to treat a wide range of diseases, and is of especial use in treating various kinds of pain.

Everyone will, at some time or another, suffer from pain or disability. Pain is an unpleasant experience associated with actual or potential tissue damage. It may arise from accident or injury, cancer, arthritis, a multitude of physical ailments or even emotional distress. It may affect the head, neck, torso or any of the extremities as well as internal organs, causing different kinds of pain, such as headache, neck pain, throat pain, shoulder pain, joint pain, abdominal pain and lower back pain.

No matter what the cause, pain, especially chronic pain, transcends simply physical hurt. It limits the activities of everyday living and can erode the sufferer's ability to function. However, pain is, in reality, nature's way of protecting the body from potential tissue damage, because it serves as a warning signal, alerting the person that something is wrong. In this sense we can say that to avoid pain is to avoid severe injury.

How do modern medicine and TCM explain the occurrence of pain? Modern medical research has discovered that pain signals are transmitted by specialised nervous system cells (receptors), which are found throughout the skin and other body tissues. These cells respond to injury, inflammation or tissue damage. Immediately after receiving these messages, the signals travel by electrical and chemical means, from receptors through sensory neurons to the spinal cord and then through interneurons in the spinal cord to the brain, where they are finally interpreted as pain. TCM takes a different view: that the body maintains a balance between the principles of Yin and Yang, and between Qi and Blood. Qi and Blood travel through the body along well-defined pathways called channels. When there is not enough Qi and Blood (Emptiness or Deficiency), or when they are stuck in one area (Fullness or Excess), there is an imbalance between Yin and Yang, the Internal organs are not functioning optimally, and illness and pain develop.

Pain, whether acute or chronic, could have a variety of causes. Acute pain is usually characterised by acute onset, a short duration, normal functioning of both the peripheral and central nervous systems, a predictable course and, in most cases, a good outcome. In terms of modern medicine, acute pain usually is the result of an injury, surgery, inflammation or medical illness. Acute pain often goes away with the healing process.

Chronic pain, however, is different; it is the kind of pain that most people worry about as it lasts beyond the expected time for healing; that is, it does not go away when it is supposed to.

3

Chronic pain is often difficult to relieve or cure completely, and may occur even if there is no tissue damage or physical cause. The exact causes of chronic pain are not fully understood, or, in other words, one could say that there is no adequate medical explanation for many chronic pain cases.

Pain can be extremely debilitating and frequently requires unique treatment approaches. In some cases it can be seen that the damaged tissues have been repaired, but nevertheless the pain continues. Besides tissue damage, there are some other clinical symptoms associated with pain, such as muscle tension, spasm, stiffness, or weakness. There could also be some degree of immobilisation of an injured part by the patient in order to avoid pain from movement. It has also been observed that, whatever the cause of chronic pain, feelings of frustration, anger and fear make the pain more intense and more difficult to treat.

In short, pain, especially chronic pain, interferes with normal life and physical activities. We could even say that such pain can often diminish the quality of people's life in terms of their psychology, sociology and physiology. It is, finally, one of the most frequent causes of suffering and disability in the world today.

Pain control by TCM

In Western medicine it is quite common to find or be told that doctors are unable to find the real cause of pain in patients even after extensive examination. Patients are often told: 'There is nothing wrong with you', or 'Sorry, we can do nothing about it, and you'll have to learn to live with it' or even 'It is all in your head'. It is poor practice, however, for a doctor to make such comments to patients; they don't have to live in pain. Fortunately, since acupuncture has acquired a very good reputation as a treatment for relieving pain, many physicians are now referring their patients for an acupuncture or herbal evaluation, or patients are starting to investigate the potential of acupuncture and herbal treatment for themselves.

In terms of pain control, the effects of Chinese herbal and acupuncture treatment include:

- to relieve pain completely, or give as much relief as possible
- to reduce pain levels
- to improve the ability to deal with pain
- to regulate the emotions
- to increase the energy
- to increase the ability to perform everyday functions

- to enhance the quality of life
- to reduce reliance on inappropriate medications.

Points from different channels are, according to TCM theory, energetically connected to specific organs and body structures. The purpose of acupuncture treatment for pain is to use selected points on these channels to activate Qi and Blood circulation, and balance Yin and Yang. During the treatment, moxibustion and point massage are also often applied simultaneously.

Acupuncture treatment for pain is varied and based largely on what is causing the patient's suffering; the treatments for acute and chronic pain are often quite different. In chronic pain patients, treatment that had proved useful for acute pain management may lose its effectiveness, be inappropriate or even be counter-productive.

The Chinese do not limit the use of Chinese herbs and acupuncture to alleviating pain; they use combinations of herbs and acupuncture to treat the whole range of diseases that are encountered in association with the pain. These include TCM therapies for hypertension, hypotension, allergy, asthma, diabetes, stomach ulcers, depression, infections, etc. It is clear that many diseases respond better to modern medicine, whereas some may respond better to Chinese herbal medicines and acupuncture. However, in the majority of cases Chinese herbal medicine and acupuncture may either be a reasonable alternative for, or be used in conjunction with modern medicine. For this reason all TCM schools and universities in China continue to offer courses and training in both TCM and modern medicine at present. During Chinese herbal and acupuncture treatment, it should be kept in mind that essential contact and communication with other specialists must be maintained, for instance with neurologists, neurosurgeons, orthopaedists, internists, radiologists, and physical and occupational therapists, so that patients receive the necessary support at their time of greatest need.

In China, increasingly acupuncturists are applying acupuncture to diminish pain directly or decrease the amount of drugs needed for the control of pain, even during surgery. This well-known practice indicates that acupuncture potentially has anaesthetic effects. After conducting thousands of experiments on both animals and people, researchers become firmly convinced that acupuncture was indeed effective in its own right for anaesthesia. In consequence, acupuncture has been used quite successfully in place of chemical anaesthesia for many types of surgery in the last 30 years in China. It has been shown to be effective in gastric (Ye Qiang et al 1984), dental (Lin Guochu et al 1984) and thyroid surgery (Zhuang Xinliang 1984). It is also potentially indicated for those patients unable to tolerate regular anaesthesia. Because of its efficiency in acupuncture anaesthesia, doctors in many hospitals, especially the affiliated hospitals of TCM universities, use acupuncture routinely in cases of thyroidectomy.

The advantages of acupuncture anaesthesia include:

- fewer side-effects than with chemical anaesthesia
- more cooperation from the patient during the operation
- a lack of disturbance of the brain and memory following anaesthesia
- the patient remaining alert during the procedure
- rapid recovery of functional activities after the operation, etc.

The disadvantages of acupuncture anaesthesia include:

- a feeling of pulling and tugging during the operation
- inadequacy with children and some senile patients
- inability to replace all kinds of chemical anaesthesia
- sometimes a need for local chemical anaesthesia, etc.

Modern research on pain control by acupuncture

Over the past thirty years, both patients and professionals have been asking questions about how acupuncture works in a modern, scientific sense? What are the mechanisms? Is there any scientific evidence that supports the effectiveness of acupuncture?

In order to reply to these questions, since the 1970s scientists and practitioners both in China and in other countries have been conducting a number of scientific studies and clinical trials, which are described in this section. This research has tended to substantiate the ancient theories of traditional Chinese medicine. Other recent research has revealed that human beings are complex bioelectric systems (Becker 1985), and on this basis the mechanics of acupuncture can now be better understood.

To date, a few theories have been suggested concerning these questions.

Transmission of pain impulses along acupuncture channels

The first theory is that most pain impulses travel along the same pathways as those of the traditional Qi circu-

lation (i.e. the channels). It is an objective fact that pain is always transmitted along certain pathways. These pathways are closely related with channel theory in TCM. An interesting observation is that when acupuncture needling is used in the treatment of pain, and when the needle sensation (Deqi) is reported along a particular channel, the greatest reduction in sensitivity to pain is be found in a line along the middle of the channel (Fujian Provincial Research Institute for Traditional Chinese Medicine 1979). This reduction in sensitivity decreases gradually as one moves from the centre of the channel to its outer boundary—that is to say, the more the needle is moved towards the central line of the channel, the less the patient feels the pain. Observation has also shown that pain transmission along the course of the channels is greatly diminished when certain methods are used to promote the circulation of the channel (Li Baojiao 1981). Pain transmission along the channels is, conversely, greatly increased when certain methods are used to block the channel circulation.

Pain-gate theory

Another theory suggests that pain impulses are blocked from reaching the spinal cord or brain at various 'gates' within the nervous system. Research studies have shown that both peripheral and central nerves are very important in pain relief by acupuncture (Lu Guowei et al 1979, Shanghai no. 1 People's Hospital 1977, Wu Jianping et al 1979).

In the peripheral nervous system acupuncture when used to treat pain can, firstly, block the conduction of sensory fibres in the algetic nerves (Lu Guowei et al 1979, Qiu Maoliang et al 1989); secondly, it can cause downward inhibition of the dorsal horn cell conduction in the spinal cord resulting from the noxious stimulation (Qiu Maoliang et al 1989). It is the peripheral nerves that receive and conduct the acupuncture 'message'; the II, III and IV fibres could all participate in the pain-relief process.

In the central nervous system the structures at various levels, including the spinal cord, brain stem, thalamus, caudate nucleus and cortex, participate in the process of pain relief by acupuncture.

SPINAL CORD

Scientific research has found that acupuncture can cause postsynaptic inhibition in the posterior horn of the spinal cord (Qiu Maoliang et al 1989). It has also been found that the acupuncture 'message' is conducted to the medulla oblongata from the anterior funiculus of the spinal cord, and then to the medial reticular structure (Qiu Maoliang et al 1989). Afterwards, it is conducted downwards to the posterior funiculus of the spinal cord, where it causes postsynaptic inhibition by depolarising the fine afferent nerve endings. This has the effect of partially blocking the afferent impulse from the fine fibres.

BRAIN STEM AND PARAFASCICULAR NUCLEUS

In the brain stem, electroacupuncture has been found to control the activity of hyperalgetic neurons in the reticular structure of the midbrain (Qiu Maoliang et al 1989). In animal experiments, it was found that electroacupuncture stimulation of the median raphe nuclei could raise the pain threshold in the animals, improving their ability to resist the pain (Qiu Maoliang et al 1989). Impairment of the locus ceruleus increased the capacity for pain relief by electroacupuncture, whereas activation and stimulation of this structure decreased its pain-relief capacity. Researches also showed that acupuncture treatment led to the release of neural impulses from the grey matter around the aqueduct of the midbrain, the giant nucleus in the medial reticular structure of the brain stem and the median raphe nuclei (Qiu Maoliang et al 1989). From here, ascending impulses inhibit electrical activity of the hyperalgetic cells in the parafascicular nucleus of the thalamus, and descending impulses inhibit the activity of neurons transmitting pain impulses in the posterior horn of the spinal cord, so relieving the pain. The parafascicular nucleus has been found to be one of the important key locations in the transmission of pain impulses.

CAUDATE NUCLEUS

Research has established that when the caudate nucleus is stimulated, the pain threshold is increased, which could increase the pain-relieving effect of electroacupuncture, whereas inhibition of the caudate nucleus decreases the pain-relieving effect (Qiu Maoliang et al 1989).

Generally speaking, when the pain impulse enters the central nervous system, it can take a circuitous route to the cerebrum. The posterior horn of the spinal cord and the parafascicular nucleus are two key locations in the reception and transmission of pain impulses. The caudate nucleus, the grey matter around the aqueduct of the midbrain, the giant nucleus in the

medial reticular structure of the brain stem and the median raphe nuclei are also very important.

Stimulation of endorphins

A third theory suggests that acupuncture stimulates the brain's production of polypeptides that reduce pain sensitivity. Scientists have discovered that one of its possible mechanisms is that it increases the release of natural pain-relieving molecules known as endorphins by the brain (Qiu Maoliang et al 1989). These are very similar to opiates (such as morphine), which are potent anaesthetic agents. In China this work was performed and directed in the 1970s by Professor Han Jisheng, an internationally known researcher of acupuncture, when a research programme to study acupuncture-induced anaesthesia was initiated during the Cultural Revolution. His studies showed that electrical stimulation of inserted acupuncture needles caused release of different amounts of endorphin compounds into the central nervous system (Han Jisheng et al 1979). This is the key mechanism that is most widely used as explanation for the effect of acupuncture treatment in relieving pain. This is not a complete explanation, however, of all of acupuncture's pain-alleviating mechanisms, because acupuncture has other physiological effects besides decreasing pain sensitivity. For instance, it often increases local blood circulation in areas of muscle spasm, and can decrease the muscular contraction that often causes or contributes to painful conditions. Thus, local actions such as decreasing tissue swelling (due to better blood circulation) and lessening muscle spasm may, in turn, release pressure on nerves or interior organs, contributing to the pain relief.

Effects on neurotransmitters

Another theory suggests a central nervous system connection that induces the production or secretion of other chemicals in the body such as neurotransmitters, hormones and lymphokines, etc. Though most of these chemicals are used up fairly quickly, clinical experience indicates that acupuncture generally has cumulative effects. Thus, acupuncture must provide some training effect in the body's autonomic mechanisms that control and regulate the physiological reactions to pain.

Acupuncture treatments have been found to affect several neurotransmitters, resulting in changes in their blood serum levels. In particular, acupuncture may bring about the following biochemical changes.

SEROTONIN CHANGES

It has been found that levels of serotonin (5-HT), one of the neurotransmitters with the greatest potential influence on sensitivity to pain, change in correspondence with the degree of pain relief reported during acupuncture treatment (Chinese Academy of Traditional Chinese Medicine 1977, Han Jisheng 1978, Jin Guozhang et al 1979). That is to say, the higher the level of 5-HT that is recorded, the greater is the level of pain relief. Acupuncture, and especially electro-acupuncture, can increase the level of 5-HT, which helps to increase the pain threshold. For instance, Yi Qingchen et al (1978) has reported that when the pain threshold is increased by acupuncture on ST-36 Zusanli in rabbits, a higher serotonin level is recorded by perfusion streaming in the ventricles of brain. Similarly, Zhu Dinger (1980) has reported that high serotonin levels can be detected in the thalamus, medulla oblongata and midbrain when electro-acupuncture is used for sedating pain.

ACETYLCHOLINE CHANGES

Other studies have shown that, when the pain threshold is raised by the use of acupuncture, a high level of acetylcholinesterase is recorded in the cerebral cortex, caudate nucleus and hypothalamus, and when the threshold is artificially decreased, a low level of acetylcholinesterase is recorded (Chinese Academy of Traditional Chinese Medicine 1976, 1978, Ge Zi et al 1983). It appears, therefore, that the level of acetylcholine (Ach) could play an important role in acupuncture pain relief.

CATECHOLAMINE (CA) CHANGES

The results of some studies indicate that noradrenaline (NA) has the opposite effect in pain relief (Han Jisheng et al 1979). That is, when the pain threshold is raised and pain relief is obtained, there is a low level of NA recorded in the cortex, hypothalamus, brain stem, spinal cord and striate body. It is also very interesting to observe that dopamine (DA) levels increase in the caudate nucleus when the pain threshold is raised by electroacupuncture, and in addition the level of homovanillic acid (HVA), one of the products of the metabolism of DA, is high in the midbrain and hind-brain.

In short, acupuncture achieves its effects by working with a the body's own chemicals, rather than the addition of synthetic chemicals. This approach has several advantages over drug-based medicine.

Psychological and cultural factors

Psychological and cultural factors are also important in pain. It is believed that many psychological modalities, including formal relaxation and distraction training as well as clear explanations before giving acupuncture treatment, may directly ameliorate pain and increase the person's positive attitude to the treatment. People who are very anxious about the acupuncture treatment and feel very nervous during it would have a lot of muscular tension generally in their body, which may directly diminish the effectiveness of acupuncture in relieving pain.

Conversely, because of cultural differences, Chinese people find it easier to undergo acupuncture treatment for pain syndrome than do Westerners, and during the treatment they also tend to cooperate more with the acupuncturist, which in turn results in less muscular tension, cramp and nervousness. All these are very important for achieving the therapeutic result.

Another contributing factor could be external suggestion. Until recently, it has been commonly believed, particularly by medical practitioners, that the effect of acupuncture on pain is a form of hypnosis, or can be explained by the 'placebo effect', but there is lack of evidence for this belief. Studies have shown, conversely, that there is no correlation between capacity to be hypnotised or belief in the treatment and the subsequent results (Qiu Maoliang et al 1989). People who receive acupuncture and do not believe that it will help are just as likely to respond to it as people with full faith in the treatment. The successful use of acupuncture to treat many animal diseases is one of the best arguments that the effect of acupuncture on pain is not a form of hypnosis.

Historical development of the pain concept

2

疼痛概念的历史沿革

It is widely known throughout the world that both acupuncture and Chinese herbal medicine can be used to treat pain. According to popular legend, about two thousand years ago an outstanding doctor named Hua Tuo had already started to use herbs and acupuncture to different kinds of pain (Hua Tuo c. AD 180). For instance, he used acupuncture successfully to treat an emperor who suffered from severe Toufeng (severe migraine headache). Dr Hua was also very skilful in using Chinese herbs that produced anaesthesia, and once opened the skull of a patient, drained some infected blood and a damaged skull fragment and finally successfully sewed up the wound. Another legend concerns a Mr Bian Que, a famous doctor of 5th century BC. He also successfully healed a son of the then emperor by opening his abdomen and removing a damaged section of the intestines.

The earliest relative systematic discussion on pain can be found in the Neijing or Yellow Emperor's Classic of Internal Medicine (1956). In this book there is a chapter devoted to the aetiology, pathology and symptoms of pain. For the first time here, Qi and Blood stagnation were considered to be the major causes of pain. The terms used in this book to describe Qi and Blood stagnation included 'retardation of Blood circulation', 'retardation of circulation in the Blood vessels', 'disorder of Qi and Blood', 'fullness of the Blood vessels', 'failure of Blood to circulate' and 'blockage of the Blood vessels', amongst others. Its theory is still applicable to clinical practice. In addition, the Neijing distinguished 13 kinds of pain; however, most of these were considered to be caused by Cold, and only one kind by Heat. Moreover, this book emphasised only the Exogenous factors as causes, so the book's treatment was incomplete or only partially correct, because there are many kinds of causative factors, both Exogenous and Internal, in addition to Cold and Heat—for instance, Deficiency may also cause pain.

During the Jin, Sui, Tang and Song dynasties, concepts about the causes of the pain continued to be based on the theory set down in the Neijing. In fact, right up until the Ming and Qing dynasties, most physicians still based their treatments on this same theory, although they made some corrections to it, to complete the known types of aetiology, pathology, symptoms and treatment. For instance, doctor Liu Hengrui mentioned in his book General discussion on experience (1998) that exogenous invasion, emotional disorders and physical trauma can all cause pain. Besides these, Deficiency may also result in pain. He wrote: 'the ancient people stated that there is no pain if there is free flow, and there is pain if there is blockage, but this refers only to the situation of Excess. If physicians followed only this theory in treating pain, this would be an error' and 'the pain is only one of many diseases; it must be treated according to the differentiation of the aetiology, thus there will be no mistakes' (p. 141).

Yu Chang (1585–1664), a famous doctor of the Qing dynasty, pointed out in his book Principle of prohibition for the medical profession (written in 1658, new edition 1999): *to promote Qi and Blood circulation is the method only for Excessive cases. In cases of Exogenous invasion, it should*

9

be combined with the method to promote sweating; in case of Excessive retention, it should be combined with purging. But the pain may be caused by Deficiency and Excess, and the treatment here is not tonification and reduction. In principle, pain with distension and fullness is caused by Excess, whereas that without distension and fullness is caused by Deficiency. Pain with a dislike of pressure is the Excessive type; pain that is relieved by pressure is the Deficient type. The pain with a preference for Cold is mostly caused by Excess; pain with a preference for warmth is mostly caused by Deficiency. Pain that becomes worse after eating is caused by Excess; pain that becomes worse with hunger is caused by Deficiency. Pain with an Excessive pulse and rough breath is due to Excess; pain with a weak pulse and shortness of breath is due to Deficiency. Acute onset of pain in young and strong people is usually due to Excess, and pain that becomes worsened after purging is due to Deficiency.

Wang Qingren (1768–1831), another famous doctor, made a great contribution to the understanding of how to treat pain. He focused mainly on the treatment of painful diseases caused by Blood stagnation. The causes of Blood stagnation were discussed in detail in his famous book *Correction on the Errors of Medical Works* (1830, new edition 1991), in which several important prescriptions for painful diseases were given. For instance, Tong Qiao Huo Xue Tang *Unblock the Orifices and Invigorate the Blood Decoction* was used to treat headache caused by Blood stagnation, Xue Fu Zhu Yu Tang *Blood Mansion Eliminating Stasis Decoction* could be used to treat chest pain due to Blood stagnation and Shao Fu Zhu Yu Tang *Drive Out Blood Stasis in the Lower Abdomen Decoction* was chosen to treat lower abdominal pain caused by Blood stagnation. These prescriptions are now widely applied to treat many painful diseases caused by Blood stagnation.

From the 1960s to 1970s, acupuncture was widely used both in preparation for and during surgery. It attracted the attention of the medical profession both in China and internationally because it could safely and effectively either reduce or entirely eliminate the pain usually associated with many operations performed on the head, chest, abdomen and in the limbs. Moreover, its use allowed the physiological functions of patients to remain at normal levels, and during the operation they remained conscious, and could therefore play an active role throughout the operation. Because most of the side-effects associated with chemical anaesthesia are avoided, the period of postoperative recovery is accelerated.

It is understandable that acupuncture is widely accepted within China. But how did acupuncture come to be so popular internationally? This was largely a result of US national media coverage of acupuncture when the People's Republic of China started opening its door to the US and other foreign countries in early 1970s. At that time the columnist James Reston went to China with the delegation of President Nixon and his Secretary of State Henry Kissinger to re-establish relationships with Mao Zedong and his government on Mainland China. James Reston wrote extensively in the popular press about the remarkable experiences he had had in China. During his visit he was taken ill with appendicitis, and his post-appendectomy pain relief was performed under acupuncture anaesthesia. His story quickly appeared in the media. Moreover, during that period visits to China by the general public became popular and during these many visitors saw demonstrations of the effectiveness of acupuncture generally. Such visits were subsequently written up in the Western media, capturing the public's imagination and rapidly increasing the popularity of acupuncture in the West. However, what interested Western physicians and people most were those aspects of acupuncture that involved anaesthesia and pain control.

Besides acupuncture, treatments with herbs, moxibustion, massage, herbal pastes, cupping and QiGong are widely applied for the pain syndromes. Currently a lot of patent herbal products are used effectively for treating many kinds of pain. For example, Su Xiao Jiu Xin Wan *Rapid Save the Heart Pill* and Su He Xiang Wan *Styrax Pill* are good at treating chest pain caused by heart disease, and Tong Jing Wan *Regulate Menses Pill* is effective for treating dysmenorrhoea. In a word, more and more new herbal products and acupuncture devices are currently being produced for use in treating pain syndromes.

Aetiology and pathology of pain

3

疼痛的病因和病机

Aetiology of pain

Exogenous factors

WIND

Wind is one of six exogenous factors, which is predominant in the spring but may also occur in any of the four seasons. When attacking the body, Wind is likely to combine with another of the pathogenic factors, such as Cold, Damp or Heat, etc., leading to retardation of Qi and Blood circulation. This causes blockage in the Zang-Fu organs, muscles, tendons, joints and channels, and pain follows.

Wind is classified as a Yang pathogenic factor because it has the characteristic of upward and outward movement. Because of this quality, it may easily invade the upper and superficial areas of the body, for instance the face, head, neck, shoulders, arms, chest, upper back, etc. So pain that is caused by Wind is found mostly in the top half of the body.

In nature Wind blows in gusts and is subject to rapid changes. Similarly, in the body it causes symptoms that are characterised by their migratory appearance. When a pain has no fixed location, but rather tends to wander around, this implies that its primary causative factor is Wind.

COLD

Cold is the predominant factor in winter. Although it can be seen in other seasons, in these its nature is not so severe. Cold invasion normally results from wearing too little clothing, exposure to Cold after sweating, being caught in rain, or wading through water in cold weather.

Cold is a Yin pathogenic factor and is likely to damage the Yang Qi of the Heart, Stomach, Spleen or Kidney. Cold includes both Exogenous and Internal Cold pathogenic factors; the former refers to Cold due to External invasion, and the latter to Cold due to Deficiency of Yang Qi. Exogenous Cold and Internal Cold may mutually influence and transform each other. For instance, Exogenous Cold may change into Internal Cold where there is prolonged persistence of the condition, resulting in damage to the Internal Yang Qi; conversely, a state of Internal Cold may easily induce invasion of Exogenous Cold.

Cold is characterised by stagnation and contraction, so Cold can easily slow the circulation of Qi and Blood. Thus, pain accompanied by a sensation of contraction, limitation of joint movement, aversion to cold and anhidrosis will be classified as being caused by Cold.

Cold may invade the body not only through the skin, mouth and nose, and drinking of cold liquids, but also through the uterus (e.g. after walking in the rain, or swimming or sex during menstruation). Moreover it can directly invade the muscles and joints, or even the Internal Zang-Fu organs if the Cold is very extreme, or the body very weak. The other opportunity for External Cold to invade is through the practice of walking barefoot. In Western countries, many people often do this inside the house, even on a cold floor, and in winter. Since the Kidney, Liver and Spleen channels all begin on the foot, External Cold may easily invade the Spleen, Kidney and Liver through these channels, especially the Kidney channel, which begins on the soles, in people who too frequently walk around barefoot on a cold floor.

Nowadays more and more homes and other buildings have air-conditioning to cool the place in the heat of summer. Consequently, many people now suffer from pain that becomes worse when they are sitting in their office equipped with air-conditioning, and they improve spontaneously once they leave the office and go out in sun. Thus they form a clear impression that cold places are bad and warm places are good for them, which is true. This is because our skin pores stay relatively open in the summer in order that we may sweat and keep our body temperature down. However, this also provides a very good opportunity for invasion of Cold, as the artificially cooled air can enter the body through the opened pores. Being characterised by contraction and stagnation, Cold may cause closure of the skin pores; this results in accumulation of Cold in the joints and muscles, so leading to pain due to Qi and Blood stagnation. Moreover, since the skin pores are now closed, Internal Heat cannot easily leave the body in sweat evaporation. So accumulated Cold can soon change into Heat, leading to symptoms of that aggravation, including redness, hotness, pain and swollen joints and muscles.

DAMP

Invasion of Exogenous Damp is usually induced by humid weather, walking in the rain, living and working too long in humid places, or not changing out of one's wet clothing after sweating. There is also a condition of Internal Damp, which is normally caused by disorder of the transportation and transformation functions of the Spleen and Stomach leading to formation of excessive water in the body. Exogenous Damp and Internal Damp often mutually influence each other in the causation of pain—that is to say, invasion of Exogenous Damp often attacks the Spleen and

Stomach, while weakness of the Spleen and Stomach with formation of Damp may easily induce invasion of External Damp.

Damp is similar to water, which is characterised by heaviness. When it attacks the body, it causes pain accompanied by a feeling of heaviness of the head, limbs and body, together with a sense as though the body is bound. Where there is invasion of the skin and muscles by External Damp, this results in a blockage of the Clear Yang and disharmony of the Nutritive and Defensive Qi, which manifests as symptoms such as soreness of the limbs and joints, numbness of the limbs and muscles, and lassitude.

Damp is also characterised by viscosity and stagnation. Following on from this principle, pain that is caused by Damp is, generally speaking, stubborn and tends to be prolonged and intractable, compared with that caused by other pathogenic factors.

Damp is a Yin pathogenic factor and easily blocks Qi circulation and impairs Yang. When Damp accumulates in the Zang-Fu organs, joints, muscles or channels it may affect the ascending and descending of the Qi, leading to symptoms such as numbness of the skin and joints, and limitation of movement.

DRYNESS

Dryness is predominant in autumn, and tends most often to impair the Lung, impeding the dispersal of Lung-Qi and causing stagnation, leading to symptoms such as throat and chest pain.

Dryness can also damage the Body Fluids, causing dryness of the skin, nose and throat. Furthermore, it may disturb and consume the Blood; then the blood vessels are not properly nourished resulting in narrowed vessels, and then the Qi and Blood stagnate, leading to painful skin.

HEAT (FIRE, WARMTH)

Fire and Heat both indicate excessive Yang Qi, thus in most cases they are interchangeable, but there is still some slight difference between them. In terms of pathology, Heat is usually caused by Exogenous invasion, for instance Wind-Heat or Damp-Heat, whereas Fire is often caused by Internal disorders, for example flaming up of Heart-Fire or hyperactivity of Liver-Fire. In terms of the physiology, Fire has a proper function, which is to warm the Zang-Fu organs and promote Qi transformation and energy production; only if it becomes excessive does it become a kind of pathogenic factor causing overconsumption of energy in the body. Heat, in contrast, is simply a pathogenic factor.

Warmth is like Fire, with a physiological role but potentially pathogenic, and is also a kind of Heat, but milder. Of the three, Fire is the most severe, and Warmth the least severe, yet they all share similar characteristics. In practice, the terms Fire-Heat and Warmth-Heat are often used interchangeably.

Heat, a Yang pathogenic factor, is characterised by flaming up, burning and hotness. When it attacks the body, it may cause abnormal Qi and Blood circulation as well as injury to the Blood Vessels, causing pain accompanied by a burning feeling, a hot sensation, or redness. When Heat disturbs the Blood, the Blood circulation will be accelerated and the Blood Vessels can be damaged, causing swelling of the joints, muscles, or even bleeding, such as epistaxis, etc. Heat may also often disturb the Heart, which houses the Mind, causing restlessness and insomnia.

Like pathogenic Wind, Heat often attacks the top half of the body because of its characteristics of flaming up and moving in an upward direction, thus a combination of Wind and Heat causation is often seen. In most case of acute inflammatory joints and muscles in the upper parts of the body, Wind-Heat is the chief causative factor, thus the main treatment principle will be to dispel Wind and clear Heat.

Emotional factors

Pain is an indication of human suffering. This suffering may frequently be rooted in emotional distress as well as physical trauma.

Mental activities relating to emotion in TCM are classified into joy, anger, melancholy, meditation, grief, fear and fright, and are known as the seven emotional factors. The seven emotional factors differ from the six Exogenous factors in that they affect the Zang-Fu organs, and the Qi and Blood, directly. For this reason, they are considered to be the chief causative factors for various kinds of pain. It is believed traditionally that different emotional factors tend to affect the circulation of Qi and Blood of various individual internal organs, resulting in retardation of Qi and Blood circulation, causing blockage to follow, and pain as the main clinical manifestation. The saying 'anger injures the Liver, joy injures the Heart, grief and melancholy injure the Lung, meditation injures the Spleen, and fear and fright injure the Kidney' (Yellow Emperor's Classic of Internal Medicine: Simple Questions 1956, p. 17) is an expression of relationship between the different emotional factors and each of the internal Zang-Fu organs.

Another saying from ancient medical texts is: 'anger causes the Qi to rise, joy causes it to move slowly, grief drastically consumes it, fear causes it to decline, fright causes it to be deranged, and worry causes it to stagnate' (Yellow Emperor's Classic of Internal Medicine: Simple Questions 1956, pp. 80–81). From this it can be seen clearly that abnormal Qi and Blood circulation is one explanation for the occurrence of pain.

In clinical practice, it has often been observed that in some patients suffering with pain their pain is aggravated or alleviated by their emotional state. Take shoulder pain, for instance: if the biceps muscle (which is in the area of the Lung channel) is involved, it is sometimes found that such patients either have suffered much grief in the past or do so at present and usually admit that when their feelings of grief recur their shoulder pain worsens. Since the Lung and Large Intestine share a pair of channels and collaterals, if the Lung channel is blocked the Large Intestine channel can also become impaired, leading to shoulder or arm pain. In this case, the points nearby (such as LU-2 Yunmen, LU-3 Tianfu, LU-5 Chize or LU-6 Kongzui) are usually found to be tender. There may also be tenderness found around LI-4 Hegu, LI-9 Shanglian and LI-10 Shousanli, as well as LI-11 Quchi. Another example is patients suffering from lower back pain, some of whom may have aggravation of pain with particular emotional states, especially anger and stress. This kind of pain can also radiate to the inguinal region, and even to the interior aspect of the leg along the Liver channel, and consequently along the Gall Bladder channel also. Conversely, if the Gall Bladder channel is primarily affected, there could be impairment of the Liver channel as well. For instance, disc herniation between L4 and L5 often manifests as pain along the Gall Bladder channel, which sometimes refers to the inguinal region. In this case, anger or stress may play a very important rule in the aggravation of the low back pain.

The causation of pain by excessive emotional activities is basically described in following sections.

EXCESSIVE JOY, FEAR OR ANXIETY

These often disturb the physiological functions of the Heart, leading to retardation of Qi and Blood circulation in the Heart, causing chest pain, heart pain, and pain in the shoulder along the Heart channel; palpitation and insomnia also occur. A point of distinct tenderness is typically found along the Heart channel, especially at HT-3 Shaohai. Needling or even simple massage at this point can greatly relieve the chest, heart or shoulder pain.

EXCESSIVE ANGER

Anger may cause dysfunction of the Liver, impeding its free flow of Qi, and leading to a condition of stagnation of Liver-Qi. In TCM anger in fact includes other emotions such as frustration and irritation, which also may cause disharmony of the Liver leading to stagnation of Liver-Qi. Liver-Qi stagnation gives rise to symptoms such as headache, hypochondriac pain and distension, depression, abdominal pain and distension, and low back pain. Such pain is characterised by being wandering and distending in nature, or intermittent, or fluctuating in intensity and location. Another characteristic is that the pain often occurs at times of strong emotion, especially anger, stress, nervousness or irritability.

Stagnation of Liver-Qi can also be traced to emotions arising from being mistreated during childhood (e.g. from being beaten, lack of love, limitation of freedom, sexual abuse, or difficulties with friends, parents, brothers or sisters). Stagnation of Liver-Qi originating in childhood may cause either conscious or subconscious blockage in the Liver, bringing on pain at a later date due to severe psychological and physiological problems.

The Liver is in charge of promoting Qi circulation both in the Liver itself and generally in the body. If there is Liver Qi stagnation, the Liver fails to maintain the free flow of Qi in the channels, muscles, and Zang-Fu organs as well. The consequences can be summarised as follows.

BLOOD STAGNATION

Because Qi is the commander of the Blood, Qi circulation leads to Blood circulation, and Qi stagnation causes Blood stagnation. Hence, Liver-Qi stagnation may finally bring about Blood stagnation, which results in a more severe pain, stabbing pain, or a constant pain with fixed location.

GENERATION OF LIVER-FIRE

Prolonged Liver-Qi stagnation may also generate Fire, leading to flaming up of Liver-Fire, and symptoms such as headache, painful ears or painful eyes. A further development of this is hyperactivity of Liver-Yang, which can develop into internal stirring of Liver-Wind which causes severe headache, facial pain, neck pain, or stiffness of the neck.

If Liver-Fire persists it eventually can consume the Yin of the Liver, and even the Yin of the Kidney, resulting in failure of the Liver and the tendons to be nourished, and consequently in hypochondriac pain, tiredness, headache, muscle pain with cramp, dizziness, constipation, or abdominal pain.

When there is Liver-Yin deficiency, the Yang of the Liver will not be properly controlled, leading to hyperactivity of Liver-Yang; thus a mixture of Deficiency and Excess appears, which is not easy to deal with.

ABNORMAL BILE CIRCULATION

Bile is stored in the Gall Bladder, but its formation depends on the normal circulation of Liver-Qi. Once bile is formed it must be distributed, with the help of Liver-Qi, into the Stomach and intestines in order to help the digestion. However, if there is Liver-Qi stagnation there is either insufficient bile secretion or abnormal bile distribution, so the digestion is disturbed, leading to stomach pain, belching, abdominal pain and distension, or constipation, etc. resulting from the dysfunction of the the digestive action of the Stomach and Intestine.

DYSFUNCTION OF SPLEEN

To produce Qi and Blood, the Spleen also needs the help from the Liver, as the latter maintains the free circulation of Qi not only in the Liver itself, but also over the whole body. Without Liver-Qi circulation, the Spleen would find it impossible to maintain its physiological function of transportation and transformation. Where there is stagnation of Liver-Qi, there could also be stagnation of Spleen-Qi. In this situation the Spleen cannot transport and transform food and water, and excessive water forms in the body, causing pain resulting from blockage of the Zang-Fu organs, channels, joints and muscles by Damp-Phlegm. Moreover, Liver-Qi stagnation often attacks the Spleen, leading to formation of so-called disharmony between the Liver and Spleen; this manifests in symptoms such as abdominal pain, loose stool or diarrhoea when nervous, or flatulence.

BLOCKAGE OF THE CHANNELS

Liver-Qi stagnation is one of the direct causes of stagnation of circulation in the channels generally. In addition, stagnation of Blood and formation of Damp-Phlegm may also impede circulation in the channels; in such cases blockage occurs in the channels, followed by numbness, pain, diminished skin and muscle sensitivity, joint pain, etc.

EXCESSIVE GRIEF AND MELANCHOLY

These may cause dysfunction of the Lung, leading to Qi and Blood stagnation in the Lung and its channel. The symptoms of this include: chest pain, shoulder pain and throat pain, accompanied by cough, difficulty in breathing out, and a sensation of oppression across the chest area.

Dysfunction of the Lung may also cause shoulder pain, which occurs in the interior aspect of the shoulder, down the biceps muscle. Patients with such pain often admit that they might have experienced enormous grief prior to the onset of the pain. Points of tenderness along the Lung channel may be found at LU-1 Zhongfu, LU-2 Yunmen, LU-3 Tianfu, LU-4 Xiabai, LU-5 Chize and LU-6 Kongzui.

EXCESSIVE MEDITATION

This brings about Qi stagnation in the Spleen and Stomach, leading to dysfunction in the functions of transportation and transformation. This may cause the following four kinds of pathological changes.

PAIN

Types of pain include epigastric pain, abdominal pain and distension with fullness, and pain that is worsened after eating.

DEFICIENCY OF QI AND BLOOD

This may cause failure to nourish the Zang-Fu organs, muscles, joints and channels.

FORMATION OF DAMP-PHLEGM

Damp-Phlegm may block the Zang-Fu organs, joints, muscles and channels. Slowing the circulation of Qi and Blood, and causing pain, swelling and numbness of muscles and joints accompanied by a heavy feeling, limitation of movement and lassitude.

ATTRACTION OF EXOGENOUS DAMP INVASION

If Damp-Phlegm accumulates in the body then it is vulnerable to External Damp invasion, leading to aggravation of the pain, and complications in treatment.

FRIGHT MAY CAUSE SUNKEN QI OF THE KIDNEY

Fright or shock gives rising to a failure of the Kidney to distribute the Kidney-Essence, which in normal circumstances produces the marrow and nourishes the Bones. Weakness of the knees and lower back, dizziness, tinnitus and other symptoms can be the result. Of course, this type of lower back pain is not often seen in practice.

From the above account, it can be concluded that it is insufficient simply to use the method of circulating the channels to treat the various kinds of pain associated with certain emotions. It is also necessary to use the method of smoothing the emotions and regulating the organs.

Miscellaneous pathogenic factors

INAPPROPRIATE FOOD INTAKE

Food is the main material from which human beings receive energy, Qi and Blood; even Kidney-Essence needs to be nourished continuously from food. Inappropriate food intake comprises three aspects: overindulgence, insufficiency and intake of unsanitary food.

In industrialised countries, insufficient food intake normally is now seldom seen; overindulgence or intake of unsuitable or unsanitary food, however, is much more common. Generally speaking, insufficient food intake causes pain of the Deficient type resulting from failure to nourish the body, joints, muscles or Zang-Fu organs. In contrast, overindulgence and intake of unsanitary food often cause pain of the Excessive type resulting from blockage of the Zang-Fu organs, meridians, joints and muscles from Qi and Blood stagnation or Phlegm and Damp accumulation.

OVEREATING OF RAW AND COLD FOOD, OR DRINKING ICE-COLD DRINKS

Raw food, cold food and cold water are Yin in nature. Generally speaking, Westerners eat far fewer vegetables than do Chinese people; moreover, many like to eat them raw, whereas Chinese people usually don't like to eat their vegetables uncooked, but rather steamed or oil-baked, for instance. In addition, in hot weather Westerners prefer to drink cooled water from the refrigerator, or even with a few pieces of ice in the glass. This is not good for the health, according to TCM, because the Spleen organ 'dislikes' cold and raw food, as it needs to spend more energy to first warm it before digesting it, compared with warm or cooked food. If Spleen, day after day, year after year, has to do this extra work, the Spleen-Yang eventually becomes impaired, causing inhibition of its functions of transportation and transformation, and Phlegm-Damp develops as a consequence. Once this is formed, it may spread throughout the body together with the Qi and Blood, causing, for instance, blockage in one of the Zang-Fu organs, or the joints, muscles or channels; Qi and Blood circulation are impeded and, as a result, pain occurs. Overeating of raw or cold food and drinking cold water is a common cause of the formation of Cold-Damp, or Cold-Phlegm.

One more fact that needs to be mentioned is that inappropriate use of some medicinal drugs or herbs may also sometimes cause damage of the Spleen and Stomach leading to formation of Cold Damp-Phlegm. In clinical practice it is often seen that some patients, and especially children, suffering from Spleen-Yang deficiency have been taking antibiotics for too long or too often frequently. People who often use Heat-clearing herbs for their Heat syndromes may also eventually damage their Spleen and Stomach-Yang. All these habits finally bring about dysfunction of the processes of digestion, transportation and transformation of the Spleen and Stomach, resulting in the development of Cold-Damp.

Addition of too much salt to food is another important pathogenic factor. This practice damages the Kidney. A certain amount of salt intake in the food is necessary for the functioning body, especially for the Kidney, because according to TCM a salty taste goes into the Kidney and can disperse Qi and promote defecation. However, overuse of salt will impair the physiological function of the Kidney—that of Qi transformation and water metabolism. As a result, Excessive Water accumulates in the body, leading to pain in the limbs and body, oedema, and a feeling of heaviness in the body generally.

OVEREATING OF FATTY AND FIERY FOOD AS WELL AS DRINKING HEATING BEVERAGES

In the West, many people have a tendency to be too Yang, probably because of the following factors:

- constitutional Yang excess or Yin deficiency from the parents
- depletion of Liver-Yin and Kidney-Yin due to too much sex, overworking, too much excitement or too much stress
- too much consumption of warming meats (e.g. pork, lamb, beef or rabbit)

- too much drinking of milk and eating milk products, such as cheese
- eating of too much sweet food (e.g. sweets, biscuits and chocolate)
- too-frequent consumption of fiery food (e.g. too much application of pepper in the cooking)
- too-frequent consumption of wine or other warming alcohol.

According to TCM theory, the constitution of the parents is largely passed on to the next generation. Constitutional Yang Excess leads to a predisposition to many diseases, and can also predispose to the invasion of External Heat, leading to the development of a mixture of Internal Heat and Exogenous Heat.

Alcohol that is warm or hot in nature can overload the Spleen and Stomach, leading to impedance of their functions of transportation and transformation, and a condition of Phlegm-Heat subsequently develops. Both white wine and red wine are equally warming by nature. However, drinking a certain amount of rice wine from time to time is healthy for the Qi, and specially the Blood, circulation—which is why there are a lot of herbal formulas to be taken at the beginning of winter that need to be decocted in a little wine, or soaked in wine. Rice wine, according to TCM, warms the interiors, dispels Cold, resolves stagnant Blood, smoothes the channels and circulates the collaterals. Many diet therapists also prescribe 10 to 20 ml of wine every day for people suffering from Qi and Yang deficiency. However, it is not advisable to give wine to people with Yin deficiency, Yang Excess, Damp-Heat accumulation, etc.

In addition, prolonged use of some pharmaceutical drugs, such as corticosteroids, may also deplete the Yin of the body, specially that of the Lung, Spleen, Liver and Kidney, leading to the concentration of Body Fluids, and the development of sticky Phlegm, which in turn would cause stagnation of Blood in the body.

INADEQUATE FOOD INTAKE

An adequate amount of food is necessary to maintain health. Eating too little food may cause malnutrition, causing pain due to undernourishment of the body. Inadequate nourishment can be caused by dysfunction of the Spleen and Stomach; this may be the result of prolonged sickness, or of undereating because of financial shortage or being on a weight-reducing diet. Of course, if it is due to prolonged sickness, different methods should be used to treat the sickness. People who have a financial shortage may need to be helped or given advice to enable them to get enough food. However, nowadays more and more people in the West, specially women, desire to become or remain slim merely by following a strict diet, ignoring inherited differences. Of course, if the overweight were purely caused by overconsumption of food and drink then a fairly strict diet would be one of the best methods to reduce the weight. However, if the cause is Spleen-Qi deficiency, causing weakness of transportation and transformation, such diets can only aggravate this deficiency, as a Damp condition would constantly be precipitated, tending to increase the weight. Once Damp blocks the channels, joints, muscles and Zang-Fu organs, pain also occurs.

INTAKE OF UNHYGIENIC FOOD

Unhygienic food includes not only poisonous food, food that has deteriorated and allergenic food, but also other contaminated food. Although it is not so difficult to avoid the first of these, it is not easy to avoid all contamination. Indeed, with industrial development, these days one can say that pollution exists everywhere—in the air, water and earth. Pollution can also be caused by nuclear weapon testing and use. So the food we eat naturally will sometimes be contaminated. Eating food with traces of contaminants disturbs the physiological functions of the Spleen and Stomach, leading to the development of Damp and Toxin accumulation, which may spread with the Qi and Blood circulation everywhere in the body, causing disorders in other Zang-Fu organs, and in the channels, joints and muscles. Generally speaking, food poisons and pollution first attack the Spleen and Stomach, and because the Spleen dominates the muscles and the limbs, pain from this cause usually occurs in the muscles and the limbs.

Drugs and hormones may be given to farm animals so as to promote their growth and shorten their developmental period. Eating the meat from such animals can, of course, disturb the person's Spleen, Stomach and especially the Kidney. So this inhibits the physiological function of these organs in transportation and transformation of water, and as a consequence Damp-Phlegm develops. That is why people who frequently eat such meats tend to suffer from body swelling, overweight, body pain, and so on.

OVERSTRESS, OVERSTRAIN OR LACK OF PHYSICAL EXERTION

STRESS

In addition to the emotions mentioned earlier, too much stress is also a causative factor in many diseases. In the industrialised countries many people work and live under enormous stress. This could include stress in any of the areas of social and work relationships, sexual relationships, family relationships, living conditions, finances, etc. According to TCM, stress may cause the following disorders:

- stagnation of the Qi of the Heart, Lung, Liver and Spleen, eventually leading to stagnation of Blood, which is a common causative factor in various kinds of pain
- depletion of the Qi and Yin, specially the Yin of the Liver and Kidney and the Qi of the Kidney. This is the causative factor that can cause pain due to deficiency of Qi and Yin, leading to undernourishment of the body.

PHYSICAL EXERTION AND EXERCISE

According to TCM theory, normal and regular physical exercises, combined with adequate rest, are very important for health, because they build up the constitution and help prevent disease. However, overstrain or excessive exercise, or indeed any excessive physical or mental activity, may deplete the energy generally, including the Qi, Blood, Yin and Yang, leading to weakening of the body's Defensive Qi. This leaves the body more vulnerable to the invasion of Exogenous factors, and to dysfunction of the Zang-Fu organs. For instance, overstudy will deplete the energy in the brain. Since according to TCM the brain substance is formed from the Marrow, which derives from the Kidney-Essence, if there is mental exhaustion then the Kidney-Essence will in turn gradually be depleted, leading to lack of nourishment of the brain and lower back and symptoms such as headache and lower back pain follow. This is the reason why many intellectuals and students suffer from chronic headaches and lower back pain even if they are very conscientious about the degree of physical exertion and sexual activity they undertake. In addition, overheavy labour or making the same physical movements for long periods may lead to weakness and strain of the muscles and tendons in the locality; Qi and Blood circulation will also be impaired. For example, builders often suffer from low back pain due to frequent lifting of too-heavy loads, and players of some sports suffer overexertion of their elbows, causing 'tennis elbow'.

The other extreme, of too little exertion, or living an excessively comfortable life with lack of physical exercise, can also be a causative factor in pain. According to TCM, this is because these habits may:

- slow down the Qi and Blood circulation
- weaken the functions of the Spleen and Stomach
- soften the muscles, tendons and bones.

All these effects may eventually cause Qi and Blood to stagnate, leading to the development of Damp, weakness in the tendon and bones, etc., and finally the appearance of pain. This situation can be seen in, for example, some people on benefits and old people who may suffer from general body pain that is made worse by more rest and sleep. Once they are advised to take some moderate physical exercise (such as slow walking, running, swimming, as well as light physical work) their pain tends to improve. The reason for this is that once they start to exercise, their Qi and Blood circulation improves, which stimulates the physiological function of the Zang-Fu organs, and the pain then diminishes. Pain caused by too little exertion can typically be seen in patients who lie for too long in bed without enough movement; their limbs can become swollen and purplish in colour, and stiff and painful as muscular atrophy with stabbing accompanying or contracting pain occurs. As soon as they begin to walk, or even do some physical movements while seated, the muscular atrophy gradually disappears, the stiff joints becomes freer and flexible, and the pain often vanishes by itself, or with the help of some simple treatment.

TRAUMATIC INJURIES

Traumatic injuries include gunshots, penetrating knife wounds, beating, falling, accidents, scalds, burns, frostbite, muscular sprain caused by sudden or frequent lifting or carrying too-heavy loads, bites by animals or insects, and so on.

WOUNDS AND JOINT INJURIES

Gunshots, incision by knives, beating, falling, accidents, etc., may directly result in muscular swelling, bleeding and haematoma, or joint dislocation or fracture involving the tendons, muscles and bones. There may also be damage to the internal Zang-Fu organs, and shock following on from sudden and severe pain.

BURNS, SCALDS AND FREEZING CONDITIONS

Scalds and burns may result from industrial chemicals, boiling water or oil, or fires. If only the superficial layer of the skin is affected then tissue damage may be confined to redness, swelling, heat and blisters, and pain may be moderate. However, if scalds or burns are severe, the tendons, deep muscles and even the bones can be damaged, resulting in severe pain.

Frostbite may also cause damage of the skin, muscles and even tendons, leading to severe pain. This often occurs in locations where the winter temperatures are very low. Frostbite may affect only the limbs, or the body generally, often attacking those who tend to have deficiency of Yang Qi with poor Blood circulation. In consequence, the body is not sufficiently warmed and protected, and Qi and Blood stagnation develop, causing contraction of the tendons, blood vessels and muscles, and pain develops.

SPRAINS

Muscle contraction or sprain due to sudden or quite frequent lifting or carrying too-heavy loads is also a common cause of pain, especially in the limbs and lower back. It leads to disorder of Qi and Blood circulation, damage to the tendons and muscles, abnormal joint movement, and hence to an alteration in the body's physical structure; this causes Qi and Blood stagnation, and pain follows. The longer stagnation of Qi and Blood persists, the more complications are seen.

OPERATIONS

Operations can be also be causative factors in pain. In the West, operations are carried out in all hospital departments, most of the time they have positive results, but sometimes the operation is a failure, or may even aggravate the problem. In any event, the operation often necessitates cutting through tissues, so almost inevitably there is some bleeding during the operation, and some blood may be left behind in the body, leading to the development of Blood stagnation.

According to the TCM viewpoint, pain after an operation can be caused by:

- disturbance of the Qi and Blood circulation
- a deleterious effect on the physiological functions of the Zang-Fu organs
- damage to or even complete blockage of channel circulation
- the persistence of excessive amounts of blood in the body from bleeding during the operation, which then becomes stagnant
- scar formation.

Pathology of pain

The main pathology: disorder of Qi and Blood circulation

From the above discussion, it can be clearly seen that there are various kinds of causative factors bringing about pain, but the main pathology is either due to blockage and obstruction, or to deficiency. The basic statement about pain, formed almost two thousand years ago, is: if there is free flow, there is no pain; however, if there is a disruption of this free flow then pain occurs. Here 'free flow' refers to the free flow of Qi and Blood. The circulation of Qi and Blood in the body should be constant, just like the continual courses of the sun and moon. According to TCM, this circulation depends upon the correct, interdependent functioning of the Zang-Fu organs, including the Lung, Heart, Liver and Kidney. The Lung disperses Qi to every part of the body, and also connects to the blood vessels, thus keeping the Qi and Blood circulating freely in the body. The Heart is in charge of promoting the circulation of Blood in their Vessels. The Liver is in charge of keeping the Qi circulating freely, which in turn keeps the Blood circulating freely. The circulation of Liver-Qi also promotes the digestive functions of the Spleen and Stomach, and this keeps the water passages clear, so preventing the accumulation of Damp in the body. The Kidney is the root of Yang Qi, which warms the Qi and Blood to maintain their free circulation. Moreover, the Kidney also produces Yuan Qi or Original Qi, which is the root energy for all the Zang-Fu organs. Where there is dysfunction of any of these organs, due to the various kinds of pathogenic factors discussed earlier, there will be retardation of the Qi and Blood circulation, eventually causing pain.

Mechanisms in the disorder of Qi and Blood circulation

DISORDER OF QI AND BLOOD CIRCULATION DUE TO EXOGENOUS FACTORS

The mechanisms causation of the disorder of Qi and Blood circulation vary according to the nature of the pathogenic factor.

When Wind, Heat and Fire, the Yang pathogenic factors, invade the body they accelerate the circulation of Qi and Blood creating an abnormal circulation and local congestion of Qi and Blood. This may cause blockage in the Qi and Blood circulation, and so pain develops.

Cold, a Yin pathogenic factor, may damage the Yang of the body, so that Excess of Yin and Cold develop in the body. Cold is characterised by Stagnation and contraction, so when Cold and Excess Cold invade the body there is a decreased Qi and Blood circulation and also spasm of the channels and Blood Vessels. This slows the circulation of Qi and Blood, and pain eventually results.

Damp is characterised by stagnation and viscosity. The presence of Damp, whether caused by Exogenous invasion or by dysfunction of the Internal Zang-Fu organs, may slow the Qi and Blood circulation because the channels and Blood Vessels become narrowed, or there may even be Qi and Blood stagnation.

Dryness may damage the Lung causing failure of the Lung to disperse the Qi and Body Fluids. As a consequence the channels and blood vessels are not properly nourished, the Qi and Blood circulation slows, and so pain follows.

DISORDER OF THE QI AND BLOOD CIRCULATION DUE TO EMOTIONAL DISTURBANCE

Emotional disorder may cause direct dysfunction in the Zang-Fu organs, disturbing in turn the Qi and Blood circulation, so that the Qi and Blood stagnate, and pain follows.

Excessive grief may slow the Qi circulation in the Lung, so the Lung cannot properly disperse the Qi and Body Fluids; this causes both stagnation of Qi and Blood and formation of Damp, and pain develops.

Too much anger, frustration, anxiety and stress may prevent the Liver from maintaining a free Qi circulation through the body, and stagnation of Qi as well as of Blood occur, as a consequence. In addition, Qi stagnation in the Liver may cause stagnation of Qi in other organs such as Lung, Heart and Spleen, leading to Blood stagnation and accumulation of Damp as well. All these situations bring about pain.

Too much meditation may cause the Qi in the Spleen to stagnate, disturbing the transportational and transformative functions of the organ, and so Damp accumulates, or Qi and Blood become deficient, any of which which may result in pain.

Fear and fright may impair the Kidney, leading to sinking of the Qi there; as a consequence the original Qi becomes weak, so it cannot properly promote Qi and Blood circulation in the body, and the Qi and Blood circulation slows.

TCM also holds that the Heart stores the Mind, and a person's emotional states are a reflection of mental stimulation caused by the External environment, thus the Heart will be affected by all kinds of emotional activities.

DISORDER OF QI AND BLOOD CIRCULATION DUE TO BAD DIET, PHYSIC TRAUMA AND ANIMAL BITES

Bad diet may disrupt the ascending and descending of Qi in the Middle Jiao, or Middle Burner. This can lead to a slowing down in the Qi circulation, thus Qi stagnates, and pain will be the result. A bad diet may also make the Qi and Blood deficient, or cause Damp to develop in the body. The former may cause under-nourishment of the Zang-Fu organs, channels, muscles, tendons, bones and Blood Vessels, and as a result pain of a deficient type may occur. The latter may cause the channels and Blood Vessels to narrow, leading in turn to stagnation of the Qi and Blood. Physic trauma and bites by animals may cause direct injury to the muscles, tendons, bones, channels, and even Internal Zang-Fu organs, also leading to stagna-tion of Qi and Blood, or damage to body tissues.

DISORDER OF QI AND BLOOD CIRCULATION DUE TO IMPROPER EXERTION

Overstrain, overindulgence in sex and excessive study may all exhaust the Qi and Blood, leading to their defi-ciency; thus pain occurs caused by undernourishment of the body. Too little physical exertion and living too luxuriously may also slow the Qi and Blood circula-tion, leading to pain resulting from a gradual stagna-tion of the Qi and Blood.

An explanation for pain resulting from disordered Qi and Blood circulation

It should now be clear that pain is mainly a result of dis-turbances in the Qi and Blood circulation, and may be caused by stagnation of Qi and Blood, or deficiency of Qi and Blood—but why does this disturbance of Qi and Blood flow cause pain? Which organ is in charge of pain? The reason was stated clearly, two thousand years ago, in the Simple question: 'all kinds of pain, itching and sores are due to Heart disorder' (Yellow Emperor's Classic of Internal Medicine: Simple Questions 1956, p. 190). Why did the ancient texts attribute pain to the Heart? This can be explained as follows.

THE HEART DOMINATES THE BLOOD AND BLOOD VESSELS

The Heart promotes normal Blood circulation in the Zang-Fu organs, Blood Vessels, channels and the

tissues. Where the Qi and Blood circulation are dis-ordered, a disturbed feedback will be sent to the Heart. In other words, one can say that the Heart is constantly sensitive to the condition of the Qi and Blood circulation.

THE HEART IS THE CONTROLLER OF THE MIND

Modern medicine considers that pain is the body's way of responding to damaged tissue. For instance, when a bone breaks, nerves send pain messages through the spinal cord to the brain, where they are interpreted. The TCM viewpoint is that pain is the reflection of the Mind (Shen) to the stimulation from the environment, and the activity of the Mind is con-sidered to be the result of physiological function of the Heart. When the Qi and Blood circulation are dis-turbed, this situation will be conveyed to the Heart, and the pain that follows is a response from the Mind to this situation. According to this viewpoint, pain is closely related to the Heart.

THE HEART IS THE ROOT CONTROLLER OF THE OTHER ZANG-FU ORGANS

How a person responds to pain is determined by many factors, of which emotional states are very important. For example, depression seems to increase a person's perception of pain and to decrease the ability to cope with both the pain and the treatment. Thus treating the depression treats the pain as well. If pain is not adequately treated, then pain impulses are more readily transmitted to the brain. Therefore, in TCM it is considered that it is more effective to prevent pain than to treat it after it occurs.

In terms of the relationship between the emotions, the interior organs and the Heart, TCM holds that the Heart dominates the emotions and is the root con-troller of other Zang-Fu organs. For instance, Ling Shu (1963) states: 'the Heart is the root controller for five Zang organs and six Fu organs, therefore the Heart will be disturbed by grief and meditation' (p. 69). In the same book Ben Shen points out in addition that: 'the Heart has the responsibility to all kinds of emo-tional stimulation' (p. 23). All these statements clearly mention that the Heart can be influenced by the dys-function of other Zang-Fu organs as well the difference emotions, and this may lead to the development of pain.

Occurrence of pain

4

疼
痛
的
发
生

According to TCM, pain occurs when there is stagnation of Qi and Blood, or deficiency of Qi and Blood, resulting from the various kinds of causative factors discussed earlier in the book. However, its occurrence also reflects the fight between the body's Wei Qi, or Defensive Qi, and the pathogenic Qi. When pain occurs and develops this indicates that the person's Defensive Qi is relative weak, or that the pathogenic factors are particularly strong. However, if pain resolves spontaneously or after the proper treatment this indicates that the Defensive Qi is stronger than the pathogenic Qi, and the proper circulation of Qi and Blood has been restored. In a word, whether pain occurs, and its time-course, relies on the state of Defensive Qi.

Generally speaking, the state of the body's Defensive Qi is determined by factors such as the person's constitution, emotional state, living environment, the diet and the amount and type of physical exercise undertaken, amongst other things.

Constitution

The constitution is composed of two basic elements: the congenital and the postnatal conditions.

Congenital condition

The congenital condition is closely related to the condition of the parents. People may inherit both positive and negative constitutions. The congenital condition may greatly influence the reaction of the body to pain in later life. TCM places some importance on the conditions of the parents immediately before pregnancy. In general, they should ensure they are in their best physical health and a good emotional state while preparing for pregnancy. They are advised to complete copulation when both partners are in orgasm, and conversely to try to avoid the woman getting pregnant when under stress or during physical sickness. This important advice is widely given at present in China because of the one-child policy. For young couples who want a pregnancy, a general physical check-up is carried out so as to try to get as healthy a baby as possible.

The situation during the pregnancy is also of importance. During this time, the woman should have abundant sleep, avoid stress and extreme emotional disturbance, quit smoking and other bad habits, avoid as far as possible taking any medical drugs, and have a sufficient intake of nutritious food, accompanied by a certain amount of physical exercise. All these steps are necessary to maintain good health so as to ensure the child has a good constitution.

Postnatal condition

The postnatal condition is also an important factor in the overall constitution; according to TCM theory this is because the Congenital Essence (or 'Pre-Heaven Essence') is nourished constantly by the Postnatal Essence (or 'Post-Heaven Essence'). If people do not take proper care of their health, the Postnatal Essence becomes deficient and the constitution will also become impaired. Excessive sex is one of the most common causes for weakness of the Kidney-Essence. It is true that a moderate amount of sex can also stimulate the production of Kidney-Essence, relieve pent-up emotions and smooth the Qi and Blood circulation. However, excessive sex may quickly exhaust the Qi and Blood, especially Kidney-Essence. As a consequence, the bone and Marrow receive no nourishment, the low back is not properly supported, and lower back pain follows.

In fact, Deficiency of Kidney-Essence can be caused not only by excessive sex, but also by the natural decline of Kidney-Essence with age. According to TCM, after middle age, which is around 45 years old, the Kidney-Essence start to decline, the body resistance becomes weaker, and thus pathogenic factors may more easily invade the body. That is why more older people tend to suffer from pain than do young people.

Emotional state

A person's emotional state constantly influences the activity of Qi and Blood as well as physiology of the Zang-Fu organs; in fact it may directly affect the state of the Upright Qi (Zheng Qi). If the person's emotions are well-balanced, the physiological function of the Zang-Fu organs will be harmonious, the Qi and Blood flow freely without any blockage, and Defensive Qi will be abundant. The physical condition as a whole will prevent pathogenic factors invading, and diseases will not be able to take hold. However, if there is emotional disturbance, and especially if this is of long duration, the result will be disharmony of the Zang-Fu organs, blockage of the Qi and Blood circulation and a weakening of Defensive Qi, and this will predispose the person to invasion of pathogenic factors and occurrence of disease.

Living conditions

The person's environment is also related to the occurrence of disease. For instance, moving around to different areas with different climates, water, food and drink may induce changes in physiological functions. Normally people can adapt to the new environment without harm to their health, but if there is a too-sudden change of living area this can cause weakness of the body, and illness as a consequence.

The living environment also includes good lifestyle habits, such as regularity in everyday activities, as this also influences the condition of Defensive Qi. In present-day society this could be one of the most important causative factors in illness.

Diet

A proper diet is the correct and sufficient intake of nutrients. It doesn't mean that the more you eat the better. Irregular eating, or overeating of certain kinds of food, or eating too little, all directly impede the function of Spleen and Stomach in digesting, transporting and transforming the food. As a consequence the Qi, Blood and Body Fluids will become deficient, which will in turn decrease the amount of Defensive Qi, and illness may follow.

Physical exercises

There is a Chinese saying that the life comes from constant moving. Here 'moving' refers to active participation in physical exercises to improve the constitution and keep the circulation of Qi and Blood smooth, so as to increase the ability of the body to resist disease. Sport, and exercises such as Qigong, Taijiquan (Tai Chi Chuan), and Wushu are good physical exercises that have been practised by Chinese people for thousands of years. In China it is common to see both old and young people, in groups or alone practising exercises in the early morning or in the evening. Such activity is especially good for retired people. Many retired people in the West stop most of their physical activities after retirement, and that is why so many old people suffer from a slow digestion after sitting or resting for a long time; their digestion would be improved if they increased their amount of physical movement.

In summary, the TCM viewpoint is that pain occurs when there is disorder of Yin and Yang, disharmony of Qi and Blood and dysfunction of the Zang-Fu organs, as a result of various kinds of pathogenic factors.

Differentiation of pain 5

疼痛的辨证

Differentiation of the location of pain

Pain generally occurs at only certain locations, and it is very important to find out where these are in order to determine which Zang-Fu organs or channels are involved, as this may help greatly in determining treatment accurately.

The Zang-Fu organs

The locations of the Zang-Fu organs are as follows:

- Upper Jiao (or Upper Burner): Heart and Lung
- Middle Jiao (Middle Burner): Spleen, Stomach, Liver and Gall Bladder
- Lower Jiao (Lower Burner): Kidney, Bladder, Uterus, Small and Large Intestine.

However, since the Internal Zang-Fu organs are closely related to each other through the channels and collaterals, it is very possible to see pain occurring in a certain place that is caused by a problem in other place, so attention also has to be paid to clinical manifestations. For instance, in a case of stagnation of Liver-Qi with invasion of the Lung by Liver-Fire, there would be chest pain, fullness of the chest, cough, blood in the phlegm, a red tip and edge of the tongue, and a thin and yellow tongue coating, and in addition hypochondriac pain, restlessness, nervousness and headache. In this case, the chest pain is nothing to do with the External invasion to the Lung, but rather with the Liver disorder. The correct treatment should be to calm the Liver, reduce the Liver-Fire, and make the Lung-Qi descend.

The channels

As to the distribution of the 14 channels, the 12 regular channels are distributed symmetrically on the left and right sides of the body. The other two major channels, the Governing Vessel (abbreviated GV, the DuMai) and the Directing (or Conception) Vessel (abbreviated CV, the Ren Mai), emerge from the perineum, and ascend respectively along the middle line of the front and back of the body.

CHANNEL DISTRIBUTION IN THE LIMBS

On the upper limbs the distribution is as follows:

- The anterior border of the medial aspect and radial end of the thumb are supplied by the Greater Yin (Tai Yin) channel of the hand.
- The middle of the medial aspect and the radial end of the middle finger are supplied by the Terminal Yin (Jue Yin) channel of the hand.
- The posterior border of the medial aspect and the radial end of the small finger are supplied by the Lesser Yin (Shao Yin) channel of the hand.
- The Bright Yang (Yang Ming) channel of the hand goes from the radial end of the index finger to the anterior border of the lateral aspect.
- The Lesser Yang (Shao Yang) channel of the hand goes from the end of the index finger to the middle of the lateral aspect.
- The Greater Yang (Tai Yang) channel of the hand goes from the ulnar end of the small finger to the posterior border of the lateral aspect.

On the lower limbs the distribution is as follows:

- The anterior border of the lateral aspect and the lateral end of the second toe are supplied by the Bright Yang (Yang Ming) channel of the foot.
- The middle of the lateral side and the lateral end of the fourth toe by the Lesser Yang (Shao Yang) channel of the foot.
- The posterior border of the lateral aspect and the lateral end of the little toe are supplied by the Greater Yang (Tai Yang) channel of the foot.
- The Greater Yin (Tai Yin) channel of the foot runs from the medial end of the great toe to the middle of the medial aspect of the lower limb and then goes round to its anterior border.
- The Terminal Yin (Jue Yin) channel of the foot goes from the lateral end of the great toe to the anterior border of the medial aspect of the lower limb and then shifts to the middle.
- The Lesser Yin (Shao Yin) channel of the foot starts under the little toe, crosses the sole and then goes along the posterior border of the medial aspect of the lower limb.

CHANNEL DISTRIBUTION IN THE TRUNK

In the thoracic and abdominal regions the Directing Vessel is situated on the middle line. The first line lateral to it is the Kidney channel–Lesser Yin channel of the foot, the second lateral line is the Stomach channel–Bright Yang channel of the foot, and the Lung channel–Greater Yin channel of the hand and the Spleen channel–Greater Yin channel of the foot correspond to the third line. The Gall Bladder channel–Lesser Yang channel of the foot is located at the lateral side of the hypochondria and the lumbar region, while the Liver channel–Terminal Yin channel of the foot is in the region of the anterior external genitalia and hypochondria.

On the back, the Governing Vessel is in the midline, while both the first and second lines lateral to it are the Bladder channel–Greater Yang channel of the foot.

CHANNEL DISTRIBUTION IN THE HEAD, FACE AND NECK

The Bright Yang channels of the hand and foot run in the facial region; and the Lesser Yang channels of the hand and foot travel in the lateral sides of the head. The Governing Vessel goes along the middle line of the neck and head, while the Bladder channel–Greater Yang channel of the foot runs on both sides of this channel.

Differentiation of the level of pain

Differentiation of the level of pain is a TCM method of recognising and diagnosing pain that is also a way of making a comprehensive analysis of the symptoms and signs obtained when applying four diagnostic methods. This method enables the clinician to differentiate whether the cause of the pain is due to invasion of external factors or to internal disorders, to Cold or Heat, to Excess or Deficiency, to Qi disorder or Blood disorder, as well as to Wind, Cold, Damp, Heat or Dryness, and so on.

Exogenous invasion or internal disorder

The categories of Exogenous invasion and Internal disorder are two principles that are used to determine the depth of the pain and to generalise the direction of its development (Table 5.1).

Generally, treatment will be relatively easy and have relatively good therapeutic results if the pain is caused by Exogenous invasion. The principles of treatment in this case are to induce sweating so as to dispel Exogenous factors, promote Qi and Blood circulation and so sedate the pain.

Table 5.1 Differentiation of pain into Exogenous and Internal types

	Exogenous	Internal
Onset	acute	gradual
Duration	short	long
Symptoms	yes	no
Tongue	normal, or no change	much change
Pulse	superficial (floating)	deep

If the pain is caused by Internal disorders, however, its treatment will be not so easy, since such disorders are often caused by factors such as emotional disturbance, bad diet, overstrain, and as a result the level of the sickness tends to be deeper than that caused by exogenous invasion. Furthermore, if the Externally derived pathogenic factors are not expelled from the Exterior of the body, they will affect the Interior, giving rise to pain due to Interior disorders. The main principles of treatment in this instance are to harmonise the Zang-Fu organs, tonify the Deficiency, eliminate the Excess, circulate Qi and Blood and so stop the pain.

Cold and Heat

Cold and Heat are the two principles used to differentiate the nature of the pain (Table 5.2).

If the pain is caused by Cold, it is usually a result of invasion of Exogenous Cold, or deficiency of Yang of the body, leading to hypofunction of Internal Zang-Fu organs. Its manifestations include aversion to cold and chills, a pale complexion, cold hands and feet, a preference for warmth, an absence of thirst, clear urine, loose stools, a white or wet tongue coating, and a slow pulse. The main principles of treatment here are to dispel the Cold, warm the Yang and stop the pain;

Table 5.2 Differentiation of pain into Cold and Hot types

	Cold	Hot
Hands and feet	cold	warm
Face	pale, or blue	red
Thirst	absent	present
Stiffness	yes	no
Urine	clear	turbid and deep yellow
Stool	mostly diarrhoea	mostly constipation
Tongue	pale tongue, white coating	red tongue, yellow coating
Pulse	slow	rapid

cupping and moxibustion are the best ways to relieve pain due to Cold.

If the pain is due to Heat, it is usually caused by invasion of Exogenous Heat, or conversion of Cold into Heat because of overlong Cold accumulation, or Excessive-Yang in the body, or the formation of Deficient-Heat resulting from Yin deficiency. Its manifestations are fever, aversion to heat, headache, thirst, deep yellow urine, a red face, warm hands and feet, restlessness, insomnia, constipation, a red tongue with yellow coating and a rapid pulse. The principles of treatment in this case are to clear the Heat, reduce the fever, cool the Blood and stop the pain.

Excess and Deficiency

Excess and Deficiency are the two principles that are used to generalise and distinguish the relative strength of the Defensive Qi and pathogenic factors (Table 5.3). Chapter 28 of the Plain questions states, 'Excess is due to hyperactivity of the pathogenic factors, and Deficiency is due to overconsumption of essential Qi' (Yellow Emperor's Classic of Internal Medicine: Simple Questions 1956, p. 62). This differentiation determines whether treatment aims at eliminating the pathogenic factors or tonifying the Defensive Qi.

Table 5.3 Differentiation of pain into Excess and Deficiency types

	Excess	Deficiency
Onset	acute	gradual
Duration	short	long
Location	fixed	moving
Response to touch	preference for pressure and massage	dislike of pressure and massage
Intensity	constant	intermittent
Pulse	excessive (full)	deficient (empty)

Qi stagnation and Blood stagnation

The main pathogenic change in pain is stagnation of Qi and Blood. However, it is very important to find out whether the situation is predominantly one of Qi stagnation, or Blood stagnation, or Qi and Blood stagnation in equal proportion. This differentiation determines whether treatment is geared towards circulating the Qi, or circulating the Blood, or circulating both Qi and Blood together (Table 5.4).

Table 5.4 Differentiation of pain into Qi stagnation and Blood stagnation types

	Qi stagnation	Blood stagnation
Location	moving	fixed
Nature	distending	stabbing
Hardness	soft	hard
Fullness	yes	no
Time of attack	daytime	night-time
Emotion	aggravating pain	no direct influence
Tongue	not purplish	purplish
Pulse	wiry	choppy

Damp and Dryness

Damp and Dryness are the two principles that are used to determine the condition of the Body Fluids (Table 5.5).

Damp, whether caused by Exogenous invasion or by disorder of Zang-Fu organs, is a pathogenic factor that easily blocks the channels, muscles and Zang-Fu organs, causing pain of the Excess type to occur. The main principles of treatment in this case are to eliminate Damp, activate the Spleen and Stomach, circulate Qi and Blood in the channels, relieve the blockage and so stop the pain.

Dryness is usually caused by Exogenous invasion, or deficiency of Yin due to Yang Excess, or excessive vomiting, diarrhoea, sweating or bleeding, or weakness of Zang-Fu organs. The pain caused by Dryness is usually due to undernourishment of the body, leading to contraction of the channels, Blood Vessels, muscles and Zang-Fu organs. The principles of treatment in this situation are to nourish Yin and Blood, promote the secretion of Body Fluids, moisten the Dryness and relieve spasm so as to stop the pain.

Table 5.5 Differentiation of pain into Damp and Dryness types

	Damp	Dryness
Lassitude	yes	no
Heaviness	yes	no
Fullness	yes	no
Appetite	disturbed	not disturbed
Mouth	watery feeling	dry mouth
Nose	nasal discharge	dry nose
Throat	phlegm in the throat	dry throat
Stool	loose, or diarrhoea	hard, or constipation
Tongue	greasy, or wet coating	dry, or peeled coating
Pulse	slippery	thready, or choppy

Wind, Cold, Damp and Heat

Where the pain is caused by Wind, Cold, Damp or Heat due to either Exogenous invasion or Internal disorders, there is often seen to be a predominance of one or two of these pathogenic factors. The differentiation of Wind, Cold, Damp and Heat is the way to distinguish whether treatment should be based on dispelling Wind, warming the Cold, eliminating Damp or clearing Heat.

PAIN DUE TO PREDOMINANCE OF WIND

Pain due to invasion of Exogenous Wind usually is not very heavy nor constant, but if the pain is caused by internal disorders, it tends to be more severe. Internal Wind can be caused by hyperactivity of Liver-Yang, formation of Wind resulting from Excessive-Heat, and formation of Wind due to deficiency of Blood. The principles of treatment for Exogenous Wind are to dispel the Wind and relieve External symptoms; for Internal disorders they are to calm the Liver, suppress the Wind, reduce the Heat and moisten the Blood Dryness.

The symptoms of Wind include the following.

- It is basically moving, wandering, erratic or migratory, coming and going like the wind. The pain is moving continuously—for instance, rheumatic pain occurs first in one joint and then in another, and a headache may occur on the left side one day and on the right the next.
- The type of symptom changes—for example, the quality of pain may sometimes be sharp, sometimes there is soreness, at another time there is numbness, later on there will be distending pain. Different sensations occur, or the sensibility varies.
- Symptoms are often abrupt, appear suddenly, and are acute or paroxysmal—for example, in migraine the headache is acute and very heavy. Wind symptoms can occur suddenly and disappear as rapidly as well.
- There is an aversion to wind and a slight fever where the pain is due to invasion of exogenous Wind.

If the pain is due to Internal Wind resulting from hyperactivity of Liver-Yang, there is restlessness, headache, thirst, nervousness, a red tongue with yellow coating and a wiry and rapid pulse. If the pain is due to accumulation of Excessive-Heat, there is a high fever, headache, much thirst, restlessness, constipation, a deep red tongue with no coating and a rapid and forceful pulse. In case the pain is due to deficiency of Blood in the Liver, there is trembling of the head and limbs, tiredness, a pale complexion, dry eyes and skin, numbness in the limbs, scanty menstruation or amenorrhoea, a pale tongue with a thin coating and a thready and weak pulse.

Besides the above characteristics, other general symptoms of Wind can occur, such as:

- fear of Wind, fear of draught, aggravation when the weather is Windy
- sweating, which is due to opening of the pores by the invasion of the Wind factor.

PAIN DUE TO PREDOMINANCE OF COLD

Pain can be caused by either invasion of Exogenous Cold or deficiency of Yang Qi in the body; the latter situation is usually a deficiency of Yang of the Heart, Spleen or Kidney. If there is Exogenous Cold invasion then the principles of treatment are to dispel the Cold and relieve the External symptoms; for Internal disorders treatment aims to warm the Interior, strengthen the Heart, activate the Spleen and tonify the Kidney.

The symptoms of Cold include the following.

- Unlike pain that is due to Wind, Coldness freezes Qi and Blood locally, so the pain is fixed, seldom moves and is well localised.
- Since Cold is contracting and blocking, it slows down any movement. If the pain is caused by Cold, then it is rather severe, and very sharp or stabbing as the Cold causes Blood stagnation.
- Another possible symptom accompanying the pain is stiffness due to the freezing effect of the Cold, as in 'frozen shoulder'.
- The pain is improved by warmth and movement, but is aggravated by cold and rest. It is also aggravated in cold weather or by using cold therapy.
- There is aversion to cold and occasionally a slight fever in cases of invasion of Exogenous Cold.

The Exogenous Cold pathogenic factor has Yin characteristics. However, invasion of the body by Exogenous Cold may cause a Yang reaction in the superficial layers of the body as the skin pores are closed, so the body is not able to sweat. Due to this, the Body Fluids try to escape out of the body through the urine, thus there is frequent discharge of large quantities of clear urine.

Besides a lack of perspiration, the person shivers to help the body maintain its temperature at a normal level. Muscular fibrillation also produces some warmth, so there can be a degree of fever, but chills and a cold feeling are predominant.

If the Heart-Yang is deficient, there is pain in the chest, an aversion to cold, cold limbs, palpitations, the spirits are low, there is a pale tongue with a thin coating and deep, slow and thready pulse.

If the Spleen-Yang is deficient, there are loose stools, or diarrhoea, abdominal pain, an aversion to cold, cold in the limbs, a feeling of tiredness, a thin and white coating, or even greasy coating, to the tongue and a thready, slow and weak pulse.

If the Kidney-Yang is deficient, there is lower back pain, weakness of the knees, frequent urination, nycturia, a feeling of tiredness, cold hands and feet, low potency, a thin and white tongue coating and a thready, slow and weak pulse.

In summary, generally, in Cold syndromes the following are noted:

- *tongue*: a thin and white coating, or a pale tongue
- *pulse*: a tight and superficial pulse if there is exogenous invasion, or a wiry and slow pulse if Yang of the Zang-Fu organs is deficient.

PAIN DUE TO PREDOMINANCE OF DAMP

Pain can be caused either by invasion of Exogenous Damp or by disorder of the Internal Zang-Fu organs, especially the Lung, Spleen or Kidney. The principles of treatment for the former are to dispel the Damp and relieve External symptoms; for the latter the aim is to restore the Zang-Fu organ function, eliminate the Damp and promote urination.

The symptoms of Damp include the following.

- The pain is very localised, and never moves as Damp, which is of the same nature as water, is characterised by heaviness and inertia, therefore there is no movement.
- There is a feeling of heaviness, tiredness and numbness, especially in the lower limbs and lower parts of the body.
- The affected parts are swollen; this swelling may be in the body or in the joints, and there may be an accumulation of liquid under the skin.
- Pain that is due to Damp is never sharp or acute; rather, it is deep, heavy and dull. Also it never appears suddenly, but slowly, gradually and chronically.
- Pain that is due to invasion of Exogenous Damp is aggravated in damp climatic conditions, such as when the weather is foggy, humid, wet or overcast. Wet places, moist walls or houses built

on swamps usually also make the pain more severe (this can be compared to miasmatic symptoms in homeopathy). Moreover, this kind of pain is mostly aggravated if it becomes complicated by Wind or Cold factors, as happens in Damp-Bi Syndrome.

- Pain that is due to Damp resulting from Internal disorder is usually aggravated by eating too-fatty and greasy food as well as by eating cold food.

In general, in Damp conditions the following are noted:

- *tongue*: the coating is thick, sticky, whitish and wet; also it is very wet and never dry, even watery
- *pulse*: this is weak-floating soft (Ru), or slippery (Hua) and a little slowed down (Huan).

PAIN DUE TO PREDOMINANCE OF HEAT

Heat can be caused either by invasion of Exogenous Heat or by accumulation of Internal Heat resulting from Yang Excess or Yin Deficiency. The principles of treatment for invasion of Exogenous Heat are to dispel the Heat, reduce the fever and relieve the External symptoms. For Yang Excess the aim is to clear the Heat, reduce the Fire and promote defecation in order to induce the Heat out of the body. For Yin Deficiency, it is to nourish Yin, clear the Heat and promote the secretion of Body Fluids.

The symptoms of Heat include the following.

- Heat, like Fire, is a Yang pathogenic factor, which may cause pain accompanied by redness and swelling of the joints and muscles.
- The joints are painful, with a feeling of warmth, and are difficult to move (as seen in acute inflammatory arthritis).

Besides these characteristics of any joint or muscle pain, the following general symptoms of Heat may be observed:

- fever, sometimes with a slight chill, although the fever and hot sensation predominate
- aversion to Heat
- thirst, dryness of the mouth
- irritability, nervousness or restlessness
- *tongue*: a red tip to the tongue, or the whole body of the tongue, and a yellowish coating; if there is Yin Deficiency a peeled or scanty coating
- *pulse*: a rapid and superficial pulse if there is invasion of exogenous Heat, rapid and forceful in Yang Excess, and rapid, thready and weak in Yin Deficiency.

At least two circumstances are required for a diagnosis of invasion of Exogenous Heat:

- predominance of Heat among Wind-Heat and Damp;
- the pre-existence of Excessive-Heat or Deficient-Heat in the body, which is usually caused by bad dietary habits, such as eating too much greasy, fatty or hot foods, or too many sweets, or drinking too much alcohol.

Emotional disturbances such as stress, frustration, excessive meditation, pent-up emotions and so on produce Liver-Qi stagnation and hyperactive Liver-Fire, which are manifested as irritability, nervousness, anger, insomnia, hot flushing, etc. Overwork, and infectious or chronic diseases, amongst other things, cause Yin deficiency with Deficient-Heat.

Invasive pathogenic factors can also be transformed into Heat (Huo Hua) if they are of prolonged duration. This transformation is generally incomplete at the beginning of the process, so a mixture of Heat, Wind, Cold and Damp are generally seen, but the Heat predominates.

Differentiation of the characteristics of pain

Sore pain

This kind of pain often occurs in all four limbs and the trunk, especially the lower back and places where there are a lot of soft muscles. It is not very severe, and is accompanied by weakness, soreness, lightness and emptiness. It is mostly caused by deficiency of Qi and Blood.

Distending pain

This type of pain often occurs in the chest and abdomen, and is mostly caused by stagnation of Qi. Because of the stagnation, it fluctuates in intensity and location, and is rather obviously influenced by emotional changes, especially by stress, anger, irritation, nervousness.

Stabbing pain

This is commonly seen in daily practice, and characteristically feels as if a needle or knife were pricking the skin or muscles. The pain occurs always in the same place, but can be worsened during the night or by lying/sitting in a still position; it is better after movement, and is accompanied by swelling or petechiae on the skin, a dislike of pressure, a purplish tongue, and sometimes petechiae on the tongue, and a choppy pulse. This type of pain is typically seen in patients with stagnation of Blood, and after physical trauma, thus to promote Blood circulation can quickly relieve the pain.

Sharp pain

This kind of pain is mostly seen to be caused by acute Qi and Blood stagnation, and especially Qi stagnation, and is due to various factors. It is greatly diminished by treating with methods that circulate the Qi and Blood; however, it is very important to discover and treat the real cause, otherwise the pain will always return.

Throbbing pain

This type of pain is characterised by its rhythmic quality, similar to beating of the pulse. It is often seen in patients with migraine, which is normally caused by hyperactivity of Liver-Yang. A throbbing pain is also found in patients with a carbuncle or furuncle of the Yang type, which is caused by invasion or accumulation of Toxic Heat in the body, and is accompanied by a feeling of heat, redness and swelling.

Burning pain

This kind of pain is characterised by pain with very hot feeling, as though the skin were burned, and is typically caused by Heat, either from invasion of exogenous Wind-Heat, Damp-Heat, Dryness-Heat or Toxic Heat, or Internal Heat from dysfunction of the Zang-Fu organs. In most cases, local redness and swelling can be observed.

Prolonged stagnation of Cold, or Qi and Blood, also may gradually produce Heat.

In contrast, in some patients who complain of a subjective burning feeling, nothing can be found physically. In this case, the burning pain is mostly caused by generation of Heat from the interior.

Colic pain

This kind of pain is usually very severe, often occurring in the internal Zang-Fu organs, such as the Small Intestine, Gall Bladder or Uterus. It is caused either by invasion of Exogenous Cold, or by accumulation of Cold, stagnation of Qi, or some substantial blockage such as stones, sand, stagnant Blood or Phlegm.

Hemialgia

This is pain that develops gradually and is confined to either the right or left side of the body. This type of pain often fluctuates in its intensity. Its causes include disharmony of the Nutritive Qi and Defensive Qi system, slowing of the Qi and Blood circulation, and disorder of Yin and Yang—for instance, it can often be seen on those who suffer from the sequelae of a cerebrovascular accident (Zhongfeng).

Pantalgia

This is pain that is experienced over the general body, but mainly in the joints and muscles. It can be caused either by Excessive factors, such as Qi and Blood stagnation or accumulation of Damp, or by deficient factors, for instance a deficiency of Qi and Blood.

Wandering pain

This is pain in the muscles and the joints that comes and goes, and fluctuates in its location. This type of pain is often seen in people suffering from Painful Obstruction Syndrome (Bi Zheng) due primarily to invasion of Wind.

Wandering pain can also be seen in the internal Zang-Fu organs, mostly in the abdomen and chest, and is caused by stagnation of Qi; it is closely related to emotional changes, which means that under conditions of stress, nervousness or anger the pain will be aggravated.

Pain with fixed location

This type of pain can be caused either by stagnation of Blood, or by invasion of Exogenous Damp, or by accumulation of Damp in the body.

If the pain is due to stagnation of Blood there is a stabbing pain, aggravation of the pain at night and when the person remains in a still position. If it is caused by invasion of Exogenous Damp there is an aversion to cold, slight sweating, a feeling of heaviness in the limbs and trunk, and headache. If it is caused by accumulation of Damp in the body there is nausea, poor appetite, loose stool or diarrhoea, a feeling of lassitude, fullness of the chest and abdomen, a greasy coating to the tongue and a slippery pulse.

Pain with spasm

This kind of pain can be caused either by invasion of Exogenous Cold, by deficient Blood in the Liver, by retardation of Blood circulation, or by formation of

Deficient-Cold. For instance, acute facial paralysis is often caused by invasion of Wind-Cold, since Cold is characterised by contraction and stagnation.

Deficiency of Blood in the Liver often causes headache with a feeling of spasm. Spasm in the legs, especially in the gastrocnemius muscle, during the night, could be caused by deficiency of Blood in the Liver accompanied by poor Blood circulation, leading to undernourishment of the tendons. This condition is often seen in elderly people.

Pain with a suffocating feeling

This kind of pain is caused by blockage of the Qi circulation due to Qi stagnation or Damp-Phlegm accumulation, often occurring in the chest or abdominal region. For example, Painful Obstruction Syndrome in the chest is usually due to mixture of Qi stagnation and Phlegm accumulation.

Pain with radiation

This kind of pain refers to conditions characterised by pain occurring mainly in one location and radiating to another. It is usually caused either by stagnation of Qi and Blood or by accumulation of stone or sand in the Zang-Fu organs. For instance, stagnation of Qi in the Liver and Gall Bladder often causes hypochondriac pain with radiation of the pain to one shoulder or the upper back. Again, stagnation of Blood in the Heart may cause chest pain radiating to the arms and neck.

Pain with contraction

Since Cold is characterised by contraction, this kind of pain is usually caused by invasion of Exogenous Cold or formation of Deficient-Cold due to deficiency of Yang.

If the pain is caused by invasion of Exogenous Cold, the pain is severe, and accompanied by an aversion to cold, slight fever, headache, anhidrosis, a runny nose with a whitish nose and throat discharge, a thin and white coating to the tongue and a superficial and tight pulse. If it is caused by formation of Deficient-Cold due to deficiency of Yang, the pain tends to be slight and intermittent, and is accompanied by an aversion to cold, a feeling of tiredness, a pale complexion, shortness of breath, cold hands and feet, a pale tongue with a thin coating and a slow and deep pulse.

Pain with heaviness

This kind of pain is normally not very severe, it often occurs in the limbs, chest, epigastric region, abdomen or head, and there is a feeling as if the limbs and the head are bound by a piece of band, or as if the person is suffocating. It is a sign of invasion of Damp or accumulation of Damp in the body.

Pain with swelling

This kind of pain often occurs in the joints and muscles, and is usually caused by stagnation of Blood after trauma, or accumulation of Damp, or of Toxic Heat.

If the cause is stagnation of Blood due to trauma, there is severe pain, limitation of joint movement, a hard swelling with distinct edges, and blue spots on the skin. If it is accumulation of Damp in the joints and muscles, the joints are painful and the muscles have a heavy feeling, there is a soft swelling with indistinct edges, and a feeling of vibration can be obtained under the skin, the tongue has a greasy coating and there is a slippery pulse. If it is accumulation of Toxic Heat, the joints and muscles are swollen and there is redness, heat and severe pain, accompanied by fever, thirst, a feeling of restlessness, a red tongue with yellow coating and a rapid and forceful pulse.

Pain with dislike of pressure and massage

This kind of pain is usually severe and constant, and is caused by Excessive factors such as Qi and Blood stagnation, accumulation of Cold, or stagnation of food. It is accompanied by aggravation of the pain according to emotional changes, or food intake, and there is also rough breathing, constipation and a wiry pulse.

Pain with preference for pressure and massage

This kind of pain is usually slight and intermittent, and is caused by Deficient factors such as deficiency of Qi and Blood, deficiency of Yin or Yang. It is accompanied by a feeling of tiredness, or a weak feeling, it is aggravated by exertion, and there is a weak and thready pulse. After pressure and massage, the pain will disappear for a bit, but then gradually returns.

In addition, in some patients a pain caused by excessive factors may also be alleviated by pressure and massage; this is because pressure and massage disperse the Qi and Blood circulation temporarily, so the pain diminishes; however, it quickly returns.

Pain with preference for warmth

When this kind of pain occurs it means that there is too much Yin and Cold in the body. This is caused either by invasion of Exogenous Cold, or by formation of

Deficient-Cold due to Yang deficiency. Because warmth can counteract and diminish Yin and Cold, the person prefers warmth.

If the pain is caused by invasion of Exogenous Cold, the onset is usually acute and relatively severe, and is accompanied by an aversion to cold, fever, headache, muscle pain with a contracting feeling, a runny nose with a whitish discharge, cough, a thin and white coating to the tongue and superficial and tight pulse. If it is caused by development of Deficient-Cold due to Yang deficiency, the onset is usually gradual, and is accompanied by an aversion to cold, a feeling of tiredness, a pale complexion, a poor appetite, there is intermittent occurrence of pain, the tongue is pale with a thin coating and there is a deep, thready and slow pulse.

Pain with preference for cold

Cold can clear Heat and reduce fever, so this kind of pain is usually caused either by invasion of Exogenous Heat, or by accumulation of Heat in the body.

If the pain is caused by invasion of Exogenous Heat, there is fever, a slight aversion to cold, a runny nose with a yellow discharge, throat pain with redness and thirst, a thin and yellow tongue coating and superficial and rapid pulse. If it is caused by accumulation of Heat in the body, there would be no External symptoms, but fever, thirst, restlessness, constipation, insomnia, yellow and dry coating, wiry and rapid pulse.

Constant pain

This kind of pain can be caused by all kinds of Excessive factors. It implies that the battle between the Defensive Qi and the pathogenic Qi is still very active and when the Defensive Qi is the stronger one, the pain level diminishes, and when it is the reverse level the pain increases. Treatment is mainly aimed at helping the Defensive Qi to eliminate the pathogenic Qi.

Intermittent pain

This kind of pain is usually caused by a deficiency of Qi, Blood, Yin or Yang, and this implies that the Defensive Qi is weak, so the battle between the Defensive Qi and the pathogenic Qi is not very active. Treatment is mainly aimed at nourishing the Defensive Qi so as to relieve the pain.

Intermittent pain, specially intermittent pain around the navel, can also be caused by accumulation of worms, and is often accompanied by vomiting, even vomiting of worms, and intermittent abdominal pain with sudden aggravation. If the worms are in the Gall Bladder, there is hypochondriac pain, nausea, vomiting, jaundice and fever.

Treatment differentiation 6

General concepts of treatment

This chapter deals with the basic principles of making a decision about which treatment methods and prescriptions to use. This decision is reached by following the guidance of the TCM holistic concepts about differentiation of the syndromes. The principle of treatment differs from the method of the treatment, as the former refers to the rules of the treatment, whereas the latter refers to the steps of the treatment, which are determined by the principle of treatment. For instance, all kinds of pain, as a rule, are caused by conflict between the Defensive Qi and pathogenic factors, so the basic principle of treatment is to regulate the Defensive Qi and eliminate the pathogenic factors. Following the guidance of this principle, the general treatment method would be to nourish the Qi, tonify the Yang, circulate the Qi and Blood, and so on. However, in practice there are various different types of pain with rather complicated pathologies, and differences in severity and intensity, as well as in the seasons, the exact circumstances and the constitution of patients, so it is impossible that just one or a few fixed treatment methods will treat all kinds of pain. The only way to obtain good therapeutic results, therefore, is to master a number of other principles of treatment, which include:

- searching for the root cause and secondary symptoms
- supporting the Defensive Qi and expelling the pathogenic factors
- regulating Yin and Yang
- determining the treatment in accordance with climate and season, geographical location and individual constitution.

Searching for the root cause and secondary symptoms

The concepts of the root cause and secondary symptoms can have different meanings, but here they mainly refer to the nature and primary aspect of the pain, and the phenomena associated with the pain. Pain should be assessed clinically to determine the primary and the secondary aspects, the root cause, the symptoms, whether acute or chronic so as to ascertain the main contradictions, and then should be treated accordingly. Generally speaking, the root cause should be treated first, and the secondary symptoms second. For instance, if a headache is caused by invasion of Exogenous Cold, the root treatment would be to dispel the Exogenous factor and promote the circulation of Qi and Blood in the head, and this would be done first of all. However, if the secondary symptoms are acute and severe, they would be treated first. Again taking headache as an example, if headache is very severe, treatment should first aim to sedate

33

the pain and only afterwards to dispel the Cold. If both the symptoms and the root cause are serious, they should be treated simultaneously.

Supporting the Defensive Qi and expelling pathogenic factors

The occurrence of pain, according to TCM theory, is an indication of a process of struggle between the Defensive Qi and pathogenic factors, so strengthening the Defensive Qi to defeat the pathogenic factors is the correct method of curing the pain. Strengthening the Defensive Qi means improving the body's resistance and building up its energy. Once resistance against pathogenic factors is increased, the pathogenic factors are naturally eliminated.

Clinically, the condition both of the Defensive Qi and of the pathogenic factors should be observed carefully, in order to determine whether to strengthen the body resistance or to eliminate the pathogenic factors first. If a patient has weak resistance but the pathogenic factors are not yet very strong, the body resistance is strengthened first. If a patient is suffering Excessive pathogenic factors but the body resistance has not yet been damaged, the primary task is to eliminate the pathogenic factors. But some patients have weak body resistance and the pathogenic factors are also overwhelming, so in these cases both methods need to be employed simultaneously.

Regulating Yin and Yang

The occurrence of pain is, fundamentally speaking, caused by an imbalance of Yin and Yang, either an excess or deficiency. So it is very clear that treatment also needs to restore the balance between Yin and Yang.

Clinically, Excess of Yin makes Yang suffer, and Excess of Yang makes Yin suffer. For such Excess of Yin or Yang, the best treatment is to reduce or remove the Excess. But whilst correcting this Excess, attention should also be paid to whether a corresponding Yin or Yang deficiency exists. If one of these is deficient, the treatment given should be either simultaneous Yang reduction and Yin reinforcement, or Yin reduction and Yang reinforcement.

Also a deficiency of Yin or Yang may cause failure of the other to be controlled, leading to a state of Deficient-Heat or Deficient-Cold. Treatment in this case should be given to reinforce either Yin or Yang so as to eliminate Deficient-Heat or Deficient-Cold. If there is a deficiency of both Yin and Yang then the treatment needs to tonify both Yin and Yang simultaneously.

Determining the treatment in accordance with climate and season, geographical location and individual constitution

CLIMATIC AND SEASONAL CONDITIONS

It was stated in the Ling Shu (1963, p. 27) that in spring the pathogenic factors are most likely to attack the superficial layer. In summer, they are most likely to attack the skin. In autumn, they are most likely to attack the muscles. In winter, they are most likely to attack the tendons and bones. When treating such disorders, the clinician should ensure that the techniques used are consistent with the seasons. Generally speaking, in spring and summer the climate is relatively warm, and the Yang Qi of the body is floating at the superficial level of the body, so shallow acupuncture is applied. If herbs are used during these seasons then herbs that are very pungent and warm and have a strong dispelling action should be avoided. But the climate in autumn and winter is colder and the skin pores are closed, so the Yang Qi of the body remains deep inside, so the deeper acupuncture is better, and if herbs are applied then those that are relatively pungent and warm and strong in their action should be prescribed in preference.

GEOGRAPHICAL LOCATION

The therapeutic method used should be appropriate to the geographical location. Climate and lifestyle vary in different regions, so do the body's physiological activities and pathological changes, therefore methods of treatment should be varied in accordance with the region. For instance, the weather in Belgium and Holland is rather cold and humid, so many people suffer from Cold Bi and Damp Bi. In this climate dispelling the Cold and elimination of the Damp are of relatively greater importance in the treatment determination. In China, very strong manipulation of the needle is often used in patients who have pain caused by Excessive factors; however, if this were used in the West it would cause a bad reaction for many patients, so the even method is used instead of strong manipulation.

INDIVIDUAL CONSTITUTION

TCM treatment also varies according to a person's age, sex and personal constitutional condition, which is quite logical. For instance, men and women are different in constitution, women have menstruation and pregnancy, so the treatment method should vary as well. Most women will not be able to stand strong herbal treatment and strong manipulation of the needle. A difference also exists between adults and children.

Therapeutic steps

In modern medicine, there are three usual methods of treating pain:

1. Remove the causes of the pain, such as an ulcer or abscess.
2. Alleviate the pain by reducing or stopping transmission of the pain impulses from the affected region—for instance, by administration of sedatives, or electricity. Antidepressants are often used as an adjunctive treatment; originally they were used only to treat depression, but studies have shown that these medications can alleviate pain in certain situations (Antkiewicz-Michaluk et al 1991, Ardid & Guilbaud 1992, Ardid et al 1992, Bank 1994, Danysz et al 1986). Furthermore, they may have the added benefit of helping the patient to sleep at night. Also antiseizure medication may help relieve certain types of pain by reducing abnormal electrical discharges in damaged nerves.
3. Reduce reception of the impression of pain in the brain by use of drugs.

Medications that are prescribed are usually of two types: painkillers and anti-inflammatory drugs. The first type includes narcotic painkillers, which are often used to treat acute pain or cancer pain and are seldom prescribed for chronic pain. The latter type includes aspirin-like drugs, which are the most commonly used medications of this type. These not only reduce swelling and irritation but can also relieve the pain.

In contrast with Western medicine, TCM practice is to take a detailed history from the patient, including sleep, emotions, diet, exercise, and any operations, and combine this with an examination of the tongue, pulse, skin colour, stool, urine, hair condition, breathing, and so on, before making a diagnosis. In treatment, herbs and acupuncture can be applied in combination or separately; they are used to stimulate the Qi and Blood circulation in the body. The treatment aim is to restore the balance between Yin and Yang in the body, and Qi and Blood circulation in the channels as a whole, thereby influencing the person's entire health and dispelling the pain. There is some similarity between the method of treating pain in TCM and in Western medicine, in that, in the latter, sedatives are used to calm the brain, and in TCM the same end is achieved by means of methods to calm the Mind (Shen). To calm the Mind is in fact to regulate the physiological function of the Heart; this is because the Heart is the root of the response to the pain.

To treat the pain successfully, simultaneous application of acupuncture and herbal medicine treatment is recommended. To achieve the therapeutic effect the following steps have to be followed:

- remove the pathogenic factors, so as to diminish or eliminate the causes of stagnation of Qi and Blood; this is an important step to avoid a vicious circle
- promote the Qi and Blood circulation, restore Qi and Blood levels and harmonise the Zang-Fu organs and channels
- calm the Mind and regulate the Heart, so as to diminish the pain
- prevent recurrence of the pain.

Treatment procedures

CAUSATIVE TREATMENT

The differentiation process should first be employed to establish the cause for each syndrome. If this step is not followed the treatment may be wrong or inaccurate. Causal treatment is the root treatment, as it is a unique way of preventing a vicious circle, and includes dispelling of Exogenous pathogenic factors, smoothing the emotions, regulating the Internal Zang-Fu organs, and avoidance of inappropriate diet, an irregular lifestyle and injury, so the Qi and Blood can circulate freely, and pain disappears. Generally speaking, in a patient with pain, the root cause should be treated first if the case is chronic, or if an acute case is not of a serious nature.

SYMPTOMATIC TREATMENT

Treatment of the symptoms, or secondary cause, is appropriate in the following circumstances:

- if the patient has a single symptom that does not appear to have any root cause, or
- if the pain is acute, or if the pain though chronic is of a serious nature.

Treatment of the root cause and symptoms at the same time is the most common approach in the treatment of pain, especially in chronic cases. This method is used particularly when the case is rather complicated.

PATHOGENIC TREATMENT

Since the main mechanism of pain is disorder of Qi and Blood circulation, it is necessary to restore this to normal. Treatment includes methods to circulate the Qi and Blood, to eliminate the Qi and Blood stagnation and to tonify the Qi and Blood. When these steps are employed to maintain the free flow of Qi and Blood, the pain vanishes.

Acupuncture and moxibustion are useful for treating local trigger points (Ah Shi points), or other points in the vicinity chosen according to the channel, because they can temporarily restore the normal circulation of Qi and Blood in the body.

TREATMENT TO CALM THE MIND

Acupuncture and herbal medicine can calm the Mind and regulate the Heart so as to inhibit nerve impulses from the disordered Qi and Blood circulation being sent to the Heart. There exist many effective points and herbs that can alleviate pain rapidly. Achievement of this effect doesn't mean that the causative pathogenic factors are totally eliminated, but rather that the sensitivity to the pain is diminished. However, it is only symptomatic treatment. Based upon this reasoning, some points that calm the Mind and tranquillise the Heart include HT-3 Shaohai, HT-7 Shenmen, PC-6 Neiguan, GB-20 Fengchi, GV-20 Baihui and Extra Sishencong, and these should be combined with the treatment for the aetiology and pathology.

PREVENTATIVE TREATMENT

TCM also emphasises the importance of the prevention of pain. For this, acupuncture and herbal medicine can be applied in combination or in separation. Each of them can regulate the level of Qi and Blood, maintain the free flow of Qi and Blood in the body, improve the body's resistance from pathogenic invasion, harmonise the internal Zang-Fu organs and smooth the emotions. All these elements of prevention of TCM significantly make it different from the treatment approach of modern medicine.

Treatment for the prevention of pain varies according to the primary cause of the pain. In headache, for instance, if the cause is Exogenous invasion, then the treatment methods used aim at raising the body's resistance. In cases of pain caused by stagnation of Qi and Blood due to too much anger, stress and frustration, the preventative treatment method used is to smooth the Liver, circulate the Qi and eliminate the Blood stagnation. If there is blockage of Clear Yang due to accumulation of Damp, the treatment used should include avoidance of eating too-rich or fatty food and elimination of alcohol so as to prevent accumulation of Damp in the body, as well as a method to activate the Spleen and Stomach so as to maintain normal transportation and transformation of food and water. Where there is deficiency of Kidney-Essence, prevention should include reducing excessive sexual intercourse in order to preserve the Essence. In cases of deficiency of Qi and Blood, a method should be used to tonify the Qi and Blood, activate the Spleen and tonify the Kidney-Essence so as to produce more Qi and Blood. In addition the patient should take regular physical exercises to activate the normal circulation of Qi and Blood, and maintain good function of the Zang-Fu organs.

Therapeutic principles

Depending on the aetiology, the clinical symptoms and the localisation of the pain, different therapeutic principles should always be taken into account so as to treat correctly. Some of the main principles are as follows.

TO DISPEL WIND AND ELIMINATE COLD (QU FENG SAN HAN)

This method is used to treat pain syndrome due to invasion of Wind-Cold, which is manifested as an aversion to cold, a slight fever, chills, general body pain, headache, toothache, abdominal pain, joint pain, a thin and white tongue coating and a superficial and tight pulse.

TO DISPERSE WIND AND CLEAR HEAT (QU FENG QING RE)

This method is indicated in pain syndrome due to invasion of Wind-Heat. The manifestations of this are a high fever, an aversion to cold, body pain, joint pain, headache, abdominal pain, a red tongue with a thin and yellow coating and a superficial and rapid pulse.

TO CLEAR HEAT AND REMOVE TOXINS (QING RE JIE DU)

This method is applied to treat pain syndrome due to invasion of Toxic Heat or accumulation of Excessive Heat in the body. The manifestations of this are fever, restlessness, insomnia, headache, thirst, constipation, or redness, hotness, swelling and pain of the face, joints, skin, and so on, a red tongue with a yellow coating and a forceful and rapid pulse.

TO DISPEL WIND AND MOISTEN DRYNESS (QU FENG RUN ZAO)

This method is used to treat pain syndrome caused by invasion of Wind-Dryness. The manifestations of this are an aversion to cold, fever, throat pain with dryness, thirst, a dry nose, chest pain, a dry cough with a non-productive cough, or a cough with blood breaks in the phlegm, dry skin and mouth, slight constipation, a thin and dry tongue coating and a superficial pulse.

TO DISPEL WIND, ELIMINATE COLD AND RESOLVE DAMP (QU FENG SAN HAN LI SHI)

This method is used to treat pain syndrome resulting from invasion of Exogenous Wind, Cold and Damp. The manifestations of this are an aversion to cold, a slight fever, generalised body pain or joint pain with heaviness, headache with a heavy feeling, or even oedema of the body or the joints, a white and greasy tongue coating and a superficial and slippery pulse.

TO DISPEL WIND, CLEAR HEAT AND RESOLVE DAMP (QU FENG QING RE LI SHI)

This method is applied to treat pain syndrome resulting from invasion of Wind, Heat and Damp, manifested as fever, thirst, painful joints and muscles with redness and hotness, limitation of joint movement, a red tongue with a yellow coating and a superficial and tight pulse.

TO SMOOTH THE LIVER AND REGULATE THE QI (SHU GAN LI QI)

This is the most important method to treat pain syndrome when there is retardation of the Qi circulation, or even stagnation of Qi and Blood. This treatment varies depending on whether Qi stagnation or Blood stagnation predominates. If Qi stagnation is the main problem, and Blood stagnation is secondary, the treatment should focus on the Qi circulation, in combination with a method to circulate the Blood. If the problem is primarily one of Blood stagnation, and Qi stagnation is of lesser importance, treatment should focus on the Blood circulation. However, if there is simultaneous stagnation of both Qi and Blood, the method should also aim to circulate Qi and Blood simultaneously.

TO ELIMINATE BLOOD STASIS AND RESOLVE PHLEGM (QU YU HUA TAN)

This method is used to treat stubborn pain in the joints, muscles, channels and Interior organs, which may persist for years, due to stagnation of Blood with accumulation of Phlegm in the collaterals. According to TCM, persistence of any sickness may cause impairment of the collateral, leading to stagnation of Blood. It manifests as severe muscle pain, joint pain, limitation of joint movement, deformity of the joints, atrophy of the muscles, swelling of the joints and muscle, heaviness of the body, purplish skin, a purplish tongue with a greasy coating and a wiry and slippery pulse. To treat this sort of pain, the only method is to ensure free circulation of the Qi and Blood in the body.

TO TONIFY THE QI AND BLOOD (BU QI YANG XUE)

This method is applied to treat pain syndrome due to lack of nourishment of the body. Because of the Qi deficiency, the power of the Qi to promote Qi and Blood circulation is weakened, leading to slowing of Qi and Blood circulation, so stagnation of Qi and Blood develops. It is obvious that this type of pain is one of deficiency. It manifests as a dull pain, a slight pain, intermittent pain, pain that is aggravated by exertion and alleviated by rest, a feeling of tiredness, shortness of breath, dizziness, poor memory, a pale complexion, a pale tongue with a thin and white coating and a deep, thready and weak pulse.

TO NOURISH THE LIVER AND KIDNEY (ZI YANG GAN SHEN)

Since the Liver stores the Blood, and the Kidney stores the Essence, the Blood and Essence can be mutually nourished, thus it is said that the Liver and Kidney are derived from the same source (Gan Shen Tong Yuan). In cases of deficiency of Liver and Kidney, the tendons and bones will not be properly nourished. This leads to chronic lower back pain, neck pain, knee pain, heel pain, or pain in other joints, weakness of the body, a feeling of tiredness, vulnerability to bone fracture, hair loss, poor concentration, dizziness, tinnitus, a thin tongue coating and a deep and weak pulse.

TO WARM THE INTERIOR AND RELIEVE PAIN (WEN LI ZHI TONG)

This method is used to treat epigastric pain, abdominal pain or lower back pain due to deficiency of the Yang of the Spleen, Stomach or Kidney. The clinical manifestations are chronic pain, alleviation with massage and pressure, a feeling of tiredness, coldness of the hands and feet, an aversion to cold, a pale complexion, diarrhoea, nycturia, lower back pain, impotence, a pale tongue with a thin and white coating and a deep, thready and slow pulse.

In practice the causative factors for different types of pain are seldom pure, but mostly mixed, so the therapeutic rules need to be adapted according to the predominant pathogenic factors.

Beside causal treatment of Wind, Cold, Damp and Heat factors, attention should be directed to the congenital or acquired constitutional factors: also, any underlying diseases must be diagnosed and treated. For example, it is very important to check for deficiency of Stomach Qi, Defensive Qi, Original Qi, the general state of the Ying Qi or Yang Qi, and so on.

In chronic cases especially, when the pain has persisted for a long time, not only is it important to circulate the Qi and Blood, or warm the channels if there is severe pain due to Cold, but also the following principle must be considered.

CHANNEL-INDUCING METHODS (YIN JING BAO SHI)

This is a complementary therapeutic method and principle, which involves the selection of particular herbs that can direct the other ingredients in a formula to work on the affected channels or sites.

The following herbs conduct the other ingredients in the formula towards particular areas:

- Gu Sui Bu *Rhizoma Drynariae* directs toward the bones and marrow
- Chuan Niu Xi *Radix Cyathulae* directs towards the lower limbs

- Chai Hu *Radix Bupleuri* directs towards the lesser Yang channel
- Bai Zhi *Radix Angelicae Dahuricae* directs towards the Bright Yang channel
- Gao Ben *Rhizoma et Radix Ligustici* directs towards the Greater Yang channel.

Channel and point palpation

TCM practitioners must carry out careful examination of the body surfaces so as to detect any abnormalities such as points of tenderness, warmth, skin eruptions and subcutaneous nodules. These phenomena are then linked to the pathology of a neighbouring channel.

Method of examination

The thumb is rubbed lightly over the skin along the course of a channel, or the thumb is used together with the index finger to knead the skin gently in order to detect alterations in the superficial cutaneous layers. A greater degree of pressure may be needed to probe the deeper layers of skin. It is important that the pressure be uniform, however, and that the clinician notes any differences between the same channel on the left and right sides of the body. Ordinarily, examination begins along the channels of the back and then proceeds to the chest, abdomen and limbs. Particular attention should be given to special points such as the Back Transporting (Shu) points, Front Collecting (Mu) points, Source (Yuan) points, and Accumulation (Xi) points.

Abnormalities

These include subcutaneous nodules, area of tenderness, hard or flaccid muscle tissue, and indentations, or discoloration of the skin or change in its temperature. Once discovered, it is necessary to determine whether the abnormality reflects symptoms of Excess or Deficiency in the related channel.

Clinical application

The following method is used in examination of the back. The thumb is pressed along the left and right sides of the spinous processes (the medial course of the Bladder channel), generally beginning beside the twelfth thoracic vertebra and working upward to the first thoracic vertebra, and then from the sacrum up to the lumbar vertebrae. When this is complete, the skin surface in the vicinity of the ilium and shoulder blades may be similarly palpated.

In addition to the abnormalities discussed above, attention should be paid to the position of the spinous processes and any abnormalities in the tissue tension of the paraspinal musculature. Such areas may be sensitive to the touch. The practitioner should also check the vertebrae to see whether they are evenly spaced or if there is any scoliosis.

If any abnormalities are found that indicate a strictly local problem these are treated accordingly. The remaining may be regarded as External manifestations of an internal disease:

- commonly, abnormalities discovered between the first and third thoracic vertebrae suggest an illness related to the Heart
- those between the first and fourth are related to the upper limbs
- those between the second and fifth are related to the Lung and bronchioles
- those between the fifth and eighth are related to the Stomach and duodenum
- those between the eighth and tenth are related to the Liver, Gall Bladder and pancreas
- those between the tenth and twelfth are related to the Stomach and intestines

- those between the twelfth and the second lumbar are related to the Kidney and urinary system
- those between the first and fourth lumbar vertebrae are related to the lower limbs
l those in the sacral region are related to the reproductive organs.

Because these lines running parallel to the spine correspond to the course of the Bladder channel, the Back Transporting points along this channel are frequently palpated for diagnostic purposes, as are the Front Collecting points on the chest and abdomen. In practice, these points are considered the primary diagnostic indicators. The acupuncture points on neighbouring channels may also be checked for reaction—for instance, the Front Collecting point LU-1 Zhongfu and the neighbouring point KI-27 Shufu may reflect the condition of the Lung and bronchioles.

When palpating points on the limbs, the Accumulation points are considered to be of primary importance, and the neighbouring points are secondary; for example, the Accumulation point ST-34 Liangqui and the neighbouring point ST-36 Zusanli may both reflect Stomach disease.

Selection and combination of acupuncture points

Selection of acupuncture points

Acupuncture treatment consists of the application of a few points at specific places on the body. Thus, the selection and combination of points in an acupuncture treatment is most important. Since selection of points along the channels is guided by the theory of Zang-Fu organs and channels, it is essential for practitioners to have a full understanding of the following so as to be able to choose the correct points:

- physiology and pathology
- the course of the channels
- the Exterior–Interior relationship of Yin and Yang
- the function, and difference and characteristics of the points.

Selection of points along the course of the channels is one of the basic principles of acupuncture treatment, and is performed according to the theory that disease is related to channels. In practice the points are selected from the channel to which the affected organ is related; or from related channels according to the relations between the Zang-Fu organs and channels; or from several channels.

There are three principles for point selection: local point selection in the vicinity of the pain, distal point selection and symptomatic point selection. Each may be used in combination, or independently of the others.

Local point selection

This is the selection of points in the locality of the pain—for instance, pain in the head, forehead, neck or arm can be treated by using the points in the vicinity. In cases of elbow pain, LI-11 Quchi and LU-5 Chize can be selected to promote the circulation of Qi and Blood in that region; CV-12 Zhongwan can be selected to treat epigastric pain; GB-20 Fengchi can be chosen to treat headache and neck pain in the occipital region.

This method also includes selection of adjacent points close to the pain. For instance, ST-21 Liangmen can be used as an adjacent point to CV-12 Zhongwan to treat stomach pain; LI-10 Shousanli can be used as an adjacent point to LI-11 Quchi to treat painful elbow. Adjacent points may be applied independently or in combination with the local points.

Distal point selection

This is the selection of points far from the sides of pain, and usually below the elbow and knees. This method is often used to treat pain caused by disorder of Internal Zang-Fu organs; for instance, ST-44 Neiting and LI-4 Hegu are used to treat toothache due to Stomach-Heat.

Special point selection

Stream points

It was stated two thousand years ago in the Neijing that Stream (Shu) points can be used to joint and limb problems. These points are indicated in painful joints, stiff joints, joint deformity, joint swelling as well as injury in the joints. Also, these points can also be used as inducing points to conduct the treatment to the affected parts of the limbs.

Source points

As the name implies, Source (Yuan) points are the points where the Original Qi resides. On the Yang channels, the Source points are the points just proximal to the Stream points. On the Yin channels, they are the same as the Stream points.

The Source points are said to be responsible for regulation of the Original Qi in both the interior organs and the channels, so they are used for the treatment of diseases that affect the organs, and problems in those channels. Generally speaking, Source points are really good only for blockage of the channels resulting from Excessive pathogenic factors. In this treatment, they are often applied together with the Connecting points. This is because the channels are subdivided into channels and collaterals, and whereas the Source points can regulate the channels, the Connecting points can harmonise the collaterals, thus both channels and collaterals are treated together.

Connecting points

The place where a Connecting Vessel splits from a main channel is called Connecting (Luo) point. Each channel has its own Connecting point—the 12 regular channels and two of the extraordinary channels, the Governing Vessel and the Directing Vessel—and there is in addition a Connecting point from the Spleen: the Spleen Connecting vessel. So, in total, there are 15 Connecting points.

Classically speaking, the Connecting points have two major applications:

- they can be used in the treatment of Interior–Exterior coupled organ problems
- they can also be used in the treatment of Connecting Vessel symptoms.

Since these points directly connect to the collateral, in fact they have a third function, which is to harmonise and promote the circulation in the collateral. It is true that not all diseases affect the channels and Interior organs. In a lot of cases, pathogenic factors may attack only the collaterals, especially in cases of pain at the superficial levels.

As was mentioned in Source points, when treating pain the Source points and Connecting points are often combined so as to regulate both the channels and collaterals.

Accumulation points

Accumulation (Xi) points (or Cleft points) are the place where Qi and Blood accumulate in the channels. These points are very important in dealing with pain, both in diagnosis and in treatment.

In terms of diagnosis, a sharp or intense pain on pressure, or redness, swelling, hardening, a tingling 'electric' feeling or the formation of nodulations indicate Excess, whereas a dull, mild, slight or intermittent pain indicates Deficiency.

In terms of treatment, these points are often used to treat stubborn and acute cases. In treating pain, these points are very effective in relieving pain involving the organs, channels or collaterals. Therefore, in some cases they can be punctured first of all, so as to sedate the pain as soon as possible. However, such treatment can only be considered as symptomatic—that is to say, it doesn't deal with the cause of the pain. A root treatment should be followed immediately after application of these points.

Eight Gathering points

The following eight points have special functions on the organ or substance for which they are named. They can be applied for pain originating from either Excess or Deficiency. They can in addition be used as the inducing points to lead the treatment to the affected areas.

BL-11 Dashu

This is the Gathering point for the Bones. In case of pain related to bone disorder, use of this point is advisable. For instance, in rheumatoid arthritis there is stabbing finger pain, bone deformity and swelling of the hand. Points should be used that promote circulation of the Blood, smooth the channels and sedate the pain. However, BL-11 should be added simultaneously in order to strengthen the bones.

GB-39 Xuanzhong

This is the Gathering point for the Marrow. This point is often applied to treat pain due to deficiency of Blood, since the Marrow produces Blood. Moreover, since the Marrow nourishes the Bones, thus this point is often combined with some other points to treat bone problems due to deficiency. For instance, lower back pain in senile people is commonly due to weakness of the Liver and Kidney, thus the points to tonify the Liver and Kidney should be used together with GB-39 in order to strengthen the bones. It is clear to see that this point is indicated only in chronic cases.

GB-34 Yanglingquan

This is the Gathering point for the Tendons. It is effective for treating pain in the Tendons originating from both Excessive and Deficient causes. For instance, in the treatment of sciatica, no matter the cause, this point should be coupled with the local point and distal points to eliminate pathogenic factors and relieve the pain. In treating acute ankle sprain, which is usually caused by stagnation of Blood in the channels, this point should be punctured first to relieve the pain, followed by needling at local and distal points to eliminate Blood stasis.

CV-17 Tanzhong

This is the Gathering point for the Qi. This point is mostly used to treat general stagnation of Qi or stagnation of Qi in the chest, Lung, Heart or Liver. So it is clear to see that this point is usually not indicated in deficiency of Qi.

BL-17 Geshu

This is the Gathering point for the Blood. It is indicated in both deficiency of Blood and stagnation of Blood. Also this point is very effective for clearing Heat in the Blood, and is indicated in the generation of Heat caused by over-to-long Blood stagnation, or invasion of Blood by Excess-Heat or Deficient-Heat.

LU-9 Taiyuan

This is the Gathering point for the vessels. Generally speaking, this point is often indicated in pain due to stagnation of Blood in the vessels.

LR-13 Zhangmen

This is the Gathering point for the Zang organs. It is indicated in pain due to disorder of the Zang organs. Of course, it should be be used together with other points to treat the affected organs. For instance, in treating pain due to Damp resulting from weakness of the Spleen, LR-13 can be applied in combination with

SP-3, SP-9 and ST-40 to activate the Spleen and resolve the Damp.

CV-12 Zhongwan

This is the Gathering point for the Fu organs. This point has the function of promoting the digestion and transportation functions in the Fu organs. However, it is particularly indicated in pain due to disorder of Stomach and Large Intestine.

Front Collecting points

The Front Collecting (Mu) points are those points that are located on the chest and abdomen where the channel Qi collects. Each Zang-Fu organ has a Front Collecting point. These points can be found directly above or near to the organ to which they are related. Generally speaking, when there is disorder of the organ, there can be found some pathogenic reaction at these points, including tenderness, lumps, hardening, redness, blistering, a hot feeling, depression and swelling. Thus the Front Collecting points can be used for diagnostic purpose to determine whether there is disorder of the interior Zang-Fu organ, or of the channels.

The Front Collecting points can also be used as therapeutic points. In this case, they should be combined with other points to treat the root causes.

Mother–Son points

This is the method expounded in the Nanjing (c. AD 198, new edition Nanjing College of Traditional Chinese Medicine, 1979) based on the combination of the theory of the Five Elements and the nature of internal Zang-Fu organs. In the treatment, the Mother points should be tonified in cases of deficiency of the interior organs, and the Son points should be reduced in cases of Excess in the Interior organs. For instance, the Lung corresponds to Metal. According to Five Element theory, Metal produces Water, so the Water point from the Lung channel is the Son point; this is LU-5 Chize. Thus, in cases of Excess in the Lung, LU-5 should be needled using the reducing method. Furthermore, according to the Five Elements, Earth is the mother of Metal, so LU-9 (the Earth point) is the Mother point. In cases of deficiency, LU-9 Taiyuan should be needled using the tonifying method.

Back Transporting points

Although the Back Transporting (Shu) points are located on the Bladder channel, they are also the places where Qi passes through all named organs. These points can be used to diagnose and to treat the organ with which they are associated. Disorder of an Interior organ can be detected by finding tenderness, swelling, hardening, blister, or some other abnormality when palpating on the corresponding point. For instance, Liver disorder can often be detected by palpating at BL-18 Ganshu; in most cases, there is tenderness, hardening or discoloration. This point can also be needled to treat disorder of Liver. The Back Transporting points are indicated in pain due to disorder of Interior organs rather than superficial complaints on the channels, skins, muscles and tendons resulting from invasion of External factors.

The four Command points

The Command points govern particular parts of the body. They include the following:

- ST-36 Zusanli commands the abdomen
- LI-4 Hegu commands the head, face and mouth
- LU-7 Lieque commands the head and neck
- BL-40 Weizhong commands the back of the body.

These points are selected when the parts of the body they command are involved in the problem. Thus they can be leading points to bring the treatment to certain parts of the body. However, they can only be applied together with other points to treat the root causes.

Eight Confluence points

The eight Confluence points are located on the limbs; each is linked with one of the eight extraordinary channels. They are: PC-6, SP-4, TE-5, GB-41, LU-7, KI-6, SI-3 and BL-62. These eight points are very important in the treatment of pain. These eight Confluence points can also be considered as the opening points and leading points of the extraordinary channels. In practice, they can be subdivided into four groups:

PC-6 Neiguan and SP-4 Gongsun. These are indicated in Heart pain, Stomach pain and chest pain. When these two points are combined, they can regulate Qi and Blood in the Heart, Stomach and chest. They can also regulate the Penetrating Vessel (Chong Mai) and cause the Qi to descend, and are indicated in belching, acid regurgitation, nausea, vomiting, and uprising of Qi from the abdomen to the chest.

SI-3 Houxi and BL-62 Shenmai. These are indicated in pain at the inner canthus, pain at the back of the neck, ear pain, shoulder pain and back pain caused either by invasion of External factors, or disorder of the Internal Zang-Fu organs. They are used only to treat pain at places where covered by the Greater Yang channels.

Since this combination can open the Governing Vessel, it is widely used to treat all kinds of back pain due to blockage of this channel.

TE-5 Waiguan and GB-41 Zulinqi. These are indicated in pain at the outer canthus, pain behind the ear, cheek pain, and pain at the side of the neck or shoulder. This combination is specially indicated in pain on the sides of the body due to invasion of external factors or stagnation of Liver-Qi and disharmony of the Gall Bladder.

LU-7 Lieque and KI-6 Zhaohai. These are indicated in chest pain, throat pain and pain at the epigastric regions. Generally speaking, this combination is very effective for treating chronic pain above the waist resulting from deficiency of the Yin of Lung and Kidney.

Six Lower Sea points

Each of the three Yang channels of hand and three Yang channels of the foot has a Lower Sea (He) point around the knee. They are:

- ST-36 Zusanli for the Stomach
- ST-37 Shangjuxu for the Large Intestine
- ST-39 Xiajuxu for the Small Intestine
- GB-34 Yanglingquan for the Gall Bladder
- BL-40 Weizhong for the Bladder
- BL-39 Weiyang for the Triple Burner.

Actually, these six Lower Sea points are a kind of symptomatic treatment points. They are usually used in combination with the corresponding Front Collecting or Back Transporting points. For instance, in cases of abdominal pain due to accumulation of Excess-Heat in the Bright Yang Fu organs manifesting as abdominal pain, constipation, thirst, a large appetite, a foul smell in the mouth, a red tongue with a yellow and dry coating and a rapid and forceful pulse, ST-37 should be applied together with ST-25 Tianshu, ST-40 Fenglong, ST-44 Neiting and LI-11 in order to clear the Heat, drain the Stomach and Large Intestine and sedate the pain.

Ah Shi points

Since these points are especially sensitive to palpation and pressing, they usually reveal blockage or disorder of channels or Interior organs. However, the practitioner should remember that a discovery of a sensitive Ah Shi point doesn't mean the problem is only in the locality, as it can also reflect some disturbance at a distal place or an Interior organ. Moreover, Ah Shi points can be used only as the symptomatic treatment. They have to be used in combination with other points that treat the root causes.

Symptomatic point selection

Selection of local and distal point is based upon the distance of the points from the site of the pain; however, some diseases are not local but systemic in nature, and can be treated at those points that have long been associated with relieving a particular disease. Such points include the eight Confluence points and the six Lower Sea points.

Certain individual points have also traditionally been found useful for treating specific symptoms. For instance. GV-14 Dazhui is used for reducing fever, GV-26 Renzhong for reviving unconscious patients, PC-6 Neiguan for relieving nausea and vomiting, ST-40 Fenglong for eliminating Damp-Phlegm in the body and ST-36 Zusanli for activating the Spleen and tonifying the Qi and Blood.

Combination of points

In addition to the method of individual point selection outlined above, there are several traditional methods of combining one point with another in an acupuncture prescription. These techniques are flexible, permitting much variation according to the particular needs of the case.

Combining local points and distal points

This method is the most popular in everyday practice. In this, a point (or points) at or near the place of the diseases (the local point(s)) would be combined with distal points that are traditionally considered to have an effect on the disordered area. For example, in Stomach disease, the local points CV-12 Zhongwan and ST-21 Liangmen, and the distal points PC-6 Neiguan and ST-36 Zusanli could be used together.

When treating pain, the practitioner is advised to use a greater number of distal points to treat acute pain, and a greater number of local points to treat chronic pain.

Combining points on the front with points on the back

The front includes both the chest and abdomen, and the back includes both the back and waist. In this method, points on both the front and back appropriate to a particular disease are used in combination. It employs simultaneous use of the Front Collecting points and Back Transporting points to increase the therapeutic effect of both. For instance, in Spleen disease, both LR-13 Zhangmen on the front and BL-20 Pishu on the back can be needled in tandem. This method of point selection is often used to treat pain due to Internal Zang-Fu organs. If, in contrast, pain is caused by channel problems, for instance channels blockage, symptomatic point selection is more often carried out.

Combining points on the Yang channels and the points on the Yin channels

Each of the channels has a paired channel, and they form a Yin and Yang relationship. By combining a point on a Yang channel with another on its paired Yin channel, the practitioner can obtain a greater effect than if needling either point separately. Examples include: combining ST-36 Zusanli on the Stomach channel with SP-4 Gongsun on the Spleen channel for Stomach disease, or combining LU-9 Taiyuan on the Lung channel with LI-4 Hegu on the Large Intestine channel for cough. The most well-known combination of this kind is between the Source point on the channel primarily affected by a disease, and the Connecting point on the channel with which the first has a Yin–Yang relationship. In this combination, the Source point is called the 'host', and the Connecting point is called the 'guest'. For example, a disease affecting the Lung channel may be treated through that channel's Source point, LU-9 Taiyuan, in combination with the Connecting point of its Yang partner the Large Intestine channel, LI-6 Pianli. Conversely, a disease affecting the Large Intestine channel could be treated by that channel's Source point, LI-4 Hegu, together with the Connecting point of the Lung channel, LU-7 Lieque.

Combining points above with points below

'Above' refers to points on the arms and above the waist, and 'below' to points on the legs and below the waist. However, this method of point combination is mostly commonly practised on the limbs. For instance, in cases of Stomach disease, PC-6 Neiguan on the arm may be combined with ST-36 Zusanli on the leg. For sore throat or toothache, LI-4 Hegu on the hand can be combined with ST-44 Neiting on the foot.

Traditionally, a distinctive use of the above–below combination was made with respect to the confluence points of the eight extraordinary channels. A confluence point on one of these channels affected by a disease above would be combined with a confluence point on another extraordinary channel below. For example, diseases of the Heart, chest and abdomen are related to the Yin Linking channel and the Penetrating channel; therefore, PC-6 Neiguan, the Confluence point of the former on the arm (above), and SP-4 Gongsun, the Confluence point of the latter on the foot (below), are selected as a combination for needling.

Combining points on the left with the diseases on the right

Because channel points are bilateral, it is common to treat diseases of the internal organs by manipulating the same points on both sides in order to strengthen the effect. For example, ST-36 Zusanli on both legs can be needled to treat diseases of the Stomach. Furthermore, because the channels on the right side intersect with those on the left, a point on the right may be chosen to treat disease or pain on the left side of the body, and vice versa. For instance, in the case of hemiplegia, the practitioner may select not only a point on the side affected by the paralysis, but also the same point on the healthy side.

Combining corresponding points

If the body is subdivided into upper and lower parts, it is clear to see that there is a correspondence between the upper and lower limbs. This implies that, for points on the shoulders, elbows, wrists and fingers in the upper limbs, there are corresponding points on the hips, knees, ankles and toes in the lower limbs—that is, there are points on the shoulders corresponding to points on the hips, elbows to knees, wrists to ankles and finally fingers to toes. Meridians in these corresponding places bear the same names, as Qi and Blood in these places can mutually influence each other.

By combining corresponding points the practitioner can treat painful areas by using points in the corresponding areas rather than in the painful area itself. For instance, in the treatment of shoulder pain along the Large Intestine channel, the practitioner can use the corresponding point from the channel that bears the same name on the hip (i.e. ST-30 Qichong), and vice versa. This method is especially indicated for treating most acute pain syndromes, and gives very good results. In some cases, if the pain is very localised and very acute, needling only one point can sedate pain. Attention should be paid here to diagnosis, as some cases of pain may have ruptured tendons or bone that are fractured or even broken. The following is a list of suggested corresponding points:

- *Shoulder to hip*: HT-1 Jiquan to KI-11 Henggu, PC-2 Tianquan to LR-12 Jimai, LU-2 Yunmen to SP-12 Chongmen; LI-15 Jianyu to ST-30 Qichong, TE-14 Jianliao to GB-30 Huantiao, SI-10 Naoshu to BL-36 Chengfu.
- *Elbow to knee*: HT-3 Shaohai to KI-10 Yingu, PC-3 Quze to LR-8 Ququan, LU-5 Chize to SP-9 Yinlingquan; LI-11 Quchi to ST-35 Dubi, TE-10 Tianjing to GB-34 Yanglingquan, SI-8 Xiaohai to BL-40 Weizhong.
- *Wrist to ankle*: HT-7 Shenmen to KI-3 Taixi, PC-7 Daling to LR-4 Zhongfeng, LU-9 Taiyuan to SP-5 Shangqiu; LI-5 Yangxi to ST-41 Jiexi, TE-4 Yangchi to GB-40 Qiuxu, SI-4 Wangu to BL-62 Shenmai.

Point prescriptions

When selecting points for a prescription, the number of points in prescription should be as few as possible. In practice, four to six points are selected to treat acute pain, or mild pain, or with persons of weak constitution. For treating severe pain, or chronic pain, since they are complicated in pathology, the practitioner should use a larger number of points (eight to ten) to produce stronger stimulation. After a few initial treatments, points may be added or subtracted as the condition requires.

When treating a nervous patient for the first time, the practitioner should needle fewer points, increasing the number in later treatment when the patient feels more accustomed to acupuncture.

Each acupuncture point has its own distinctive characteristics, yet those on the same channel or in the same locality can produce certain effects in common. It is wrong to needle the same point for too many times in the same treatment series, as the efficacy of these points will diminish. Rather, other points with similar characteristics should be substituted, or a similar prescription made up of different points should be used instead.

Frequency of treatment

A small number of cases of acute pain require more than one treatment in a single day. Most cases of chronic pain are treated once every 1 to 3 days, or even once a week. After giving acupuncture treatment for a period of weeks, treatment should be suspended temporarily to rest the patient.

Part 2

Generalised body pain 周身疼痛

Pain in the entire body 8

周
身
疼
痛

This chapter deals with the occurrence of pain affecting the entire body, including joints, tendons and muscles, which may be accompanied by an aversion to cold, fever, sweating or lack of sweating, fatigue or even dysfunction of the limbs. Pain throughout the body can, according to TCM, be caused by disorders in the Internal organs and disturbance of the channels. There are many factors that may lead to this. They are differentiated in the following way: invasion of External Wind-Cold, invasion of External Wind-Damp, invasion of External Damp-Heat, stagnation of Liver-Qi, stagnation of Qi and Blood in the channels, deficiency of Qi and Blood, deficiency of Liver-Yin and Kidney-Yin and deficiency of Kidney-Yang. Entire body pain may be attributed to any of the following disorders in Western medicine: the common cold, influenza, leptospirosis, poliomyelitis, polymyalgia rheumatica, chronic fatigue syndrome (CFS), and fibromyalgia, etc.

Aetiology and pathology

Invasion of External Wind-Cold

Invasion of External Wind-Cold is one of the most common causative factors of pain throughout the body. The nature of Cold is contracting, so it may depress the Defensive Qi and lead to obstruction in the channels, muscles and tendons. Wind exists in every season, being able to invade the superficial layers and the upper part of the human body easily. When there is an invasion of External Wind-Cold in the body, the Qi and Blood will not be able to circulate freely to nourish the body and there will be contraction of the channels, muscles and tendons, leading to stagnation of Qi and Blood. This may cause pain throughout the body. Exposure to a cold environment without proper clothing and a direct invasion of Wind-Cold in people who sweat during the course of their work or from playing sports are the major causes.

Invasion of external Wind-Damp

Wind is a Yang pathogenic factor that frequently attacks the human body. It is often combined with other pathogenic factors. Damp is a substantial Yin pathogen; it has a heavy and sticky nature, easily blocking and damaging the circulation of Qi in the muscles. When Wind and Damp are combined together, they may obstruct the circulation of Qi and Blood and pain in the entire body follows.

49

Invasion of External Damp-Heat

An invasion of Exterior Damp may cause stagnation in the circulation of Qi, and persistence of Damp may cause transformation of Damp into Damp-Heat. Living or working in warm and humid conditions can lead to a direct invasion of External Damp-Heat into the human body. The External Damp-Heat may block the Qi circulation in the channels and muscles, leading to pain in the entire body.

Also, eating too much high-fat and sweet food and dairy products, or drinking too much alcohol, may damage the Spleen and Stomach, leading to the formation of Damp-Heat in the Middle Burner.

Stagnation of Liver-Qi

The Liver plays an important role in the emotions. It also regulates the Qi circulation and stores the Blood. Negative emotions, such as overstress and frustration, may cause stagnation of Liver-Qi, which in turn causes poor circulation of Blood and Body Fluids. In this way, the muscles and tendons as well as the channels will not be nourished sufficiently and pain in the entire body occurs.

Stagnation of Qi and Blood in the channels

Prolonged persistence of chronic diseases, incomplete dispelling of Wind-Cold, too much emotional disturbance, imbalance between warmth and cold and accumulation of Damp-Phlegm, may all cause a slowing down of the circulation of Blood, leading to Blood stagnation. Too little exercise may also result in stagnation of Qi and Blood. Physical strain and inappropriate operations may directly damage the muscles, tendons and channels, leading to stagnation of Blood. When Blood stasis blocks the muscles, tendons and channels, pain in the entire body occurs.

Deficiency of Qi and Blood

Excessive physical work as well as mental work may cause Spleen-Qi and Kidney-Qi to be consumed. When Spleen-Qi is not strong enough to produce Blood, this may result in deficiency of Blood. In women, chronic excessive blood loss during menstruation may immediately lead to deficiency of Blood. Chronic diseases could also cause a gradual consumption of Qi and Blood, leading to their deficiency. Moreover, excessive sexual activity or giving birth to several children may decrease Kidney-Essence, leading directly to a deficiency of Qi and Blood. In all these conditions, the muscles and tendons will not be nourished properly, leading to pain in the entire body.

Deficiency of Yin of the Liver and Kidney

Chronic febrile disease, improper treatment with hot herbs and even overeating spicy and hot food may gradually consume the Yin in the body. Poor constitution, old age and excessive sexual activities may also cause consumption of the Qi and Yin of the Kidney. The Liver and Kidney share the same origin, so deficiency of Kidney-Yin may cause deficiency of Liver-Yin. Where there is Yin deficiency, there will also be deficiency of Blood, thus the muscles, tendons and channels will not be properly nourished and pain in the entire body will follow.

Deficiency of Kidney-Yang

Long-standing Cold diseases or excessive use of Cold herbs may damage Kidney-Yang. A weak constitution, ageing, too many operations, as well as chronic sickness, may all induce the damage of Kidney-Yang, gradually leading to deficiency. Cold has the characteristics of stagnation and contraction. If there is deficiency of Kidney-Yang, the Qi and Blood in the body will stagnate, the body temperature will decrease and pain in the entire body will follow.

Treatment based on differentiation

Differentiation

Differentiation of External or Internal origin

Entire body pain can be caused either by invasion of external pathogenic factors or by internal disorder.

— If it is caused by invasion of External pathogenic factors, it is usually acute, and accompanied by External symptoms such as headache, fever, an aversion to cold, runny nose, coughing, etc.
— If it is caused by disorder of internal organs, it is chronic in nature and has no External symptoms.

Differentiation of character of the pain

— Entire body pain with an acute onset, fever and aversion to cold is usually caused by External pathological factors, such as Wind-Cold, Wind-Damp or Damp-Heat.
— If entire body pain is accompanied by acute occurrence of severe headache, stiff neck, slight fever, aversion to cold and no sweating, it is often due to invasion of Wind-Cold.

— Acute occurrence of entire body pain with an obvious heavy sensation in the body generally, soreness and numbness of the muscles and joints, fever, an aversion to cold, a poor appetite and loose stools, is usually caused by invasion of Wind-Damp.

— Entire body pain with a hot and heavy sensation, swelling of the joints, a poor appetite with bitter taste, fever, an aversion to cold, a thick yellow tongue coating and a slippery and rapid pulse, is usually caused by invasion of Damp-Heat.

— Chronic entire body pain with a wandering nature, which is aggravated by stress or emotional upset, with insomnia, irritability, palpitations, dull stomach or overeating, is caused by stagnation of Liver-Qi.

— Chronic pain in the body with a fixed location, or stabbing pain, history of trauma or operation, with aggravation of the pain at night, is caused by stagnation of Blood.

— Chronic pain in the entire body, soreness of the muscles, fatigue and dizziness is often due to Deficiency. Patients usually have a weak constitution and a history of chronic disease. If the main cause is deficiency of Qi and Blood, there will be shortness of breath, a poor appetite, a pale complexion, and so on. If it is deficiency of Kidney-Yin, there will be a sensation of heat in the palms and the soles of the feet, lower back pain with soreness, a low-grade fever, night sweating, and so on. If it is deficiency of Kidney-Yang, there will be a cold sensation, lassitude, an aversion to cold, cold limbs, a pale complexion, oedema, lower back pain with soreness, and so on.

Treatment

INVASION OF WIND-COLD

Symptoms and signs

Pain in the entire body with an acute onset, headache, stiff neck, back pain, joint pain, aversion to cold, fever, lack of sweating, lack of thirst, clear urine, a pale tongue with a white coating and a floating and tense pulse.

Principle of treatment

Dispel External Cold, promote sweating and relieve the pain.

HERBAL TREATMENT

Prescription

MA HUANG TANG
Ma Huang Combination
Ma Huang *Herba Ephedrae* 10 g
Gui Zhi *Ramulus Cinnamomi* 10 g
Xing Ren *Semen Armeniacae* 10 g
Qiang Huo *Rhizoma seu Radix Notopterygii* 10 g
Du Huo *Radix Angelicae Pubescentis* 10 g
Zhi Gan Cao *Radix Glycyrrhizae Praeparata* 6 g

Explanations

- Ma Huang promotes sweating and dispels Cold.
- Gui Zhi helps Ma Huang to dispel Cold and warm the channels.
- Xing Ren helps Ma Huang to regulate the circulation of Lung-Qi in order to eliminate the external Cold.
- Qiang Huo and Du Huo dispel Wind-Cold to relieve the superficial symptoms and stop the pain in the entire body.
- Zhi Gan Cao harmonises the actions of the other herbs in the prescription.

Modifications

1. If there is sweating, remove Ma Huang, and add Bai Shao *Radix Paeoniae Alba* 10 g, Sheng Jiang *Rhizoma Zingiberis Recens* 10 g and Da Zao *Fructus Ziziphi Jujubae* 10 g to harmonise Yin and Yang and to relieve the pain.
2. If there is headache, add Chuan Xiong *Radix Ligustici Chuanxiong* 10 g and Bai Zhi *Radix Angelicae Dahuricae* 10 g to eliminate Wind-Cold in the head in order to relieve the headache.
3. If there is a stiff neck, add Ge Gen *Radix Puerariae* 10 g and Bai Shao *Radix Paeoniae Alba* 12 g to nourish the tendons and regulate the circulation of Qi.
4. If there is severe pain with a cold sensation, add Gan Jiang *Rhizoma Zingiberis* 10 g and Yan Hu Suo *Rhizoma Corydalis* 12 g to warm the channels and relieve the pain.

Patent remedy

Jing Fang Bai Du Pian *Schizonepeta and Ledebouriella Tablets to Overcome Pathogenic Toxin*

ACUPUNCTURE TREATMENT

LI-4 Hegu, TE-5 Waiguan, GB-40 Qiuxu, BL-40 Weizhong, BL-60 Kunlun and ST-36 Zusanli. Reducing method is applied for these points. The points on the leg can be treated with moxibustion.

Explanations

- LI-4, the Source point of the Large Intestine channel, regulates the Qi circulation in the channels and relieves pain.
- TE-5, the Connecting (Luo) point of the Triple Burner channel, regulates the Qi circulation in the entire body and relieves the pain.
- GB-40, the Source point of the Gall Bladder channel, regulates the Qi circulation and relieves pain along this channel.
- BL-40, the Sea point of the Bladder channel, promotes the Qi circulation. BL-60, the River point, regulates the circulation of Qi. (These two points are used to relieve the pain along the Bladder channel.)
- ST-36, the Sea point of the Stomach channel, tonifies the Stomach-Qi and relieves pain along the Stomach channel.
- Moxibustion on acupuncture points on the legs may warm the channels and dispel External Wind-Cold and in this way relieve the pain.

Modifications

1. If there is headache, add GB-20 and LU-7 to regulate the Qi circulation and to relieve the headache.
2. If there is a stiff neck, add GB-21 and BL-10 to promote the Qi circulation and to relieve the pain.
3. If there is back pain, add BL-58, the Connecting point, and BL-63, the Accumulating point of the Bladder channel, to regulate the Qi circulation and to relieve the pain.
4. If there is joint pain, add some local Ah Shi points to regulate the Qi circulation and to relieve the pain. Treatment with moxa on these points is recommended.
5. If there is a fever and an aversion to cold, add GV-14 and LI-11 to induce sweating and to reduce fever.

Case history

A 33-year-old woman complained of pain in her entire body that had persisted for 15 days. The pain started after she caught a cold 2 weeks previously. When she visited her doctor he had prescribed some painkillers. She had had no relief of the pain, however, so she asked for acupuncture treatment. When she came to the acupuncture department, she had a low fever, an aversion to cold with no sweating, pain and soreness in the entire body, headache, low back pain, joint pain, cold limbs, a pale tongue with a white coating and a superficial pulse.

Diagnosis
Invasion of Cold in the channels.

Principle of treatment
Dispel External Cold, warm the channels and relieve body pain.

Acupuncture treatment
The points LI-4, LU-7, GB-20, GB-34 and BL-58 were needled daily with reducing method.

Explanations

- LI-4, the Source point of the Large Intestine channel, and LU-7, the Connecting point of the Lung channel, regulate the circulation of the Liver and promote sweating in order to dispel External Wind-Cold from the channels.
- GB-20, the meeting point of the Gall Bladder channel and the Yang Linking channel, promotes the circulation of Qi, dispels External Cold and relieves the headache.
- GB-34, the Gathering point of the tendons, promotes the Qi circulation and relieves the pain.
- BL-58, the Connecting point of the Bladder channel, regulates the Qi circulation and relieves the pain.

After the first treatment, the patient sweated slightly and felt relief of the pain. The pain disappeared completely after the third treatment. Upon consultation a year later she reported having been free of pain since the treatment.

INVASION OF WIND-DAMP

Symptoms and signs

Pain in the entire body with a heavy sensation, soreness and numbness of the muscles, headache with a heavy feeling, painful and swollen joints, low fever, a poor appetite, a thirst without a desire to drink, loose and sticky stools, a white and sticky tongue coating and a deep and slippery pulse.

Principle of treatment

Dispel Wind, eliminate Damp and relieve the pain.

HERBAL TREATMENT

Prescription

QIANG HUO SHENG SHI TAN
Notopterygium Dispelling Dampness Decoction
Qiang Huo *Rhizoma seu Radix Notopterygii* 10 g
Du Huo *Radix Angelicae Pubescentis* 10 g
Gao Ben *Rhizoma et Radix Ligustici* 10 g
Fang Feng *Radix Ledebouriellae* 10 g

Chuan Xiong *Rhizoma Ligustici Chuanxiong* 10 g
Man Jing Zi *Fructus Viticis* 15 g
Zhi Gan Cao *Radix Glycyrrhizae Praeparata* 6 g

Explanations

- Qiang Huo, Du Huo, Fang Feng, Man Jing Zi and Gao Ben promote sweating, dispel Wind and eliminate Damp in order to relieve the pain.
- Chuan Xiong invigorates the circulation of Blood and promotes the circulation of Qi in the channels.
- Zhi Gan Cao harmonises the actions of the other herbs in the prescription.

Modifications

1. If there is headache, add Bai Zhi *Radix Angelicae Dahuricae* 10 g and Bo He *Herba Menthae* 6 g to dispel the Wind and relieve the headache.
2. If there is swelling of the joints, add Fang Ji *Radix Stephaniae Tetrandrae* 10 g and Fu Ling *Poria* 15 g to eliminate the Damp and promote urination.
3. If there is soreness of the muscles, add Mu Gua *Fructus Chaenomelis* 10 g and Yi Yi Ren *Semen Coicis* 10 g to eliminate the Damp and regulate the Qi circulation.
4. If there is heavy sensation in the body, add Can Sha *Excrementum Bombycis Mori* 10 g and Ze Xie *Rhizoma Alismatis* 15 g to promote urination and eliminate the Damp.
5. If there is a low fever, add Huo Xiang *Herba Agastachis* 6 g and Pei Lan *Herba Eupatorii* 6 g to promote sweating and reduce the fever.
6. If there is a poor appetite, add Ban Xia *Rhizoma Pinelliae* 10 g and Sha Ren *Fructus Amomi* 6 g to dry the Damp and improve the appetite.

Patent remedies

Tian Ma Qu Feng Bu Pian *Gastrodia Dispel Wind Formula Tablet*
Feng Shi Pian *Wind-Damp Tablet*

ACUPUNCTURE TREATMENT

LU-7 Lieque, TE-6 Zhigou, SP-6 Sanyinjiao, SP-9 Yinlingquan, ST-36 Zusanli, GB-34 Yanglingquan and BL-60 Kunlun. Reducing method is applied on these points.

Explanations

- LU-7, the Connecting point of the Lung channel, promotes the Qi circulation and dispels the Wind-Damp.
- TE-6 dispels the Wind, promotes urination and eliminates the Damp.
- SP-6, the crossing point of the Spleen, Kidney and Liver channels, and SP-9, the Sea point of the Spleen channel, eliminate the Damp and activate the Spleen.
- ST-36, the Lower Sea point of the Stomach regulates the Stomach-Qi and eliminates the Damp.
- GB-34, the Sea point of the Gall Bladder channel and the Gathering point for the tendons, regulates the Qi circulation and relieves pain in the tendons.
- BL-60, the River point of the Bladder channel, promotes the circulation of Qi and eliminates the Wind-Damp.

Modifications

1. If there is a low fever, add LI-4 and BL-20 to promote sweating, to eliminate the Wind-Damp and reduce the fever.
2. If there is joint pain, add BL-11, the Gathering point for the bones, BL-20 and local Ah Shi points to regulate the Qi circulation and relieve the pain.
3. If there is headache, add GV-20 and Extra Taiyang to promote sweating and relieve the headache.
4. If there is a poor appetite, add CV-12, the Front Collecting point, and BL-20, the Back Transporting point of the Stomach, to promote the Qi circulation and improve the appetite.
5. If there is numbness in the muscles, add SP-4, the Connecting point, to activate the Spleen and Stomach and reduce the numbness.

INVASION OF DAMP-HEAT

Symptoms and signs

Pain in the entire body with an acute onset, or chronic pain with an acute aggravation, a hot and heavy sensation in the entire body, swelling of the body, aggravation of the pain by heat, alleviation of the pain by cold, lumbago, scanty and yellow urine, constipation, fever and an aversion to cold, headache, a bitter taste in mouth, thirst, a red tongue with a thick yellow coating and a slippery and rapid pulse.

Principle of treatment

Clear Heat and eliminate Damp.

HERBAL TREATMENT

Prescription

BAI HU JIA GUI ZHI TANG
White Tiger Ramulus Cinnamomi Decoction
Shi Gao *Gypsum Fibrosum* 30 g
Zhi Mu *Rhizoma Anemarrhenae* 10 g
Gui Zhi *Ramulus Cinnamomi* 10 g
Qiang Huo *Rhizoma seu Radix Notopterygii* 10 g
Du Huo *Radix Angelicae Pubescentis* 10 g
Jing Mi *Semen Oryzae* 15 g
Zhi Gan Cao *Radix Glycyrrhizae Praeparata* 6 g

Explanations

- Shi Gao and Zhi Mu clear the Heat and reduce the Fire.
- Gui Zhi dispels the Wind and eliminates the Damp.
- Qiang Huo and Du Huo help Gui Zhi eliminate the Wind and relieve the pain in the body.
- Jing Mi and Zhi Gan Cao tonify the Qi and protect the Stomach-Qi from being damaged by the other Cold herbs. Also, Zhi Gan Cao harmonises the actions of the other herbs in the prescription.

Modifications

1. If there are swollen and painful joints, add Qing Feng Teng *Caulis Sinomenii* 20 g, Hu Zhang *Rhizoma Polygoni Cuspidati* 15 g and Luo Shi Teng *Caulis Trachelospermi* 15 g to dispel the Wind, to eliminate the Damp-Heat and relieve the pain.
2. If there is fever, add Sheng Ma *Rhizoma Cimicifugae* 10 g and Chai Hu *Radix Bupleuri* 12 g to clear the Heat and relieve the pain.
3. If there is swelling of the body, add Ku Shen *Radix Sophorae Flavescentis* 10 g, Lian Qiao *Fructus Forsythiae* 10 g and Jin Yin Hua *Flos Lonicerae* 10 g to eliminate the Damp-Heat and relieve the swelling.
4. If there is constipation, add Da Huang *Radix et Rhizoma Rhei* 10 g and Mang Xiao *Natrii Sulfas* 10 g to clear the Fire and promote defecation.

Patent remedy

Gan Lu Xiao Du Dan *Sweet Dew Special Pill to Eliminate Toxin*

ACUPUNCTURE TREATMENT

LI-4 Hegu, LU-7 Lieque, TE-5 Waiguan, LR-4 Zhongfeng, SP-9 Yinlingquan and GB-34 Yanglingquan. Reducing method is used on these points.

Explanations

- LI-4, the Source point of the Large Intestine channel, eliminates the Damp-Heat by promoting sweating.
- LU-7, the Connecting point of the Lung channel, regulates the Lung-Qi in order to eliminate the Damp-Heat.
- TE-5, the Connecting point of the Triple Burner channel, promotes the circulation of Qi and relieves the pain.
- LR-4, the River point of the Liver channel, eliminates the Damp-Heat in this channel.
- SP-9, the Sea point of the Spleen channel, removes the Damp-Heat by promoting urination.
- GB-34, the Sea point of the Gall Bladder channel and the Gathering point for the tendons, regulates the Qi circulation and eliminates the Damp-Heat in order to relieve the pain.

Modifications

1. If there is fever, add LI-11 and GV-14 to clear the Damp-Heat and to lower the fever by inducing sweating.
2. If there is swelling of the muscles, add SP-6 and TE-6 to eliminate the Damp-Heat and reduce the swelling.
3. If there are painful joints, add BL-11, BL-40 and some local Ah Shi points to remove the Qi stagnation in order to relieve pain.
4. If there is headache, add GV-20 and GB-20 to regulate the Qi circulation and relieve the headache.
5. If there is constipation, add ST-25, the Front Collecting point of the Large Intestine and ST-37, the Lower Sea point of the Large Intestine, to promote defecation.
6. If there is lumbago, add BL-23 and BL-58 to strengthen the lower back and to relieve the pain.

STAGNATION OF LIVER-QI

Symptoms and signs

Chronic pain in the entire body, accompanied by a distending sensation, aggravated by negative emotions, with a headache, dizziness, insomnia, irritability, palpitations, irregular menstruation, a poor appetite, a dull stomach, pain in the lower abdomen, a red tongue with white coating and a wiry pulse.

Principle of treatment

Regulate Liver-Qi, remove Qi stagnation and relieve the pain.

HERBAL TREATMENT

Prescription

XIAO YAO SAN
Free and Relaxed Powder
Chai Hu *Radix Bupleuri* 10 g
Bo He *Herba Menthae* 3 g
Dang Gui *Radix Angelicae Sinensis* 10 g
Yan Hu Suo *Rhizoma Corydalis* 12 g
Bai Shao *Radix Paeoniae Alba* 20 g
Bai Zhu *Rhizoma Atractylodis Macrocephalae* 10 g
Fu Ling *Poria* 15 g
Sheng Jiang *Rhizoma Zingiberis Recens* 5 g
Gan Cao *Radix Glycyrrhizae* 5 g

Explanations

- Chai Hu and Bo He regulate and promote the circulation of Liver-Qi in order to remove the Qi stagnation in the Liver.
- Bai Shao and Dang Gui nourish the Blood and strengthen the Liver. These two herbs can also relieve body pain directly.
- Yan Hu Suo regulates the Blood circulation and relieves the pain.
- Bai Zhu, Fu Ling and Sheng Jiang tonify the Spleen and Stomach.
- Gan Cao harmonises the actions of the other herbs in the prescription.

Modifications

1. If there is headache or dizziness, add Chuan Xiong *Radix Ligustici Chuanxiong* 10 g and Qiang Huo *Rhizoma seu Radix Notopterygi* 10 g to regulate the Qi circulation and relieve the headache and dizziness.
2. If there is bad temper, add Xinag Fu *Rhizoma Cyperi* 10 g and Yu Jin *Radix Curcumae* 10 g to promote the circulation of Liver-Qi and remove Qi stagnation.
3. If there is irregular menstruation, add Huai Niu Xi *Radix Achyranthis Bidentatae* 10 g and Yi Mu Cao *Herba Leonuri* 10 g to regulate the menstruation.

Patent remedies

Xiao Yao Wan *Free and Relaxed Pill*
Shu Gan Wan *Soothe Liver Pill*

ACUPUNCTURE TREATMENT

LR-3 Taichong, BL-18 Ganshu, PC-6 Neiguan, GV-20 Baihui, LI-4 Hegu, SP-6 Sanyinjiao and ST-36 Zusanli. Even method is used on these points.

Explanations

- LR-3, the Source point and the Stream point of the Liver channel, regulates the Liver-Qi to relieve pain in the entire body.
- BL-18, the Back Transporting point of the Liver, can regulate the Liver-Qi to remove Qi stagnation in the Liver.
- PC-6, the Connecting point of the Pericardium channel and the Confluence point of the Yin Linking Vessel, regulates the Qi circulation and calms down the Mind.
- GV-20 is the patent point to calm down the Mind and regulate the Qi circulation.
- LI-4, the Source point of the Large Intestine channel, regulates the Qi circulation to relieve the pain.
- SP-6, the crossing point of three Yin channels of the leg, can remove Liver-Qi stagnation and calm down the Mind.
- ST-36, the Sea point of the Stomach channel, tonifies the Stomach-Qi and relieves the pain in the leg.

Modifications

1. If there is headache or dizziness, add GB-20 and TE-4 to calm the Liver and to stop the headache.
2. If there is a poor appetite, add CV-12 and SP-3 to strengthen the Spleen and Stomach and improve the appetite.
3. If there is irregular menstruation, add CV-6 and KI-3 to regulate the menstruation.
4. If there is insomnia, add BL-15 and HT-7 to calm down the Mind and improve the sleep.
5. If there is irritability, add LR-2 and HT-8 to regulate the Qi circulation, to calm down the Mind and improve the mood.

Case history

A 52-year-old woman had suffered pain in the entire body for 6 months. She had the pain, which was movable and changeable, especially when she got angry or distressed. She was diagnosed with menopausal syndrome in a hospital. In addition to Western medical treatment, she asked for acupuncture. Besides pain in her whole body, she mentioned she had irregular menstruation, lumbago, sweating with a hot or cold sensation, dizziness, palpitations, irritability and a poor appetite. Her tongue was red and had a thin coating and she had a wiry pulse.

Diagnosis
Stagnation of Liver-Qi and deficiency of Kidney-Yin.

Principle of treatment
Regulate Liver-Qi, remove Qi stagnation and nourish Kidney-Yin.

Herbal treatment

XIAO YAON SAN *Free and Relaxed Powder* for Liver-Qi regulation

Chai Hu *Radix Bupleuri* 10 g
Dang Gui *Radix Angelicae Sinensis* 10 g
Bai Shao *Radix Paeoniae Alba* 20 g
Bai Zhu *Rhizoma Atractylodis Macrocephalae* 10 g
Fu Ling *Poria* 15 g
Gan Cao *Radix Glycyrrhizae* 5 g
Yan Hu Suo *Rhizoma Corydalis* 15 g
Yu Jin *Radix Curcumae* 10 g
Chuan Xiong *Radix Ligustici Chuanxiong* 6 g
LIU WEI DI HUANG WAN *Six-Flavour Rehmanniae Pill* for Kidney-Yin nourishment, 10 pills, 3 × day

Explanations

- Chai Hu and Chuan Xiong regulate and promote the circulation of Liver-Qi in order to remove Qi stagnation in the Liver.
- Bai Shao and Dang Gui nourish the Blood and strengthen the Liver. These two herbs can also relieve the body pain directly.
- Bai Zhu and Fu Ling tonify the Spleen and Stomach.
- Yan Hu Suo and Yu Jin regulate the circulation of Liver-Qi and relieve the pain.
- Gan Cao harmonises the actions of the other herbs in the prescription.
- Liu Wei Di Huang Wan nourishes Kidney-Yin and calms down Liver-Yang.

The patient took the herbal decoction Xiao Yao San *Free and Relaxed Powder* and a patent pill of Liu Wei Di Huang Wan daily. After 50 days of treatment, her body pain had disappeared. Upon consultation 2 years later she reported being free of pain since completing the herbal treatment.

STAGNATION OF BLOOD

Symptoms and signs

History of trauma or operation, long duration of pain in the body with a fixed location, sharp pain with a stabbing sensation, joint pain, pain in the entire body induced by a change of posture or movement, aggravation of the pain at night, thirst without much drinking, a purplish tongue with a white coating and a deep and choppy pulse.

Principle of treatment

Promote Blood circulation, remove Blood stagnation and sedate the pain.

HERBAL TREATMENT

Prescription

SHEN TONG ZHU YU TANG
Meridian Passage

Qin Jiao *Radix Gentianae Macrophyllae* 10 g
Hong Hua *Flos Carthami* 10 g
Gan Cao *Radix Glycyrrhizae* 5 g
Qiang Huo *Rhizoma seu Radix Notopterygii* 10 g
Xiang Fu *Rhizoma Cyperi* 10 g
Huai Niu Xi *Radix Achyranthis Bidentatae* 10 g
Tao Ren *Semen Persicae* 10 g
Mo Yao *Resina Myrrhae* 6 g
Dang Gui *Radix Angelicae Sinensis* 12 g
Chuan Xiong *Radix Ligustici Chuanxiong* 6 g
Wu Ling Zhi *Faeces Trogopterorum* 9 g
Di Long *Lumbricus* 10 g

Explanations

- Qin Jiao, Qiang Huo and Xiang Fu promote the circulation of Qi and relieve the pain.
- Tao Ren, Hong Hua, Chuan Xiong, Huai Niu Xi and Dang Gui remove the Blood stagnation and relieve the pain.
- Mo Yao, Wu Ling Zhi and Di Long promote the circulation of Blood and remove the Blood stagnation in order to relieve the pain.
- Gan Cao harmonises the herbs in the prescription.

Modifications

1. If there is sharp pain, add Yan Hu Suo *Rhizoma Corydalis* 10 g and Pu Huang *Pollen Typhae* 10 g to increase the pain-relieving effect.
2. If there is aggravation of pain at night, add Gui Zhi *Ramulus Cinnamomi* 6 g and Xi Xin *Herba Asari* 3 g to warm the channels and relieve the pain.
3. If the joints are painful, add Chuan Shan Long *Rhizoma Dioscoreae* 20 g and Jiang Huang *Rhizoma Curcumae Longae* 10 g to regulate the Qi circulation in the channels and relieve the joint pain.

Patent remedies

Yan Hu Suo Pian *Rhizoma Corydalis Tablet*
Xiao Huo Luo Dan *Minor Invigorate the Collaterals Special Pill*

ACUPUNCTURE TREATMENT

LI-4 Hegu, LR-3 Taichong, SP-10 Xuehai, BL-17 Geshu, GB-34 Yanglingquan and ST-36 Zusanli. Reducing method is used on these points.

Explanations

- LI-4, the Source point of the Large Intestine channel, promotes the circulation of Qi and relieves pain in the entire body.

- LR-3 is the Stream and Source point of the Liver channel. Qi is the guide for Blood, so improvement of the circulation of Qi leads to a better Blood circulation. SP-10 is the patent point to treat Blood stasis and to relieve pain in the body. BL-17 is the Gathering point for the Blood. These two points are used to promote the circulation of Blood and to remove the Blood stasis.
- GB-34, the Gathering point for the tendons, relieves pain. ST-36, the Sea point of the Stomach channel, tonifies the Qi and promotes the circulation of Blood. These two points are also used to relieve local pain in the knee.

Modifications

1. If there is sharp pain, add PC-6 and SP-6 to promote the Qi circulation and to relieve the pain.
2. If there is joint pain, add some local Ah Shi points and the Accumulation points of the channels that are involved, to promote the local circulation of Blood and eliminate the Blood stasis.
3. If there is pain induced by movement, add TE-5 and GB-39 to activate the local Qi circulation and stop the pain.
4. If there is aggravation of the pain at night, add HT-7 and KI-6 to promote the circulation of Qi and Blood and remove Blood stasis.

DEFICIENCY OF QI AND BLOOD

Symptoms and signs

Chronic pain in the entire body, soreness of the muscles, fatigue, shortness of breath, dizziness, spontaneous sweating on exertion, an aversion to wind, a poor appetite, a pale complexion, diarrhoea with loose stools, a pale tongue with a white coating and a weak and thready pulse.

Principle of treatment

Tonify Qi and Blood and relieve the pain.

HERBAL TREATMENT

Prescription

BU ZHONG YI QI TANG
Tonifying the Middle and Benefiting Qi Decoction
Huang Qi *Radix Astragali seu Hedysari* 20 g
Zhi Gan Cao *Radix Glycyrrhizae Praeparata* 5 g
Ren Shen *Radix Ginseng* 10 g

Dang Gui *Radix Angelicae Sinensis* 10 g
Ju Pi *Pericarpium Citri Reticulatae* 6 g
Sheng Ma *Rhizoma Cimicifugae* 3 g
Chai Hu *Radix Bupleuri* 3 g
Qin Jiao *Radix Gentianae Macrophyllae* 10 g
Fang Feng *Radix Ledebouriellae* 10 g
Bai Zhu *Rhizoma Atractylodis Macrocephalae* 10 g

Explanations

- Ren Shen, Huang Qi, Bai Zhu and Zhi Gan Cao strengthen the Spleen and tonify the Spleen-Qi and Stomach-Qi.
- Sheng Ma and Chai Hu raise the Yang-Qi.
- Dang Gui aids Chai Hu to regulate the Liver-Qi in order to tonify the Blood.
- Ju Pi promotes the Qi circulation and strengthens the Spleen and Stomach.
- Qin Jiao and Fang Feng dispel the Wind and relieve the body pain.

Modifications

1. If there is muscle pain, add Qiang Huo *Rhizoma seu Radix Notopterygii* 10 g and Du Huo *Radix Angelicae Pubescentis* 10 g to regulate the circulation of Qi and relieve the pain.
2. If there is dizziness, add Tian Ma *Rhizoma Gastrodiae* 10 g and Man Jing Zi *Fructus Viticis* 10 g to regulate the circulation of Qi in order to relieve the dizziness.
3. If there is a poor appetite, add Sha Ren *Fructus Amomi* 6 g and Mu Xiang *Radix Aucklandiae* 10 g to promote the Spleen-Qi and improve the appetite.

Patent remedy

Shi Quan Da Bu Wan *Ten Inclusive Great Tonifying Pill*

ACUPUNCTURE TREATMENT

GV-20 Baihui, SP-6 Sanyinjiao, CV-6 Qihai, BL-20 Pishu, BL-23 Shenshu and ST-36 Zusanli. Reinforcing method is used on these points. Moxibustion treatment is recommended.

Explanations

- GV-20, the crossing point of the Governing Vessel and the Bladder channel, can raise the Yang-Qi and reinforce the Internal organs.
- CV-6 tonifies the Spleen-Qi and produces the Blood.
- BL-20 is the Back Transporting point of the Spleen and BL-23 is the Back Transporting point of the

Kidney. These two points in combination can tonify the Qi of Spleen and Kidney.

- SP-6, the crossing point of the three Yin channels of the foot, and ST-36, the Sea point of the Stomach channel, tonify the Qi and produce the Blood.

Modifications

1. If the appetite is poor, add CV-12 and SP-3 to regulate the Spleen-Qi and improve the appetite.
2. If there is dizziness, add CV-4 and GB-39 to reinforce the Qi, to tonify the Blood and relieve the dizziness.
3. If there is fatigue, add moxibustion on CV-8 to tonify the Spleen and warm the Yang.
4. If there is muscle soreness, add LI-4 and GB-34 to regulate the Qi circulation and relieve the pain.
5. If there is diarrhoea, add ST-25 and SP-9 to reinforce the Qi and stop the diarrhoea.

DEFICIENCY OF KIDNEY-YIN

Symptoms and signs

Chronic pain in the entire body, a hot sensation in the palms and soles, lumbago with soreness, a slight fever, night sweating, a dry mouth, thirst, a poor appetite, restlessness, insomnia, lassitude, tinnitus, constipation, a deep red tongue with a thin or no coating and a threadly and rapid pulse.

Principle of treatment

Nourish Kidney-Yin and relieve the pain.

HERBAL TREATMENT

Prescription

LIU WEI DI HUANG WAN
Six-Flavour Rehmanniae Pill
Shu Di Huang *Radix Rehmanniae Praeparata* 24 g
Shan Zhu Yu *Fructus Corni* 12 g
Shan Yao *Rhizoma Dioscoreae* 12 g
Fu Ling *Poria* 9 g
Mu Dan Pi *Cortex Moutan Radicis* 9 g
Ze Xie *Rhizoma Alismatis* 9 g
Fang Feng *Radix Ledebouriellae* 10 g
Dang Gui *Radix Angelicae Sinensis* 10 g

Explanations

- Shu Di Huang, Shan Zhu Yu and Shan Yao tonify the Blood and tonify the Essence of the Liver and Kidney.

- Ze Xie promotes urination and clears Deficient-Heat.
- Mu Dan Pi cools the Blood and activates the Blood circulation.
- Fu Ling strengthens the Spleen and drains the Damp.
- Dang Gui nourishes the Blood and relieves the pain.
- Fang Feng dispels the Wind and relieves the pain.

Modifications

1. If there is insomnia, add Suan Zao Ren *Semen Ziziphi Spinosae* 10 g and Wu Wei Zi *Fructus Schisandrae* 10 g to calm the Mind and improve the sleep.
2. If there is severe pain, add Fang Ji *Radix Stephaniae Tetrandrae* 10 g and Lao Guan Cao *Herba Erodii seu Cenanii* 20 g to relieve the pain.
3. If there is lower back pain, add Xu Duang *Radix Dipsaci* 10 g, Sang Ji Sheng *Ramulus Loranthi* 10 g and Bai Shao *Radix Paeoniae Alba* 10 g to strengthen the Kidney and relieve the lower back pain.
4. If there is constipation, add Sheng Di Huang *Radix Rehmanniae* 15 g and Xuan Shen *Radix Scrophulariae* 12 g to tonify the Kidney-Yin and lubricate the Large Intestine in order to relieve the constipation.

Patent remedies

Liu Wei Di Huang Wan *Six-Flavour Rehmanniae Pill*
Qi Ju Di Huang Wan *Lycuim Fruit, Chrysanthemum and Rehmannia Pill*

ACUPUNCTURE TREATMENT

LR-3 Taichong, KI-3 Taixi, KI-7 Fuliu, SP-6 Sanyinjiao, CV-3 Zhongji, BL-18 Ganshu and BL-23 Shenshu. Reinforcing method is used on these points.

Explanations

- LR-3, the Stream and Source point of the Liver channel, nourishes the Liver Yin and relieves pain.
- KI-3, the Stream and Source point of the Kidney channel, and KI-7, the River and Metal point, nourish the Kidney-Yin and relieve the pain.
- CV-3, the Front Collecting point of the Bladder channel and the crossing point of the Directing Vessel and the three Yin channels of the foot, is often used in the treatment for reinforcement.
- SP-6, the crossing point of the Spleen, Kidney and Liver channels, can nourish the Yin and clear the Deficient-Fire.

- BL-18, the Back Transporting point of the Liver, and BL-23, the Back Transporting point of the Kidney, nourish the Yin of the Kidney and Liver.

Modifications

1. If there is lumbago with soreness, add BL-36, BL-58 and BL-62 to strengthen the lower back and relieve the pain.
2. If there is dizziness and lassitude, add SP-3, GV-20 and CV-4 to strengthen the body and relieve the dizziness.
3. If there is insomnia, add HT-7 and GV-20 to tranquillise the Mind and to improve the sleep.
4. If there is a poor appetite, add CV-12 and SP-3 to activate the Spleen and Stomach, regulate the Qi in the Middle Burner and improve the appetite.
5. If there is constipation, add BL-25, the Back Transporting point of the Large Intestine channel, and ST-37, the Lower Sea point of the Large Intestine channel, to regulate the Qi in the Large Intestine and to promote defecation.

DEFICIENCY OF KIDNEY-YANG

Symptoms and signs

A weak constitution or chronic disease, pain in the entire body with a cold sensation, lassitude, an aversion to cold, cold limbs, a pale complexion, frequent urination, especially at night, lower back pain with soreness, a pale tongue with a white coating and a deep and thready pulse.

Principle of treatment

Tonify Kidney, warm the channels and relieve the pain.

HERBAL TREATMENT

Prescription

FU ZI TANG
Prepared Aconite Decoction
Zhi Fu Zi *Radix Aconiti Praeparata* 10 g
Bai Shao *Radix Paeoniae Alba* 30 g
Fu Ling *Poria* 15 g
Bai Zhu *Rhizoma Atractylodis Macrocephalae* 10 g
Ren Shen *Radix Ginseng* 10 g
Sang Ji Sheng *Ramulus Loranthi* 12 g

Explanations

- Zhi Fu Zi and Sang Ji Sheng tonify the Kidney-Yang and warm the channels as well as relieve the pain.
- Fu Ling and Bai Zhu strengthen the Spleen and eliminate the Damp.
- Bai Shao and Ren Shen tonify the Qi and improve energy.

Modifications

1. If there is pain with a cold sensation, add Wu Zhu Yu *Fructus Evodiae* 10 g and Gui Zhi *Ramulus Cinnamomi* 10 g to warm the Kidney-Yang and relieve the pain.
2. If there is lower back pain with soreness, add Xu Duan *Radix Dipsaci* 12 g and Tu Si Zi *Semen Cuscutae* 10 g to tonify the Kidney-Yang and relieve the pain in the lower back.
3. If there is an aversion to cold, add Gan Jiang *Rhizoma Zingiberis* 10 g and Rou Gui *Cortex Cinnamomi* 5 g to warm the channels and dispel the Cold.

Patent remedy

Jin Gui Shen Qi Wan *Kidney Qi Pill*

ACUPUNCTURE TREATMENT

KI-3 Taixi, BL-23 Shenshu, CV-4 Guanyuan, CV-6 Qihai, ST-36 Zusanli and GV-20 Baihui. Reinforcing method is used for these points. Moxibustion is recommended.

Explanations

- KI-3 is the Stream and Source point of the Kidney channel. BL-23 is the Back Transporting point of the Kidney. These two points are used to tonify Kidney-Yang, to warm the channels and to relieve the pain.
- CV-4 and CV-6 tonify the Yang, warm the body and remove the Cold from the interior.
- ST-36, the Sea point of the Stomach channel, tonifies the Qi and relieves the pain.
- GV-20 raises the Yang-Qi and improves the energy.
- Moxibustion treatment has a strong effect in warming the Yang and promotes the circulation of Qi in order to relieve the pain in the entire body.

Modifications

1. If there is pain with a cold sensation, add moxibustion on CV-8 to warm the channels, to dispel the Cold and relieve the pain.
2. If there is lower back pain with soreness, add BL-25 and BL-58 to harmonise the collateral and relieve the lower back pain.
3. If there is dizziness, add GB-20 and GB-39 to tonify the Blood and relieve the dizziness.
4. If there is lassitude, add SP-3 and BL-20 to tonify the Qi and strengthen the body.
5. If there is a poor appetite, add CV-12 and SP-4 to reinforce the Stomach-Qi, regulate the Spleen-Qi and improve the appetite.

Unilateral pain 9

半
身
疼
痛

Unilateral pain is pain at one side of the body, including that in the joints, tendons and muscles; it may be accompanied by restlessness, insomnia, sweating, fatigue or even hemiplegia. According to TCM, unilateral pain can be caused by disorder of the internal organs or by disturbance of the channels. Many factors may lead to pain at one side of the body, including invasion of the channels by External Wind, blockage of Wind and Phlegm, stagnation of Liver Qi, deficiency of Qi and stagnation of Blood, and deficiency of Yin of the Liver and Kidney.

Unilateral pain may be attributed to any of the the following disorders in Western medicine: the common cold, influenza, poliomyelitis, polymyalgia, rheumatism, depression, chronic fatigue syndrome, cerebral infarction and cerebral haemorrhage.

Aetiology and pathology

Invasion of the channels by External Wind

External Wind is one of the most common causative factors in unilateral pain. Wind exists as a pathogenic factor that may quickly invade the body in any season. When it invades the body, it induces disharmony between the Defensive and Nutritive Qi systems. The result of this is that the Defensive Qi cannot distribute the Body Fluids evenly, so the Body Fluids are unable to remain completely within the channels. Therefore the Qi and Blood cannot circulate freely to nourish the body and unilateral pain follows. Moreover, an invasion of External Wind may cause stagnation of Qi in the channels, muscles and tendons, which could at a later stage cause stagnation of Blood, resulting in unilateral pain.

Blockage of Wind and Phlegm

Eating too much sweet or greasy food may damage the Spleen and Stomach, easily leading to the formation of internal Damp-Phlegm. Phlegm is a substantial Yin pathogenic factor, which may circulate together with Qi, thus reaching everywhere in the body. Phlegm can also block Qi circulation and cause stagnation of Qi in the channels, tendons and muscles.

Wind is a Yang pathogenic factor that easily attacks the superficial levels of the human body. When Wind attacks in combination with Phlegm, the circulation of Qi and Blood will often be blocked, resulting in stagnation of Qi and Blood, and so unilateral pain occurs.

Stagnation of Liver-Qi

The Liver regulates the Qi circulation and stores the Blood. The emotions are closely related with the function of the Liver, and negative emotions, such as anger, stress and frustration, may cause stagnation of the Liver-Qi, which may in turn cause dysfunction of the circulation of Blood. When the tendons and muscles are not nourished properly, unilateral pain occurs.

Deficiency of Qi and stagnation of Blood

Multiple birth, chronic diseases and physical overexertion consume the Qi and may cause Qi deficiency. Qi is the power that promotes the free flow of Blood in the body, and if it is insufficient, the Blood circulation will slow, and later on eventually stagnate, and so unilateral pain occurs.

Deficiency of Yin of Liver and Kidney

Weak constitution, old age and sexual overactivity may cause consumption of the Kidney-Yin. As the Liver and Kidney share the same source, deficiency of Kidney-Yin may cause deficiency of Liver-Yin. As a result, there is insufficient Yin and Blood in the channels to nourish the tendons and muscles, and so pain occurs. Many chronic cases with unilateral pain are due to deficiency of the Yin of the Liver and Kidney.

Treatment based on differentiation

Before a differentiation is made, it is important to make a general examination of the patient. Special attention should be paid to the following characteristics of the unilateral pain: the quality, the accompanying symptoms and the factors that cause the pain to start, to increase or to decrease.

Differentiation

Differentiation of the quality of the pain

— Acute pain with an aversion to cold is usually due to an invasion of External Wind.
— Stagnation of Liver-Qi usually causes chronic pain with distension and migration.
— Stabbing pain with fixed locations and palpable nodulation or masses is usually due to stagnation of Blood.

— Pain with numbness and a heavy sensation is usually caused by Wind-Phlegm.
— A mild pain with a burning sensation is usually due to deficiency of Yin.

Differentiation of occurrence, aggravation and relief of unilateral pain

— A pain that starts or is aggravated when the patient feels cold or after sweating is usually due to an invasion of External Wind.
— A pain that occurs during the menstruation period is usually caused by stagnation or deficiency of Blood.
— If a pain starts or is aggravated when the patient feels warm or is in a hot environment, deficiency of Yin is usually the cause.
— If the pain starts or gets worse under stressful or other emotional conditions, it is usually due to stagnation of Liver-Qi.
— Stagnation of Qi and Blood. A pain that starts after trauma, operations, strokes or other diseases is usually caused by stagnation of Qi and Blood.
— If the pain occurs or gets worse at night, it is usually due to stagnation of Blood or to deficiency of Yin.

Differentiation of accompanying symptoms

— A pain accompanied by fever, an aversion to cold and pain in the limbs is usually due to an invasion of External Wind.
— Pain with irritability or bad mood is usually due to stagnation of Liver-Qi.
— Pain accompanied by numbness and a heavy feeling is usually caused by Wind-Phlegm.
— When the pain is combined with fatigue, palpitation and pale lips, it is usually due to deficiency of Qi.
— Deficiency of Yin usually causes pain with a hot sensation and dizziness. Pain with a sharp or stabbing sensation is usually due to stagnation of Blood.

Treatment

INVASION OF CHANNELS BY EXTERNAL WIND

Symptoms and signs

Fever, an aversion to cold, sweating or lack of sweating, a unilateral pain in the trunk, headache, a stiff neck, a unilateral joint pain in the extremities, back pain, a lack of thirst, clear urine, a pale tongue with a white coating and a floating and wiry pulse.

Principle of treatment

Dispel External Wind, regulate Defensive and Nutritive Qi and relieve the pain.

HERBAL TREATMENT

Prescription

GUI ZHI TANG
Cinnamon Twig Decoction
Gui Zhi *Ramulus Cinnamomi* 10 g
Bai Shao *Radix Paeoniae Alba* 10 g
Zhi Gan Cao *Radix Glycyrrhizae Praeparata* 6 g
Sheng Jiang *Rhizoma Zingiberis* 10 g
Da Zao *Fructus Ziziphi Jujubae* 6 g
Qiang Huo *Rhizoma seu Radix Notopterygii* 10 g

Explanations

- Gui Zui warms the channels, dispels Wind and strengthens the Defensive Qi. Bai Shao nourishes the Blood, dries the Body Fluids and tonifies the Yin in the Nutritive system. These two herbs in combination harmonise the Defensive and the Nutritive Qi.
- Qiang Huo helps Gui Zhi to promote sweating and dispel Wind-Cold.
- Sheng Jiang aids Gui Zhi to dispel the External Wind and strengthen the function of the Stomach.
- Da Zao aids Gui Zhi to nourish the Yin and Blood. It may also strengthen the Spleen and promote the Spleen-Qi.
- Zhi Gan Cao harmonises the functions of the other herbs used in the prescription.

Modifications

1. If there is headache, add Chuan Xiong *Radix Ligustici Chuanxiong* 6 g to eliminate the Wind in the head.
2. If there is a stiff neck, add Ge Gen *Radix Puerariae* 15 g to nourish the tendons and regulate the circulation of Qi.
3. If there is a severe pain with a cold sensation, add Gan Jiang *Rhizoma Zingiberis Officinalis* 10 g and Yan Hu Suo *Rhizoma Corydalis* 10 g to warm the channels and relieve the pain.
4. If there is joint pain, add Du Huo *Radix Angelicae Pubescentis* 10 g and Chuan Shan Long *Rhizoma Dioscoreae Nipponicae* 20 g to eliminate the External Wind and relieve the pain.

Patent remedy

Jing Fang Bai Du Pian *Schizonepeta and Ledebouriella Tablet to Overcome Pathogenic Influences*

ACUPUNCTURE TREATMENT

LI-4 Hegu, TE-5 Waiguan, GB-34 Yanglingquan, ST-36 Zusanli, BL-58 Feiyang, BL-60 Kunlun and BL-63 Jinmen. Reducing method is used on these points.

Explanations

- LI-4, the Source point of the Large Intestine channel, regulates the Qi and promotes sweating. TE-5, the Connecting point of the Triple Burner channel, regulates the Qi circulation and relieves the pain. These two points in combination relieve pain in the arm.
- GB-34, the Sea point of the Gall Bladder channel, relieves pain along the channel. It is also the Gathering point of the tendons, regulating the circulation of Qi in the tendons.
- ST-36, the Sea point of the Stomach channel, regulates the circulation of Qi and relieves the pain. BL-60, the River point, regulates the circulation of Qi in the Bladder channel, dispels the external Wind and relieves the pain.
- BL-58, the Connecting point of the Bladder channel, and BL-63, the Accumulation point, promote the circulation of Qi in the channel and relieve the pain.

Modifications

1. If there is fever, add GV-14 and LI-11 to promote sweating and lower the fever.
2. If there is a stiff neck, add GB-20 and BL-10 to promote the circulation of Qi and relieve the pain.
3. If the joints are painful and swollen, add GB-34 and SP-9 to eliminate the Damp and relieve the swelling.
4. If there is headache, add GV-20 and LU-7 to promote the Qi circulation and relieve the headache.
5. If there is back pain, add GB-21 and BL-23 to regulate the Qi circulation and relieve the pain.

BLOCKAGE OF WIND AND PHLEGM

Symptoms and signs

Unilateral pain with a heavy sensation, awkward or even paralysed limbs on the same side of the·body, soreness or numbness of the muscles, dizziness with a heavy feeling, nausea, painful and swollen joints, a poor appetite, fullness of the stomach, loose and sticky faeces, a tongue with a white and greasy coating and a wiry and slippery pulse.

Principle of treatment

Dispel Wind, eliminate Phlegm and relieve the pain.

HERBAL TREATMENT

Prescription

BAN XIA BAI ZHU TIAN MA TANG
Pinellia–Atractylodes–Gastrodia Decoction
Tian Ma *Rhizoma Gastrodiae* 10 g
Bai Zhu *Rhizoma Atractylodis Macrocephalae* 10 g
Ban Xia *Rhizoma Pinelliae* 10 g
Qiang Huo *Rhizoma seu Radix Notopterygii* 10 g
Chen Pi *Pericarpium Citri Reticulatae* 10 g
Fu Ling *Poria* 20 g
Gan Cao *Radix Glycyrrhizae* 5 g
Sheng Jiang *Rhizoma Zingiberis Recens* 6 g
Da Zao *Fructus Ziziphi Jujubae* 6 g

Explanations

- Tian Ma pacifies the Liver and eliminates the Wind-Phlegm.
- Ban Xia, Bai Zhu and Fu Ling strengthen the Spleen, dry the Damp and resolve the Phlegm.
- Qiang Huo eliminates the Damp-Phlegm in the muscles and resolves soreness and numbness of the muscles.
- Chen Pi regulates the Qi and resolves the Phlegm.
- Sheng Jiang, Gan Cao and Da Zao reinforce the Spleen and Stomach.

Modifications

1. If there is dizziness, add Man Jing Zi *Fructus Viticis* 10 g and Chuan Xiong *Rhizoma Ligustici Chuanxiong* 10 g to pacify the Liver-Wind and relieve the dizziness.
2. If there is swelling of the limbs, add Tong Cao *Medulla Tetrapanacis* 10 g and Gui Zhi *Ramulus Cinnamomi* 6 g to warm the channels and eliminate the Phlegm.
3. If there is soreness and numbness of the limbs, add Chang Pu *Rhizoma Acori Graminei* 10 g and Yuan Zhi *Radix Polygalae* 10 g to eliminate the Wind-Phlegm and regulate the circulation of Qi in the channels.

4. If there is nausea or even vomiting, add Guang Mu Xiang *Radix Saussureae Lappae* 10 g and Dan Nan Xing *Arisaema cum Bile* 10 g to resolve the Phlegm and cause the Stomach-Qi to descend.
5. If there is paralysis of the limbs, add Dang Gui *Radix Angelicae Sinensis* 10 g, Tao Ren *Semen Persicae* 10 g and Shui Zhi *Hirudo* 6 g to remove the Blood stagnation.

Patent remedy

Tian Ma Qu Feng Bu Pian *Gastrodia Dispel Wind Formula Tablet*

ACUPUNCTURE TREATMENT

L1-4 Hegu, PC-6 Neiguan, GB-20 Fengchi, SP-6 Sanyinjiao, LR-3 Taichong, ST-36 Zusanli and GB-34 Yanglingquan. Reducing method is used on these points.

Explanations

- LI-4, the Source point of the Large Intestine channel, regulates the Qi and eliminates the Phlegm to relieve the pain.
- PC-6, the Connecting point of the Pericardium channel, promotes the circulation of Qi.
- GB-20, the crossing point of the Gall Bladder and the Yang Linking Vessel, is very effective for dispelling Wind in the Upper Burner.
- SP-6, the crossing point of the Spleen, Kidney and Liver channels, regulates the circulation of Qi and Blood and eliminates the Phlegm.
- LR-3, the Stream and Source point of the Liver channel, promotes the circulation of Qi and eliminates the Phlegm in order to stop the pain.
- ST-36, the Lower Sea point of the Stomach channel, tonifies the Stomach-Qi and eliminates the Phlegm.
- GB-34, the Gathering point of the tendons, regulates the circulation of Qi and relieves the pain.

Modifications

1. If there is dizziness, add GV-20 and ST-8 to promote the circulation of Qi and eliminate the Wind.
2. If there is swelling of the limbs, add TE-6, SP-9 and ST-39 to promote the Qi circulation, to eliminate the Damp and relieve the swelling.
3. If there is a feeling of dullness or fullness of the Stomach, add CV-12, the Front Collecting point of

the Stomach channel, and SP-4, the Connecting point of the Spleen channel, to promote the circulation of Qi and to improve the appetite.

4. If there is soreness and numbness of the limbs, add SP-1 and SP-21 to promote the circulation of Qi and to eliminate the Wind-Phlegm.
5. If there is a poor appetite, add SP-3 and BL-20 to activate the Spleen and to improve the appetite.
6. If there is nausea or vomiting, add BL-21 and ST-40 to regulate the Qi circulation in the Stomach channel and stop vomiting.

STAGNATION OF LIVER-QI

Symptoms and signs

Unilateral pain with a distending sensation is not palpable. The pain starts after an emotional disturbance and can be aggravated by a bad mood. Insomnia, irritability, migraine, irregular menstruation, a poor appetite, a dull feeling in the stomach, lower abdominal pain, a red tongue with a white coating and a wiry pulse.

Principle of treatment

Soothe the Liver, regulate the Liver-Qi and relieve the pain.

HERBAL TREATMENT

Prescription

XIAO YAO SAN
Free and Relaxed Powder
Chai Hu *Radix Bupleuri* 10 g
Dang Gui *Radix Angelicae Sinensis* 10 g
Bai Shao *Radix Paeoniae Alba* 20 g
Bai Zhu *Rhizoma Atractylodis Macrocephalae* 10 g
Fu Ling *Poria* 15 g
Gan Cao *Radix Glycyrrhizae* 5 g
Bo He *Herba Menthae* 5 g
Sheng Jiang *Rhizoma Zingiberis Recens* 5 g

Explanations

- Bai Shao and Dang Gui nourish the Blood in the Liver and smooth and strengthen the Liver, to strengthen its physiological function.
- Chai Hu and Bo He regulate and promote the circulation of Liver-Qi and remove the stagnation of Qi in the Liver. These two herbs may also relieve body pain directly.
- Bai Zhu, Fu Ling and Sheng Jiang tonify the Spleen and Stomach.

- Gan Cao harmonises the actions of the other herbs in the prescription.

Modifications

1. If there is migraine, add Chuan Xiong *Rhizoma Ligustici Chuanxiong* 10 g and Xiang Fu *Rhizoma Cyperi* 10 g to regulate the Liver-Qi and relieve the pain.
2. If there is a sharp pain, add Yan Hu Suo *Rhizoma Corydalis* 10 g and Mo Yao *Resina Myrrhae* 10 g to heighten the effectiveness of the prescription in relieving the pain.
3. If there is lower abdominal pain, add Wu Yao *Radix Linderae* 5 g and Ju He *Semen Citri Reticulatae* 10 g to regulate the Qi circulation in the lower abdomen and relieve the pain.
4. If there is irregular menstruation, add Xiang Fu *Rhizoma Cyperi* 10 g, Huai Niu Xi *Radix Achyranthis Bidentatae* 10 g and Yi Mu Cao *Herba Leonuri* 10 g to promote the circulation of Qi and regulate the circulation of Blood.

Patent remedies

Xiao Yao Wan *Free and Relaxed Pill*
Shu Gan Wan *Soothe Liver Pills*

ACUPUNCTURE TREATMENT

TE-5 Waiguan, PC-6 Neiguan, BL-18 Ganshu, SP-6 Sanyinjiao, LR-3 Taichong and GB-41 Zulinqi. Even method is used for these points.

Explanations

- TE-5, the Connecting point, and GB-41, the Confluence point, of the Governing Vessel, promote the Qi circulation in the Lesser Yang channels and relieve the unilateral pain.
- PC-6, the Connecting point of the Pericardium channel and Confluence point of the Yin Linking Vessel, regulates the circulation of Qi and removes the Qi stagnation.
- BL-18, the Back Transporting point of the Liver, regulates the circulation of Qi and removes the Qi stagnation.
- SP-6, the crossing point of the three Yin channels of the foot, regulates the Qi and removes the Qi stagnation.
- LR-3, the Source and Stream point of the Liver channel, may regulate the Liver-Qi and relieve the pain.

Modifications

1. If there is hypochondriac pain, add LR-14, the Front Collecting point of the Liver, and GB-40 to regulate the Qi circulation and to relieve the pain.
2. If there is lower abdominal pain, add ST-29 and SP-8, the Accumulation point of the Spleen channel, to regulate the Qi circulation and to relieve the pain.
3. If there is irregular menstruation, add SP-9 and KL-3 to regulate the menstruation.
4. If there is insomnia, add GV-20, HT-7 and BL-15 to calm the Mind and improve sleep.
5. If there is irritability, add LR-2 and HT-6 to regulate the Liver and to clear the Heat in the Liver, to improve the mood.

Case history

A 41-year-old woman had been suffering from unilateral pain for 2 years. She complained of pain with numbness on the right side of her body when she felt stressed or angry. Sometimes the pain occurred before menstruation. She had many check-ups; however, no organic disease was found. As well as the unilateral pain, she had headache, irregular menstruation, a poor appetite and numbness on her tongue. Her tongue was red with a white coating. Her pulse was wiry.

Diagnosis
Stagnation of Liver Qi.

Principle of treatment
Regulate Liver Qi and remove the Qi stagnation in the channels.

Herbal treatment
Prescription
XIAO YAO SAN
Free and Relaxed Powder
Chai Hu *Radix Bupleuri* 10 g
Dang Gui *Radix Angelicae Sinensis* 10 g
Bai Shao *Radix Paeoniae Alba* 20 g
Bai Zhu *Rhizoma Atractylodis Macrocephalae* 10 g
Fu Ling *Poria* 15 g
Gan Cao *Radix Glycyrrhizae* 5 g
Bo He *Herba Menthae* 3 g
Yu Jin *Radix Curcumae* 10 g
Yan Hu Suo *Rhizoma Corydalis* 10 g

Explanations

- Chai Hu and Bo He regulate and promote the circulation of Liver Qi and remove the Qi stagnation in the Liver.
- Bai Shao and Dang Gui nourish the Blood and strengthen the Liver. These two herbs can also relieve body pain directly.
- Bai Zhu and Fu Ling tonify the Spleen and Stomach.

- Yu Jin helps Chai Hu to regulate Liver Qi and relieve the pain.
- Yan Hu Suo regulates the circulation of Qi and Blood and relieves the pain.
- Gan Cao harmonises the actions of the other herbs used in this prescription.

After the herbal treatment, the pain in the right side of her body was relieved within 5 weeks. Two years later, she reported that the problem had not recurred.

DEFICIENCY OF QI AND STAGNATION OF BLOOD

Symptoms and signs

Half-body pain with weakness, numbness and soreness of the limbs, sometimes stabbing pain in the muscles, hemiplegia, joint rigidity, muscle atrophy, low back pain, palpitation, headache, dizziness, fatigue, shortness of breath, a poor appetite, loose stool or diarrhoea, a pale tongue with a white coating and a deep and thready pulse.

Principle of treatment

Tonify Qi, promote Blood circulation and remove Blood stasis.

HERBAL TREATMENT

Prescription

BU YANG HUAN WU TANG
Tonify the Yang to Restore Five-tenths Decoction
Huang Qi *Radix Astragali seu Hedysari* 30 g
Dang Gui *Radix Angelicae Sinensis* 12 g
Chi Shao *Radix Paeoniae Rubrae* 10 g
Chuan Xiong *Radix Ligustici Chuanxiong*
Tao Ren *Semen Persicae* 10 g
Hong Hua *Flos Carthami* 10 g
Di Long *Lumbricus* 10 g

Explanations

- Huang Qi with heavy dosage tonifies the Qi and promotes the Qi and circulation.
- Chuan Xiong helps Huang Qi to promote the Qi and Blood circulation.
- Dang Gui, Chi Shao, Tao Ren, Hong Hua and Di Long invigorate the Blood circulation, remove the Blood stasis and relieve the pain.

Modifications

1. If there is hemiplegia, add Du Zhong *Cortex Eucomiae* 10 g, Dan Shen *Radix Salviae Miltiorrhizae* 10 g and Rou Gui *Cortex Cinnamomi* 10 g to tonify the Kidney and strengthen the limbs.
2. If there is fatigue and dizziness, add Gou Ji *Rhizoma Cibotii Barometz* 10 g and Dang Shen *Radix Codonopsis Pilosulae* 10 g to tonify the Qi and nourish the Yin to relieve the dizziness.
3. If there is joint pain, add Gui Zhi *Ramulus Cinnamomi* 10 g, Yan Hu Suo *Rhizoma Corydalis* 10 g and Sang Zhi *Ramulus Mori* 10 g to promote the Qi circulation and relieve the pain.
4. If there is a poor appetite, add Chen Pi *Pericarpium Citri Reticulatae* 10 g and Mu Xiang *Radix Aucklandiae* 10 g to regulate the Stomach-Qi and improve the appetite.

Patent remedy

Xiao Huo Luo Dan *Minor Invigorate the Collaterals Special Pill*

ACUPUNCTURE TREATMENT

LI-4 Hegu, TE-5 Waiguan, BL-17 Geshu, CV-12 Zhongwan, ST-36 Zusanli, LR-3 Taichong and SP-10 Xuehai. Reinforcing method is used on these points.

Explanations

- LI-4, the Source point, regulates the Qi circulation and relieves the pain.
- TE-5, the Connecting point, promotes the Qi circulation and removes Blood stagnation.
- BL-17, the Gathering point of the Blood, promotes the Blood circulation and removes the Blood stagnation.
- CV-12, the Gathering point for the Fu organs, promotes the Blood circulation and removes the Blood stagnation.
- ST-36, the Lower Sea point of the Stomach, tonifies the Qi and promotes the Blood circulation.
- LR-3 is the Stream and Source point of the Liver channel; Qi is the guide for Blood, so LR-3 is used to regulate the Qi circulation so as to promote the Blood circulation in turn.
- SP-10 is the patent point for treating Blood stasis and relieving the pain.

Modifications

1. If there is headache or dizziness, add GV-20 and GB-20 to regulate the Qi circulation and relieve the pain or dizziness.

2. If there is numbness in the limbs, add SP-3 and SP-6 to regulate the Qi circulation and relieve the numbness.
3. If there is fatigue, add CV-4 and CV-6 to tonify the Qi and Blood and increase the energy.
4. If there are palpitations, add PC-6 and HT-3 to promote the Qi circulation and calm the Mind.
5. If there is hemiplegia, add LI-11, GB-30 and GB-34 to promote the Qi and Blood circulation in the region.
6. If there is a poor appetite, add SP-4 to regulate the Qi circulation and improve the appetite.

Case history

A 66-year-old man had experienced a cerebral infarction 3 months previously. Since then he had suffered hemiplegia with pain on the left side of his body. His left limbs were numb and there was slight swelling. Also, he felt weak, dizzy and was tired especially after exercise. His tongue was enlarged and was a pale colour with a white coating. He had a deep and thready pulse.

Diagnosis
Deficiency of Qi and stagnation of Blood.

Principle of treatment
Tonify Spleen-Qi, promote Qi and Blood circulation and remove Blood stagnation.

Acupuncture treatment
The points LI-4, TE-5, CV-12, ST-36, SP-6, LR-3 and BL-17 were selected. Treatment was given once every other day. Even method was used on these points.

Explanations

- LI-4 is the Source point of the Large Intestine channel. TE-5 is the Connecting point of the Triple Burner channel. These two points in combination promote the circulation of Qi and relieve pain in the left arm.
- CV-12 is the Front Collecting point of the Fu organs. ST-36 is the Lower Sea point of the Stomach. These two points in combination tonify the Spleen-Qi and promote the Qi and Blood circulation.
- SP-6 is a crossing point of three Yin channels of the foot. LR-3 is the Stream and Source point of the Liver channel. These two points in combination promote the Blood circulation and remove the Blood stagnation so as to relieve the pain in the leg on the left side.
- BL-17, the Gathering point for the Blood, regulates the Blood circulation and removes the Blood stagnation.

After 2 months of treatment, the pain on the left side of the patient's body had gone. He was visited a year later and he said he had had no pain after the acupuncture treatment.

DEFICIENCY OF YIN OF LIVER AND KIDNEY

Symptoms and signs

Half-body pain with soreness, dizziness, palpitations, a low fever, night sweating, lassitude, insomnia, tinnitus, numbness of the limbs, hemiplegia, lumbago with soreness, a dry mouth, night sweating, a poor appetite, constipation, scanty menstruation with a pale colour, a red tongue with a thin coating, and a thready and rapid pulse.

Principle of treatment

Nourish the Yin of Liver and Kidney and relieve the pain.

HERBAL TREATMENT

Prescription

QI JU DI HUANG WAN
Lycuim Fruit, Chrysanthemum and Rehmannia Pill
Gou Ji Zi *Fructus Lycii* 10 g
Ju Hua *Flos Chrysanthemi* 6 g
Shu Di Huang *Radix Rehmanniae Praeparata* 20 g
Shan Zhu Yu *Fructus Corni* 12 g
Shan Yao *Rhizoma Dioscoreae* 12 g
Fu Ling *Poria* 9 g
Mu Dan Pi *Cortex Moutan Radicis* 9 g
Ze Xie *Rhizoma Alismatis* 9 g

Explanations

- Gou Ji Zi and Ju Hua nourish the Yin of the Liver and pacify the Liver-Fire.
- Shu Di Huang, Shan Zhu Yu and Shan Yao tonify the Blood and the Essence of the Liver and Kidney.
- Ze Xie promotes urination, eliminates the Damp and clears the Heat.
- Mu Dan Pi cools the Blood and activates the Blood circulation.
- Fu Ling strengthens the Spleen and drains the Damp.

Modifications

1. If there is dizziness, add Chuan Xiong *Rhizoma Ligustici Chuanxiong* 10 g and Gou Teng *Ramulus Uncariae cum Uncis* 6 g to promote the Qi circulation and pacify the Liver-Wind.
2. If there is hemiplegia, add Dan Shen *Radix Salviae Miltiorrhizae* 10 g and Di Long *Lumbricus* 10 g to promote the Blood circulation and remove the Blood stasis.
3. If there is insomnia, add Suan Zao Ren *Semen Ziziphi Spinosae* 10 g and Wu Wei Zi *Fructus Schisandrae* 10 g to calm down the Mind.
4. If there are palpitations, add Suan Zao Ren *Semen Ziziphi Spinosae* 10 g and Bai Zi Ren *Semen Biotae* 10 g to calm down the Mind and relieve the palpitations.
5. If there is lower back pain, add Xu Duang *Radix Dipsaci* 10 g, Sang Ji Sheng *Ramulus Loranthi* 10 g and Bai Shao *Radix Paeoniae Alba* 10 g to strengthen the Kidney and relieve the pain.
6. If there is constipation, add Sheng Di Huang *Radix Rehmanniae* 10 g and Xuan Shen *Radix Scrophulariae* 10 g to nourish the Kidney-Yin and lubricate the Large Intestine so as to relieve the constipation.

Patent remedy

Qi Ju Di Huang Wan *Lycuim Fruit, Chrysanthemum and Rehmannia Pill*

ACUPUNCTURE TREATMENT

LI-4 Hegu, PC-6 Neiguan, LR-3 Taichong, KI-3 Taixi, KI-7 Fuliu, CV-6 Qihai, SP-6 Sanyinjiao and BL-23 Shenshu. Reinforcing method is used on these points.

Explanations

- LI-4, the Source point, promotes the Qi circulation and relieves the pain.
- PC-6, the Connecting point of the Pericardium channel, nourishes the Yin and relieves the pain.
- LR-3, the Stream and Source point of the Liver channel, promotes the circulation of Qi and nourishes the Liver-Yin.
- KI-3, the Stream and Source point, and KI-7, the Metal point, enhance the effect of the Yin tonification.
- CV-3, the Front Collecting point of the Bladder, and a crossing point of the Directing Vessel and the three Yin channels of the foot, is often used for tonification.
- SP-6, the crossing point of the Spleen, Kidney and Liver channels of the foot, can nourish the Yin and clear the Fire to relieve pain.
- BL-23, the Back Transporting point of the Kidney, may be used to nourish the Kidney-Yin so as to nourish the Liver-Yin indirectly.

Modifications

1. If there is dizziness or headache, add GB-20 and TE-8 to relieve the headache or dizziness.
2. If there are palpitations, add HT-7 and BL-15 to regulate the Qi and calm the Mind.
3. If there is restlessness and insomnia, add GV-20 and HT-8 to clear the Heat and calm the Mind.
4. If there is a poor appetite and lassitude, add ST-36, CV-12 and SP-3 to promote the Qi circulation in the Middle Burner and improve the appetite.
5. If there is constipation, add ST-37 and ST-25 to nourish the Yin and promote defecation.
6. If there is hemiplegia, add TE-5, LI-11, GB-34 and ST-40 to promote the Qi circulation and remove the Blood stagnation.

Pain due to cancer 10

癌
症
疼
痛

Pain due to cancer is one of the most important topics in the field of pain research. Pain caused by cancer may occur in many different parts of the body. It is often seen in patients suffering from cancer in its medium and later stages. More than 80% of patients with late-stage cancer may suffer from pain.

In Western medicine, it is believed that the growing of cancer or its metastases may invade or press on nerves, vessels, bones and adjacent tissues. The fast-growing cancer cells cause pressure on the nerves. The tumour growth may also severely compress or stretch normal tissue, which by itself causes pain. These conditions may lead to poor blood supply, infection or necrosis, also causing pain.

The TCM viewpoint is that pain due to cancer is usually the result of invasion of the channels by the cancer toxin or blockage of the circulation of Qi and Blood in the channels and internal organs, because of tissue damage. In the development of cancer, TCM stresses the importance of interior imbalance, such as disorders of the Zang-Fu organs, Yin and Yang, Qi and Blood with accumulation of Phlegm, Damp, stagnant Blood, and so on. In short, cancer results from a mixture of Deficiency and Excess.

There are many publications, both ancient and recent, on TCM in the field of cancer, covering the aetiology, pathology, differentiation, treatment and prognosis of cancer. Many ancient descriptions of its aetiology, pathology and treatment are still very helpful and effective in modern clinical practice.

The ancient TCM literature on cancer (e.g. Qi Kun 1665, new edition 1997) covered many different kinds of cancers, including that of the tongue, the stomach, the oesophagus, the large intestine, the liver, the uterus and the bladder. In antiquity, TCM practitioners described cancer as diseases characterised by masses found on the skin or in the body, which are unsmooth on the surface, as hard as stones and rocks and cause severe pain (e.g. Ren Zhai Zhi Zhi 1982). The word 'cancer' dates back to the time when the Chinese characters were first formed, which strongly implies that even at that time cancers and pain due to cancer were one of the biggest pathogenic causes in daily life and endangered many people.

Over the past few decades, prevention and treatment of cancer and pain due to cancer have become one of the most important subjects in medical treatment. In TCM, comprehensive theories about cancer and pain due to cancer have been elaborated, departments of cancer research and treatment have been set up in many universities and hospitals, and many scientific reports and books have been published (e.g. Lei Yongzhong 1982, Liu Jiaxiang 1981). Great progress has been made in this field—in China, research has been carried out not only on the effects of herbal medicine, but also on those of acupuncture, Qigong, diet, massage, lasers, injections and infusions. For instance, some reports on acupuncture treatment for different kinds of cancers mention the points ST-36, SP-6, GB-34, LR-13 and LR-14 as being effective for treating severe pain due to Liver cancer. Some practitioners use electroacupuncture, which can produce heat in order to kill cancer cells, to treat many kinds of cancer on the superficial part of the human body with satisfying results.

According to TCM, pain caused by cancer reflects the many pathological changes in channels, internal organs, Qi and Blood and the clinical manifestations vary with the different kinds of cancer. When the cancer occurs in the brain then headache, dizziness and vomiting are among the symptoms. Patients suffering from oesophagus cancer often have chest pain and difficulty in swallowing and vomiting. Patients with Stomach cancer often have stomach pain, nausea and a hard mass in the upper abdomen. Cancer in the Large Intestine may cause abdominal pain, constipation or diarrhoea with blood. Patients suffering from cancer in the Bladder may have bloody urine and lumbago. Patients with Lung cancer often have upper back pain, chest pain and sputum with blood.

Although pain due to cancer varies in nature—for instance, it can be stabbing, distending, a swollen feeling, a colic pain, pain with a feeling of contraction or pressure, there are common characteristics:

1. long history of pain
2. rapid aggravation of the pain
3. rapid deterioration of the general physical condition
4. the pain appears at a place near to the tumour area
5. there are hard masses on the skin or in the abdomen, which are palpable
6. cancers in deep parts of the body, such as brain or chest, can be detected by modern medical techniques.

Aetiology and pathology

There are many causes of cancer pain. Here only the major causes are discussed, which include invasion of pathogenic factors, disorders of diet and emotions, weakness of constitution, stagnation of Liver-Qi, stagnation of Blood, accumulation of Toxic Fire, accumulation of Damp-Phlegm, and deficiency of Qi and Blood, and Yin and Yang.

Invasion of External pathogenic factors

Persistence of any External pathogenic factors may cause blockage of the channels in the body, which leads to stagnation of Qi and Blood or disorders of the internal Zang-Fu organs. In the Ling Shu, it was pointed out that invasion and accumulation of Wind in the body might cause blockage of the channels (Ling Shu, 1963, p. 145). The same book also mentioned that cancer could be triggered by Cold. Of course, due to limitation of understanding of the aetiology and pathology two thousand years ago, the Classics could not discover all the causes for cancer. However, in the book Zhu Bing Yuan Hou Lun—general treatise on the causes and symptoms of diseases (611, new edition 1955), the author Chao Yuanfang detailed some causative factors, and pointed out that the major causes of the pain associated with cancer were disharmony between Yin and Yang, and weakness and Cold of the internal Zang-Fu organs leading to invasion of External Wind (p. 105). From this description, it can be seen clearly that invasion of Wind and Cold were considered to be causative factors.

However, invasion and accumulation of these External pathogenic factors are only triggering factors; Interior disorders are the key causes. In the Ling Shu, it also states that cancers of the Large Intestine are due to accumulation of some Toxin in the Intestine first, which subsequently predisposes the person to invasion of External factors (Ling Shu, 1963, p. 89). Thus the primary cause is disease of the Intestines and the Stomach, and cancer occurs secondarily. Moreover, accumulation of Cold in the Spleen and Stomach with invasion and accumulation of External factors may cause stagnation, thus the cancer is stimulated. In the book Jing Yue Quan Shu—Complete works of Zhang Jingyue (1624, new edition 1991) it was stated that invasion of External Wind and Cold may mix with the Phlegm and stagnant food in the Spleen and Stomach, leading to formation of cancers in the Stomach and the Intestines (p. 479).

Disorder of emotions

TCM also stresses the role of the emotions in the development of cancer. For instance, the Neijing stated that sudden and strong grief may cause dysphasia, which is actually a preliminary form of oesophageal cancer. Again, in the case of breast cancer, Dr Chen Shigong described in his book Wai Ke Zheng Zong—Orthodox manual of external diseases (1617, new edition 1997) that excessive grief and depression may cause impairment of the Liver, excessive meditation may damage the Spleen, and too much thinking may disturb the Heart, and these pathogenic factors may result in weakening of the circulation in the channels leading to the formation of nodules, and so breast cancer follows (p. 435). It is very clearly stated in TCM theory that disorder of the seven emotions may cause disturbance of the interior organs, bringing about invasion of external pathogenic factors based on weakness of the organs. Also, emotional disorders could also directly cause slowing down of the circulation of the Qi and Blood in the channels and the internal Zang-Fu organs, thus cancer occurs.

Disorder of diet

Unhealthy diets may cause impairment of the Spleen and Stomach, leading to weakening of their functions of transportation and transformation, thus the production of Qi and Blood is damaged and deficiency of Qi and Blood follows. External invasion may easily take place under such conditions. Moreover, weakness of the Spleen and Stomach may cause retention of food and water, leading to formation of Damp-Phlegm, which in its turn could block the circulation of Qi and Blood. A mixture of Phlegm and stagnant Qi and Blood may slow down the circulation in the channels and weaken the functioning of the Zang-Fu organs, which makes the formation of cancer more likely.

Unhealthy diet includes overeating of fatty and greasy food, and of milky products, sweet foods, highly flavoured food, too pungent food, as well as drinking too much alcohol, leading to the formation of Damp-Heat. Overeating of cold food and raw food may also cause damage of Spleen-Yang, resulting in the formation of Cold-Damp.

Also included is the intake of Toxic food, including contaminated food and unhygienic food, which causes formation of Toxin in the body, leading to stagnation of Qi and Blood, dysfunction of the Zang-Fu organs and blockage of the channels, thus predisposing to cancer development.

Stagnation of Qi and Blood

Stagnation of Qi and Blood is the result of pathogenic changes; however, when it develops it becomes a pathogenic factor in itself. Most of the pain due to cancer, especially at a later stage, is caused by this kind of pathogenic factor. When stagnation of Blood develops, besides causing pain it may further block the channels, and disturb the physiological functions of the Internal Zang-Fu organs and the nourishing function of the Blood, resulting in emaciation, dry skin and hair, tiredness, bleeding, formation of masses, damage of veins, purplish tongue, and a thready and unsmooth pulse.

Generally speaking, stagnation of Qi and Blood may be caused by:

- too-strong emotion and prolonged emotion
- invasion of External pathogenic factors
- deficiency of Qi and Yang

- deficiency of Yin
- accumulation of Heat
- accumulation of Damp-Phlegm
- physical trauma
- inappropriate operations
- interior bleeding
- inappropriate injection, infusion or vaccination
- inappropriate intake or prolonged intake of some medications
- insufficient physical activity.

So when there is a Stagnation of Qi and Blood, except for treating the pain, it is necessary to search for its cause and to try to get rid of it.

Weakness of constitution

Old age, constitutional weakness, prolonged sickness, and weakness of the Spleen and Kidney may cause disorders of Yin and Yang, dysfunction of the Zang-Fu organs and slowing down of the circulation of Qi and Blood. This situation creates an opportunity for the invasion of External pathogenic factors and uprising of internal pathogenic factors, such as Phlegm, Damp, toxin, Fire and so on, leading to formation of cancer blocking the Zang-Fu organs and channels, so pain develops. Formation of cancer in the body may also further consume Qi, Blood, Yin and Yang, resulting in weakening of the Defensive Qi and aggravating the stagnation of Qi and Blood and the accumulation of Damp-Phlegm. In some cases, inheritance of some pathogenic factors also plays a very important role in the occurrence of cancer.

Unhealthy lifestyle

Smoking, drinking too much alcohol and taking drugs may cause dysfunction of the internal Zang-Fu organs, leading to the stagnation of Qi and Blood, and accumulation of Damp-Phlegm, so cancer may develop and pain follows.

Hyperactivity of Toxic Fire

Toxin may invade the body from outside; however, it may also be formed internally because of dysfunction of the Zang-Fu organs. For instance, persisting stagnation of Qi and Blood and accumulation of stagnant Damp-Phlegm may cause formation of Toxin in the body. If this process continues over a long period, the result would be generation of Toxic Fire. Hyperactivity of Toxic Fire burns the Zang-Fu organs, muscles and other body tissues, thus high fever, severe pain, bleeding, erosions and ulceration follow.

In summary, the causative factors for cancer are actually a mixture of several kinds of pathogenic factors, including invasion of External factors, disordered emotions, unhealthy diets and lifestyle and a weak constitution.

Diagnosis

Pain due to cancer usually occurs in the later stage of the disease. Whether the pain is due to cancer or to other causes may be easily differentiated by modern technology, such as X-ray, computed tomography (CT) scan, echo, blood test, marrow puncture, etc. However, by means of a differentiation of the symptoms and signs, TCM may also predict whether the pain is due to cancer or to another cause. The key points are as follows.

1. Cancer may occur at any age; however, most diseased people are middle-aged or elderly, owing to weakness of the Defensive Qi and a lowered resistance.

2. Most of the patients suffer from prolonged emotional disorders, especially too-intensive emotions, which may lead to impairment of mentality, stagnation of Qi and Blood, and blockage of the channels.

3. Bad dietary habits, including smoking too much, drinking too much alcohol, overeating of highly flavoured food and deep-fried food, and eating contaminated food, resulting in injury of the Spleen and Stomach with formation of Damp-Phlegm in the body.

4. Symptoms include prolonged high- or low-grade fever, fixed pain, no clear origin of bleeding, and progressive emaciation.

5. A hardening mass forms that grows progressively.

Treatment based on differentiation

Differentiation

Differentiation of location

When pain due to cancer occurs, it is very necessary to differentiate its location in order to discover which organ (or organs) is affected. Palpation of the painful areas and the course of the channels and differentiation of the clinical symptoms and signs may give a clear suggestion. For instance, in case of chest pain due to lung cancer, there would be cough, shortness of breath and expectoration of phlegm mixed with blood clots or pure haemoptysis; there could be tenderness at BL-13 Feishu, LU-1 Zhongfu and LU-5 Chize. If pain is caused by oesophageal cancer or stomach cancer, there would be painful swallowing, inability to swallow, vomiting after eating, and haematemesis, and tenderness in the epigastric region (e.g. at ST-34 Liangqiu and ST-42 Chongyang).

Differentiation of Excess and Deficiency

Pain due to cancer differs according to whether it is caused by Excess or Deficiency.

— A distending pain, stabbing pain, colic pain, sharp pain, contracting pain or constant pain are usually due to Excess.
— A slight pain, intermittent pain or empty pain are usually caused by Deficiency.
— More often the pain caused by cancer is Excessive pain.

Differentiation of Yin and Yang

— The Yin type of cancer has the following characteristics: slight pain due to cancer on the surface of the body, a lack of itching, a diffuse swelling without clear delimitation, local hardening, erosion, necrosis, and a purplish colour to the tumour or a lack of colour change in the area. Accompanying symptoms can include an aversion to cold, cold hands and feet, a lack of thirst, tiredness, a pale complexion, listlessness, low voice, shortness of breath, palpitations, a pale tongue and a thready and weak pulse.
— The Yang type of cancer has the following characteristics: severe pain due to cancer on the surface of the body, redness, swelling, heat, a foul smell, erosion and necrosis with yellowing oozing. These symptoms are accompanied by fever, restlessness, a bitter taste in the mouth, thirst, constipation and a red tongue.

Differentiation of tongue and pulse

Differentiation of the tongue and pulse characteristics is a very important step in making an accurate diagnosis and in distinguishing between Excess and Deficiency.

— A pale tongue, swollen tongue, or small tongue, tooth marks, a wet tongue coating and a peeled coating indicate Deficiency syndrome.
— A red tongue, purplish tongue, or even black tongue and a greasy coating indicate Excess.
— A big pulse, wiry pulse, slippery pulse, forceful pulse, tight pulse and choppy pulse indicate Excess.

— A thready pulse, weak pulse, slow pulse, deep pulse, intermittent pulse and floating pulse indicate Deficiency.

Treatment

STAGNATION OF LIVER-QI

Symptoms and signs

Local distension and pain, formation of masses that are soft in nature, hypochondriac pain and distension, aggravation of the pain by emotional upset, much stress, depression, headache, irritability, nervousness, a thin and white tongue coating, or a thin and yellow coating, and a wiry and tight pulse.

Principle of treatment

Smooth the Liver and circulate the Liver-Qi, harmonise the collateral and sedate the pain.

HERBAL TREATMENT

Prescription

XIAO YAO SAN
Free and Relaxed Powder
Chai Hu *Radix Bupleuri* 10 g
Dang Gui *Radix Angelicae Sinensis* 10 g
Bai Shao *Radix Paeoniae Alba* 20 g
Bai Zhu *Rhizoma Atractylodis Macrocephalae* 10 g
Fu Ling *Poria* 15 g
Gan Cao *Radix Glycyrrhizae* 5 g
Bo He *Herba Menthae* 3 g
Sheng Jiang *Rhizoma Zingiberis Recens* 5 g

Explanations

- Chai Hu and Bo He regulate and promote the Liver-Qi circulation and remove Qi stagnation in the Liver.
- Bai Shao and Dang Gui nourish the Blood and strengthen the Liver. These two herbs can also relieve pain directly.
- Bai Zhu, Fu Ling and Sheng Jiang tonify the Spleen and Stomach.
- Gan Cao harmonises the actions of the other herbs.

Modifications

1. If there is low abdominal pain, add Wu Yao *Radix Linderae* 5 g and Ju He *Semen Citri Reticulatae* 10 g to regulate the Qi circulation and relieve the pain.

2. If there is sharp pain, add Yan Hu Suo *Rhizoma Corydalis* 15 g and Mo Yao *Resina Myrrhae* 10 g to relieve the pain.

3. If there is irritability and nervousness, add Yu Jin *Radix Curcumae* 10 g and Chuan Xiong *Radix Ligustici Chuanxiong* 10 g to regulate the circulation of Qi and Blood and smooth the Liver.

4. If there is a poor appetite, add Shan Zha *Fructus Crataegi* 20 g and Mai Ya *Fructus Hordei Germinatus* 20 g to promote the circulation of Qi and improve the appetite.

5. If there is fullness in the stomach, add Zhi Shi *Fructus Aurantii Immaturus* 10 g and E Zhu *Rhizoma Zedoariae* 10 g to promote the circulation of Qi and Blood and relieve the fullness.

6. If there is constipation, add Da Huang *Radix et Rhizoma Rhei* 6 g and Mang Xiao *Natrii Sulfas* 15 g to promote defecation and remove the stagnation of Qi and Blood.

Patent remedies

Xiao Yao Wan *Free and Relaxed Pill*
Shu Gan Wan *Soothe Liver Pill*

ACUPUNCTURE TREATMENT

LR-3 Taichong, LR-5 Ligou, LR-14 Qimen, PC-6 Neiguan, CV-17 Tanzhong and GB-20 Fengchi. Reducing method is used on these points.

Explanations

- The Liver is in charge of promoting free flow of Qi in the body. If there is prolonged persistence of emotional disturbance the Liver is impaired, so stagnation of Liver-Qi occurs. In fact, stagnation of Liver-Qi may cause stagnation of Qi in the other Zang-Fu organs, such as the Lung, Stomach and Large Intestine. The key treatment therefore is to promote the circulation of Liver-Qi.
- LR-3, the Source point of the Liver channel, and LR-14, the Front Collecting point of the Liver, regulate the Liver, smooth the Liver and promote the free flow of Liver-Qi.
- LR-5, the Connecting point of the Liver channel, harmonises the collateral and sedates pain.
- PC-6, the Connecting point of the Pericardium channel and the point connecting to the Yin Linking Vessel, and CV-17, the Gathering point for the Qi, harmonise the Qi circulation, relax the chest, soothe the emotions, and relieve the blockage in the chest.

- GB-20 calms the Mind and the Liver and sedates headache.

Modifications

1. If there is stagnation of Qi in the Stomach and oesophagus, add ST-21 and CV-12 to promote Qi circulation in the Stomach and to sedate the pain.
2. If there is pain in the abdomen, add ST-25 and ST-28 to circulate Qi in the abdomen and to sedate the pain.
3. If there is coughing and chest pain due to stagnation of Qi in the Lung, add LU-5 and BL-13 to circulate the Qi in the Lung, to cause the Lung-Qi to descend and to relieve the cough.
4. If there is pain in the groin or perineum, add LR-11 and LR-12 to harmonise the collaterals and to sedate pain.
5. If there is irritability and nervousness, add GV-20 and LR-2 to clear the Heat in the Liver and to suppress the Liver.
6. If there is insomnia and restlessness, add HT-3 and HT-8 to calm the Heart and to tranquillise the Mind.
7. If there is a poor appetite, belching and nausea, add SP-4, ST-36 and ST-40 to cause the Stomach-Qi to descend and to improve the appetite.
8. If there is constipation, add TE-6 and LI-4 to promote defecation.

STAGNATION OF BLOOD

Symptoms and signs

Stabbing pain with a fixed location, aggravation of the pain at night or by immobility, alleviation of the pain with activity, hard swelling, hard masses, bleeding with purplish blood, a dark complexion, a purplish tongue and a choppy pulse.

Principle of treatment

Promote the circulation of Qi and Blood, eliminate the Blood stasis and sedate the pain.

HERBAL TREATMENT

Prescription

GE XIA ZHU YU TANG
Drive out Blood Stasis Below the Diaphragm Decoction
Tao Ren *Semen Persicae* 9 g
Hong Hua *Flos Carthami* 9 g
Yan Hu Suo *Rhizoma Corydalis* 6 g

Wu Ling Zhi *Faeces Trogopterorum* 9 g
Chuan Xiong *Rhizoma Ligustici Chuanxiong* 9 g
Dang Gui *Radix Angelicae Sinensis* 9 g
Dan Pi *Cortex Moutan Radicis* 6 g
Chi Shao *Radix Paeoniae Rubra* 6 g
Xiang Fu *Rhizoma Cyperi* 9 g
Zhi Qiao *Fructus Aurantii* 6 g
Wu Yao *Radix Linderae* 6 g
Gan Cao *Radix Glycyrrhizae* 6 g
Chen Pi *Pericardium Citri Reticulatae* 9 g
Sha Ren *Fructus Amomi* 6 g

Explanations

- This formula is suitable for upper abdominal pain radiating to the hypochondriac region. The herbs can be divided into two groups.
- One group of herbs invigorates the Blood and dispels Blood stasis. Tao Ren, Hong Hua, Yan Hu Suo, Wu Ling Zhi, Chuan Xiong, Dang Gui, Chi Shao and Dan Pi are commonly used herbs for invigorating the Blood and relieving the pain. But there are some differences among them.
- Tao Ren and Hong Hua are pungent and warm, breaking up and dispersing the stagnant Blood; they can be used for Blood stagnation in different regions of the body, especially for abdominal pain or swelling and pain of the limbs after trauma or operation.
- Yan Hu Suo can regulate both Qi and Blood and is very effective for stopping the pain. It can be used alone or in combination with other herbs.
- Wu Ling Zhi can break up Blood stasis, but will not consume the Blood nor disturb its normal circulation. Dang Gui can tonify and move the Blood. Both of these are especially suitable for Blood stagnation in deficiency syndrome.
- Chuan Xiong has a very strong effect on activating the circulation of Blood. It reaches all parts of the body and is very effective in stopping the pain.
- Chi Shao and Dan Pi can clear Heat in the Blood.
- Another group of herbs regulates the Qi: Xiang Fu, Zhi Qiao, Wu Yao, Sha Ren, Chen Pi and Gan Cao.
- Xiang Fu, Zhi Qiao and Wu Yao particularly regulate the Liver-Qi; they treat pain at the sides of the abdomen.
- Sha Ren regulates the Spleen-Qi and treats pain in the middle or lower abdomen.
- Chen Pi regulates the Stomach-Qi as well as the Spleen-Qi and treats the pain in the upper and middle abdomen.
- Gan Cao harmonises the actions of other herbs in the formula that work on different levels and in different directions. It can also protect the Spleen-Qi.

- All the herbs together are used to remove the stagnation of Blood and Qi in order to stop the pain. This formula can be used in the early stage of cirrhosis of the liver, trauma, adhesions and tumours.

Modifications

1. If there is irritability and restlessness, add Chai Hu *Radix Bupleuri* 5 g to diffuse the Liver-Qi and Dan Shen *Radix Salviae Miltiorrhizae* 10 g to clear the Heat in the Heart.
2. If there is severe pain of a cramping nature, add Bai Shao *Radix Paeoniae Alba* 10 g to smooth the muscles and tendons in order to relieve the cramp.
3. If there are palpable, immobile masses, add the herbs to soften the hardness, such as Xuan Shen *Radix Scrophulariae* 10 g, Zhe Bei Mu *Bulbus Fritillariae Thunbergii* 10 g, Mu Li *Concha Ostreae* 20 g, Shan Zha *Fructus Crataegi* 10 g, Ji Nei Jin *Endothelium Galli Corneum Gigeriae* 10 g, San Leng *Rhizoma Sparganii* 10 g and E Zhu *Rhizoma Zedoariae* 10 g.
4. If there is deficiency of Liver-Yin and Liver-Qi stagnation, add Bai Shao *Radix Paeoniae Alba* 10 g, Sheng Di Huang *Radix Rehmanniae Recens* 10 g and Chuan Lian Zi *Fructus Meliae Toosendan* 10 g to nourish the Yin and to promote the circulation of Qi.

Patent remedy

Bie Jia Jian Wan *Turtle Shell Pill*

ACUPUNCTURE TREATMENT

LR-3 Taichong, LR-5 Ligou, PC-6 Neiguan, SP-6 Sanyinjiao, SP-10 Xuehai, BL-17 Geshu and LI-4 Hegu. Reducing method is used on these points.

Explanations

- LR-3 and PC-6 promote the circulation of Qi in order to regulate the circulation of Blood.
- LI-4, SP-6, SP-10 and BL-17 promote the circulation of Blood, eliminate Blood stasis and sedate the pain.
- LR-5, the Connecting point of the Liver channel, harmonises the collateral and sedates the pain.

Modifications

1. If there is severe pain, add LR-6 and some other Accumulation points on the channels that are related to the affected organs to harmonise the collateral and sedate the pain.
2. If there is restlessness and insomnia, add HT-3 and HT-7 to calm the Mind and benefit sleep.
3. If there is bleeding with purplish blood, add SP-1 to stop the bleeding.
4. If there is weakness of the body, tiredness and poor appetite, add ST-36 and SP-3 to improve the appetite and raise the Yang and the Qi in the body.
5. If there is constipation, add ST-25 and ST-40 to promote defecation.

ACCUMULATION OF TOXIC FIRE

Symptoms and signs

Acute or subacute pain in the body, which is usually fixed at one place, but can also be throughout the body, formation of masses on the skin or within the body, erosion and necrosis with foul smell, discharge of yellow and sticky liquid from the masses, high fever, restlessness, thirst, a bitter taste in the mouth, deep yellow urine, constipation, a red tongue with a yellow and greasy coating and a wiry, slippery and rapid pulse.

Treatment principle

Cool Heat and remove Toxin, reduce Fire and sedate the pain.

HERBAL TREATMENT

Prescription

GAN LU XIAO DU DAN
Special Sweet Dew Pill to Eliminate Toxin
Hua Shi *Talcum* 10 g
Yin Chen *Herba Artemisiae Capillaris* 10 g
Huang Qin *Radix Scutellariae* 10 g
Shi Chang Pu *Rhizoma Acori Graminei* 10 g
Mu Tong *Caulis Akebiae* 5 g
Chuan Bei Mu *Bulbus Fritillariae Cirrhosae* 10 g
She Gan *Rhizoma Belamcandae* 10 g
Lian Qiao *Fructus Forsythiae* 10 g
Bo He *Herba Menthae* 5 g
Bai Kou Ren *Semen Amomi Rotundus* 10 g
Huo Xiang *Herba Agastachis* 10 g

Explanations

- Huang Qin, Lian Qiao and Chuan Bei Mu clear Heat and eliminate the Toxin.
- Lian Qian, Chuan Bei Mu and She Gan disperse stagnation, reduce the swelling and stop the pain.

- Mu Tong, Hua Shi and Yin Chen clear Heat and dry up Damp.
- Yin Chen can relieve jaundice.
- Huo Xiang, Shi Chang Pu, Bai Kou Ren and Bo He are aromatic herbs to resolve turbidity and Damp and to promote the circulation of Qi.

Modifications

1. If there is severe Heat Toxin in the Intestines, manifesting as constipation and abdominal pain, add Yin Hua *Flos Lonicerae* 10 g, Ma Chi Xian *Herba Portulacae* 10 g and Da Huang *Radix et Rhizoma Rhei* 10 g to clear the Heat and to remove the Toxicity.
2. If there is blood and mucus in the stools, but the blood predominates, add Zi Cao *Radix Arnebiae seu Lithospermi* 10 g, Dan Pi *Cortex Moutan Radicis* 10 g, Huai Hua *Flos Sophorae* 10 g and Di Yu *Radix Sanguisorbae* 10 g to cool the Blood and stop bleeding.
3. If the mucus predominates, add Fu Ling *Poria* 10 g, Yi Yi Ren *Semen Coicis* 10 g to transform the Damp.
4. If there is pronounced tenesmus, add Bai Shao *Radix Paeoniae Alba* 10 g to moderate the Qi in the Intestines.
5. If there is weakness of the Spleen, manifesting as poor appetite, tiredness and loose stools, add Dang Shen *Radix Codonopsis Pilosulae* 10 g, Bai Zhu *Rhizoma Atractylodis Macrocephalae* 10 g and Fu Ling *Poria* 10 g to tonify the Spleen and to transform the Damp.
6. If there is stagnation of the Liver-Qi, manifesting as depression, fullness of the chest and hypochondriac pain, add Xiang Fu *Rhizoma Cyperi* 10 g and Chai Hu *Radix Bupleuri* 5 g to promote the circulation of Liver-Qi.

Patent remedy

Gan Lu Xiao Du Dan *Special Sweet Dew Pill to Eliminate Toxin*

ACUPUNCTURE TREATMENT

LI-4 Hegu, LI-11 Quchi, TE-6 Zhigou, ST-37 Shangjuxu, ST-40 Fenglong, ST-44 Neiting, SP-21 Dabao, SP-2 Dadu, SP-6 Sanyinjiao, SP-10 Xuehai and LR-2 Xingjian. Reducing method is used on these points.

Explanations

- LI-4 and LI-11, the Source and Sea points from the Large Intestine channel, and ST-44, the Spring (Ying) point from the Stomach channel, clear the Heat, reduce Fire and remove Toxin.
- TE-6 promotes discharge of Fire and eliminates Toxin.
- ST-37, the Lower Sea point of the Large Intestine, and ST-40, the Connecting point of the Stomach channel, promote defecation in order to clear Heat and to remove Toxin.
- LR-2 and SP-2, the Spring points from the Liver and Spleen channel respectively, cool the Heat and reduce Toxic Fire.
- SP-6 and SP-10 cool toxic Fire at the Blood level and prevent Blood stagnation due to the accumulation of Heat in the Blood.
- SP-21, the great Connecting point of the Spleen channel, circulates Qi and Blood in the whole body and sedates body pain.

Modifications

1. If there is high fever and restlessness, add HT-8 and PC-8, the Spring points, to eliminate the Toxin, reduce the Fire and calm the Mind.
2. If there is discharge of blood with pus from the masses, add BL-17 to reduce the Heat in the Blood and cool the Blood.
3. If there is profuse discharge of pus, add SP-9 to eliminate the Toxic Damp.
4. If the person is only semiconscious, add HT-8 and GV-26 to waken the patient.

ACCUMULATION OF DAMP-PHLEGM

Symptoms and signs

Prolonged persistence of dull pain, sometimes pain with a distending and heavy feeling, lassitude, poor appetite, loose stools, formation of tumours that are soft in nature, gradual occurrence of erosions, discharge of white and sticky phlegm from the tumours, nausea, vomiting, a pale and swollen tongue with a white and greasy coating, and a slippery pulse.

Principle of treatment

Eliminate Phlegm and resolve Damp, disperse hardness and sedate the pain.

HERBAL TREATMENT

Prescription

DI TAN TANG
Scour Phlegm Decoction

Huang Qin *Radix Scutellariae* 10 g
Huang Lian *Rhizoma Coptidis* 10 g
Ge Gen *Radix Prerariae* 15 g
Yin Hua *Flos Lonicerae* 10 g
Mu Tong *Caulis Akebiae* 5 g
Fu Ling *Poria* 15 g
Che Qian Zi *Semen Plantaginis* 10 g

Explanations

- Huang Qin and Huang Lian, Cold and bitter in nature, enter the Large Intestine channel, are effective in clearing Heat and drying up Damp in the Intestines.
- Ge Gen, pungent and Cold in nature, enters the Bright Yang channels, and can not only clear the Heat, but can also cause the clear Spleen-Qi to ascend in order to stop the diarrhoea.
- Yin Hua can enhance the action of Huang Qin and Huang Lian to reduce Heat.
- Mu Tong, Fu Ling and Che Qian Zi increase urination and eliminate Damp.

Modifications

1. If there is a poor appetite, add Huo Xiang *Herba Agastachis* 10 g and Pei Lan *Herba Eupatorii* 10 g to eliminate the Damp and Phlegm and improve the appetite.
2. If there is nausea or vomiting, add Zhi Ban Xia *Rhizoma Pinelliae Praeparata* 10 g and Chen Pi *Pericarpium Citri Reticulatae* 10 g to dry the Damp and regulate the Qi circulation.
3. If there are loose stools, add Cang Zhu *Rhizoma Atractylodis* 10 g to help Fu Ling eliminate the Damp.
4. If there is severe diarrhoea, add Ze Xie *Rhizoma Alismatis* 10 g to promote urination and eliminate the Damp.

Patent remedy

Xiang Sha Liu Jun Wan *Six-Gentleman Pill with Aucklandia and Amomum*

ACUPUNCTURE TREATMENT

LI-4 Hegu, LI-11 Quchi, ST-39 Xiajuxu, SP-9 Yinlingquan, SP-6 Sanyinjiao, ST-25 Tianshu and CV-6 Qihai. Reducing method is used on these points.

Explanations

- LI-4, the Source point and LI-11, the Sea point, can clear Heat in the Large Intestine channel. They can also expel the Wind-Heat and reduce fever in an Exterior syndrome.
- ST-39, the Lower Sea point of the Small Intestine, and SP-9, the Sea point of the Spleen channel, are able to reduce the Heat, to transform the Damp in the Middle and Lower Burners and to stop the abdominal pain.
- SP-6 is an important point to resolve Damp and to stop pain in the lower abdomen.
- ST-25, the Front Collecting point of the Large Intestine, regulates the function of the Large Intestine.
- CV-6, the point where the Qi gathers, is used to regulate the Qi and open the obstructions in order to stop the abdominal pain.
- When all the points are used together, the Damp-Heat can be eliminated, the diarrhoea stops and the abdominal pain will disappear.

Modifications

1. If there is exterior syndrome, add TE-5 to expel the Wind-Heat.
2. If there is high fever, add GV-14 and ST-44 to reduce the fever.
3. If there is indigestion, add CV-12 and ST-44 to reduce the Heat and regulate the Large Intestine.

Part 3

Sense organ pain 五官疼痛

Facial pain 11

面
部
疼
痛

The face is the place where all the Yang channels meet; facial pain can be caused by a disturbance of one or more of these channels. Pain may occur at one side or on both sides of the face, but it is most commonly confined to one side.

Facial pain is often caused, according to TCM, by invasion of External factors, also by flaring up of Liver-Fire, accumulation of Heat in the Bright Yang Fu organs, or of Wind-Phlegm in the channels, deficiency of Qi, or stagnation of Qi and Blood. Facial pain may be attributed to any of the following disorders in Western medicine: primary or secondary trigeminal neuralgia, mumps, rhinitis, caries, trauma, post-facial operation, herpes zoster and its sequelae, and acute facial dermatitis.

Aetiology and pathology

Invasion of External factors

Overexposure to Wind, Cold or Heat may cause these pathogenic factors to invade the face. Cold is characterised by contraction and stagnation. In Wind-Cold invasion, there is a contraction of the channels and muscles on the face, leading to stagnation of Qi and Blood, and pain follows. Heat is characterised by uprising and burning. In Wind-Heat invasion, Qi and Blood in the channels, especially the Bright Yang channels, will be disturbed, leading to accumulation of Qi and Blood in local regions, then swelling, redness and pain occur.

Furthermore, an invasion of the face by Toxic Heat or insect bites may also cause an accumulation of Toxin in the channels, and stagnation of Qi and Blood occurs, leading to facial pain.

Flaring up of Liver-Fire

Overstress, overstrain, excessive anger or anxiety, or too much meditation, may also cause disharmony of the Liver and impede its function of promoting Qi circulation, leading to stagnation of Qi in the Liver. If this stagnation persists for a long time, this may generate Liver-Fire, causing flaring up of Liver-Fire to the face, and facial pain occurs.

Accumulation of Heat in the Bright Yang channels

Overeating of pungent, sweet or fatty food, or drinking too much alcohol, may cause Heat accumulation in the Bright Yang Fu organs, leading to constipation, a big appetite, bleeding of the gums, a foul smell in the mouth and thirst. This Heat may also ascend along the Bright Yang channels to the face and disturb the Qi and Blood circulation, so causing facial pain.

Accumulation of Wind-Phlegm in the channels

If External Wind invasion is not completely expelled, it may accumulate in the channels. When Phlegm accumulates in the body then Wind might mix with this Phlegm and block the channels, causing facial pain.

Deficiency of Qi

Overstrain or prolonged sickness may cause consumption of Qi, leading to Qi deficiency, then the face is not properly nourished, and this causes facial pain.

Stagnation of Qi and Blood

Qi and Blood should be freely circulated on the face. If Qi and Blood stagnate owing to various causes, the channels become blocked, causing pain. Physical trauma or inappropriate facial surgery may directly damage the channels and muscles leading to stagnation of Qi and Blood, and causing pain.

Treatment based on differentiation

Differentiation

Differentiation of External or Internal origin

— Acute onset of facial pain, mild in intensity, accompanied by External symptoms such as an aversion to cold, fever, muscle pain, a runny nose, cough and superficial pulse, is usually caused by invasion of External factors.
— A chronic history of facial pain, mild or severe in intensity, associated with diet, emotional state or other physical conditions, is usually caused by disorders of the Internal Zang-Fu organs.

Differentiation of character of the pain

— Acute sharp facial pain with a burning sensation, a thin and yellow tongue coating, together with some External symptoms, is usually caused by invasion of Wind-Heat.

— Acute sharp facial pain, together with some External symptoms, such as an aversion to cold, low-grade fever, muscle pain, absence of thirst, is usually caused by invasion of Wind-Cold.
— Acute sharp facial pain with a burning sensation, swelling of the face, redness, heat, fever, a thick or thin and yellow coating on the tongue, together with some symptoms caused by Toxic Heat, such as an aversion to cold, headache, throat pain and swelling, restlessness and constipation, etc., is usually caused by invasion of Toxic Heat.
— Chronic sharp facial pain with a burning sensation, redness and pain of the eyes, with aggravation of the pain by emotional upset, nervousness or dizziness, is usually caused by flaring-up of Liver-Fire.
— Chronic sharp facial pain with a burning sensation, redness of the face, aggravation of facial pain by consumption of some pungent food, a foul smell in the mouth, thirst and constipation is usually caused by accumulation of Excessive-Heat in the Bright Yang channels.
— Stabbing facial pain with a fixed location, which gets worse at night, with a purplish colour of the tongue, is usually caused by stagnation of Blood.
— Slight intermittent facial pain, with aggravation by exertion and during the day, poor vision, tiredness, an aversion to cold, cold hands and feet, a pale tongue with a thin, white and slight greasy coating, and a thready and weak pulse, is usually caused by deficiency of Qi.
— Chronic facial pain with numbness or a tingling feeling, intermittent facial pain, spasm of the facial muscles, local swelling on the face, mostly on one side, tic in the face, a thin, white and greasy tongue coating, and a wiry and slippery pulse, is usually caused by accumulation of Wind-Phlegm in the channels.

Treatment

INVASION OF WIND-HEAT

Symptoms and signs

Facial pain with a burning sensation, or a prickling sensation, or a sharp pain, constant pain, redness of the face, sweating, aggravation of pain by exposing to warmth, alleviation of pain by cold, thirst or fever, deep yellow urine, a red tip to the tongue and a thin and yellow coating, and a superficial and rapid pulse.

Principle of treatment

Dispel Wind, clear Heat and calm the pain.

HERBAL TREATMENT

Prescription

XIONG ZHI SHI GAO TANG
Cnidium, Angelica and Gypsum Decoction
Chuan Xiong *Rhizoma Ligustici Chuanxiong* 10 g
Bai Zhi *Radix Angelicae Dahuricae* 10 g
Shi Gao *Gypsum Fibrosum* 20 g
Sang Ye *Folium Mori* 10 g
Ju Hua *Flos Chrysanthemi* 10 g
Jin Ying Hua *Flos Lonicerae* 10 g
Man Jing Zi *Fructus Viticis* 10 g
Cang Er Zi *Fructus Xanthii* 10 g
Sheng Di Huang *Radix Rehmanniae* 10 g

Explanations

- Sang Ye, Jin Yin Hua and Ju Hua dispel the Wind and clear the Heat.
- Man Jing Zi and Cang Er Zi dispel the Wind-Heat and sedate the pain.
- Bai Zhi and Chuan Xiong sedate the pain on the face.
- Shi Gao clears the Heat and reduces the fever.
- Sheng Di Huang cools the Heat and removes the Toxin from the face.

Modifications

1. If there is a high fever, add Da Qing Ye *Folium Isatidis* 10 g and Ban Lan Gen *Radix Isatidis* 10 g to reduce the fever.
2. If there is redness and swelling on the face, add Pu Gong Ying *Herba Taraxaci* 10 g and Zi Hua Di Ding *Herba Violae* 10 g to clear the Heat, remove the Toxin and reduce the swelling.
3. If there is throat pain, add Xuan Shen *Radix Scrophulariae* 10 g to benefit the throat and relieve the throat pain.
4. If there is cough and expectoration of yellow phlegm add Sang Bai Pi *Cortex Mori Radicis* 10 g, and Zhe Bei Mu *Bulbus Fritillariae Thunbergii* 10 g to clear the Heat and eliminate the Phlegm.
5. If there is blocked nose with running nose, add Er Bu Shi Cao *Herba Centipedae* 10 g to open the nose and relieve the blockage in the nose.

Patent remedies

Yin Qiao Pian *Honeysuckle and Forsythia Tablet*

Yin Qiao Jie Du Pian *Honeysuckle and Forsythia Tablet to Overcome Toxins*

ACUPUNCTURE TREATMENT

LI-4 Hegu, LI-11 Quchi, TE-5 Waiguan, ST-6 Jiache, ST-7 Xiaguan, GB-20 Fengchi. Reducing method is used for all these points.

Explanations

- LI-4 and LI-11 are used to clear Heat, especially in the Bright Yang channel of the hand. These two points are suitable for pain around the nose since the Large Intestine channel ends at the nose. Besides, these two points can dispel the Wind-Heat and reduce fever. If there is a blocked nose, add LI-20, LU-7, LU-10 and Extra Bitong to circulate the channel and open the nasal orifice.
- ST-6 and ST-7 are used especially to circulate the channel and sedate the pain to treat pain in the cheek region since the Stomach channel passes through this region. In fact, Stomach channel disturbance is one of the main causes of facial pain. In this case, ST-4 and ST-5 should be used together to sedate the pain. ST-34, ST-40 and ST-42 can be prescribed at the same time. ST-34 is the Accumulation point of the Stomach channel, which has a good effect on relieving the pain in the Stomach channel. ST-40 is the Connecting point, which is effective for harmonising the collateral. ST-42 is the Source point, being effective for circulating the channel and stopping the pain.
- GB-20 is used to dispel the Wind-Heat and stop the pain. This point is prescribed especially for pain occurring near the ear that refers to the neck, causing a painful and stiff neck. This point also relieves headache, and in this case it would be best to combine it with TE-5, since this is the point that connects to the Yang Linking Vessel. And it is also the Connecting point of the Triple Burner, so it is effective in relieving pain on the side of the head. TE-5 is also effective for dispelling Wind and clearing Heat.

Modifications

1. If there is a fever, add GV-14, and ST-44, the Spring point of the Stomach channel, to reduce fever.
2. If there is throat pain and swelling, add LU-10 to relieve the pain and reduce the swelling.

3. If there is headache, add Extra Taiyang and Extra Yintang to sedate the headache.
4. If there is a swollen face with redness add ST-44 and LI-1 to clear the Heat and reduce the swelling.

Case history

A 30-year-old man had been suffering from facial pain with a burning feeling for 5 days. At the beginning, he had fever, throat pain, headache, an aversion to cold and runny nose with a white discharge, so he went to his general practitioner and took antibiotics for 3 days. Generally his symptoms improved slightly, but the burning facial pain remained. He also had general body pain, a tidal fever and aversion to cold, a slight thirst, a dry mouth, a red tip to his tongue, and thin and slightly yellow coating, and a superficial and slightly rapid pulse.

Diagnosis
This case was clearly a condition of facial pain due to invasion of Wind-Heat. The key symptoms of external invasion of Wind-Heat were: he was a young man who had never complained about these symptoms before, it was an acute attack, it was facial pain with a burning feeling, fever, an aversion to cold, throat pain, and the conditions of the tongue and pulse.

Principle of treatment
Dispel Wind, clear Heat, harmonise the collateral and sedate the pain.

Acupuncture treatment
LI-4 Hegu, TE-5 Waiguan, ST-3 Juliao, ST-7 Xiaguan, SI 18 Quanliao, GB-20 Fengchi. Reducing method was used on these points. Treatment was given once every other day.

Explanations
- LI-4 and TE-5 dispel Wind-Heat in general. Also, LI-4 and GB-20 can dispel Wind-Heat in the upper body, especially the face.
- ST-3, ST-7 and SI-18, all local points, are used to harmonise the collateral and sedate the facial pain.
- Normally, LI-11 is recommended to be added to the prescription; however, in this case there was not much fever, so this point can be omitted.

Due to the short duration of his problem, the facial pain was under control in 2 weeks.

INVASION OF TOXIC HEAT

Symptoms and signs

Acute occurrence of facial pain, redness, swelling and burning feeling on the face, formation of pus on the face, itching, fever, thirst, constipation, deep yellow urine, restlessness, a poor appetite, a red tongue with a yellow and dry coating and a rapid and wiry pulse.

Principle of treatment

Clear Heat, reduce Fire and eliminate Toxin.

HERBAL TREATMENT
Prescription

PU JI XIAO DU YIN
Universal Benefit Decoction to Eliminate Toxin
Huang Qin *Radix Scutellariae* 10 g
Huang Lian *Rhizoma Coptidis* 10 g
Xuan Shen *Radix Scrophulariae* 6 g
Zhi Zi *Fructus Gardeniae* 10 g
Ban Lan Gen *Radix Isatidis* 6 g
Lian Qiao *Fructus Forsythiae* 3 g
Ma Bo *Lasiosphaerae seu Calvatiae* 3 g
Niu Bang Zi *Fructus Arctii* 3 g
Bo He *Herba Menthae* 3 g
Jiang Can *Bombyx Batryticatus* 3 g
Sheng Ma *Rhizoma Cimicifugae* 3 g
Gan Cao *Radix Glycyrrhizae* 6 g
Da Qing Ye *Folium Isatidis* 10 g
Zhe Bei Mu *Bulbus Fritillariae Thunbergii* 10 g

Explanations

- Huang Qin, Huang Lian and Zhi Zi clear Heat, reduce the swelling and eliminate the Toxin.
- Ma Bo and Xuan Shen eliminate the Toxin.
- Ban Lan Gen, Lian Qiao, Bo He, Sheng Ma and Da Qing Ye dispel the Heat, reduce the fever and clear the toxin.
- Niu Bang Zi, Jiang Can and Zhe Bei Mu resolve the Phlegm and harmonise the collateral on the face.
- Gan Cao harmonises the herbs in the prescription and eliminates the Toxin.

Modifications

1. If there is fever due to flaring up of Fire-Heat, add Shi Gao *Gypsum Fibrosum* 20 g and Zhi Mu *Rhizoma Anemarrhenae* 10 g to clear Heat and reduce the fever.
2. If there is nasal bleeding due to invasion of the Lung system by Heat, add Sheng Di Huang *Radix Rehmanniae Recens* 10 g and Sang Bai Pi *Cortex Mori Radicis* 10 g to clear Heat in the Lung system and stop the bleeding.
3. If there is redness and swelling of the eyes with yellow secretion due to invasion of Heat into the Liver channel, add Xia Ku Cao *Spica Prunellae* 10 g and Long Dan Cao *Radix Gentianae* 5 g to clear Heat in the eyes and reduce the swelling.
4. If there is restlessness due to invasion of the Heart channel by Heat, add Dan Zhu Ye *Herba Lophatheri* 10 g to clear Heat from the Heart.

5. If there is nausea due to the penetration of Toxic Heat from the channel to the Stomach organ, add Xuan Fu Hua *Flos Inulae* 10 g to harmonise the Stomach and cause the Stomach-Qi to descend.
6. If there is constipation due to blockage of the Large Intestine by Heat, add Da Huang *Radix et Rhizoma Rhei* 10 g to promote defecation so as to clear the Heat.

Patent remedies

Niu Huang Jie Du Wan *Cattle Gallstone Pill to Resolve Toxin*
Yin Qiao Jie Du Wan *Honeysuckle and Forsythia Pill to Overcome Toxins*

ACUPUNCTURE TREATMENT

LI-2 Erjian, LI-4 Hegu, LI-11 Quchi, ST-5 Daying, ST-7 Xiaguan, ST-36 Zusanli, ST-42 Changyang, and ST-44 Neiting. Reducing method is used on these points.

Explanations

- In most cases when there is invasion of toxic Heat, the Bright Yang channel is affected, thus the points from the Large Intestine channel and Stomach channel are usually selected.
- LI-2 and ST-44 are two important points here in this case, because LI-2 and ST-44, the Spring points of these two channels, are able to clear Heat and reduce Fire, so as to eliminate the redness and swelling. Besides, they are the Water points according to the Five Element theory, and Water controls Fire, so it is appropriate to use these two points.
- LI-4, the Source point, and LI-11, the Sea point, clear Heat and circulate the channel so as to sedate pain. In most cases of invasion of Toxic Heat, there could be fever. When these two points are applied together, they will be more effective in reducing the fever.
- ST-42 and ST-36, which are the same as LI-4 and LI-11, the Source point and Sea point respectively, have a function in clearing Heat in the foot Bright Yang channel and sedating the pain.
- ST-5, ST-6 and ST-7 dispel Heat and harmonise the collateral, so they treat the pain in the locality.

Modifications

1. If there is fever due to flaring-up of Fire-Heat, add GV-14 to clear Heat and reduce the fever.

2. If there is nasal bleeding due to invasion of the Lung system by Heat, add LU-6 and LU-10 to clear Heat in the Lung system and stop the bleeding.
3. If there is redness and swelling of the eyes with yellow secretion due to invasion of Heat to the Liver channel, add LR-2 and Extra Taiyang to clear Heat in the eyes and reduce the swelling.
4. If there is restlessness due to invasion of the Heart channel by Heat, add HT-3 and HT-8 to clear Heat from the Heart.
5. If there is nausea due to penetration of toxic Heat from the channel to the Stomach organ, add PC-6 and CV-12 to harmonise the Stomach and cause the Stomach-Qi to descend.
6. If there is constipation due to blockage of the Large Intestine by Heat, add ST-25 and ST-37 to promote defecation so as to clear the Heat.

INVASION OF WIND-COLD

Symptoms and signs

Sharp pain at the face with spasm feeling, aggravation of pain after exposure to cold, alleviation with warmth, a purplish face or slight blue colour on the face, a thin and white tongue coating, and a superficial and tight pulse.

Principle of treatment

Dispel Wind, eliminate Cold, and promote circulation of the collateral and sedate the pain.

HERBAL TREATMENT

Prescription

CHUAN XIONG CHA TIAO SAN
Ligusticum–Green Tea Regulating Powder
Chuan Xiong *Rhizoma Ligustici Chuanxiong* 6 g
Jing Jie *Herba Schizonepetae* 6 g
Fang Feng *Radix Ledebouriellae* 6 g
Bai Zhi *Radix Angelicae Dahuricae* 6 g
Yan Hu Suo *Rhizoma Corydalis* 10 g
Man Jing Zi *Fructus Viticis* 10 g
Dang Gui *Radix Angelicae Sinensis* 10 g
Xi Xin *Herba Asari* 3 g
Gan Cao *Radix Glycyrrhizae* 5 g
Qiang Huo *Rhizoma seu Radix Notopterygii* 6 g

Explanations

- Jing Jie and Fang Feng dispel Wind and eliminate Cold.

- Chuan Xiong, Xi Xin, Bai Zhi and Qiang Huo dispel Wind-Cold and sedate the facial pain.
- Man Jing Zi and Yan Hu Suo arrest the facial pain.
- Dang Gui tonifies Blood and strengthens the Liver so as to harmonise the collateral.
- Gan Cao harmonises the prescription.

Modifications

1. If there is a runny nose with white discharge and sneezing due to invasion of the Lung system by Wind-Cold, add Cang Er Zi *Fructus Xanthii* 10 g and Cong Bai *Bulbus Allii Fistulosi* 10 g to dispel the Wind-Cold.
2. If there is headache due to stagnation of Qi and Blood in the head resulting from invasion of Wind-Cold, add Gao Ben *Rhizoma et Radix Ligustici* 10 g to eliminate the Wind-Cold in the head and sedate the headache.
3. If there is an aversion to cold and the hands and feet are cold because of impairment of the Yang-Qi by Cold, add Gui Zhi *Ramulus Cinnamomi* 10 g and Gan Jiang *Rhizoma Zingiberis* 5 g to warm the Yang and dispel the Cold.
4. If there is spasm of facial muscles due to Cold accumulation, add Bai Fu Zi *Rhizoma Typhonii* 5 g to relieve the muscle spasm.

Patent remedy

Chuan Xiong Cha Tiao Wan *Ligusticum–Green Tea Regulating Pill*

ACUPUNCTURE TREATMENT

LU-7 Lieque, LI-4 Hegu, TE-5 Waiguan, GB-20 Fengchi, ST-7 Xiaguan and SI-18 Quanliao. Reducing method is used. Moxibustion should also be used.

Explanations

- LU-7 and LI-4 are two important points in treating facial pain due to invasion of Wind-Cold. Wind-Cold often attacks the superficial parts of the face, and LU-7 opens the skin pores and relieves external invasion. LI-4 is a key point for treating problems on the head and face. When they are used together, they can promote the dispelling of Wind-Cold and the sedation of pain in the face.
- TE-5, the Connecting point of the Triple Burner and the Confluent point of the Yang Linking Vessel, is effective in relieving External invasion especially in the Lesser Yang channel causing pain around the ears. In this case, TE-5 is often combined with GB-20 in order to dispel Wind-Cold from the Lesser Yang channels. In fact, GB-20 can also be used with other points to dispel External invasion.
- ST-7 is the local point selected, as it has the function of circulating the collateral and sedating pain. This point is especially useful when there is an invasion of the Stomach channel by Wind-Cold causing pain at the mandible region; it is often combined with ST-5, ST-6 and ST-40 to promote circulation of the Stomach channel and relieve pain.
- SI-18 is used when there is an invasion of the Small Intestine channel by Wind-Cold causing pain around the cheek mandibular region; it is often combined with SI-4, SI-6 and SI-7, to circulate the Small Intestine and sedate the pain.

Modifications

1. If there is a runny nose with white discharge and sneezing due to invasion of the Lung system by Wind-Cold, add BL-12 and BL-13 to dispel the Wind-Cold.
2. If there is headache due to stagnation of Qi and Blood in the head resulting from invasion of Wind-Cold, add GV-16 to relieve Wind-Cold in the head and sedate the headache.
3. If there is an aversion to cold and cold hands and feet due to the impairment of the Yang-Qi by Cold, add ST-36 with moxibustion to warm the Yang and dispel the Cold.
4. If there is spasm of the facial muscles due to Cold accumulation, add SP-3 and LR-3 to relieve the muscle spasm.

Case history

A 40-year-old woman had suffered from facial pain for 2 weeks. For the first 4 to 5 days, she felt contractions or spasms in the face, which were alleviated with warmth (she used a warm towel and took showers), slight general body pain, aversion of cold, and slight fever. She rested for a couple of days at home and all the symptoms went away except for the facial problems. She was very afraid of her face being paralysed. When she came for consultation, her tongue was thin and white, and her pulse was superficial and tight.

Diagnosis
Blockage of the collateral due to uncompleted disappearance of Wind-Cold.

Principle of treatment
Harmonise the collateral and dispel Wind-Cold.

Acupuncture treatment
LI-4 Hegu, LU-7 Lieque, ST-3 Juliao, ST-7 Xiaguan, ST-40 Fenglong and SI-7 Zhizheng. Moxibustion was prescribed on LI-4, ST-3, ST-7 and ST-40. Reducing method was used. Treatment was given once every other day.

Explanations
- Moxibustion warms the channels and dispels Cold in the collateral.
- LI-4 and LU-7 dispel Wind-Cold, especially on the face.
- ST-3 and ST-7 regulate the Qi and Blood circulation on the face and sedate the facial pain.
- ST-40, the Connecting point of the Stomach channel, and SI-7, the Connecting point of the Small Intestine channel, harmonise the collateral on the face.

After a 10 day treatment, her facial pain disappeared.

FLARING UP OF LIVER-FIRE

Symptoms and signs

Painful face with burning feeling, aggravation of the pain by emotional upset and nervousness, restlessness, irritability, fullness of the chest, insomnia, headache, a bitter taste in the mouth, constipation, a red tongue with a yellow coating and a wiry and rapid pulse.

Principle of treatment

Clear Heat, reduce Fire, and sedate the pain.

HERBAL TREATMENT

Prescription

LONG DAN XIE GAN TANG
Gentiana Draining the Liver Decoction
Long Dan Cao *Radix Gentianae* 6 g
Huang Qin *Radix Scutellariae* 9 g
Zhi Zi *Fructus Gardeniae* 9 g
Ze Xie *Rhizoma Alismatis* 12 g
Mu Tong *Caulis Akebiae* 9 g
Xiao Ku Cao *Spica Prunellae* 10 g
Dang Gui *Radix Angelicae Sinensis* 3 g
Sheng Di Huang *Radix Rehmanniae Recens* 9 g
Sang Ye *Folium Mori* 10 g

Explanations

- Long Dan Cao, Sang Ye and Xia Ku Cao clear the Heat in the Liver and reduce the Liver-Fire.
- Mu Tong and Ze Xie clear the Heat by means of urination.

- Zhi Zi and Huang Qin clear the Heat and reduce the Fire in the body.
- Sheng Di Huang cools the Heat and eliminates the toxin in the Liver.
- Dang Gui harmonises the Liver.

Modifications

1. If there is emotional upset or depression due to stagnation of Liver-Qi, add Bai Shao *Radix Paeoniae Alba* 10 g and Chai Hu *Radix Bupleuri* 5 g to promote the Liver-Qi circulation and relieve depression.
2. If there is stomach pain due to the invasion of the Stomach by Liver-Fire, add Qing Dai *Indigo Naturalis* 5 g and Yan Hu Suo *Rhizoma Corydalis* 10 g to clear the Heat in the Stomach and sedate the pain.
3. If there is a headache due to disturbance of Clear Yang in the head by Liver-Fire, add Gou Teng *Ramulus Uncariae cum Uncis* 10 g to suppress the Liver-Fire and relieve the headache.
4. If there is restlessness, palpitations and insomnia due to disturbance of the Mind by Liver-Fire, add Huang Lian *Rhizoma Coptidis* 5 g and Long Gu *Os Draconis* 15 g to clear the Heat in the Heart and tranquillise the Mind.
5. If there is a bitter taste in the mouth with vomiting due to uprising of the Gall Bladder-Qi, add Yin Chen Hao *Herba Artemisiae Capillaris* 10 g and Xuan Fu Hua *Flos Inulae* 10 g to cause the Gall Bladder-Qi to descend and relieve the vomiting.
6. If there is constipation, add Da Huang *Radix et Rhizoma Rhei* 10 g to promote defecation and clear Heat in the Bright Yang Fu organs.

Patent remedy

Long Dan Xie Gan Wan *Gentiana Draining the Liver Pill*

ACUPUNCTURE TREATMENT

LI-4 Hegu, LR-3 Taichong, LR-2 Xingjian, LR-8 Ququan, GV-20 Baihui, GB-2 Tinghui, GB-20 Fengchi and GB-43 Xiaxi. Reducing method is used on all the points except LR-8 and GB-2; even method should be used on these last points.

Explanations

- This case is mostly caused by a prolonged persistence of emotional disturbance, including stress, frustration, anger, depression, upset, etc. If there is facial pain due to flaring of Liver-Fire, the side of the face is often affected, thus the points from the Liver and Gall Bladder channel are mainly selected. In case of invasion of the Stomach by Liver-Fire, points from the Stomach channel can also be applied.

- LI-4 and LR-3, the so-called 'four gate points', are effective in subduing Excessive-Fire and Wind, and reducing the pain and subduing the Liver-Fire.
- LR-2, the Spring point of the Liver channel, and GB-43, the Spring point of the Gall Bladder channel, together with GV-20 and GB-20, cool the face, reduce the Fire and clear the Heat, so as to treat the root cause.
- LR-8, the Water point from the Liver channel, nourishes Water so as to control the Liver-Fire. Also, this point is the Sea point from the Liver channel, and is good for treating Liver disorders generally.
- GB-2 treats facial pain at the side of the face. This point is also good for relieving tinnitus and ear pain, since flaring up of Liver-Fire often causes these two symptoms.

Modifications

1. If there is emotional upset or depression due to stagnation of Liver-Qi, add BL-18 and LR-14 to promote the Liver-Qi circulation and relieve the depression.
2. If there is pain occurring around the Stomach channel (i.e. in the cheek region) due to invasion of the Stomach by Liver-Fire, add SP-6, ST-7 and ST-44 to clear the Heat in the Stomach channel and sedate the pain.
3. If there is headache due to disturbance of clear Yang in the head by Liver-Fire, add GB-1 and GV-19 and GV-21 to suppress the Liver-Fire and relieve the headache.
4. If there is restlessness, and palpitations and insomnia, due to disturbance of the Mind by Liver-Fire, add HT-3 and PC-8 to clear the Heat in the Heart and tranquillise the Mind.
5. If there is a bitter taste in the mouth with vomiting due to uprising of Gall Bladder-Qi, add GB-34 and PC-6 to cause the Gall Bladder-Qi to descend and relieve the vomiting.

Case history

A 65-year-old man was suffering from time to time with facial pain. This lasted for more than 4 years. His facial pain could be greatly influenced by his emotions and alcoholic drinking. He would easily lose his temper and drink one to two glasses of red wine every day. Besides this, he liked pungent food very much. When he was young, he had suffered from hepatitis B. As he came for consultation, his face was red and slightly sweating, restless, his blood pressure was 170/100 mmHg, and he also had insomnia, sometimes a headache at the vertex, red eyes, a constant feeling of warmth over the body, occasional ear pain, constipation, thirst, a red tongue, (especially at the edges) with a yellow, thick and slight dry tongue coating and a wiry and rapid pulse.

Diagnosis
Flaring-up of Liver-Fire and accumulation of Heat in the Bright Yang channel.

Principle of treatment
Calm the Liver, reduce Fire and clear Heat in the Bright Yang channel.

Acupuncture treatment
LR-2 Xingjian, LR-8 Ququan, GB-20 Fengchi, GB-43 Xiaxi, LI-4 Hegu, ST-3 Juliao, ST-7 Xiaguan and ST-44 Neiting. Reducing method was used. Treatment was given once a week.

Explanations

- LR-2, the Spring point of the Liver channel, clears Heat in the Liver and reduces Liver-Fire. LR-8, the Sea point and Water point of the Liver channel, controls Liver-Fire to treat the root cause.
- GB-20 suppresses Liver-Fire and clears Heat in the head. GB-43, the Spring point of the Gall Bladder channel, cools the Gall Bladder so as to reduce the Fire in the Liver.
- LI-4 and ST-44 clear Heat in the Large Intestine and Stomach.
- ST-3 and ST-7 harmonise the collateral and sedate the pain.

In addition to above treatment, a herbal prescription based upon Long Dan Xie Gan Tang *Gentiania Draining the Liver Portfolio* was given. Drinking of alcoholic and eating of pungent foods were forbidden during the treatment. After a 4 month treatment, his facial pain was under control.

ACCUMULATION OF EXCESSIVE-HEAT IN THE BRIGHT YANG CHANNELS

Symptoms and signs

Gradual occurrence of facial pain, a hot feeling in the face, toothache, headache, thirst, constipation, a lot of hunger, a foul smell in the mouth, a red tongue with a yellow and dry coating, and a rapid and forceful pulse.

Principle of treatment

Clear Heat, reduce Fire and regulate the Bright Yang Fu organ.

HERBAL TREATMENT

Prescription

LIANG GE SAN
Cool the Diaphragm Powder
Da Huang *Radix et Rhizoma Rhei* 10 g
Mang Xiao *Natrii Sulfas* 10 g
Gan Cao *Radix Glycyrrhizae* 5 g
Zhi Zi *Fructus Gardeniae* 10 g
Huang Qin *Radix Scutellariae* 10 g
Lian Qiao *Fructus Forsythiae* 10 g
Bo He *Herba Menthae* 5 g
Sang Ye *Folium Mori* 10 g
Ju Hua *Flos Chrysanthemi* 10 g
Bai Zhi *Radix Angelicae Dahuricae* 10 g

Explanations

- Da Huang and Mang Xiao promote defecation and clear the Heat in the Bright Yang Fu organs.
- Zhi Zi, Bo He, Sang Ye, Ju Hua, Lian Qiao and Huang Qin clear the Heat.
- Gan Cao harmonises the prescription and clears the Heat.
- Bai Zhi arrests the facial pain.

Modifications

1. If there is gum bleeding due to flaring up of Stomach-Fire, add Sheng Di Huang *Radix Rehmanniae Recens* 10 g and Xuan Shen *Radix Scrophulariae* 10 g to clear the Heat and reduce the Fire.
2. If there is severe constipation due to accumulation of Heat in the Intestine, add Huo Ma Ren *Fructus Cannabis* 10 g to promote defecation and relieve the constipation.
3. If there is thirst due to consumption of Body Fluids by Bright Yang Fire, add Tian Hua Fen *Radix Trichosanthis* 10 g to promote secretion of Body Fluids.
4. If there is stomach ache due to accumulation of Heat in the Stomach, add Bai Shao *Radix Paeoniae Alba* 10 g and Yan Hu Suo *Rhizoma Corydalis* 10 g to relieve the stomach pain.
5. If there is a foul smell from the mouth, add Sha Ren *Fructus Amomi* 5 g to harmonise the Stomach and relieve the foul smell.
6. If there is nausea and vomiting, add Xuan Fu Hua *Flos Inulae* 10 g to cause the Stomach-Qi to descend and relieve the vomiting.

Patent remedy

Wei Te Ling *Stomach Especially Effective Remedy*

ACUPUNCTURE TREATMENT

ST-3 Juliao, ST-6 Jiache, ST-7 Xiaguan, ST-34 Liangqiu, ST-44 Neiting, LI-4 Hegu and LI-11 Quchi. Reducing method is used on these points.

Explanations

- This type of facial pain is often due to bad diet, especially overeating of pungent, sweet, fatty food, as well as drinking too much alcohol. However, it can also be caused by invasion of the Stomach by Liver-Fire. Once the Stomach is affected, the Large Intestine will be involved as well, and vice versa. No matter what the cause, points from both the Stomach channel and Large Intestine channel with reducing method should be mainly used, thus all the above points are selected from the Bright Yang channels.
- ST-3, ST-6 and ST-7 harmonise the local region and relieve pain in the area.
- ST-34, the Accumulation point from the Stomach channel, relieves pain and harmonises the Stomach.
- ST-44, the Spring point from the Stomach channel, clears Heat and reduces Excessive-Fire, which is the root treatment of this case.
- LI-4, the Source point, and LI-11, the Sea point, all from the Large Intestine channel, are able to clear Heat and reduce Fire in the intestine.

Modifications

1. If there is gum bleeding due to flaring up of Stomach-Fire, add ST-45, the son point of the Stomach channel, to clear the Heat and reduce the Fire.
2. If there is constipation due to accumulation of Heat in the intestine, add ST-25, the front Collecting point of the Large Intestine, and ST-37, the Lower Sea point of the Large Intestine, to promote Qi circulation in the Large Intestine and relieve the constipation.
3. If there is thirst due to consumption of Body Fluids by Bright Yang Fire, add SP-6 to promote secretion of Body Fluids.
4. If there is stomach pain due to accumulation of Heat in the Stomach, add CV-12, the Front Collecting point of the Stomach, to relieve the stomach pain.

ACCUMULATION OF WIND-PHLEGM IN THE CHANNELS

Symptoms and signs

Intermittent occurrence of facial pain, spasm of the facial muscles, mostly on one side of the face, tic in the face, aggravation of the situation by emotions, especially by anger, numbness of the face, a thin, white and greasy tongue coating and a wiry and slippery pulse.

Principle of treatment

Suppress Wind, resolve Phlegm and sedate the pain.

HERBAL TREATMENT

Prescription

QIAN ZHENG SAN
Lead to Symmetry Powder
Bai Fu Zi *Rhizoma Typhonii* 5 g
Zhi Ban Xia *Rhizoma Pinelliae Praeparata* 10 g
Gui Zhi *Ramulus Cinnamomi* 10 g
Dan Nan Xing *Rhizoma Arisaematis cum Felle bovis* 5 g
Chuan Xiong *Rhizoma Ligustici Chuanxiong* 10 g
Bai Zhi *Radix Angelicae Dahuricae* 10 g

Explanations

- Bai Fu Zi and Dan Nan Xing dispel Wind and sedate the facial pain.
- Ban Xia resolves Phlegm in the collateral.
- Gui Zhi warms the channels and harmonises the collateral on the face.
- Chuan Xiong promotes circulation of Blood on the face and sedates the pain.
- Bai Zhi arrests the facial pain.

Modifications

1. If there is spasm on the face, add Bai Shao *Radix Paeoniae Alba* 10 g and Zhi Gan Cao *Radix Glycyrrhizae Praeparata* 5 g to relieve the spasm and smooth the muscles on the face.
2. If there is severe pain, add Xi Xin *Herba Asari* 5 g to arrest the pain.
3. If there is dizziness, add Tian Ma *Rhizoma Gastrodiae* 10 g and Gou Teng *Ramulus Uncariae cum Uncis* 10 g to calm the Liver and subdue the Wind.
4. If there is an aversion to cold, add Gan Jiang *Rhizoma Zingiberis* 10 g to warm the body and relieve the Cold.
5. If there is nervousness, add Xia Ku Cao *Spica Prunellae* 10 g to clear Heat and calm the Liver.
6. If there is a white, thick and greasy tongue coating, add Cang Zhu *Rhizoma Atractylodis* 10 g to resolve Damp and eliminate the Phlegm.

ACUPUNCTURE TREATMENT

LR-3 Taichong, LR-5 Ligou, LR-6 Zhongdu, LI-4 Hegu, GB-3 Shangguan, GB-20 Fengchi, ST-40 Fenglong and SP-6 Sanyinjiao. Reducing method is used.

Explanations

- Since external Wind has entered the body and mixed already with Phlegm, it will be absolutely incorrect to use only points to dispel external Wind. The correct treatment should be to suppress the Wind and resolve the Phlegm, thus the above points are prescribed.
- LI-4 and LR-3, the four gate points, together with GB-20, check the Wind and sedate the pain.
- LR-5, the Connecting point, LR-6, the Accumulation points, all from the Liver channel, harmonise the Liver channel and collateral, and resolve Phlegm in the collateral so as to relieve the pain.
- GB-3 treats pain in the local area.
- ST-40 and SP-6, the crossing point of three Yin channels of the foot, eliminate the Phlegm in the body as well as in the collateral. Since ST-40 is also the Connecting point from the Stomach channel, it can sedate the pain on the face simultaneously.

Modifications

1. If there is a tic at the corner of the mouth due to Wind-Phlegm in the Stomach collateral, add ST-3 and ST-4 to relieve the tic.
2. If there is a tic at the corner of the eye due to Liver-Wind stirring inside, add Extra Taiyang and GB-14 to relieve the tic.
3. If there is an aversion to cold on the face due to a blockage of the Yang-Qi in the channel by Phlegm, apply moxibustion on the face, and add ST-36 with moxibustion to promote the Yang-Qi circulation and relieve the blockage.
4. If there is depression, nervousness, irritability and emotional instability due to stagnation of Liver-Qi, add BL-15, BL-17 and BL-18 to circulate the Liver-Qi and harmonise the emotions.

DEFICIENCY OF QI

Symptoms and signs

Persistence of facial pain with a heavy feeling, aggravation of pain with tiredness, a pale complexion, facial oedema, a poor appetite, loose stool, shortness of breath, an aversion to cold, spontaneous sweating, a low voice, a pale tongue with a thin, white and greasy coating and a thready and weak pulse.

Principle of treatment

Tonify Qi, eliminate Damp and circulate the collateral.

HERBAL TREATMENT

Prescription

BU ZHONG YI QI TANG
Tonifying the Middle and Benefiting Qi Decoction
Huang Qi *Radix Astragali seu Hedysari* 20 g
Shan Yao *Rhizoma Dioscoreae* 10 g
Huang Jing *Rhizoma Polygonati* 10 g
Gan Cao *Radix Glycyrrhizae* 5 g
Dang Shen *Radix Codonopsis Pilosulae* 10 g
Dang Gui *Radix Angelicae Sinensis* 10 g
Chen Pi *Pericarpium Citri Reticulatae* 6 g
Sheng Ma *Rhizoma Cimicifugae* 3 g
Chai Hu *Radix Bupleuri* 3 g
Bai Zhu *Rhizoma Atractylodis Macrocephalae* 10 g

Explanations

- Dang Shen, Bai Zhu, Huang Jing and Shan Yao activate the Spleen and tonify the Qi.
- Dang Gui nourishes Blood so as to support the Qi.
- Huang Qi tonifies Qi and lifts the Qi to the face.
- Sheng Ma and Chai Hu, prescribed in small dosage, are used to help Huang Qi lift up the Qi to the face.
- Chen Pi harmonises the stomach.
- Gan Cao tonifies the Qi and harmonises the prescription.

Modifications

1. If there is a swollen face, add Fu Ling *Poria* 10 g and Ze Xie *Rhizoma Alismatis* 10 g to promote water discharge and eliminate swelling in the face.
2. If there is a poor appetite, add Shan Zha *Fructus Crataegi* 15 g and Mai Ya *Fructus Hordei Germinatus* 15 g to activate the Stomach and Spleen and improve the appetite.
3. If there is diarrhoea, add Ge Gen *Radix Puerariae* 10 g to raise the Clear Yang-Qi and stop the diarrhoea.
4. If there is numbness on the face, add Ban Xia *Rhizoma Pinelliae* 10 g, Chuan Xiong *Rhizoma Ligustici Chuanxiong* 5 g and Di Long *Lumbricus* 10 g to eliminate the Damp-Phlegm and promote circulation in the collateral.

Patent remedy

Bu Zhong Yi Qi Wan *Tonifying the Middle and Benefiting Qi Pill*

ACUPUNCTURE TREATMENT

ST-6 Jiache, ST-7 Xiaguan, ST-34 Liangqiu, ST-36 Zusanli, ST-42 Chongyang, SP-3 Taibai, SP-6 Sanyinjiao, GV-20 Baihui and CV-6 Qihai. Reinforcing method is used on all these points except ST-34. Even method is used on ST-34. Moxibustion is advisable for use on ST-36, CV-6, SP-3 and GV-20.

Explanations

- This type of facial pain is often caused by overstrain and prolonged sickness. Furthermore, it is seen in elderly people who have a gradual depletion of their energy, especially in the Spleen and Stomach. Thus their production of Qi and Blood will be impaired.
- ST-36, the Sea point, ST-42, the Source point from the Stomach channel, and SP-3, the Source point from the Spleen channel, are able to activate the Spleen and Stomach and reinforce the Qi.
- ST-40, the Connecting point from the Stomach channel, harmonises the collateral and sedates the pain.
- SP-6 and CV-6 tonify Blood of the general body. GV-20 lifts up the Qi to the face so as to nourish the channels and collateral on the face.
- ST-34, the Accumulation point of the Stomach channel, harmonises the collateral and sedates the pain.
- ST-6 and ST-7 are used to relieve the pain in the local area.

Modifications

1. If there is chronic tiredness due to deficiency of general Qi, add CV-4 with moxibustion to tonify the Yuan Qi and relieve the tiredness.
2. If there is shortness of breath due to deficiency of Lung-Qi, add LU-9, the Source point, and PC-6, the Confluence point of the Yin Linking Vessel and the Connecting point of the Pericardium channel, to tonify the Lung-Qi and relieve the shortness of breath.
3. If there is a poor appetite and loose stool due to weakness of the Stomach and Spleen, add CV-12, the Front Collecting point of the Stomach, and SP-9, the Sea point of the Spleen channel, to activate the Spleen and Stomach and relieve the loose stool.

4. If there is numbness on the face due to deficiency of Qi, use Plum-Blossom needling to improve the numbness.

STAGNATION OF QI AND BLOOD

Symptoms and signs

Long duration of facial pain with fixed location, inter-mittent stabbing pain, aggravation of the pain at night, a purplish colour of the face, a purplish tongue with a thin coating and wiry and unsmooth pulse.

Principle of treatment

Circulate Qi and Blood, smooth the collateral and sedate the pain.

HERBAL TREATMENT

Prescription

TONG QIAO HUO XUE TANG

Unblock the Orifices and Invigorate the Blood Decoction
Chuan Xiong *Rhizoma Ligustici Chuanxiong* 10 g
Chi Shao *Radix Paeoniae Rubra* 10 g
Dang Gui *Radix Angelicae Sinensis* 10 g
Dan Shen *Radix Salviae Miltiorrhizae* 10 g
Hong Hua *Flos Carthami* 10 g
Bai Zhi *Radix Angelicae Dahuricae* 10 g
Xiang Fu *Rhizoma Cyperi* 10 g
Qing Pi *Pericarpium Citri Reticulatae Viride* 5 g
Zhi Qiao *Fructus Aurantii* 10 g

Explanations

- Chuan Xiong, Chi Shao, Dan Shen and Hong Hua all eliminate Blood stasis and promote its circulation. Also, Chuan Xiong is very good for inducing the other herbs to reach the head.
- Dang Gui promotes the circulation of Blood and harmonises it so as not to harm the Blood circulation.
- Since the circulation of Qi promotes the circulation of Blood, some herbs to promote the circulation of Qi are prescribed here as well, such as Qing Pi, Zhi Qiao and Xiang Fu.
- Bai Zhi goes to the face and sedates the facial pain.

Modifications

1. If there is severe facial pain or aggravation of pain at night due to stagnation of Blood, add Pu Huang *Pollen Typhae* 10 g and San Leng *Rhizoma Sparganii* 10 g to promote the Blood circulation strongly and overcome the Blood stasis.
2. If there is a swollen face with purplish colour on the face due to stagnation of Blood, add Wu Ling Zhi *Faeces Trogopterorum* 10 g and Mo Yao *Resina Myrrhae* 5 g to promote Blood circulation and reduce the swelling.
3. If there is numbness on the face, add Di Long *Lumbricus* 10 g to smooth the collateral and relieve numbness.

Patent remedies

Chuan Xiong Cha Tiao Pian *Ligusticum–Green Tea Regulating Tablet*
Xiao Huo Luo Dan *Minor Invigorate the Collaterals Special Pill*

ACUPUNCTURE TREATMENT

LI-4 Hegu, LR-3 Taichong, SP-6 Sanyinjiao, ST-3 Juliao, ST-6 Jiache, ST-7 Xiaguan, ST-40 Fenglong and SI-18 Quanliao. Reducing method is used on these points.

Explanations

- This type of facial pain is often due to incomplete elimination of external factors, inappropriate facial surgery, severe emotional disturbance, trauma, as well as prolonged persistence of above types of facial pain, thus the collaterals on the face are blocked leading to stagnation of Blood. The points selected can promote the circulation of Qi and Blood and eliminate the Blood stasis to sedate the pain.
- Qi is the guide for Blood; LI-4 and LR-3 regulate the circulation of Qi so as to lead the circulation of Blood.
- SP-6 promotes the circulation of Blood and relieves the pain.
- ST-3, ST-6 and ST-7 are applied here to harmonise the collateral of the Stomach on the face to sedate the pain in the local region. These three points are especially used when there is pain around the cheek or mandibular region related to the Stomach channel.
- SI-18, the meeting point of the hand Lesser Yang channel and hand Taiyang channel, is used to treat facial pain occurring around the mandibular region.
- ST-40, the Connecting point of the Stomach channel, harmonises the collateral and relieves the pain.

Modifications

1. If there is pain around the mouth due to stagnation of Blood in the Stomach channel, add ST-4 and ST-42 to promote the Blood circulation in the Stomach channel and relieve the pain around the mouth.

2. If there is aggravation of pain at night due to severe stagnation of Blood, add BL-17 to regulate Blood circulation and eliminate the Blood stasis.

3. If there is pain around the ear due to stagnation of Blood in the Lesser Yang channel, add GB-2 and TE-21 to activate the Qi and Blood circulation in the Lesser Yang channel and arrest the pain.

Eye pain 12

眼
睛
疼
痛

Eye pain includes pain at the eyelid, orbit, canthus, eyeball, and over the whole eye. It may occur in one or in both eyes. The types of eye pain include distending pain, sour pain, stabbing pain, severe pain, slight pain, constant pain and intermittent pain.

According to TCM, the following pathogenic factors may cause eye pain: invasion of External pathogenic factors, stagnation of Qi or Blood, Flaring up of Liver-Fire, hyperactivity of Liver-Yang, deficiency of Qi, deficiency of Blood in the Liver and deficiency of Yin of the Liver and Kidney.

Eye pain may be attributed to any of the following diseases in Western medicine: haematopsia, xerophthalmia, posterior staphyloma, blepharospasm, ophthalmospasm, orbital neuralgia, endophthalmitis, herpes zoster on the eyelid, dacryocystitis, conjunctivitis, scleritis, keratitis, iritis, trachoma and glaucoma.

Aetiology and pathology

Invasion of External pathogenic factors

Overexposure to strong Wind, Cold, Heat or Dryness may cause an invasion of pathogenic factors to the eyes, leading to stagnation of Qi and Blood in the eye, and causing eye pain as a consequence.

Furthermore, working for too long in bright sunlight, studying for too long in artificial light that is too strong, or not strong enough, staring for too long at a TV or VDU screen, or working or walking in fog, may weaken the eyes and bring about the slowing of Qi and Blood circulation. This leaves the eyes vulnerable to the invasion of External pathogenic factors, causing eye pain.

Emotional disturbance

The eye is related with the interior Zang-Fu organs. If there is persistent emotional disturbance this leads to stagnation of Qi and Blood, causing a slowing down of the circulation of Qi and Blood in the eye, and so eye pain follows. For instance, excessive anger, stress and frustration will cause the Qi of the Liver to stagnate, inhibiting the Liver's function in opening the orifice. So stagnation of Qi in the eye develops and eye pain follows. Also, where there is excessive grief with a lot of crying, the Lung-Qi stagnates, leading to a stagnation of Qi in the eyes because the Lung fails to disperse Qi to the eyes, causing eye pain.

Moreover, when Qi stagnation persists in the body for a long time, excessive Fire is generated, causing Fire to flare up the eyes, which causes eye pain—for example, Liver-Qi stagnation may generate Liver-Fire, which could flare up to disturb the eye and eye pain follows. Long-lasting stagnation of Liver-Qi and flaring up of Liver-Fire can also cause a failure to comfort the Liver-

Yang, leading to eye pain due to hyperactivity of Liver-Yang.

Unhealthy diets

The eye needs to be nourished by Qi and Blood. The Spleen and Stomach are the centres for production of Qi and Blood. Overconsumption of fatty, sweet and pungent food, or of alcohol, causes injury to the Spleen and Stomach, which causes food to accumulate in the body, generating Damp-Heat and forming Damp-Phlegm. In contrast, overconsumption of raw and cold food causes Cold-Damp to form in the Spleen and Stomach so that, instead of sending Qi and Blood to the eye, the Spleen sends Damp-Phlegm, Damp-Heat, or Cold-Damp up to the eye. This causes blockage in the eye and eye pain will be the result. Moreover, disturbance of the Spleen and Stomach may cause a poor production of Qi and Blood, leading to malnourishment of the eye, and eye pain follows.

Overstrain or prolonged sickness

The eye is connected with the five interior Zang organs. If there is dysfunction of the interior Zang-Fu organs, the eye is not sufficiently nourished by the Qi and Blood, and eye pain of the deficient type follows. Too much physical work, too much study and mental work, or too much sex may cause consumption of the Qi and Blood, leading to deficiency of Kidney-Essence.

Also, prolonged sickness or congenital weakness may cause an insufficiency of Qi, Blood and Essence in the eye, and eye pain follows. Finally, if there is deficiency of Kidney-Yin then the Liver is not properly nourished, which leads to hyperactivity of Liver-Fire, and again eye pain follows.

Treatment based on differentiation

Differentiation

Differentiation of External or Internal origin

— Acute onset of eye pain, mild in intensity, accompanied by External symptoms, such as an aversion to cold, fever, muscle pain, runny nose, cough, or superficial pulse, is usually caused by invasion of External factors.
— A chronic history of eye pain, mild or severe in intensity, and association of the pain with diet,

emotion and other physical conditions, is usually caused by disorders of the Internal Zang-Fu organs.

Differentiation of character of the pain

— Acute sharp eye pain, together with External symptoms, such as an aversion to cold, slight fever, muscle pain or absence of thirst, is usually caused by invasion of Wind-Cold.
— Acute sharp eye pain with a burning sensation, a thin and yellow tongue coating, together with some external symptoms, is usually caused by invasion of Wind-Heat.
— Chronic sharp eye pain, which is related to the emotional state, is usually caused by stagnation of Qi.
— Stabbing eye pain, which worsens at night, with a purplish colour of the tongue, is usually caused by stagnation of Blood.
— Slight eye pain, which is intermittent, or aggravated by exertion and during the day, with poor vision, tiredness, an aversion to cold, cold hands and feet, a pale tongue with a thin, white and slight greasy coating, and a thready and weak pulse, is usually caused by deficiency of Qi.
— Chronic eye pain with a burning sensation, restlessness, nervousness, irritability, a bitter taste in the mouth, thirst, constipation, a red tongue with a yellow and dry coating, and a wiry, forceful and rapid pulse, is usually caused by hyperactivity of Liver-Fire.
— Chronic eye pain with slight burning and a sensation of dryness, thirst, night sweating, dry mouth and throat, a red tongue with a thin coating, and a deep, thready, rapid and weak pulse, is usually caused by deficiency of the Yin of Liver and Kidney.
— Eye pain with poor vision, dryness of the eyes, a pale complexion, dry hair, loss of hair and skin, tiredness, dry stools, a pale tongue with a thin coating and a thready and weak pulse, is usually caused by deficiency of Blood in the Liver.

Treatment

EYE PAIN CAUSED BY EXTERNAL FACTORS

INVASION OF WIND-COLD

Symptoms and signs

Acute onset of eye pain, aggravation of eye pain with exposure to wind and cold, no redness or swelling of the eyelids, a slight fever, an aversion to wind and cold, headache with a contracting sensation that is referred to the neck and the back of the body, an absence of thirst, accompanied by stuffiness of the nose with a nasal discharge, a thin and white tongue coating and a superficial and tense pulse.

Principle of treatment

Dispel Wind and eliminate Cold.

HERBAL TREATMENT

Prescription

CHUAN XIONG CHA TIAO SAN
Ligusticum–Green Tea Regulating Powder
Chuan Xiong *Rhizoma Ligustici Chuanxiong* 6 g
Jing Jie *Herba Schizonepeta* 6 g
Fang Feng *Radix Ledebouriellae* 6 g
Bai Zhi *Radix Angelicae Dahuricae* 6 g
Xi Xin *Herba Asari* 3 g
Gan Cao *Radix Glycyrrhizae* 5 g
Qiang Huo *Rhizoma seu Radix Notopterygii* 6 g
Cha Ye *Folium Camelliae Sinensis* 3 g

Explanations

- Chuan Xiong and Qiang Huo dispel Wind, relieve the eye pain and sedate the headache.
- Bai Zhi and Xi Xin work as assistants to relieve the eye pain and headache.
- Jing Jie and Fang Feng dispel Wind and release the External symptoms.
- Cha Ye dispels Wind, calms the Mind and benefits the eye.
- Gan Cao is used to harmonise the actions of the other herbs.

Modifications

1. If there is fever caused by Wind-Cold invasion, add Chai Hu *Radix Bupleuri* 5 g and Gui Zhi *Ramulus Cinnamomi* 10 g to eliminate Wind-Cold and reduce the fever.
2. If there is a stiff neck due to stagnation of Qi in the Bladder channels, add Ge Gen *Radix Puerariae* 10 g to regulate Qi circulation and relieve the stiff neck.
3. If there is a blocked nose, add Cang Er Zi *Fructus Xanthii* 10 g and Xin Yi *Flos Magnoliae* 10 g to dispel Wind and clear the nose.
4. If there is a headache, add Wu Zhu Yu *Fructus Evodiae* 5 g to warm channel, dispel Wind-Cold and relieve the headache.

Patent remedy

Chuan Xiong Cha Tiao Wan *Ligusticum–Green Tea Regulating Pill*

ACUPUNCTURE TREATMENT

BL-2 Zanzhu, ST-2 Sibai, ST-3 Juliao, LI-4 Hegu, TE-5 Waiguan, GB-20 Fengchi and LU-7 Lieque. Reducing method is used on these points. When puncturing at GB-20, the tip of the needle should point to the opposite eye.

Explanations

- BL-2, ST-2 and ST-3 the local points, dispel Wind-Cold, promote circulation in the collateral of the eye and relieve the eye pain.
- LI-4, the Source point, and LU-7, the Connecting point, are indicated in complaints of the face and eyes. They can open the skin pores and promote sweating so that Wind-Cold is expelled. LI-4 also regulates the Qi and Blood circulation in the eye, enhancing the effect of reducing the eye pain.
- TE-5, the Connecting point, dispels Wind-Cold and harmonises the Lesser Yang channel and the collateral of the Triple Burner. Besides this it connects with the Yang Linking Vessel, which dominates the superficial parts of the body. When TE-5 is punctured with a reducing method, the Yang Linking Vessel is stimulated, which diminishes the External symptoms due to invasion of Wind-Cold.
- GB-20 dispels Wind-Cold out of the head. Since the tip of the needle points towards the opposite eye, this strongly enhances the effect of dispelling Wind-Cold.

Modifications

1. If there is pain at the eye orbit, add Extra Yuyao and GB-14 to harmonise the collateral and sedate eye pain.
2. If there is pain at the external eye corner, add Extra Taiyang and TE-23 to dispel Wind-Cold and relieve the pain.
3. If there is eye pain at the inner eye corner, add BL-1 and Extra Yintang to relieve Wind-Cold in the collateral and stop the pain.
4. If there is headache due to an invasion of Wind-Cold, add GB-8 and GV-23 to harmonise the collateral and relieve the headache.
5. If there is an aversion to cold and general body pain, add BL-58 and BL-63 to dispel Wind-Cold, harmonise the collateral and relieve the pain.

6. If there is a runny nose, cough and expectoration of white phlegm, add LU-5, the Sea point and BL-13, the Back Transporting point of the Lung, to dispel Wind-Cold and relieve the cough.
7. If there is a fever, add GV-14 to dispel Wind and reduce the fever.
8. If there is a blocked nose, add LI-20 to dispel Wind-Cold and clear the blockage in the nose.

INVASION OF WIND-HEAT

Symptoms and signs

Acute occurrence of eye pain, redness and swelling of the eye with a burning sensation, aggravation of pain on exposure to wind and heat, formation of pus in the eye, fever, an aversion to cold, thirst, a distending headache, constipation, a red tip to the tongue, a yellow tongue coating and a superficial and rapid pulse.

Principle of treatment

Dispel Wind and clear Heat.

HERBAL TREATMENT

Prescription

XIE PI CHU RE YIN
Reduce the Spleen and Clear Heat Decoction
Chong Wei Zi *Fructus Leonuri* 10 g
Fang Feng *Radix Ledebouriellae* 6 g
Huang Qin *Radix Scutellariae* 10 g
Xuan Shen *Radix Scrophulariae* 10 g
Zhi Zi *Fructus Gardeniae* 10 g
Shi Gao *Gypsum Fibrosum* 18 g
Da Huang *Radix et Rhizoma Rhei* 6 g
Zhi Mu *Rhizoma Anemarrhenae* 6 g
Huang Bai *Cortex Phellodendri* 6 g
Ju Hua *Flos Chrysanthemi* 6 g

Explanations

- Chong Wei Zi and Huang Qin clear Wind-Heat in the Liver channels to improve the eyesight and stop the eye pain.
- Fang Feng and Zhi Zi eliminate Wind-Heat and relieve pain and itching in the eyes.
- Shi Gao and Zhi Mu clear Heat in the Upper Burner.
- Xuan Shen nourishes the Liver-Yin and clears Heat.
- Huang Bai and Ju Hua clear Liver-Fire.
- Da Huang eliminates Internal Heat by promoting defecation.

Modifications

1. If there is pus in the eye, add Pu Gong Ying *Herba Taraxaci* 10 g and Ye Ju Hua *Flos Chrysanthemi Indici* 10 g to clear Heat and eliminate the Toxin.
2. If there is a headache caused by Wind-Heat, add Chuan Xiong *Rhizoma Ligustici Chuanxiong* 10 g and Bo He *Herba Menthae* 5 g to clear Wind-Heat and relieve the headache.
3. If there is fever, add Chai Hu *Radix Bupleuri* 5 g and Ban Lan Gen *Radix Isatidis* 10 g to clear Heat and lower the fever.
4. If there is constipation, add Lu Hui *Pasta Aloes* and Mang Xiao *Natrii Sulfas* to clear the Heat and promote defecation.

Patent remedies

Yin Qiao Jie Du Pian *Honeysuckle and Forsythia Tablet to Overcome Toxins*
Yin Qiao Pian *Honeysuckle and Forsythia Tablet*

ACUPUNCTURE TREATMENT

BL-2 Zanzhu, ST-2 Sibai, Extra Taiyang, LI-2 Erjian, LI-4 Hegu, LU-7 Lieque, TE-2 Yemen, LI-5 Yangxi and GB-20 Fengchi. A reducing method is used on these points. The bleeding method is used on LI-2 and TE-2. When needling GB-20, the tip of the needle should point towards to the opposite eye.

Explanations

- BL-2, ST-2 and Extra Taiyang, the local points, dispel Wind, clear Heat, promote the circulation of the collateral in the eye and relieve the pain.
- LI-2 and TE-2, the Spring points, clear Heat, relieve redness, reduce swelling and stop the pain.
- LI-4, the Source point, and LU-7, the Connecting point, promote sweating and dispel Wind-Heat in the face and eye.
- TE-5, the Connecting point, dispels Wind-Heat and harmonises the Lesser Yang channel and the collateral of the Triple Burner, and relieves External symptoms.
- GB-20 dispels Wind-Heat out of the head and sedates the eye pain.

Modifications

1. If there is pain at the eye orbit, add Extra Yuyao and GB-14 to harmonise the collateral and sedate the pain.

2. If there is pain at the external eye corner, add Extra Taiyang and TE-23 to dispel Wind-Heat and relieve the pain.
3. If there is eye pain at the inner eye corner, add BL-1 and Extra Yintang to relieve Wind-Cold in the collateral and stop the pain.
4. If there is a headache due to the invasion of Wind-Heat, add GB-8 and GV-23 to harmonise the collateral and relieve the headache.
5. If there is a high fever, add GV-14 and LI-11 to clear Heat and reduce the fever.
6. If there is a runny nose, cough and expectoration of yellow phlegm, add LU-5, the Sea point, and LU-10, the Spring point, to dispel Wind-Heat and relieve the cough.
7. If there is a blocked nose, add LI-20 to dispel Wind-Heat and clear the blockage in the nose.

EYE PAIN CAUSED BY INTERNAL DISORDERS

EYE PAIN CAUSED BY STAGNATION OF QI

Symptoms and signs

Eye pain with a sensation of pressure and tension, which starts or gets worse under stress or emotional disturbance, with depression, distension and pain in the hypochondriac region, dizziness, irregular menstruation, a poor appetite or overeating, a thin and white tongue coating and a wiry pulse.

Principle of treatment

Smooth the Liver, promote Liver-Qi circulation and relieve the headache.

HERBAL TREATMENT

Prescription

XIAO YAO SAN
Free and Relaxed Powder
Chai Hu *Radix Bupleuri* 10 g
Dang Gui *Radix Angelicae Sinensis* 10 g
Bai Shao *Radix Paeoniae Alba* 20 g
Bai Zhu *Rhizoma Atractylodis Macrocephalae* 10 g
Fu Ling *Poria* 15 g
Gan Cao *Radix Glycyrrhizae* 5 g
Bo He *Herba Menthae* 3 g
Chuan Xiong *Rhizoma Ligustici Chuanxiong* 10 g
Huang Qin *Radix Scutellariae* 10 g

Explanations

- Chai Hu and Bo He regulate and promote the Liver-Qi circulation so as to remove Qi stagnation in the Liver.
- Bai Shao and Dang Gui nourish the Blood in the Liver, harmonise the Liver and relieve the hypochondriac pain.
- Chuan Xiong regulates Liver-Qi and relieves the headache.
- Bai Zhu and Fu Ling strengthen the Spleen and Stomach.
- Huang Qin clears internal Heat resulting from stagnation of Liver-Qi.
- Gan Cao harmonises the actions of the other herbs.

Modifications

1. If there is severe eye pain and headache, add Yan Hu Suo *Rhizoma Corydalis* 10 g and Bai Zhi *Radix Angelicae Dahuricae* 10 g to promote the circulation of Qi in the head and relieve the eye pain and headache.
2. If there is hypochondriac pain, add Yu Jin *Radix Curcumae* 10 g and Ju He *Semen Citri Reticulate* 10 g to regulate the circulation of Qi and relieve the pain.
3. If there is irregular menstruation or dysmenorrhoea, add Huai Niu Xi *Radix Achyranthis Bidentatae* 10 g and Yi Mu Cao *Herba Leonuri* 10 g to regulate the menstruation.
4. If there is a poor mood, add Xiang Fu *Rhizoma Cyperi* 10 g and Gou Teng *Ramulus Uncariae cum Uncis* 10 g to regulate the Liver-Qi and improve the mood.
5. If there is insomnia, add Long Gu *Os Draconis* 15 g to calm the Heart and tranquillise the Mind.
6. If there is a poor appetite, add Mai Ya *Fructus Hordei Germinatus* 15 g and Yu Jin *Radix Curcumae* 10 g to remove Qi stagnation and improve the appetite.

Patent remedies

Xiao Yao Wan *Free and Relaxed Pill*
Shu Gan Wan *Soothe Liver Pill*

ACUPUNCTURE TREATMENT

ST-1 Chengqi, ST-2 Sibai, BL-2 Zanzhu, LR-3 Taichong, PC-6 Neiguan, LI-4 Hegu and SP-6 Sanyinjiao. Even method is used on ST-1, ST-2 and BL-2. Reducing method is used on the rest of the points.

Explanations

- LR-3, the Stream and Source point of the Liver channel, regulates the Liver-Qi and removes Qi stagnation.
- PC-6, the Connecting point of the Pericardium channel, regulates the circulation of Qi and calms the Mind.
- LI-4, the Source point of the Large Intestine channel, regulates the circulation of Qi and relieves the eye pain and headache.
- SP-6, the crossing point of the three Yin channels of the foot, regulates the Liver-Qi circulation and removes Qi stagnation.
- ST-1, ST-2 and BL-2 harmonise the collateral and improve the circulation of Qi and Blood and so stop the eye pain.

Modifications

1. If there is dizziness, add GB-8 to relieve dizziness.
2. If there is depression, add HT-3 and BL-18 to regulate the circulation of Qi, calm the Mind and improve the emotional state.
3. If there is insomnia, add HT-3 and HT-7 to calm the Mind and improve the sleep.
4. If there is hypochondriac pain, add LR-5, the Connecting point, and LR-1, the Front Collecting point, to promote Liver-Qi circulation, harmonise the collateral and relieve the pain.
5. If there is a poor appetite or overeating, add CV-12 to harmonise the Stomach-Qi and improve the appetite.
6. If there are loose stools when nervous, and abdominal pain and cramp due to invasion of the Spleen by the Liver, add LR-13 and SP-3 to promote the circulation of Liver-Qi and strengthen the Spleen.
7. If there is irregular menstruation or dysmenorrhoea, add ST-28 and KI-10 to promote the circulation of Qi and Blood and regulate the menstruation.

EYE PAIN CAUSED BY STAGNATION OF BLOOD

Symptoms and signs

Prolonged persistence of stabbing eye pain, or eye pain with fixed location, which is aggravated at night, before or during menstruation, accompanied by dark and purplish menstruation with clots, a history of physical trauma or operation, insomnia, a purplish tongue or purplish spots on the tongue and a thready or choppy pulse.

Principle of treatment

Promote circulation of Blood, eliminate Blood stasis and relieve the headache.

HERBAL TREATMENT

Prescription

TONG QIAO HUO XUE TANG
Unblock the Orifices and Invigorate the Blood Decoction
Chuan Xiong *Rhizoma Ligustici Chuanxiong* 10 g
Chi Shao *Radix Paeoniae Rubra* 10 g
Dang Gui *Radix Angelicae Sinensis* 10 g
Dan Shen *Radix Salviae Miltiorrhizae* 10 g
Hong Hua *Flos Carthami* 10 g
Bai Zhi *Radix Angelicae Dahuricae* 10 g
Xiang Fu *Rhizoma Cyperi* 10 g
Qing Pi *Pericarpium Citri Reticulatae Viride* 5 g
Zhi Qiao *Fructus Aurantii* 10 g

Explanations

- Chuan Xiong, Chi Shao, Dan Shen and Hong Hua all promote the circulation of Blood and eliminate Blood stasis. Also, Chuan Xiong is a very good herb for inducing the other herbs to reach the head to treat the eye pain.
- Dang Gui promotes the circulation of Blood and harmonises the Blood to ensure the Blood-circulating herbs do not harm the Blood.
- Since the circulation of Qi promotes the circulation of Blood, some herbs to promote the circulation of Qi are also prescribed here, such as Qing Pi, Zhi Qiao and Xiang Fu.
- Bai Zhi together with Chuan Xiong and Dang Gui relieve the eye pain.

Modifications

1. If there is severe eye pain or aggravation of the eye pain at night or related to the menstruation, add Pu Huang *Pollen Typhae* 10 g and San Leng *Rhizoma Sparganii* 10 g to promote the circulation of Blood strongly and remove the Blood stasis.
2. If there are swollen eyes, add Wu Ling Zhi *Faeces Trogopterorum* 10 g and Mo Yao *Resina Myrrhae* 5 g to promote the circulation of Blood, reduce swelling and relieve the eye pain.
3. If there is dizziness, add Di Long *Lumbricus* 10 g and Tian Ma *Rhizoma Gastrodiae* 10 g to relieve this.

4. If there is dysmenorrhoea, add Yan Hu Suo *Rhizoma Corydalis* 10 g to promote the circulation of Blood and relieve the dysmenorrhoea.

5. If there is insomnia, add Suan Zao Ren *Semen Ziziphi Spinosae* 10 g and Bai Zi Ren *Semen Biotae* 10 g to calm the Mind and improve the sleep.

6. If there is a poor memory, add Shi Chang Pu *Rhizoma Acori Graminei* 10 g to improve the memory.

Patent remedy

Yan Hu Suo Zhi Tong Pian *Corydalis Stop Pain Tablet*

ACUPUNCTURE TREATMENT

ST-1 Chengqi, ST-2 Sibai, BL-2 Zanzhu, GB-20 Fengchi, LI-4 Hegu, BL-17 Geshu, SP-6 Sanyinjiao, LR-3 Taichong and Ah Shi points. Reducing method is used on these points.

Explanations

- Qi is the guide for Blood. LI-4 and LR-3 regulate the circulation of Qi so as to lead the circulation of Blood.
- SP-6, the crossing point of three Yin channels of the foot, and BL-17, the Gathering point for the Blood, promote the circulation of Blood and relieve pain.
- GB-20, the crossing point of the foot Lesser Yang channel and the Yang Linking Vessel, promotes the circulation of Qi and Blood in the head and relieves the eye pain.
- ST-1, ST-2 and BL-2 harmonise the collateral and improve the circulation of Qi and Blood so as to stop the eye pain.
- The Ah Shi points promote the circulation of Qi and Blood in the head to relieve the headache.

Modifications

1. If there is severe eye pain at night, add SI-3 to promote the circulation of Qi and Blood and relieve the headache.

2. If there is headache, add the Ah Shi points in the painful area to promote the circulation of Qi and Blood and eliminate Blood stasis.

3. If there is dysmenorrhoea with clots, add ST-28 and SP-8 to promote the circulation of Blood and relieve the dysmenorrhoea.

4. If there is insomnia, add HT-3 to regulate the circulation of Qi and Blood and calm the Mind.

5. If there is neck pain, add BL-10 to promote the circulation of Blood and relieve the neck pain.

6. If there is a poor memory, add GV-20 and Extra Sishencong to promote the circulation of Qi and Blood.

EYE PAIN CAUSED BY FLARING-UP OF LIVER-FIRE

Symptoms and signs

Sharp or distending eye pain, with redness of the eyes, irritability, a bitter taste in the mouth, restlessness, insomnia, irregular menstruation, a poor appetite, deep yellow urine, constipation, a red tongue and a rapid and wiry pulse.

Principle of treatment

Reduce Liver-Fire, calm the Mind and relieve the pain.

HERBAL TREATMENT

Prescription

LONG DAN XIE GAN TANG
Gentiana Draining the Liver Decoction
Long Dan Cao *Radix Gentianae* 10 g
Huang Qin *Radix Scutellariae* 10 g
Zhi Zi *Fructus Gardeniae* 10 g
Ze Xie *Rhizoma Alismatis* 12 g
Chuan Xiong *Rhizoma Ligustici Chuanxiong* 10 g
Xia Ku Cao *Spica Prunellae* 10 g
Che Qiang Zi *Semen Plantaginis* 10 g
Dang Gui *Radix Angelicae Sinensis* 10 g
Sheng Di Huang *Radix Rehmanniae Recens* 12 g
Chai Hu *Radix Bupleuri* 10 g
Gan Cao *Radix Glycyrrhizae* 6 g

Explanations

- Long Dan Cao, Huang Qin, Xia Ku Cao and Zhi Zi reduce Liver-Fire.
- Ze Xie and Che Qian Zi promote urination and induce Fire out of the body through urination.
- Dang Gui, Chuan Xiong and Chai Hu promote the Liver-Qi circulation and relieve the headache.
- Sheng Di Huang clears Heat and nourishes the Yin of Liver and Kidney.
- Gan Cao harmonises the actions of the other herbs in the formula.

Modifications

1. If the eyes are red, add Cao Jue Ming *Semen Cassiae* 12 g to clear Liver-Fire and relieve the redness.

2. If there is irritability, add Zhi Mu *Rhizoma Anemarrhenae* 10 g to regulate the Liver-Qi and clear Liver-Fire.
3. If there is insomnia and restlessness, add Suan Zao Ren *Semen Ziziphi Spinosae* 15 g and Zhen Zhu Mu *Concha Margaritifera Usta* 20 g to calm the Mind and improve sleep.
4. If there is hypochondriac pain, add Yu Jin *Radix Curcumae* 10 g to promote the circulation of Liver-Qi and relieve the pain.
5. If there is painful urination, add Ku Shen *Radix Sophorae Flavescentis* 10 g and Che Qian Zi *Semen Plantaginis* 10 g to clear Liver-Fire and promote urination.
6. If there is irregular menstruation or dysmenorrhoea, add Chi Shao *Radix Paeoniae Rubra* 10 g to regulate the circulation of Blood and harmonise the menstruation.
7. If there is night sweating, add Huang Bai *Cortex Phellodendri* 10 g to clear Deficient-Heat and stop the sweating.
8. If there is constipation, add Da Huang *Radix et Rhizoma Rhei* 6 g and Mang Xiao *Natrii Sulfas* 12 g to clear Liver-Fire and promote defecation.

Patent remedy

Long Dan Xie Gan Wan *Gentiana Draining the Liver Pill*

ACUPUNCTURE TREATMENT

ST-1 Chengqi, ST-2 Sibai, BL-2 Zanzhu, Extra Taiyang, GV-20 Baihui, TE-6 Zhigou, SP-6 Sanyinjiao, LR-2 Xingjian and GB-43 Xiaxi. All the points are needled with reducing method.

Explanations

- Extra Taiyang and GV-20 tranquillise the Mind and calm Liver-Fire.
- LR-2, the Spring point of the Liver channel, clears Liver-Fire and relieves the eye pain.
- GB-43, the Spring point of the Gall Bladder channel, clears Heat, regulates the circulation of Qi in the Gall Bladder channel and relieves eye pain.
- TE-6 promotes the function of the Triple Burner, regulates the circulation of Qi, clears Fire in the Triple Burner and reduces Liver-Fire.
- SP-6, the crossing point of the three Yin channels of the foot, clears Liver-Fire and regulates the circulation of Qi in the Liver.
- ST-1, ST-2 and BL-2 harmonise the collateral and improve the circulation of Qi and Blood and so stop the eye pain.

Modifications

1. If the eyes are red, add GB-1 to subdue Liver-Fire and reduce the redness.
2. If there is neck pain with stiffness, add GB-21 and TE-5 to harmonise the collateral and relieve the neck pain.
3. If there is irritability, add Extra Sishencong to calm the Mind and relieve the irritability.
4. If there is insomnia, add HT-8 to clear Heat in the Heart and improve the sleep.
5. If there is a poor appetite, add CV-12 to promote the Stomach-Qi and improve the appetite.
6. If there is a bitter taste in the mouth, add GB-40 to clear Heat in the Liver and Gall Bladder and remove the taste.
7. If there are loose stools when nervous, and abdominal pain and cramp owing to invasion of the Spleen by the Liver, add LR-13 and SP-3 to promote the Liver-Qi circulation and strengthen the Spleen.
8. If there is constipation, add ST-25 to promote defecation and relieve the constipation.
9. If there is irregular menstruation, add SP-10 and ST-28 to promote the circulation of Qi and Blood and regulate the menstruation.

EYE PAIN CAUSED BY HYPERACTIVITY OF LIVER-YANG

Symptoms and signs

Severe and frequent eye pain and headache with a distending sensation, with dizziness, restlessness, irritability, shaking of the head and hands, insomnia, hypochondriac pain and distension, red face and eyes, a red tongue with a thin and yellow coating and a wiry pulse.

Principle of treatment

Calm the Liver, subdue Liver-Yang and relieve the headache.

HERBAL TREATMENT

Prescription

TIAN MA GOU TENG YIN
Gastrodia and Uncaria Decoction
Tian Ma *Rhizoma Gastrodiae* 10 g
Gou Teng *Ramulus Uncariae cum Uncis* 10 g
Shi Jue Ming *Concha Haliotidis* 15 g
Huang Qin *Radix Scutellariae* 10 g
Chuan Niu Xi *Radix Cyathulae* 10 g

Sang Ji Sheng *Ramulus Loranthi* 10 g
Ye Jiao Teng *Caulis Polygoni Multiflori* 15 g
Chuan Xiong *Rhizoma Ligustici Chuanxiong* 10 g
Ju Hua *Flos Chrysanthemi* 10 g

Explanations

- Tian Ma and Gou Teng smooth the Liver and subdue the Liver-Yang so as to relieve eye pain and headache.
- Chuan Xiong and Ju Hua assist Tian Ma to regulate the Liver-Qi circulation and relieve eye pain.
- Shi Jue Ming and Chuan Niu Xi subdue the Liver-Yang and guide it downward.
- Huang Qin clears Heat in the Liver.
- Ye Jiao Teng calms the Mind and improves sleep.
- Sang Ji Sheng nourishes the Yin of Liver and Kidney and calms the Liver-Yang.

Modifications

1. If there is severe headache, add Quan Xie *Scorpio* 1.5 g and Bai Jiang Can *Bombyx Batryticatus* 10 g to subdue Liver-Wind and sedate the headache.
2. If there is irritability, add Huang Lian *Rhizoma Coptidis* 10 g to clear Liver-Fire and relieve the irritability.
3. If there is hypochondriac pain, add Qing Pi *Pericarpium Citri Reticulatae Viride* 10 g and Chuan Lian Zi *Fructus Meliae Toosendan* 10 g to regulate the circulation of Qi and stop the pain.
4. If there is insomnia, add Suan Zao Ren *Semen Ziziphi Spinosae* 10 g to calm the Mind and improve the sleep.
5. If there is a bitter taste in mouth, add Zhi Zi *Fructus Gardeniae* 10 g to clear Heat in the Liver and Gall Bladder.
6. If there is abdominal pain, add Yan Hu Suo *Rhizoma Corydalis* 10 g and Bai Shao *Radix Paeoniae Alba* 15 g to promote the circulation of Qi and Blood and stop the pain.
7. If there is a feeling of warmth in the head, add Mu Dan Pi *Cortex Moutan Radici* 10 g to clear Heat in the head.

Patent remedy

Jiang Ya Ping Pian *Subdue Internal Wind Tablet*

ACUPUNCTURE TREATMENT

ST-1 Chengqi, ST-2 Sibai, BL-2 Zanzhu, GB-20 Fengchi, GB-43 Xiaxi, Extra Taiyang, GV-20 Baihui, LI-4 Hegu, SP-6 Sanyinjiao, KI-2 Rangu, LR-2 Xingjian and LR-8 Ququan.

Explanations

- GB-20, the crossing point of the foot Lesser Yang channel and the Yang Linking Vessel, and GV-20 clear Heat in the head, subdue the Liver-Yang and relieve the eye pain and headache.
- Extra Taiyang clears Heat and relieves the eye pain.
- SP-6, the crossing point of the three Yin channels of the foot, regulates the Liver and clears Heat in the Liver.
- LI-4, the Source point of the Large Intestine channel, promotes the circulation of Qi, clears Heat in the head and relieves the headache.
- GB-43, KI-2 and LR-2, all Spring points, clear Heat and subdue Liver-Yang.
- LR-8, the Water point, clears Heat in the Liver and subdues Liver-Yang.
- ST-1, ST-2 and BL-2 harmonise the collateral and improve the circulation of Qi and Blood so as to stop the eye pain.

Modifications

1. If the face and eyes are red, add ST-44 and GB-1 to clear Heat and relieve the redness.
2. If there is irritability, add HT-3 and PC-6 to calm the Mind and relieve the irritability.
3. If there is a bitter taste in the mouth, add GB-40 to clear Heat in the Gall Bladder.
4. If there is hypochondriac pain, add LR-14 to promote the circulation of Qi and relieve the pain.
5. If there is insomnia, add HT-8 to clear Heat in the Heart, calm the Mind and relieve the insomnia.

EYE PAIN CAUSED BY QI DEFICIENCY

Symptoms and signs

Slight eye pain, intermittent aggravation of eye pain, or aggravation of eye pain by exertion or during the day, poor vision, tiredness, an aversion to cold, cold hands and feet, shortness of breath, a pale complexion, spontaneous sweating, a low voice, weakness of the limbs, a poor appetite, loose stools, a pale tongue with a thin, white and slight greasy coating, and a thready and weak pulse.

Principle of treatment

Tonify Qi, activate the Spleen and Stomach and benefit the eyes.

HERBAL TREATMENT

Prescription

BU ZHONG YI QI TANG
Tonifying the Middle and Benefiting Qi Decoction
Huang Qi *Radix Astragali seu Hedysari* 20 g
Gan Cao *Radix Glycyrrhizae* 5 g
Ren Shen *Radix Ginseng* 10 g
Dang Gui *Radix Angelicae Sinensis* 10 g
Ju Pi *Pericarpium Citri Reticulatae* 6 g
Sheng Ma *Rhizoma Cimicifugae* 3 g
Chai Hu *Radix Bupleuri* 3 g
Bai Zhu *Rhizoma Atractylodis Macrocephalae* 10 g
Tian Ma *Rhizoma Gastrodiae* 10 g

Explanations

- Ren Shen, Huang Qi, Bai Zhu and Gan Cao strengthen the Spleen and tonify the Qi of the Spleen and Stomach.
- Sheng Ma and Chai Hu lift the Yang-Qi.
- Dang Gui aids Chai Hu to regulate the Liver-Qi and tonify the Blood.
- Tian Ma coordinates the circulation of Qi and improves the eyesight.
- Ju Pi promotes the circulation of Qi and strengthens the Spleen and Stomach.

Modifications

1. If there are cold limbs, add Gui Zhi *Ramulus Cinnamomi* 10 g and Gan Jiang *Rhizoma Zingiberis* 5 g to warm the Middle Burner.
2. If there is a pale complex, add Sang Shen Zi *Fructus Mori* 10 g and Huang Jing *Rhizoma Polygonati* 10 g to tonify the Qi and Blood.
3. If there is poor vision, add He Shou Wu *Radix Polygoni Multiflori* 10 g and Ju Hua *Flos Chrysanthemi* 10 g to tonify the Blood and nourish the eyes.
4. If there is a poor appetite, add Sha Ren *Fructus Amomi* 5 g and Mu Xiang *Radix Aucklandiae* 10 g to activate the Spleen and improve the appetite.

Patent remedy

Bu Zhong Yi Qi Wan *Tonifying the Middle and Benefiting Qi Pill.*

ACUPUNCTURE TREATMENT

ST-2 Sibai, BL-2 Zanzhu, GB-1 Tongziliao, GV-20 Baihui, LR-3 Taichong, ST-36 Zusanli and SP-6 Sanyinjiao. Even method is used on ST-2, BL-2 and GB-1; a reinforcing method is used on the rest of the points.

Explanations

- ST-2, BL-2 and GB-1 harmonise the collateral in the local areas and relieve the eye pain.
- ST-36 and SP-6 activate the Spleen and Stomach and promote the production of Qi.
- LR-3 tonifies the Liver and benefits the eyes.
- GV-20 lifts up Qi to the head and benefits the eyes.

Modifications

1. If there is pain at the eye orbit, add Extra Yuyao and GB-14 to harmonise the collateral and sedate the pain.
2. If there is pain at the external eye corner, add Extra Taiyang and TE-23 to dispel Wind-Heat and relieve the pain.
3. If there is pain at the inner eye corner, add BL-1 and Extra Yintang to relieve Wind-Cold in the collateral and stop the pain.
4. If there is headache, add GB-8 and GV-23 to harmonise the collateral and relieve the headache.
5. If there is general tiredness, aversion to cold, and dizziness due to deficiency of Qi, add CV-4 and CV-6 and use moxa to tonify the Qi and to warm the body and dispel the Cold.
6. If there is shortness of breath on exertion, a vulnerability to catching colds and a slight cough due to deficiency of Qi of the Lung and Kidney, add KI-3 and LU-9, two Source points, to tonify the Qi and aid respiration.
7. If there is a poor appetite, nausea and loose stools due to weakness of the Spleen and Stomach, add SP-3, the Source point, SP-4, the Confluence point of the Penetrating Vessel, and CV-12, the Front Collecting point of the Stomach, to harmonise the Stomach, activate the Spleen and resolve Damp in the body.

EYE PAIN CAUSED BY DEFICIENCY OF BLOOD IN THE LIVER

Symptoms and signs

Eye pain with dryness, tired eyes, blurred vision, black spots in front of the eyes, night blindness, aggravation of eye pain by reading and studying, a slight headache, dizziness, a pale complexion, a slight pain in the hypochondriac region, a pale tongue with a thin and white coating and a thready and weak pulse.

Principle of treatment

Reinforce Blood, nourish the eye and sedate the pain.

HERBAL TREATMENT

Prescription

QI JU DI HUANG WAN
Lycuim Fruit, Chrysanthemum and Rehmannia Pill
Gou Qi Zi *Fructus Lycii* 12 g
Ju Hua *Flos Chrysanthemi* 10 g
Shu Di Huang *Radix Rehmanniae Praeparata* 24 g
Shan Zhu Yu *Fructus Corni* 12 g
Shan Yao *Rhizoma Dioscoreae* 12 g
Fu Ling *Poria* 9 g
Mu Dan Pi *Cortex Moutan Radicis* 9 g
Ze Xie *Rhizoma Alismatis* 9 g
Nu Zhen Zi *Fructus Ligustri Lucidi* 10 g
Han Lian Cao *Herba Ecliptae* 10 g

Explanations

- Shu Di Huang, Shan Zhu Yu and Shan Yao tonify the Blood and the Essence of the Liver and the Kidney.
- Since the Blood belongs to the Yin, deficiency of Blood in the Liver may cause deficiency of Yin, leading to formation of Deficient-Heat. Ze Xie promotes urination and clears Heat in the Liver. Mu Dan Pi cools the Blood, clears Deficient-Heat and activates the circulation of Blood.
- Fu Ling strengthens the Spleen and drains Damp.
- Nu Zhen Zi, Han Lian Cao and Gou Qi Zi nourish the Blood in the Liver and improve the eyesight.
- Ju Hua clears internal Heat and relieves eye pain.

Modifications

1. If there is blurred vision, add He Shou Wu *Radix Polygoni Multiflori* 10 g and Wu Wei Zi *Fructus Schisandrae* 10 g to nourish the Blood and improve the eyesight.
2. If there is dizziness, add Dang Gui *Radix Angelicae Sinensis* 10 g and Tian Ma *Rhizoma Gastrodiae* 10 g to nourish the Yin and Blood, calm the Liver and relieve Liver-Wind.
3. If there is hypochondriac pain, add Bai Shao *Radix Paeoniae Alba* 10 g and Chuan Lian Zi *Fructus Meliae Toosendan* 10 g to promote Qi circulation in the Liver and relieve the pain.
4. If there is night blindness, add He Zi Ma *Semen Sesami* 10 g to improve the eyesight at night.
5. If there is constipation, add Xuan Shen *Radix Scrophulariae* 10 g and Da Huang *Radix et Rhizoma*

Rhei 10 g to nourish the Kidney-Yin and lubricate the Large Intestine in order to relieve the constipation.

Patent remedy

Qi Ju Di Huang Wan *Lycuim Fruit, Chrysanthemum and Rehmannia Pill*

ACUPUNCTURE TREATMENT

ST-1 Chengqi, ST-2 Sibai, BL-2 Zanzhu, BL-18 Ganshu, ST-36 Zusanli, SP-6 Sanyinjiao, LR-3 Taichong and LR-8 Ququan. Even method is used on ST-1, ST-2 and BL-2; reinforcing method is used on the rest of the points.

Explanations

- The Liver opens into the eyes. If there is Blood deficiency in the Liver, the eyes will not be properly nourished, leading to eye pain of the Deficient type.
- LR-3, the Source point, LR-8, the Sea point, and BL-18, the Back Transporting point of the Liver, all tonify the Liver and reinforce the Blood in the Liver so as to nourish the eyes. This is the basic treatment for this condition.
- ST-36, the Sea point, and SP-6, the crossing point of three Yin channels of the foot, activate the Spleen and Stomach and reinforce Qi and Blood production so as to tonify the Liver-Blood.
- ST-1, ST-2 and BL-2 harmonise the collateral and improve the Qi and Blood circulation and so stop the pain.

Modifications

1. If there is dizziness, an empty feeling in the head, blurred vision and black spots in front of the eyes resulting from Blood deficiency in the Liver, add GB-20 and GV-20 with reinforcing method to lift up the Blood to nourish the brain and relieve the emptiness in the head.
2. If there is general tiredness, scanty menstruation and a pale complexion due to Blood deficiency, add CV-4, CV-6 and KI-3 to tonify the Kidney-Essence, reinforce the Blood and regulate the menstruation.
3. If there is insomnia due to deficiency of Blood in the Heart, add HT-3 and HT-7 to tonify the Heart and tranquillise the Mind.
4. If there is hypochondriac pain due to weakness of the Liver with stagnation of Liver-Qi, add LR-14

and GB-24 to regulate the Liver and relieve the pain.

EYE PAIN CAUSED BY DEFICIENCY OF YIN OF THE LIVER AND KIDNEY

Symptoms and signs

Dull pain in the eyes with dryness, aggravation of the pain by studying and reading, blurred vision, a hollow sensation in the head, dizziness, listlessness, lumbago, weakness of the knees, tinnitus, night sweating, thirst, dry stools, insomnia, a red tongue with a thin and peeled coating and thready, weak and rapid pulse, specially at both Liver and Kidney positions.

Principle of treatment

Benefit the Kidney and reinforce Liver-Yin.

HERBAL TREATMENT

Prescription

MING MU DI HUANG WAN
Improve Vision Pill with Rehmannia
Sheng Di Huang *Radix Rehmanniae Recens* 15 g
Shu Di Huang *Radix Rehmanniae Praeparata* 15 g
Chuan Niu Xi *Radix Cyathulae* 10 g
Zhi Qiao *Fructus Aurantii* 10 g
Fang Feng *Radix Ledebouriellae* 6 g
Xin Ren *Semen Armeniacae* 6 g
Shi Hu *Herba Dendrobii* 10 g
Ju Hua *Flos Chrysanthemi* 10 g
Han Lian Cao *Herba Ecliptae* 10 g

Explanations

- Sheng Di Huang, Shi Hu and Shu Di Huang nourish the Yin of the Kidney and the Liver.
- Han Lian Cao and Ju Hua nourish the Liver-Yin and improve the eyesight.
- Fang Feng and Xin Ren clear the internal Heat caused by deficiency of Yin.
- Chuan Niu Xi conducts Heat downward and relieves pain.
- Zhi Qiao regulates the circulation of Qi and moderates the effects of the strong-smelling and greasy herbs.

Modifications

1. If there is dizziness, add Tian Ma *Rhizoma Gastrodiae* 10 g and Chuan Xiong *Rhizoma Ligustici Chuanxiong* 10 g to regulate the Liver-Qi and relieve the dizziness.
2. If there is blurred vision, add Shan Zhu Yu *Fructus Corni* 10 g and Qian Li Guang *Herba Senecionis Scandentis* 10 g to nourish the Liver-Yin and improve the eyesight.
3. If there is night sweating, add Wu Wei Zi *Fructus Schisandrae* 10 g and Mu Li *Concha Ostreae* 10 g to arrest the sweating at night.
4. If there is insomnia, add Suan Zao Ren *Semen Ziziphi Spinosae* 10 g and Bai Zi Ren *Semen Biotae* 10 g to nourish the Heart-Blood and calm the Mind.
5. If there are dry stools, add Xuan Shen *Radix Scrophulariae* 10 g and Lu Hui *Pasta Aloes* 5 g to nourish the Liver-Yin, clear the Liver-Fire and soften the stools in order to relieve the constipation.

Patent remedy

Ming Mu Di Huang Wan *Improve Vision Pill with Rehmannia*

ACUPUNCTURE TREATMENT

ST-2 Sibai, BL-1 Jingming, BL-18 Ganshu, SP-6 Sanyinjiao, LR-8 Ququan, KI-3 Taixi, KI-7 Fuliu and KI-10 Yingu. Even method is used on ST-2 and BL-1; reinforcing method is used on the rest of the points.

Explanations

- The Liver opens into the eyes and nourishes the eyes; the Liver stores Blood and the Kidney stores Essence. Liver-Blood and Kidney-Essence are mutually nourishing. Deficiency of one of them will cause weakness in the other.
- If there is Yin deficiency of the Liver and Kidney, the eyes will not be properly nourished, leading to eye pain of the Deficient type.
- LR-3, the Source point, LR-8, the Sea point, and BL-18, the Back Transporting point of the Liver, tonify the Liver and reinforce the Liver-Yin so that they will nourish the eyes.
- KI-3, the Source point, KI-7, the Metal point and KI-10, the Sea point, all tonify the Kidney and nourish the basic Yin of the body. When the Yin of the Liver and Kidney is reinforced, the eyes are nourished and eye pain will disappear spontaneously.
- SP-6, the crossing point of the three Yin channels of the foot, activates the Spleen and Stomach, and

reinforces Blood so that the Liver and Kidney are tonified.
- ST-2 and BL-1 harmonise the collateral and improve the Qi and Blood circulation to stop the pain.

Modifications

1. If there is pain at the eye orbit, add Extra Yuyao and GB-14 to harmonise the collateral and sedate the pain.
2. If there is pain at the external eye corner, add Extra Taiyang and TE-23 to dispel Wind-Heat and relieve the pain.
3. If there is pain at the inner eye corner, add Extra Yintang to relieve Wind-Cold in the collateral and stop the pain.
4. If there is a headache, add GB-8 and GV-23 to harmonise the collateral and relieve the headache.
5. If there is distension of the eyes, nervousness and headache due to hyperactivity of Liver-Yang resulting from deficiency of Liver-Yin, add LR-2, the Spring point, and LI-4, the Source point, to subdue the Liver-Yang and relieve distension of the eyes.
6. If there is dizziness and empty feeling in the head resulting from Essence deficiency of the Liver and Kidney, add GB-20 and GV-20 with reinforcing method to lift up Essence to nourish the brain and relieve the emptiness of the head.
7. If there is general tiredness and scanty menstruation due to Essence deficiency of the Liver and Kidney, add CV-4 and CV-6 to tonify the Kidney-Essence, reinforce the Blood and regulate menstruation.
8. If there is insomnia and night sweating due to Yin deficiency of the Heart with hyperactivity of Deficient-Fire, add HT-3 and HT-6 to tonify the Heart and clear the Deficient-Fire.
9. If there is lower back pain and weakness of the knees due to deficiency of the Kidney, add BL-58 and GV-4 to tonify the Kidney and regulate the collateral.

Case history

A 61-year-old woman had been suffering from left eye pain for 4 months. She complained of eye pain with a dry sensation when she was watching something or reading longer than half an hour. She had been diagnosed as having chronic trachoma a year previously. However, there was no improvement after eyedrop treatment. Also, she had a slight headache in her temple area at both sides, especially on the left side. Sometimes she was dizzy, had an aversion to strong light, and night sweating, a dry mouth and dry stools. Her tongue was red with little coating. Her pulse was deep and wiry.

Diagnosis
Deficiency of Yin of Liver and the Kidney.

Principle of treatment
Nourish the Yin of the Liver and the Kidney and benefit the eyes.

Acupuncture treatment
LR-3 Taichong, KI-3 Taixi, SP-6 Sanyinjiao, GB-20 Fengchi, BL-1 Jingming, ST-2 Sibai and Extra Taiyang were selected. Reinforcing method was used on these points, every other day and for 1 month.

Explanations
- KI-3 is the Stream and Source point of Kidney channels. It is used to nourish the Kidney-Yin and nourish Liver-Yin indirectly.
- LR-3, the Stream and Source point of Liver channel, tonifies the Liver, smoothes the Liver and benefits the eyes. SP-6 is the crossing point of three Yin channels of feet. These two points in combination to nourish Yin and regulate the circulation of Liver-Qi.
- GB-20 is an empirical point to regulate Qi, relieve headache and improve the eyesight.
- BL-1, ST-2 and Extra Taiyang are local points to regulate Qi circulation and relieve the eye pain and headache.

After 30 days of treatment the eye pain was relieved. One year later, when the patient returned to the clinic to get treatment for her lower back pain, she said she had had no more eye pain since the last treatment.

Ear pain 13

耳部疼痛

The term 'ear pain' encompasses pain both in and on the ear, including the auricle, the external auditory canal and the drum membrane. Most of the time ear pain is unilateral, but sometimes bilateral ear pain is observed. Ear pain is usually accompanied by swelling, redness, tinnitus, deafness, headache, dizziness, a pussy discharge from the ear, or even a mixture of pus and blood discharged from the ear.

According to TCM, ear pain is usually considered to be caused by an invasion of external pathogenic factors, accumulation of Excessive-Heat in the Liver and Gall Bladder, or stagnation of Blood due to trauma. Ear pain might be attributed to any of the following diseases in Western medicine: inflammation, abscess or infection of the external auditory canal, acute or chronic otitis media, or mastoiditis. It also includes some diseases that occur in the vicinity of *near* the ears, such as acute tonsillitis, peritonsillar abscess, disorders of the temperomandibular joint (TMJ), such as inflammation, and so on.

The ear is the opening orifice of the Kidney. If there is sufficient Kidney-Essence, the ears will be properly nourished and hearing will be normal. However, if there is any weakness of the Kidney, and deficiency of Kidney-Essence, the ear will not be nourished, leading to the appearance of symptoms such as dizziness, tinnitus, and even ear pain.

Generally speaking, the Heart opens into the tongue. However, the tongue is not an orifice. In fact, according to TCM the Heart also secondarily opens into the ear. This means that if there is harmony between Heart and Kidney there is balance between Water and Fire, and the ear will function normally. However, where disharmony develops between the Heart and Kidney, the ear will not stop functioning properly, and this leads to ear pain with poor hearing and deafness. Therefore, deficiency of Blood in the Heart, for instance due to excessive grief, thinking or meditation, may also cause ear pain.

The Liver promotes the free flow of Qi circulation in the body. In cases of prolonged periods of stress or emotional overstimulation, the Liver will fail to maintain the free flow of Qi, and this leads to the stagnation of Liver-Qi. Uprising of Liver-Qi may follow, or uprising of Liver-Fire resulting from stagnation of Liver-Qi, and cause disturbances of the ear leading to ear pain. Also, the Gall Bladder is attached to the Liver, and they share a pair of channels and a collateral. A branch from the Gall Bladder channel reaches the middle of the ear and comes out in front of the ear. If there is stagnation of Liver-Qi, or hyperactivity of Liver-Fire, or accumulation of Damp-Heat in the Liver, the Gall Bladder will be disturbed, blocking the free flow of Qi in the Gall Bladder channel, and ear pain occurs.

The Spleen is in charge of transportation and transformation, which maintain the production of Qi and Blood. If the ear is properly nourished by these, it will perform its normal physiological function. However, when there is insufficient nourishment from Qi and Blood ear pain will occur. Moreover, if the Spleen fails to transport Damp and Water properly then Damp-Phlegm will form, which leads to a blockage in the ear, causing ear pain.

Aetiology and pathology

Invasion of External factors

The ear is a clear orifice and located at the upper part of the body, and is therefore easily attacked by External invasion. Among the External factors, invasion of Wind-Heat, or Wind-Heat and toxin, or Damp-Heat are those most often seen in the daily practice. Heat or Damp-Heat may disturb the Qi and Blood circulation as well as causing stagnation of Qi and Blood, so swelling, redness and pain occur.

In some cases, a painful ear can also be caused by the invasion of Wind-Cold. Since Cold is characterised by contraction and stagnation, a painful ear, purplish ear, discoloration of the ear, aversion to cold, etc. might occur.

Accumulation of Excessive-Heat in the Liver and Gall Bladder

The Gall Bladder channel descends behind the ears, enters them and then travels anterior to them. Its sinews also follow behind the ear. Since the Liver and Gall Bladder share a pair of channels and a collateral and influence each other physiologically and pathologically, disorders of the Liver may cause a dysfunction of the Gall Bladder in turn. Excessive anger, stress, frustration or agitation, may cause Qi to stagnate in the Liver and Gall Bladder, leading to generation of Fire there that ascends and disturbs the ear, causing pain. Stagnation of Liver and Gall Bladder-Qi may also cause the Blood to stagnate, blocking the collateral of the ears, so ear pain develops.

Furthermore, overeating of fatty, sweet or pungent food, and drinking too much alcohol, may cause a dysfunction in the Spleen and Stomach, leading to the formation of Damp-Heat in the body. If Damp-Heat invades the Liver and Gall Bladder it blocks the ears, and pain develops.

Physical trauma and insect bites

Physical trauma in or around the ears may directly injure the channels and collateral, damaging the ear tissues and bringing about stagnation of the Qi and Blood, causing a painful ear.

Insect bites may cause Toxic Heat to invade the ear, leading to sudden ear pain with redness, swelling and heat, and even fever or headache.

Treatment based on differentiation

Differentiation

Differentiation of pain

— Acute onset of ear pain, a mild pain, a feeling of fullness in the ear, diminished hearing, throat pain, or redness in the throat and ear tube, is usually caused by invasion of Wind-Heat.
— A history of chronic ear pain, mild pain, fullness and distension in the ear, tinnitus or poor hearing, without any pus discharge from the ear, is usually caused by deficiency of the Liver and Kidney, or weakness of the Spleen.
— Long-standing mild ear pain, with a slight discharge of white and diluted pus from the ear, poor hearing, is usually caused by weakness of the Spleen with formation of Damp.
— Severe ear pain occurring deep inside the ear, a throbbing or drilling pain, swelling, redness, fever or thirst is usually caused by hyperactivity of Fire from the Liver and Gall Bladder, or accumulation of Damp-Heat in the Liver and Gall Bladder.
— Sudden aggravation of ear pain, with a profuse yellow pus discharge from the ear, high fever, nausea, vomiting, or even semiconsciousness or delirium, is caused by invasion of Toxic Heat with blockage of the Pericardium channel, which is very serious.
— Redness, swelling and heat of the auricle, with a dislike of touch or aggravation of ear pain when sleeping on the affected side, is usually caused by invasion of Toxic Heat.

Differentiation of pus

— Acute onset of ear pain with a slight amount of yellow and sticky pus is usually caused by hyperactivity of Fire from the Liver and Gall Bladder.
— A gradual onset of profuse yellow pus with a foul smell is usually caused by accumulation of Damp-Heat in the Liver and Gall Bladder.
— Persistent dilute white pus, whether in small or profuse amounts, is usually caused by weakness of the Spleen with formation of Damp-Phlegm.
— Long-standing discharge of pus containing white and yellow piece fragments, and a foul smell, is usually caused by Kidney weakness with accumulation of stubborn Damp-Heat.

Differentiation of tinnitus and deafness

— Sudden onset of tinnitus that is high or sharp in tone, and gradual occurrence of poor hearing, is usually caused by hyperactivity of Fire from the Liver and Gall Bladder.
— Deficiency of Liver and Kidney usually causes a gradual onset of tinnitus with low tones and a poor hearing.
— Sudden occurrence of deafness is usually caused by invasion of Wind, Cold, Damp or Heat. Stagnation of Liver-Qi resulting from emotional upset can also cause this. A gradually developing deafness is usually caused by weakness in the Liver, Kidney and Spleen.
— Deficiency of Qi and Blood also usually cause gradual occurrence of deafness, with a lack of any history of pus formation in the ear.
— Deafness with pus discharge is usually caused by invasion of toxic Heat, accumulation of Damp-Heat, or formation of Damp-Phlegm resulting from weakness of the Spleen and Stomach.

Treatment

INVASION OF WIND-HEAT

Symptoms and signs

Severe pain at the ears, redness and swelling of the ears, aggravation of pain on speaking, a yellow discharge from the ears, fever, an aversion to cold, headache, thirst, throat pain, coughing, expectoration of yellow phlegm, a red tongue with a thin and yellow coating and a superficial and rapid pulse.

Principle of treatment

Dispel Wind, clear Heat and eliminate Toxin.

HERBAL TREATMENT

Prescription

YIN QIAO SAN
Honeysuckle and Forsythia Powder
Jin Yin Hua *Flos Lonicerae* 10 g
Lian Qiao *Fructus Forsythiae* 10 g
Jie Geng *Radix Platycodi* 6 g
Bo He *Herba Menthae* 6 g
Dan Dou Chi *Semen Sojae Praeparetum* 10 g
Zhu Ye *Herba Lophatheri* 10 g
Gan Cao *Radix Glycyrrhizae* 6 g
Jing Jie Sui *Spica Schizonepetae* 6 g

Niu Bang Zi *Fructus Arctii* 10 g
Lu Gen *Rhizoma Phragmitis* 10 g

Explanations

- Jin Yin Hua and Lian Qiao clear Heat and eliminate toxin.
- Bo He, Jing Jie Sui and Dan Dou Chi promote sweating, release the exterior and dispel Heat.
- Niu Bang Zi, Jie Geng and Gan Cao eliminate toxin, dissolve nodules, benefit the throat and stop pain.
- Zhu Ye and Lu Gen clear Heat and promote the production of Body Fluids so as to relieve thirst.

Modifications

1. If there is redness and swelling of the ear due to the invasion of Toxic Heat, add Pu Gong Ying *Herba Taraxaci* 10 g and Xia Ku Cao *Spica Prunellae* 10 g to clear the Heat, eliminate the Toxin and reduce the swelling.
2. If there is discharge of yellow liquid from the ear due to invasion of Toxic Damp-Heat, add Long Dan Cao *Radix Gentianae* 5 g and Ku Seng *Radix Sophorae Flavesentis* 10 g to eliminate the Toxin and the Damp and clear the Heat.
3. If there is fever due to the predominance of Heat invasion, add Chai Hu *Radix Bupleuri* 5 g and Shen Ma *Rhizoma Cimicifugae* 5 g to clear the Heat and reduce the fever.
4. If there is headache due to the disturbance of the Clear Yang in the head by Wind-Heat, add Chuan Xiong *Rhizoma Ligustici Chuanxiong* 10 g and Man Jing Zi *Fructus Viticis* 10 g to dispel Wind-Heat and sedate the headache.
5. If there is a cough and expectoration of yellow phlegm due to invasion of the Lung by Wind-Heat, add Qian Hu *Radix Peucedani* 10 g and Zhe Bei Mu *Bulbus Fritillariae Thunbergii* 10 g to disperse the Lung-Qi and dispel the Wind-Heat.

Patent remedies

Yin Qiao Pian *Honeysuckle and Forsythia Tablet*
Yin Qiao Jie Du Pian *Honeysuckle and Forsythia Tablet to Overcome Toxins*

ACUPUNCTURE TREATMENT

LI-4 Hegu, TE-5 Waiguan, TE-17 Yifeng, TE-21 Ermen, GB-2 Tinghui, GB-8 Shuaigu and GB-20 Fengchi. Reducing method is used on these points.

Explanations

- LI-4, the Source point, opens the skin pores and promotes sweating so as to dispel Wind, clear Heat and eliminate Toxin.
- TE-5 dispels Wind, clears Heat and relieves pain.
- TE-17, TE-21, GB-2 and GB-8 are all local points around the ear, and are able to circulate Qi and Blood and harmonise the collateral so as to stop the pain.
- GB-20 dispels Wind, clears Heat and relieves the ear pain.

Modifications

1. If there is redness and swelling of the ear due to invasion of Toxic Heat, add TE-2 and LI-11 to clear Heat, eliminate the Toxin and reduce the swelling.
2. If there is discharge of yellow liquid from the ear due to invasion of Toxic Damp-Heat, add GB-34, and TE-6 to eliminate the Toxin, eliminate the Damp and clear the Heat.
3. If there is fever due to predominance of Heat invasion, add GV-14 to clear the Heat and reduce the fever.
4. If there is headache due to disturbance of the Clear Yang in the head by Wind-Heat, add Extra Taiyang to dispel Wind-Heat and sedate the headache.
5. If there is cough and expectoration of yellow phlegm due to invasion of the Lung by Wind-Heat, add LU-7 and BL-13 to disperse the Lung-Qi and dispel the Wind-Heat.

INVASION OF WIND-COLD

Symptoms and signs

Painful ears, a slight purplish or blue colour to the ears, ear pain referring to the head, headache, an aversion to cold, a slight fever, a runny nose with a white discharge, a cough with expectoration of white phlegm, a thin and white tongue coating and a superficial and wiry pulse.

Principle of treatment

Dispel Wind, eliminate Cold and relieve the pain.

HERBAL TREATMENT

Prescription

DANG GUI SI NI TANG
Angelica Four Rebellious Decoction
Gui Zhi *Ramulus Cinnamomi* 10 g
Dang Gui *Radix Angelicae Sinensis* 10 g

Bai Shao *Radix Paeoniae Alba* 20 g
Mu Tong *Caulis Akebiae* 6 g
Xi Xin *Herba Asari* 3 g
Gan Cao *Radix Glycyrrhizae* 5 g
Da Zao *Fructus Ziziphi Jujubae* 10 g

Explanations

- Gui Zhi and Dang Gui promote the Blood circulation so as to remove Qi stagnation in the channels. Bai Shao and Dang Gui nourish the Blood and remove Qi stagnation to relieve the pain.
- Gui Zhi and Xi Xin warm the channels to relieve pain.
- Mu Tong regulates the circulation of Qi in the channels to remove Qi stagnation.
- Da Zao tonifies the Qi and Blood. Gan Cao harmonises the actions of the other herbs in the formula.

Modifications

1. If there is spasm of the face due to the predominance of Cold invasion, add Bai Zhi *Radix Angelicae Dahuricae* 10 g and Bai Fu Zi *Rhizoma Typhonii* 10 g to eliminate the Cold and relieve the spasm.
2. If there is stiffness of the neck and headache due to slowing down of the Qi and Blood circulation as a result of Wind-Cold invasion, add Qiang Huo *Rhizoma seu Radix Notopterygii* 10 g and Ge Gen *Radix Puerariae* 10 g to relieve the stiff neck and headache.
3. If there is cough and expectoration of white phlegm due to invasion of the Lung by Wind-Cold, add Ban Xia *Rhizoma Pinelliae* 10 g and Chen Pi *Pericarpium Citri Reticulatae* 10 g to disperse the Lung-Qi, dispel the Wind-Cold and relieve the cough.
4. If there is headache due to Wind-Cold invasion, add Chuan Xiong *Rhizoma Ligustici Chuanxiong* 10 g and Qiang Huo *Rhizoma seu Radix Notopterygii* 10 g to dispel the Wind-Cold and relieve the headache.

Patent remedy

Jing Fang Bai Du Pian *Schizonepeta and Ledebouriella Tablet to Overcome Pathogenic Influences*

ACUPUNCTURE TREATMENT

LI-4 Hegu, LU-7 Lieque, TE-17 Yifeng, GB-2 Tinghui, GB-8 Shuaigu and BL-12 Fengmen. Reducing method is used on these points. Moxibustion should be applied on LI-4, TE-5, TE-17 and GB-2.

Explanations

- Actually this group of acupuncture points is almost the same as those for invasion of Wind-Heat; the only slight difference is the application of moxibustion so as to warm the ear, dispel Wind-Cold and relieve the pain.
- Cold has the characteristics of contraction and stagnation; thus those points that have a strong ability in dispelling Cold and opening the skin pores—LI-4, the Source point, and LU-7, the Connecting point—are used to open the skin pores and promote sweating so as to dispel Wind-Cold.
- BL-12 dispels Wind, eliminates Cold and relieves External symptoms.
- TE-17 and GB-2 are local points around the ear, and are able to circulate the Qi and Blood and harmonise the collateral so as to stop the pain.

Modifications

1. If there is spasm of the face due to predominance of Cold invasion, add ST-6 and ST-7 with moxibustion to eliminate the Cold and relieve the spasm.
2. If there is stiffness of the neck and headache due to slowing down of the Qi and Blood circulation resulting from invasion of Wind-Cold, add SI-3, the Confluence point of the Governing Vessel, and BL-62, the Confluence point of the Yang Heel Vessel, to relieve the stiff neck and headache.
3. If there is cough and expectoration of white phlegm due to invasion of the Lung by Wind-Cold, add LU-1, the Front Collecting point, and BL-13, the Back Transporting point of the Lung to disperse the Lung-Qi, dispel the Wind-Cold and relieve the cough.

Case history

A 51-year-old woman had been suffering from pain in her right ear for 2 weeks. She had a painful ear and stiff neck when she woke up one winter morning. She received massage treatment, which got rid of the neck pain but the painful ear remained. Therefore she came to the acupuncturist for treatment. When she arrived at the clinic, she had right ear pain with spasm sensation, and slight rigidity in her neck, which always got worse when she went outdoors. She wore a heavy scarf all the time when she left the house. Her tongue was white and wet, and her pulse was wiry.

Diagnosis

Invasion of External Cold. The key symptoms of this case were the ear pain caused by improper exposition to Cold. The pain was acute and with a cold sensation. The white tongue coating and wiry pulse were also due to External Cold syndrome.

Principle of treatment

Warm the Gall Bladder channels and eliminate External Cold to relieve the ear pain.

Acupuncture treatment

SI-19 Tinggong, TE-17 Yifeng, TE-5 Waiguan, GB-2 Tinghui and GB-20 Fengchi were needled with reducing method. Treatment was given every other day.

Explanations

- TE-5 is the Connecting point of the Triple Burner channel. It is needled to promote the Qi circulation in the Triple Burner channel, to dispel the external Cold in the channels. GB-20 is a key point to treat Wind-Cold disorders in the head area. It can be used to dispel Wind-Cold to treat a painful ear. This point was also warmed with moxa stick after needling.
- GB-2, TE-17 and SI-19 are local points to treat ear pain.

Ten days later, the ear pain was relieved completely.

INVASION OF TOXIN OR INSECT BITES

Symptoms and signs

Sudden swelling and pain of the ear, mostly at one side, itching, redness, a hot or even burning sensation, restlessness, or fever, a thirst, constipation, a red tongue with a thin and yellow coating and a wiry and rapid pulse.

Principle of treatment

Clear Heat, remove Toxin, reduce swelling and relieve the pain.

HERBAL TREATMENT

Prescription

WU WEI XIAO DU YIN
Five-Ingredient Decoction to Eliminate Toxin
Jin Yin Hua *Flos Lonicerae* 20 g
Ye Ju Hua *Flos Chrysanthemi Indici* 15 g
Pu Gong Ying *Herba Taraxaci* 30 g
Zi Hua Di Ding *Herba Violae* 30 g
Zi Bei Tian Kui *Herba Begonia Fibristipulatae* 15 g

Explanations

- Jin Yin Hua and Pu Gong Ying are used to clear Heat and eliminate toxin to relieve the pain and itching.
- Ye Ju Hua, Zi Hua Di Ding and Zi Bei Tian Kui are used to eliminate Toxin and cool the Blood to relieve swelling in the ears and skin ulcer.

Modifications

1. If there is obvious redness and swelling of the ear due to severe Toxin invasion, add Huang Lian *Rhizoma Coptidis* 10 g and Da Qing Ye *Folium Isatidis* 10 g to clear the Heat, eliminate the Toxin and reduce the swelling.
2. If there is fever due to invasion of Toxic Heat, add Chai Hu *Radix Bupleuri* 5 g and Sheng Ma *Rhizoma Cimicifugae* 5 g to clear the Heat and reduce the fever.
3. If there is headache due to disturbance of the Clear Yang in the head by Toxic Heat, add Man Jing Zi *Fructus Viticis* 10 g and Bo He *Herba Menthae* 5 g to dispel the Wind-Heat and sedate the headache.
4. If there is restlessness and insomnia due to failure of the Heart to house the Mind, resulting from disturbance of the Heart by Toxic Heat, add Huang Lian *Rhizoma Coptidis* 10 g and Zhu Ye *Herba Lophatheri* 10 g to clear the Heat and calm the Mind.
5. If there is fever with thirst, add Shi Gao *Gypsum Fibrosum* 20 g and Zhi Mu *Rhizoma Anemarrhenae* 10 g to clear the Heat and relieve the thirst.
6. If there is constipation, add Da Huang *Radix et Rhizoma Rhei* 10 g and Mang Xiao *Natrii Sulfas* 10 g to clear the Fire and promote defecation.

Patent remedies

Niu Huang Jie Du Pian *Cattle Gallstone Tablet to Resolve Toxin*
Huang Lian Shang Qing Wan *Coptis Pill to Clear Heat of Upper Burner*

ACUPUNCTURE TREATMENT

BL-17 Geshu, GV-10 Lingtai, LI-2 Erjian, LI-4 Hegu, TE-6 Zhigou, TE-21 Ermen and GB-3 Shangguan. Reducing method is used on these points.

Explanations

- This condition is usually caused by a Toxic Heat invasion resulting from insect bites; thus some points to clear the Heat and remove the Toxin from the Blood should be used, as well as some points to clear Heat in the Qi stage.
- BL-17 and GV-10 clear Heat and remove toxin from the Blood as well as reducing swelling.
- LI-2, the Spring point, and LI-4, the Source point, clear Heat, eliminate Toxin, reduce swelling and relieve the pain.

- TE-6 clears Heat and drains Toxin downward.
- TE-21 and GB-3 are the local points around the ear; they are able to circulate the Qi and Blood and harmonise the collateral so as to stop the pain.

Modifications

1. If there is obvious redness and swelling of the ear due to severe Toxin, add TE-2 and GB-43 to clear Heat, eliminate the Toxin and reduce the swelling.
2. If there is fever due to invasion of Toxic Heat, add GV-14 and LI-11 to clear Heat and reduce the fever.
3. If there is headache due to disturbance of the Clear Yang in the head by Toxic Heat, add Extra Taiyang to dispel Wind-Heat and sedate the headache.
4. If there is restlessness and insomnia due to failure of the Heart to house the Mind resulting from disturbance of the Heart by Toxic Heat, add HT-3 to clear the Heat and calm the Mind.

INVASION OF TOXIC HEAT WITH BLOCKAGE OF THE PERICARDIUM

Symptoms and signs

Gradual onset of ear pain with sudden aggravation, a profuse discharge of yellow pus from the ear, high fever, restlessness, severe headache, nausea, vomiting, delirium or even semiconsciousness, a thirst, constipation, a deep red tongue with a thick, yellow and greasy coating and a wiry, rapid and forceful pulse.

Principle of treatment

Clear Heat, reduce fever, remove Toxin and relieve the blockage.

HERBAL TREATMENT

Prescription

HUANG LIAN JIE DU TANG
Coptis Decoction to Relieve Toxicity
Huang Lian *Rhizoma Coptidis* 5 g
Huang Qin *Radix Scutellariae* 10 g
Huag Bai *Cortex Phellodendri* 10 g
Zhi Zi *Fructus Gardeniae* 10 g

plus:

DA CHENG QI TANG
Major Order the Qi Decoction
Da Huang *Radix et Rhizoma Rhei* 10 g
Mang Xiao *Natrii Sulfas* 10 g

Hou Po *Cortex Magnoliae Officinalis* 10 g
Zhi Shi *Fructus Aurantii Immaturus* 10 g
Pu Gong Ying *Herba Taraxaci* 10 g
Long Dan Cao *Radix Gentianae* 10 g
Zhi Gan Cao *Radix Glycyrrhizae Praeparata* 3 g

Explanations

- The first formula is used to clear Heat and eliminate the Toxin.
- The second formula is used to promote defecation and eliminate the Toxin by means of defecation.
- Pu Gong Ying and Long Dan Cao are prescribed together with other two formulas to strengthen the effect of elimination of Heat and Toxin.
- Zhi Gan Cao harmonises the actions of all the other herbs in the prescription.

Modifications

1. If there is obvious redness and swelling of the ear, add Sheng Di Huang *Radix Rehmanniae* 10 g and Tu Fu Ling *Rhizoma Smilacis Glabrae* 10 g to clear the Heat, eliminate the toxin and reduce the swelling.
2. If there is fever, add Shi Gao *Gypsum Fibrosum* 30 g to clear the Heat and reduce the fever.
3. If there is headache, add Man Jing Zi *Fructus Viticis* 10 g and Bo He *Herba Menthae* 5 g to dispel the Wind-Heat and sedate the headache.
4. If there is restlessness and insomnia, add Zhu Ye *Herba Lophatheri* 10 g to clear the Heat and calm the Mind.
5. If there is delirium, add An Gong Niu Huang Wan, one pill every day to clear Heat and wake the patient.
6. If there is nausea and vomiting, add Xuan Fu Hua *Flos Inulae* 10 g to cause the Stomach Qi to descend and relieve the vomiting.

Patent remedies

Niu Huang Jie Du Pian *Cattle Gallstone Tablet to Resolve Toxin*
An Gong Niu Huang Wan *Calm the Palace Pill with Cattle Gallstone*

ACUPUNCTURE TREATMENT

BL-15 Xinshu, GV-10 Lingtai, LI-2 Erjian, LI-4 Hegu, LI-11 Quchi, TE-6 Zhigou, TE-21 Ermen, HT-3 Shaohai and ST-44 Neiting. Reducing method is used on these points.

Explanations

- BL-15 and HT-3 clear Heat from the Heart and calm the Mind.
- GV-10 clears Heat and removes Toxin from the Blood as well as reducing swelling in the ear.
- LI-2, the Spring point of the Large Intestine channel, LI-4, the Source point, and LI-11, the Sea point, as well as ST-44, the Spring point of the Stomach channel, are prescribed here to clear Heat, eliminate the Toxin, reduce the swelling and relieve the pain.
- TE-6 clears Heat and drains toxin downward.
- TE-21 is able to circulate the Qi and Blood and harmonise the collateral so as to stop the pain.

Modifications

1. If there is severe redness and swelling of the ear, add TE-2 and GB-43, the Spring points, to clear the Heat, eliminate the toxin and reduce the swelling.
2. If there is a high fever, add GV-14 to clear the Heat and reduce the fever.
3. If there is headache, add Extra Taiyang and Extra Yintang to sedate the headache.
4. If there is restlessness and insomnia, add HT-7, the Source point, to clear the Heat and calm the Mind.
5. If there is semiconsciousness, add GV-26 to regulate the Mind and wake the patient.
6. If there is expectoration of profuse yellow phlegm, add LU-5 and ST-40 to resolve the Phlegm and cause the Lung-Qi to descend.
7. If there is nausea or vomiting, add CV-12 and PC-6 to cause the Stomach-Qi to descend and relieve the vomiting.
8. If there is constipation, add ST-25, the Front Collecting point of the Large Intestine, to promote defecation and relieve the constipation.

STAGNATION OF QI

Symptoms and signs

Pain in one or both ears, which moves up and down, aggravation of the pain by emotional upset, and alleviation by relaxation, depression, nervousness, headache, a feeling of fullness in the chest and ears, a slight purplish tongue with a thin and white coating, and a wiry pulse.

Principle of treatment

Smooth the Liver, promote Qi circulation and relieve the pain.

HERBAL TREATMENT

Prescription

XIAO YAO SAN
Free and Relaxed Powder
Xiang Fu *Rhizoma Cyperi* 10 g
Chi Shao *Radix Paeoniae Rubrae* 10 g
Chuan Xiong *Rhizoma Ligustici Chuanxiong* 6 g
Yu Jin *Radix Pruni* 10 g
Ju Hua *Flos Chrysanthemi* 10 g
Xia Ku Cao *Spica Prunellae* 10 g
Chai Hu *Radix Bupleuri* 10 g
Dang Gui *Radix Angelicae Sinensis* 10 g
Bai Shao *Radix Paeoniae Alba* 20 g

Explanations

- This type of ear pain is often seen in patients with explosive anger, or a long-standing period of stress, frustration or emotional upset, leading to slowing down of the Liver-Qi, blocking the circulation in the channels, causing ear pain.
- Chai Hu, Xiang Fu and Bai Shao smooth and promote Qi circulation in the Liver.
- Dang Gui tonifies the Liver-Blood and harmonises the Liver.
- Since Qi stagnation may cause Blood stagnation, Chuan Xiong, Yu Jin and Chi Shao promote Blood circulation and eliminate Blood stagnation in the channels.
- Stagnation of Liver Qi may cause generation of Liver Fire, thus Xia Ku Cao and Ju Hua are prescribed here to clear Heat in the Liver and cool the Liver.

Modifications

1. If there is severe ear pain due to stagnation of Liver-Qi, add Tan Xiang *Lignum Santali* 3 g and Bing Pian *Borneolum Syntheticum* 2 g (as infusion) to increase of Qi circulation and stop the pain.
2. If there is fullness of ears with distension, add Cong Bai *Bulbus Allii Fistulosi* 5 g and Qing Pi *Pericarpium Citri Reticulatae Viride* 5 g to induce the formula to ascend to the ears and promote Qi circulation there.
3. If there is headache, add Man Jing Zi *Fructus Viticis* 10 g and Jue Ming Zi *Semen Cassiae* 10 g to sedate the headache and harmonise the collateral in the head.
4. If there are unstable emotions, nervousness and insomnia add Long Gu *Os Draconis* 20 g and Huang Lian *Rhizoma Coptidis* 3 g to calm the Liver and Heart, and tranquillise the Mind.
5. If there is fullness of the chest, add Zhi Qiao *Fructus Aurantii* 10 g and Gua Lou Pi *Pericarpium Trichosanthis* 10 g to relax the chest and promote the Qi circulation in the chest.
6. If there is poor appetite, add Shan Zha *Fructus Crataegi* 10 g and Shen Qu *Massa Fermentata Medicinalis* 15 g to improve the appetite and promote digestion.
7. If there is diarrhoea and nervousness, add Mu Xiang *Radix Aucklandiae* 10 g and Ge Gen *Radix Puerariae* 10 g to cause the Clear Spleen-Qi to ascend and stop the diarrhoea.

Patent remedies

Shu Gan Wan *Soothe Liver Pill*
Xiao Yao Wan *Free and Relaxed Pill*

ACUPUNCTURE TREATMENT

LI-4 Hegu, LR-3 Taichong, SI-19 Tinggong, GB-8 Shuaigu, GB-12 Wangu, TE-17 Yifeng and TE-21 Ermen. Reducing method is used on these points, except SI-19, GB-8 and TE-21, on which even method should be employed.

Explanations

- LI-4 is indicated in all the problems on the head, as it promotes Qi and Blood circulation and relieves ear pain. LR-3, the Stream point from the Liver channel, smoothes the Liver and promotes the circulation of Qi. These two points are often prescribed simultaneously for relief of Qi stagnation so as to increase the therapeutic result.
- The Lesser Yang channel of the hand and Lesser Yang channel of the foot are two important channels passing and circulating around the ears. These two channels are frequently impaired in Qi stagnation leading to the occurrence of ear pain. GB-8, GB-12, TE-17 and TE-21, the local points, harmonise the channels, promote the circulation of Qi in the channels and in the ears and sedate the ear pain.
- SI-19, another local point, is prescribed to circulate the Qi and Blood, harmonise the collateral and stop the ear pain.

Modifications

1. If there is severe ear pain, add GB-41 and TE-5 to increase the effect on the Qi circulation and stop the ear pain.

2. If there is aggravation of ear pain by emotional upset and nervousness, add PC-6 and GB-20 to smooth the emotions, promote the Qi circulation and clear the Heat in the Liver.
3. If there is headache, add Extra Taiyang and Extra Yintang to harmonise the collateral in the head and arrest the headache.
4. If there is insomnia, add HT-3 and Extra Anmian to calm the Heart and tranquillise the Mind.
5. If there is depression and a feeling of fullness in the chest, add CV-17 and Extra Sishencong to relax the chest and relieve the depression.
6. If there is nausea, or stomach pain during periods of nervousness, add CV-12 and ST-34 to cause the Stomach-Qi to descend and relieve the stomach pain.
7. If there are loose stools or diarrhoea during periods of nervousness, add ST-25, the Front Collecting point of the Large Intestine, and LR-13, the Front Collecting point of the Spleen, to activate the Spleen and relieve the diarrhoea.
8. If there is a bitter taste in the mouth, and a yellow and slight greasy tongue coating, add GB-34, the Sea point, to regulate the Gall Bladder and cause the Turbid Qi to descend.

HYPERACTIVITY OF FIRE OF LIVER AND GALL BLADDER

Symptoms and signs

Acute onset of pain, or a chronic onset with acute aggravation, or discharge of yellow liquid from the ear, tinnitus, heat in the ear, irritability, nervousness, headache, a bitter taste in the mouth, a red tongue with a yellow and greasy tongue coating, and a wiry and rapid pulse.

Principle of treatment

Clear Heat in the Liver and Gall Bladder and reduce Fire.

HERBAL TREATMENT

Prescription

LONG DAN XIE GAN TANG
Gentianae Decoction to Drain the Liver
Long Dan Cao *Radix Gentianae* 6 g
Huang Qin *Radix Scutellariae* 9 g
Zhi Zi *Fructus Gardeniae* 9 g
Ze Xie *Rhizoma Alismatis* 12 g
Mu Tong *Caulis Akebiae* 9 g

Che Qian Zi *Semen Plantaginis* 9 g
Dang Gui *Radix Angelicae Sinensis* 3 g
Sheng Di Huang *Radix Rehmanniae Recens* 9 g
Chai Hu *Radix Bupleuri* 6 g
Gan Cao *Radix Glycyrrhizae* 6 g

Explanations

- Long Dan Cao and Huang Qin clear Heat and dry up Damp.
- Zhi Zi, Mu Tong, Ze Xie and Che Qian Zi clear Heat, promote urination and eliminate Damp.
- Dang Gui and Sheng Di Huang nourish the Yin and Blood and prevent the actions of the other herbs from injuring the Yin.
- Chai Hu regulates the Liver-Qi removes Qi stagnation.
- Gan Cao harmonises the actions of the other herbs in the formula.

Modifications

1. If there is redness and swelling of the ear due to hyperactivity of Fire from the Liver and Gall Bladder, add Ku Shen *Radix Sophorae Flavescentis* 10 g and Huang Bai *Cortex Phellodendri* 10 g to clear the Heat, suppress the Fire, eliminate the toxin and reduce the swelling.
2. If there is discharge of yellow liquid from the ear due to accumulation of Damp-Heat in the Liver and Gall Bladder, add Tu Fu Ling *Rhizoma Smilacis Glabrae* 10 g and Che Qian Zi *Semen Plantaginis* 10 g to eliminate the Damp and clear the Heat.
3. If there is nervousness, irritability and headache due to hyperactivity of Liver-Yang, add Gou Teng *Ramulus Uncariae cum Uncis* 10 g and Yu Jin *Radix Curcumae* 10 g to calm the Liver and subdue the Liver-Yang.
4. If there is a bitter taste in the mouth due to disharmony of the Gall Bladder, add Zhi Zi *Fructus Gardeniae* 10 g and Dan Pi *Cortex Moutan Radicis* 10 g to harmonise the Gall Bladder and promote normal bile distribution.
5. If there is hypochondriac pain due to stagnation of Qi and Blood in the Liver, add Ju He *Semen Citri Reticulatae* 10 g and Bai Shao *Radix Paeoniae Alba* 10 g to promote the Qi and Blood circulation and relieve the pain.

Patent remedies

Long Dan Xie Gan Wan *Gentianae Pill to Drain the Liver*
Niu Huang Jie Du Wan *Cattle Gallstone Pill to Resolve Toxin*

ACUPUNCTURE TREATMENT

LI-4 Hegu, TE-6 Zhigou, GB-2 Tinghui, GB-8 Shuaigu, GB-41 Zulinqi, GB-43 Xiaxi and LR-2 Xingjian. Reducing method is used on these points.

Explanations

- LI-4 and TE-6 clear Heat and drain Fire by means of promoting defecation and regulating the Triple Burner.
- GB-2 and GB-8, the local points around the ear, are able to clear Heat in the collateral of the Gall Bladder and circulate the Qi and Blood so as to stop the pain.
- LR-2 and GB-43, both being the Spring points, clear Heat and reduce Fire in the Liver and Gall Bladder so as to reduce the swelling.
- GB-41 clears Heat in the Gall Bladder and harmonises the Liver and Gall Bladder.

Modifications

1. If there is redness and swelling in the ear, add LR-8, the Water point, to clear the Heat, suppress the Fire, eliminate the toxin and reduce the swelling.
2. If there is discharge of yellow liquid from the ear due to accumulation of Damp-Heat in the Liver and Gall Bladder, add GB-34 and SP-9 to eliminate the Damp and clear the Heat.
3. If there is pain in front of the ear, add GB-3 to reduce the Fire and harmonise the collateral of the Gall Bladder.
4. If there is nervousness, irritability and headache due to hyperactivity of Liver-Yang, add GV-20 and GB-20 to calm the Liver and subdue the Liver-Yang.
5. If there is a bitter taste in the mouth due to disharmony of the Gall Bladder, add GB-40 to harmonise the Gall Bladder and promote normal bile distribution.
6. If there is hypochondriac pain due to stagnation of Qi and Blood in the Liver, add LR-14 to promote Qi and Blood circulation and relieve the pain.

Case history

A 14-year-old boy had been suffering from pain in his left ear pain for 2 weeks, and an acute otitis about 20 days previously. He was treated with antibiotics to reduce his ear inflammation. His swelling and reddish ear had improved but his left ear was still feeling painful. When he came to the clinic there was a slight reddish glow on his left ear, and some yellow liquid in his otic tract. His other symptoms were tinnitus, constipation, a red tongue with yellow coating and a wiry pulse.

Diagnosis
External Toxic Heat invasion in the Liver and Gall Bladder channels.

Principle of treatment
Clear Heat and eliminate Toxin to relieve the pain.

Acupuncture treatment
LI-4 Hegu, TE-6 Zhigou, TE-17 Yifeng, GB-2 Tinghui, GB-8 Shuaigu and LR-2 Xingjian were needled with reducing method. Treatment was given every other day and the treatment series lasted for 10 days.

Explanations

- LR-3 is the Spring point, used to clear Fire in the Liver channel. LI-4 is the Source point of the Large Intestine channel, used to clear Excessive-Fire in the face area.
- TE-6 is the River point of the Triple Burner channel, used to reduce Fire.
- TE-17, GB-2 and GB-8 are local points to eliminate Heat and Toxin indirectly.

After 20 days' treatment, the boy's ear pain had disappeared completely.

STAGNATION OF BLOOD

Symptoms and signs

Stabbing pain in the ears, aggravation of the pain at night, headache, a purplish colour to the ears and tongue, a thin tongue coating and a wiry and a choppy pulse.

Principle of treatment

Circulate Qi and Blood, eliminate Blood stasis and relieve the pain.

HERBAL TREATMENT

Prescription

TONG QIAO HUO XUE TANG
Unblock the Orifices and Invigorate the Blood Decoction
Chi Shao *Radix Paeoniae Rubra* 10 g
Chuan Xiong *Rhizoma Ligustici Chuanxiong* 10 g
Tao Ren *Semen Persicae* 10 g
Hong Hua *Flos Carthami* 10 g
Cong Bai *Herba Allii Fistulosi* 10 g
Sheng Jiang *Rhizoma Zingiberis Recens* 6 g
Da Zao *Fructus Ziziphi Jujubae* 6 g
She Xiang *Moschus* 0.1 g (for infusion)

Explanations

- Chuan Xiong and Chi Shao promote the circulation of Blood in the upper part of the human body including the head and sense organs such the ears. They are also effective for relieving the pain.
- Tao Ren and Hong Hua assist the first two herbs to promote the circulation of Blood and remove its stagnation.
- She Xiang and Cong Bai open the orifice and promote the circulation of Blood so as to relieve the pain.
- Sheng Jiang and Da Zao regulate the Qi and Blood circulation.

Modifications

1. If there is severe ear pain due to the stagnation of Blood, add Yan Hu Suo *Rhizoma Corydalis* 10 g and Mo Yao *Resina Myrrhae* 5 g to strengthen the Blood circulation and stop the pain.
2. If there is stagnation of Blood resulting from Qi stagnation, add Qing Pi *Pericarpium Citri Reticulatae Viride* 5 g and Xiao Hui Xiang *Fructus Foeniculi* 3 g to relieve the Qi stagnation and promote the Blood circulation.
3. If there is headache due to stagnation of Blood, add Tian Ma *Rhizoma Gastrodiae* 10 g and Chai Hu *Radix Bupleuri* 5 g to harmonise the collateral in the head and eliminate the Blood stasis so as to arrest the headache.

Patent remedy

Yan Hu Suo Zhi Tong Pian *Corydalis Stop Pain Tablet*

ACUPUNCTURE TREATMENT

LI-4 Hegu, LR-3 Taichong, SP-6 Sanyinjiao, SI-19 Tinggong, GB-2 Tinghui, GB-8 Shuaigu and TE-21 Ermen. Reducing method is used on these points, except SI-19, GB-2 and TE-21, on which even method is used.

Explanations

- LI-4, indicated in all the problems on the head caused by Excessive pathogenic factors, promotes the Qi and Blood circulation and relieves the pain. When this point is used to promote Qi circulation, LR-3 is usually combined with it to increase the therapeutic effect.
- SP-6 promotes the Blood circulation and eliminates Blood stasis.

- TE-21, SI-19, GB-8 and GB-2 are all local points around the ear to circulate Qi and Blood, harmonise the collateral and stop the pain.

Modifications

1. If there is severe ear pain due to stagnation of Blood, add BL-17 to increase the Blood circulation and stop the pain.
2. If there is stagnation of Blood resulting from Qi stagnation, add PC-6 and CV-17 to relieve the Qi circulation and promote the Blood circulation.
3. If there is headache due to stagnation of Blood, add SI-3 and GB-20 to harmonise the collateral in the head and eliminate the Blood stasis so as to arrest the headache.

DEFICIENCY OF QI AND BLOOD

Symptoms and signs

Gradual onset of ear pain, a feeling of slight fullness in the ear, diminished hearing, tiredness, dizziness, tinnitus, hair loss, a pale complexion, a poor appetite, loose stools, weakness of the muscles and limbs, shortness of breath, tendency to sweat easily, a pale tongue with a thin and white coating and a deep, thready and weak pulse.

Principle of treatment

Activate the Spleen and Stomach, and tonify Qi and Blood.

HERBAL TREATMENT

Prescription

SHI QUAN DA BU TANG
All-Inclusive Great Tonifying Decoction
Ren Shen *Radix Ginseng* 10 g
Bai Zhu *Rhizoma Atractylodis Macrocephalae* 10 g
Huang Qi *Radix Astragali seu Hedysari* 10 g
Sheng Ma *Rhizoma Cimicifugae* 5 g
Bai Shao *Radix Paeoniae Alba* 5 g
Dang Gui *Radix Angelicae Sinensis* 5 g
Shu Di Huang *Radix Rehmannia Praeparata* 5 g
Chuan Xiong *Rhizoma Ligustici Chuanxiong* 10 g
Huang Jing *Rhizoma Polygonati* 10 g
Zhi Gan Cao *Radix Glycyrrhizae Praeparata* 10 g

Explanations

- Ren Shen and Bai Zhu activate the Spleen and Stomach and tonify the Qi.

- Huang Jing and Huang Qi tonify the Qi generally; also, Huang Qi and Sheng Ma lift the Qi to the head.
- Dang Gui and Shu Di nourish the Blood so as to support the Qi.
- Bai Shao and Chuan Xiong harmonise the Blood and prevent its stagnation.
- Zhi Gan Cao tonifies the Qi and harmonises the prescription.

Modifications

1. If there is a feeling of fullness in the ear, add Shi Chang Pu *Rhizoma Acori Graminei* 10 g and Hong Hua *Flos Carthami* 5 g to promote the Qi and Blood circulation in the ears and relieve the fullness.
2. If there is tinnitus, add Ci Shi *Magnetitum* 15 g and Chai Hu *Radix Bupleuri* 3 g to relieve the tinnitus.
3. If there is a discharge of white and diluted phlegm from the ear, add Ban Xia *Rhizoma Pinelliae* 10 g and Cang Zhu *Rhizoma Atractylodis* 10 g to resolve Damp and eliminate the phlegm.
4. If the appetite is poor, add Gu Ya *Fructus Oryze Germinatus* 10 g to activate the Stomach and Spleen and improve the appetite.
5. If there is diarrhoea, add Ge Gen *Radix Puerariae* 10 g to raise the Clear Yang-Qi and stop the diarrhoea.
6. If the face is numb, add Ban Xia *Rhizoma Pinelliae* 10 g, and Di Long *Lumbricus* 10 g to eliminate the Damp-Phlegm and promote circulation in the collateral.
7. If the hands and feet are cold, add Rou Gui *Cortex Cinnamomi* 5 g to warm the interior and dispel the Cold.

Patent remedies

Shi Quan Da Bu Wan *All-Inclusive Great Tonifying Pill*
Bu Zhong Yi Qi Wan *Tonify the Middle and Augment the Qi Pill*

ACUPUNCTURE TREATMENT

ST-7 Xiaguan, ST-36 Zusanli, ST-42 Chongyang, SP-3 Taibai, SP-6 Sanyinjiao, GV-20 Baihui, GB-2 Tinghui and TE-21 Ermen. Reinforcing method is used on all these points except GB-2 and TE-21, on which even method is used. Use of moxibustion is advisable on SP-36, SP-3 and GV-20.

Explanations

- This type of ear pain is often caused by overstrain, prolonged sickness, or occurs in an elderly person with gradual depletion of the energy, especially in the Spleen and Stomach, leading to deficiency of Qi and Blood, so the ear is not properly nourished.
- ST-36, the Sea point, SP-42, the Source point of the Stomach channel, and SP-3, the Source point of the Spleen, are able to activate the Spleen and Stomach and reinforce the Qi.
- SP-6 tonifies the Blood in general.
- GV-20 lifts up the Qi to the head so as to nourish the ears.
- GB-2, TE-21 and SP-7 are used to promote the Qi and Blood circulation and harmonise the collateral in the vicinity in order to relieve the ear pain.

Modifications

1. If there is severe ear pain, add GB-8 and TE-17 to sedate the pain.
2. If there is chronic fatigue due to a general deficiency of Qi, add CV-6 with moxibustion to tonify the Original Qi and relieve the tiredness.
3. If there is shortness of breath due to deficiency of Lung-Qi, add LU-9, the Source point, to tonify the Lung-Qi and relieve the shortness of breath.
4. If there is a pale complexion, dizziness and scanty menstruation due to deficiency of Blood, add BL-18, the Back Transporting point of the Liver, and GB-39, the Gathering point for the Marrow, to increase the production of Blood.
5. If there is a poor appetite and loose stool due to weakness of the Stomach and Spleen, add CV-12, the Front Collecting point of the Stomach channel, and SP-9, the Sea point of the Spleen, to activate the Spleen and Stomach and relieve the loose stool.

DEFICIENCY OF LIVER AND KIDNEY

Symptoms and signs

Gradual onset of a slight ear pain that is usually deep inside the ear tract, and moves up and down. Aggravation of the pain when tired, a feeling of slight fullness in the ear, diminished hearing or even deafness, tiredness, dizziness, tinnitus, hair loss, poor concentration, lower back pain, poor vision, a thin tongue coating and a deep and weak pulse.

Principle of treatment

Tonify Liver and Kidney and benefit Essence.

HERBAL TREATMENT

Prescription

LIU WEI DI HUANG WAN
Six-Ingredient Pill with Rehmannia
Huang Jing *Rhizoma Polygonati* 10 g
Nu Zhen Zi *Fructus Ligustri Lucidi* 10 g
Sha Yuan Ji Li *Semen Astragali Complanati* 10 g
Dang Gui *Radix Angelicae Sinensis* 10 g
He Shou Wu *Radix Polygoni Multiflori* 10 g
Zhi Gan Cao *Radix Glycyrrhizae Praeparata* 10 g
Shu Di Huang *Radix Rehmanniae Praeparata* 10 g
Shan Zhu Yu *Fructus Corni* 12 g
Shan Yao *Radix Dioscoreae* 12 g
Fu Ling *Poria* 9 g

Explanations

- Shu Di and Shan Zhu Yu nourish the Liver and Kidney and tonify the Kidney Essence.
- Shan Yao, Fu Ling and Huang Jing activate the Spleen and tonify the Qi so as to increase the production of Blood and Essence.
- Dang Gui and He Shou Wu tonify the Blood and supply the source of Blood production.
- Nu Zhen Zi and Sha Yuan Ji Li tonify the Kidney-Essence and benefit the vision.
- Zhi Gan Cao tonifies the Qi and harmonises the prescription.

Modifications

1. If there is a feeling of slight fullness in the ear, add Shi Chang Pu *Rhizoma Acori Graminei* 10 g to open the ear orifice and relieve the fullness.
2. If there is tinnitus, add Ci Shi *Magnetitum* 15 g to relieve the tinnitus.
3. If the vision is poor, add Qing Xiang Zi *Semen Celosiae* 10 g and Gou Qi Zi *Fructus Lycii* 10 g to nourish the Liver and benefit the eyes.
4. If there is an aversion to cold, and cold hands and feet, add Zhi Fu Zi *Radix Aconiti Praeparata* 10 g and Rou Gui *Cortex Cinnamomi* 5 g to warm the Kidney and dispel the Cold.
5. If there is oedema, add Ze Xie *Rhizoma Alismatis* 10 g and Chuan Niu Xi *Radix Cyathulae* 10 g to eliminate the excessive water and relieve the oedema.
6. If there is heat in the body and night sweating, add Zhi Mu *Rhizoma Anemarrhenae* 10 g and Huang Bai *Cortex Phellodendri* 10 g to nourish the Yin and reduce Deficient-Heat.
7. If there is dizziness and headache, add Gou Teng *Ramulus Uncariae cum Uncis* 10 g and Tian Ma *Rhizoma Gastrodiae* 10 g to suppress the Liver and subdue Interior Wind.
8. If there is nervousness and irritability, add Xia Ku Cao *Spica Prunellae* 10 g to calm the Liver and clear the Fire.

Patent remedy

Qi Ju Di Huang Wan *Lycuim Fruit, Chysanthemum and Rehmannia Pill*

ACUPUNCTURE TREATMENT

SP-6 Sanyinjiao, LR-3 Taichong, KI-3 Taixi, BL-18 Ganshu, BL-23 Shenshu, CV-6 Qihai, GB-2 Tinghui and TE-21 Ermen. Reinforcing method is used on all these points except GB-2 and TE-21, on which even method is employed.

Explanations

- LR-3 and KI-3, BL-18 and BL-23, the Source points and Back Transporting points of the Liver and Kidney respectively, tonify the Liver and Kidney and benefit the Essence.
- SP-6 tonifies Blood in the body generally and benefits the Liver and Kidney.
- CV-6 tonifies the Liver and Kidney and nourishes the Essence.
- GB-2 and TE-21 are used to promote the Qi and Blood circulation and harmonise the collateral in the vicinity in order to relieve the ear pain.

Modifications

1. If there is severe ear pain, add SI-19 and TE-17 to sedate the pain.
2. If there is tinnitus, add GB-10 and TE-18 to harmonise the collateral and relieve the tinnitus.
3. If there is a feeling of slight fullness in the ear, add SI-4 to open the ear orifice and relieve the fullness.
4. If the vision is poor, add GB-37 and ST-2 to nourish the Liver and benefit the eyes.
5. If there is an aversion to cold, and cold hands and feet, add CV-4 with moxibustion to warm the Kidney and dispel the Cold.
6. If there is oedema, add CV-9 and SP-9 to eliminate the excessive water and relieve the oedema.
7. If there is heat in the body and night sweating, add KI-2 and HT-6 to nourish the Yin and reduce the Deficient-Heat.

8. If there is dizziness and headache, add GB-20 to suppress the Liver and subdue the interior Wind.

9. If there is nervousness and irritability, add LR-2 to calm the Liver and clear the Fire.

10. If there is a discharge of yellow phlegm from the ear due to accumulation of Damp-Heat, add GB-43 and TE-2 to clear the Heat and eliminate the Damp.

Nasal pain 14

鼻
部
疼
痛

Nasal pain is characterised by pain occurring on or inside the nose, usually accompanied by symptoms such as headache, stuffiness of the nose, loss of the sense of smell, nasal discharge and a cough. The nature of the pain varies, and may be burning, distending, stabbing, pain with dryness, or pain with itching.

The nose is the opening orifice of the Lung, being in charge of smelling, assisting speech and respiration, and so on. The head is the place where all the Yang channels meet, and the nose is situated in the centre of the face, the so-called Yang point in the Yang place. So, according to TCM, nasal pain can be caused not only by disorder of the Lung, but also by that of the other interior organs. Nasal pain may be attributed to any of the following diseases in Western medicine: acute and chronic sinusitis, rhinitis, nasal vestibulitis, nasopharyngitis, conchitis, tumour of the nose, nasal mucosal ulceration, and carbuncle on the nose.

The nose is related especially to the Lung, of which it is the opening orifice, Spleen, Gall Bladder and Kidney Zang-Fu organs. It is connected with the Lung through the throat. Its main physiological function is the sense of smell. This function completely depends upon the physiological function of the Lung, so if the Lung is functioning well the nose will also function properly in detecting smells. If there is deficiency of Lung-Qi, however, the body is vulnerable to invasion of External pathogenic factors through the nose, leading to a nasal disorder, and pain may develop as a consequence.

The Lung is in charge of respiration, and the Kidney holds the respiration. If the Kidney is functioning properly, the Lung can also perform its physiological function normally, thus the nose can smell and protect the body from being invaded by external pathogenic factors. If there is deficiency of the Qi or Yin of the Kidney, however, the nose will also be affected, leading to disorder of the nose, and nasal pain.

The Heart is situated together with the Lung in the Upper Burner. If there is harmony between the Heart and Lung then the nose functions normally in smelling and assisting respiration. However, if there is a disorder of the Heart, the physiological function of the nose will be impaired, so External factors may invade, or there may be an uprising of interior Fire, and nasal pain follows.

The Spleen is in charge of Qi and Blood production as well as housing the Blood. The physiological function of the nose relies on the physiological function of the Spleen, as the nose needs to be nourished by Qi and Blood. If there is weakness of the Spleen the Qi and Blood production will decrease, and the nose will fail to be nourished, so causing nasal pain. The Gall Bladder is a Fu organ. Its Qi reaches the head, and its channel circulates above the nose and distributes in the occipital regions. In practice, harmony of Qi in the Gall Bladder keeps the head and nose healthy. However, if there is accumulation of Heat in the Gall Bladder, this pathogenic factor may ascend and block the nose, causing nasal pain.

The following channels and collateral reach or meet the nose: the Stomach, the Large Intestine, the Bladder and the Small Intestine, and the Governing, Directing and Yang Heel Vessels.

Aetiology and pathology

Invasion of External pathogenic factors

The Lung dominates respiration and opens into the nose. Since the nose is the start of the corridor of respiration, External invasion usually takes place through the nasal passage. Of the External pathogenic factors, Wind-Heat, Wind-Cold and Toxic Heat are most often seen. When invading the nasal orifice, these pathogenic factors may cause failure of the Lung to disperse Qi and cause the Qi to descend, leading to a blocked nose, which causes nasal pain. If there is invasion of Wind-Heat, or Toxic Heat, then pathogenic Heat will burn the nasal muscle and mucosa, and concentrate Body Fluids into Phlegm, causing discharge of yellow phlegm from the nose and nasal pain.

Unhealthy diet

Overeating of fatty, sweet, greasy or pungent food, drinking too much alcohol, and excessive intake of milk products, may all cause dysfunction of the Spleen and Stomach, leading to the formation of Damp-Heat in the body.

Since the Stomach channel begins on the face and nose, Damp-Heat may flow with Qi up to the nose and block the orifice, causing the Qi and Blood to stagnate in the channel and collateral, and nose pain is a consequence. Also, pathogenic Heat may burn the muscle and mucosa of the nose, causing deterioration of the muscle, and hence nasal pain.

Accumulation of Excessive-Heat in the Lung and Stomach

Incomplete disappearance of External pathogenic factors from the Lung, excessive grief, or smoking over a long period may cause the formation of Excessive-Heat in the Lung. Overconsumption of sweet or fatty food or alcohol may cause Excessive-Heat to form in the Stomach. The Stomach and Large Intestine are both Bright Yang Fu organs, and the Lung and Large Intestine form a pair of channels and a collateral, so Excessive-Heat accumulating in the Stomach may affect the Lung, leading to accumulation of Excessive-Heat in the Lung also. The formation of Excessive-

Heat in other Zang-Fu organs attacking the Lung may also trigger the accumulation of Heat in the Lung; for instance, Liver-Fire can attack the Lung, the so-called 'invasion of Metal by Wood Fire'.

When there is accumulation of Excessive-Heat in the Lung and Stomach, the Lung will fail to disperse Qi, the nose will be blocked, the nasal mucosa and muscle will be burned, and nasal pain will occur.

Hyperactivity of Fire of Liver and Gall Bladder

The Qi of the Liver and the Gall Bladder prefers to move freely. The Liver and the Gall Bladder share a pair of channels and a collateral. If there is excessive stress and frustration, the function of the Liver and Gall Bladder will be impaired, leading to stagnation of Qi here. Prolonged Qi stagnation will gradually generate Excessive-Fire, resulting in hyperactivity of Fire. When this Fire reaches the nose, the nose will be burned, deterioration of muscle and mucosa occurs, and there will be nasal pain, with a yellow discharge.

Stagnation of Qi and Blood

Qi and Blood circulation should be maintained constantly in the nose. The formation of Damp-Heat, accumulation of Heat in the Lung and Stomach, hyperactivity of Fire of Liver and Gall Bladder and incomplete disappearance of External factors in the nose will all impair the Qi and Blood circulation in the nose, causing stagnation of Qi and Blood, and pain will follow. Qi deficiency in the Lung will also cause slowing of the Qi circulation in the nose, so stagnation of Qi follows, resulting in turn in stagnation of Blood.

Overstrain and prolonged sickness

Since the Lung opens into the nose, and the Kidney holds respiration, deficiency of the Qi and Yin of Lung or Kidney will cause malnutrition of the nose, and consequently nasal pain.

Old age, too much physical work, too much sex, constitutional weakness, frequent colds, and too much speaking and singing, may all deplete the Qi and Yin of the Lung and Kidney, leading to deficiency of Qi and Yin of the Lung and Kidney. Weakness of the Spleen and Stomach due to an unhealthy diet may also result in Qi deficiency, so the Kidney and Lung are not properly nourished, and deficiency of Lung and Kidney Qi follows.

Treatment based on differentiation

Differentiation

Differentiation of pain

— Acute onset of nasal pain, a mild pain, a burning feeling in the nose, throat pain, and redness inside the nose is usually caused by an invasion of Wind-Heat.

— Acute onset of nasal pain, mild in intensity, a cold feeling in the nose, a pale nose and headache is usually caused by an invasion of Wind-Cold.

— A chronic history of nasal pain, mild in intensity, a feeling of fullness and distension in the nose and discharge of phlegm is usually caused by deficiency of Qi and Blood resulting from weakness of the Spleen.

— A mild nasal pain over a long period, with a slight discharge of white and dilute phlegm from the nose, a poor appetite and loose stools, is usually caused by a weakness of the Spleen with formation of Damp.

— Severe nasal pain occurring deep inside the nose, throbbing or drilling pain, headache, redness in the nose, thirst and cough with expectoration of yellow phlegm, is usually caused by hyperactivity of Phlegm-Fire in the Lung, or accumulation of Damp-Heat in the Gall Bladder. Redness, swelling and heat in the nose, with a dislike of touch, are usually caused by an invasion of Toxic Heat.

Differentiation of pus

— Acute onset of a nasal pain with slight white phlegm, headache and generalised body pain, is usually caused by an invasion of Wind-Cold.

— Gradual onset of a profuse amount of yellow pus that has a foul smell, with headache, is usually caused by accumulation of Damp-Heat in the Gall Bladder.

— Prolonged existence of white and diluted pus, whether a small or profuse amount, is usually caused by weakness of the Spleen with formation of Damp-Phlegm.

— A discharge of yellow pus with a foul smell over a long period of time, with headache, is usually caused by weakness of the Spleen and Lung with accumulation of stubborn Damp-Heat.

Differentiation of smelling

— Sudden loss of smell, slight redness of the mucous membrane in the nose, a runny nose with white discharge, and headache, is usually caused by an invasion of Wind-Heat or Toxic Heat.

— A gradual onset of poor smelling, and a swollen and whitish mucous membrane in the nose, is usually caused by deficiency of the Spleen and Lung-Qi.

— Gradual onset of a loss of smell, swelling and a purplish mucous membrane in the nose, with a stabbing nasal pain, is usually caused by stagnation of Qi and Blood with blockage of the collateral in the nose.

— Gradual loss of smell, discharge of sticky phlegm from the nose, cough, expectoration of phlegm, is usually caused by accumulation of Phlegm with stagnation of Qi and Blood.

Differentiation of nasal bleeding

— Nasal bleeding, with the loss of a small amount of fresh red-coloured blood, fever and an aversion to cold is usually caused by invasion of Wind-Heat, or Toxic Heat.

— Profuse nasal bleeding, with fresh red-coloured blood, thirst, constipation, nervousness, headache, a red tongue and a wiry pulse is usually caused by hyperactivity of Fire of the Liver or Stomach.

— Intermittent nasal bleeding, with slightly fresh red-coloured blood, aggravation of nasal bleeding at night, night sweating, thirst, a dry nose, throat and lip, dry stools, tiredness and a thready, weak and rapid pulse, is usually caused by deficiency of Yin of the Liver and Kidney with hyperactivity of Deficient-Fire.

— Intermittent nasal bleeding, with light red-coloured blood, aggravation of nasal bleeding by tiredness, spontaneous sweating, loose stools and shortness of breath is usually caused by deficiency of Spleen and Lung-Qi.

Treatment

INVASION OF WIND-COLD

Symptoms and signs

Acute onset of nasal pain, a stuffed-up nose, a diminished sense of smell, or a complete disappearance of it, an aversion to cold, a slight fever, runny nose with a white discharge, headache, a cough with expectoration of white phlegm, chest pain, a thin and white tongue coating and a superficial and tight pulse, specially at the Lung position.

Principle of treatment

Dispel Wind and eliminate Cold, disperse Lung-Qi and relieve the blockage in the nose.

HERBAL TREATMENT

Prescription

MA HUANG TANG
Ephedra Decoction
Ma Huang *Herba Ephedrae* 10 g
Gui Zhi *Ramulus Cinnamomi* 6 g
Xing Ren *Semen Armeniacae* 10 g
Zhi Gan Cao *Radix Glycyrrhizae Praeparata* 6 g
Xi Xin *Herba Asari* 3 g
Jie Gen *Radix Platycodi* 6 g

Explanations

- Ma Huang and Gui Zhi, pungent and warm in nature, promote sweating so as to dispel the Exogenous Wind and Cold.
- Ma Huang and Xing Ren disperse the Lung-Qi and cause it to descend so as to relieve cough and low fever.
- Xi Xin promotes the Lung-Qi circulation and dispels Wind-Cold.
- Jie Gen disperses the Lung-Qi and eliminates Phlegm from the nose.
- Zhi Gan Cao harmonises the actions of the other herbs in the prescription.

Modifications

1. If there is a stuffed-up nose, add Bai Zhi *Radix Angelicae Dahuricae* 10 g to eliminate the Cold and relieve the blockage.
2. If there is fever and an aversion to cold, add Qiang Huo *Rhizoma seu Radix Notopterygii* 10 g and Chai Hu *Radix Bupleuri* 5 g to promote sweating and dispel the Wind.
3. If there is a cough and expectoration of white phlegm due to the invasion of the Lung by Wind-Cold, add Ban Xia *Rhizoma Pinelliae* 10 g and Chen Pi *Pericarpium Citri Reticulatae* 5 g to disperse the Lung-Qi, dispel the Wind-Cold and relieve the cough.
4. If there is headache, add Chuan Xiong *Rhizoma Ligustici Chuanxiong* 10 g and Qiang Huo *Rhizoma*

seu Radix Notopterygii 10 g to dispel the Wind-Cold and relieve the headache.

Patent remedy

Chuan Xiong Cha Tiao Wan *Ligusticum and Green Tea Regulating Pill*

ACUPUNCTURE TREATMENT

LI-4 Hegu, LI-20 Yingxiang, LU-7 Lieque, LU-6 Kongzui, BL-2 Zanzhu, BL-12 Fengmen, BL-13 Feishu and BL-64 Jinggu. Reducing method is used on these points.

Explanations

- LI-4 and LU-7 open the skin pores and promote sweating so as to dispel Wind-Cold. Also, these two points relieve problems on the face, including nasal problems. Since the Large Intestine channel ends at the nose, LI-4, the Source point, promotes circulation of Qi and Blood in the channel so as to relieve the blockage.
- LU-7, the Connecting point, opens the nasal orifice and eliminates blockage in the nose.
- LI-20, BL-2 and BL-64 promote the physiological function of the nose, relieve blockage and sedate the pain.
- LU-6, the Accumulation point, promotes Qi circulation in the Lung channel and arrests pain in the nose.
- BL-12 and BL-13 dispel Wind-Cold and relieve the symptoms from disorder of the Lung system.

Modifications

1. If there is an aversion to cold, coldness of the nose and chills due to heavy invasion of Cold, apply moxibustion on LI-4, LI-20, LU-7, BL-12 and BL-13 to warm the body and dispel the Cold.
2. If there is severe cough with expectoration of white phlegm, due to failure of the Lung to disperse Qi, add LU-1 and LU-5 to disperse the Lung-Qi and relieve the cough.
3. If there is expectoration of profuse phlegm, add SP-6 and ST-40 to activate the Spleen and Stomach and resolve the Phlegm.
4. If there is a diminishment or lack of the sense of smell due to nasal blockage and the Lung is failing to disperse Lung-Qi properly, add SI-18 and ST-36 to clear the nasal passage and tonify the Lung-Qi.

5. If there is chest pain due to stagnation of Lung-Qi, add CV-17 to promote the Qi circulation in the chest and relieve the pain.

Case history

A 53-year-old man had complained of nose pain with a blocked nose for 10 days, when he had caught a cold. The doctor diagnosed a cold and rhinitis and gave him some tablets for the cold. There had been some improvement in his headache and fever, but not the nasal pain, so he had requested acupuncture treatment. When he arrived in the acupuncture department, he had a slight headache, an aversion to cold, a stiff neck, a clear nasal discharge and a cold sensation on his limbs besides the nose pain. His tongue was thin and white, and pulse was superficial and wiry, especially at the first level of the right Cun position.

Diagnosis
Invasion of External Cold.

Principle of treatment
Promote Lung-Qi circulation, dispel Wind-Cold and relieve the nasal pain.

Acupuncture treatment
LI-4 Hegu, LI-20 Yingxiang, LU-7 Lieque, BL-2 Zanzhu, BL-7 Tongtian and GB-20 Fengchi were needled with reducing method. One treatment was given every day.

Explanations

- LI-4 is the Source point of the Large Intestine channel. LU-7 is the Connecting point of the Lung channel. These two points in combination regulate Lung-Qi and dispel External Cold in the Lung channels, as well as clearing the blocked nose. When the pathogenic factors are dispelled, nasal pain will disappear.
- CB-20 is the patent point to regulate the Qi and improve the sense of smell. Here it can also serve as a point to dispel Wind-Cold and relieve external symptoms.
- BL-7 warms the channels and regulates the Qi circulation in the vicinity, especially for nasal disorders.
- LI-20 and BL-2 increase the circulation of Qi in the nose so as to relieve the pain.

After being treated for 1 week, the nasal pain had completely resolved.

Half year later he was followed up, and had experienced no more nasal pain since the end of the acupuncture treatment.

INVASION OF WIND-HEAT

Symptoms and signs

Acute nasal pain, redness and swelling of the nose, a yellow nasal discharge, fever, a slight aversion to cold, headache, a thirst, a cough with yellow expectoration, redness and pain of the throat, a red tongue, especially at the tip, with a thin and yellow coating and a superficial and rapid pulse, especially at the Lung position.

Principle of treatment

Dispel Wind, clear Heat and disperse the Lung-Qi.

HERBAL TREATMENT

Prescription

SANG JU YIN
Mulberry Leaf and Chrysanthemum Decoction
Sang Ye *Folium Mori* 6 g
Ju Hua *Flos Chrysanthemi* 6 g
Jie Geng *Radix Platycodi* 5 g
Lian Qiao *Fructus Forsythiae* 10 g
Xing Ren *Semen Armeniacae Amarum* 10 g
Bo He *Herba Menthae* 6 g
Gan Cao *Radix Glycyrrhizae* 6 g
Lu Gen *Rhizoma Phragmitis* 15 g

Explanations

- Sang Ye, Ju Hua and Bo He clear Heat and dispel Wind-Heat in the Upper Burner.
- Lian Qiao clears Heat, releases Toxin and dispels Wind-Heat.
- Jie Geng and Xing Ren cause the Lung-Qi to descend so as to stop cough and resolve Phlegm.
- Lu Gen clears Heat and promotes the production of Body Fluids so as to relieve thirst.
- Gan Cao harmonises the actions of other herbs in the prescription.

Modifications

1. If the nose is red and swollen, add Pu Gong Ying *Herba Taraxaci* 10 g and Zhi Zi *Fructus Gardeniae* 10 g to clear the Heat, eliminate the Toxin and reduce the swelling.
2. If there is a discharge of yellow liquid from the nose, add Huang Qin *Radix Scutellariae* 10 g and Zi Hua Di Ding *Herba Violae* 15 g to eliminate the Toxin and clear the Heat.
3. If there is fever due to predominance of Heat invasion, add Chai Hu *Radix Bupleuri* 5 g and Shen Ma *Rhizoma Cimicifugae* 5 g to clear the Heat and reduce the fever.
4. If there is headache due to disturbance of the clear Yang in the head by Wind-Heat, add Chuan Xiong *Rhizoma Ligustici Chuanxiong* 10 g and Man Jing Zi

Fructus Viticis 10 g to dispel the Wind-Heat and sedate the headache.

5. If there is a cough and expectoration of yellow phlegm due to invasion of the Lung by Wind-Heat, add Qian Hu *Radix Peucedani* 10 g and Zhe Bei Mu *Bulbus Fritillariae Thunbergii* 10 g to disperse the Lung-Qi and dispel the Wind-Heat.

Patent remedies

Yin Qio Pian *Honeysuckle and Forsythia Tablet*
Yin Qiao Jie Du Pian *Honeysuckle and Forsythia Tablet to Overcome Toxins*

ACUPUNCTURE TREATMENT

LI-4 Hegu, LI-20 Yingxiang, LU-6 Kongzui, LU-7 Lieque, LU-10 Yuji, BL-2 Zanzhu, BL-12 Fengmen, BL-13 Feishu and BL-64 Jinggu. Reducing method is used on these points.

Explanations

- LI-4 and LU-7 open the skin pores and promote sweating so as to relieve invasion of Wind-Heat, LI-4, the Source point, promotes circulation of Qi and Blood in this channel so as to relieve the blocked nose. LU-7, the Connecting point, opens the nasal orifice and unblocks the nose.
- LI-20, BL-2 and BL-64 promote the physiological function of the nose and clear the blockage.
- LU-6, the Accumulation point, promotes Qi circulation in the Lung channel and arrests the nasal pain.
- LU-10, the Spring point, clears Heat, reduces the swelling and relieves the nasal pain.
- BL-12 and BL-13 dispel Wind-Heat and relieve the symptoms of Lung channel disorder.

Modifications

1. If there is fever due to severe invasion of Heat, add GV-14 and LI-11 to clear the Heat and reduce the fever.
2. If there is a cough with expectoration of yellow phlegm due to invasion of Lung by Wind-Heat, add LU-5, the Sea point, and ST-40 to disperse the Lung-Qi, clear the Heat and resolve the Phlegm.
3. If there is a thirst due to consumption of the Body Fluids by Wind-Heat, add LU-8, the Metal point, to promote the secretion of Body Fluids and relieve the thirst.
4. If there is headache due to disturbance of the clear Yang by Wind-Heat, add GB-20 and Extra Taiyang to dispel the Wind-Heat and relieve the headache.

INVASION OF TOXIC HEAT

Symptoms and signs

Acute onset of nasal pain, redness, heat and swelling in the nose, a yellow discharge, fever, a slight aversion to cold, headache, thirst, a cough with yellow expectoration, redness and pain in the throat, a red tongue, specially the tip, with a thin and yellow coating, and a superficial and rapid pulse, specially at the Lung position.

Principle of treatment

Clear Heat, remove toxin and stop pain.

HERBAL TREATMENT

Prescription

WU WEI XIAO DU YIN
Five-Ingredient Decoction to Eliminate Toxin
Jin Yin Hua *Flos Lonicerae* 20 g
Ye Ju Hua *Flos Chrysanthemi Indici* 15 g
Pu Gong Ying *Herba Taraxaci* 30 g
Zi Hua Di Ding *Herba Violae* 30 g
Zi Bei Tian Kui *Herba Begonia Fibristipulatae* 15 g
Jie Gen *Radix Platycodi* 6 g
Xin Yi *Flos Magnoliae* 6 g

Explanations

- Jin Yin Hua and Pu Gong Ying clear Heat and eliminate Wind to relieve pain in the nose.
- Ye Ju Hua, Zi Hua Di Ding and Zi Bei Tian Kui eliminate Toxin and cool the Blood to relieve the nasal pain.
- Jie Gen disperses the Lung-Qi and eliminates Phlegm.
- Xin Yi promotes the circulation of Qi and opens the nasal orifice.

Modifications

1. If there is a high fever and an aversion to cold, add Cai Hu *Radix Bupleuri* 5 g and Shen Ma *Rhizoma Cimicifugae* 5 g to clear the Heat and lower the body temperature.
2. If there is a headache, add Shi Gao *Gypsum Fibrosum* 30 g and Chuan Xiong *Rhizoma Ligustici Chuanxiong* 10 g to clear the Toxic Heat and relieve the pain.
3. If there is a fever with thirst, add Huang Lian *Rhizoma Coptidis* 5 g, Da Qing Ye *Folium Isatidis* 10 g and Zhi Mu *Rhizoma Anemarrhenae* 10 g to clear the Heat and relieve the thirst.

4. If there is constipation, add Da Huang *Radix et Rhizoma Rhei* 10 g and Mang Xiao *Natrii Sulfas* 10 g to clear the Fire by promoting defecation.

5. If there is a yellow discharge, add Niu Bang Zi *Fructus Arctii* 10 g and Dan Nan Xing *Arisaema cum Bile* 10 g to clear the Heat and resolve the Phlegm.

Patent remedy

Niu Huang Jie Du Pian *Cattle Gallstone Tablet to Resolve Toxin*

ACUPUNCTURE TREATMENT

LI-4 Hegu, LI-11 Quchi, LI-20 Yingxiang, LU-5 Chize, LU-7 Lieque, LU-10 Yuji, ST-3 Juliao, ST-44 Neiting, SP-6 Sanyinjiao and GV-10 Lingtai. Reducing method is used on these points.

Explanations

- LI-14 and LI-11 clear Heat, remove toxin and reduce fever.
- LI-20 and ST-3 clear Heat and toxin in the nose.
- LU-5, LU-10 and LU-7 clear Heat, disperse Lung-Qi and relieve cough. Also, they promote the opening of the nose.
- ST-44, SP-6 and GV-10 clear Heat, remove toxin and reduce swelling of the nose.

Modifications

1. If there is a fever, add GV-14 to clear the Heat and reduce the fever.
2. If there is a headache due to disturbance of the Clear Yang by Wind-Heat, add Extra Taiyang and TE-2 to clear the Heat and relieve the headache.
3. If there is restlessness due to invasion of Heart by toxic Heat, add HT-3 and HT-7 to clear the Heat and calm the Mind.
4. If there is a cough with yellow phlegm, add LU-1 and ST-40 to disperse the Lung-Qi and resolve the Phlegm.

ACCUMULATION OF DAMP-HEAT IN THE SPLEEN AND STOMACH

Symptoms and signs

Chronic onset of nasal pain, redness of the nasal mucosa, slight redness and swelling of the nose, a loss of the sense of smell, itching in the nose, a yellow nasal discharge, a feeling of fullness in the abdomen, a poor appetite, loose stools, a red tongue with a yellow and greasy coating and a slippery and rapid pulse.

Principle of treatment

Activate the Spleen and Stomach, eliminate Damp and clear Heat.

HERBAL TREATMENT

Prescription

SAN REN TANG
Three-Nut Decoction
Xing Ren *Semen Armeniacae* 10 g
Hua Shi *Talcum* 10 g
Yi Yi Ren *Semen Coicis* 15 g
Hou Po *Cortex Magnoliae Officinalis* 10 g
Bai Kou Ren *Semen Amomi Rotundus* 6 g
Ban Xia *Rhizoma Pinelliae* 10 g
Tong Cao *Medulla Tetrapanacis* 10 g
Zhu Ye *Herba Lophatheri* 10 g
Jie Gen *Radix Platycodi* 6 g

Explanations

- Xing Ren and Jie Gen disperse the Lung-Qi to eliminate Damp.
- Bai Kou Ren promotes the circulation of Spleen-Qi circulation and eliminates Damp.
- Ban Xia and Hou Po regulate the circulation of Spleen-Qi circulation and dry Damp.
- Yi Yi Ren, Hua Shi and Tong Cao promote urination and eliminate Damp.
- Zhu Ye is used to clear the Internal Heat.

Modifications

1. If there is no sense of smell, add Xin Yi *Flos Magnoliae* 10 g and Cang Er Zi *Fructus Xanthii* 10 g to promote the Qi circulation and improve the sense of smell.
2. If there is a yellow discharge from the nose, add Ku Shen *Radix Sophorae Flavesentis* 10 g and Dong Gua Zi *Semen Benincasae* 10 g to dry the Damp and clear the Heat.
3. If the appetite is poor, add Sha Ren *Fructus Amomi* 10 g to promote the Spleen-Qi circulation and improve the appetite.
4. If there are loose stools, add Cang Zhu *Rhizoma Atractylodis* 10 g to dry the Damp and promote the Spleen-Qi circulation.

Patent remedy

Xiang Sha Yang Wei Wan *Nourish the Stomach Pill with Aucklandia and Amomum*

ACUPUNCTURE TREATMENT

LI-4 Hegu, LI-20 Yingxiang, ST-3 Juliao, ST-34 Liangqiu, ST-40 Fenglong, ST-44 Neiting, SP-6 Sanyinjiao and SP-9 Yinlingquan. Reducing method is used on these points.

Explanations

- The Large Intestine channel and the Stomach channel meeting at the nose. If there is accumulation of Damp-Heat in the Spleen and Stomach, Damp-Heat may flow with the Qi circulation in the channel to the nose, causing a blocked nose, so pain follows.
- LI-4 promotes Qi and Blood circulation and relieves nasal pain.
- LI-20 and ST-3, the local points, open the nasal orifice and relieve blockage in the nose by Damp-Heat.
- ST-34, the Accumulation point, and ST-40, the Connecting point, harmonise the collateral and clear blockage in the Stomach channel.
- ST-44, the Spring point, SP-6, the crossing point of the three Yin channels of the foot, and SP-9, the Sea point, clear Heat and eliminate Damp.

Modifications

1. If there is discharge of yellow phlegm from the nose and cough due to accumulation of Phlegm-Heat in the Lung, add LU-5, the Sea point, and LU-10, the Spring point, to clear the Heat, eliminate the Phlegm and relieve the cough.
2. If there is loss of smell, add SI-18 and BL-2, the local points, to open the nasal orifice and promote the physiological function of the nose.
3. If the nose is red and swollen, add LI-2, the Spring point, and LI-11, the Sea point, to clear the Heat and reduce the swelling.
4. If there is fullness of the abdomen, poor appetite and loose stools, add SP-3, the Source point, and SP-4, the Connecting point and the Confluence point of the Penetrating Vessel, to activate the Spleen and improve the digestion.

Case history

A 14-year-old boy had been suffering from a painful nose for about 10 days. He was ill with acute sinusitis. He had been given Western medical treatment with antibiotics when he went to clinic. The nasal swelling and blockage had improved but his nose was still painful. When he arrived at the acupuncture clinic he had a slightly blocked nose. He also had other symptoms, such as a yellow discharge from the nose, a dulled sense of smell, a bitter taste in the mouth, a poor appetite, a red tongue with a white greasy coating and a deep wiry pulse.

Diagnosis
Accumulation of Damp-Heat in the Spleen channel.

Principle of treatment
Clear Damp-Heat and relieve the pain.

Acupuncture treatment
LI-4 Hegu, LI-20 Yingxiang, ST-40 Fenglong and SP-6 Sanyinjiao were needled with a reducing method. Treatment was given every other day for a period of 10 days.

Explanations

- LI-4, the Source point of the Large Intestine channel, clears Damp-Heat and regulates Qi circulation in the Large Intestine channel.
- ST-40, the Connecting point of the Stomach channel, clears Damp-Heat.
- SP-6, the crossing point of the three Yin channels of the feet, promotes urination and so clears Damp-Heat.
- LI-20 is the local point to promote Qi circulation and improve the sense of smell.
- After 20 days of treatment, the pain had disappeared completely. A year later, he was followed up and he reported he had had no pain in the nose since the last treatment.

ACCUMULATION OF EXCESSIVE-HEAT IN THE LUNG AND STOMACH

Symptoms and signs

Gradual onset of nose pain with a burning sensation, epistaxis, tenderness adjacent to the nose, chest pain, thirst, a tendency to hunger, a foul smell in the mouth, constipation, a red tongue with a yellow coating and a rapid and wiry pulse.

Principle of treatment

Clear Heat, promote defecation and relieve the pain.

HERBAL TREATMENT

Prescription

BAI HU TANG
White Tiger Decoction
Shi Gao *Gypsum Fibrosum* 30 g
Zhi Mu *Rhizoma Anemarrhenae* 12 g
Gan Cao *Radix Glycyrrhizae* 6 g

Jing Mi *Semen Oryzae* 30 g
Xin Yi *Flos Magnoliae* 10 g
Pu Gong Ying *Herba Taraxaci* 10 g

Explanations

- Shi Gao and Zhi Mu clear Heat, replenish the Yin and relieve the thirst.
- Essence Mi and Gan Cao tonify the Qi and prevent the first two herbs from injuring the Stomach by Cold.
- Pu Gong Ying clears Fire and removes Toxin.
- Xin Yi promotes the circulation of Lung-Qi and improves the sense of smell.

Modifications

1. If there is thirst, add Sheng Ma *Rhizoma Cimicifugae* 5 g and Da Qing Ye *Folium Isatidis* 10 g to clear the Heat and relieve the thirst.
2. If there is nose bleeding, add Zhu Ye *Herba Lophatheri* 10 g and Ou Jie *Nadus Nelumbinis Rhizomatis* 10 g to clear the Heat and stop the bleeding.
3. If there is a foul smell in the mouth, add Jin Yin Hua *Flos Lonicerae* 10 g and Zhi Zi *Fructus Gardeniae* 10 g to clear the Heat in the Stomach.
4. If there is constipation, add Da Huang *Radix et Rhizoma Rhei* 10 g and Mang Xiao *Natrii Sulfas* 10 g to clear the Fire in the Stomach and promote defecation.

Patent remedy

Qing Fei Yi Huo Pian *Clear Lungs Restrain Fire Tablet*

ACUPUNCTURE TREATMENT

LI-4 Hegu, LI-11 Quchi, LI-20 Yingxiang, LU-5 Chize, LU-10 Yuji, ST-3 Juliao, ST-40 Fenglong and ST-44 Neiting. Reducing method is used on these points.

Explanations

- Since the Large Intestine and the Stomach channel are both Bright Yang channels, and the Lung and the Large Intestine share a pair of channels and collateral, they may influence each other. If there is an accumulation of Heat in the Stomach or in the Lung, then there will be Heat in the Large Intestine as well. In other words, clearing Heat from the Large Intestine will also reduce Heat in the Lung and Stomach.

- LI-4, the Source point, and LI-11, the Sea point, clear Heat, promote defecation and cool the Lung and Stomach.
- LI-20 and ST-3, the local points, open the nasal orifice and relieve the nasal pain.
- LU-5, the Sea point and Water point, and LU-10, the Spring point, clear Heat in the Lung and disperse the Lung-Qi.
- ST-40, the Connecting point, and ST-44, the Spring point, clear Heat in the Stomach and harmonise the collateral to arrest the nasal pain.

Modifications

1. If there is a cough and expectoration of yellow phlegm, add LU-1, the Front Collecting point of the Lung, and BL-13, the Back Transporting point of the Lung, to clear the Heat in the Lung and relieve the cough.
2. If the nose is dry, add LU-8, the Metal point, and SP-6 to promote secretion of Body Fluids and relieve the Dryness.
3. If there is constipation, add ST-25, the Front Collecting point of the Large Intestine, and ST-37, the Lower Sea point of the Large Intestine, to promote defecation and relieve constipation.
4. If there is a tendency to frequent hunger, add CV-12, the Front Collecting point of the Stomach, to clear the Heat in the Stomach and relieve the hungry feeling.

HYPERACTIVITY OF FIRE OF LIVER AND GALL BLADDER

Symptoms and signs

Gradual onset of nose pain with a burning feeling, a discharge of yellow and sticky phlegm from the nose with a foul smell, a diminished sense of smell, headache, a sense of distension of the head, nervousness, red eyes, a bitter taste in the mouth, tinnitus, a red tongue with a yellow coating and a rapid and wiry pulse.

Principle of treatment

Clear Heat, reduce Fire and relieve the pain.

HERBAL TREATMENT

Prescription

LONG DAN XIE GAN TANG
Gentianae Decoction to Drain the Liver
Long Dan Cao *Radix Gentianae* 6 g
Huang Qin *Radix Scutellariae* 9 g

Zhi Zi *Fructus Gardeniae* 9 g
Ze Xie *Rhizoma Alismatis* 12 g
Mu Tong *Caulis Akebiae* 9 g
Che Qian Zi *Semen Plantaginis* 9 g
Dang Gui *Radix Angelicae Sinensis* 3 g
Sheng Di Huang *Radix Rehmanniae Recens* 9 g
Chai Hu *Radix Bupleuri* 6 g
Gan Cao *Radix Glycyrrhizae* 6 g
Xin Yi *Flos Magnoliae* 10 g

Explanations

- Long Dan Cao and Huang Qin clear Heat and dry Damp.
- Zhi Zi, Mu Tong, Ze Xie and Che Qian Zi clear Heat and eliminate Damp through urination.
- Dang Gui and Sheng Di Huang nourish the Yin and Blood and prevent the actions of the other herbs from injuring the Yin.
- Chai Hu regulates the Liver-Qi and removes Qi stagnation.
- Xin Yi promotes the circulation of Qi and improves the sensory function of the nose.
- Gan Cao harmonises the actions of the other herbs in the formula.

Modifications

1. If there is a yellow discharge from the nose, add Zhi Mu *Rhizoma Anemarrhenae* 10 g, Dan Nan Xing *Rhizoma Arisaematis preparation Cum Fell Bovis* 10 g and Bo He *Herba Menthae* 3 g to clear the Heat and eliminate the Phlegm.
2. If there is headache, add Chai Hu *Radix Bupleuri* 5 g and Chuan Xiong *Rhizoma Ligustici Chuanxiong* 10 g to regulate the Liver-Qi and relieve the pain.
3. If there is a foul smell in the mouth, add Shi Gao *Gypsum Fibrosum* 30 g and Huang Lian *Rhizoma Coptidis* 5 g to clear the Heat and improve the taste.
4. If there is nervousness, add Yu Jin *Radix Curcumae* 10 g and Chai Hu *Radix Bupleuri* 5 g to regulate the Liver-Qi and calm the emotions.
5. If there is constipation, add Da Huang *Radix et Rhizoma Rhei* 10 g and Mang Xiao *Natrii Sulfas* 10 g to clear the Fire by promoting defecation.

Patent remedy

Long Dan Xie Gan Wan *Gentianae Pill to Drain the Liver*

ACUPUNCTURE TREATMENT

LI-4 Hegu, LI-11 Quchi, LI-20 Yingxiang, GB-15 Toulinqi, GB-16 Muchuang, GB-20 Fengchi and LR-2 Xingjian. Reducing method is used on these points.

Explanations

- LI-4 and LI-11 clear Heat and reduce Fire in the body.
- LI-20 promotes the opening of the nasal orifice and relieves the nasal pain.
- GB-15 and GB-16 clear Heat and reduce Fire from the Gall Bladder. Also, these two points have a function in clearing the nasal passage and relieving blockage, to stop the nasal pain.
- GB-20 and LR-2 clear Heat and reduce Fire from the Liver and Gall Bladder.

Modifications

1. If there is a stuffed-up nose, add Extra Bitong and BL-2 to clear the nasal passage.
2. If the nose is red and swollen, add SI-18 and ST-3 to clear Heat and reduce the swelling.
3. If there is headache and nervousness, add GV-20 to calm the Liver and subdue the Liver-Fire.
4. If there is discharge of yellow phlegm from the nose with a foul smell and a diminished sense of smell, add LU-5 to clear Phlegm in the nose and promote smelling.

DEFICIENCY OF QI AND YIN OF LUNG AND KIDNEY

Symptoms and signs

Minor nasal pain, diminished or loss of sense of smell, a tendency to catch colds easily, a frequent white nasal discharge, cough, an aversion to cold, shortness of breath by exertion, lower back pain, poor memory, tiredness, heat in the palms and soles of the feet, thirst, red tongue with a thin and white coating and a deep, thready and weak pulse.

Principle of treatment

Tonify Qi, nourish Yin and benefit the nose.

HERBAL TREATMENT

Prescription

LIU WEI DI HUANG WAN
Six-Flavour Rehmanniae Pill
Mai Dong *Radix Ophiopogonis* 12 g
Wu Wei Zi *Fructus Schisandrae* 10 g
Shu Di Huang *Radix Rehmanniae Praeparata* 24 g
Shan Zhu Yu *Fructus Corni* 12 g
Shan Yao *Radix Dioscoreae* 12 g
Fu Ling *Poria* 9 g

Mu Dan Pi *Cortex Moutan Radicis* 9 g
Ze Xie *Rhizoma Alismatis* 9 g

Explanations

- Mai Dong nourishes the Lung-Yin. Wu Wei Zi strengthens the deficient Qi and Yin.
- Shu Di Huang, Shan Zhu Yu and Shan Yao tonify the Blood and the Essence of the Liver and Kidney.
- Ze Xie promotes urination and clears Heat.
- Mu Dan Pi cools the Blood and activates its circulation.
- Fu Ling strengthens the Spleen.

Modifications

1. If there is shortness of breath, add Ren Sen *Radix Ginseng* 10 g to tonify the Lung-Qi and improve the breathing.
2. If there is aversion to Cold, add Huang Qi *Radix Astragali seu Hedysari* 10 g to tonify the Qi.
3. If there is a white discharge from the nose, add Fang Feng *Radix Ledebouriellae* 10 g and Dang Gui *Radix Angelicae Sinensis* 10 g to dry up the discharge from the nose.
4. If there is lower back pain, add Gou Qi Zi *Fructus Lycii* 10 g and Yan Hu Suo *Rhizoma Corydalis* 10 g to tonify the Qi and regulate its circulation to relieve the pain.
5. If there is thirst add Sheng Di Huang *Radix Rehmanniae Recens* 12 g and Xuan Shen *Radix Scrophulariae* 10 g to nourish the Kidney-Yin and increase the Body Fluids to relieve the thirst.

Patent remedy

Liu Wei Di Huang Wan *Six-Flavour Rehmanniae Pill*

ACUPUNCTURE TREATMENT

LU-5 Chize, LU-8 Jingqu, LU-9 Taiyuan, LI-20 Yingxiang, SI-18 Quanliao, ST-3 Juliao, ST-36 Zusanli, SP-6 Sanyinjiao and KI-3 Taixi. Reinforcing method is used on these points, except for LI-20, ST-3 and SI-18, on which even method is employed.

Explanations

- LU-5, the Sea point, tonifies the Qi and Yin of the Lung and promotes the physiological function of the nose.
- LU-8, the Metal point, nourishes the Yin of the Lung and promotes the secretion of Body Fluids.

- LU-9, the Source point, reinforces the Lung-Qi, opens the nasal orifice and activates the circulation of Qi in the Lung channel so as to reinforce the Qi and Yin of the Lung.
- LI-20, SI-18 and ST-3, the local points, open the nasal orifice and promote the physiological function of the nose.
- ST-36, the Sea point of the Stomach channel, tonifies the Qi of the general body.
- SP-6 and KI-3 tonify the Qi and Yin of the Kidney.

Modifications

1. If there is a tendency to catch colds easily, add LU-7, the Connecting point, and BL-13, the Back Transporting point, with reinforcing method to consolidate the skin and prevent a cold invasion.
2. If there is a diminished or no sense of smell, add BL-2 and GV-24 to open the nasal orifice and improve the sense of smell.
3. If there is general tiredness, shortness of breath on exertion and lower back pain, add KI-10 and BL-23 to tonify the Kidney and benefit the Kidney-Essence.
4. If the nose is dry and the palms and soles of the feet are hot owing to deficiency of Yin, add KI-2 and KI-7 to clear the Deficient-Heat and nourish the Kidney-Yin.

STAGNATION OF BLOOD

Symptoms and signs

Stabbing pain in the nose, aggravation of the pain at night, a purplish colour to the nose, a swollen nose, headache, insomnia, chest pain, depression, a purplish tongue with a thin and white tongue and a wiry pulse.

Principle of treatment

Smooth the Liver, circulate the Qi and Blood and eliminate Blood stasis.

HERBAL TREATMENT

Prescription

TAO HONG SI WU TANG
Four-Substance Decoction with Safflower and Peach Pit
Dang Gui *Radix Angelicae Sinensis* 10 g
Sheng Di Huang *Radix Rehmanniae Recens* 12 g
Chi Shao *Radix Paeoniae Rubra* 10 g

Chuan Xiong *Rhizoma Ligustici Chuanxiong* 6 g
Tao Ren *Semen Persicae* 10 g
Hong Hua *Flos Carthami* 10 g
Jie Gen *Radix Platycodi* 6 g

Explanations

- Sheng Di Huang and Chi Shao tonify the Blood and nourish the fluid in the Large Intestine.
- Chuan Xiong and Hong Hua promote the Blood circulation and eliminate Blood stagnation.
- Dang Gui and Tao Ren regulate the Blood circulation and eliminate Blood stagnation; also, these two herbs may lubricate the Large Intestine if there is a hard stool.
- Jie Gen promotes the circulation of Lung-Qi and improves the sensitivity of the nose.

Modifications

1. If the nose is swollen, add Fang Feng *Radix Ledebouriellae* 10 g and Xi Xin *Herba Asari* 3 g to promote the Qi circulation and improve the sense of smell in the nose.
2. If there is headache, add Bai Zhi *Radix Angelicae Dahuricae* 10 g and Qiang Huo *Rhizoma seu Radix Notopterygii* 10 g to regulate the Qi circulation and relieve the pain.
3. If there is depression, add Chai Hu *Radix Bupleuri* 5 g and Yu Jin *Radix Curcumae* 10 g to promote the Qi circulation and improve the emotional state.
4. If there is insomnia, add Suan Zao Ren *Semen Ziziphi Spinosae* 10 g and Dan Shen *Radix Salviae Miltiorrhizae* 10 g to calm down the Mind and improve the sleep.

Patent remedy

Xiao Huo Luo Dan *Minor Invigorate the Collaterals Special Pill*

ACUPUNCTURE TREATMENT

LI-4 Hegu, LI-20 Yingxiang, LU-5 Chize, LU-7 Lieque, SI-18 Quanliao, BL-2 Zanzhu, BL-17 Geshu, LR-3 Taichong and SP-6 Sanyinjiao. Reducing method is used on these points.

Explanations

- LI-4 and LR-3 promote circulation of the Qi so as to increase the Blood circulation and arrest nasal pain.
- Since the Lung opens into the nose, LU-5 and LU-7 are used here to promote the opening of the nasal orifice and activate the Qi and Blood circulation in the Lung channel.
- LI-20, SI-18 and BL-2, the local points, promote the physiological function of the nose and relieve nasal pain.
- SP-6 and BL-17 promote the circulation of Blood and eliminate its stasis.

Modifications

1. If there is headache, add GB-20 and Extra Taiyang to circulate the Qi and Blood in the head and relieve the headache.
2. If there is restlessness and insomnia, add HT-3 and BL-15 to calm the Mind and improve sleep.
3. If there is chest pain and depression due to stagnation of Liver-Qi, add LR-14, CV-17 and PC-6 to smooth the Liver, circulate the Liver-Qi and relieve the depression.

口
唇
疼
痛

Lip pain is often seen together with toothache or tongue pain. However, it can also occur by itself. Lip pain may be attributed to any of the following diseases in Western medicine: herpes labialis, cracked lip, cheilitis, herpes zoster, fever sores, aphtosis, aphthous stomatitis, aphthous ulcer, angular stomatitis and canker sore.

Aetiology and pathology

Invasion of External factors and Toxin

The lip connects with the mouth, and the mouth is the opening of the Stomach and the passage of respiration dominated by the Lung. Since the mouth and lips are exposed to the external environment, there are many opportunities for External pathogens to invade. Invasion of the lips by Wind-Cold, Wind-Heat, Damp-Heat, or Toxic Heat, are often causes of lip pain resulting from disturbance of Qi and Blood on the lips. For instance, herpes zoster is often due to invasion of one of the above pathogenic factors. Generally speaking, careless living habits, overstrain or prolonged illness are the underlying causes for invasion of External pathogenic factors. Insect bites are also a common cause for lip pain.

Accumulation of Heat in the Spleen and Stomach

The lip is the external reflection of the Spleen, and the Stomach channel reaches the mouth and circulates around the lips. If a person eats too much pungent, sweet or fatty food or dairy products, or drinks too much alcohol, the Spleen and Stomach will be impaired, leading to the formation of Excessive-Heat and Fire in the body. If there is uprising of Heat and Fire to the lips, then lip pain will occur.

Stagnation of Qi and Blood

Excessive emotionality, prolonged stress, invasion of External Cold that persists for a long time in the body, exposure to Cold for too long, or even deficiency of Qi, may cause poor circulation of the Qi and Blood, leading to a blockage of the channels and collateral around the mouth and lips, and lip pain will appear here.

Moreover, inappropriate surgery and physical trauma to the lips may directly cause stagnation of Qi and Blood and damage of the collateral, and lip pain may result.

Hyperactivity of Deficient-Fire

Prolonged febrile diseases, chronic diarrhoea or vomiting, or excessive sweating, excessive emotionality with generation of Fire, overstrain with lack of proper rest, excessive intake of warming herbs, or prolonged bleeding during menstruation or from haemorrhoids, may all cause consumption of the Yin. This situation could lead to a deficiency of Yin with the formation of Deficient-Fire.

When there is hyperactivity of Deficient-Fire, the Heat goes up and disturbs the collateral around the lips and lip pain occurs.

Treatment based on differentiation

Differentiation

Differentiation of External or Internal origin

— Acute onset of lip pain, mild in intensity, accompanied by External symptoms, such as an aversion to cold, fever, muscle pain, runny nose, cough or a superficial pulse, is usually caused by invasion of External factors.
— A chronic history of lip pain, mild or severe pain in intensity, association of the lip pain with diet, emotional state and other physical conditions, is usually caused by disorder of the Internal Zang-Fu organs.

Differentiation of character of the pain

— Acute sharp lip pain with a burning sensation, a thin and yellow tongue coating, together with some External symptoms, is usually caused by invasion of Wind-Heat.
— Acute sharp lip pain with a cold sensation, accompanied by External symptoms, such as an aversion to cold, slight fever, muscle pain or absence of thirst, is usually caused by invasion of Wind-Cold.
— Acute sharp lip pain with a burning sensation and swelling of the lip, redness and heat in the lip, fever, an aversion to cold, headache, throat pain and swelling, restlessness and constipation, is usually caused by invasion of Toxic Heat.
— Chronic sharp lip pain with a burning sensation, redness of the face, aggravation of the pain by consumption of pungent food, constipation, a foul smell in the mouth, or thirst, is usually caused by accumulation of Heat in the Spleen and Stomach.
— Chronic sharp or stabbing lip pain, which is related with emotional upsets, or is aggravated at night, with purplish lips, is usually caused by stagnation of Qi and Blood.
— Chronic sharp facial pain with a slight burning sensation and dryness, redness of the face, aggravation of the pain by exertion, night sweating, dry stools, or a peeled tongue coating, is usually caused by hyperactivity of Deficient-Fire.

Treatment

INVASION OF WIND-COLD

Symptoms and signs

Sudden onset lip pain after catching cold, a cold feeling on the face and lips, a purplish colour around the lips, aggravation of lip pain on exposure to cold, an aversion to cold, a slight fever, headache, generalised body pain, a lack of thirst, a cough with expectoration of white phlegm, a thin white tongue coating and a superficial and tight pulse.

Principle of treatment

Dispel Wind, eliminate Cold and remove the Toxin.

HERBAL TREATMENT

Prescription

JING FANG BAI DU SAN
Schizonepeta and Ledebouriella Powder to Overcome Pathogenic Influences
Jing Jie *Herba Schizonepetae* 10 g
Fang Feng *Radix Ledebouriellae* 10 g
Zi Su Ye *Folium Perillae* 10 g
Bai Zhi *Radix Angelicae Dahuricae* 10 g
Chuan Xiong *Radix Ligustici Chuanxiong* 10 g
Qiang Huo *Rhizoma et Radix Notopterygii* 10 g
Cong Bai *Bulbus Allii* 5 g
Sheng Jiang *Rhizoma Zingiberis Recens* 5 g

Explanations

● Jing Jie and Fang Feng promote sweating, dispel Wind and eliminate Cold.
● Chuan Xiong regulates the Qi and Blood circulation and relieves the lip pain.

- Zi Su Ye dispels Wind-Cold and relieves cough.
- Qiang Huo and Bai Zhi dispel Wind-Cold and relieve body pain.
- Cong Bai and Sheng Jiang dispel Wind-Cold and help the above herbs to relieve External symptoms.

Modifications

1. If the lips are swollen, add Qing Dai *Indigo Naturalis* 5 g to eliminate the toxin and reduce the swelling.
2. If there is an aggravation of lip pain on exposure to cold, add Gan Jiang *Rhizoma Zingiberis* 5 g and Gui Zhi *Ramulus Cinnamomi* 5 g to warm the interior and dispel the Cold.
3. If the lips are a purplish colour, add Chi Shao *Radix Paeoniae Rubra* 10 g and Dan Shen *Radix Salviae Miltiorrhizae* 10 g to promote the Blood circulation and reduce the purplish colour.
4. If there is headache, add Man Jing Zi *Fructus Viticis* 10 g to dispel the Wind-Cold and sedate the headache.
5. If there is a cough and expectoration of white phlegm Ban Xia *Rhizoma Pinelliae* 10 g and Bai Jie Zi *Semen Sinapis Albae* 10 g to dispel the Cold in the Lung and relieve the cough.

Patent remedies

Jing Fang Bai Du Pian *Schizonepeta and Ledebouriella Tablet to overcome Pathogenic Influences*
Chuan Xiong Cha Tiao Pian *Ligusticum and Green Tea Regulating Powder*

ACUPUNCTURE TREATMENT

LI-4 Hegu, LU-7 Lieque, BL-12 Fengmen, TE-5 Waiguan, CV-24 Chengjiang and ST-4 Dicang. Reducing method is used on these points.

Explanations

- LI-4, the Source point, and LU-7, the Connecting point, promote sweating, dispel Wind, and eliminate Cold and Toxin.
- TE-5 dispels Wind, and eliminates and relieves the lip pain.
- BL-12 dispels Wind-Cold and relieves the general symptoms due to invasion of Wind-Cold.
- CV-24 and ST-4, the local points, promote the circulation in the collateral, reduce the swelling and relieve the lip pain.

Modifications

1. If there is severe lip pain, add ST-34 and SP-8, the Accumulation points, to eliminate the Toxin and relieve the lip pain.
2. If the lips are swollen, add ST-40, the Connecting point, to reduce the swelling and relieve the lip pain.
3. If there are insect bites, add SP-6 and GV-10 to eliminate the toxin and reduce the swelling.
4. If there is aggravation of the lip pain on exposure to cold, add moxibustion on LI-4, TE-5 and CV-6 to warm the interior and dispel the Cold.
5. If there is headache, add GB-20 to dispel the Wind-Cold and sedate the headache.
6. If there is cough and expectoration of white phlegm due to invasion of Wind-Cold in the Lung, add LU-5, the Sea point of the Lung, and BL-13, the Back Transporting point, to disperse the Lung-Qi, dispel the Wind-Cold and relieve the cough.

INVASION OF WIND-HEAT

Symptoms and signs

Sudden onset of lip pain with a burning feeling, yellow blisters on the lips, red and swollen lips, fever, a slight aversion to cold, headache, thirst, cough, a red-tipped tongue with a thin and yellow coating, and a superficial and rapid pulse.

Principle of treatment

Dispel Wind, clear Heat and remove the Toxin.

HERBAL TREATMENT

Prescription

YIN QIAO SAN
Honeysuckle and Forsythia Powder
Jin Yin Hua *Flos Lonicerae* 6 g
Lian Qiao *Fructus Forsythiae* 10 g
Zhu Ye *Herba Lophatheri* 6 g
Pu Gong Ying *Herba Taraxaci* 10 g
Ban Lan Gen *Radix Isatidis* 10 g
Huang Qin *Radix Scutellariae* 10 g
Zhi Gan Cao *Radix Glycyrrhizae Praeparata* 5 g

Explanations

- Jin Yin Hua and Lian Qiao dispel Wind, clear Heat and eliminate Toxin.
- Pu Gong Ying and Ban Lan Gen clear Heat, reduce fever and eliminate Toxin.

- Zhu Ye clears Heat and promotes the production of Body Fluids so as to relieve External symptoms.
- Huang Qin clears Heat in the Upper Burner, causes the Lung-Qi to descend and relieves pain.
- Zhi Gan Cao eliminates Toxin, removes nodules, benefits the throat and stops the pain.

Modifications

1. If there are yellow blisters on the lips, add Long Dan Cao *Radix Gentianae* 5 g and Zi Hua Di Ding *Herba Violae* 10 g to clear the Heat and eliminate the Toxin.
2. If the lips are swollen, add Huang Lian *Rhizoma Coptidis* 5 g and Chi Shao *Radix Paeoniae Rubra* 10 g to reduce the swelling.
3. If there are insect bites, add Ban Bian Lian *Herba Lobeliae Radicantis* 10 g to clear the Heat, eliminate the Toxin and reduce the swelling.
4. If the lips are dry, or cracked, add Lu Gen *Rhizoma Phragmitis* 10 g and Yu Zhu *Rhizoma Polygonati Odorati* 10 g to promote the secretion of Body Fluids and relieve the Dryness.
5. If there is fever, add Ye Ju Hua *Flos Chrysanthemi Indici* 10 g to clear the Heat and reduce the fever.
6. If there is headache, add Man Jing Zi *Fructus Viticis* 10 g to dispel the Wind-Heat and sedate the headache.
7. If there is a cough and expectoration of yellow phlegm due to invasion of the Lung by Wind-Heat, add Zhe Bei Mu *Bulbus Fritillariae Thunbergii* 10 g to dispel the Wind-Heat and relieve the cough.

Patent remedies

Yin Qiao Pian *Honeysuckle and Forsythia Tablet*
Yin Qiao Jie Du Pian *Honeysuckle and Forsythia Tablet to Overcome Toxins*

ACUPUNCTURE TREATMENT

LI-2 Erjian, LI-4 Hegu, LU-7 Lieque, LU-10 Yuji, TE-5 Waiguan, CV-24 Chengjiang, ST-4 Dicang and GV-28 Yinjiao. Reducing method is used on these points.

Explanations

- LI-2 and LU-10, the Spring points from the Large Intestine and Lung channels respectively, clear Heat, reduce fever, reduce swelling and stop the lip pain.
- LI-4, the Source point, and LU-7, the Connecting point, promote sweating, dispel Wind, clear Heat and eliminate Toxin.

- TE-5 dispels Wind, clears Heat and relieves the lip pain.
- CV-24, ST-4 and GV-28, the local points, clear Heat and reduce the swelling.

Modifications

1. If there are many blisters with yellow discharge owing to the invasion of Toxic Damp-Heat, add GB-43 and ST-44 to eliminate the Toxin, eliminate the Damp and clear the Heat.
2. If the lips are swollen, add ST-40, the Connecting point, to reduce the swelling and diminish the lip pain.
3. If there are insect bites, add SP-6 and GV-10 to clear the Heat, eliminate the Toxin and reduce the swelling.
4. If there is fever, add GV-14 to clear Heat and reduce the fever.
5. If there is a headache, add GB-20 to dispel the Wind-Heat and sedate the headache.
6. If there is a cough and expectoration of yellow phlegm due to invasion of Wind-Heat in the Lung, add BL-12 and BL-13 to disperse the Lung-Qi and dispel the Wind-Heat.

Case history

A 10-year-old girl had suffered from lip pain for 8 days. She was ill with acute cheilitis on her arrival from south China 10 days previously. She had been given Western medical treatment with antibiotics for 10 days. After this treatment, her lip swelling had improved, but the pain remained.

When she arrived at the clinic, she still had slightly swollen lips, especially the lower lip. The pain was constant with a slightly burning feeling. Besides painful lips, she had a slight aversion to cold, a fever (38.4°C), thirst, a dry mouth and sore throat, constipation, a red tip to her tongue and a dry yellow coating, and a floating and rapid pulse.

Diagnosis
Invasion of Wind-Heat.

Principle of treatment
Clear Heat, dispel Wind and relieve the pain.

Acupuncture treatment
LI-2 Erjian, LI-4 Hegu, LU-7 Lieque, TE-5 Waiguan and ST-25 Tianshu were needled with reducing method. Treatment was given daily, over a period of 6 days.

Explanations
- LI-2, the Spring point, clears Fire in the Bright Yang channels and cools the Large Intestine channel, which has an Internal and External relationship with the Lung.

- LI-4, the Source point of the Large Intestine channel, promotes sweating, clears Heat and reduces Fire.
- LU-7, the Connecting point of the Lung channels, dispels Wind-Heat and reduces Fire.
- TE-5, the Connecting point of the Triple Burner channel, dispels Wind-Heat, regulates the circulation of Qi and reduces Heat.
- ST-25, the Front Collecting point of the Large Intestine, regulates the circulation of Qi in the local area to relieve constipation.

After being treated for 5 days, the girl's painful lips had resolved completely. Three months later her mother was visited for follow-up. She stated that the girl had had no pain since her last treatment.

ACCUMULATION OF HEAT IN THE SPLEEN AND STOMACH

Symptoms and signs

Lip pain with redness and swelling, cracked lips, or ulceration on the lips or tongue, thirst, a preference for cold drinks, a tendency to feel hungry, toothache, a foul smell from the mouth, constipation, stomach pain, sometimes gum bleeding, a red tongue with a yellow and dry coating and a rapid and forceful pulse.

Principle of treatment

Clear Heat, reduce Fire and arrest the pain.

HERBAL TREATMENT

Prescription

QING WEI SAN
Clear Heat in the Stomach Powder
Huang Lian *Rhizoma Coptidis* 10 g
Dang Gui *Radix Angelicae Sinensis* 6 g
Sheng Di Huang *Radix Rehmanniae* 15 g
Sheng Ma *Rhizoma Cimicifugae* 10 g
Mu Dan Pi *Cortex Moutan Radicis* 10 g
Shi Gao *Gypsum Fibrosum* 20 g
Zhi Mu *Rhizoma Anemarrhenae* 10 g
Huang Qin *Radix Scutellariae* 10 g

Explanations

- Huang Lian, Huang Qin and Sheng Ma clear Heat, eliminate toxin and heal ulceration.
- Sheng Di Huang and Mu Dan Pi clear Heat and cool the Blood.
- Dang Gui nourishes the Blood, increases the circulation of Blood and reduces swelling.
- Shi Gao and Zhi Mu clear Stomach-Fire and nourish the Body Fluids.

Modifications

1. If the lips are ulcerated and swollen, add Chi Shao *Radix Paeoniae Rubra* 10 g and Zhi Zi *Fructus Gardeniae* 10 g to clear the Fire, cool the Blood and reduce the swelling.
2. If there is thirst, add Xuan Shen *Radix Scrophulariae* 10 g and Zhu Ye *Herba Lophatheri* 10 g to clear the Fire and nourish the Body Fluids.
3. If the gums are bleeding, add Bai Mao Gen *Rhizoma Imperatae* 10 g to clear the Stomach-Fire and stop the bleeding.
4. If there is stomach ache, add Yan Hu Suo *Rhizoma Corydalis* 10 g and Bai Shao *Radix Paeoniae Alba* 10 g to regulate the Stomach-Qi and relieve the pain.
5. If there is constipation, add Da Huang *Radix et Rhizoma Rhei* 10 g and Mang Xiao *Natrii Sulfas* 10 g to eliminate Heat through defecation.

Patent remedy

Wei Te Ling *Stomach Especially Effective Remedy*

ACUPUNCTURE TREATMENT

ST-3 Juliao, ST-4 Dicang, GV-28 Yinjiao, ST-42 Chongyang, ST-44 Neiting, ST-45 Lidui, SP-2 Dadu, LI-4 Hegu and LI-11 Quchi. Reducing method is used on these points.

Explanations

- ST-42, the Source point, clears Heat and harmonises the Stomach.
- ST-44, the Spring-point and the Water point of the Stomach channel, can clear Heat in the Stomach directly, suppress Stomach-Fire and reduce pain.
- ST-45, the Son point of the Stomach channel, eliminates Heat from the Stomach.
- SP-2, the Spring and Fire point of the Spleen channel, is capable of clearing Heat in the Spleen and reducing Fire.
- Since both the Stomach and Large Intestine are Bright Yang Fu organs, having a mutual influence on each other especially in Excessive cases, LI-4, the Source point and LI-11, the Sea point, clear Heat in the Large Intestine and promote defecation so as to drain Heat from the Stomach.
- ST-3, ST-4 and GV-28, the local points, clear Heat, harmonise the collateral and stop the lip pain.

Modifications

1. If the tongue and lips are ulcerated, with a foul smell in the mouth, owing to Excessive-Heat in the Stomach, add SP-6 and ST-40 to clear the Heat and reduce the Fire.
2. If the gums are bleeding owing to disturbance of the blood vessels by hyperactivity of Stomach-Fire, add SP-10 to clear the Heat and cool the Blood.
3. If there is stomach pain due to disturbance of the Stomach by Excessive-Heat, add CV-12, the Front Collecting point, and BL-21, the Back Transporting point of the Stomach, to clear the Heat and harmonise the Stomach.
4. If there is thirst and the lips and mouth are dry owing to consumption of Body Fluids in the Stomach and Spleen by Heat, add SP-5, the Metal point, to promote secretion of Body Fluids and relieve the thirst.
5. If there is constipation due to Heat in the Large Intestine, add ST-25, the Front Collecting point of the Large Intestine, to clear the Heat and promote defecation.

STAGNATION OF QI AND BLOOD

Symptoms and signs

Intermittent occurrence of painful lips, closely related to the emotional state, sometimes a stabbing pain, tic or numbness of the lips, purplish lips, a purplish tongue with a thin coating, and a wiry pulse.

Principle of treatment

Circulate Qi and Blood and sedate the pain.

HERBAL TREATMENT

Prescription

TAO HONG SI WU TANG plus **SHI XIAO SAN**
Four-Substance Decoction with Safflower and Peach Pit plus *Sudden Smile Powder*
Chai Hu *Radix Bupleuri* 5 g
Bai Shao *Radix Paeoniae Alba* 10 g
Xiang Fu *Rhizoma Cyperi* 10 g
Yu Jin *Radix Curcumae* 10 g
Dang Gui *Radix Angelicae Sinensis* 10 g
Sheng Di Huang *Radix Rehmanniae Recens* 12 g
Chi Shao *Radix Paeoniae Rubra* 10 g
Chuan Xiong *Rhizoma Ligustici Chuanxiong* 6 g
Tao Ren *Semen Persicae* 10 g
Hong Hua *Flos Carthami* 10 g

Pu Huang *Pollen Typhae* 10 g
Wu Ling Zhi *Faeces Trogopterorum* 5 g

Explanations

- Chai Hu smoothes the Liver and promotes the Qi circulation in the Liver.
- Bai Shao harmonises and relaxes the Liver and relieves the lip pain.
- Xiang Fu promotes the Qi circulation so as to promote Blood circulation.
- Sheng Di Huang and Chi Shao regulate the Blood and promote its circulation.
- Chuan Xiong, Yu Jin, Tao Ren and Hong Hua promote the Blood circulation and remove its stagnation.
- Dang Gui regulates the Blood circulation and tonifies the Blood.
- Pu Huang and Wu Ling Zhi remove Blood stagnation and relieve the pain.

Modifications

1. If there is emotional upset, add Xia Ku Cao *Spica Prunellae* 10 g to cool the Liver and reduce the Liver-Fire.
2. If the lips are numb, add Tian Ma *Rhizoma Gastrodiae* 10 g and Chan Tui *Pertostracum Cicadae* 10 g to calm the Liver and suppress the Liver-Wind.
3. If the lips are purplish in colour, add Mo Yao *Resina Myrrhae* 10 g to promote the Blood circulation and remove Blood stagnation.
4. If there is a stabbing pain, add Dan Shen *Radix Salviae Miltiorrhizae* 10 g and Yan Hu Suo *Rhizoma Corydalis* 10 g to remove Blood stagnation and relieve the lip pain.

Patent remedy

Xiao Huo Luo Dan *Minor Invigorate the Collaterals Special Pill*

ACUPUNCTURE TREATMENT

ST-4 Dicang, CV-24 Chengjiang, GV-28 Yinjiao, LI-4 Hegu, LR-3 Taichong, SP-6 Sanyinjiao and SP-10 Xuehai. Even method is used on CV-24 and GV-28. Reducing method is employed on the other points.

Explanations

- Stagnation of Qi and Blood may cause rather severe lip pain.

- LI-4, indicated in all facial problems caused by Excessive pathogenic factors, promotes the Qi and Blood circulation on the face and mouth, harmonises the collateral and relieves the lip pain.
- It would be incorrect to treat stagnation of Blood without applying some points to promote the circulation of Qi, since Qi circulation leads to Blood circulation. Thus LR-3 is prescribed to circulate the Qi and relieve pain in the lips. When LR-3 is used together with LI-4, the effectiveness in promoting Qi circulation will be increased.
- SP-6 and SP-10 promote the circulation of Blood and relieve its stagnation so as to stop the lip pain.
- ST-4, CV-24 and GV-28 are the local points, but also good points in treating the lip pain. Bleeding method can be applied on GV-28 to achieve better therapeutic results.

Modifications

1. If the lips are obviously swollen, add BL-17 to promote the Blood circulation and eliminate the Blood stasis.
2. If there is emotional upset, add LR-2, the Spring point, and LR-14, the Front Collecting point, to smooth and calm the Liver.
3. If there is pain and spasm of the facial muscles owing to stagnation of Blood, add ST-5 and ST-6 to harmonise the collateral and arrest the pain and spasm.
4. If there are tics of the lips, add GB-20 to calm the Liver and subdue the Wind.
5. If the tongue is painful owing to stagnation of Blood, add HT-5, the Connecting point, and HT-6, the Accumulation point, to circulate the Blood, eliminate the Blood stasis and relieve the painful tongue.
6. If there is a generalised stabbing pain in the body owing to stagnation of Blood, add ST-40 and SP-21 to promote circulation of the Blood and relieve the pain.

HYPERACTIVITY OF DEFICIENT-FIRE

Symptoms and signs

Dry and painful lips, cracked lips, hot flushes, night sweating, thirst, restlessness, insomnia, dry stools or constipation, a red tongue with a scanty or peeled coating and a deep, thready and rapid pulse.

Principle of treatment

Nourish Yin, descend Deficient-Fire and sedate the pain.

HERBAL TREATMENT

Prescription

ZHI BAI DI HUANG WAN
Anemarrhena, Phellodendron and Rehmannia Pill
Shu Di Huang *Radix Rehmanniae Praeparata* 24 g
Shan Zhu Yu *Fructus Corni* 12 g
Shan Yao *Radix Dioscoreae* 12 g
Fu Ling *Poria* 9 g
Mu Dan Pi *Cortex Moutan Radicis* 9 g
Ze Xie *Rhizoma Alismatis* 9 g
Zhi Mu *Rhizoma Anemarrhenae* 10 g
Huang Bai *Cortex Phellodendri* 6 g
Sha Shen *Radix Adenophorae* 15 g

Explanations

- Shu Di Huang, Shan Zhu Yu and Shan Yao tonify the Blood and nourish the Yin of the Liver and Kidney.
- Ze Xie promotes urination and clears the Heat.
- Mu Dan Pi cools the Blood and activates its circulation.
- Fu Ling strengthens the Spleen, drains Damp and promotes Qi and Blood production.
- Sha Shen nourishes the Yin and clears Internal Heat.
- Zhi Mu and Huang Bai nourish the Yin, clear Deficient-Fire and stop hot flushes.

Modifications

1. If the lips are cracked, add Sheng Di Huang *Radix Rehmanniae Recens* 10 g and Xuan Shen *Radix Scrophulariae* 10 g to nourish the Yin and promote the secretion of Body Fluids so as to lubricate the lips.
2. If there is insomnia, add Suan Zao Ren *Semen Ziziphi Spinosae* 10 g and Wu Wei Zi *Fructus Schisandrae* 10 g to calm the Heart and tranquillise the Mind.
3. If there is night sweating, add Mu Li *Concha Ostreae* 15 g and Lian Xu *Stamen Nelumbinis* 10 g to stop the night sweating.
4. If there is restlessness, add Huang Lian *Rhizoma Coptidis* 5 g to clear the Heat in the Heart and calm the Mind.
5. If there is constipation, add Xuan Shen *Radix Scrophulariae* 10 g and Da Huang *Radix et Rhizoma Rhei* 10 g to promote defecation.

Patent remedy

Zhi Bai Di Huang Wan *Anemarrhena, Phellodendron and Rehmannia Pill*

ACUPUNCTURE TREATMENT

KI-2 Rangu, KI-3 Taixi, KI-7 Fuliu, KI-10 Yingu, SP-2 Dadu, SP-6 Sanyinjiao, CV-24 Chengjiang and ST-4 Dicang.

Even method is used on KI-2, CV-24, ST-4 and SP-2. Reinforcing method is employed on KI-3, KI-7, KI-10 and SP-6.

Explanations

- The mouth and lips are the opening orifices of the Spleen, and the Kidney-Yin is the root Yin of the body. Thus some points from the Kidney and Spleen channels are applied.
- KI-2 and SP-2, the Spring points of the Kidney channel and Spleen respectively, clear Deficient-Heat and reduce Deficient-Fire.
- KI-7, the Metal point, promotes the secretion of Body Fluids in the Kidney channel and nourishes the Kidney-Yin so as to control Deficient-Fire.
- KI-3, the Source point, and KI-10, the Sea point, are applied to tonify the Kidney and regulate its physiological function so as to treat Kidney deficiency. Also, KI-10 is the Water point of the Kidney channel, being able to nourish the Yin directly and promote the secretion of Body Fluids in the Kidney.
- SP-6, the crossing point for the three Yin channels of the foot, nourishes the Yin in general and tonifies the Kidney.
- ST-4 and CV-24, the local points, circulate the Qi and Blood in the area and harmonise the collateral to arrest the pain.

Modifications

1. If there is lower back pain and weakness of the knees due to deficiency of the Kidney-Yin, add BL-23, the Back Transporting point of the Kidney, and BL-58, the Connecting point of the Bladder channel, to tonify the Kidney, harmonise the collateral and sedate the lower back pain.
2. If there is nocturia due to weakness of the Kidney-Qi, add CV-4 and KI-6 to tonify the Kidney and relieve the nocturia.
3. If there is insomnia and dream-disturbed sleep due to disharmony between the Kidney and Heart, add HT-3 and HT-8 to calm the Heart, nourish the Heart-Yin and reduce the Deficient-Fire.

4. If there is thirst and a dry mouth, add LU-8, the Metal point, and Extra Jinjin and Extra Yuye, to promote the secretion of Body Fluids and relieve the thirst.
5. If there is constipation due to deficiency of Body Fluids in the Large Intestine, add ST-25, the Front Collecting point of the Large Intestine, to promote defecation and relieve the constipation.

Case history

A 39-year-old woman had been suffering from lip pain for 6 months. She complained of lip pain with a dry sensation when she was tired or angry for some reason. She was diagnosed with chronic aphthous ulcer. Besides lip pain, she had a dry mouth, thirst but with little desire for drinking, a poor appetite and a dry stool. Her tongue was red with a scanty coating. Her pulse was thready, and weak, but wiry at the Liver position.

Diagnosis
Yin deficiency of the Liver and the Stomach with a hyperactivity of Deficient-Fire.

Principle of treatment
Nourish Yin, clear Fire and relieve the pain.

Acupuncture treatment
SP-6 Sanyinjiao, KI-3 Taixi, LR-3 Taichong, LI-4 Hegu, ST-3 Juliao, ST-42 Chongyang, ST-44 Neiting and CV-24 Chengjiang were selected. Reinforcing method was used for SP-6, KI-3, LR-3 and ST-42. ST-3 and CV-24 were needled with even method. LI-4 and ST-44 were needled with reducing method. Treatment was given every other day, for a period of one month.

Explanations
- SP-6, the crossing point of the three Yin channels of the foot to nourish the Yin, regulates the Qi circulation and relieves the pain.
- ST-42, the Source point, nourishes the Yin of the Stomach and clears Deficient-Fire.
- LR-3, the Source point, calms the Liver and nourishes the Yin of the Liver.
- KI-3, the Stream and Source point of the Kidney channel, nourishes the Yin of the body generally.
- LI-4, the Source point of the Large Intestine channel, and ST-44, the Spring point of the Stomach channel, clear Stomach-Heat and relieve the lip pain.
- ST-3 and CV-24 are used as local points to regulate the Qi circulation and relieve the pain.

After 30 days of treatment, her lip pain was relieved. One year later, she was visited and she said she had not had painful lips since then.

Tooth pain 16

牙
齿
疼
痛

Toothache is a complaint that is commonly encountered in daily practice. In mild cases, besides the toothache there is an increased sensitivity of the teeth to sour, cold and hot food. However, severe cases may also be accompanied by headache, swollen cheeks, bleeding gums, difficulty in eating, fever, chills, or even insomnia and restlessness. According to TCM, toothache is normally caused by invasion of Wind-Heat, uprising of Stomach-Fire, hyperactivity of Deficient-Fire from the Kidney, deficiency of Kidney-Yang or bacterial infection of the teeth.

Aetiology and pathology

Invasion of Wind

The head is located at the top of the body, where all the Yang channels meet. When External Wind invades it first attacks the upper parts of the body, so the teeth can be involved. Invasion of Wind-Heat and that of Wind-Cold are two common factors leading to the onset of toothache. If there is invasion of Wind-Heat then Qi and Blood circulation in the mouth will be accelerated and disturbed, resulting in an accumulation of Heat. If there is invasion of Wind-Cold, it may block the Qi and Blood circulation, causing toothache.

Uprising of Stomach Fire

Both the Bright Yang channels of hand and foot are related to the teeth; the Large Intestine channel enters the upper teeth, and the Stomach channel enters the lower teeth. If there is overindulgence in pungent, sweet or fatty food, or milk products, or alcohol, Excessive-Heat may accumulate in the Bright Yang channels, leading to toothache pain. As well as the toothache, there will be other symptoms such as a foul smell in the mouth, thirst, bleeding or swollen gums, constipation and deep red urine.

Weakness of the Kidney

According to TCM theory, the Kidney dominates the Bones, and the teeth are considered to be 'an extension of the bones', so the state of the Kidney energy influences greatly the condition of the teeth. If there is deficiency of Kidney-Essence without specific deficiency of Yin or of Yang, the teeth are merely loose or may be lost, but there is no pain. However, if there is hyperactivity of Deficient-Fire from the Kidney, the teeth will be disturbed by this, which leads to symptoms such as intermittent toothache over a long period, red and swollen gums, loose teeth,

145

sweating and feeling too warm at night, heat in the palms and soles and lower back pain, etc. Deficiency of Kidney-Yin is often caused by too much sex and masturbation, ageing, overstrain with lack of sufficient rest, too much study, prolonged sickness, too much blood loss during menstruation, haemorrhoids, chronic nasal and gum bleeding, drinking too much alcohol as well as prolonged use of corticosteroid drugs. It may also be caused by congenital weakness of the Kidney derived from the parents.

Toothache can also be caused by deficiency of Kidney-Yang. This may be caused by ageing, chronic illness, eating too little, especially too little nutritious food or overstrain, as these may cause interior Cold to form. Cold is characterised by contraction and stagnation, and if there is a state of interior Cold due to deficiency of Kidney-Yang, this may affect the teeth through the Kidney channel, bringing about stagnation of the Qi and Blood in the channel, so causing toothache.

Bacterial infection of the teeth

Overeating of sweet, fatty food, incorrect tooth brushing and lack of oral hygiene may all cause accumulation of turbid and dirty matter in the mouth and on the teeth, which provides the opportunity for bacteria to invade the teeth, so toothache follows.

Treatment based on differentiation

Differentiation

Differentiation of External or Internal origin

— Acute onset of tooth pain, sharp or with a cold sensation, aggravation of the pain by exposure of the teeth to cold or heat, and accompanied by External symptoms, is usually caused by invasion of External factors.
— A chronic history of tooth pain, mild or severe in intensity, association of the pain with diet, emotional state and other physical conditions, is usually caused by disorder of the Internal Zang-Fu organs.

Differentiation of character of the pain

— Acute sharp tooth pain with a cold sensation, accompanied by External symptoms, such as an aversion to cold, slight fever, muscle pain,

absence of thirst, is usually caused by invasion of Wind-Cold.
— Acute sharp tooth pain with a burning sensation, an aversion to cold, fever, throat pain, a cough, thin and yellow tongue coating and a superficial and rapid pulse, is usually caused by invasion of Wind-Heat.
— Chronic sharp tooth pain, or chronic tooth pain with acute aggravation, with a burning sensation, redness of the face and gums, aggravation of the tooth pain by consumption of pungent food, constipation, a foul smell in the mouth, or thirst, is usually caused by accumulation of Heat in the Stomach.
— Chronic tooth pain, which is intermittent, is dull in nature with a slight burning pain, with loose teeth, slight redness of the gums, swelling of the gums, thirst, night sweating, dry stool, or lower back pain, is usually caused by hyperactivity of Deficient-Fire in the Kidney.
— Chronic intermittent tooth pain, alleviation of the pain by warmth, with loose teeth, lack of redness and swelling of the gums, an aversion to cold, cold hands and feet, much salivation, or lower back pain, is usually caused by deficiency of Kidney-Yang.
— Tooth pain with caries, intermittent toothache, aggravation by touch, chewing, or contact with sour food, is usually caused by bacterial infection.

Treatment

INVASION OF WIND-HEAT

Symptoms and signs

Acute onset of toothache, aggravation of the pain on eating hot food, and its alleviation with cold food and cold drinks, swollen gums with slight bleeding, fever, an aversion to cold, a cough, throat pain, thirst, constipation, a red tip to the tongue and a thin and yellow coating, and a superficial and rapid pulse.

Principle of treatment

Dispel Wind, clear Heat and remove the Toxin.

HERBAL TREATMENT

Prescription

YIN QIAO SAN
Honeysuckle and Forsythia Powder
Jin Yin Hua *Flos Lonicerae* 10 g
Lian Qiao *Fructus Forsythiae* 10 g
Jie Geng *Radix Platycodi* 6 g

Bo He *Herba Menthae* 6 g
Dan Dou Chi *Semen Sojae Praeparetum* 10 g
Zhu Ye *Herba Lophatheri* 10 g
Gan Cao *Radix Glycyrrhizae* 6 g
Jing Jie Sui *Spica Schizonepetae* 6 g
Niu Bang Zi *Fructus Arctii* 10 g
Lu Gen *Rhizoma Phragmitis* 10 g

Explanations

- Jin Yin Hua and Lian Qiao clear Heat and eliminate Toxin.
- Bo He, Jing Jie Sui and Dan Dou Chi promote sweating, dispel Heat and release the External symptoms.
- Niu Bang Zi, Jie Geng and Gan Cao eliminate Toxin, benefit the throat and stop the pain.
- Zhu Ye and Lu Gen clear Heat and promote the production of Body Fluids so as to relieve the thirst.

Modifications

1. If there is fever due to Wind-Heat invasion, add Ban Lan Gen *Radix Isatidis* 10 g and Huang Qin *Radix Scutellariae* 10 g to clear the Heat and reduce the fever.
2. If the gums are swollen, add Pu Gong Ying *Herba Taraxaci* 12 g and Ye Ju Hua *Flos Chrysanthemi Indici* 12 g to clear the Heat, eliminate the Toxin and reduce the swelling.
3. If there is headache, add Chuan Xiong *Rhizoma Ligustici Chuanxiong* 6 g and Man Jing Zi *Fructus Viticis* 10 g to dispel the Wind-Heat and sedate the headache.
4. If there is cough due to invasion of the Lung by Wind-Heat, add Qian Hu *Radix Peucedani* 10 g and Zhe Bei Mu *Bulbus Fritillariae Thunbergii* 10 g to disperse the Lung-Qi and dispel the Wind-Heat.
5. If there is constipation, add Da Huang *Radix et Rhizoma Rhei* 10 g and Dong Gua Ren *Semen Benincasae* 10 g to clear the Heat and promote the defecation.

Patent remedies

Yin Qiao Pian *Honeysuckle and Forsythia Tablet*
Yin Qiao Jie Du Pian *Honeysuckle and Forsythia Tablet to Overcome Toxins*

ACUPUNCTURE TREATMENT

LI-2 Erjian, LI-4 Hegu, LI-5 Yangxi, Lu-7 Lieque, ST-6 Jiache, ST-7 Xiaguan and TE-5 Waiguan. Reducing method is used on these points.

Explanations

- LI-2, the Spring point, clears and dispels External Heat and sedates toothache.
- LI-4, the Source point, and LI-5, the River point, are able to dispel Wind, clear Heat and relieve the pain. LI-4 is especially used to treat External invasion in the upper body. Moreover, this point is effective for relieving the pain due to Excessive factors.
- LU-7, the Connecting point, dispels Wind and relieves External symptoms as well as stopping toothache. When this point is prescribed together with LI-4, it increases its effect of promoting the opening of the skin pores so as to relieve External invasion. Also, LU-7 is another good point for treating facial and tooth problems.
- ST-6 and ST-7 are the local points, and can relieve External invasion and promote the Qi circulation so as to sedate the toothache.
- TE-5, the Connecting point and the Confluence point with the Yang Linking Vessel, is able to disperse external Wind-Heat invasion and relieve toothache.

Modifications

1. If there is fresh gum bleeding due to the disturbance of the blood vessels by Wind-Heat, add ST-44 and SP-10 to clear the Heat and cool the Blood. It is advisable to employ the bleeding method on LI-2 to reduce the Heat quickly and stop the bleeding.
2. If there is fever due to the invasion of Wind-Heat, add GV-14 and LI-11 to clear the Heat and reduce the fever.
3. If there is headache, add GB-20 to relieve the Wind-Heat and sedate the headache.
4. If there is a painful and swollen throat due to the invasion of Toxic Heat, add LU-10 to clear the Heat and eliminate the Toxin.
5. If there is thirst due to the consumption of Body Fluids by External Heat, add CV-23 and LU-8 to promote the secretion of Body Fluids and relieve the thirst.
6. If there is cough and expectoration of yellow phlegm due to the invasion of Wind-Heat to the Lung, add BL-12 and BL-13 to dispel the Wind-Heat from the Lung and relieve the cough.

INVASION OF WIND-COLD

Symptoms and signs

Acute onset of toothache, pain with a contracting feeling, aggravation of toothache on eating cold food or cold drinks, and its alleviation on eating warm food or drinks, an aversion to cold, a slight fever, a lack of thirst, a thin and white tongue coating, and a superficial and tight pulse.

Principle of treatment

Dispel Wind, eliminate Cold and sedate the pain.

HERBAL TREATMENT

Prescription

JING FANG BAI DU SAN

Schizonepeta and Ledebouriella Powder to Overcome Pathogenic Influences
Jing Jie *Herba Schizonepetae* 6 g
Fang Feng *Radix Ledebouriellae* 6 g
Qiang Huo *Rhizoma seu Radix Notopterygii* 6 g
Du Huo *Radix Angelicae Pubescentis* 6 g
Chai Hu *Radix Bupleuri* 6 g
Zhi Qiao *Fructus Aurantii* 6 g
Chuan Xiong *Rhizoma Ligustici Chuanxiong* 5 g
Gan Cao *Radix Glycyrrhizae* 5 g
Xi Xin *Herba Asari* 3 g

Explanations

- Jing Jie and Fang Feng dispel Wind-Cold and relieve External symptoms.
- Qiang Huo and Du Huo are pungent and Warm herbs, and promote sweating, dispel pathogenic Wind-Cold and relieve the pain.
- Chai Hu and Zhi Qiao promote the Qi circulation and relieve toothache due to stagnation of Qi resulting from Wind-Cold invasion.
- Chuan Xiong invigorates the Blood circulation and promotes Qi circulation so as to stop the toothache.
- Xi Xin, a pungent herb going to all the channels, promotes the Qi circulation and relieves toothache.
- Gan Cao is used to harmonise the actions of the other herbs in the formula.

Modifications

1. If the gums are swollen, add Ban Xia *Rhizoma Pinelliae* 10 g and Qing Pi *Pericarpium Citri Reticulatae Viride* 10 g to reduce the swelling.
2. If there is headache, add Ge Gen *Radix Puerariae* 12 g to regulate the Qi circulation and sedate the headache.
3. If there is a cough due to the invasion of the Lung by Wind-Cold, add Bai Qian *Rhizoma Cynanchi Stauntonii* 10 g to eliminate Phlegm and relieve the cough.

Patent remedy

Jing Fang Bai Du Pian *Schizonepeta and Ledebouriella Pill to Overcome Pathogenic Influences*

ACUPUNCTURE TREATMENT

LI-4 Hegu, LI-20 Yingxiang, LU-7 Lieque, ST-6 Jiache, ST-7 Xiaguan and ST-40 Fenglong. Reducing method is used on these points.

Explanations

- As mentioned above, when LI-4, the Source point, and LU-7, the Connecting point, are applied together, their effect in opening the skin pores will be heightened, increasing their effectiveness in dispersing the External invasion. They also have a function in stopping the toothache.
- LI-20, together with SP-6 and ST-7, are all local points, regulating the Qi circulation in the vicinity and stopping the pain.
- SP-40, the Connecting point, harmonises the collateral of the Stomach to relieve the toothache.

Modifications

1. If there is an obvious aversion to cold and spasm of the face due to the predominance of the invasion of Cold, apply moxibustion on the points on the face, and add TE-5 to strengthen the effectiveness in dispersing the Cold.
2. If there is headache due to slowing down of the Qi and Blood circulation in the head caused by invasion of Wind-Cold, add GB-20 and GV-16 to dispel the Wind-Cold, promote the Qi and Blood circulation in the head and relieve the headache.
3. If there is throat pain due to the accumulation of Cold in the throat, add CV-23 to eliminate the Cold and relieve the throat pain.
4. If there is a cough and expectoration of white phlegm due to failure of the Lung to disperse the Lung-Qi resulting from invasion of Wind-Cold, add BL-12 and BL-13 to disperse the Lung-Qi and relieve the cough.

ACCUMULATION OF HEAT IN THE STOMACH

Symptoms and signs

Toothache, swollen and red or bleeding gums, thirst, a dry mouth, a preference for cold drinks, a foul smell in the mouth, constipation, a tendency to get hungry, abdominal pain, restlessness, a red tongue with a yellow and dry coating and a rapid and forceful pulse.

Principle of treatment

Clear Heat, promote defecation and consolidate the teeth.

HERBAL TREATMENT

Prescription

QING WEI SAN
Clear Heat in the Stomach Powder
Huang Lian *Rhizoma Coptidis* 10 g
Dang Gui *Radix Angelicae Sinensis* 6 g
Sheng Di Huang *Radix Rehmanniae* 15 g
Sheng Ma *Rhizoma Cimicifugae* 10 g
Mu Dan Pi *Cortex Moutan Radicis* 10 g
Shi Gao *Gypsum Fibrosum* 15 g
Zhi Mu *Rhizoma Anemarrhenae* 10 g
Da Huang *Radix et Rhizoma Rhei* 10 g

Explanations

- Huang Lian and Sheng Ma clear Heat, eliminate toxin and reduce swelling.
- Sheng Di Huang and Mu Dan Pi clear Heat and cool the Blood.
- Dang Gui nourishes the Blood, invigorates the circulation of Blood and relieves swelling.
- Shi Gao and Zhi Mu clear Stomach-Heat and relieve toothache.
- Da Huang clears Heat and promotes defecation.

Modifications

1. If the gums are swollen, add Chi Shao *Radix Paeoniae Rubra* 10 g and Zhi Zi *Fructus Gardeniae* 10 g to clear the Fire and cool the Blood.
2. If there is thirst, add Xuan Shen *Radix Scrophulariae* 12 g and Zhu Ye *Herba Lophatheri* 10 g to clear the Fire and nourish the Body Fluids.
3. If the gums are bleeding, add Xuan Shen *Radix Scrophulariae* 10 g and Bai Mao Gen *Rhizoma Imperatae* 10 g to clear the Stomach-Fire, cool the Blood and stop the bleeding.
4. If there is abdominal pain, add Yan Hu Suo *Rhizoma Corydalis* 10 g and Bai Shao *Radix Paeoniae Alba* 10 g to regulate the Stomach-Qi and relieve the pain.
5. If there is severe constipation, add Mang Xiao *Natrii Sulfas* 10 g to eliminate the Heat and promote defecation.

Patent remedy

Wei Te Ling *Stomach Especially Effective Remedy*

ACUPUNCTURE TREATMENT

ST-5 Daying, ST-6 Jiache, ST-7 Xiaguan, ST-42 Chongyang, ST-44 Neiting, ST-45 Lidui, SI-18 Quanliao, LI-4 Hegu and LI-11 Quchi. Reducing method is used on these points.

Explanations

- Toothache may occur in the upper or lower teeth. Since the Stomach channel contacts the the upper teeth, if the pain is there then ST-7 and SI-18 are used together with LI-4 as local points to circulate the Qi and Blood, clear the Heat and harmonise the collateral so as to arrest the pain.
- If the toothache is in lower teeth, this area is dominated by the Large Intestine channel, so LI-4, the Source point, is used together with ST-5 and ST-6 to clear the Heat, reduce the Fire and stop the pain. Conventionally, LI-4 is a major point for treating toothache due to Excessive factors.
- ST-42, the Source point, is able to clear the Heat and harmonise the Stomach.
- ST-44, the Spring-point and the Water point of the Stomach channel, can directly clear Heat in the Stomach, subdue the Stomach-Fire and reduce the toothache.
- ST-45, the Son point of the Stomach channel, clears Heat from the Stomach. Since the Stomach and Large Intestine are both Bright Yang Fu organs, having a mutual influence on each other especially in Excessive cases, LI-11 is used to clear Heat in the Large Intestine and promote defecation so as to drain Heat from the Stomach.

Modifications

1. If the gums are bleeding because of the disturbance of the blood vessels resulting from a hyperactivity of Stomach-Fire, add SP-6 and SP-10 to clear the Heat and cool the Blood.
2. If there is a foul smell in the mouth, and stomach pain due to a disturbance of the Stomach by Excessive-Heat, add CV-12, the Front Collecting point of the Stomach, and BL-21, the Back Transporting point of the Stomach, to clear the Heat, improve the digestion and harmonise the Stomach.
3. If there is nausea and vomiting due to the uprising of Stomach-Qi, add PC-6, the Connecting point

with the Yin Linking Vessel, and SP-4, the Connecting point with the Penetrating Vessel, to cause the Stomach-Qi to descend and relieve the vomiting.

4. If there is constipation due to Heat in the Large Intestine, add ST-25, the Front Collecting point of the Large Intestine, to clear the Heat and promote defecation.

Case history

A 34-year-old man had suffered from a severe toothache for 5 days. He was ill with acute odontitis and had received Western medicine, in the form of antibiotics cefalexin and painkiller tablets. His swollen gum had been improved but his toothache had not. When he arrived at the clinic he had a slightly swollen gum in the upper left side of his mouth. His left cheek was also a little swollen and painful. His other symptoms included thirst, a bitter taste in the mouth, constipation, a red tongue with a dry and yellow coating and a rapid pulse.

Diagnosis
Accumulation of Excessive-Fire in the Stomach.

Principle of treatment
Clear Fire and eliminate Toxin.

Acupuncture treatment
ST-6 Jiache, ST-7 Xiaguan, ST-42 Chongyang, LI-4 Hegu and CV-12 Zhongwan were needled with reducing method. Treatment was given daily, over a period of 10 days.

Explanations
- ST-42, the Source point, clears Fire in the Stomach.
- ST-6 and ST-7, the local points, regulate the circulation of Qi and relieve toothache. LI-4, the Source point of the Large Intestine channel, reduces Fire and relieves the pain.
- CV-12, the Front Collecting point of the Stomach and the Gathering point for the Fu organs, reduces Stomach-Fire and regulates the Qi circulation so as to relieve the toothache.

After 8 days of treatment, the patient had got rid of the dental pain completely. He was visited 6 months later and he had experienced no more toothache after the accupuncture treatment.

HYPERACTIVITY OF DEFICIENT-FIRE FROM THE KIDNEY

Symptoms and signs

Chronic toothache, intermittent aggravation of pain, toothache that is dull in nature with a slight burning pain, loose teeth, slightly red and swollen gums, thirst, a red throat, night sweating, dry stools, lower back pain, weakness in the knees, restlessness, insomnia, a red tongue with a scanty coating and a thready and rapid pulse that is weak at the Stomach and Kidney positions.

Principle of treatment

Nourish Yin and bring down the Deficient-Fire.

HERBAL TREATMENT

Prescription

ZHI BAI DI HUANG WAN
Anemarrhena, Phellodendron and Rehmannia Pill
Zhi Mu *Rhizoma Anemarrhenae* 10 g
Huang Bai *Cortex Phellodendron* 10 g
Shu Di Huang *Radix Rehmanniae Praeparata* 15 g
Shan Zhu Yu *Fructus Corni* 12 g
Shan Yao *Rhizoma Dioscoreae* 12 g
Fu Ling *Poria* 9 g
Mu Dan Pi *Cortex Moutan Radicis* 9 g
Ze Xie *Rhizoma Alismatis* 9 g
Gui Ban *Plastrum Testudinis* 10 g

Explanations

- Shu Di Huang, Shan Zhu Yu and Shan Yao tonify the Blood and the Essence of the Liver and Kidney.
- Ze Xie promotes urination and reduces Deficient-Fire.
- Mu Dan Pi cools the Blood, activates the Blood circulation and clears Deficient-Fire.
- Fu Ling activates the Spleen so as to increase the production of Kidney-Essence.
- Zhi Mu, Huang Bai and Gui Ban nourish the Yin and clear Deficient-Fire.

Modifications

1. If there is night sweating, add Sang Piao Xiao *Ootheca Mantidis* 10 g and Mu Li *Concha Ostreae* 15 g to stop the sweating.
2. If there is insomnia, add Suan Zao Ren *Semen Ziziphi Spinosae* 10 g and Wu Wei Zi *Fructus Schisandrae* 10 g to calm the Mind.
3. If there is heat in the palms and soles, add Hu Huang Lian *Rhizoma Picrorhizae* 10 g and Qing Hao *Herba Artemisiae Chinghao* 10 g to clear the Deficient-Fire.
4. If the mouth is dry, add Sheng Di Huang *Radix Rehmanniae Recens* 15 g and Xuan Shen *Radix Scrophulariae* 12 g to nourish the Kidney Yin and relieve the thirst.

5. If there is lower back pain, add Sang Ji Sheng *Ramulus Loranthi* 10 g and Bai Shao *Radix Paeoniae Alba* 10 g to strengthen the Kidney and relieve the pain.
6. If there is constipation, add Sheng Di Huang *Radix Rehmanniae* 15 g and Xuan Shen *Radix Scrophulariae* 12 g to tonify the Yin and lubricate the Large Intestine to relieve the constipation.

Patent remedy

Zhi Bai Di Huang Wan *Anemarrhena, Phellodendron and Rehmannia Pill*

ACUPUNCTURE TREATMENT

KI-2 Rangu, KI-3 Taixi, KI-7 Fuliu, KI-10 Yingu, SP-6 Sanyinjiao, ST-6 Jiache and ST-7 Xiaguan. Reducing method is used on KI-2. Even method is used on ST-6 and ST-7. Reinforcing method is employed on the other points.

Explanations

- KI-2, the Spring point, clears Deficient-Heat and reduces Deficient-Fire.
- KI-7, the Metal point, promotes the secretion of Body Fluids in the Kidney channel, and nourishes the Kidney-Yin so as to control Deficient-Fire.
- KI-3, the Source point, and KI-10, the Sea point, are applied to tonify the Kidney and regulate its physiological function so as to treat Kidney deficiency. KI-10 is also the Water point of the Kidney channel, being able to nourish the Yin directly and promote the secretion of Body Fluids in the Kidney channel.
- SP-6 nourishes the Yin generally and tonifies the Kidney.
- ST-6 and ST-7 are local points, applied to circulate the Qi and Blood in the area and harmonise the collateral so as to arrest the toothache.

Modifications

1. If there is lower back pain and weakness of the knees due to deficiency of the Kidney-Yin, add BL-23, the Back Transporting point of the Kidney, and BL-58, the Connecting point of the Bladder channel, to tonify the Kidney, harmonise the collateral and sedate the lower back pain.
2. If there is nocturia due to weakness of the Kidney-Qi, add KI-6 to tonify the Kidney and stop the nocturia.

3. If there is general tiredness due to deficiency of Kidney-Essence, add CV-4 and CV-6 to tonify the Kidney and benefit the Kidney-Essence.
4. If there is insomnia and dream-disturbed sleep due to a disharmony between the Kidney and the Heart, add HT-3 and HT-8 to calm the Heart, to nourish Heart-Yin and to reduce the Deficient-Fire.

DEFICIENCY OF KIDNEY-YANG

Symptoms and signs

Chronic toothache with intermittent aggravation, alleviation of the pain by warmth, loose teeth, a lack of redness and swelling in the gums, an aversion to cold, cold hands and feet, excessive salivation, lower back pain, impotence, profuse clear urine, a pale tongue with tooth marks and a thin and wet coating, and a deep, thready and slow pulse, especially at the Kidney-Yang position.

Principle of treatment

Tonify Yang, eliminate Cold and sedate the pain.

HERBAL TREATMENT

Prescription

MA HUANG FU ZI XI XIN TANG
Ephedra, Asarum and Prepared Aconite Decoction
Ma Huang *Herba Ephedrae* 6 g
Fu Zi *Radix Aconiti Carmichaeli Praeparata* 10 g
Xi Xin *Herba Asari* 3 g
Bu Gu Zhi *Fructus Psoraleae* 10 g
Qiang Huo *Rhizoma seu Radix Notopterygii* 10 g

Explanations

- Ma Huang, a pungent and Warm herb, promotes the Lung-Qi circulation and dispels External Cold. Fu Zi, a Hot and Warm herb, reinforces the Kidney-Yang and relieves the toothache.
- Xi Xin and Qiang Huo, two pungent and Warm herbs, promote the Qi circulation and relieve the toothache.
- Bu Gu Zhi tonifies the Kidney-Yang and helps Fu Zi to relieve the toothache.

Modifications

1. If there is aversion to cold, add Wu Zhu Yu *Fructus Evodiae* 10 g and Rou Gui *Cortex Cinnamomi* 10 g to warm Kidney-Yang so as to relieve the pain.

2. If there is excessive salivation, add Yi Zhi Ren *Fructus Alpiniae Oxyphyllae* 10 g and Sang Piao Xiao *Ootheca Mantidis* 10 g to tonify the Kidney-Yang and reduce the salivation.
3. If there is lower back pain with soreness, add Xu Duan *Radix Dipsaci* 10 g and Sang Ji Sheng *Ramulus Loranthi* 10 g to tonify the Kidney-Yang to relieve the pain.
4. If there is impotence, add Dang Gui *Radix Angelicae Sinensis* 10 g and Yin Yang Huo *Herba Epimedii* 10 g to warm the Kidney-Yang and promote the Blood circulation.

Patent remedy

Jin Gui Shen Qi Wan *Kidney Qi Pill*

ACUPUNCTURE TREATMENT

KI-3 Taixi, KI-10 Yingu, SP-3 Taibai, ST-6 Jiache, ST-7 Xiaguan, ST-36 Zusanli and CV-4 Guangyuan. Even method is used on ST-6 and ST-7. Reinforcing method is employed on the other points; moxibustion should also be used on these.

Explanations

- KI-3, the Source point, and KI-10, the Sea point, tonify the Kidney and regulate its physiological function so as to treat deficiency of Kidney-Yang.
- SP-3, the Source point, and ST-36, the Sea point, tonify the Spleen and Stomach so as to promote the production of Qi and Yang in the body.
- CV-4 reinforces the Original Qi to tonify the Kidney, warm the Interior and eliminate Cold.
- ST-6 and ST-7 are the local points, applied to circulate the Qi and Blood in the area and harmonise the collateral so as to arrest the toothache.
- When moxibustion is used on these points, the effect in arresting pain and eliminating Interior Cold will be greater.

Modifications

1. If there is lower back pain, weakness in the knees and nocturia due to deficiency of the Kidney-Yang, add BL-23, the Back Transporting point of the Kidney, and BL-58, the Connecting point of the Bladder channel, with moxibustion to reinforce the Kidney-Yang, harmonise the collateral and sedate the lower back pain.
2. If there is general tiredness, dizziness and a poor memory due to deficiency of Kidney-Yang, add CV-6 with moxibustion to tonify the Kidney-Yang and relieve the tiredness.
3. If there is water retention with swollen legs and face due to failure of the Kidney-Yang to control water metabolism, add CV-7 and SP-9 to eliminate the excessive water and relieve the oedema.

Case history

A 69-year-old man had been ill with chronic periodontitis 6 years previously, and since that time he had experienced toothache from time to time. Besides this, he had loose teeth, and suffered from dizziness and tiredness, especially after exertion, and had an aversion to cold and cold limbs. His tongue was enlarged and pale with a white coating, and he had a deep and thready pulse.

Diagnosis
Deficiency of Kidney-Yang.

Principle of treatment
Tonify Kidney-Yang, warm the channel and relieve the pain.

Herbal treatment
MA HUANG FU ZI XI XIN TANG (modified)
Ephedra, Asarum and Prepared Aconite Decoction (modified)
Ma Huang *Herba Ephedrae* 6 g
Fu Zi *Radix Aconiti Praeparata* 10 g
Xi Xin *Herba Asari* 3 g
Bu Gu Zhi *Fructus Psoraleae* 10 g
Xu Duan *Radix Dipsaci* 10 g
Rou Gui *Cortex Cinnamomi* 10 g
Wu Zhu Yu *Fructus Evodiae* 10 g
Yin Yang Huo *Herba Epimedii* 10 g

Explanations
- Ma Huang warms the channels and dispels External Cold.
- Fu Zi warms the Kidney-Yang and relieves toothache.
- Xi Xin and Wu Zhu Yu promote the circulation of Qi in the channels so as to relieve toothache.
- Bu Gu Zhi, Xu Duan and Yin Yang Huo tonify the Kidney-Yang, strengthen the teeth and relieve the toothache.
- Rou Gui helps Fu Zi to warm the Kidney and relieve the toothache.

After 1 month of treatment, his toothache was relieved completely. He was followed up a year later and he stated he had experienced no toothache after this treatment.

BACTERIAL INFECTION

Symptoms and signs

Toothache and caries, intermittent toothache, aggravation of the toothache with touch, chewing or contact with sour food, a red tongue with a thin and yellow coating and a rapid pulse.

Principle of treatment

Clear Heat, kill the bacteria and sedate the pain.

HERBAL TREATMENT

Chuan Jiao in powder mixed with honey to form some small pills. Insert the pill into the holes on the teeth to kill the bacteria and arrest the pain.

Patent remedy

Niu Huang Jie Du Wan *Cattle Gallstone Pill to Resolve Toxin*

ACUPUNCTURE TREATMENT

LI-4 Hegu, LI-20 Yingxiang, SI-18 Quanliao, ST-6 Jiache and ST-7 Xiaguan. Reducing method is used on these points.

Explanations

- LI-4 circulates the Qi and Blood and arrests toothache.
- LI-20, SI-18, together with ST-6 and ST-7, are local points, regulating the Qi circulation in the vicinity and stopping the pain.

Modifications

1. If there is restlessness due to the pain, add HT-3 and HT-7 to calm the Heart and tranquillise the Mind.
2. If there is a craving for sweet food, due to accumulation of Heat in the Spleen and Stomach, add ST-44 and SP-2, the Spring points, to clear the Heat and reduce the desire for sweet food.
3. If there is constipation due to accumulation of Heat in the Large Intestine, add ST-25, the Front Collecting point of the Large Intestine, and ST-37, the Lower Sea point of the Large Intestine, to promote defecation and relieve the constipation.

Tongue pain 17

舌
头
疼
痛

Tongue pain may be of various types, including a burning pain, pricking pain or stabbing pain, and may be located in different regions of the tongue—including the tip, the middle area, the edges, the back, or even over the whole tongue. As well as the pain, other symptoms such as swelling, erosion, stiffness and ulceration can be seen in conjunction, and these may cause difficulty in swallowing, drinking or speaking. In some cases, tongue pain can also be induced by ulceration due to careless biting or chewing during eating.

In general, according to TCM, tongue pain can be caused by External invasion or by disorder of the Internal Zang-Fu organs, including invasion of Wind-Heat, hyperactivity of Excessive-Heat, hyperactivity of Deficient-Fire and accumulation of Damp in the Spleen. It may be attributed to any of the following conditions in Western medicine: lingual papillitis, lingual ulcer, hypoglossiadenitis, hypoglossitis, periglossitis, glossopyrosis, tongue abscess and even carcinoma of tongue.

Aetiology and pathology

Invasion of External factors

Invasion of External factors, especially Wind-Heat, Dryness-Heat and Wind-Cold, may cause accumulation of pathogenic factors on the tongue, resulting in stagnation of Qi and Blood and blockage of the collateral, so tongue pain follows.

Accumulation of Excessive-Heat in the Interior

Incomplete expelling of External factors in the Lung may cause disorder of the Lung so it cannot disperse Qi properly, leading to Qi stagnation in the Lung, which in turn results in the generation of Lung-Fire. The tongue is in the mouth, and the mouth is an opening to the respiratory passages, which are dominated by the Lung. If there is an uprising of Lung-Fire, the tongue will be impaired, and pain in the tongue follows.

Overeating of pungent, fatty and sweet food, and overindulgence in alcohol, may cause food to stagnate in the Spleen and Stomach, leading to the formation of Damp-Heat in the Spleen or of Stomach-Fire. The mouth is the opening passage of the Spleen, and the Stomach and Spleen form a pair of Zang-Fu organs. If there is accumulation of Damp-Heat in the Spleen, or hyperactivity of Stomach-Fire, the mouth will be affected, leading to disorders of the tongue, and so tongue pain occurs.

Accumulation of Cold-Phlegm in the Spleen

Bad eating habits, for instance, eating too much of cold and raw food, drinking too many cold drinks or taking too many cooling herbs, may damage the Yang of the Spleen, leading to poor transportation and transformation and therefore the formation of Cold-Phlegm. Once the collaterals related to the tongue are blocked by this pathogenic factor then tongue pain will follow.

Excessive emotional stimulation

Prolonged emotional disorder may cause dysfunction of the Zang-Fu organs, leading to generation of Heat or Fire in the Interior. For instance, excessive grief may cause blockage in the Lung channel, resulting in stagnation of Qi there, and gradually Lung-Fire is generated. Once this is formed, it may flow upward and cause tongue pain. Excessive thinking may cause Qi to stagnate in the Heart, leading to the formation of Heart-Fire. If there is hyperactivity of Heart-Fire, the tongue—the opening orifice of the Heart—will be burned and impaired, thus tongue pain happens.

Excessive meditation may cause stagnation of Qi in the Spleen, leading to poor transportation and transformation, and then Damp-Heat forms. When this disturbs and impairs the tongue, it causes tongue pain.

Excessive anger, stress, frustration or other emotional upset, may cause Liver-Qi to stagnate, leading to the generation of Liver-Fire. Fire is characterised by uprising and flaring; when the tongue is burned by Liver-Fire, tongue pain occurs.

Prolonged fear and fright, or sudden extreme fear and fright, may cause Qi to sink in the Kidney, leading to uprising of Kidney-Fire. The Kidney channel roots in the tongue, so this causes tongue pain.

Overstrain and prolonged sickness

Too much physical or mental work, as well as prolonged sickness, may consume the Yin of the body, leading to failure of the Fire to be controlled by Water, so hyperactivity of Deficient-Fire occurs, which ascends and burns the tongue, causing tongue pain.

Treatment based on differentiation

Differentiation

Differentiation of External or Internal origin

— Acute onset of tongue pain, mild in intensity, accompanied by External symptoms, such as an aversion to cold, fever, muscle pain, runny nose, cough, or superficial pulse, is usually caused by invasion of External factors.
— A chronic history of tongue pain, mild or severe in intensity, associated with diet, emotional state and other physical conditions, is usually caused by disorder of the Internal Zang-Fu organs.

Differentiation of character of the pain

— Acute sharp tongue pain with stiffness of the tongue, together with External symptoms, such as an aversion to cold, slight fever, muscle pain or absence of thirst, is usually caused by invasion of Wind-Cold.
— Acute sharp tongue pain with a burning sensation, a thin and yellow tongue coating, together with External symptoms, is usually caused by invasion of Wind-Heat.
— Acute tongue pain with dryness on the tongue and in the mouth and throat, and thirst, together with External symptoms, is usually caused by invasion of Wind-Dryness
— Chronic sharp tongue pain, which is related to the emotional state, is usually caused by stagnation of Qi.
— Stabbing tongue pain, which worsens at night, and a purplish colour of the tongue, is usually caused by stagnation of Blood.
— Chronic tongue pain with a burning sensation, restlessness, nervousness, thirst, constipation, a red tongue with a yellow and dry coating, and a forceful and rapid pulse, is usually caused by accumulation of Excessive-Fire from the Zang-Fu organs.
— Chronic tongue pain with a slight burning sensation, thirst, night sweating, dry mouth and throat, a red tongue with a thin coating, and a deep, thready, rapid and weak pulse, is usually caused by hyperactivity of Deficient-Fire from Zang-Fu organs.
— Tongue pain with swelling and a burning sensation, a bitter taste in the mouth, constipation, a yellow and greasy tongue coating and a slippery and rapid pulse, is usually caused by hyperactivity of Phlegm-Fire.
— Tongue pain with swelling, numbness on the tongue, tastelessness or nausea, is usually caused by accumulation of Damp in the Spleen.

Differentiation of tongue colour

— If the tongue pain is caused by invasion of Wind-Cold, the tongue colour is usually slightly red, or slightly purplish-red, or there are no tongue colour changes. The tongue coating is usually thin and white.

— If the tongue pain is caused by invasion of Wind-Heat, the tongue colour is usually red, especially at the tip of the tongue, or slightly purplish-red. The tongue coating is usually thin and yellow.

— If the tongue pain is caused by invasion of Wind-Dryness, the tongue colour is usually slightly red, or there are no tongue colour changes. The tongue coating is usually thin and dry.

— If the tongue pain is caused by accumulation of Damp in the Spleen, the tongue colour is usually pale, with tooth marks. The tongue is usually swollen and big. The coating is usually white and greasy.

Treatment

INVASION OF EXTERNAL FACTORS

Symptoms and signs

Tongue pain, fever, an aversion to cold and headache are the most common symptoms where the tongue pain is caused by invasion of External factors.

If it is an invasion of Wind-Heat, there is a red and swollen tongue, erosions on the tongue, thirst, a red tongue with a thin and yellow coating and a superficial and rapid pulse.

If it is an invasion of Dryness-Heat, the throat is dry, there is thirst, and the tongue has a yellow and dry coating.

If it is an invasion of Wind-Cold, the tongue is stiff, and there is a lack of thirst, spasm of the facial muscles, a thin and white tongue coating and a superficial and tight pulse.

Principle of treatment

Dispel Wind, dispel External factors and relieve the tongue pain.

HERBAL TREATMENT

a. Prescription for invasion of Wind-Heat

YIN QIAO SAN
Honeysuckle and Forsythia Powder
Jin Yin Hua *Flos Lonicerae* 10 g
Lian Qiao *Fructus Forsythiae* 10 g
Jie Geng *Radix Platycodi* 6 g
Bo He *Herba Menthae* 6 g
Dan Dou Chi *Semen Sojae Praeparatum* 10 g

Zhu Ye *Herba Lophatheri* 10 g
Gan Cao *Radix Glycyrrhizae* 6 g
Jing Jie Shui *Spica Schizonepetae* 6 g
Niu Bang Zi *Fructus Arctii* 10 g
Lu Gen *Rhizoma Phragmitis* 10 g

Explanations

- Jin Yin Hua and Lian Qiao clear Heat and eliminate Toxin.
- Bo He, Jing Jie Shui and Dan Dou Chi promote sweating, release the Exterior and dispel Heat.
- Niu Bang Zi, Jie Geng and Gan Cao eliminate toxin, benefit the throat and stop the pain.
- Zhu Ye and Lu Gen clear the Heat and increase the production of Body Fluids so as to relieve the thirst.

b. Prescription for invasion of Dryness-Heat

SANG XING TANG
Mulberry Leaf and Apricot Kernal Decoction
Sang Ye *Folium Mori* 6 g
Xing Ren *Semen Armeniacae Amarum* 10 g
Sha Shen *Radix Adenophorae* 10 g
Zhe Bei Mu *Bulbus Fritillariae Thunbergii* 10 g
Dan Dou Chi *Semen Sojae Praeparatum* 10 g
Zhi Zi Pi *Pericarpium Gardeniae* 10 g
Li Pi *Exocarpium Pyrus* 10 g

Explanations

- Sang Ye and Zhi Zi Pi clear Dry-Heat.
- Dan Dou Chi dispels Wind and relieves Exterior syndrome.
- Sha Shen and Li Pi nourish the Lung-Yin.
- Xing Ren and Zhe Bei Mu disperse the Lung-Qi and stop the cough.

c. Prescription for invasion of Wind-Cold

JING FANG BAI DU SAN
Schizonepeta and Ledebouriella Powder to Overcome Pathogenic Influences
Jing Jie *Herba Schizonepetae* 6 g
Fang Feng *Radix Ledebouriellae* 6 g
Ren Shen *Radix Ginseng* 6 g
Qiang Huo *Rhizoma seu Radix Notopterygii* 6 g
Du Huo *Radix Angelicae Pubescentis* 6 g
Qian Hu *Radix Peucedani* 6 g
Chai Hu *Radix Bupleuri* 6 g
Jie Geng *Radix Platycodi* 5 g
Zhi Qiao *Fructus Aurantii* 6 g
Fu Ling *Poria* 6 g
Chuan Xiong *Rhizoma Ligustici Chuanxiong* 5 g
Gan Cao *Radix Glycyrrhizae* 5 g

Explanations

- Jiang Jie, Qiang Huo and Du Huo are pungent and Warm herbs used to promote sweating and dispel pathogenic Wind-Cold.
- Chai Hu and Bo He are pungent and Cold herbs, used for dispersing Heat.
- Chuan Xiong invigorates the Blood circulation and promotes the Qi circulation so as to stop the pain.
- Jie Geng and Qian Hu promote the circulation of Lung-Qi and stop the cough.
- Fu Ling and Sheng Jiang resolve the Phlegm and eliminate Damp.
- Zhi Qiao promotes the Qi to relax the chest.
- Gan Cao harmonises the actions of the other herbs in the formula.

Modifications

1. If the tongue is red and swollen owing to invasion of Wind-Heat, add Pu Gong Ying *Herba Taraxaci* 10 g and Zhu Ye *Herba Lophatheri* 10 g to clear the Heat and reduce the swelling.
2. If there is thirst due to invasion of Dryness-Heat, add Mai Dong *Radix Ophiopogonis* 10 g and Xuan Shen *Radix Scrophulariae* 10 g to nourish the Yin of the Lung and the Stomach and relieve the thirst.
3. If there is fever due to the predominance of Heat invasion, add Huang Qin *Radix Scutellariae* 10 g to clear the Heat and reduce the fever.
4. If there is headache, add Man Jing Zi *Fructus Viticis* 10 g to dispel the Wind-Heat and sedate the headache.
5. If there is a cough and expectoration of yellow phlegm owing to invasion of the Lung by Wind-Heat, add Qian Hu *Radix Peucedani* 10 g and Zhe Bei Mu *Bulbus Fritillariae Thunbergii* 10 g to disperse the Lung-Qi and dispel the Wind-Heat.

Patent remedy

Jing Fang Bai Du Pian *Schizonepeta and Ledebouriella Tablet to Overcome Pathogenic Influences*

ACUPUNCTURE TREATMENT

Lu-7 Lieque, LI-4 Hegu, GB-20 Fengchi, TE-5 Waiguan, GV-15 Yamen and CV-23 Lianquan. Reducing method is used on all these points.

Explanations

- Among the External factors causing tongue pain, invasion of Wind-Heat and invasion of Wind-

Dryness are the most common. All the above-mentioned points have the function of dispelling external invasion; however, LU-7 is used especially when there are symptoms from the Lung, including cough, expectoration of phlegm, chest pain and throat pain.
- LI-4 is used especially to dispel Wind invasion, including Wind-Heat, Wind-Dryness and Wind-Cold, since this point has a function in opening the skin pores so as to induce sweating. Since it is also the point from the Large Intestine channel, it is able to clear Heat and reduce a fever.
- GB-20 is used to dispel the Wind and relieve the headache. When this point is punctured towards the tip of the nose, it has also the function of treating problems in the mouth, including tongue pain.
- TE-5 is applied to relieve External symptoms. Also, this point is connected with the Yang Linking Vessel, which ends at GV-15. GV-15 is a good point to relieve stiffness of the tongue and neck. CV-23 is a good point for treating tongue problems, including tongue pain. When this point is punctured, the direction of the needle should be toward the root of the tongue to achieve the best therapeutic result.

Modifications

1. If the throat and tongue are red, with a burning feeling on the tongue due to invasion of Wind-Heat, add LI-2, the Spring point, and LI-11, the Sea point, to clear the Heat strongly and stop the pain.
2. If there is a high fever due to predominance of Heat, add GV-14 to clear the Heat and reduce the fever.
3. If the throat and tongue are dry, with a thirst due to invasion of Wind-Dryness, add LU-8 and SP-6 to promote secretion of the Body Fluids and moisten the Dryness.
4. If there is tongue pain and spasm of the face due to invasion of Wind-Cold, add ST-6 and ST-40 to relieve the tongue pain and muscular spasm in the face.

ACCUMULATION OF EXCESSIVE-HEAT

EXCESSIVE-HEAT IN THE HEART

Symptoms and signs

Tongue pain, especially on the tip with a burning, packing sensation and red spots, restlessness, insomnia, deep yellow urine, even painful urination, a red tongue with a yellow coating and a rapid and wiry pulse, specially at the Heart region.

Principle of treatment

Clear Heat and calm the Heart.

HERBAL TREATMENT

Prescription

DAO CHI SAN
Guide Out the Red Powder
Mu Tong *Caulis Akebiae* 6 g
Sheng Di Huang *Radix Rehmanniae* 12 g
Zhu Ye *Herba Lophatheri* 10 g
Gan Cao *Radix Glycyrrhizae* 5 g
Zhi Zi *Fructus Gardeniae* 10 g
Huang Lian *Rhizoma Coptidis* 10 g

Explanations

- Sheng Di Huang clears the Heat, cools the Blood and nourishes the Yin.
- Mu Tong and Zhu Ye promote urination and conduct the Heart-Fire downward to flow to the Small Intestine.
- Gan Cao reduces Fire and stops tongue pain.
- Huang Lian and Zhi Zi clear Heart-Fire and relieve the pain.

Modifications

1. If there is severe ulceration of the mouth and on the tongue, add Qing Dai *Indigo Naturalis* 5 g and Dan Shen *Radix Salviae Miltiorrhizae* 5 g to clear the Heart-Fire, eliminate the Toxin and relieve the ulceration.
2. If urination is painful, add Xiao Ji *Herba Cephalanoploris* 10 g and Zhi Zi *Fructus Gardeniae* 10 g to clear the Heart-Fire and relieve the pain.
3. If there is insomnia, add Suan Zao Ren *Semen Ziziphi Spinosae* 10 g and Deng Xin Cao *Medulla Junci* 10 g to clear the Heart-Fire and tranquillise the Mind.
4. If there is restlessness, add Long Gu *Os Draconis* 20 g and Ci Shi *Magnetitum* 15 g to clear the Heat and calm the Mind.

Patent remedy

Dao Chi Pian *Guide Out the Red Tablet*

ACUPUNCTURE TREATMENT

HT-3 Shaohai, HT-6 Yinxi, HT-7 Shenmen, HT-8 Shaofu, PC-8 Laogong, SI-2 Qiangu and SI-4 Wangu. Reducing method is used on these points, except HT-3 and HT-7, on which even method is employed.

Explanations

- The tongue is the opening orifice of the Heart channel. When there is Excessive-Heat in the Heart, this Heat may flow up through the channel to the tongue, and cause tongue pain.
- HT-8 and PC-8, the Spring points, are able to clear Heat and relieve pain. They are particularly indicated in tongue pain resulting from Heart-Heat, or Heart-Fire.
- HT-3, the Sea point, and HT-7, the Source point, are able to regulate the function of the Heart and to treat the basic causes of Heart-Heat. This also calms the Mind, which will relieve the insomnia and restlessness due to Heat in the Heart.
- HT-6, the Accumulation point, relieves the pain in the tongue.
- SI-2, the Spring point, and SI-4, the Source point, are applied here to promote urination so as to clear up the Heat in the Heart. This method is called 'reducing the son so as to treat the Excessive mother'.

Modifications

1. If there is insomnia and restlessness due to failure of the Heart to house the Mind, add GV-20 and Extra Sishencong to calm the Mind and improve the sleep.
2. If urination is painful owing to shifting of Heart-Heat to the Small Intestine, add ST-39 the Lower Sea point of the Small Intestine, and SI-8, the Sea point, to clear the Heat in the Small Intestine and promote urination.
3. If there is constipation due to the accumulation of Heat in the Large Intestine, add ST-25, the Front Collecting point of the Large Intestine, and LI-4, the Source point, to clear the Heat in the Large Intestine and promote defecation.

EXCESSIVE-HEAT IN THE LUNG

Symptoms and signs

Tongue pain, especially on the tip of the tongue, with a burning, pricking sensation and red spots, a dry cough or a cough with yellow phlegm, chest pain, a dry nose, epistaxis, thirst, dry stools, throat pain, a red tongue with a yellow coating and a rapid and superficial pulse.

Principle of treatment

Clear Heat and disperse Lung-Qi.

HERBAL TREATMENT

Prescription

XIE BAI SAN
Drain the White Powder
Di Gu Pi *Cortex Lycii Radicis* 10 g
Sang Bai Pi *Cortex Mori Radicis* 10 g
Gan Cao *Radix Glycyrrhizae* 6 g
Jing Mi *Semen Oryzae* 10 g
Shi Gao *Gypsum Fibrosum* 20 g
Huang Qin *Radix Scutellariae* 10 g

Explanations

- Sang Bai Pi reduces Heat in the Lungs to relieve pain.
- Di Gu Pi clears Heat in the Lung.
- Jing Mi and Gan Cao harmonise the Stomach-Qi and strengthen the Stomach.
- Shi Gao and Huang Qin clear Heat and relieve pain.

Modifications

1. If there is a dry cough, add Chuan Bei Mu *Bulbus Fritillariae Cirrhosae* 10 g and Xuan Shen *Radix Scrophulariae* 10 g to nourish the Lung-Yin and stop the cough.
2. If there is a cough with yellow phlegm, add Zhu Ru *Caulis Bambusae in Taeniam* 10 g and Gua Lou *Fructus Trichosanthis* 10 g to clear the Heat and eliminate the Heat-Phlegm.
3. If there is chest pain, add Bai Shao *Radix Paeoniae Alba* 10 g and Zhi Qiao *Fructus Aurantii* 10 g to regulate the Qi circulation and relieve the pain.
4. If there is nasal bleeding, add Bai Mao Gen *Rhizoma Imperatae* 15 g and Chi Shao *Radix Paeoniae Rubra* 10 g to cool the Blood and stop the bleeding.

Patent remedy

Qing Fei Yi Huo Pian *Clear Lungs Restrain Fire Tablet*

ACUPUNCTURE TREATMENT

LU-5 Chize, LU-6 Kongzui, LU-10 Yuji, LI-4 Hegu, LI-11 Quchi and CV-23 Lianquan. Reducing method is used on these points, except for CV-23, on which even method is employed.

Explanations

- The mouth is an opening of the Lung. Therefore, when there is accumulation of Excessive-Heat in the Lung, it may ascend and affect the mouth, leading to tongue pain.
- LU-5, the Sea point, clears Heat in the Lung and causes the Lung-Qi to descend so as to restore the physiological function of the Lung. This point is also the Son point of the Lung channel, so is indicated for eliminating Excessive pathogenic factors from the Lung.
- LU-10, the Spring point, is applied here to clear Heat in the Lung and relieve the pain due to Heat. Also, this point can relieve the redness and pain in the throat.
- LU-6, the Accumulation point, is indicated in acute tongue pain due to accumulation of Heat in the Lung.
- LI-4, the Source point, and LI-11, the Sea point, clear Heat and promote defecation (this is the meaning of clearing Heat from the Lung by means of draining the Large Intestine).
- CV-23, the local point, clears Heat on the tongue directly, and also induces effects to the tongue.

Modifications

1. If there is nasal bleeding due to uprising of Lung-Heat, add LI-20 and LU-11 to clear the Heat and stop the bleeding.
2. If there is a cough due to dysfunction of the Lung in dispersing Qi and causing Lung-Qi to descend, add LU-1, the Front Collecting point of the Lung, and BL-13, the Back Transporting point of the Lung, to disperse the Lung-Qi and cause it to descend.
3. If there is expectoration of yellow phlegm due to concentration of Body Fluids by Heat in the Lung, add ST-40 to clear the Heat and resolve the Phlegm.

EXCESSIVE-HEAT IN THE STOMACH

Symptoms and signs

Tongue pain, especially over the whole tongue body or the middle of the tongue, thirst, a dry mouth, a preference for cold drinks, a foul smell in the mouth, constipation, swelling and redness or bleeding of the gums, a tendency to be frequently hungry, abdominal pain, restlessness, red tongue with a yellow and dry coating and a rapid and forceful pulse.

Principle of treatment

Clear Heat and promote defecation.

HERBAL TREATMENT

Prescription

QING WEI SAN
Clear Heat in the Stomach Powder
Huang Lian *Rhizoma Coptidis* 10 g
Dang Gui *Radix Angelicae Sinensis* 6 g
Sheng Di Huang *Radix Rehmanniae* 15 g
Sheng Ma *Rhizoma Cimicifugae* 10 g
Mu Dan Pi *Cortex Moutan Radicis* 10 g
Shi Gao *Gypsum Fibrosum* 20 g
Zhi Zi *Fructus Gardeniae* 10 g

Explanations

- Huang Lian and Sheng Ma clear Heat and eliminate Toxin.
- Sheng Di Huang and Mu Dan Pi clear Heat and cool the Blood.
- Dang Gui nourishes the Blood, invigorates its circulation and relieves the swelling.
- Shi Gao and Zhi Zi clear Heat and relieve pain.

Modifications

1. If the tongue is ulcerated and swollen, add Chi Shao *Radix Paeoniae Rubra* 10 g and Zhi Zi *Fructus Gardeniae* 10 g to clear the Fire and cool the Blood.
2. If there is a thirst, add Xuan Shen *Radix Scrophulariae* 15 g and Zhu Ye *Herba Lophatheri* 10 g to clear the Fire and nourish the Body Fluids.
3. If the gums are swollen, add Shi Gao *Gypsum Fibrosum* 20 g and Zhi Mu *Rhizoma Anemarrhenae* 10 g to clear the Stomach-Fire and reduce the swelling.
4. If there is abdominal pain, add Yan Hu Suo *Rhizoma Corydalis* 10 g and Bai Shao *Radix Paeoniae Alba* 10 g to regulate the Stomach-Qi and relieve the pain.
5. If there is constipation, add Da Huang *Radix et Rhizoma Rhei* 10 g and Mang Xiao *Natrii Sulfas* 10 g to eliminate the Heat, promote defecation and relieve the constipation.

Patent remedy

Wei Te Ling *Stomach Especially Effective Remedy*

ACUPUNCTURE TREATMENT

ST-40 Fenglong, ST-42 Chongyang, ST-44 Neiting, ST-45 Lidui, LI-4 Hegu and LI-11 Quchi. Reducing method is used on these points.

Explanations

- ST-42, the Source point and ST-40, the Connecting point of the Stomach channel, are able to clear Heat and harmonise the Stomach.
- ST-44 is the Spring point of the Stomach channel, being able to clear Heat in the Stomach directly and reduce the tongue pain.
- ST-45, the Son point of the Stomach channel, is applied here to eliminate Heat from the Stomach.
- Since the Stomach and Large Intestine are both Bright Yong-Fu organs, having a mutual influence on each other, especially in Excessive cases, LI-4 and LI-11 are used here to clear Heat in the Large Intestine and promote defecation so as to reduce Heat from the Stomach.

Modifications

1. If there is stomach pain due to disturbance of the Stomach by Excessive-Heat, add CV-12, the Front Collecting point of the Stomach, and BL-21, the Back Transporting point of the Stomach, to clear the Heat and harmonise the Stomach so as to relieve the pain.
2. If there is nausea and vomiting due to uprising of Stomach-Qi, add PC-6, the connecting point with the Yin Linking Vessel, and SP-4, the connecting point with the Penetrating Vessel channel, to descend the Stomach-Qi and relieve the vomiting.
3. If there is constipation due to the Heat in the Large Intestine, add ST-25, the Front Collecting point of the Large Intestine, to promote defecation and relieve the constipation.

Case history

A 9-year-old girl had been suffering from tongue pain for 9 days. She was ill with an acute periglossitis and had received Western medical treatment with painkiller tablets. When she came to the clinic she had a slight swollen tongue with ulcers on the edges. She suffered with thirst, a sore throat, irritability and constipation. Her tongue was red with a dry and yellow coating and her pulse was rapid.

Diagnosis
Hyperactivity of Stomach-Fire.

Principle of treatment
Clear Stomach-Fire and relieve the pain.

Acupuncture treatment
ST-40 Fenglong, ST-42 Chongyang, SP-6 Sanyinjiao, LI-4 Hegu and CV-23 Lianquan were needled with reducing method. She got daily treatment during 12 days.

Explanations
● ST-40 is the Connecting point of the Stomach channel, being able to clear Stomach-Fire and relieve the pain.
● ST-42 is the Source point of the Stomach channel, being able to reduce Fire and relieve the tongue pain. SP-6 is the crossing point of the three Yin channels of the foot, and is able to conduct Fire downward.
● LI-4 is the Source point of the Large Intestine channel, and is used to regulate the Qi circulation and relieve the tongue pain.
● CV-23 Lianquan is a local point, used to regulate the Qi and relieve the tongue pain.

After 12 days of treatment, the tongue pain had disappeared. She was followed up 6 months later and she stated that she had experienced no tongue pain since the last treatment.

EXCESSIVE-HEAT IN THE LIVER

Symptoms and signs

Tongue pain, especially at the edges, irritability, nervousness, headache, insomnia, painful eyes, a tendency to get emotionally upset easily, a red tongue with a yellow coating and a wiry and rapid pulse.

Principle of treatment

Clear Heat and cool the Liver.

HERBAL TREATMENT

Prescription

LONG DAN XIE GAN TANG
Gentianae Decoction to Drain the Liver
Long Dan Cao *Radix Gentianae* 6 g
Xia Ku Cao *Spica Prunellae* 10 g
Huang Qin *Radix Scutellariae* 9 g
Zhi Zi *Fructus Gardeniae* 9 g
Ze Xie *Rhizoma Alismatis* 12 g
Dang Gui *Radix Angelicae Sinensis* 3 g
Sheng Di Huang *Radix Rehmanniae Recens* 9 g
Chai Hu *Radix Bupleuri* 6 g
Gan Cao *Radix Glycyrrhizae* 6 g

Explanations

● Long Dan Cao, Xia Ku Cao and Huang Qin clear Heat and dry Damp.

● Zhi Zi and Ze Xie clear Heat, promote urination and eliminate Damp through urination.
● Dang Gui and Sheng Di Huang nourish the Yin and Blood and prevent the actions of the other herbs from injuring the Yin.
● Chai Hu regulates the Liver-Qi to remove Qi stagnation.
● Gan Cao harmonises the actions of the other herbs in the formula.

Modifications

1. If there is irritability, add Gou Teng *Radix Uncariae cum Uncis* 10 g to calm the Liver and clear the Liver-Fire.
2. If there is a headache, add Ju Hua *Flos Chrysanthemi* 10 g and Tian Ma *Rhizoma Gastrodiae* 10 g to suppress the Liver and relieve the pain.
3. If there is insomnia, add Suan Zao Ren *Semen Ziziphi Spinosae* 10 g and Zhi Zi *Fructus Gardeniae* 10 g to calm the Heart and calm the Mind.
4. If there is hypochondriac pain, add Yan Hu Suo *Rhizoma Corydalis* 10 g and Zhi Qiao *Fructus Aurantii* 10 g to regulate the Liver-Qi and relieve the pain.

Patent remedy

Long Dan Xie Gan Wan *Gentianae Pill to Drain the Liver*

ACUPUNCTURE TREATMENT

LR-2 Xingjian, LR-8 Ququan, GB-40 Qiuxu, GB-41 Zulinqi, GB-43 Xiaxi and LI-4 Hegu. Reducing method is used on these points.

Explanations

● LR-2, the Spring point, is able to clear Heat in the Liver and reduce Liver-Fire. Besides, this is also the Son point of the Liver channel, indicated in treating Excessive cases of the Liver.
● LR-8, the Water point of the Liver channel, is able to extinguish Liver-Fire. Meanwhile, this point is also the Sea point, being able to regulate the function of the Liver and clear Heat in the Liver, which is the root treatment for this case.
● The Gall Bladder and Liver share a pair of channels and a collateral. If there is accumulation of Heat in the Liver, the Gall Bladder will be affected as well. Conversely, to clear Heat in the Gall Bladder can also reduce Heat in the Liver, thus GB-40, the Source point, and GB-43, the Spring point, are used here to clear Heat in the Gall Bladder in order to reduce Heat in the Liver.

- GB-41 is a special point in this case. Since a branch of the Gall Bladder channel runs from this point to connect with the Liver channel, needling at this point can achieve the effect of regulating the Gall Bladder and Liver simultaneously.

Modifications

1. If the eyes are red, painful or burning, owing to uprising of Liver-Fire, add Extra Taiyang and GB-14 to reduce the Liver-Fire and benefit the eyes.
2. If there is nervousness or a headache due to hyperactivity of Liver-Yang, add GV-20 to calm the Liver and suppress the Liver-Yang.
3. If there is dizziness due to Liver-Wind stirring inside, add GB-20 to sedate the Liver-Wind and clear up the dizziness.

STAGNATION OF QI AND BLOOD

Symptoms and signs

A severe stabbing pain in the tongue, which might relate to emotional situations, aggravation of tongue pain during night, sometimes numbness of the tongue, a purplish tongue with a thin coating and a wiry and unsmooth pulse.

Principle of treatment

Circulate Qi and Blood and sedate the pain.

HERBAL TREATMENT

Prescription

TAO HONG SI WU TANG plus **SHI XIAO SAN**
Four-Substance Decoction with Safflower and Peach Pit plus *Sudden Smile Powder*
Dang Gui *Radix Angelicae Sinensis* 10 g
Sheng Di Huang *Radix Rehmanniae Recens* 12 g
Chi Shao *Radix Paeoniae Rubra* 10 g
Chuan Xiong *Rhizoma Ligustici Chuanxiong* 6 g
Tao Ren *Semen Persicae* 10 g
Hong Hua *Flos Carthami* 10 g
Pu Huang *Pollen Typhae* 10 g
Wu Ling Zhi *Faeces Trogopterorum* 5 g
Yan Hu Suo *Fructus Corydalis* 10 g

Explanations

- Chuan Xiong, Chi Shao and Hong Hua promote the circulation of Blood and remove the Blood stagnation.

- Dang Gui and Tao Ren regulate the circulation of Blood and remove the Blood stagnation; also, these two herbs may lubricate the Large Intestines to relieve hard stools.
- Pu Huang, Wu Ling Zhi and Yan Hu Suo are used to remove the Blood stasis and relieve the pain.
- Long-standing stagnation of Blood may cause Heat to form in the Blood, so Sheng Di Huang is used here to clear Heat in the Blood and prevent further Heat formation in the Blood due to Blood stagnation.

Modifications

1. If the tongue is stiff, add Tian Ma *Rhizoma Gastrodiae* 10 g and Chan Tui *Pertostracum Cicadae* 5 g to calm down the Liver-Wind and relax the tongue.
2. If the tongue is purplish, add Dan Shen *Radix Salviae Miltiorrhizae* 10 g and Mo Yao *Resina Myrrhae* 7 g to promote the circulation of Blood and remove the Blood stagnation.
3. If there is a severe stabbing pain on the tongue, add E Zhu *Rhizoma Zedoariae* 10 g to remove the Blood stagnation and relieve the pain.
4. If the emotions are unstable, add Chai Hu *Radix Bupleuri* 10 g and Xiang Fu *Rhizoma Cyperi* 10 g to promote the Liver-Qi circulation and regulate the emotions.

Patent remedy

Xiao Huo Luo Dan *Minor Invigorate the Collaterals Special Pill*

ACUPUNCTURE TREATMENT

HT-3 Shaohai, HT-5 Tongli, HT-6 Yinxi, HT-7 Shenmen, LI-4 Hegu, LR-3 Taichong, SP-6 Sanyinjiao and SP-10 Xuehai. Reducing method is used on these points.

Explanations

- If there is tongue pain due to the stagnation of Blood, treatment should be mainly focused on promoting Blood circulation. The tongue is the opening orifice of the Heart, and the Heart is in charge of regulating the Blood circulation, thus the majority of the points prescribed here are on the Heart channel.

- HT-7, the Source point, and HT-3, the Sea point, are applied to regulate the physiological function of the Heart, promote the Blood circulation, calm the Mind and arrest the pain.
- HT-5, the Connecting point, and HT-6, the Accumulation point, are able to harmonise the collateral, eliminating the Blood stasis and stopping the pain.
- LI-4, indicated in all the problems on the head caused by Excessive pathogenic factors, is used here to promote the Qi and Blood circulation and relieve the tongue pain.
- It is very common to apply some points to promote Qi circulation to treat stagnation of Blood, since Qi circulation leads to Blood circulation. LR-3 is prescribed to circulate the Qi and arrest the pain. When LR-3 is used together with LI-4, the effect of the Liver in promoting Qi circulation will be increased.
- SP-6 and SP-10 promote the circulation of Blood and relieve its stagnation so as to stop the pain.

Modifications

1. If there are palpitations, pressure over the chest, or even heart pain due to stagnation of Blood in the Heart, add BL-14, the Back Transporting point of the Pericardium, BL-15, the Back Transporting point of the Heart, and PC-4, the Accumulation point, to circulate the Blood, eliminate the Blood stasis and relieve the pain.
2. If there is pain and spasm of the facial muscles due to stagnation of Blood, add ST-5 and ST-6 to harmonise the collateral and arrest the pain and spasm.
3. If there is a stabbing pain in the general body due to stagnation of Blood, add BL-17 and SP-21 to promote the circulation of Blood and relieve the pain.

HYPERACTIVITY OF PHLEGM-FIRE

Symptoms and signs

Tongue pain, especially over the whole body of the tongue, swelling and sometimes numbness of the tongue, nausea, a poor appetite, a purplish tongue with a greasy coating and slippery pulse.

Principle of treatment

Reduce Fire and resolve Phlegm.

HERBAL TREATMENT

Prescription

MENG SHI GUN TAN WAN
Chlorite-Schist Pill for Chronic Phlegm Syndrome
Da Huang *Radix et Rhizoma Rhei* 6 g
Huang Qin *Radix Scutellariae* 10 g
Duan Meng Shi *Lapis Chloriti Usta* 15 g
Chen Xiang *Lignum Aquilariae Resinatum* 5 g
Dan Nan Xing *Rhizoma Arisaematis Praeparatum Cum Felle Bovis* 10 g
Tian Zhu Huang *Concretio Silicea Bambusae* 10 g

Explanations

- Da Huang eliminates Fire in the Middle Burner and the Lower Burner by promoting defecation.
- Huang Qin clears Heat in Upper Burner and resolves Damp.
- Duan Meng Shi eliminates Heat-Phlegm, especially in the Heart channel, so as to remove the blockage caused by Damp-Phlegm.
- Accumulation of Damp-Phlegm in the channels may cause stagnation of Qi, so Chen Xiang is used to promote the Qi circulation and eliminate the Phlegm.
- Dan Nan Xing and Tian Zhu Huang clear Phlegm-Fire and relieve the pain.

Modifications

1. If there is severe tongue pain, add Mu Tong *Caulis Akebiae* 6 g and Sheng Di Huang *Radix Rehmanniae* 15 g to cool the Blood and relieve the pain.
2. If the tongue is numb, add Quan Xie *Scorpio* 3 g and Zhu Ye *Herba Lophatheri* 10 g to clear the Fire and eliminate the Wind-Phlegm.
3. If there is a poor appetite, add Bai Kou Ren *Semen Amomi Rotundus* 10 g and Ban Xie *Rhizoma Pinelliae* 10 g to resolve the Phlegm and improve the appetite.
4. If there is nausea, add Zhu Ru *Caulis Bambusae in Taeniam* 10 g and Chen Pi *Exocarpium Citri Grandis* 10 g to regulate the Qi, resolve the Phlegm and disperse the Stomach-Qi.

Patent remedy

Meng Shi Gun Tan Wan *Chlorite-Schist Pill for Chronic Phlegm Syndrome*

ACUPUNCTURE TREATMENT

HT-3 Shaohai, HT-5 Tongli, HT-8 Shaofu, ST-40 Fenglong, ST-44 Neiting, LI-4 Hegu and SP-9 Yinlingquan. Reducing method is used on these points.

Explanations

- If the tongue pain is caused by Phlegm-Fire, the Heart, Stomach and Spleen are usually involved. The Heart, the Fire organ, opens into the tongue. The Stomach and Spleen, the Earth organs, transport Damp and Water through the body. If there is dysfunction of the Heart, Spleen and Stomach, Phlegm-Fire will be produced, leading to blockage of the opening orifices, causing tongue pain.
- HT-3, the Sea point, is applied here to calm the Heart and regulate the its function.
- HT-5, the Connecting point, is able to circulate the collateral of the Heart and eliminate the blockage there due to Damp-Phlegm.
- HT-8, the Spring point, clears the Heat and reduces the Fire in the Heart as well as relieving the tongue pain.
- ST-40, the Connecting point, is applied here to harmonise the collateral of the Stomach and eliminate the Phlegm. ST-44, the Spring point, is used to clear the Heat and reduce the Fire.
- LI-4 promotes defecation and clears the Heat in the Bright Yang Fu organs.
- SP-9, the Sea point, activates the Spleen and Stomach and eliminates the Damp-Phlegm.

Modifications

1. If there is restlessness and insomnia due to hyperactivity of Heart-Fire, add PC-6 and HT-7 to calm the Heart and the Mind.
2. If there is a bitter taste in the mouth, dizziness, nausea and an uncomfortable feeling in the hypochondriac area owing to disturbance of the Gall Bladder by Phlegm-Fire, add GB-20, GB-40 and GB-41 to clear the Phlegm-Fire in the Gall Bladder.
3. If there is nausea, poor appetite and epigastric distension due to the accumulation of Phlegm in the Stomach, add CV-12, the Front Collecting point of the Stomach, and SP-4, the Confluence point of the Penetrating Vessel, to activate the Stomach and cause the Stomach-Qi to descend.

HYPERACTIVITY OF DEFICIENT-FIRE

DEFICIENT-FIRE IN THE HEART

Symptoms and signs

Tongue pain, aggravation of the pain at night, thirst, a dry mouth, dry stools, night sweating, heat in the palms and soles, restlessness, palpitation, insomnia, a red tip of the tongue with a thin or peeled coating, a deep, thready and rapid pulse.

Principle of treatment

Nourish Yin and reduce Deficient-Heat.

HERBAL TREATMENT

Prescription

HUANG LIAN E JIAO TANG
Coptis and Ass-hide Gelatin Decoction
Huang Lian *Rhizoma Coptidis* 6 g
Huang Qin *Radix Scutellariae* 6 g
Bai Shao *Radix Paeoniae Alba* 10 g
E Jiao *Colla Corii Asini* 10 g
Ji Zi Huang *Fresh yolk* 1 piece
Zhu Ye *Herba Lophatheri* 10 g

Explanations

- Huang Lian and Huang Qin clear the Fire in the Upper Burner.
- Bai Shao nourishes the Yin and relieves the tongue pain.
- E Jiao and Ji Zi Huang nourish the Yin and Blood to reduce the Fire. Also, they can also nourish the Heart-Yin and calm the Mind.
- Zhu Ye clears the Heart-Fire and calms the Mind.

Modifications

1. If there is thirst, add Tian Hua Fen *Radix Trichosanthis* 10 g and Sheng Di Huang *Radix Rehmanniae Recens* 10 g to nourish the Yin and relieve the thirst.
2. If there are palpitations, add Zhu Fu Shen *Lignum Pini Poriaferum* 10 g and Ye Jiao Teng *Caulis Polygoni Multiflori* 15 g to calm the Mind and relieve the palpitations.
3. If there is night sweating, add Wu Wei Zi *Fructus Schisandrae* 10 g and Mu Li *Concha Ostreae* 15 g to stop the sweating.
4. If there is insomnia, add Suan Zao Ren *Semen Ziziphi Spinosae* 10 g and Bai Zi Ren *Semen Biotae* 10 g to nourish Heart-Blood and calm the Mind.
5. If there are dry stools, add Xuan Shen *Radix Scrophulariae* 15 g and Lu Hui *Pasta Aloes* 5 g to nourish the Liver-Yin and clear the Liver-Fire to soften the stools.

Patent remedy

Tian Wang Bu Xin Dan *Emperor of Heaven's Special Pill to Tonify the Heart*

ACUPUNCTURE TREATMENT

HT-3 Shaohai, HT-4 Lingdao, PC-3 Quze, PC-5 Jianshi, BL-15 Xinshu and SP-6 Sanyinjiao. Even method is used on HT-4 and PC-5. Reinforcing method is employed on the rest of the points.

Explanations

- HT-3 and PC-3, the Sea points of the Heart channel and Pericardium channel respectively, tonify the Heart and regulate its physiological function. Moreover, these are all Water points, so are able to promote the secretion of Body Fluids in the Heart so as to extinguish the Deficient-Fire.
- HT-4 and PC-5, the Metal points of the Heart channel and Pericardium channel respectively, promote the secretion of Body Fluids in the Heart so as to nourish the Yin and clear the Deficient-Fire.
- BL-15, the Back Transporting point of the Heart, nourishes the Yin of the Heart and reduces the Deficient-Fire.
- SP-6 nourishes the Yin in general so as to regulate the Heart as well.

Modifications

1. If there are palpitations and insomnia due to failure of the Heart to house the Mind, add Extra Anmian and Extra Sishencong to calm the Heart and tranquillise the Mind.
2. If there is night sweating due to hyperactivity of Deficient-Fire in the Heart, add HT-6, the Accumulation point, to reduce the Deficient-Fire and relieve the sweating.
3. If there is ulceration on the tongue and restlessness due to uprising of Deficient-Fire in the Heart, add HT-8, the Spring point, to clear the Heat and reduce the Deficient-Fire.

DEFICIENT-FIRE IN THE LUNG

Symptoms and signs

Tongue pain, with aggravation at night, thirst, a dry mouth, dry stools, night sweating, heat in the palms and soles of the feet, restlessness, a dry cough, throat pain, chest pain, sometimes nasal bleeding, a tongue with a red tip and a thin or peeled coating, and a deep, thready and rapid pulse.

Principle of treatment

Nourish Yin and cool the Lung.

HERBAL TREATMENT

Prescription

BAI HE GU JIN TANG
Lily Bulb Decoction to Preserve the Metal
Shu Di Huang *Radix Rehmanniae Praeparata* 10 g
Sheng Di Huang *Radix Rehmanniae Recens* 10 g
Zhe Bei Mu *Bulbus Fritillariae Thunbergii* 6 g
Bai He *Bulbus Lilii* 10 g
Mai Dong *Radix Ophiopogonis* 10 g
Xuan Shen *Radix Scrophulariae* 10 g
Dang Gui *Radix Angelicae Sinensis* 6 g
Bai Shao *Radix Paeoniae Alba* 6 g
Gan Cao *Radix Glycyrrhizae* 6 g
Jie Geng *Radix Platycodi* 6 g

Explanations

- Sheng Di Huang and Shu Di Huang nourish the Kidney-Yin, which is the root Yin of the body.
- Zhe Bei Mu and Jie Geng promote the Qi circulation in the Lungs and remove the Phlegm.
- Bai He, Xuan Shen and Mai Dong nourish the Lung-Yin and stop the cough.
- Dang Gui and Bai Shao regulate the Blood circulation and relieve the tongue pain.
- Gan Cao harmonises the actions of the other herbs.

Modifications

1. If there is a dry mouth, add Shi Hu *Herba Dendrobii* 10 g to nourish Kidney-Yin and relieve the thirst.
2. If there is restlessness, add Suan Zao Ren *Semen Ziziphi Spinosae* 10 g and Wu Wei Zi *Fructus Schisandrae* 10 g to calm the Heart and tranquillise the Mind.
3. If there is heat in the palms and soles, add Hu Huang Lian *Rhizoma Picrorhizae* 10 g and Qing Hao *Herba Artemisiae Chinghao* 10 g to clear the Deficient-Fire.
4. If there is a dry cough, add Bo He *Herba Menthae* 6 g and Wu Wei Zi *Fructus Schisandrae* 10 g to dispel the Wind-Heat and arrest the Lung-Qi and relieve the cough.
5. If there is night sweating, add Sang Piao Xiao *Ootheca Mantidis* 10 g and Mu Li *Concha Ostreae* 15 g to arrest the sweating.

Patent remedy

Liu Wei Di Huang Wan *Six-Flavour Rehmanniae Pill*

ACUPUNCTURE TREATMENT

LU-5 Chize, LU-8 Jingqu, LU-10 Yuji, BL-13 Feishu, CV-23 Lianquan and SP-6 Sanyinjiao. Even method is used on LU-8 and CV-23. Reinforcing method is used on the other points.

Explanations

- LU-5, the Sea point, and BL-13, the Back Transporting point of the Lung, are able to nourish the Yin of the Lung and clear the Deficient-Fire in this channel. Also, LU-5 is the Water point of the Lung channel, being able to promote the secretion of Body Fluids here so as to extinguish the Deficient-Fire in the Lung.
- LU-8, the Metal point, is capable of promoting the secretion of Body Fluids in the Lung and relieving the tongue pain.
- LU-10, the Spring point, is used here to reduce the Deficient-Fire and relieve the tongue pain.
- SP-6 nourishes the Yin generally so as to tonify the Yin of the Lung.
- CV-23, the local point, can be used here to relieve the tongue pain.

Modifications

1. If there is nasal bleeding, add LU-6 and LU-11 to clear Heat in the Lung and stop the bleeding.
2. If there is chest pain, add CV-17 and PC-6 to relieve the chest pain.
3. If there is constipation, add LI-4 to promote defecation.

DEFICIENT-FIRE IN THE STOMACH

Symptoms and signs

Tongue pain, with aggravation at night, thirst, a dry mouth, dry stools, night sweating, heat in the palms and soles of the feet, a burning sensation in the stomach, a poor appetite, sometimes gum bleeding, a red tongue with a thin or peeled coating in the middle, and a deep, thready and rapid pulse, specially at the Stomach position.

Principle of treatment

Nourish Yin and reduce Stomach-Fire.

HERBAL TREATMENT

Prescription

YU NU JIAN
Jade Woman Decoction

Shi Gao *Gypsum Fibrosum* 15 g
Shu Di Huang *Radix Rehmanniae Praeparata* 10 g
Mai Dong *Radix Ophiopogonis* 10 g
Zhi Mu *Rhizoma Anemarrhenae* 10 g
Huai Niu Xi *Radix Achyranthis Bidentatae* 10 g
Zhu Ye *Herba Lophatheri* 10 g
Xuan Shen *Radix Scrophulariae* 12 g

Explanations

- Shi Gao and Zhi Mu clear the Fire strongly and relieve the pain.
- Shu Di Huang, Xuan Shen and Mai Dong nourish the Yin and clear the Fire indirectly.
- Huai Niu Xi nourishes the Yin, conducts the Blood downward and causes the descent of the attacking Fire.
- Zhu Ye clears the Heat and relieves the pain.

Modifications

1. If there is a dry mouth and thirst, add Sheng Di Huang *Radix Rehmanniae* 15 g to nourish the Kidney-Yin and relieve the thirst.
2. If there is night sweating, add Sang Piao Xiao *Ootheca Mantidis* 10 g and Mu Li *Concha Ostreae* 15 g to stop night sweating.
3. If there is a poor appetite, add Dan Pi *Cortex Moutan Radicis* 10 g and Zhi Zi *Fructus Gardeniae* 10 g to clear Fire.
4. If there is heat in the palms and soles, add Hu Huang Lian *Rhizoma Picrorhizae* 10 g and Qing Hao *Herba Artemisiae Chinghao* 10 g to clear Deficient-Fire.
5. If there is gum bleeding, add Ce Bai Ye *Cacumen Biotae* 10 g and Xiao Ji *Herba Cephalanoploris* 10 g to cool the Blood and stop the bleeding.

Patent remedy

Wei Te Ling *Stomach Especially Effective Remedy*

ACUPUNCTURE TREATMENT

ST-36 Zusanli, ST-40 Fenglong, ST-42 Chongyang, ST-44 Neiting, ST-45 Lidui and SP6 Sanyinjiao. Reducing method is used on ST-40, even method is used on ST-44 and ST-45 and reinforcing method is used on ST-36, ST-42 and SP-6.

Explanations

- ST-40, the Connecting point, is able to circulate and harmonise the collateral of the Stomach and resolve a blockage in the Stomach.

- ST-36, the Sea point, ST-42, the Source point, and SP-6 nourish the Yin and tonify the Stomach.
- ST-44, the Spring point, is capable of clearing Heat and reducing Deficient-Fire in the Stomach. Moreover, this point is also the Water point of the Stomach channel, being able to nourish the Yin. Thus even method is applied here.
- ST-45, the Well point and Metal point, promotes the secretion of Body Fluids and relieves a painful tongue.

Modifications

1. If there is epigastric pain due to deficiency of Stomach-Yin, add ST-34, the Accumulation point, to sedate the epigastric pain.
2. If there is a poor appetite due to weakness of the Stomach, add CV-12, the Front Collecting point of the Stomach, and BL-21, the Back Transporting point of the Stomach, to activate the Stomach and improve the digestion.
3. If there is constipation due to failure of the Large Intestine to be nourished by Yin, add ST-37, the Lower Sea point of the Large Intestine, to increase the secretion of Body Fluids and promote defecation.
4. If there is nausea or vomiting due to the uprising of the Stomach-Qi, add PC-6, the Confluence point of the Yin Linking Vessel, and SP-4, the Confluence point of the Penetrating Vessel, to harmonise the Stomach and cause the Stomach-Qi to descend so as to relieve the vomiting.

DEFICIENT-FIRE IN THE LIVER

Symptoms and signs

Tongue pain, with aggravation at night, thirst, a dry mouth, dry stools, night sweating, heat in the palms and soles, irritability, blurred vision, hypochondriac pain, tiredness, a red tongue with a thin peeled coating at the edges, and a deep, thready, weak and wiry pulse at the Liver position.

Principle of treatment

Nourish Yin and reduce Liver-Fire.

HERBAL TREATMENT

Prescription

YI GUAN JIAN
Linking Decoction
Sha Shen *Radix Adenophorae* 10 g

Mai Dong *Radix Ophiopogonis* 10 g
Dang Gui *Radix Angelicae Sinensis* 6 g
Sheng Di Huang *Radix Rehmanniae Recens* 15 g
Gou Qi Zi *Fructus Lycii* 6 g
Chuang Lian Zi *Fructus Meliae Toosendan* 6 g
Zhi Zi *Fructus Gardeniae* 10 g

Explanations

- Dang Gui activates the Blood, removes the Blood stagnation and stops the pain.
- Gou Qi Zi helps Dang Gui to nourish the Blood and Yin.
- Sheng Di Huang, Mai Dong and Sha Shen nourish the Blood and tonify the Yin.
- Chuan Lian Zi promotes the Qi circulation and also aids the Liver in dispersing the Qi.
- Zhi Zi clears the Fire to relieve the pain.

Modifications

1. If there is night sweating, add Sang Piao Xiao *Ootheca Mantidis* 10 g and Mu Li *Concha Ostreae* 15 g to stop the sweating.
2. If there is irritability, add Suan Zao Ren *Semen Ziziphi Spinosae* 15 g and Mu Li *Concha Ostreae* 15 g to nourish the Yin and calm the Mind.
3. If there is heat in the palms and soles of the feet, add Hu Huang Lian *Rhizoma Picrorhizae* 10 g and Qing Hao *Herba Artemisiae Chinghao* 10 g to clear the Deficient-Fire.
4. If there is hypochondriac pain, add Zhi Qiao *Fructus Zurantii* 10 g and Bai Shao *Radix Paeoniae Alba* 12 g to regulate the Liver-Qi and relieve the pain.
5. If there is a dry mouth, add Sheng Di Huang *Radix Rehmanniae* 15 g and Xuan Shen *Radix Scrophulariae* 15 g to nourish the Kidney-Yin and relieve the thirst.
6. If the vision is blurred, add Han Lian Cao *Herba Ecliptae* 12 g and Nu Zhen Zi *Fructus Ligustri Lucidi* 12 g to nourish the Liver-Blood and improve the eyesight.

Patent remedy

Qi Ju Di Huang Wan *Lycium Fruit, Chrysanthemum and Rehmannia Pill*

ACUPUNCTURE TREATMENT

LR-2, Xingjian, LR-3 Taichong, LR-5 Ligou, LR-8 Ququan, KI-3 Taixi and SP-6 Sanyinjiao. Reducing method is used on LR-2. Reinforcing method is used on the other points.

Explanations

- LR-2, the Spring point, nourishes the Yin of the Liver and reduces the Deficient-Fire.
- LR-3 and KI-3, the Source points, and LR-8, the Sea point, tonify the Liver and regulate the physiological function of both Liver and Kidney so as to control the Deficient-Fire. LR-8 is also the Water point of the Liver channel, being able to nourish the Yin and promote the secretion of Body Fluids in the Liver.
- LR-5, the Connecting point, harmonises the collateral and relieves the pain.
- SP-6, the crossing point of the three Yin channels of the foot, nourishes the Yin generally and tonifies the Liver and Kidney.

Modifications

1. If there is a headache, add GB-20 to calm the Liver and relieve the headache.
2. If there is nervousness, add GV-20 to calm the Liver and relieve the nervousness.
3. If there is a feeling of oppression over the chest, add CV-17 and PC-6 to promote the Qi circulation in the chest and relieve the feeling of oppression.
4. If there is abdominal pain and diarrhoea due to nervousness, add ST-25 and LR-13 to harmonise the Liver and Spleen so as to relieve the diarrhoea.
5. If there is insomnia, add HT-8 to clear the Heat in the Heart and calm the Mind.

DEFICIENT-FIRE IN THE KIDNEY

Symptoms and signs

Tongue pain, with aggravation at night, thirst, a dry mouth, dry stools, night sweating, heat in the palms and soles of the feet, hair loss, lower back pain, tinnitus, tiredness, a red tongue with a thin or peeled coating at the back, and a deep, thready, weak and wiry pulse at the left Kidney position.

Principle of treatment

Nourish Yin and reduce Deficient-Fire.

HERBAL TREATMENT

Prescription

ZHI BAI DI HUANG WAN
Anemarrhena, Phellodendron and Rehmannia Pill
Shu Di Huang *Rhizoma Rehmanniae Praeparata* 24 g
Shan Zhu Yu *Fructus Corni* 12 g
Shan Yao *Rhizoma Dioscoreae* 12 g
Fu Ling *Poria* 9 g
Mu Dan Pi *Cortex Moutan Radicis* 9 g
Ze Xie *Rhizoma Alismatis* 9 g
Zhi Mu *Rhizoma Anemarrhenae* 6 g
Huang Bai *Cortex Phellodenron* 6 g
Han Lian Cao *Herba Ecliptae* 10 g

Explanations

- Shu Di Huang, Han Lian Cao, Shan Zhu Yu and Shan Yao tonify the Blood and benefit the Essence of the Liver and Kidney.
- Ze Xie promotes urination and induces the downward flow of Deficient-Fire.
- Mu Dan Pi cools the Blood, activates the Blood circulation and clears the Deficient-Fire.
- Fu Ling strengthens the Spleen and tonifies the Qi so as to promote the production of Kidney-Essence.
- Zhi Mu and Huang Bai clear the Deficient-Fire.

Modifications

1. If there is night sweating, add Sang Piao Xiao *Ootheca Mantidis* 10 g and Mu Li *Concha Ostreae* 15 g to stop the sweating.
2. If there is insomnia, add Suan Zao Ren *Semen Ziziphi Spinosae* 12 g and Wu Wei Zi *Fructus Schisandrae* 12 g to calm the Mind.
3. If there is heat in the palms and soles of the feet, add Hu Huang Lian *Rhizoma Picrorhizae* 10 g and Qing Hao *Herba Artemisiae Chinghao* 10 g to clear the Deficient-Fire.
4. If there is lower back pain, add Xu Duan *Radix Dipsaci* 10 g and Sang Ji Sheng *Ramulus Loranthi* 10 g to strengthen the Kidney and relieve the pain.
5. If there is a dry mouth, add Sheng Di Huang *Radix Rehmanniae* 12 g and Xuan Shen *Radix Scrophulariae* 12 g to nourish the Kidney-Yin and relieve the thirst.

Patent remedy

Zhi Bai Di Huang Wan *Anemarrhena, Phellodendron and Rehmannia Pill*

ACUPUNCTURE TREATMENT

KI-2 Rangu, KI-3 Taixi, KI-7 Fuliu, KI-10 Yingu and SP-6 Sanyinjiao. Reducing method is used on KI-2. Reinforcing method is used on the other points.

Explanations

- KI-2, the Spring point, and KI-7, the Metal point, nourish the Yin of the Kidney and reduce the Deficient-Fire.

- KI-3, the Source point, and KI-10, the Sea point, are used here to tonify the Kidney and regulate its physiological function so as to control the Deficient-Fire. KI-10 is also the Water point of the Kidney channel, being able to nourish the Yin and promote the secretion of Body Fluids in the Kidney.
- SP-6, the crossing point of the three Yin channels of the foot, nourishes the Yin generally and tonifies the Kidney.

Modifications

1. If there is lower back pain and weakness in the knees due to deficiency of the Kidney-Yin, add BL-23, the Back Transporting point of the Kidney, and BL-58, the Connecting point of the Bladder channel, to tonify the Kidney, harmonise the collateral and sedate the lower back pain.
2. If there is nocturia due to weakness of Kidney-Qi, add KI-6 to tonify the Kidney and relieve the nocturia.
3. If there is general tiredness due to deficiency of Kidney-Essence, add CV-4 and CV-6 to tonify the Kidney and benefit the Essence.
4. If there is insomnia and dream-disturbed sleep due to disharmony between the Kidney and the Heart, add HT-3 and HT-8 to calm the Heart, nourish the Heart-Yin and reduce the Deficient-Fire.

ACCUMULATION OF DAMP IN THE SPLEEN

Symptoms and signs

Tongue pain with numbness and swelling, ulceration on the tongue, no sense of taste, excessive salivation, tiredness, a poor appetite, abdominal pain with a cold feeling, loose stools, somnolence, a pale and swollen tongue with a white and greasy coating and a slippery and weak pulse.

Principle of treatment

Activate the Spleen and resolve Damp.

HERBAL TREATMENT

Prescription

SHEN LING BAI ZHU SAN
Ginseng–Poria–Atractylodis Powder
Ren Shen *Radix Ginseng* 6 g

Fu Ling *Poria* 12 g
Bai Zhu *Rhizoma Atractylodis Macrocephalae* 6 g
Bai Bian Dou *Semen Dolichoris* 10 g
Shan Yao *Rhizoma Dioscoreae* 10 g
Lian Zi *Semen Nelumbinis* 10 g
Sha Ren *Fructus Amomi* 6 g
Yi Yi Ren *Semen Coicis* 10 g
Jie Geng *Radix Platycodi* 5 g
Gan Cao *Radix Glycyrrhizae* 5 g

Explanations

- Ren Shen, Bai Zhu and Fu Ling tonify the Spleen-Qi and remove the Phlegm.
- Shan Yao and Lian Zi tonify the Spleen-Qi and improve the appetite.
- Bai Bian Dou, Sha Ren and Yi Yi Ren eliminate the Damp and promote urination.
- Jie Geng and Gan Cao promote the Lung-Qi circulation and resolve the Phlegm.

Modifications

1. If the tongue is swollen, add Si Gua Luo *Retinervus Luffae Fructus* 10 g to promote the Qi circulation and remove the Phlegm in the channels.
2. If the tongue is ulcerated, add Bai Zhi *Radix Angelicae Dahuricae* 10 g to dispel the Wind and heal the ulceration.
3. If the appetite is poor, add Zhi Qiao *Fructus Aurantii* 10 g to promote the Stomach-Qi circulation and improve the appetite.
4. If there is abdominal pain, add Mu Xiang *Radix Aucklandiae* 10 g and Chen Pi *Pericarpium Citri Reticulatae* 10 g to regulate the Qi circulation and relieve the pain.
5. If there are loose stools, add Cao Guo *Fructus Tsaoko* 10 g and Cang Zhu *Rhizoma Atractylodis* 10 g to dry the Damp and improve the stool.

Patent remedy

Xiang Sha Liu Jun Wan *Six-Gentleman Pill with Aucklandia and Amomum*

ACUPUNCTURE TREATMENT

ST-36 Zusanli, ST-40 Fenglong, SP-6 Sanyinjiao, SP-9 Yinlingquan, CV-12 Zhongwan, LI-4 Hegu and LR-3 Taichong. Reinforcing method is used on ST-36 and

SP-6. Even method is used on CV-12. Reducing method is used on ST-40, SP-9, LI-4 and LR-3.

Explanations

- ST-36, the Sea point of the Stomach channel, and SP-6 activate the Spleen and Stomach, which is the basic treatment for accumulation of Damp in the body.
- CV-12, the Front Collecting point of the Stomach and the Gathering point for the Fu organs, harmonises the Stomach and resolves Damp in the body.
- ST-40, the Connecting point of the Stomach channel, and SP-9, the Sea point of the Spleen channel, eliminate and resolve the Phlegm.
- Accumulation of Damp-Phlegm will easily cause stagnation of Qi, so LI-4 and LR-3 are used to promote the Qi circulation and relieve the tongue pain.

Modifications

1. If there is nausea and vomiting due to uprising of Stomach-Qi resulting from accumulation of Damp in the Stomach, add PC-6, the Connecting point with the Yin Linking Vessel, to harmonise the Stomach and cause the Stomach-Qi to descend.
2. If there is a poor appetite due to the blockage of the Stomach by Damp-Phlegm, add ST-42, the Source point, to activate the Stomach and improve the appetite.
3. If there are loose stools or diarrhoea due to dysfunction of the transportation and transformation of the Spleen, resulting from an accumulation of Damp in the Spleen add SP-9 and SP-3 to activate the spleen and stop diarrhoea.

Case history

A 46-year-old woman had been ill with a lingual ulcer for 4 months. Since then she had been suffering from tongue pain and numbness. Also, she had a sensation of heaviness in her tongue, a poor appetite, a feeling of dullness in the stomach and loose and sticky stools. Her tongue was pale, with a white greasy coating. Her pulse was deep and slippery.

Diagnosis
Accumulation of Damp in Spleen.

Principle of treatment
Promote Qi circulation and eliminate Damp.

Herbal treatment
SHEN LING BAI ZHU SAN
Panax–Poria–Atractylodis Powder (modified)
Ren Shen *Radix Ginseng* 6 g
Fu Ling *Poria* 12 g
Bai Zhu *Rhizoma Atractylodis Macrocephalae* 6 g
Mu Xiang *Radix Aucklandiae* 10 g
Si Gua Luo *Retinervus Luffae Fructus* 10 g
Sha Ren *Fructus Amomi* 6 g
Chen Pi *Pericarpium Citri Reticulatae* 10 g
Yi Yi Ren *Semen Coicis* 10 g
Cang Zhu *Rhizoma Atractylodis* 10 g
Gan Cao *Radix Glycyrrhizae* 5 g

Explanations

- Ren Shen, Bai Zhu and Fu Ling tonify the Spleen-Qi and remove the Phlegm.
- Sha Ren and Yi Yi Ren eliminate the Damp by drying and promoting urination.
- Cang Zhu and Si Gua Luo eliminate the Damp and relieve the pain.
- Mu Xiang and Chen Pi promote Qi circulation and help above herbs resolve Damp.
- Gan Cao harmonises the prescription.

The patient received daily treatment with a herbal decoction. After 1 month of treatment, her tongue pain resolved completely. Two years later she was followed up by telephone and her painful tongue had not recurred.

Part 4

Head and neck pain 头颈疼痛

Headache 18

头
痛

Headache is a subjective symptom, which can be induced by various acute and chronic disorders. It may occur on one side, on both sides, or over the whole of the head area. It is one of the most common conditions seen in clinical practice.

According to TCM, all six Yang channels traverse the head area. The Governing Vessel and Liver channel also connect to or are distributed through the head. The Kidney is the most important organ for producing Marrow and the Brain is the Sea of Marrow. The Spleen transforms the Essence of food into Qi and Blood, which nourish the brain. The Lung disperses the Qi to all the parts of the body, including the head. The Heart dominates the Blood circulation and is in charge of mental activity. Blood is the basic energetic source for the physiological activity of the brain. Disorders in any of these channels or internal organs will influence the Qi and Blood circulation in the head, leading to headache.

Headache might be attributed to any of the following disorders in Western medicine: nasosinusitis, trigeminal neuralgia, neurosis, vascular and neurotic headache, sequela of concussion of brain. Headache may accompany hypertension, cephalitis, glaucoma or tumour, and if these are diagnosed they must be treated in combination with Western medicine.

Aetiology and pathology

The head is the place where all the Yang channels of hand and foot meet, and the Qi and Blood of the five Zang organs and six Fu organs all flow upward to the head. Both exogenous and endogenous factors may cause headache by bringing about derangement of the Qi and Blood in the head and by slowing the circulation of Qi in the channels that distribute to the head.

Generally speaking, headache with an acute onset is probably caused by invasion of Exogenous pathogen. Wind is the most common cause; it exists in every season and often combines with one or more of the other pathogenic factors, e.g. Cold, Heat and Damp. When it attacks in combination with Cold, then contraction of the channels, muscles and tendons may result in a disordered circulation of Qi and Blood causing headache. Wind combined with Heat is also commonly seen, and often occurs in spring and summer. Thirdly, Wind easily mixes with Damp to block the channels in both body and head, causing headache.

Dysfunction of the Liver is a common cause for headache due to Endogenous factors. A function of the Liver is to coordinate the Qi circulation, which is very important both emotionally and physically. Bad mood, excessive anger, distress and other mental upsets may disturb the Liver-Qi circulation and cause the Qi to stagnate. A prolonged period of Qi stagnation may then induce formation of Liver-Fire. Extreme anger may also cause the uprising of Liver-Fire and hyperactivity of Liver-Yang; in fact, the latter is one of the commonest causes of headache.

A bad diet may also cause headache. Eating too much spicy or hot food or drinking too much alcohol may cause the formation of Heat in the Stomach, and even the formation of Stomach-Fire. This Stomach-Fire burns the Stomach-Yin, disturbs the Qi circulation and induces stomach pain and headache. Eating too much fat, sweet or salty food may also damage the function of the Spleen, leading to failure of the Spleen to transport and transform the food and Damp. Damp-Phlegm consequently forms, and this may block the Qi circulation in the channels, and headache follows.

Deficiency of Qi and Blood is another cause of headache. Qi and Blood deficiency can be caused by chronic diseases, overwork, excessive bleeding in menstruation, or blood loss in trauma or during operation and so on: these lead to the failure of the brain to be sufficiently nourished by the Qi and Blood, and headache follows.

Deficiency of Kidney-Essence will also result in headache. Deficiency of Kidney-Essence can be caused by a hereditary defect, excessive sex, multiple birth and chronic sickness. As a result, the Kidney-Essence fails to produce sufficient Marrow, leading to a feeling of emptiness in the brain, and causing headache.

Finally, physical trauma to the brain, inappropriate surgery to the head, and some chronic diseases may cause blockage of the Blood circulation in the head, and therefore headache.

Invasion of Wind-Cold

External Wind-Cold is one of the most common factors causing headache, as it exists in every season. When it invades the human body, it usually attacks the superficial parts and the upper parts of the body. The head is the top of the body, so is easily invaded by External Wind-Cold.

Cold is characterised by contraction. If invasion of Wind-Cold is causing the headache, there will be contraction of the channels, muscles and tendons. Cold is also characterised by stagnation, so invasion of Wind-Cold may cause the slowing down of the Qi and Blood circulation in the head, causing a headache. Overexposure to windy and cold surroundings generally, standing around in a wind or a cold environment when sweating after sport or physical work, and careless living habits such as wearing too little clothing are all common causes of Wind-Cold invasion.

The headache caused by invasion of Wind-Cold is usually acute and accompanied by other External symptoms such as an aversion to cold, muscular pain, a cough with white expectoration, a runny nose, a thin and white tongue coating and a superficial pulse. Repeated invasions of Wind-Cold may also give rise to chronic headaches and stiffness of the neck and shoulders.

Invasion of Wind-Heat

In late spring or early summer, because of the strong sunlight and hot surroundings, Wind-Heat often causes headache. Wind-Heat usually attacks the Upper Burner through the mouth and nose. Wind and Heat are Yang pathological factors; when they invade they often attack the upper body leading to disturbance of the channels and disordered Qi and Blood circulation in the head, so headache occurs. This type of headache is frequently accompanied by fever, an aversion to cold, generalised body pain, a red face and eyes, a yellow nasal discharge, a sore throat, a cough with yellow phlegm, a red tongue with a thin and yellow coating and a superficial and rapid pulse.

Attack of Toxic Fire

In late spring or summer, especially in summer, hot weather can act as a kind of pathogenic Toxic Fire, which may easily attack and accumulate in the body. Toxic Fire is a strong Yang pathological factor; when it flares up to the head it may disturb the Qi and Blood circulation on the head and damage the channels and blood vessels there, causing a headache with swollen, red nodules or even erosions on the head, fever, restlessness, a red tongue with a yellow and dry coating and a rapid pulse. Insect bites may cause Toxin to invade the body directly, leading to the formation of Toxic Fire.

Invasion of Wind-Damp

Wind is a Yang pathological factor that always attacks the Upper Burner of the human body. If often combines with other pathological factors. A combination of Wind with Cold or Heat is often seen, as discussed above. A combination of Wind and Damp is another common cause for headache due to external invasion.

Damp is a substantial Yin pathogenic factor, which mainly exists in late summer in China, especially in the southern and south-eastern areas. It is characterised by viscosity, heaviness and stagnation. When Wind-Damp invades the body, it may block the Qi and Blood circulation in the head, muscles and tendons, leading to headache, generalised body pain and joint pain with stiffness and heaviness.

Invasions of Wind-Damp may also easily affect the Middle Burner, disturbing the ascent of clear Yang-Qi to the head and descending of Turbid Qi, so the head and Clear Orifices are blocked by turbid Qi and not properly nourished by Clear Yang-Qi, and headache follows.

Stagnation of Liver-Qi

Liver plays an important role in the emotions. It regulates Qi circulation and stores Blood. Too much stress, resentment or frustration may cause a slowing down of the Liver-Qi circulation, so the Liver-Qi stagnates. Once stagnation of Liver-Qi takes place, this may influence the circulation in the head, causing stagnation of Qi and Blood, and so headache occurs. This kind of headache is quite often seen in everyday practice.

The most important way to differentiate a headache caused by stagnation of Liver-Qi from that caused by other pathogenic factors is that a headache caused by stagnation of Liver-Qi could be greatly influenced by the emotional state, whereas other kinds of headache are not. Headache caused by stagnation of Liver-Qi is also often located at the top of the head or in the temple areas.

Flaring up of Liver-Fire

Qi is a kind of Yang energy, which should be in the state of constant movement. If there is a prolonged stagnation of the Liver-Qi, this may cause the gradual formation of Liver-Fire. Excessive anger and stress may accelerate this process. Fire is characterised by uprising and burning, so when Liver-Fire forms in the body, it may rise up to the head disturbing the Qi and Blood circulation and burning the channels on the head, causing headache. This is usually accompanied by a feeling of distension of the head, a red face and eyes, swelling in the eyes, nervousness, irritability, insomnia, a bitter taste in the mouth, a red tongue with a thin and yellow coating and a rapid and wiry pulse.

Headache caused by stagnation of Liver-Fire is usually located in the temples or over the whole head.

Hyperactivity of Liver-Yang

If the flaring of Liver-Fire persists it may cause hyperactivity of Liver-Yang, leading to a severe headache or migraine. Long-lasting flaring of Liver-Fire may also gradually consume the Yin of the Liver and Kidney, leading to deficiency of the Yin of Liver and Kidney, and here the Liver-Yang is not controlled by the Yin of Liver and Kidney, and hyperactivity of the Liver-Yang occurs. Chronic states of anxiety, distress and excessive mental activity may also consume Kidney-Essence leading to deficiency of Kidney-Yin, and so to hyperactivity of Liver-Yang. Constitutional weakness and

chronic sickness play an important role in the development of Kidney-Yin deficiency.

Uprising of Stomach-Fire

The Bright Yang channel ends on the head. Eating too much pungent, sweet or fatty food, excessive intake of milk products, or drinking too much alcohol, will cause Excessive-Heat to accumulate in the Bright Yang Fu organs and channels, and this in turn disturbs the Qi and Blood circulation and burns the channels on the head, causing a headache. This kind of headache is usually accompanied by a red face, thirst, constipation, a large appetite, a foul smell in the mouth, fever, swollen gums, a red tongue with a yellow and dry coating and a rapid and forceful pulse.

Headache caused by uprising of Stomach-Fire is usually located on the forehead or over the whole head.

Accumulation of Damp-Phlegm

The Spleen has the function of transport and transforming food and liquids. If the person has a bad diet—for instance, overeating sweet, fatty, greasy or pungent food, or drinking too much alcohol—the physiological function of the Spleen and Stomach is impaired, resulting in formation of the Damp-Phlegm. When the head is blocked by Damp-Phlegm, Clear Yang-Qi cannot rise and Turbid Qi cannot descend, so the Qi and Blood circulation in the head stagnates and headache occurs.

Deficiency of Qi and Blood

The Spleen is the source of Nutritive Qi and Blood production, so dysfunction of the Spleen and Stomach in turn causes deficiency of Qi and Blood, so the head is not properly nourished, causing headache.

Irregular eating habits, an unhealthy diet and eating too little may impair the Spleen's function of transportation and transformation, causing the Qi and Blood production to be impaired in turn and finally a deficiency of Qi and Blood. Prolonged sickness, prolonged heavy bleeding during menstruation and excessive amounts of physical or mental work may also cause deficiency of Qi and Blood, leading in turn to headache.

Deficiency of Kidney-Essence

The Kidney is the congenital energetic source for the human being. Kidney produces Essence and dominates Marrow, and the Brain is the Sea of Marrow. If there is a deficiency of Kidney-Essence then the Marrow will also be deficient, resulting in the brain not being properly nourished, then the physiological function of the head is impaired, and headache occurs.

A frail constitution, prolonged sickness, senility, and excessive sexual activity as well as giving birth to multiple infants may cause weakness or consumption of the Kidney-Essence. Also, chronic states of anxiety and fear deplete the Kidney-Essence, causing headache. Another common cause of deficiency of Kidney-Essence is weakness of the Spleen and Stomach, leading to poor levels of Qi and Blood production.

Deficiency of Kidney-Essence may be either deficiency of Kidney-Yin or deficiency of Kidney-Yang.

Stagnation of Blood

There is a saying in TCM that prolonged persistence of any disorder causes stagnation of Blood in the collateral. Indeed, a lengthy sickness, even of headache itself, may produce Blood stagnation. Improper head movement may also cause Qi and Blood stagnation, as may physical trauma, such as car accident, falling down and stroke, as well as inappropriate surgery on the head and neck, which may all directly damage the channels and muscles.

Headache caused by stagnation of Blood is characterised by headache at a fixed location that is stabbing in nature, and is often aggravated at night. As to the tongue and pulse, it is not necessary to see purplish tongue and unsmooth pulse before making a definite diagnosis of Blood stagnation, because if Blood stagnation is confined to the collateral and is not in the body as a whole, the tongue and pulse would not be able to reflect it.

Treatment based on differentiation

Differentiation

In order to understand the key points for the differentiation of headache, special attention should be paid to the quality and location of headache, and other factors that may alleviate or aggravate it.

Differentiation of the quality of headache

— Generally, a dull pain indicates Deficiency condition, while a sharp pain indicates an Excessive condition, according to the Eight Principles perspective.

— A sudden onset tends to indicate an Exterior invasion, whilst a gradual onset tends to indicate an Interior disorder.

— Dull headache indicates deficiency of Qi and Blood or deficiency of Kidney-Essence.

— Sharp headache indicates stagnation of Liver-Qi, flaring-up of Liver-Fire, hyperactivity of Liver-Yang, Stomach-Fire or Toxic Fire.

— A headache with a feeling of heaviness is usually caused by accumulation of Damp-Phlegm. This is because when the head is blocked by Damp-Phlegm there is a mixture of Clear Yang-Qi and Turbid Yin Qi in the head. Beside heaviness in the head, the head feels muzzy and as if it is wrapped in a cloth, with poor concentration and memory. There may additionally be nausea, vomiting, phlegm, obesity or diarrhoea.

— A headache with a feeling of distension has a 'swollen', 'throbbing', 'bursting' or 'pulsating' sensation. This kind of headache is usually caused by a Liver disorder, such as flaring-up of Liver-Fire or hyperactivity of Liver-Yang. Headache with distension could also be caused by invasion of Wind-Heat, flaring-up of Stomach-Fire, or Toxic Fire.

— A headache with pronounced stiffness of the occiput usually indicates an invasion of exterior Wind-Cold, and usually occurs suddenly.

— A chronic headache with stiffness of the neck usually indicates hyperactivity of Liver-Yang with formation of Liver-Wind. This kind of headache often occurs at the occipital region.

— A headache with pulling sensation also indicates formation of Liver-Wind.

— A headache with a stabbing pain, fixed in one place and worse at night or before menstruation indicates stagnation of Blood.

— A headache with a sensation of emptiness of the head indicates deficiency of Kidney-Essence.

Differentiation of location of the painful areas on the head

Top of the head

— Headache at the top of the head is also called vertex headache. A branch from the Liver channel reaches the vertex of the head internally. Vertex headache is usually caused by disorders of the Liver, due to either deficiency of Liver-Blood or hyperactivity of Liver-Yang. It will be dull in character if caused by deficiency of Liver-Blood, and sharp in character if caused by hyperactivity of Liver-Yang. Moreover, if caused by deficiency

of Liver-Blood, there will be intermittent headache, aggravation during menstruation, tiredness, poor vision, hair loss, a pale tongue and a thready pulse. If caused by hyperactivity of Liver-Yang, there will be nervousness, irritability, distension in the head, dizziness, vertigo, a red tongue and a rapid and wiry pulse.
— If there is vertex headache during invasion of external factors, it is usually blockage of the Bladder channel, which is not related to Liver disorder.

The back of the head

— The back of the head is also called the occipital area. If it is an acute case, it is usually caused by invasion of external factors, such as Wind, Cold and Damp, and this invasion often attacks the Bladder channel, leading to blockage and obstruction in the channel. If it is a chronic case, it is usually caused by accumulation of Damp-Phlegm, deficiency of Kidney-Essence or hyperactivity of Liver-Yang.
— If an occipital headache is caused by invasion of external factors, there will be other external symptoms, such as fever, an aversion to cold, muscle pain, a runny nose, a thin tongue coating and a superficial pulse.
— If it is caused by accumulation of Damp-Phlegm, the headache will be accompanied by a feeling of heaviness, dizziness, nausea, heaviness in the body, a greasy tongue coating and a slippery pulse, etc.
— If it is caused by deficiency of Kidney-Essence, there will also be general tiredness and poor concentration, lower back pain, weakness in the knees, a thin tongue coating and a thready and weak pulse.
— If it is caused by hyperactivity of Liver-Yang, there will also be nervousness, irritability, a feeling of distension in the head, dizziness, vertigo, a red tongue and a rapid and wiry pulse.

The sides of the head

Headache at the side of the head is generally caused either by external factors invading the Gall Bladder channel or by a disorder of the Gall Bladder and Liver.

— If it is caused by invasion of external factors, there will also be External symptoms, and it is usually acute.
— If it is caused by a disorder of the Gall Bladder and Liver, it is usually chronic. In everyday practice, accumulation of Damp-Heat or stones in the Gall Bladder, or stagnation of Liver-Qi, or

flaring-up of Liver-Fire, or hyperactivity of Liver-Yang are the most common causes. If the cause is accumulation of Damp-Heat, the headache is often dull or heavy in character. If the problem is accumulation of stones in the Gall Bladder, or stagnation of Liver-Qi, or flaring-up of Liver-Fire, or hyperactivity of Liver-Yang, the headache is often sharp and throbbing in character. If it is on one side only, it is usually caused by flaring-up of Liver-Fire or by hyperactivity of Liver-Yang.

The forehead

Headache in the forehead area is usually caused by disorder of internal organs. Going by the location of channels, headache in this part of the head is usually caused by a disorder of the Stomach or Gall Bladder, mostly the former.

— If headache is caused by deficiency of Stomach-Qi, the pain is dull.
— If it is caused by flaring-up of Stomach-Fire, the pain is sharp.
— If it is caused by Damp-Phlegm, the pain is dull with a heavy sensation in the head.

Behind the eyes

Headache behind the eyes is usually due to disorder of the Liver, which may include deficiency of Liver-Blood, stagnation of Liver-Qi, stagnation of Blood, flaring of Liver-Fire and hyperactivity of Liver-Yang. It often occurs during migraine, and this type of headache usually occurs on one side only, seldom on both.

— If the cause is deficiency of Liver-Blood, the pain is dull.
— If it is stagnation of Liver-Qi, the pain is distending.
— If it is stagnation of Blood, the pain is stabbing.
— If it is flaring of Liver-Fire, the pain is burning.
— If it is hyperactivity of Liver-Yang, the pain is sharp and throbbing, and often quite severe.

The whole head

Headache over the whole head may be acute or chronic.

— Acute headache affecting the whole head is usually caused by invasion of External factors, such as Wind-Cold, Wind-Heat and Wind-Damp. The pain is often constant, severe and sharp in character, and accompanied by External symptoms such as fever, an aversion to cold, muscular pain, a runny nose, a thin tongue coating and a superficial pulse, etc.

— Chronic headache of this type is usually caused by deficiency of Kidney-Essence, which results in a failure to nourish the brain properly. The pain is dull and intermittent, its occurrence closely related to the menstrual cycle and general levels of energy. The patients with this kind of headache often have a feeling of emptiness in the head.

Differentiation of other factors

Weather

— Aggravation of a headache in hot weather is usually due to flaring-up of Liver-Fire, hyperactivity of Liver-Yang, or flaring-up of Stomach-Fire.
— Aggravation in cold weather is usually due to deficiency of Yang Qi or deficiency of Blood.
— Aggravation in humid weather is usually due to accumulation of Damp-Phlegm.

Emotions

— Headache that worsens with stress and improves with relaxation is usually due to stagnation of Liver-Qi.
— If it worsens with anger and improves with relaxations it is usually due to flaring-up of Liver-Fire or hyperactivity of Liver-Yang.
— If it worsens with fear it is usually due to deficiency of Kidney-Essence.
— If it worsens with worry it is usually due to deficiency of Spleen-Qi.

Sexual activity

— Headache that worsens after sexual activity is usually due to deficiency of Kidney-Essence.
— If it is alleviated after sexual activity then it is probably due to stagnation of Liver-Qi or flaring-up of Liver-Fire.

Food

— If a headache is aggravated on eating fatty, greasy, sweet food or dairy products it is usually due to accumulation of Damp-Phlegm.
— If it worsens on drinking alcohol or eating pungent food it is usually due to flaring-up of Stomach-Fire or of Liver-Fire.
— Headache that is alleviated after eating cold food is usually due to flaring-up of Stomach-Fire.
— If alleviated after eating warm food then it is usually due to deficiency of Qi and Blood.

Posture

— Headache that is alleviated on lying down is usually due to deficiency of Qi and Blood, or of Kidney-Essence.
— Headache that worsens on lying down and improves on standing is usually due to an Excess condition.

Menstruation

— Aggravation of headache before the onset of or during menstruation is usually due to stagnation of Liver-Qi, or of Blood, or hyperactivity of Liver-Yang.
— Aggravation of headache at the end of the menstruation is usually due to deficiency of Blood or of Kidney-Essence.

Pressure

— Headache that is alleviated with pressure is usually due to deficiency of Qi and Blood, or of Kidney-Essence.
— If it worsens with pressure it is usually due to an Excess condition.

Treatment

INVASION OF WIND-COLD

Symptoms and signs

Headache with a contracting sensation, aggravation of the headache in windy or cold conditions, an aversion to wind and cold, fever, cold limbs, an absence of sweat, an absence of thirst, a stuffed-up nose with a white nasal discharge, a stiff neck, joint or body pain, a thin and white tongue coating and a superficial and tense pulse.

Principle of treatment

Dispel Wind, eliminate Cold and relieve the headache.

HERBAL TREATMENT

Prescription

CHUAN XIONG CHA TIAO SAN
Ligusticum and Green Tea Regulating Powder
Chuan Xiong *Rhizoma Ligustici Chuanxiong* 6 g
Jing Jie *Herba Schizonepetae* 6 g
Fang Feng *Radix Ledebouriellae* 6 g
Bai Zhi *Radix Angelicae Dahuricae* 6 g

Xi Xin *Herba Asari* 3 g
Gan Cao *Radix Glycyrrhizae* 5 g
Qiang Huo *Rhizoma seu Radix Notopterygii* 6 g
Cha Ye *Folium Camelliae Sinensis* 3 g

Explanations

- Chuan Xiong and Qiang Huo are used to dispel Wind-Cold, regulate the Qi circulation and sedate the headache.
- Bai Zhi and Xi Xin are used to help the two herbs above to relieve the headache.
- Jing Jie and Fang Feng are used to dispel Wind and release the External symptoms.
- Cha Ye is used to dispel Wind and calm the Mind to relieve the pain.
- Gan Cao is used to harmonise the actions of the other herbs.

Modifications

1. If there is a strong aversion to cold, add Wu Zhu Yu *Fructus Evodiae* 5 g and Gui Zhi *Ramulus Cinnamomi* 10 g to warm the channels and dispel the Wind-Cold.
2. If there is fever, add Chai Hu *Radix Bupleuri* 15 g and Ma Huang *Herba Ephedrae* 10 g to promote sweating, regulate the Qi circulation and dispel the Cold to reduce the fever.
3. If there is body pain, add Du Huo *Radix Angelicae Pubescentis* 12 g and Xi Xin *Herba Asari* 3 g to promote the Qi circulation and relieve the pain.
4. If there is a stiff neck due to stagnation of Qi in the Bladder channel, add Ge Gen *Radix Puerariae* 10 g to regulate the Qi circulation and relieve the stiffness.
5. If the nose is stuffed up, with a discharge, add Cang Er Zi *Fructus Xanthii* 10 g and Xin Yi *Flos Magnoliae* 10 g to dispel the Wind and clear the nasal passage.

Patent remedy

Chuan Xiong Cha Tiao Wan *Ligusticum and Green Tea Regulating Pill*

ACUPUNCTURE TREATMENT

GB-20 Fengchi, GB-21 Jianjing, BL-10 Tianzhu, LU-7 Lieque, LI-4 Hegu, TE-5 Waiguan and some Ah Shi points. All the points are needled with reducing method.

Explanations

- GB-20 is the crossing point of the foot Lesser Yang channel and Yang Linking Vessel. It is one of the patent points to dispel Wind and regulate the Qi circulation. It is good at treating the headache caused by Wind-Cold.
- GB-21, the crossing point of the hand and foot Lesser Yang channel and Yang Linking Vessel, dispels Wind-Cold, regulates the circulation of Qi and relieves headache.
- BL-10, a local point, regulates the circulation of Qi and relieves the headache in the Bladder channel distribution area.
- LU-7, the Connecting point of the Lung channel, dispels Wind-Cold and relieves the headache.
- LI-4, the Source point of the Large Intestine channel, regulates Qi circulation and relieves the headache.
- TE-5, the Connecting point of the Triple Burner channel, regulates Qi circulation and relieves the headache.
- The Ah Shi points promote the circulation of Qi on the head to relieve the headache.

Modifications

1. If there is an aversion to cold, add ST-36 with moxibustion to warm the channels and dispel the Cold.
2. If there is a fever, add GV-14 to dispel the Wind and reduce the fever.
3. If there is body pain, add LR-3 and BL-60 to promote the circulation of Qi, dispel the Wind and relieve the pain.
4. If there is a stiff neck, add SI-3 and BL-62 to promote the circulation of Qi and relieve the stiff neck.
5. If there is a stuffed-up nose with a discharge, add LI-20 and GV-23 to dispel the Wind and clear the nasal passage.

Case history

A 39-year-old man had suffered from occipital headache for 2 weeks. The pain developed after he had caught a cold. It was diagnosed as neurotic headache in a hospital and he was given some painkillers. He had no relief from this, so he asked for TCM treatment.

When he arrived at the clinic, he had severe headache in the occipital region, a stiff neck, a slight aversion to cold, a poor appetite, and a stuffed-up nose with a clear discharge. His tongue was white, and his pulse was superficial and wiry.

Diagnosis
Headache due to invasion of Wind-Cold.

Principle of treatment
Warm channels, eliminate External Cold and relieve the headache.

Herbal treatment
CHUAN XIONG CHA TIAO SAN
Ligusticum and Green Tea Regulating Powder
Chuan Xiong *Rhizoma Ligustici Chuanxiong* 10 g
Jing Jie *Herba Schizonepetae* 6 g
Fang Feng *Radix Ledebouriellae* 6 g
Bai Zhi *Radix Angelicae Dahuricae* 6 g
Xi Xin *Herba Asari* 3 g
Gan Cao *Radix Glycyrrhizae* 5 g
Qiang Huo *Rhizoma Seu Radix Notopterygii* 10 g
Cha Ye *Folium Camelliae Sinensis* 3 g
Gui Zhi *Ramulus Cinnamomi* 10 g
Ge Gen *Radix Puerariae* 10 g

Explanations

- Chuan Xiong, Ge Gen and Qiang Huo dispel Wind-Cold and sedate headache.
- Gui Zhi, Bai Zhi and Xi Xin work as assistants to warm the channels and relieve the headache.
- Jing Jie and Fang Feng dispel Wind and release the external symptoms.
- Cha Ye dispels Wind and calms the Mind.
- Gan Cao harmonises the actions of the other herbs in the formula.

The patient received daily herbal treatment. He had recovered from headache after 1 week of treatment. Two years later, he was followed up and he stated that he completely recovered after the herbal treatment.

INVASION OF WIND-HEAT

Symptoms and signs

Distending headache with hot or burning feeling, fever, an aversion to wind, red face and eyes, thirst, nasal obstruction, a runny nose with a yellow discharge, a sore throat, constipation, a red tip of the tongue and a yellow coating, a superficial and rapid pulse.

Principle of treatment

Dispel Wind, clear Heat and relieve the headache.

HERBAL TREATMENT

Prescription

SANG JU YIN
Mulberry Leaf and Chrysanthemum Decoction
Sang Ye *Folium Mori* 10 g
Ju Hua *Flos Chrysanthemi* 10 g
Jie Geng *Radix Platycodi* 6 g
Lian Qiao *Fructus Forsythiae* 10 g
Bo He *Herba Menthae* 6 g
Man Jing Zi *Fructus Viticis* 15 g
Lu Gen *Rhizoma Phragmitis* 20 g
Gan Cao *Radix Glycyrrhizae* 6 g

Explanations

- Sang Ye and Ju Hua dispel Wind-Heat and promote the Qi circulation.
- Jie Geng promotes the Lung-Qi circulation and dispels Wind.
- Man Jing Zi and Bo He promote the Qi circulation and relieve headache.
- Lian Qiao and Lu Gen clear Wind-Heat and increase the Body Fluids.
- Gan Cao harmonises the function of the other herbs in the formula.

Modifications

1. If there is a severe headache, add Chuan Xiong *Rhizoma Ligustici Chuanxiong* 6 g to dispel the Wind-Heat and sedate the headache.
2. If there is a stiff neck, add Ge Gen *Radix Puerariae* 15 g to dispel the Wind and relieve the neck stiffness.
3. If there is a high fever, add Shi Gao *Gypsum* 15 g to clear the Heat and reduce the fever.
4. If the throat is red and painful, add Zhe Bei Mu *Bulbus Fritillariae Thunbergii* 10 g and Pu Gong Ying *Herba Taraxaci* 10 g to disperse the Lung-Qi, clear the Heat and benefit the throat.
5. If there is a cough, add Qian Hu *Radix Peucedani* 10 g and Niu Bang Zi *Fructus Arctii* 10 g to disperse the Lung-Qi and relieve the cough.
6. If there is thirst, add Zhu Ye *Herba Lophatheri* 10 g to clear the Heat in the Upper Burner and relieve the thirst.
7. If there is constipation, add Da Huang *Radix et Rhizoma Rhei* 6 g to clear the Heat, promote defecation and so relieve the constipation.

Patent remedy

Huang Lian Shang Qing Pian *Coptis Tablet to Clear Heat of Upper Jia*.

ACUPUNCTURE TREATMENT

ST-8 Touwei, Extra Taiyang, GV-23 Shangxing, LI-4 Hegu, LI-11 Quchi and TE-5 Waiguan. All the points needled with reducing method.

Explanations

- ST-8 is the crossing point of the Gall Bladder channel of the foot Lesser Yang and Bright Yang. It is used to promote the Qi circulation and relieve the headache.
- Extra Taiyang clears Heat, regulates the circulation of Qi and relieves the headache.

- GV-23 is good at clearing Heat and regulating circulation of Qi in the head so as to relieve the headache.
- LI-4, the Source point of the Large Intestine channel, regulates the circulation of Qi, clears Heat and relieves the headache.
- LI-11, the Sea point of the Large Intestine channel, reduces Heat, reduces fever and relieves the headache.
- TE-5, the Connecting point, dispels Wind-Heat, promotes circulation of Qi and relieves the headache.

Modifications

1. If there is a severe headache, add GB-20 to dispel the Wind-Heat and sedate the headache.
2. If there is fever, add GV-14 to clear the Heat and reduce the fever.
3. If there is obstruction in the nose, add LU-7 to disperse the Lung-Qi and relieve the nasal obstruction.
4. If there is a runny nose with much nasal yellow discharge, add LI-20 and BL-2 to clear the Heat and clear the nasal passage.
5. If there is thirst, add SP-6 to clear the Heat, nourish the Yin and relieve the thirst.
6. If there is a sore throat, add LU-10 to clear the Heat and relieve the throat pain.
7. If there is constipation, add ST-25 and ST-37 to promote defecation and so relieve the constipation.

INVASION OF TOXIC FIRE

Symptoms and signs

Severe headache that is sharp or with a sense of distension, a red face, high fever, thirst, irritability or even coma, a stiff neck, convulsion, delirium, constipation, deep yellow urine, a dark reddish purple tongue and a rapid pulse.

Principle of treatment

Clear toxic Fire, cool Blood and relieve the headache.

HERBAL TREATMENT

Prescription

QING WEN BAI DU YIN
Clear Epidemics and Overcome Toxin Decoction
Shi Gao *Gypsum Fibrosum* 30 g
Sheng Di Huang *Radix Rehmanniae Recens* 15 g
Huang Lian *Rhizoma Coptidis* 10 g
Zhi Mu *Anemarrhenae* 10 g
Chi Shao *Radix Paeoniae Rubra* 10 g

Lian Qiao *Fructus Forsythiae* 10 g
Gan Cao *Radix Glycyrrhizae* 5 g
Dan Pi *Cortex Moutan Radicis* 10 g
Zhi Zi *Fructus Gardeniae* 10 g
Huang Qin *Radix Scutellariae* 10 g
Zhu Ye *Herba Lophatheri* 10 g
Jie Geng *Radix Platycodi* 5 g

Explanations

- Shi Gao, Huang Lian and Zhi Mu clear toxic Fire and reduce fever.
- Lian Qiao, Zhi Zi, Huang Qin and Zhu Ye clear toxic Fire in the Upper Burner.
- Sheng Di Huang, Dan Pi and Chi Shao clear Heat in the Blood and cool the Blood.
- Jie Geng and Gan Cao regulate the Qi circulation and remove Phlegm.

Modifications

1. If there is coma, add An Gong Niu Huang Wan *Calm the Palace Pill with Cattle Gallstone* (patent pill, 1 pill a day) to the recipe to open the Heart orifice and revive the patient.
2. If there is high fever, add Zi Xue Dan *Purple Snow Special Pill* (patent pill, 1 pill a day) to the recipe to clear the Heat and reduce the fever.
3. If there is convulsion, add Gou Teng *Ramulus Uncariae cum Uncis* 10 g and Jiang Can *Bombyx Batryticatus* 10 g to subdue the Liver-Wind and relieve the convulsion.
4. If there is thirst, add Mai Dong *Radix Ophiopogonis* 10 g and Xuan Shen *Radix Scrophulariae* 10 g to nourish the Body Fluids and relieve the thirst.
5. If the face is swollen, add Jin Yin Hua *Flos Lonicerae* 10 g and Tian Hua Fen *Radix Trichosanthis* 15 g to eliminate the Toxin and reduce the swelling.

Patent remedy

Niu Huang Jie Du Pian *Cattle Gallstone Tablet to Resolve Toxin*

ACUPUNCTURE TREATMENT

GV-20 Baihui, GB-20 Fengchi, LI-4 Hegu, LI-11 Quchi, TE-6 Zhigou, SP-6 Sanyinjiao, SP-10 Xuehai and LR-2 Taichong. All the points are needled with reducing method.

Explanations

- GV-20, the crossing point of the foot Greater Yang channel and Governing Vessel Channel, and GB-20, the crossing point of the foot Lesser Yang channel and Yang Linking Vessel, clear Heat in the head, and calm the headache.

- LI-4, the Source point, and LI-11, the Sea point, of the Large Intestine channel, together with TE-6, clear the Heat, eliminate Toxin, reduce fever and relieve the headache.
- SP-6, the crossing point of the three Yin channels of the foot, and SP-10 clear Heat in the Blood, eliminate toxin and relieve the headache.
- LR-2, the Spring point, clears Heat in the Liver, suppresses the Liver-Yang and relieves the headache.

Modifications

1. If there is a high fever, add GV-14 to clear the Heat and reduce the fever.
2. If there is a stiff neck, add SI-3 to regulate the Qi and Blood circulation and relieve the neck stiffness.
3. If there is restlessness, add HT-8 and PC-8 to clear the Heat in the Heart and calm the Mind.
4. If there is coma, add GV-26 and KI-1 to clear the Heat and revive the patient.
5. If there is thirst, add KI-6 to clear the Fire and nourish the Yin.
6. If there is constipation, add ST-25 and SP-9 to nourish the Yin, clear the Fire and promote defecation.

INVASION OF WIND-DAMP

Symptoms and signs

Headache with a heavy sensation, a feeling as though the head is wrapped in a piece of cloth, an aversion to cold, slight fever, lassitude, a sense of fullness in the chest, generalised body pain with a sensation of heaviness, a poor appetite, a sense of fullness in the stomach, a white and greasy tongue coating and a slippery and superficial pulse.

Principle of treatment

Dispel Wind, eliminate Damp and relieve the headache.

HERBAL TREATMENT

Prescription

QIANG HUO SHENG SHI TANG
Notopterygium Dispelling Dampness Decoction
Qiang Huo *Rhizoma seu Radix Notopterygii* 10 g

Du Huo *Radix Angelicae Pubescentis* 10 g
Gao Ben *Rhizoma et Radix Ligustici* 10 g
Fu Ling *Poria* 15 g
Chuan Xiong *Rhizoma Ligustici Chuanxiong* 10 g
Gan Cao *Radix Glycyrrhizae* 6 g
Fang Feng *Radix Ledebouriellae* 6 g
Zhi Ban Xia *Rhizoma Pineiliae Praeparata* 10 g
Man Jing Zi *Fructus Viticis* 10 g

Explanations

- Qiang Huo and Du Huo can dispel Wind-Cold-Damp from the upper body so as to relieve External symptoms.
- Fang Feng dispels Wind-Cold and relieves the headache.
- Chuang Xiong expels Wind and promotes the Qi and Blood circulation so as to relieve the headache.
- Gao Ben dispels Wind-Damp and relieves the headache.
- Man Jing Zi eliminates Wind and relieves the headache.
- Zhi Ban Xia and Fu Ling dry up Damp and eliminate Phlegm.
- Gan Cao coordinates the effects of the other herbs in the recipe.

Modifications

1. If there is a heavy sensation in the body, add Cang Zhu *Rhizoma Atractylodis* 10 g to dry the Damp and relieve the pain.
2. If there is lassitude, add Xiang Ru *Herba Elsholtziae seu Moslae* 10 g and Hou Po *Cortex Magnoliae Officinalis* 10 g to promote the Qi circulation in the body and dry the Damp.
3. If there is a sense of fullness in the chest, add Huo Xiang *Herba Agastachis* 12 g and Bai Kou Ren *Semen Amomi* 5 g to promote the Qi circulation in the chest and relieve the fullness in the chest.
4. If there is a poor appetite, add Ji Nei Jin *Endothelium Corneum Gigeriae Galli* 15 g and Mai Ya *Fructus Hordei Germinatus* 30 g to improve the appetite and promote the digestion.
5. If there are loose stools, add Cang Zhu *Rhizoma Atractylodis* 10 g and Hou Po *Cortex Magnoliae Officinalis* 10 g to activate the Spleen and dry the Damp.

Patent remedy

Qiang Huo Sheng Shi Pian *Notopterygium Dispelling Dampness Tablet*

ACUPUNCTURE TREATMENT

LU-7 Lieque, TE-4 Yangchi, TE-6 Zhigou, LI-4 Hegu, GB-20 Fengchi, SP-6 Sanyinjiao and Ah Shi points on the head. All the points are needled with even method.

Explanations

- LU-7, the Connecting point of the Lung channel, promotes the circulation of Qi, eliminates Damp in the Upper Burner and relieves the headache.
- TE-4, the Source point of the Triple Burner channel, together with TE-6, dispels Wind-Damp, promotes urination and relieves the headache.
- LI-4, the Source point of the Large Intestine channel, dispels Wind-Damp, regulates the circulation of Qi and relieves the headache.
- GB-20, the crossing point of the foot Lesser Yang channel and Yang Linking Vessel, dispels External pathogenic factors, promotes the circulation of Qi and relieves the headache.
- SP-6, the crossing point of three Yin channels of the foot, promotes the circulation of Qi and eliminates Damp.
- The Ah Shi points regulate the Qi circulation, harmonise the local collateral and relieve the headache.

Modifications

1. If there is a sense of heaviness in the body, add SP-3 and SP-9 to activate the Spleen and eliminate the Damp.
2. If there is lassitude, add ST-36 to activate the Spleen and Stomach, eliminate the Damp and relieve the lassitude.
3. If there is a sense of fullness in the chest, add PC-6 and CV-17 to regulate the Qi circulation in the chest and relieve the sense of fullness.
4. If there is a poor appetite, add CV-12 to regulate the Qi circulation in the Stomach and improve the appetite.
5. If there are loose stools, add ST-25 to eliminate the Damp and regulate the Large Intestine.

STAGNATION OF LIVER-QI

Symptoms and signs

Headache with sensation of pressure and tension, which starts or gets worse under stress or emotional disturbance, depression, distension and pain in the hypochondriac region, dizziness, irregular menstru- ation, a poor appetite or excessive eating, a thin and white tongue coating and a wiry pulse.

Principle of treatment

Smooth the Liver, promote Liver-Qi circulation and relieve the headache.

HERBAL TREATMENT

Prescription

XIAO YAO SAN
Free and Relaxed Powder
Chai Hu *Radix Bupleuri* 10 g
Dang Gui *Radix Angelicae Sinensis* 10 g
Bai Shao *Radix Paeoniae Alba* 20 g
Bai Zhu *Rhizoma Atractylodis Macrocephalae* 10 g
Fu Ling *Poria* 15 g
Gan Cao *Radix Glycyrrhizae* 5 g
Bo He *Herba Menthae* 3 g
Chuan Xiong *Rhizoma Ligustici Chuanxiong* 10 g
Huang Qin *Radix Scutellariae* 10 g

Explanations

- Chai Hu and Bo He regulate and promote Liver-Qi circulation so as to remove Qi stagnation in the Liver.
- Bai Shao and Dang Gui nourish the Blood in the Liver, harmonise the Liver and relieve the hypochondriac pain.
- Chuan Xiong regulates the Liver-Qi and relieves the headache.
- Bai Zhu and Fu Ling strengthen the Spleen and Stomach.
- Huang Qin clears Internal Heat resulting from stagnation of Liver-Qi.
- Gan Cao harmonises the actions of the other herbs.

Modifications

1. If there is a severe headache, add Yan Hu Suo *Rhizoma Corydalis* 10 g and Bai Zhi *Radix Angelicae Dahuricae* 10 g to promote Qi circulation in the head and relieve the headache.
2. If there is hypochondriac pain, add Yu Jin *Radix Curcumae* 10 g and Ju He *Semen Citri Reticulatae* 10 g to regulate the Qi circulation to relieve pain.
3. If there is irregular menstruation or dysmenorrhoea, add Huai Niu Xi *Radix Achyranthis Bidentatae* 10 g and Yi Mu Cao *Herba Leonuri* 10 g to regulate the menstruation.

4. If there is a low mood, add Xiang Fu *Rhizoma Cyperi* 10 g regulate the Liver-Qi and improve the mood.
5. If there is insomnia, add Long Gu *Os Draconis* 15 g to calm the Heart and tranquillise the Mind.
6. If there is a poor appetite, add Mai Ya *Fructus Hordei Germinatus* 15 g and Yu Jin *Radix Curcumae* 10 g to remove the Qi stagnation and improve the appetite.

Patent remedies

Xiao Yao Wan *Free and Relaxed Pill*
Shu Gan Wan *Soothe Liver Pill*

ACUPUNCTURE TREATMENT

GV-20 Baihui, Extra Sishencong, LR-3 Taichong, PC-6 Neiguan, LI-4 Hegu and SP-6 Sanyinjiao. All points are needled with even method.

Explanations

- GV-20, the crossing point of the foot Greater Yang channel and the Governing Vessel, promotes the Liver-Qi circulation and relieves the headache.
- Extra Sishencong helps GV-20 to regulate the Liver-Qi, calms the Mind and relieves the headache.
- LR-3, the Stream and Source point of the Liver channel, regulates the Liver-Qi and removes Qi stagnation.
- PC-6, the Connecting point of the Pericardium channel, regulates the circulation of Qi and calms the Mind.
- LI-4, the Source point of the Large Intestine channel, regulates the circulation of Qi and relieves the headache.
- SP-6, the crossing point of the three Yin channels of the foot, regulates the Liver-Qi circulation and removes Qi stagnation.

Modifications

1. If there is dizziness, add GB-8 to relieve this.
2. If there is depression, add HT-3 and BL-18 to regulate the Qi circulation, calm the Mind and improve the emotional state.
3. If there is insomnia, add HT-3 and HT-7 to calm the Mind and improve sleeping.
4. If there is hypochondriac pain, add LR-5, the Connecting point, and LR-14, the Front Collecting point, to promote the Liver-Qi circulation, harmonise the collateral and relieve the pain.
5. If there is a poor appetite, add CV-12 to harmonise the Stomach-Qi and improve the appetite.
6. If there are loose stools when nervous and abdominal pain and cramp due to invasion of the Spleen by the Liver, add LR-13 and SP-3 to promote the Liver-Qi circulation and strengthen the Spleen.
7. If there is irregular menstruation or dysmenorrhoea, add ST-28 and KI-10 to promote the Qi and Blood circulation and regulate the menstruation.

FLARING-UP OF LIVER-FIRE

Symptoms and signs

Headache with a sharp or distending pain, red eyes, irritability, a bitter taste in the mouth, restlessness, insomnia, irregular menstruation, a poor appetite, deep yellow urine, constipation, a red tongue and a rapid and wiry pulse.

Principle of treatment

Reduce Liver-Fire, calm down Mind and relieve the pain.

HERBAL TREATMENT

Prescription

LONG DAN XIE GAN TANG
Gentianae Decoction to Drain the Liver
Long Dan Cao *Radix Gentianae* 10 g
Huang Qin *Radix Scutellariae* 10 g
Zhi Zi *Fructus Gardeniae* 10 g
Ze Xie *Rhizoma Alismatis* 12 g
Chuan Xiong *Rhizoma Ligustici Chuanxiong* 10 g
Xia Ku Cao *Spica Prunellae* 10 g
Che Qiang Zi *Semen Plantaginis* 10 g
Dang Gui *Radix Angelicae Sinensis* 10 g
Sheng Di Huang *Radix Rehmanniae Recens* 12 g
Chai Hu *Radix Bupleuri* 10 g
Gan Cao *Radix Glycyrrhizae* 6 g

Explanations

- Long Dan Cao, Huang Qin, Xia Ku Cao and Zhi Zi reduce Liver-Fire.
- Ze Xie and Che Qian Zi promote urination and induce Fire out of the body through urination.

- Dang Gui, Chuan Xiong and Chai Hu promote the Liver-Qi circulation and relieve the headache.
- Sheng Di clears Heat and nourishes the Yin of the Liver and Kidney.
- Gan Cao harmonises the actions of the other herbs in the formula.

Modifications

1. If the eyes are red, add Cao Jue Ming *Semen Cassiae* 12 g to clear the Liver-Fire and relieve the redness in the eyes.
2. If there is irritability, add Zhi Mu *Rhizoma Anemarrhenae* 10 g to regulate the Liver-Qi and clear the Liver-Fire.
3. If there is insomnia and restlessness, add Suan Zao Ren *Semen Ziziphi Spinosae* 15 g and Zhen Zhu Mu *Concha Margaritifera Usta* 20 g to calm the Mind and improve sleep.
4. If there is hypochondriac pain, add Yu Jin *Radix Curcumae* 10 g to promote the Liver-Qi circulation and relieve the pain.
5. If there is painful urination, add Ku Shen *Radix Sophorae Flavescentis* 10 g and Che Qian Zi *Semen Plantaginis* 10 g to clear the Liver-Fire and promote urination.
6. If there is irregular menstruation or dysmenorrhoea, add Chi Shao *Radix Paeoniae Rubra* 10 g to regulate the Blood circulation and harmonise the menstruation.
7. If there is night sweating, add Huang Bai *Cortex Phellodendri* 10 g to clear the Deficient-Heat and stop the sweating.
8. If there is constipation, add Da Huang *Radix et Rhizoma Rhei* 6 g and Mang Xiao *Natrii Sulfas* 12 g to clear the Liver-Fire and promote defecation.

Patent remedy

Long Dan Xie Gan Wan *Gentianae Pill to Drain the Liver*

ACUPUNCTURE TREATMENT

Extra Taiyang, GV-20 Baihui, GB-8 Shuaigu, TE-6 Zhigou, SP-6 Sanyinjiao, LR-2 Xingjian and GB-43 Xiaxi. All the points are needled with reducing method.

Explanations

- Extra Taiyang and GB-8 treat the headache at the sides of the head.
- GV-20 tranquillises the Mind and calms Liver-Fire.

- LR-2, the Spring point of the Liver channel, clears Liver-Fire and relieves the headache.
- GB-43, the Spring point of the Gall Bladder channel, clears Heat, regulates the circulation of Qi in the Gall Bladder channel and relieves the headache.
- TE-6 promotes the function of the Triple Burner, regulates the circulation of Qi, clears Fire in the Triple Burner and reduces Liver-Fire.
- SP-6, the crossing point of three Yin channels of the foot, clears Liver-Fire and regulates the circulation of Qi in the Liver.

Modifications

1. If there is neck pain with stiffness, add GB-21 and TE-5 to harmonise the collateral and relieve the neck pain.
2. If the eyes are red, add GB-1 to reduce the Liver-Fire and alleviate the redness.
3. If there is irritability, add Extra Sishencong to calm the Mind and relieve irritability.
4. If there is insomnia, add HT-8 to clear the Heat in the Heart and improve the sleep.
5. If there is a poor appetite, add CV-12 to promote the Stomach-Qi and improve the appetite.
6. If there is a bitter taste in the mouth, add GB-40 to clear the Heat in the Liver and Gall Bladder and relieve the bitter taste in the mouth.
7. If there are loose stools when nervous and abdominal pain and cramp due to invasion of the Spleen by the Liver, add LR-13 and SP-3 to promote the Liver-Qi circulation and strengthen the Spleen.
8. If there is constipation, add ST-25 to promote defecation and relieve the constipation.
9. If there is irregular menstruation, add SP-10 Xuehai and ST-28 to promote the Qi and Blood circulation and regulate the menstruation.

HYPERACTIVITY OF LIVER YANG

Symptoms and signs

Severe and frequent headache accompanied by hypochondriac pain or with a sensation of distension, dizziness, restlessness, irritability, shaking of the head and hands, insomnia, red face and eyes, a red tongue with a thin and yellow coating and a wiry pulse.

Principle of treatment

Calm the Liver, subdue Liver-Yang and relieve the headache.

HERBAL TREATMENT

Prescription

TIAN MA GOU TENG YIN
Gastrodia and Uncaria Decoction
Tian Ma *Rhizoma Gastrodiae* 10 g
Gou Teng *Ramulus Uncariae cum Uncis* 10 g
Shi Jue Ming *Concha Haliotidis* 15 g
Huang Qin *Radix Scutellariae* 10 g
Chuan Niu Xi *Radix Cyathulae* 10 g
Sang Ji Sheng *Ramulus Loranthi* 10 g
Ye Jiao Teng *Caulis Polygoni Multiflori* 15 g
Chuan Xiong *Rhizoma Ligustici Chuanxiong* 10 g
Ju Hua *Flos Chrysanthemi* 10 g

Explanations

- Tian Ma and Gou Teng smooth the Liver and suppress the Liver-Yang so as to relieve the headache.
- Chuan Xiong and Ju Hua assist Tian Ma to regulate the Liver-Qi circulation and relieve the headache.
- Shi Jue Ming and Chuan Niu Xi suppress the Liver-Yang and bring the Liver-Yang downward.
- Huang Qin clears Heat in the Liver.
- Ye Jiao Teng calms the Mind and improves the sleep.
- Sang Ji Sheng nourishes the Yin of the Liver and Kidney and calms the Liver-Yang.

Modifications

1. If there is a severe headache, add Quan Xie *Scorpio* 1.5 g and Bai Jiang Can *Bombyx Batryticatus* 10 g to subdue the Liver-Wind and sedate the headache.
2. If there is irritability, add Huang Lian *Rhizoma Coptidis* 10 g to clear the Liver-Fire and relieve the irritability.
3. If there is hypochondriac pain, add Qing Pi *Pericarpium Citri Reticulatae Viride* 10 g and Chuan Lian Zi *Fructus Meliae Toosendan* 10 g to regulate the Qi circulation and stop the pain.
4. If there is insomnia, add Suan Zao Ren *Semen Ziziphi Spinosae* 10 g to calm the Mind and improve the sleep.
5. If there is a bitter taste in the mouth, add Zhi Zi *Fructus Gardeniae* 10 g to clear the Heat in the Liver and Gall Bladder.
6. If there is abdominal pain, add Yan Hu Suo *Rhizoma Corydalis* 10 g and Bai Shao *Radix Paeoniae Alba* 15 g to promote the Qi and Blood circulation and stop the pain.

7. If there is a warm feeling in the head, add Mu Dan Pi *Cortex Moutan Radici* 10 g to clear the Heat in the head.

Patent remedy

Jiang Ya Ping Pian *Lower (Blood) Pressure Calming Tablet*

ACUPUNCTURE TREATMENT

GB-20 Fengchi, GB-43 Xiaxi, Extra Taiyang, GV-20 Baihui, LI-4 Hegu, SP-6 Sanyinjiao, KI-2 Rangu, LR-2 Xingjian and LR-8 Ququan.

Explanations

- GB-20, the crossing point of the foot Lesser Yang channel and the Yang Linking Vessel, and GV-20 clear Heat in the head, subdue the Liver-Yang and relieve the headache.
- Extra Taiyang clears Heat and relieves the headache.
- SP-6, the crossing point of the three Yin channels of the foot, regulates the Liver and clears Heat in it.
- LI-4, the Source point of the Large Intestine point, promotes the Qi circulation, clears Heat in the head and relieves the headache.
- GB-43, KI-2 and LR-2, the Spring points, clear Heat and suppress the Liver-Yang.
- LR-8, the Water point, clears Heat in the Liver and subdues the Liver-Yang.

Modifications

1. If there is irritability, add HT-3 and PC-6 to calm the Mind and relieve the irritability.
2. If the face and eyes are red, add ST-44 and GB-1 to clear the Heat and relieve the redness in the face and eyes.
3. If there is hypochondriac pain, add LR-14 to promote the Qi circulation and relieve the pain.
4. If there is insomnia, add HT-8 to clear the Heat in the Heart, calm the Mind and relieve the insomnia.
5. If there is a bitter taste in the mouth, add GB-40 to clear the Heat in the Gall Bladder.

UPRISING OF STOMACH-FIRE

Symptoms and signs

Headache mainly in the forehead, a red face, profuse sweating, aggravation of headache on exposure to warmth, and alleviation on contact with cold or drinking of cold liquids, a feverish feeling, thirst, a sore throat, painful gums, constipation, deep yellow urine, a red tongue with a yellow and dry coating and a rapid and forceful pulse.

Principle of treatment

Clear Stomach-Fire, regulate Qi and relieve the headache.

HERBAL TREATMENT

Prescription

YU NU JIAN
Jade Woman Decoction
Shi Gao *Gypsum Fibrosum* 20 g
Zhi Mu *Rhizoma Anemarrhenae* 10 g
Chuan Xiong *Rhizoma Ligustici Chuanxiong* 6 g
Bai Zhi *Radix Angelicae Dahuricae* 10 g
Huang Lian *Rhizoma Coptidis* 5 g
Ju Hua *Flos Chrysanthemi* 10 g
Man Jing Zi *Fructus Viticis* 10 g
Sheng Di Huang *Radix Rehmanniae Recens* 10 g

Explanations

- Shi Gao and Zhi Mu clear Stomach-Fire and reduce fever.
- Sheng Di Huang cools Heat and removes Fire in body.
- Ju Hua clears Heat in the Upper Burner.
- Huang Lian clears Heat in the Stomach and relieves the headache.
- Man Jing Zi, Bai Zhi and Chuan Xiong promote Qi circulation and relieve the headache.

Modifications

1. If there is a feverish feeling, add Mu Dan Pi *Cortex Moutan* 10 g to clear the Heat and relieve the feverish feeling.
2. If the gums are swollen, add Da Qing Ye *Folium Isatidis* 10 g to clear the Heat and eliminate the toxin.
3. If there is thirst, add Tian Hua Fen *Radix Trichosanthis* 15 g to increase the Body Fluids and relieve the thirst.
4. If the throat is painful, add Pu Gong Ying *Herba Taraxaci* 10 g to clear the Heat, eliminate the Toxin, benefit the throat and relieve the throat pain.
5. If there is constipation, add Da Huang *Radix et Rhizoma Rhei* 10 g and Mang Xiao *Natrii Sulfas* 10 g to clear the Heat and promote defecation.

Patent remedy

Wei Te Ling *Stomach Especially Effective Remedy*

ACUPUNCTURE TREATMENT

LI-2 Erjian, LI-4 Hegu, TE-6 Zhigou, ST-8 Touwei, ST-44 Neiting, CV-12 Zhongwan and GB-20 Fengchi. Reducing method is used on all these points.

Explanations

- LI-2, the Spring point, and LI-4, the Source point, clear Heat, especially in the Large Intestine, and relieve the headache.
- TE-6 promotes the physiological function of the Triple Burner and clears Heat in the body.
- ST-8, the crossing point of foot Lesser Yang and Bright Yang channels, regulates the circulation of Qi and relieves the headache.
- ST-44, the Spring point, and CV-12, the Front Collecting point, clear Heat in the Stomach.
- GV-20 clears Heat in the head and relieves the headache.

Modifications

1. If there is a severe headache in the forehead, add ST-42, the Source point, and Extra Yuyao to clear the Heat in the Stomach and relieve the headache.
2. If there is toothache, add ST-6 and ST-7 to promote the Qi circulation and reduce the pain.
3. If there is pain and swelling in the throat, add LU-10 and CV-23 to relieve the pain and reduce the swelling.
4. If there is thirst, add LU-7 and KI-6 to regulate the Yin and relieve the thirst.
5. If there is constipation, add ST-25 Tianshu to promote defecation and relieve the constipation.

Case history

A 43-year-old man had suffered from headache for 3 months. At first, he had a fever, headache, a swollen gum on right side and toothache. He went to see a dentist, who diagnosed odontitis, so he took some antibiotics for a week. His general symptoms had improved slightly, but he still had headache over the forehead, toothache, thirst, a dry mouth, a foul smell in the mouth, constipation, a red tongue with a slight yellow and dry coating and a superficial and slight rapid pulse.

Diagnosis
Headache due to uprising of Stomach-Fire.

Principle of treatment
Clear Stomach-Fire, harmonise the collateral and sedate the pain.

Acupuncture treatment
LI-2 Erjian, LI-4 Hegu, TE-6 Zhigou, ST-6 Jiache, ST-7 Xiaguan, ST-8 Touwei, ST-44 Neiting and GB-20 Fengchi. Reducing method is used on all these points. Treatment was given once every other day.

Explanations

- LI-2, the Spring point, and LI-4, the Source point, clear Heat, especially in the Large Intestine, and relieve the headache.
- TE-6 promotes the physiological function of the Triple Burner and clears Heat in the body.
- ST-6 and ST-7, the local points, clear Heat and relieve the toothache.
- ST-8, the crossing point of the foot Lesser Yang and Bright Yang channels, regulates the circulation of Qi and relieves the headache.
- ST-44, the Spring point, and CV-12, the Front Collecting point, clear Heat in the Stomach.
- GV-20 clears Heat in the head and relieves the headache.

The patient's headache was under control in 3 weeks. He had three more treatments to stabilise the effects. One year later, he was followed up and he stated he had completely recovered since the acupuncture treatment.

ACCUMULATION OF DAMP-PHLEGM

Symptoms and signs

Headache with a sensation of heaviness, dizziness, a feeling of fullness in the chest and epigastric region, nausea, vomiting, poor appetite, phlegm, a white and greasy tongue coating and a slippery, or wiry and slippery, pulse.

Principle of treatment

Eliminate Damp, resolve Phlegm and sedate the headache.

HERBAL TREATMENT

Prescription

BAN XIA BAI ZHU TIAN MA TANG
Pinellia, Atractylodes Macrocephala and Gastrodia Decoction
Ban Xia *Rhizoma Pinelliae* 10 g
Bai Zhu *Rhizoma Atractylodis Macrocephalae* 10 g
Tian Ma *Rhizoma Gastrodiae* 10 g

Fu Ling *Poria* 15 g
Chen Pi *Pericarpium Citri Reticulatae* 10 g
Man Jing Zi *Fructus Viticis* 10 g
Gan Cao *Radix Glycyrrhizae* 5 g

Explanations

- Ban Xia and Chen Pi dry Damp and resolve Phlegm in the Middle Burner.
- Fu Ling and Bai Zhu activate the Spleen and eliminate Damp.
- Tian Ma and Man Jing Zi eliminate Damp in the head and relieve the headache.
- Gan Cao harmonises the functions of other herbs in the formula.

Modifications

1. If there is dizziness, add Chang Pu *Rhizoma Acori Graminei* 10 g to eliminate the Damp, resolve the Phlegm and relieve the dizziness.
2. If there is a headache over the forehead, a runny nose with a white discharge and loss of the sense of smell, add Gao Ben *Rhizoma et Radix Ligustici* 10 g and Cang Er Zi *Fructus Xanthii* 10 g to clear the nose, eliminate the Phlegm and relieve the headache.
3. If there is phlegm, add Chen Pi *Pericarpium Citri Reticulate* 10 g and Bai Jie Zi *Semen Sinapis Albae* 10 g to regulate the Qi and eliminate the Phlegm.
4. If there is a poor appetite, add Cang Zhu *Rhizoma Atractylodis* 10 g and Yu Jin *Radix Curcumae* 10 g to promote the Qi circulation, eliminate the Phlegm and improve the appetite.
5. If there is a sensation of fullness in the stomach, add Hou Po *Cortex Magnoliae Officinalis* 10 g to eliminate the Damp and regulate the Stomach-Qi.
6. If there is nausea or vomiting, add Zhu Ru *Caulis Bambusae in Taeniam* 10 g and Zhi Shi *Fructus Aurantii Immaturus* 10 g to cause the Stomach-Qi to descend and relieve the vomiting.

Patent remedies

Ban Xia Bai Zhu Tian Ma Pian *Pinellia, Atractylodes Macrocephala and Gastrodia Tablet*
Xiang Sha Liu Jun Wan *Six-Gentleman Pill with Aucklandia and Amomum*

ACUPUNCTURE TREATMENT

GB-20 Fengchi, ST-8 Touwei, CV-12 Zhongwan, LI-4 Hegu, ST-40 Fenglong, SP-6 Sanyinjiao, SP-9

Yinlingquan and Ah Shi points. All the points are needled with even method.

Explanations

- GB-20 and ST-8, the crossing point of the foot Lesser Yang channel and the Yang Linking Vessel, promote the circulation of Qi and eliminate Damp-Phlegm in the head so as to relieve the headache.
- CV-12, the Front Collecting point of the Stomach and the Gathering point for the Fu organs, promotes the circulation of Qi in the Middle Burner, removes Damp and resolves Phlegm.
- LI-4, the Source point of the Large Intestine channel, promotes the circulation of Qi and relieves the headache.
- SP-6, the crossing point of the three Yin channels of the foot, and SP-9, the Sea point, activate the Spleen and eliminate Damp-Phlegm.
- The Ah Shi points promote the circulation of Qi and relieve the headache.

Modifications

1. If there is dizziness, add GB-8 to eliminate the Damp, resolve the Phlegm and relieve the dizziness.
2. If there is a headache over the forehead, a runny nose with a white discharge and loss of the sense of smell, add BL-2 and Extra Yintang to clear the nose, eliminate the Phlegm and relieve the headache.
3. If there is a loss of the sense of smell, add GV-23 to clear the nose and improve the ability to smell.
4. If there is Phlegm, add LU-5 to regulate the Lung-Qi and eliminate the Phlegm.
5. If there is a poor appetite, add PC-6 to promote the Qi circulation, eliminate the Phlegm and improve the appetite.
6. If there is a sensation of fullness in the Stomach, add LR-13, which is the Front Collecting point of the Spleen, to eliminate the Damp and regulate the Spleen-Qi.
7. If there is nausea or vomiting, add SP-4, the Confluence point for the Penetrating Vessel, to cause the Stomach-Qi to descend and relieve the vomiting.

DEFICIENCY OF QI

Symptoms and signs

Headache with a sensation of lightness, an aggravation of the headache after physical exertion, tiredness, a pale complexion, an aversion to cold, cold hands, shortness of breath, loose stools, poor appetite, low voice, pale tongue with tooth marks and a thin and white coating, and a slow and deep pulse.

Principle of treatment

Activate the Spleen and Stomach, reinforce Qi and relieve headache.

HERBAL TREATMENT

Prescription

BU ZHONG YI QI TANG
Tonify the Middle and Augment the Qi Decoction
Dang Shen *Radix Codonopsis Pilosulae* 9 g
Bai Zhu *Rhizoma Atractylodis Macrocephalae* 9 g
Fu Ling *Poria* 12 g
Zhi Gan Cao *Radix Glycyrrhizae Praeparata* 6 g
Huang Qi *Radix Astragali seu Hedysari* 10 g
Chen Pi *Pericarpium Citri Reticulatae* 6 g
Mu Xiang *Radix Aucklandiae* 9 g
Sha Ren *Fructus Amomi* 6 g

Explanations

- Dang Shen, Bai Zhu, Fu Ling and Zhi Gan Cao, known as Si Jun Zi Tang—Four Gentlemen Decoction, can activate the Spleen and tonify the Spleen-Qi.
- Huang Qi tonifies the Spleen-Qi and lifts up Qi to the head.
- Chen Pi harmonises the Stomach-Qi.
- Mu Xiang and Sha Ren promote the movement of Qi in the Middle Burner.

Modifications

1. If there are cold hands and feet, an aversion to cold and a slow pulse, add Gan Jiang *Rhizoma Zingiberis* 10 g to warm the Middle Burner and dispel Interior Cold.
2. If there is a poor appetite, add Gu Ya *Fructus Oryzae Germinatus* 9 g and Mai Ya *Fructus Hordei Germinatus* 9 g to promote the digestion and improve the appetite.
3. If there is nausea, add Zhi Ban Xia *Rhizoma Pinelliae Praeparata* 6 g to harmonise the Stomach and relieve the nausea.

Patent remedy

Bu Zhong Yi Qi Wan *Tonify the Middle and Augment the Qi Pill*

ACUPUNCTURE TREATMENT

BL-20 Pishu, BL-21 Weishu, ST-3 Juliao, SP-6 Sanyinjiao and SP-3 Taibai. Reinforcing method and moxibustion are used on these points.

Explanations

- BL-20 Pishu and BL-21 Weishu, the Back Transporting point of the Spleen and Stomach, tonify the Spleen and Stomach and regulate their physiological functions.
- ST-36, the Lower Sea point of the Stomach, and SP-3, the Source point, strengthen the Spleen-Qi, tonify the Stomach, transform Damp and promote digestion.
- SP-6 strengthens the Spleen and tonifies the Qi and Blood.

Modifications

1. If there are cold hands and feet, an aversion to cold and a slow pulse, add GV-4 and moxibustion on ST-36, GV-4 and SP-3 Taibai to warm the Middle Burner and dispel Interior Cold.
2. If there is aggravation of headache by stress, add BL-18 to smooth the Liver and regulate the Liver-Qi.
3. If there is a poor appetite, add SP-9, the Sea point, to activate the Spleen, promote digestion and improve the appetite.
4. If there is nausea, add SP-4 to harmonise the Stomach and relieve the nausea.
5. If there is abdominal pain due to food stagnation, add BL-25 to regulate the Large Intestine and promote digestion.
6. If there is chronic diarrhoea, add ST-36 to transform Damp and relieve the diarrhoea.

DEFICIENCY OF BLOOD

Symptoms and signs

Headache with a hollow sensation, aggravation of the headache after physical exertion and alleviation by rest, dizziness, hair loss, palpitations, listlessness, insomnia, a pale complexion, a poor appetite, dry stools, a pale tongue with a thin and white coating and a thready and weak pulse.

Principle of treatment

Reinforce Blood and sedate the headache.

HERBAL TREATMENT

Prescription

SI WU TANG
Four-Substance Decoction
Dang Gui *Radix Angelicae Sinensis* 10 g
Shu Di Huang *Radix Rehmanniae Praeparata* 15 g
Chuan Xiong *Rhizoma Ligustici Chuanxiong* 10 g
Bai Shao *Radix Paeoniae Alba* 10 g
Man Jing Zi *Fructus Viticis* 10 g
Ju Hua *Flos Chrysanthemi* 10 g

Explanations

- Dang Gui and Chuan Xiong nourish the Blood and relieve the headache.
- Shu Di Huang tonifies the Kidney-Essence so as to promote Blood production.
- Bai Shao nourishes the Blood, harmonises the Liver and relieves the dizziness.
- Man Jing Zi and Ju Hua regulate the circulation of Qi and relieve the headache.

Modifications

1. If there is dizziness, add Tian Ma *Rhizoma Gastrodiae* 10 g and Gou Teng *Ramulus Uncariae cum Uncis* 10 g to subdue the Liver-Wind and relieve the dizziness.
2. If there are palpitations, add Dan Shen *Radix Salviae Miltiorrhizae* 10 g to nourish the Blood and calm the Mind.
3. If there is a poor appetite, add Chen Pi *Pericarpium Citri Reticulatae* 10 g and Shan Zha *Fructus Crataegi* 10 g to promote the digestion and improve the appetite.
4. If there is insomnia, add Suan Zao Ren *Semen Ziziphi Spinosae* 10 g and Wu Wei Zi *Fructus Schisandrae* 10 g to nourish the Blood and improve the sleep.
5. If there are dry stools, and Xuan Shen *Radix Scrophulariae* 10 g and Shou Wu *Radix Polygoni Multiflori* 10 g to nourish the Blood, smooth the Large Intestine and promote defecation.

Patent remedy

Ren Shen Shou Wu Jing *Ginseng, and Polygonum Extract*
Gui Pi Wan *Restore the Spleen Pill*

ACUPUNCTURE TREATMENT

GV-20 Baihui, HT-5 Tongli, PC-6 Neiguan, ST-36 Zusanli, SP-6 Sanyinjiao, KI-3 Taixi and GB-39

Xuanzhong. All the points are needled with reinforcing method.

Explanations

- GV-20, the crossing point of the foot Taiyang channel and the Governing Vessel, lifts up the Qi and Blood to the head and relieves headache.
- HT-5, the Connecting point of the Heart channel, regulates the circulation of Blood and calms the Mind.
- PC-6, the Connecting point of the Pericardium channel, regulates the Qi circulation and relieves the headache.
- ST-36, the Sea point of the Stomach channel, and SP-6, the crossing point of the three Yin channels of the foot, activate the Spleen and Stomach, tonify the Qi and Blood and relieve the headache.
- KI-3, the Source point, and GB-39, the Gathering point for the Marrow, promote the production of Blood and tonify it.

Modifications

1. If there is dizziness, add Extra Sishencong and LR-3 to tonify and regulate the Qi to relieve the dizziness.
2. If there is a poor appetite, add CV-12, the Front Collecting point of the Stomach, to regulate the Qi circulation in the Stomach and improve the appetite.
3. If there are palpitations, add HT-3 to relieve the palpitations.
4. If there is insomnia, add HT-7 and Extra Anmian to calm the Mind and improve the sleep.
5. If there are dry stools, add ST-37 to promote defecation.

STAGNATION OF BLOOD

Symptoms and signs

Prolonged persistence of a stabbing headache with fixed location, aggravation of the headache at night, before or during menstruation, dark and purplish menstruation with clots, a history of physical trauma and other cerebral diseases, insomnia, a purplish tongue, or purplish spots on the tongue, and a thready or choppy pulse.

Principle of treatment

Promote circulation of Blood, eliminate Blood stasis and relieve the headache.

HERBAL TREATMENT

Prescription

TONG QIAO HUO XUE TANG
Unblock the Orifices and Invigorate the Blood Decoction
Chuan Xiong *Rhizoma Ligustici Chuanxiong* 10 g
Chi Shao *Radix Paeoniae Rubra* 10 g
Dang Gui *Radix Angelicae Sinensis* 10 g
Dan Shen *Radix Salviae Miltiorrhizae* 10 g
Hong Hua *Flos Carthami* 10 g
Bai Zhi *Radix Angelicae Dahuricae* 10 g
Xiang Fu *Rhizoma Cyperi* 10 g
Qing Pi *Pericarpium Citri Reticulatae Viride* 5 g
Zhi Qiao *Fructus Aurantii* 10 g

Explanations

- Chuan Xiong, Chi Shao, Dan Shen and Hong Hua all promote the circulation of Blood and eliminate its stasis. Also, Chuan Xiong is a very good herb to induce the other herbs to ascend to the head to treat the headache.
- Dang Gui promotes the circulation of Blood and harmonises it so as not to harm the Blood when using Blood-circulating herbs.
- Since the Qi circulation promotes the Blood circulation, some herbs to promote the Qi circulation are prescribed here as well, such as Qing Pi, Zhi Qiao and Xiang Fu.
- Bai Zhi together with Chuan Xiong and Dang Gui relieves the headache.

Modifications

1. If there is a severe headache, or an aggravation of pain at night or the pain is related to menstruation, add Pu Huang *Pollen Typhae* 10 g, and San Leng *Rhizoma Sparganii* 10 g to strongly promote the Blood circulation and break the Blood stasis.
2. If there is a swollen spot on the head, or a brain tumour, add Wu Ling Zhi *Faeces Trogopterorum* 10 g and Mo Yao *Resina Myrrhae* 5 g to promote the Blood circulation, sedate the swelling and relieve the headache.
3. If there is dizziness, add Di Long *Lumbricus* 10 g and Tian Ma *Rhizoma Gastrodiae* 10 g to relieve this.
4. If there is dysmenorrhoea, add Yan Hu Suo *Rhizoma Corydalis* 10 g to promote the Blood circulation and so relieve the dysmenorrhoea.
5. If there is insomnia, add Suan Zao Ren *Semen Ziziphi Spinosae* 10 g and Bai Zi Ren *Semen Biotae* 10 g to calm the Mind and improve the sleep.

6. If the memory is poor, add Shi Chang Pu *Rhizoma Acori Graminei* 10 g to improve the memory.

Patent remedy

Yan Hu Suo Zhi Tong Pian *Corydalis Stop Pain Tablet*

ACUPUNCTURE TREATMENT

GB-20 Fengchi, LI-4 Hegu, PC-6 Neiguan, BL-17 Geshu, SP-6 Sanyinjiao, LR-3 Taichong, LR-5 Ligou and Ah Shi points. Reducing method is used on these points.

Explanations

- Qi is the guide for Blood. LI-4 and LR-3 are used to regulate the Qi circulation so as to lead the Blood circulation.
- SP-6, the crossing point of the three Yin channels of the foot, and BL-17, the Gathering point for the Blood, promote the Blood circulation and relieve the pain.
- GB-20, the crossing point of the foot Lesser Yang channel and the Yang Linking Vessel, promotes the Qi and Blood circulation in the head and relieves the headache.
- PC-6, the Connecting point of the Pericardium channel, regulates the circulation of Qi so as to promote the circulation of Blood.
- LR-3, the Stream and Source point, and LR-5, the Connecting point, promote the circulation of Qi, harmonise the collateral and relieve the headache.
- The Ah Shi points promote the Qi and Blood circulation in the head to relieve the headache.

Modifications

1. If there is a severe headache at night, add SI-3 to promote the Qi and Blood circulation and relieve the headache.
2. If there are painful spots on the head, add Ah Shi points in the painful areas to promote the Qi and Blood circulation and eliminate the Blood stasis.
3. If there is dysmenorrhoea with clots, add ST-28 and SP-8 to promote the circulation of Blood and relieve the dysmenorrhoea.
4. If there is insomnia, add HT-3 to regulate the Qi and Blood circulation and calm the Mind.
5. If there is neck pain, add BL-10 to promote the circulation of Blood and relieve the neck pain.
6. If the memory is poor, add GV-20 and Extra Sishencong to promote the Qi and Blood circulation.

DEFICIENCY OF KIDNEY-ESSENCE

Symptoms and signs

Headache with a hollow sensation, dizziness, listlessness, lower back pain, weakness of the knees, seminal emission, tinnitus, poor hearing, insomnia, poor memory, hair loss, loose teeth, irregular menstruation or amenorrhoea, a thin tongue coating and a thready and weak pulse, especially at the Liver and Kidney positions.

Principle of treatment

Tonify the Kidney and benefit Kidney-Essence.

HERBAL TREATMENT

Prescription

GUI SHEN WAN
Return to the Kidney Pill
Shu Di Huang *Radix Rehmanniae Praeparata* 15 g
Shan Yao *Rhizoma Dioscoreae* 10 g
Shan Zhu Yu *Fructus Corni* 10 g
Gou Qi Zi *Fructus Lycii* 10 g
Dang Gui *Radix Angelicae Sinensis* 10 g
Ge Gen *Radix Pueraria* 10 g
Gui Ban *Plastrum Testudinis* 10 g
Sang Ji Sheng *Ramulus Loranthi* 10 g

Explanations

- Shu Di Huang, Shan Yao, Gou Qi Zi and Shan Zhu Yu reinforce and tonify the Kidney and benefit the Kidney-Essence.
- Sang Ji Sheng tonifies the Kidney-Essence and strengthens the Bones.
- Gui Ban nourishes the Liver and Kidney.
- The Blood is stored and regulated in the Liver. Since the Liver and Kidney are derived from the same source, abundant Blood in the Liver benefits the Kidney-Essence, so Dang Gui is used to tonify the Blood in the Liver and promote the Blood circulation to prevent obstructions caused by the nourishing herbs.
- Ge Gen lifts the Kidney-Essence to the head and relieves the headache.

Modifications

1. If the memory is poor, add Shi Chang Pu *Rhizoma Acori Graminei* 10 g and Sha Yuan Ji Li *Semen Astragali Complanati* 10 g to nourish the Essence and improve the memory.

2. If there is tinnitus, add Ci Shi *Magnetitum* 15 g and Ji Xue Teng *Caulis Spatholobi* 15 g to relieve this.

3. If there is dizziness, add Gou Teng *Ramulus Uncariae cum Uncis* 10 g and Tian Ma *Rhizoma Gastrodiae* 10 g to subdue the interior Wind and relieve the dizziness.

4. If there is lower back pain, add Bu Gu Zhi *Fructus Psoraleae* 10 g and Lu Jiao Jiao *Colla Cornus Cervi* 10 g to tonify the Kidney and relieve the pain.

5. If there is insomnia, add Suan Zao Ren *Semen Ziziphi Spinosae* 10 g and Bai Zi Ren *Semen Biotae* 10 g to calm the Mind and improve the sleep.

6. If there is an aversion to cold, cold hands and feet, impotency a pale tongue with a wet coating and slow pulse caused by deficiency of Kidney-Yang, add Du Zhong *Cortex Eucommiae* 10 g and Zhi Fu Zi *Radix Aconiti Carmichaeli Praeparata* 10 g to tonify the Kidney-Yang and dispel the Interior Cold.

7. If there is night sweating, hot flushing, warmth in the palms and soles of the feet, thirst, a red tongue with a scanty coating and a thready and rapid pulse due to deficiency of Kidney-Yin, add Han Lian Cao *Herba Ecliptae* 10 g, Nu Zhen Zi *Fructus Ligustri* 10 g and Zhi Mu *Rhizoma Anemarrhenae* 10 g to nourish the Kidney-Yin and clear the Deficient-Heat.

Patent remedy

Ge Jie Da Bu Wan *Gecko Great Tonifying Pill*

ACUPUNCTURE TREATMENT

BL-11 Dashu, GB-39 Xuanzhong, KI-3 Taixi, LR-3 Taichong, ST-36 Zusanli and BL-23 Shenshu. All the points are needled with reinforcing method.

Explanations

- The Kidney dominates the Bones and Marrow. If the brain is insufficiently nourished by the Kidney-Essence owing to a deficiency of the Kidney, a headache occurs. KI-3, the Source point, and SP-6, the crossing point of the three Yin channels of the foot, tonify the Kidney-Essence and benefit the brain.

- BL-11, the Gathering point for the Bones, and GB-39, the Gathering point for the Marrow, nourish the Bones and benefit the Marrow so as to nourish the brain and stop pain.

- LR-3, the Stream and Source point of the Liver channel, is used to nourish Liver-Yin.

- ST-36, the Sea point of the Stomach channel, is used to tonify the Qi so as to strengthen the Kidney.

- BL-23, the Back Transporting point of the Kidney, is used to tonify the Kidney-Essence.

Modifications

1. If there is dizziness, and a poor memory and poor concentration, add GB-20 and GV-20 to raise the Yang Qi and the Kidney-Essence to the head so as to relieve the dizziness.

2. If there is lower back pain and weakness in the knees, add CV-4 and KI-10 to tonify the Kidney and benefit the knees.

3. If there is a general tiredness, a feeling of cold in the hands and feet and shortness of breath on exertion due to deficiency of the Kidney-Yang, add CV-4 and CV-6 with moxibustion to tonify the Original Qi and warm the Interior.

4. If there is night sweating, heat in the palms and soles of the feet, thirst and a dry mouth and throat due to deficiency of Kidney-Yin, add KI-2, KI-6 and KI-7 to nourish the Kidney-Yin and clear the Deficient-Heat.

Case history

A 70-year-old woman had been suffering from headache for 3 years. She complained of headache with a light feeling in the head, dizziness, stiffness and a pain in her neck. She had been diagnosed as having cervical spondylosis 3 years previously. A few months previously, she had received physiotherapy treatment; however, there was no improvement afterwards. Beside headache and dizziness, she had tenderness in the neck, poor memory, lower back pain with soreness, sometimes hot flushing, night sweating, a dry mouth and dry stools. Her tongue was red with a scanty coating, and her pulse was deep, thready and rapid.

Diagnosis
Deficiency of the Kidney-Yin.

Principle of treatment
Tonify the Kidney, nourish the Yin and relieve the headache.

Acupuncture treatment
LR-3 Taichong, LR-8 Ququan, KI-3 Taixi, KI-10 Yingu, SP-6 Sanyinjiao, GB-20 Fengchi, BL-11 Dashu, GB-39 Xuanzhong, SI-3 Houxi and BL-62 Shenmai. Reinforcing method was used on these points. Treatment was given every other day for 1 month.

Explanations

- LR-3, the Source point, and LR-8, the Sea point and Water point, tonify the Liver, smoothe the Liver and clear Heat in the Liver.

- KI-3, the Source point, and KI-10, the Sea point and Water point, nourish the Kidney-Yin, clear Deficient-Heat and relieve the headache.
- SP-6, the crossing point of the three Yin channels of the foot, regulates and tonifies the Liver and Kidney and clears Deficient-Heat.
- GB-20 calms the Liver and relieves the headache.
- BL-11, the Gathering point for the Bones, and GB-39, the Gathering point for the Marrow, are used to nourish the Bones and Marrow so as tonify the Liver and Kidney and relieve neck stiffness.
- SI-3 and BL-62 are used to open the Governing Vessel and promote the Qi and Blood circulation to the head so as to relieve neck pain and stiffness.

After 30 days' treatment, her headache was much improved. Another 10 treatment sessions were arranged for her in order to strengthen the effect. Half a year later, she was followed up and she stated that she had not suffered from headaches after this treatment.

Neck pain 19

颈

痛

Neck pain is one of the common complaints encountered in daily practice as, due to the stresses of modern life, people have more and more tension, both physical and mental. Delays in treatment, or improper treatment of neck pain may lead to further damage.

Neck pain may occur either on one side or on both sides of the neck, and includes stabbing, burning and contracting pain, and pain with stiffness. According to TCM, it is usually caused by a bad sleeping position, invasion of external pathogenic factors, stagnation of Qi and Blood, overstrain, physic trauma or inappropriate surgery. Neck pain might be attributed to any of the following diseases in Western medicine: carbuncle, local skin infection, degeneration of the cervical vertebrae, herniation of a cervical disc, osteoarthritis, cervical spondylosis, trachelokyphosis, spontaneous subluxation of cervical vertebrae, trachelagra, trachelomyitis, carotid arteritis and injury of the soft tissues of the neck.

Aetiology and pathology

Invasion of External pathogenic factors

Bad daily habits, such as standing in the wind, exposure to wind after heavy sweating, or after heavy physical exertion, or insufficient covering when sleeping, may leave the person vulnerable to invasion of External pathogenic factors, leading to stagnation of Qi and Blood in the channels and the collateral, and then neck pain follows.

Attack of Toxic Fire

When the neck is attacked by Toxic Fire, the result may be stagnation of Qi and Blood in the channels. An attack by severe Toxic Fire can even cause deterioration of the muscles, and then redness, swelling, formation of pus and pain in the neck can occur.

Attack by Toxic Fire includes both the invasion of External Toxic Heat and attack by Internal Fire. The former is usually due to existence of too-strong pathogenic Heat and bad personal hygiene; the latter includes attack by the Fire of the Liver, Lung and Stomach. If there is hyperactivity of Liver-Fire, there is a neck pain together with rigidity, occurring mostly at the back or sides of the neck, which may be accompanied by headache, nervousness, dizziness or irritability. If the pain is due to hyperactivity of the Fire of Lung and Stomach, it often occurs at the front of the neck, and refers to the sides, and may be accompanied by fever, throat pain, redness and swelling in the throat, difficulty in swallowing, cough, thirst or constipation.

Emotional disturbance

Excessive stress, frustration or depression may cause stagnation of Liver-Qi. Habital anger, indignation, animosity, or a feeling of being insulted, and rage, may cause the generation of Liver-Fire and Liver-Yang hyperactivity. The Liver and Gall Bladder share a pair of channels and a collateral. If there is stagnation of Liver-Qi, there will also be stagnation of Qi in the Gall Bladder, the Lesser Yang channel of the Gall Bladder will be blocked, and neck pain then occurs. Stagnation of Liver-Qi may also cause formation of Blood stagnation, which may aggravate the neck pain.

Physical injury

This may result from bad neck posture when reading, studying, working, driving or sleeping. It may also be caused by falling down, physical trauma, inappropriate surgery or manipulation, sudden turning of the neck, overloading of the neck, or excessive physical strain of the neck. All these factors may slow down the Qi and Blood circulation, and cause disharmony of the collateral, obstruction of the tendons and impairment of the muscles, leading to stagnation of the Qi and Blood, and so neck pain follows.

Poor constitution

Congenital weakness, excessive physical or mental work, prolonged sickness, excessive sexual activity, multiple births and a bad diet may all cause weakness of the Qi and Blood, leading to undernourishment of the neck. It may also result in Kidney weakness, leading to deficiency of Kidney-Essence, in which the neck bones are not properly nourished, and neck weakness with pain follows.

Treatment based on differentiation

Differentiation

Differentiation of External or Internal origin

— Acute onset of neck pain, sharp pain, aggravation of the pain by exposure of the neck to cold, heat or damp, accompanied by External symptoms, is usually caused by invasion of External factors.
— Acute onset of neck pain, sharp pain, aggravation of the pain by pressure and movement, and history of bad sleeping, is usually caused by stagnation of Qi or Blood in the channels.

— A chronic history of neck pain, mild or severe in intensity, associated with exertion, the emotional state and other physical conditions, is usually caused by disorder of the Internal Zang-Fu organs.

Differentiation of character of the pain

— Acute sharp neck pain with a cold sensation and contraction, accompanied by External symptoms, such as an aversion to cold, slight fever, muscle pain, absence of thirst, or superficial and tight pulse, is usually caused by invasion of Wind-Cold, or Wind, Cold and Damp.
— Acute sharp neck pain with a burning sensation, an aversion to cold, fever, throat pain, a cough, a thin and yellow tongue coating and a superficial and rapid pulse, is usually caused by invasion of Wind-Heat.
— Chronic sharp neck pain, or chronic neck pain with acute aggravation, with aggravation of neck pain by emotional stress, depression, insomnia or headache, is usually caused by stagnation of Liver-Qi.
— Chronic sharp neck pain with a burning sensation, or chronic neck pain with acute aggravation, with aggravation of the neck pain by emotional upset, nervousness, irritability, severe headache, red eyes or dizziness, is usually caused by hyperactivity of Liver-Yang.
— Neck pain occurring at the front side of neck with a burning sensation, referring to the sides of the neck, accompanied by fever, throat pain, difficulty in swallowing, cough, formation of pus in the throat or tonsils, thirst or constipation, is usually caused by hyperactivity of Fire of Lung and Stomach.
— Stabbing pain in the neck with a fixed location, aggravation of the neck pain at night, difficulty in neck movement, dislike of pressure, or history of physical trauma or operation, is usually caused by stagnation of Blood.
— Chronic slight neck pain which is worsened by exertions and often occurs in old people, with a feeling of weakness in the neck, tiredness, weakness of the knees, or lower back pain, is usually caused by deficiency of Kidney-Essence.

Treatment

INVASION OF WIND-COLD

Symptoms and signs

Acute neck pain with stiffness and cold feeling, an aversion to cold and wind, alleviation of the pain with warmth and aggravation with cold. Other symptoms include a slight fever, runny nose with a white discharge, headache, absence of sweat, generalised body pain, a thin and white tongue coating and a superficial and tight pulse.

Principle of treatment

Dispel Wind, eliminate Cold, warm the channel and relieve the pain.

HERBAL TREATMENT

Prescription

GE GEN TANG
Pueraria Decoction
Ge Gen *Radix Puerariae* 15 g
Ma Huang *Herba Ephedrae* 10 g
Gui Zhi *Ramulus Cinnamomi* 10 g
Bai Shao *Radix Paeoniae Alba* 10 g
Da Zao *Fructus Ziziphi Jujubae* 6 g
Sheng Jiang *Rhizoma Zingiberis Recens* 10 g
Qiang Huo *Rhizoma seu Radix Notopterygii* 10 g
Gan Cao *Radix Glycyrrhizae* 6 g

Explanations

- Ma Huang and Gui Zhi promote sweating and dispel Wind-Cold.
- Ge Gen and Bai Shao are used to regulate the Qi circulation, nourish the Body Fluids and relieve neck pain.
- Qiang Huo dispels Wind and relieves neck pain.
- Sheng Jiang and Da Zao dispel Wind-Cold and harmonise the Nutritive and Defensive Qi so as to relieve External symptoms.
- Gan Cao tonifies the Qi and harmonises the function of the other herbs in the prescription.

Modifications

1. If there is a headache, add Chuan Xiong *Rhizoma Ligustici Chuanxiong* 10 g and Bai Zhi *Radix Angelicae Dahuricae* 10 g to dispel the Wind-Cold, regulate the Qi circulation and relieve the pain.
2. If there is a fever, add Chai Hu *Radix Bupleuri* 15 g and Qian Hu *Radix Peucedani* 10 g to regulate the Qi circulation and reduce the fever.
3. If there is a clear nasal discharge, add Jie Geng *Radix Platycodi* 10 g and Fang Feng *Radix Ledebouriellae* 10 g to dispel the Wind and open the nasal orifice.
4. If there is an aversion to cold, add Xi Xin *Herba Asari* 3 g and Fu Zi *Radix Aconiti* 10 g to warm the channels and dispel the Cold.

Patent remedy

Jing Fang Bai Du Pian *Schizonepeta and Ledebouriella Tablet to Overcome Pathogenic Influences*

ACUPUNCTURE TREATMENT

TE-5 Waiguan, LI-4 Hegu, BL-12 Fengmen, GB-20 Fengchi and LU-7 Lieque. Reducing method is used on these points. Moxibustion should be used on the first three points.

Explanations

- LI-4 and LU-7 are used to open the skin pores and promote sweating so as to dispel Wind-Cold. LU-7 is also a good point for treating neck pain due to invasion of External factors. Conventionally, it is often used to treat neck pain where there is difficulty in turning the neck to the left and right.
- TE-5, BL-12 and GB-20 are applied to dispel Wind and eliminate Cold so as to relieve External symptoms. Moreover, GB-20 and TE-5 can arrest pain at the sides of the neck.

Modifications

1. If there is neck pain with stiffness and difficulty in turning the neck, add SI-3, the Confluence point of the Governing Vessel, to open the Vessel and harmonise the collateral.
2. If there is upper back pain with a cold feeling due to invasion of Wind-Cold to the Bladder channel, add BL-58, the Connecting point, and BL-62, the Confluentce point of Yang Heel Vessel, to dispel the Wind-Cold and relieve the pain.
3. If there is neck pain at the side of the neck due to disharmony of the Lesser Yang channels resulting from invasion of Wind-Cold, add GB-1 and TE-23 to remove the blockage in the channel and harmonise the collateral so as to arrest the pain.
4. If there is neck pain referring to the back of the shoulder, add SI-4, the Source point, SI-7, the Connecting point, and SI-12 to dispel the Cold, harmonise the collateral and relieve the pain.
5. If there is a headache, add Extra Yintang and GV-16 to dispel the Wind-Cold and stop the headache.
6. If there is a cough with a white nasal discharge due to failure of the Lung to disperse the Qi, add BL-13, the Back Transporting point of the Lung,

and LU-1, the Front Collecting point of the Lung, to disperse the Lung-Qi and relieve the cough.

Case history

A 41-year-old woman had complained of neck pain for 6 days. She had developed an acute neck pain when she woke up one morning in an air-conditioned room in the summer. The pain was mainly located on the right side. A doctor gave her some painkillers and asked her to stay at home. After taking painkillers for 1 day, there had been some relief of pain but it was not completely gone, so she asked for TCM treatment.

On her arrival at the acupuncture clinic, she had neck pain with a rigid sensation, limitation of movement, an aversion to cold and a slight upper back pain. Her tongue was white and wet, and her pulse was superficial and wiry.

Diagnosis
Neck pain due to invasion of External Cold with blockage of the channels.

Principle of treatment
Warm the channels, eliminate External Cold and relieve the neck pain.

Herbal treatment
GE GEN TANG
Pueraria Decoction
Ge Gen *Radix Puerariae* 15 g
Ma Huang *Herba Ephedrae* 6 g
Gui Zhi *Ramulus Cinnamomi* 6 g
Bai Shao *Radix Paeoniae Alba* 15 g
Da Zao *Fructus Ziziphi Jujubae* 6 g
Sheng Jiang *Rhizoma Zingiberis Recens* 10 g
Qiang Huo *Rhizoma seu Radix Notopterygii* 10 g
Chuan Xiong *Rhizoma Ligustici Chuanxiong* 10 g
Bai Zhi *Radix Angelicae Dahuricae* 10 g
Gan Cao *Radix Glycyrrhizae* 6 g

Explanations
- Ma Huang and Gui Zhi promote sweating and dispel Wind-Cold.
- Ge Gen regulates the Qi circulation, nourishes the Body Fluids and relieves the neck pain.
- Qiang Huo and Bai Zhi dispel Wind, promote the circulation of Qi and relieve the headache.
- Chuan Xiong promotes the Qi and Blood circulation and relieves the neck pain.
- Sheng Jiang and Da Zao dispel Wind-Cold and harmonise the Nutritive and Defensive Qi so as to relieve External symptoms.
- Bai Shao and Gan Cao relieve tension in the tendons to relieve the neck pain.

Acupuncture treatment
TE-5 Waiguan, LI-4 Hegu, BL-12 Fengmen, BL-58 Feiyang, GV-16 Fengfu, GB-20 Fengchi and LU-7 Lieque. Reducing method was used on these points.

Moxibustion should be used on the first three points. Treatment was given once every 2 days.

Explanations
- LI-4 and LU-7 open the skin pores and promote sweating so as to dispel the Wind-Cold. LU-7 is also a good point for treating neck pain due to invasion of External factors. Conventionally, it is often used to treat neck pain where there is difficulty in turning the neck.
- TE-5, BL-12 and GB-20 dispel Wind and eliminate Cold so as to relieve External symptoms. Moreover, GB-20 and TE-5 have the function of arresting neck pain at the sides of the neck.
- GV-16 dispels Wind-Cold in the upper back and relieves the neck pain.
- BL-58, the Connecting point, harmonises the collateral, dispels Wind-Cold and relieves the neck pain.

Her neck pain disappeared after 1 week of treatment. She was followed up 6 months later and she stated she had experienced no neck pain since the treatment.

INVASION OF WIND-HEAT

Symptoms and signs

Acute neck pain with stiffness and a burning feeling, aggravation of the pain on exposure to warmth and alleviation on exposure to cold, a slight aversion to cold and wind, fever, a runny nose with a yellow discharge, headache, sweating, thirst, restlessness, generalised body pain, a thin and yellow tongue coating and a superficial and rapid pulse.

Principle of treatment

Dispel Wind, clear Heat, harmonise the collateral and relieve the pain.

HERBAL TREATMENT

Prescription

CHAI GE JIE JI TANG
Bupleurum and Kudzu Decoction to Release the Muscle Layer
Chai Hu *Radix Bupleuri* 10 g
Ge Gen *Radix Puerariae* 15 g
Gan Cao *Radix Glycyrrhizae* 5 g
Huang Qin *Radix Scutellariae* 10 g
Qiang Huo *Rhizoma seu Radix Notopterygii* 10 g
Bai Zhi *Radix Angelicae Dahuricae* 10 g
Bai Shao *Radix Paeoniae Alba* 15 g
Jie Geng *Radix Platycodi* 10 g
Shi Gao *Gypsum Fibrosum* 20 g

Explanations

- Chai Hu and Ge Gen dispel Wind-Heat, regulate the Qi circulation and relieve the pain.
- Qiang Huo and Bai Zhi are used to promote the Qi circulation, dispel Wind and relieve the neck pain and headache.
- Shi Gao and Huang Qin clear Heat and eliminate Wind.
- Jie Geng is used to promote the Qi circulation in the Upper Burner.
- Bai Shao is used to regulate the Qi circulation, nourish the Body Fluids and relieve neck pain.
- Gan Cao harmonises the herbs in the formula.

Modifications

1. If there is headache, add Chuan Xiong *Rhizoma Ligustici Chuanxiong* 10 g and Man Jing Zi *Fructus Viticis* 10 g to dispel the Wind-Heat, regulate the Qi circulation and relieve the pain.
2. If there is fever, add Chai Hu *Radix Bupleuri* 15 g and Qian Hu *Radix Peucedani* 10 g to regulate the Qi circulation and reduce the fever.
3. If there is a yellow nasal discharge, add Jin Yin Hua *Flos Lonicerae* 10 g and Fang Feng *Radix Ledebouriellae* 10 g to dispel the Wind and clear the nasal passage.
4. If there is thirst, add Zhi Mu *Rhizoma Anemarrhenae* 10 g and Xuan Shen *Radix Scrophulariae* 10 g to clear the Heat and nourish the Yin.
5. If there is restlessness, add Huang Lian *Rhizoma Coptidis* 10 g and Zhi Zi *Fructus Gardeniae* 10 g to clear the Fire and calm the Mind.

Patent remedy

Huang Lian Shang Qing Wan *Coptis Upper Clearing Tablet*

ACUPUNCTURE TREATMENT

TE-5 Waiguan, LI-4 Hegu, LI-11 Quchi, BL-12 Fengmen, GB-20 Fengchi, LU-7 Lieque and GV-14 Dazhui. Reducing method is used on these points.

Explanations

- LI-4, LI-11 and GV-14 dispel Wind, clear Heat and reduce fever.
- LU-7 dispels Wind-Heat from the Lung channel and relieves cough. Also, LU-7 is a good point for treating neck pain where there is difficulty in turning the neck.

- TE-5, BL-12 and GB-20 dispel Wind and clear Heat so as to relieve external symptoms. Moreover, GB-20 and TE-5 arrest pain at the side of the neck.

Modifications

1. If there is neck pain with stiffness and difficulty in turning the neck, add SI-3, the Confluence point of the Governing Vessel, to open the vessel and harmonise the collateral.
2. If there is upper back pain with a burning feeling due to invasion of Wind-Heat to the Bladder channel, add BL-58, the Connecting point, BL-62, the Confluence point of Yang Heel Vessel, and BL-66, the Spring point, to dispel the Wind, clear the Heat, harmonise the collateral and relieve the pain.
3. If there is pain at the sides of the neck due to disharmony of the Lesser Yang channels resulting from invasion of Wind-Heat, add GB-1, GB-21 and TE-23 to open the channels and harmonise the collateral so as to arrest the pain.
4. If there is neck pain referring to the back of the shoulder, add SI-4, the Source point, SI-7, the Connecting point, and SI-12 to harmonise the collateral and relieve the pain.
5. If there is a headache, add Extra Yintang and GV-16 to dispel the Wind-Heat and stop the headache.
6. If there is a cough with a yellow nasal discharge due to failure of the Lung to disperse the Qi, add BL-13, the Back Transporting point of the Lung, and LU-5, the Water point, to disperse the Lung-Qi and relieve the cough.
7. If there is a throat pain with redness and swelling, add LU-10 and LI-2, the Spring points, to clear the Heat, reduce the swelling and relieve the pain.

INVASION OF WIND, COLD AND DAMP

Symptoms and signs

Neck pain with soreness, a feeling of heaviness in the neck, aggravation of the pain in rainy, humid, windy and cold weather, an aversion to cold, a cold feeling at the neck, a preference for warmth and alleviation by massage, headache, a heavy feeling to the body, a thin, white and greasy tongue coating and a superficial and slippery pulse.

Principle of treatment

Dispel Wind, eliminate Cold, resolve Damp, warm the channel and relieve the pain.

HERBAL TREATMENT

Prescription

QIANG HUO SHENG SHI TANG
Notopterygium Dispelling Dampness Decoction
Qiang Huo *Rhizoma seu Radix Notopterygii* 10 g
Du Huo *Radix Angelicae Pubescentis* 10 g
Gao Ben *Rhizoma et Radix Ligustici* 10 g
Fang Feng *Radix Ledebouriellae* 10 g
Chuan Xiong *Rhizoma Ligustici Chuanxiong* 10 g
Zhi Gan Cao *Radix Glycyrrhizae Praeparata* 6 g
Man Jing Zi *Fructus Viticis* 15 g
Ge Gen *Radix Puerariae* 15 g

Explanations

- Qiang Huo, Du Huo, Fang Feng, Man Jing Zi, Gao Ben and Chuan Xiong promote sweating, dispel Wind, eliminate Damp and relieve the pain.
- Chuan Xiong invigorates the circulation of Blood and promotes the circulation of Qi in the Channels.
- Ge Gen dispels Wind, promotes the circulation of Qi and relieves the neck pain.
- Zhi Gan Cao harmonises the actions of the other herbs in the prescription.

Modifications

1. If there is a headache, add Bai Zhi *Radix Angelicae Dahuricae* 10 g and Huo Xiang *Herba Agastachis* 6 g to dispel the Wind and relieve the headache.
2. If there is a heavy sensation in the body, add Fu Ling *Poria* 15 g and Han Fang Ji *Radix Stephaniae Tetrandrae* 10 g to promote urination and eliminate the Damp.
3. If the appetite is poor, add Ban Xia *Rhizoma Pinelliae* 10 g, Yi Yi Ren *Semen Coicis* 10 g and Sha Ren *Fructus Amomi* 6 g to dry Damp and improve the appetite.

Patent remedy

Feng Shi Pian *Wind-Damp Tablet*

ACUPUNCTURE TREATMENT

BL-11 Dashu, BL-12 Fengmen, BL-58 Feiyang, BL-62 Shenmai, SI-3 Houxi, TE-5 Waiguan, GB-20 Fengchi, GV-16 Fengfu and SP-9 Yinlingquan. Reducing method is used on these points.

Explanations

- Invasion of Wind, Cold and Damp with long duration in the body usually occurs in the Bladder channel, Governing Vessel and Triple Burner channel, so points from these three channels are often used. Moreover, the Bladder channel is the longest channel in the body, and covers the most exterior parts of the body, so, relatively speaking, more points are prescribed from the Bladder channel.
- TE-5, GB-20, GV-16, BL-12 and BL-58 dispel Wind, Cold and Damp, promote the Qi and Blood circulation in these three channels and harmonise the collateral. Moreover, TE-5, the Connecting point of the Triple Burner channel and the Confluence point of the Yang Linking Vessel, and BL-58, the Connecting point of the Bladder channel, are effective in arresting the neck pain.
- SI-3 and BL-62 open the Governing Vessel and relieve the neck pain.
- Prolonged invasion of Wind, Cold and Damp may cause problems in the muscles and bones of the neck, so BL-11, the Gathering point for the Bones, and SP-9, the Sea point, are used to consolidate the bones and resolve Damp in the muscles.

Modifications

1. If there is a wandering pain at the neck due to the predominance of Wind invasion, add LU-7 to dispel the Wind and relieve the pain.
2. If there is a fixed pain with a heavy feeling due to the predominance of Damp invasion, add TE-6 and SP-3 to activate the Spleen and eliminate the Damp.
3. If there is a severe pain with cold feeling due to the predominance of Cold invasion, add moxibustion on BL-11, BL-12, TE-5 and BL-58 to warm the channels and dispel the Cold.
4. If there is neck pain at the side of the neck due to disharmony of Lesser Yang channels resulting from invasion of Wind, Cold and Damp, add GB-1, GB-21 and TE-23 to open the channels and harmonise the collateral so as to arrest the pain.
5. If there is neck pain referring to the back of the shoulder, add SI-4, the Source point, SI-7, the Connecting point, and SI-12 to harmonise the collateral and relieve the pain.
6. If there is a headache, add Extra Yintang and GB-8 to sedate the headache.

STAGNATION OF LIVER-QI

Symptoms and signs

Spasm, tension and pain at one side or both sides of the neck, pain in the occipital and temple regions, pain that moves up and down, and is related to the emotional situation, depression, stress, a feeling of oppression over the chest, headache, a bitter taste in the mouth, insomnia, a tongue with a slight purplish colour, and a thin coating, and a wiry pulse.

Principle of treatment

Smooth the Liver, circulate Qi, harmonise the Gall Bladder and relieve the pain.

HERBAL TREATMENT

Prescription

XIAO YAO SAN
Free and Relaxed Powder
Chai Hu *Radix Bupleuri* 10 g
Dang Gui *Radix Angelicae Sinensis* 10 g
Bai Shao *Radix Paeoniae Alba* 20 g
Bai Zhu *Rhizoma Atractylodis Macrocephalae* 10 g
Fu Ling *Poria* 15 g
Gan Cao *Radix Glycyrrhizae* 5 g
Bo He *Herba Menthae* 3 g
Ge Gen *Radix Puerariae* 15 g
Yan Hu Suo *Rhizoma Corydalis* 12 g

Explanations

- Chai Hu and Bo He regulate and promote circulation of the Liver-Qi so as to remove Qi stagnation in the Liver.
- Ge Gen promotes the circulation of Qi and relieves the neck pain.
- Bai Shao and Dang Gui nourish the Blood, strengthen the Liver and remove the Qi stagnation. These two herbs can also help Ge Gen to relieve the neck pain directly.
- Bai Zhu and Fu Ling tonify the Spleen and Stomach.
- Yan Hu Suo regulates the circulation of Blood and relieves the neck pain.
- Gan Cao is used to harmonise the other herbs in the prescription.

Modifications

1. If there is a headache, add Chuan Xiong *Radix Ligustici Chuanxiong* 10 g and Qiang Huo *Rhizoma et Radix Notopterygii* 10 g to regulate the Qi circulation and relieve the headache.
2. If the emotions are unstable, add Xiang Fu *Rhizoma Cyperi* 10 g and Yu Jin *Radix Curcumae* 10 g to promote the Liver-Qi circulation and remove Qi stagnation.

3. If there is insomnia, add Dan Shen *Radix Salviae Miltiorrhizae* 10 g and Huang Lian *Rhizoma Coptidis* 5 g to calm the Mind and improve the sleep.
4. If there is irritability, add Huang Qin *Radix Scutellariae* 10 g and Zhi Zi *Fructus Gardeniae* 10 g to clear Liver-Fire and smooth the Liver.

Patent remedies

Xiao Yao Wan *Free and Relaxed Pill*
Shu Gan Wan *Soothe Liver Pill*

ACUPUNCTURE TREATMENT

LR-3 Taichong, GB-20 Fengchi, GB-21 Jianjing, GB-35 Yangjiao, GB-36 Waiqiu, GB-41 Zulinqi, PC-6 Neiguan and TE-5 Waiguan. Reducing method is used on these points.

Explanations

- Since stagnation of Liver-Qi with disharmony of the Gall Bladder is the root cause for this kind of neck pain, smoothing the Liver and promoting circulation of the Liver-Qi is the principal aim of this treatment. LR-3, the Source point of the Liver channel, fulfils this function.
- PC-6, the Connecting point of the Pericardium channel and the Confluence point of the Yin Linking Vessel, helps LR-3 circulate the Liver-Qi and regulate the emotions. It also improves the sleep.
- GB-20 and GB-21 calm the Liver and harmonise the Gall Bladder channel. These two local points are very important points for treating neck pain due to emotional disorders.
- GB-35 and GB-36, the Accumulation points of the Yang Linking Vessel and the Gall Bladder channel respectively, are used to sedate the neck pain.
- GB-41 and TE-5, a special point combination, harmonise the Lesser Yang channels and relieve the neck pain.

Modifications

1. If there is neck pain referring to the back of the shoulder, add SI-4, the Source point, and SI-7, the Connecting point, and SI-12 to harmonise the collateral and relieve the pain.
2. If there is a headache, add GV-20 to calm the Liver and suppress the Liver-Yang so as to sedate the headache.
3. If there is insomnia, dream-disturbed sleep, or restlessness due to hyperactivity of Heart-Fire,

add HT-3, the Sea point, and Extra Sishencong to calm the Mind and improve the sleep.

4. If there is depression, and a sense of fullness and pain in the chest due to stagnation of Liver-Qi, add LR-14, the Front Collecting point of the Liver, and CV-17, the Gathering point for the Qi, to smooth the Liver, circulate the Liver-Qi and relieve the depression.

5. If there is irritability, add LR-2 and GB-43, the Spring points of the Liver and Gall Bladder channels respectively, to clear Heat from the Liver.

6. If there is a bitter taste in the mouth, poor appetite and constipation due to stagnation of Qi in the Gall Bladder channel, add GB-40, the Source point, and TE-6 to regulate the Lesser Yang channel and relieve the stagnation in the Gall Bladder.

HYPERACTIVITY OF LIVER-YANG

Symptoms and signs

Spasm, pain and rigidity of the neck, a burning feeling in the neck, aggravation of the pain with nervousness, headache, dizziness, irritability, insomnia, a red tongue, especially at the edges, with a yellow coating and a wiry and rapid pulse.

Principle of treatment

Calm the Liver, subdue Liver-Yang and relieve the pain.

HERBAL TREATMENT

Prescription

TIAN MA GOU TENG YIN
Gastrodia and Uncaria Decoction
Tian Ma *Rhizoma Gastrodiae* 10 g
Gou Teng *Ramulus Uncariae cum Uncis* 10 g
Shi Jue Ming *Concha Haliotidis* 15 g
Zhi Zi *Fructus Gardeniae* 10 g
Huang Qin *Radix Scutellariae* 10 g
Chuan Niu Xi *Radix Cyathulae* 10 g
Du Zhong *Cortex Eucommiae* 10 g
Zhu Fu Shen *Sclerotium Poriae Pararadicis* 10 g
Ge Gen *Radix Puerariae* 15 g
Sang Ji Sheng *Ramulus Loranthi* 10 g
Ye Jiao Teng *Caulis Polgoni Multiflori* 10 g

Explanations

- Tian Ma and Gou Teng calm the Liver and relieve the pain.
- Shi Jue Ming and Ye Jiao Teng subdue the Liver-Yang.

- Huang Qin and Zhi Zi may clear Liver-Fire and relieve the pain.
- Du Zhong and Sang Ji Sheng tonify the Kidney and relieve the pain.
- Chuan Niu Xi subdues the Liver-Yang.
- Ge Gen regulates the Qi circulation and relieves the neck pain.
- Fu Shen calms the mind and improves sleep.

Modifications

1. If there is irritability, add Chai Hu *Radix Bupleuri* 10 g and Bai Shao *Radix Paeoniae Alba* 10 g to regulate the Liver-Qi.

2. If there is a headache, add Chuan Xiong *Rhizoma Ligustici Chuanxiong* 10 g and Xiang Fu *Rhizoma Cyperi* 10 g to regulate the Liver-Qi and relieve the headache.

3. If there is a poor appetite, add Yu Jin *Radix Curcumae* 10 g and Mai Ya *Fructus Hordei Germinatus* 10 g to regulate the Qi and improve the appetite.

4. If there is insomnia, add Suan Zao Ren *Semen Ziziphi Spinosae* 10 g and Bai Zi Ren *Semen Biotae* 10 g to calm the Mind and improve the sleep.

5. If there is dizziness, add Ju Hua *Flos Chrysanthemi* 6 g, Nu Zhen Zi *Fructus Ligustri Lucidi* 10 g and Han Lian Cao *Herba Ecliptae* 10 g to nourish the Yin and reduce the Heat.

6. If there is constipation, add Gua Lou Ren *Semen Trichosanthis* 10 g and Huo Ma Ren *Fructus Cannabis* 10 g to moisten the Intestine and promote bowel movement.

Patent remedy

Jiang Ya Ping Pian *Lower (Blood) Pressure Calming Tablet*

ACUPUNCTURE TREATMENT

GV-20 Baihui, GB-20 Fengchi, GB-21 Jianjing, GB-44 Zuqiaoyin, LR-2 Xingjian and LR-8 Ququan. Reducing method is used on these points.

Explanations

- This kind of neck pain is usually characterised by stiffness of neck with much muscle spasm, which is related to the emotional situations. GV-20 calms the Mind, suppresses the Liver-Yang and relieves nervousness.

- LR-2, the Spring point and the son point of the Liver channel, and LR-8, the Water point, cool the Liver, clear Heat and suppress the Liver-Yang, which is the root treatment in this condition.

- The Liver and Gall Bladder share a pair of channels and a collateral. Hyperactivity of Liver-Yang may cause disturbance of Gall Bladder, thus GB-20 and GB-21 are used to clear Heat in Gall Bladder and relieve the spasm and tension in the Gall Bladder channel so as to stop the neck pain.

Modifications

1. If there is a headache, add Extra Taiyang and GV-21 to calm the Liver and suppress the Liver-Yang.
2. If there is night sweating, heat in the palms and soles of the feet, tiredness and a red tongue with a scanty coating due to deficiency of the Yin of Liver and Kidney, add KI-3, KI-7 and SP-6, the crossing point of the three Yin channels of the foot, to nourish the Yin and clear Deficient-Heat.
3. If there is depression, fullness and pain in the chest due to stagnation of the Liver-Qi, add LR-14, the Front Collecting point of the Liver, and PC-6, the Connecting point, to smooth the Liver, circulate the Liver-Qi and relieve the depression.
4. If there is irritability, add HT-3, the Sea point, and GB-40, the Source point, to calm the Mind and clear Heat from the Liver.
5. If there is insomnia and palpitations, add HT-7, the Source point, and HT-8, the Spring point, to clear Heat from the Heart and tranquillise the Mind.

HYPERACTIVITY OF FIRE OF LUNG AND STOMACH

Symptoms and signs

Pain occurring at the front of the neck and referring to the sides, accompanied by fever, pain, redness and swelling in the throat, difficulty in swallowing, cough, formation of pus in the throat, or tonsils, thirst and constipation, red tongue, with a yellow and dry coating, and a rapid and forceful pulse.

Principle of treatment

Clear Heat, remove Toxin, reduce swelling and relieve the pain.

HERBAL TREATMENT

Prescription

LIANG GE SAN plus **YIN QIAO SAN**
Cool the Diaphragm Powder plus *Honeysuckle and Forsythia Powder*
Da Huang *Radix et Rhizoma Rhei* 6 g

Gan Cao *Radix Glycyrrhizae* 6 g
Zhi Zi *Fructus Gardeniae* 10 g
Huang Qin *Radix Scutellariae* 10 g
Bo He *Herba Menthae* 6 g
Lian Qiao *Fructus Forsythiae* 10 g
Zhu Ye *Herba Lophatheri* 10 g
Mang Xiao *Natrii Sulfas* 10 g
Yin Hua *Flos Lonicerae* 10 g
Ge Gen *Radix Puerariae* 10 g
Jing Jie Sui *Spica Schizonepetae* 6 g
Lu Gen *Rhizoma Phragmitis* 10 g

Explanations

- Yin Hua and Lian Qiao clear Lung-Heat and remove Toxin.
- Bo He and Jing Jie Sui promote the Qi circulation and dispel Heat.
- Zhu Ye and Lu Gen clear Heat and promote the production of Body Fluids so as to relieve the thirst.
- Zhi Zi, Huang Qin and Gan Cao clear Fire in the Upper Burner.
- Da Huang and Mang Xiao clear Stomach-Fire by means of promoting defecation.
- Ge Gen regulates the Qi and relieves the neck pain.

Modifications

1. If the throat is swollen and painful, add Pu Gong Ying *Herba Taraxaci* 10 g and Zhe Bei Mu *Bulbus Fritillariae Thunbergii* 10 g to clear Heat, eliminate Toxin and reduce the swelling.
2. If there is fever due to the predominance of invasion of Heat, add Chai Hu *Radix Bupleuri* 15 g and Shen Ma *Rhizoma Cimicifugae* 10 g to clear the Heat and reduce the fever.
3. If there is headache due to disturbance of the clear Yang in the head by Wind-Heat, add Chuan Xiong *Rhizoma Ligustici Chuanxiong* 10 g and Man Jing Zi *Fructus Viticis* 15 g to dispel the Wind-Heat and sedate the headache.
4. If there is thirst, add Sheng Di *Radix Rehmanniae Recens* 15 g and Xuan Shen *Radix Scrophulariae* 10 g to nourish the Yin and relieve the thirst.

Patent remedy

Wei Te Ling *Stomach Especially Effective Remedy*

ACUPUNCTURE TREATMENT

LU-5 Chize, LU-6 Kongzui, LU-10 Yuji, BL-13 Feishu, ST-42 Chongyang, ST-44 Neiting, LI-4 Hegu and CV-23 Lianquan. Reducing method is used on these points.

Explanations

- Since this kind of neck pain is caused by interior Heat, it starts gradually with symptoms arising from the Lung and Stomach. Also, this kind of neck pain often occurs at the front of the neck, and refers to one or both sides.
- The throat is the passage of respiration, which is dominated by the Lung, therefore points from the Lung channel should mainly be used. LU-10, the Spring point, and LU-5, the Sea point and the Water point from the Lung channel, clear Heat and descend the Lung-Qi, which is the root treatment for reducing Fire in the Lung.
- BL-13, the Back Transporting point of the Lung, clears Heat in the Lung and regulates its physiological function so as to stop the throat pain and neck pain.
- ST-42, the Source point, and ST-44, the Spring point on the Stomach channel, clear Heat from the Stomach and reduce Fire.
- LI-4, the Source point from the Large Intestine channel, clears Heat, reduces Fire and promotes defecation so as to eliminate Excessive-Fire in the Bright Yang Fu organs.
- CV-23 clears Heat in the throat and reduces swelling to relieve the throat pain and neck pain.

Modifications

1. If there is difficulty in swallowing, add CV-22 to reduce the swelling and relieve the pain.
2. If there is a cough with much expectoration of yellow phlegm, add ST-40, the Connecting point, and CV-17, the Gathering point for Qi, to resolve the Phlegm and cause the Lung-Qi to descend.
3. If there is a fever and headache, add LI-11, the Sea point, and GV-14, the meeting point of all Yang channels, to clear Heat and reduce the fever.
4. If there is constipation, add ST-25, the Front Collecting point of the Large Intestine, to promote defecation and relieve the constipation.
5. If there is a severe thirst, add LU-8, the Metal point, and LI-2, the Spring point, to promote secretion of Body Fluids and relieve the thirst.

STAGNATION OF BLOOD

Symptoms and signs

Stabbing pain at the neck with a fixed location, occurring mostly along the middle line of the back, aggravation of the pain at night, difficulty in neck movement and dislike of pressure. Some sufferers might have had cervical operations, any may have had a history of physical trauma. In some cases, there is a dark complexion, a purple tongue or purple spots on the borders and a choppy, deep, wiry or tight pulse.

Principle of treatment

Circulate Blood, eliminate Blood stasis, harmonise the collateral and arrest the pain.

HERBAL TREATMENT

Prescription

DA HUO LUO DAN
Greater Invigorate the Collaterals Special Pill
This is a patent remedy, which comes in the form of big pills. Take one pill once a day.

Patent remedies

Da Huo Luo Dan *Greater Invigorate the Collaterals Special Pill*
Xiao Huo Luo Dan *Minor Invigorate the Collaterals Special Pill*
Yan Hu Suo Pian *Corydalis Tablet*

ACUPUNCTURE TREATMENT

GV-13 Taodao, GV-14 Dazhui, LI-4 Hegu, SP-6 Sanyinjiao, SI-3 Houxi, TE-5 Waiguan, BL-58 Feiyang, BL-62 Shenmai, GB-20 Fengchi and GB-35 Yangjiao. Reducing method is used on these points.

Explanations

- Long-standing existence of pathogenic factors in the body may cause stagnation of the Blood, leading to blockage of the collateral and retardation of circulation in the channels, and causing a stabbing pain in the neck. LI-4 promotes the circulation of Qi and Blood in the upper body.
- SP-6 circulates the Blood, eliminates Blood stasis and relieves the pain.
- GV-13, GV-14 and GB-20 regulate the circulation of Qi in the channels and eliminate stagnation and blockage so as to relieve the neck pain.
- SI-3 and BL-62, a special combination of points, open the Governing Vessel and relieve the blockage in the neck.
- Since the Yang Linking Vessel goes to the neck, TE-5, the Confluence point of this vessel and the Connecting point of the Triple Burner channel, can

harmonise the Lesser Yang channel and stop the pain.

- Besides, GB-35, the Accumulation point of the Yang Linking Vessel, promotes the Qi and Blood circulation in this Vessel. This enhances the effect of arresting the neck pain.
- BL-58, the Connecting point of the Bladder channel, harmonises the collateral and circulates the Qi and Blood in the channel to stop the neck pain.

Modifications

1. If there is severe neck pain that is aggravated at night, add BL-17 to circulate the Blood, eliminate Blood stasis and stop the pain.
2. If the neck is stiff, add GB-34, the Gathering point for the tendons, to relax the tendons and relieve the stiffness.
3. If the neck is swollen owing to stagnation of Blood, add GB-21 and SI-14 to promote the circulation of Blood and reduce the swelling.
4. If there is restlessness due to severe neck pain, add BL-15 and HT-3 to calm the Heart and tranquillise the Mind.
5. If there is pain at the side of the neck, add GB-1 and TE-23 to open the collateral of the Lesser Yang channels and arrest the pain.

DEFICIENCY OF KIDNEY-ESSENCE

Symptoms and signs

Chronic slight neck pain that is worsened by exertion, a feeling of weakness in the neck, tiredness, dizziness, tinnitus, poor memory, weakness in the knees, lower back pain, a pale tongue with a thin and white coating and a slow pulse, or a red tongue with a peeled coating and a rapid pulse.

Principle of treatment

Tonify the Kidney and benefit the Bones.

HERBAL TREATMENT

Prescription

YOU GUI YIN
Restore the Right Kidney Decoction
Shu Di Huang *Radix Rehmanniae Praeparata* 15 g
Shan Yao *Rhizoma Dioscoreae* 12 g
Shan Zhu Yu *Fructus Corni* 15 g

Gou Qi Zi *Fructus Lycii* 15 g
Du Zhong *Cortex Eucommiae* 12 g
Tu Si Zi *Semen Cuscutae* 12 g
Dang Gui *Radix Angelicae Sinensis* 12 g
Ge Gen *Radix Puerariae* 15 g
Gui Ban *Plastrum Testudinis* 10 g
Sang Ji Sheng *Ramulus Loranthi* 10 g

Explanations

- Shu Di, Shan Yao, Shan Zhu Yu and Gou Qi Zi reinforce the Kidney-Essence.
- Sang Ji Sheng and Du Zhong tonify the Kidney-Essence and strengthen the Bones.
- Tu Si Zi and Gui Ban nourish the Liver and Kidney.
- Dang Gui promotes the Qi and Blood circulation and prevents obstructions in the Blood circulation.
- Ge Gen is used to regulate the Qi circulation and relieve the neck pain.

Modifications

1. If the memory is poor, add Shi Chang Pu *Rhizoma Acori Graminei* 10 g and Sha Yuan Qi Li *Semen Astragali Complanati* 10 g to nourish the Kidney-Essence and improve the memory.
2. If there is tinnitus, add Ci Shi *Magnetitum* 15 g Ji Xue Teng *Caulis Spatholobi* 15 g to relieve the tinnitus.
3. If there is dizziness and headache, add Gou Teng *Ramulus Uncariae cum Uncis* 10 g and Tian Ma *Rhizoma Gastrodiae* 10 g to suppress the Liver and subdue Interior Wind.
4. If there is lower back pain, add Bu Gu Zhi *Fructus Psoraleae* 10 g and Lu Jiao Jiao *Colla Cervi Cornus* 10 g to tonify the Kidney and relieve the pain.

Patent remedy

Ge Jie Da Bu Wan *Gecko Great Tonifying Pill*

ACUPUNCTURE TREATMENT

BL-11 Dashu, GB-39 Xuanzhong, KI-3 Taixi, GV-14 Dazhui, SP-6 Sanyinjiao, SI-3 Houxi and BL-62 Shenmai. Reinforcing method is used on these points.

Explanations

- The Kidney dominates the Bones and Marrow. If the neck bones fail to be nourished by

Kidney-Essence due to deficiency in the Kidney, weakness of the neck with pain occurs.

- KI-3, the Source point, and SP-6, the crossing point of the three Yin channels of the foot, tonify the Kidney-Essence and benefit the bones of the neck. This is the root treatment.
- BL-11, the Gathering point for the Bones, and GB-39, the Gathering point for the Marrow, nourish the Bones and benefit the Marrow so as to strengthen the neck bones and stop the pain.
- GV-14, the meeting point of all the Yang channels, promotes the circulation of Yang-Qi in the channels and relieves the neck pain.
- SI-3 and BL-62 open the Governing Vessel and sedate the neck pain.

Modifications

1. If there is dizziness, poor memory and poor concentration, add GB-20 and GV-20 to raise the Yang Qi and cause the Kidney-Essence to ascend to the head so as to relieve the dizziness.
2. If there is lower back pain and weakness in the knees, add BL-23, GV-4 and ST-36 to tonify the Kidney and benefit the knees.
3. If there is general tiredness, cold hands and feet and shortness of breath on exertion due to deficiency of the Kidney-Yang, add CV-4 and CV-6 with moxibustion to tonify the Original Qi and warm the Interior.
4. If there is night sweating, heat in the palms and soles of the feet, thirst and a dry mouth and throat due to deficiency of Kidney-Yin, add KI-2, KI-6 and KI-7 to nourish the Kidney-Yin and clear Deficient-Heat.

Case history

A 65-year-old man had been suffering from neck pain for 2 years. He complained of neck pain with dizziness. He had been diagnosed as having cervical spondylosis 3 years previously. However, he did not improve after physiotherapy. Also, he had a slight headache over the back of his head. Sometimes he had dizziness, lower back pain with soreness, night sweating, a dry mouth and dry stools. His tongue was red with a thin coating. His pulse was deep and wiry.

Diagnosis
Deficiency of Yin of Liver and Kidney.

Principle of treatment
Nourish Yin of Liver and Kidney and relieve the pain.

Acupuncture treatment
BL-11 Dashu, GB-20 Fengchi, GB-39 Xuanzhong, KI-3 Taixi, GV-14 Dazhui, SP-6 Sanyinjiao, SI-3 Houxi, BL-23 Shenshu and BL-62 Shenmai. Reinforcing method is used on these points.

Explanations

- KI-3, the Source point, BL-23, the Back Transporting point of the Kidney, and SP-6, the crossing point of the three Yin channels of the foot, tonify the Kidney-Essence and benefit the bones of the neck.
- BL-11, the Gathering point for the Bones, and GB-39, the Gathering point of the Marrow, nourish the Bones and benefit the Marrow so as to strengthen the neck bones and stop the pain.
- GB-20 is a patent point to regulate the circulation of Qi, and relieve the neck pain and headache.
- GV-14, the meeting point of all the Yang channels, promotes circulation of the Yang Qi in the channels and relieves the neck pain.
- SI-3 and BL-62 open the Governing Vessel and sedate the neck pain.

After 30 days of treatment, his neck pain was relieved. One year later, when he returned to the clinic for treatment for his lower back pain, he stated he had experienced no more neck pain since the last treatment.

Throat pain 20

咽
喉
疼
痛

Throat pain may be acute or chronic, and is often accompanied by dryness in the throat, a dry cough, expectoration of phlegm, a feeling of blockage in the throat, hoarseness, difficulty in speaking, or fever. There may also be breathlessness or an inability to swallow and drink. When such symptoms appear, treatment based on a combination of Western medicine and TCM is generally the best solution.

The throat includes the pharynx and larynx. The former is a musculomembranous sac consisting of the nasopharynx and the oropharynx, through which the nasal cavity connects with the larynx and the oral cavity with the oesophagus. The latter is the vocal organ, and also forms one of the upper parts of the air passages; it is located high up in the front of the neck, and there forms a considerable prominence on the surface.

Based on anatomy, TCM stresses that the throat has a very close relationship with the Lung and Stomach, so any disorders of the Stomach or Lung may cause throat pain. Throat pain may be attributed to any of the following diseases in Western medicine: acute laryngitis, chronic laryngitis, acute pharyngitis, chronic pharyngitis, acute tonsillitis, chronic tonsillitis, laryngeal polyp, fibroma of the larynx, laryngotyphoid, perilaryngitis, laryngeal oedema, laryngo-vestibulitis, laryngoxerosis, pharyngospasm, laryngopharyngitis and diphtheria.

Aetiology and pathology

Since the throat is connected with the oral cavity and the nose, as well as the Stomach and Lung, either invasion of External factors or imbalance in the Stomach or Lung can cause pain in the throat. Nevertheless, invasion of external pathogenic factors, Toxic Heat, a bad diet, excessive smoking, excessive strain, emotional disturbance and constitutional weakness or Excess may cause disorders of the Stomach, Lung, Liver or Kidney, leading to throat pain.

Invasion of External factors

The Lung is in charge of the skin and opens into the nose, and the throat connects to the nose. Thus External invasion may directly attack the throat. Wind-Heat, Wind-Cold and Wind-Dryness are common causes of External invasion. Wind-Heat burns and damages the throat, Wind-Cold blocks the channels in the throat, and Wind-Dryness consumes the Body Fluids in the throat and makes it dry, so throat pain follows.

External pathogens may also invade the Lung through the skin and nose, causing disturbance of the Lung's function of dispersing Qi, so that these External factors accumulate in and block

209

the throat, and throat pain occurs. Other pathogenic factors include:

- environmental prevalence of Toxic Heat (epidemics)
- living for too long time in a place equipped with central heating
- working for a long time in a dusty place, or in a place where there are many chemical products creating a chemical smell.

Inhalation of Toxic air

Inhalation of some Western medicines, such as Ventolin, may lead to burning and deterioration of the throat tissue, causing throat pain.

Hyperactivity of Fire of Stomach and Lung

This condition could be caused by the following factors:

1. *Incomplete elimination of External pathogenic factors.* External factors may invade the superficial levels of the body through the skin, nose and throat, causing External symptoms. When these pathogenic factors are not eliminated in time and completely, they may cause further invasion to the Lung and Stomach. As these factors accumulate in the Stomach and Lung over a long time, they may turn to Heat.
2. *Intake of the wrong food.* Overeating of pungent, sweet or fatty food, as well as overconsumption of alcohol, may cause impairment of transportation and transformation by the Spleen and Stomach leading to the development of Excessive-Heat.
3. *Excessive smoking.*
4. *Constitutional Yang Excess.* It is mainly caused by Yang Excess from the parents.

All these factors may accumulate, bringing about hyperactivity of Fire, in the Lung and Stomach, which flares up to the throat and causes stagnation of Qi and Blood, in turn causing throat pain. Also, this flaring up of Excessive-Fire may cause deterioration of the muscles and the collateral in the throat, and so pus is formed.

Bad diet

Overeating of very cold food and drinking too many cold drinks may damage the Yang of the Spleen and Stomach, leading to the formation of Cold and Damp. Overeating of pungent, sweet or fatty food, as well as drinking too much alcohol, may cause the formation of Damp and Heat. Irregular food intake, whether in quantity or time, may disturb the transportation and transformation in the Stomach and Spleen, and Damp-Phlegm forms. When Damp accumulates in the throat,

it blocks the Qi and Blood circulation in the body as well as in the throat, causing throat pain.

Emotional disturbance

Excessive stress, frustration and anger over a long period of time may cause depression of the Liver-Qi, leading to its stagnation, excessive thinking may cause stagnation of the Heart-Qi, and excessive sadness may suppress the Lung, bringing about stagnation of Lung-Qi. Once the Qi stagnates, it blocks the circulation in the channels in the body and throat, so causing throat pain. Moreover, prolonged stagnation of Qi may trigger Fire that flares up and burns the throat. Obviously, a long-standing stagnation of Qi may result in stagnation of Blood, also causing throat pain.

Excessive worrying may cause stagnation of Qi in the Spleen, impeding the function of the Spleen in transportation and transformation, causing Damp to form. When Damp-Phlegm blocks the throat, it causes throat pain.

Weakness of constitution

Congenital weakness, impairment of the Defensive Qi owing to prolonged sickness, or overstrain for a long time may lead to consumption of the Qi and Blood. So the throat is insufficiently nourished by the Qi and Blood, and throat pain occurs. Weakness of the constitution may also result in disturbance of water metabolism, leading to formation of Damp-Phlegm. This may be a weakness of the Spleen and Stomach in transporting Damp, weakness of the Lung in dispersing and descending water, or weakness of the Kidney in transforming Qi for water. When Damp-Phlegm is formed, it may go upwards and block the throat, thus causing throat pain.

Excessive sexual activity, prolonged febrile diseases, excessive singing, and excessive intake of some TCM medicines may cause the consumption of Yin in the Lung, Liver or Kidney, leading to failure of the throat to be nourished, and causing throat pain.

Treatment based on differentiation

Differentiation

Before giving treatment, differentiation should be firstly made in order to determine whether the throat pain has resulted from External invasion or from

Internal disorders, and whether it is due to Excess or Deficiency, and so on.

Differentiation of External invasion and internal disorder

— External invasion is characterised by an acute onset, short duration, a severe pain accompanied by External symptoms such as an aversion to cold, fever, generalised body pain, stiffness in the neck, cough, a thin tongue coating, and a superficial pulse.
— Internal disorder is characterised by a chronic onset, long duration, a pain that is usually not very severe, accompanied by symptoms relating to the Interior Zang-Fu organs, a lack of External symptoms, and many changes in the tongue and pulse.

Differentiation of Excess and Deficiency

— Excess is characterised by a pain that is relatively severe and constant, and aggravated by unhealthy foods and emotions, constipation, a red tongue with a greasy coating and a wiry and forceful pulse.
— Deficiency is characterised by a slight pain that moves up and down, and is aggravated by tiredness and exertion, a low voice, poor appetite, or dryness in the throat, night sweating, lower back pain, a red tongue with a thin coating or lack of coating and a thready and weak pulse.

Treatment

INVASION OF WIND-COLD

Symptoms and signs

Acute pain with a feeling of spasm in the throat, and aggravation with cold, a cough with expectoration of white phlegm, difficulty in swallowing, a light red colour and a slight swelling in the throat. This kind of throat pain is usually accompanied by aversion to cold and wind, a slight fever, a runny nose with a white discharge, headache, absence of sweat, generalised body pain, a thin and white tongue coating and a superficial and tight pulse.

Principle of treatment

Dispel Wind, eliminate Cold, disperse Lung-Qi and relieve the pain.

HERBAL TREATMENT

Prescription

JING FANG BAI DU SAN
Schizonepeta and Ledebouriella Powder to Overcome Pathogenic Influences
Jing Jie *Herba Schizonepetae* 6 g
Fang Feng *Radix Ledebouriellae* 6 g
Qiang Huo *Rhizoma seu Radix Notopterygii* 6 g
Chen Pi *Pericarpium Citri Reticulatae* 10 g
Qian Hu *Radix Peucedani* 6 g
Chai Hu *Radix Bupleuri* 6 g
Jie Geng *Radix Platycodi* 5 g
Zhi Qiao *Fructus Aurantii* 6 g
Chuan Xiong *Rhizoma Ligustici Chuanxiong* 5 g
Gan Cao *Radix Glycyrrhizae* 5 g

Explanations

● Qiang Huo and Fang Feng are used to promote sweating and dispel pathogenic Wind-Cold.
● Chai Hu and Chuan Xiong invigorate the Qi and Blood circulation and stop the pain.
● Jie Geng and Qian Hu disperse the Lung-Qi and stop the cough.
● Sheng Jiang resolves Phlegm and eliminates Damp.
● Zhi Qiao and Chen Pi promote the Qi circulation in the chest.
● Gan Cao harmonises the actions of the other herbs in the formula.

Modifications

1. If there is swelling in the throat, add Bai Bu *Radix Stemmonae* 10 g and Jiang Can *Bombys Batryticatus* 10 g to regulate the Qi and reduce the swelling.
2. If there is an aversion to cold, add Ma Huang *Herba Ephedrae* 10 g and Xi Xin *Herba Asari* 3 g to disperse the Lung-Qi and dispel Wind-Cold.
3. If there is a fever, add Gui Zhi *Ramulus Cinnamomi* 10 g to dispel Cold and reduce the fever.
4. If there is a headache, add Bai Zhi *Radix Angelicae Dahuricae* 10 g and Man Jing Zi *Fructus Viticis* 10 g to dispel Wind-Cold and sedate the headache.
5. If there is a cough and expectoration of white phlegm due to invasion of the Lung by Wind-Cold, add Zi Wan *Radix Asteris* 10 g and Xing Ren *Semen Armeniacae Amarum* 10 g to disperse the Lung-Qi and dispel the Wind-Cold.

Patent remedy

Jing Fang Bai Du Pian *Schizonepeta and Ledebouriella Tablet to Overcome Pathogenic Influences*

ACUPUNCTURE TREATMENT

TE-5 Waiguan, LI-4 Hegu, BL-12 Fengmen, BL-13 Feishu, GB-20 Fengchi and LU-7 Lieque. Reducing method is used on these points. Moxibustion should be used on the first three points.

Explanations

- LI-4, the Source point, and LU-7, the Connecting point, open the skin pores and promote sweating so as to dispel Wind-Cold. Also, LU-7 is a good point to disperse the Lung-Qi and benefit the throat, and is indicated in throat pain due to invasion of External factors. Conventionally, LU-7 is a very good point for treating all problems due to disturbance of the Lung system resulting from invasion of External factors.
- TE-5, the Connecting point, BL-12 and GB-20 dispel Wind and eliminate Cold so as to relieve External symptoms.
- BL-13, the Back Transporting point of the Lung, disperses Lung-Qi, relieves External invasion and benefits the throat.

Modifications

1. If there is a severe pain and swelling in the throat, and difficulty in swallowing and speaking, add CV-22 and CV-23 in order to reduce the swelling and relieve the throat pain.
2. If there is a cough with white phlegm due to invasion of Wind-Cold to the Lung, add LU-1 to disperse the Lung-Qi and relieve the cough.
3. If there is a stuffed-up nose and white nasal discharge, add LI-20 and BL-2 to clear the nasal passage and relieve the blockage.
4. If the throat is red, add LU-10, the Spring point, to clear Heat in the throat.
5. If there is generalised body pain with a cold feeling, add BL-58, the Connecting point, and BL-62, the Confluence point of the Yang Heel Vessel, to dispel Wind-Cold and relieve the body pain.
6. If there is hoarseness, add LU-11 and CV-21 to open the collateral of the Lung and improve the voice.
7. If there is headache, add Extra Yintang and GV-16 to dispel Wind-Cold and stop the headache.

Case history

A 34-year-old man had been suffering from throat pain for about 2 weeks. He was diagnosed in the hospital as having acute laryngitis, and was given injections of antibiotics. The throat swelling improved, but his throat was still painful. When he arrived at the clinic he had a slight fever, and other symptoms, such as aversion to cold, a cough with itching in the throat, a poor appetite, a red tongue with a dry, yellow coating and a rapid pulse.

Diagnosis
Invasion of External Wind-Cold.

Principle of treatment
Promote Qi circulation, dispel Wind and Cold and relieve the pain.

Herbal treatment
JING FANG BAI DU SAN
Schizonepeta and Ledebouriella Powder to Overcome Pathogenic Influences
Jing Jie *Herba Schizonepetae* 6 g
Fang Feng *Radix Ledebouriellae* 6 g
Qiang Huo *Rhizoma seu Radix Notopterygii* 6 g
Chen Pi *Pericarpium Citri Reticulatae* 10 g
Su Ye *Folium Perillae* 10 g
Chai Hu *Radix Bupleuri* 6 g
Jiang Can *Bombyx Batryticatus* 10 g
Jie Geng *Radix Platycodi* 5 g
Xing Ren *Semen Armeniacae Amarum* 10 g
Zhi Qiao *Fructus Aurantii* 6 g
Gan Cao *Radix Glycyrrhizae* 5 g

Explanations
- Jing Jie, Fang Feng and Qiang Huo promote sweating and dispel pathogenic Wind-Cold.
- Chai Hu invigorates the Qi and Blood circulation and stops the pain.
- Jie Geng and Xing Ren disperse the Lung-Qi and stop the cough.
- Su Ye and Jiang Can dispel Wind, arrest itching and stop the cough.
- Zhi Qiao and Chen Pi promote the circulation of Qi in the chest.
- Gan Cao harmonises the actions of the other herbs in the formula.

After 10 days of treatment, the cough and throat pain disappeared.

INVASION OF WIND-HEAT

Symptoms and signs

Acute pain with a burning feeling, obvious swelling and redness in the throat, accompanied by a slight aversion to cold and wind, fever, a runny nose with a yellow discharge, headache, sweating, thirst, restlessness, generalised body pain, a thin and yellow tongue coating and a superficial and rapid pulse.

Principle of treatment

Dispel Wind, clear Heat, reduce swelling and relieve the pain.

HERBAL TREATMENT

Prescription

YIN QIAO SAN
Honeysuckle and Forsythia Powder
Jin Yin Hua *Flos Lonicerae* 10 g
Lian Qiao *Fructus Forsythiae* 10 g
Jie Geng *Radix Platycodi* 6 g
Bo He *Herba Menthae* 6 g
Dan Dou Chi *Semen Sojae Praeparatum* 10 g
Zhu Ye *Herba Lophatheri* 10 g
Gan Cao *Radix Glycyrrhizae* 6 g
Jing Jie Sui *Spica Schizonepetae* 6 g
Niu Bang Zi *Fructus Arctii* 10 g
Lu Gen *Rhizoma Phragmitis* 10 g

Explanations

- Jin Yin Hua and Lian Qiao are used to clear Heat and dispel Wind.
- Bo He, Jing Jie Sui and Dan Dou Chi are used to promote sweating, relieve external symptoms and dispel Heat.
- Niu Bang Zi, Jie Geng and Gan Cao are used to regulate the Qi in the Lung, eliminate Phlegm, benefit the throat and stop the pain.
- Zhu Ye and Lu Gen are used to clear Heat and promote the production of Body Fluids so as to relieve the thirst.

Modifications

1. If the throat is red and swollen owing to invasion of Wind-Heat, add Pu Gong Ying *Herba Taraxaci* 10 g and Ban Lan Gen *Radix Isatidis* 15 g to clear the Heat, eliminate Toxin and reduce the swelling.
2. If there is a cough and expectoration of yellow phlegm due to invasion of the Lung by Wind-Heat, add Qian Hu *Radix Peucedani* 10 g and Zhe Bei Mu *Bulbus Fritillariae Thunbergii* 10 g to disperse the Lung-Qi and dispel the Wind-Heat.
3. If there is a fever, add Chai Hu *Radix Bupleuri* 15 g and Shen Ma *Rhizoma Cimicifugae* 10 g to clear Heat and reduce the fever.
4. If there is a headache, add Chuan Xiong *Rhizoma Ligustici Chuanxiong* 10 g and Man Jing Zi *Fructus Viticis* 15 g to dispel Wind-Heat and sedate the headache.
5. If there is thirst, add Xuan Shen *Radix Scrophulariae* 15 g and Mai Dong *Radix Ophiopogonis* 10 g to nourish the Yin and relieve the thirst.

Patent remedy

Yin Qiao Jie Du Pian *Honeysuckle and Forsythia Tablet to Overcome Toxins*

ACUPUNCTURE TREATMENT

LI-2 Erjian, LI-4 Hegu, LI-11 Quchi, BL-12 Fengmen, LU-7 Lieque, LU-10 Yuji and GV-14 Dazhui. Reducing method is used on these points.

Explanations

- LI-4, the Source point, LI-11, the Sea point, and GV-14, the meeting point of all the Yang channels, dispel Wind, clear Heat and reduce fever.
- BL-12 dispels Wind and clears Heat so as to relieve External symptoms.
- LU-7, the Connecting point, dispels Wind-Heat from the Lung system, harmonises the collateral and relieves the throat pain.
- LI-2 and LU-10, the Spring points, clear Heat in the throat strongly and reduce swelling so as to relieve the throat pain.

Modifications

1. If there is a high fever and severe throat pain, then bleeding, add LI-1 and LU-11, the Well (Jing) points, to clear Heat, reduce the fever, and relieve the throat pain.
2. If there is difficulty in speaking and swallowing due to a swelling in the throat, add CV-21 and CV-22 to reduce the swelling and benefit the throat strongly.
3. If there is a cough with a yellow nasal discharge due to failure of the Lung in dispersing Qi, add BL-13, the Back Transporting point of the Lung, LU-1, the Front Collecting point of the Lung, and LU-5, the Sea point and Water point, to disperse the Lung-Qi and relieve the cough.
4. If there is a blocked nose, add LI-20 and BL-2 to clear the nose and relieve the blockage.
5. If there is a headache, add Extra Yintang and GV-16 to dispel Wind-Heat and stop the headache.

INVASION OF WIND-DRYNESS

Symptoms and signs

Invasion of Wind-Dryness comprises two types: Wind-Heat-Dryness and Wind-Cold-Dryness. Most of the basic symptoms are the same: acute throat pain with an obvious dry feeling, a slight swelling and redness in the throat, accompanied by a slight aversion to cold, a low-grade fever, thirst, a dry cough, scanty phlegm expectoration, a slight headache, a thin and dry tongue coating and a superficial pulse.

Principle of treatment

Dispel Wind and moisten Dryness, reduce the swelling and relieve the pain.

HERBAL TREATMENT

a. Prescription for Wind-Cold-Dryness

XING SU SAN
Apricot Kernel and Perilla Leaf Powder
Su Ye *Folium Perillae* 6 g
Ban Xia *Rhizoma Pinelliae* 10 g
Gan Cao *Radix Glycyrrhizae* 5 g
Qian Hu *Radix Peucedani* 10 g
Jie Geng *Radix Platycodi* 6 g
Zhi Qiao *Fructus Aurantii* 10 g
Chen Pi *Pericarpium Citri Reticulatae* 10 g
Xing Ren *Semen Armeniacae Amarum* 10 g
Fu Ling *Poria* 10 g

Explanations

- Su Ye and Qian Hu dispel Wind-Cold-Dryness and promote the Qi circulation.
- Ban Xia and Fu Ling promote the Qi circulation and remove Phlegm.
- Jie Geng and Xing Ren promote the Qi circulation and resolve Phlegm.
- Zhi Qiao and Chen Pi promote the Qi circulation and relieve the pain.
- Gan Cao harmonises the herbs in the formula.

Modifications

1. If the throat is swollen, add Jiang Can *Bombyx Batyticatus* 10 g and Chan Yi *Periostracum Cicadae* 6 g to dispel Wind and reduce the swelling.
2. If there is thirst or a dry mouth, add Mai Dong *Radix Ophiopogonis* 10 g and Xuan Shen *Radix Scrophulariae* 10 g to nourish the Yin of the Lung and the Stomach and relieve the thirst.
3. If there is a fever, add Chai Hu *Radix Bupleuri* 10 g and Sheng Ma *Rhizoma Cimicifugae* 10 g to clear Heat and reduce the fever.
4. If there is a headache, add Chuan Xiong *Rhizoma Ligustici Chuanxiong* 10 g and Man Jing Zi *Fructus Viticis* 10 g to dispel Wind and sedate the headache.

5. If there is a dry cough with itching in the throat, add Tian Hua Fen *Radix Trichosanthis* 10 g and Chuan Bei Mu *Bulbus Fritillariae Cirrhosae* 10 g to disperse the Lung-Qi, nourish the Yin and dispel Dryness.

b. Prescription for Wind-Heat-Dryness

SANG XING TANG
Mulberry Leaf and Apricot Kernel Decoction
Sang Ye *Folium Mori* 6 g
Xing Ren *Semen Armeniacae Amarum* 10 g
Sha Shen *Radix Adenophorae* 10 g
Zhe Bei Mu *Bulbus Fritillariae Thunbergii* 10 g
Dan Dou Chi *Semen Sojae Praeparatum* 10 g
Zhi Zi Pi *Pericarpium Gardeniae* 10 g
Li Pi *Exocarpium Pyrus* 10 g
Bo He *Herba Menthae* 6 g
Gan Cao *Radix Glycyrrhizae* 6 g

Explanations

- San Ye and Zhi Zi Pi clear Dry-Heat.
- Sang Ye and Dan Dou Chi dispel Wind and relieve External symptoms.
- Sha Shen and Li Pi nourish the Lung-Yin.
- Xing Ren and Zhe Bei Mu disperse the Lung-Qi and stop the cough.
- Gan Cao harmonises the herbs and tonifies the Lung-Qi.

Modifications

1. If the throat is red and swollen, add Pu Gong Ying *Herba Taraxaci* 10 g and Zhu Ye *Herba Lophatheri* 10 g to clear Heat and reduce the swelling.
2. If there is thirst due to invasion of Wind-Dry-Heat, add Mai Dong *Radix Ophiopogonis* 10 g and Xuan Shen *Radix Scrophulariae* 10 g to nourish the Yin of the Lung and the Stomach and relieve the thirst.
3. If there is a fever, add Chai Hu *Radix Bupleuri* 10 g and Sheng Ma *Rhizoma Cimicifugae* 10 g to clear Heat and reduce the fever.
4. If there is a headache, add Ju Hua *Flos Chrysanthemi* 10 g and Man Jing Zi *Fructus Viticis* 10 g to dispel Wind-Dry-Heat and sedate the headache.
5. If there is a cough and expectoration of yellow phlegm due to invasion of the Lung by Wind-Dry-Heat, add Gua Lou *Fructus Trichosanthis* 10 g and Zhe Bei Mu *Bulbus Fritillariae Thunbergii* 10 g to disperse the Lung-Qi and dispel the Wind-Dryness-Heat.

6. If there is constipation, add Gua Lou Ren *Semen Trichosanthis* 15 g and Sheng Di Huang *Radix Rehmanniae Recens* 15 g to nourish the Large Intestine and promote defecation.

Patent remedy

Qing Fei Yi Huo Pian *Clear Lungs Restrain Fire Tablet*

ACUPUNCTURE TREATMENT

LI-4 Hegu, BL-12 Fengmen, TE-5 Waiguan, LU-7 Lieque, LU-8 Jingqu and LU-5 Chize. Reducing method is applied on these points except LU-8 and LU-5, on which tonifying method is used.

Explanations

- LI-4, the Source point, BL-12 and TE-5, the Connecting point, dispel External pathogenic factors in order to relieve External symptoms.
- LU-7, the Connecting point, dispels External factors from the Lung system, harmonises the collateral of the Lung and relieves the throat pain.
- LU-8, the Metal point, and LU-5, the Water point, on the Lung channel are used here to promote secretion of Body Fluids in the Lung system and to moisten the throat and relieve Dryness so as to relieve the throat pain.

Modifications

1. If there is a fever and severe throat pain due to invasion of Wind-Heat-Dryness, add LU-10 and LI-2, the Spring points, to clear Heat and reduce the fever and swelling.
2. If the throat is obviously swollen, then use bleeding method at LI-1 and LU-11 to clear Heat, reduce fever and relieve the throat pain.
3. If there is difficulty in speaking and swallowing due to swelling in the throat, add CV-21 and CV-22 to reduce the swelling and benefit the throat strongly.
4. If there is a cough with a yellow nasal discharge due to failure of Lung to disperse the Qi, add BL-13, the Back Transporting point of the Lung, and LU-1, the Front Collecting point of the Lung, and LU-5, the Water point, to disperse the Lung-Qi and relieve the cough.
5. If the nose is blocked, add LI-20 and BL-2 to clear the nose and relieve the blockage.
6. If there is a feeling of spasm or blockage in the throat due to invasion of Wind-Cold-Dryness, add CV-23 and moxibustion on LI-4, LU-7, BL-12 and BL-13 to dispel the Wind-Cold and Dryness and warm the collateral.

Case history

A 41-year-old woman had been suffering from throat pain for a month. She had complained of throat pain with a dry sensation when she caught a cold one month previously. She had suffered from chronic bronchitis 1 year before this and was treated with antibiotics. She generally catches colds very easily. Also, she had a low-grade fever, dizziness, a dry cough with itching in her throat, a dry mouth, dry stools, tiredness and a pale complexion. Her tongue was red with a dry yellow coating. Her pulse was superficial and weak at Lung position.

Diagnosis
Deficiency of Qi and Yin with invasion of Wind-Heat-Dryness.

Principle of treatment
Nourish the Qi and Yin, clear Heat, moisten Dryness and relieve the pain.

Acupuncture treatment
KI-6, SP-6, GB-20, LU-7, LI-4 and CV-23 Lianquan. Even method was used for these points. Treatment was given every other day for a week.

Explanations

- KI-6, the Confluence point of the Yin Heel Vessel, and LU-7, the Connecting point of the Lung channel and the Confluence point of the Directing Vessel, are used to promote the Qi circulation in the Lung, nourish the Qi and Yin, benefit the throat and relieve the throat pain.
- SP-6, the crossing point of the three Yin channels of the foot, nourishes the Yin and benefits the throat.
- GB-20 is a patent point to dispel Wind, Heat and Dryness and relieve the throat pain.
- LI-4, the Source point of the Large Intestine channel, is used to relieve the throat pain.
- CV-23 Lianquan is the patent point to regulate the Qi circulation in the throat and relieve the throat pain.

After 3 weeks of treatment, her throat pain was relieved. One year later when she returned to the clinic she stated that she had suffered no more throat pain since the last treatment.

INVASION OF TOXIC HEAT

Symptoms and signs

Acute severe throat pain with a burning feeling, a high fever, obvious swelling and redness with formation of pus in the throat, difficulty in swallowing, accompanied by severe headache, a heavy cough, sweating, extensive thirst, constipation, restlessness, generalised body pain, a thick and yellow tongue coating and a superficial and rapid pulse.

Principle of treatment

Clear Heat, eliminate Toxin, reduce swelling and relieve the pain.

HERBAL TREATMENT

Prescription

PU JI XIAO DU YIN
Universal Benefit Decoction to Eliminate Toxin
Huang Qin *Radix Scutellariae* 15 g
Huang Lian *Rhizoma Coptidis* 15 g
Xuan Shen *Radix Scrophulariae* 6 g
Chai Hu *Radix Bupleuri* 6 g
Ban Lan Gen *Radix Isatidis* 6 g
Jie Geng *Radix Platycodi* 6 g
Lian Qiao *Fructus Forsythiae* 3 g
Ma Bo *Fructificatio Lasiosphaerae seu Calvatiae* 3 g
Niu Bang Zi *Fructus Arctii* 3 g
Bo He *Herba Menthae* 3 g
Jiang Can *Bombyx Batryticatus* 3 g
Sheng Ma *Rhizoma Cimicifugae* 3 g
Gan Cao *Radix Glycyrrhizae* 6 g

Explanations

- Huang Qin, Huang Lian, Ma Bo and Ban Lan Gen clear Heat and remove Toxin.
- Chai Hu, Sheng Ma and Bo He regulate the Liver-Qi circulation and relieve pain.
- Xuan Shen, Jie Geng and Gan Cao nourish the Yin and reduce the swelling.
- Lian Qiao, Niu Bang Zi and Jiang Can dispel Wind and clear Liver-Fire.

Modifications

1. If there is a high fever, add Shi Gao *Gypsum Fibrosum* 20 g, Da Qing Ye *Folium Isatidis* 10 g and Zhi Mu *Rhizoma Anemarrhenae* 10 g to clear Fire and reduce the fever.
2. If there is severe swelling and pain, add Pu Gong Ying *Herba Taraxaci* 10 g and Ye Ju Hua *Flos Chrysanthemi* 10 g to eliminate Toxin and reduce the swelling.
3. If there is constipation, add Mang Xiao *Natrii Sulfas* 10 g and Da Huang *Radix et Rhizoma Rhei* 10 g to clear excess Fire, eliminate Toxin and promote defecation.

4. If there is thirst, add Sheng Di Huang *Radix Rehmanniae Recens* 15 g and Mai Dong *Radix Ophiopogonis* 15 g to nourish the Yin and relieve the thirst.
5. If there is a cough, add Gua Lou *Fructus Trichosanthis* 10 g and Qian Hu *Radix Peucedani* 10 g to regulate the Qi, eliminate Phlegm and stop the cough.

Patent remedy

Niu Huang Jie Du Pian *Cattle Gallstone Tablet to Resolve Toxin*

ACUPUNCTURE TREATMENT

LI-2 Erjian, LI-4 Hegu, LI-11 Quchi, LU-5 Chize, LU-10 Yuji, GV-14 Dazhui, CV-22 Tiantu and CV-23 Lianquan. Reducing method is used on these points.

Explanations

- LI-4, the Source point, LI-11, the Sea point, and GV-14, the meeting point of all the Yang channels, clear Heat, remove Toxin and reduce the fever.
- LI-2 and LU-10, the Spring points of the Large Intestine and Lung channels respectively, strongly clear Heat and eliminate Toxin. They can also reduce the swelling in the throat.
- LU-5, the Sea point of the Lung channel, clears Heat in the Lung and causes the Lung-Qi to descend. It is also the Water point, which serves to distinguish Fire and eliminate Toxin so as to relieve the throat pain.
- CV-22 and CV-23 reduce the swelling, relieve the pain and eliminate the blockage in the throat.

Modifications

1. If there is a high fever, add ST-44, the Spring point, to clear Heat and reduce the fever.
2. If there is severe throat pain, then use bleeding method at LI-6 and LU-7, the Connecting points, to harmonise the collateral and relieve the pain.
3. If there is a severe cough with expectoration of yellow and sticky phlegm, add CV-17, the Gathering point for Qi, and LU-1, the Front Collecting point of the Lung, to cause the Lung-Qi to descend and relieve the cough.
4. If there is constipation, add ST-25, the Front Collecting point of the Large Intestine, and ST-40, the Connecting point, to promote bowel movement and defecation.

5. If there is formation of pus in the throat, add LU-11 and LI-1, the Well points, to clear Heat and eliminate Toxin.

6. If there is headache, add Extra Yintang and GV-16 to dispel Toxic Heat and stop the headache.

HYPERACTIVITY OF FIRE OF LUNG AND STOMACH

Symptoms and signs

Gradual onset of a pain that moves up and down and redness in the throat with a burning feeling, difficulty in swallowing, aggravation of the pain with smoking, drinking alcohol and eating sweet, fatty or highly flavoured food. Other accompanying symptoms include coughing, expectoration of yellow phlegm, thirst, constipation, a foul smell from the mouth, bleeding and swollen gums, sometimes pus in the throat, a red tongue with a yellow and dry coating and a rapid pulse.

Principle of treatment

Clear Heat, promote defecation, reduce the swelling and relieve the pain.

HERBAL TREATMENT

Prescription

Liang Ge San
Cool the Diaphragm Powder
Da Huang *Radix et Rhizoma Rhei* 6 g
Gan Cao *Radix Glycyrrhizae* 6 g
Zhi Zi *Fructus Gardeniae* 10 g
Huang Qin *Radix Scutellariae* 10 g
Bo He *Herba Menthae* 6 g
Lian Qiao *Fructus Forsythiae* 10 g
Zhu Ye *Herba Lophatheri* 10 g
Mang Xiao *Natrii Sulfas* 10 g
Yin Hua *Flos Lonicerae* 10 g
Lu Gen *Rhizoma Phragmitis* 10 g

Explanations

- Yin Hua and Lian Qiao clear Lung-Heat and eliminate Toxin.
- Bo He promotes the Qi circulation and dispels Heat.
- Zhu Ye and Lu Gen clear Heat and promote the production of Body Fluids so as to relieve the thirst.
- Zhi Zi, Huang Qin and Gan Cao clear Fire in the Upper Burner.

- Da Huang and Mang Xiao may clear Stomach-Fire and promote defecation.

Modifications

1. If the throat is swollen and painful, add Pu Gong Ying *Herba Taraxaci* 10 g to clear Heat, eliminate toxin and reduce the swelling.

2. If there is a fever, add Chai Hu *Radix Bupleuri* 15 g and Sheng Ma *Rhizoma Cimicifugae* 10 g to clear Heat and reduce the fever.

3. If there is thirst, add Sheng Di Huang *Radix Rehmanniae Recens* 15 g and Xuan Shen *Radix Scrophulariae* 10 g to nourish the Yin and relieve the thirst.

4. If there is a bitter taste in the mouth, add Zhu Ru *Caulis Bambusae in Taeniam* 10 g and Zhi Shi *Fructus Aurantii Immaturus* 10 g to disperse the Stomach-Qi and clear Heat.

5. If there is constipation, add Mu Xiang *Radix Aucklandiae* 10 g and Bing Lang *Semen Arecae* 10 g to increase the Qi circulation and promote defecation.

Patent remedies

Wei Te Ling *Stomach Especially Effective Remedy*
Qing Fei Yi Huo Pian *Clear Lungs Restrain Fire Tablet*

ACUPUNCTURE TREATMENT

LU-5 Chize, LU-6 Kongzui, LU-10 Yuji, BL-13 Feishu, ST-42 Chongyang, ST-44 Neiting, LI-4 Hegu and CV-23 Lianquan. Reducing method is used on these points.

Explanations

- Since this kind of throat pain is caused by interior Heat in the Lung and Stomach, it starts gradually. It also moves up and down, and is closely related to living habits such as smoking, eating and drinking.
- The throat is part of the respiratory passage, which is dominated by the Lung; therefore, points from the Lung channel should be mainly selected. LU-5, the Water point and Sea point, and LU-10, the Spring point from the Lung channel, clear Heat and cause the Lung-Qi to descend, which is the root treatment for reducing Fire in the Lung.
- BL-13, the Back Transporting point of the Lung, clears Heat in the Lung and regulates its physiological function so as to stop the throat pain.

- ST-42, the Source point, and ST-44, the Spring point of the Stomach channel, clear Heat from the Stomach and reduce Fire.
- LI-4, the Source point from the Large Intestine channel, clears Heat, reduces Fire and promotes defecation so as to eliminate Excessive-Fire in the Bright Yang Fu organs.
- CV-23 clears Heat in the throat and reduces the swelling to relieve the throat pain.

Modifications

1. If there is difficulty in swallowing, add CV-22 to reduce swelling and enable swallowing.
2. If there is a cough with a lot of expectoration of yellow phlegm, add ST-40, the Connecting point, and CV-17, the Gathering point for the Qi, to resolve Phlegm and cause the Lung-Qi to descend so as to stop the cough.
3. If there is fever, add LI-11, the Sea point, and GV-14, the meeting point of all the Yang channels, to clear Heat and reduce the fever.
4. If there is severe constipation, add ST-25, the Front Collecting point of the Large Intestine, to promote defecation and relieve the constipation.
5. If there is a severe thirst, add LU-8, the Metal point, and LI-2, the Spring point, to promote secretion of Body Fluids and relieve the thirst.

STAGNATION OF QI

Symptoms and signs

Gradual onset of throat pain, with spasm and a feeling of tension, which moves up and down, and is closely related with the emotional situation, a feeling as if there is a plum stone in the throat, depression, stress, a feeling of oppression over the chest, headache, a bitter taste in the mouth, insomnia, a poor appetite, a slightly purplish tongue with a thin coating, and a wiry pulse.

Principle of treatment

Smooth the Liver, circulate the Qi, harmonise the emotions and relieve the pain.

HERBAL TREATMENT

Prescription

XIAO YAO SAN
Free and Relaxed Powder
Chai Hu *Radix Bupleuri* 10 g
Dang Gui *Radix Angelicae Sinensis* 10 g
Bai Shao *Radix Paeoniae Alba* 20 g

Bai Zhu *Rhizoma Atractylodis Macrocephalae* 10 g
Fu Ling *Poria* 15 g
Gan Cao *Radix Glycyrrhizae* 5 g
Bo He *Herba Menthae* 3 g
Su Ye *Folium Perillae* 6 g
Yan Hu Suo *Rhizoma Corydalis* 12 g

Explanations

- Chai Hu and Bo He regulate and promote the Liver-Qi circulation so as to remove Qi stagnation in the Liver.
- Bai Shao and Dang Gui nourish the Blood and strengthen the Liver.
- Bai Zhu, Fu Ling and Sheng Jiang tonify the Spleen and Stomach.
- Yan Hu Suo regulates the Blood circulation and relieves the pain.
- Su Ye may regulate the Qi circulation in Upper Burner and relieve the throat pain.
- Gan Cao harmonises the actions of the other herbs in the formula.

Modifications

1. If there is headache or dizziness, add Chuan Xiong *Radix Ligustici Chuanxiong* 10 g and Qiang Huo *Rhizoma seu Radix Notopterygii* 10 g to regulate the Qi circulation and relieve the headache or dizziness.
2. If there is a poor mood, add Xiang Fu *Rhizoma Cyperi* 10 g and Yu Jin *Radix Curcumae* 10 g to promote the Liver-Qi circulation and remove Qi stagnation.
3. If there is a plum-stone feeling in the throat, add Ban Xia *Rhizoma Pinelliae* 10 g and Hou Po *Cortex Magnoliae Officinalis* 10 g to disperse the Qi and remove Qi stagnation.
4. If there is irritability, add Huang Lian *Rhizoma Coptidis* 10 g and Gou Teng *Ramulus Uncariae cum Uncis* 10 g to clear Liver-Fire and calm the Mind.
5. If the appetite is poor, add Yu Jin *Radix Curcumae* 10 g and Mai Ya *Fructus Hordei Germinatus* 10 g to promote the Qi circulation and improve the appetite.

Patent remedies

Xiao Yao Wan *Free and Relaxed Pill*
Shu Gan Wan *Soothe Liver Pill*

ACUPUNCTURE TREATMENT

LR-3 Taichong, GB-20 Fengchi, PC-6 Neiguan, CV-12 Zhongwan, CV-17 Tanzhong and CV-23 Lianquan. Reducing method is used on these points.

Explanations

- In all kinds of Qi stagnation, stagnation of the Liver-Qi is generally the root cause. So treatment for stagnation of Qi will be focused on alleviating the stagnation of Liver-Qi.
- LR-3, the Source point from the Liver channel, fulfils the above function.
- PC-6, the Connecting point of the Pericardium channel and the Confluence point of the Yin Linking Vessel, and CV-17, the Gathering point for the Qi, help LR-3 circulate the Liver-Qi and regulate the emotions. They also promote the circulation of Qi in the Heart and Spleen.
- GB-20 calms the Mind and relieves spasm and tension in the body.
- CV-12, the Gathering point for the Fu organs, promotes their physiological function and eliminates Damp-Phlegm.
- CV-23, the local point, relieves throat pain.

Modifications

1. If there is depression, a sensation of fullness and pain in the chest due to stagnation of Liver-Qi, add LR-14, the Front Collecting point of the Liver, to smooth the Liver, circulate the Liver-Qi and relieve the depression.
2. If there is irritability, add LR-2 and GB-43, the Spring points, to clear Heat from the Liver and relieve the irritability.
3. If there is a headache, add GV-20 to calm the Liver and subdue the Liver-Yang so as to sedate the headache.
4. If there is a poor appetite, abdominal fullness, flatulence and belching due to stagnation of Spleen-Qi, add LR-13, the Front Collecting point, and BL-20, the Back Transporting point of the Spleen, to smooth the Spleen and relieve stagnation.
5. If there is insomnia, dream-disturbed sleep and sighing due to stagnation of Heart-Qi, add HT-3 and Extra Sishencong to regulate the Heart and calm the Mind.
6. If there is a bitter taste in the mouth, constipation due to stagnation of Qi in the Lesser Yang channel, add GB-40, the Source point, and TE-6 to regulate the Lesser Yang channel and relieve stagnation.

ACCUMULATION OF DAMP-PHLEGM IN THE THROAT

Symptoms and signs

Gradual onset of a slight throat pain, with no redness in the throat, but a slight swelling, itching and prick-ing feeling, and aggravation after eating fatty or sweet food. The pain is also accompanied by diminishment or loss of the sense of smell and taste, a nasal discharge, cough, occasional expectoration of phlegm from the throat, a feeling of fullness in the abdomen, a poor appetite, loose stools, a thick and greasy tongue coating and a slippery pulse.

Principle of treatment

Activate the Spleen and Stomach, eliminate Damp and resolve Phlegm.

HERBAL TREATMENT

Prescription

DAO TAN TANG
Guide Out Phlegm Decoction
Zhi Ban Xia *Rhizoma Pinelliae Praeparata* 10 g
Chen Pi *Pericarpium Citri Reticulatae* 10 g
Fu Ling *Poria* 10 g
Gan Cao *Radix Glycyrrhizae* 5 g
Zhi Shi *Fructus Aurantii Immaturus* 10 g
Zhi Nan Xing *Rhizoma Arisaematis Praeparata* 10 g
Jie Geng *Radix Platycodi* 10 g

Explanations

- Zhi Ban Xia and Zhi Nan Xing dry Damp and resolve Phlegm.
- Fu Ling activates the Spleen and Stomach and eliminates Damp.
- Chen Pi and Zhi Shi promote the circulation of Qi and eliminate Damp and Phlegm.
- Jie Geng disperses the Lung-Qi and eliminates Phlegm.
- Gan Cao harmonises the actions of the other herbs in the formula.

Modifications

1. If there is a sensation of fullness in the stomach, add Mu Xiang *Radix Aucklandiae* 10 g and Bin Lang *Semen Arecae* 10 g to promote the Qi circulation and relieve the fullness.
2. If there is thick phlegm in the throat, add Yuan Zhi *Radix Polygalae* 10 g and Qing Pi *Pericarpium Citri Reticulatae Viride* 10 g to promote the Qi circulation and eliminate the phlegm.
3. If the appetite is poor, add Cang Zhu *Rhizoma Atractylodis* 10 g and Sha Ren *Fructus Amomi* 10 g to dry Damp and improve the appetite.
4. If there is a cough with phlegm, add Bai Jie Zi *Semen Sinapis Albae* 10 g and Lai Fu Zi *Semen*

Raphani 10 g to resolve Phlegm and disperse the Lung-Qi.

5. If there are loose stools, add Cang Zhu *Rhizoma Atractylodis* 10 g and Bai Zhu *Rhizoma Atractylodis Macrocephalae* 10 g to dry Damp in the Middle Burner.

Patent remedies

Er Chen Wan *Two-Cured Pill*
Qing Qi Hua Tan Wan *Clear the Qi and Transform Phlegm Pill*

ACUPUNCTURE TREATMENT

ST-40 Neiting, SP-6 Sanyinjiao, SP-9 Yinlingquan, LU-5 Chize, LU-7 Lieque, BL-2 Zanzhu, CV-12 Zhongwan and CV-23 Lianquan. Reducing method is used on these points.

Explanations

- This kind of throat pain is mainly due to formation of Damp-Phlegm in the body and throat, which has blocked the collateral in the throat causing the throat pain. Based on such pathology, treatment should focus on eliminating the Damp, resolving the Phlegm and relieving the blockage in the throat.
- In order to resolve Damp-Phlegm, some points should be applied to activate the Spleen and Stomach, since this kind of Damp-Phlegm is not caused by External invasion but by Internal disorder from the Spleen and Stomach.
- ST-40, the Connecting point on the Stomach channel, SP-6, the crossing point of the three Yin channels of the foot, and SP-9, the Sea point from the Spleen channel, are prescribed here together to activate the Spleen and Stomach strongly, eliminate the Damp and resolve the Phlegm. This is the root treatment.
- CV-12, the Gathering point for the Fu organs, helps the above points to harmonise the Fu organs and resolve the Damp-Phlegm in the body.
- Since the throat is dominated by the Lung, accumulation of Damp-Phlegm in the Lung and throat causes throat pain. Thus LU-5, the Sea point, is used to eliminate Phlegm in the Lung and promote its physiological function. LU-7, the Connecting point, is prescribed to disperse the Lung-Qi and harmonise the collateral in the throat so as to relieve the pain.
- CV-23 resolves the blockage in the throat and relieves the throat pain.

- In practice, it is very often seen that this kind of chronic throat pain can also be caused by accumulation of Phlegm in the nose, leading to downward flow of Damp-Phlegm behind the nose to the throat. In such cases, BL-2 is used to clear the nose and resolve the Phlegm in the nose.

Modifications

1. If there is a discharge of yellow phlegm from the nose and cough due to accumulation of Phlegm-Heat in the Lung, add LU-10, the Spring point, and LI-4 to clear Heat, eliminate Phlegm and relieve the cough.
2. If there is a loss of the sense of smell and taste, add SI-18 and LI-20 and Extra Bitong, the local points, to clear the nose and promote its physiological function.
3. If the throat is red and swollen, add LI-2, the Spring point, and LU-11, the Well point, to clear Heat and reduce the swelling.
4. If there is a feeling of fullness in the abdomen, a poor appetite and loose stools due to weakness of the Spleen and Stomach, add SP-3, the Source point, and SP-4, the Connecting point and the Confluence point of the Penetrating Vessel, to activate the Spleen and improve the digestion.
5. If there is an accumulation of Cold-Phlegm, manifested as a white and greasy tongue coating, a slippery and slow pulse, expectoration and nasal discharge of white phlegm, add BL-13, the Back Transporting point of the Lung, with moxibustion to warm the Lung and resolve Cold-Phlegm.

STAGNATION OF BLOOD

Symptoms and signs

Prolonged persistence of throat pain with a stabbing feeling, aggravation of the pain at night, swelling in the throat and a purplish colour, difficulty in speaking and swallowing, hoarseness, bleeding from the throat, or expectoration of phlegm with blood breaks, coughing and shortness of breath. Some patients might have had surgical operations for throat cancer. In some cases, there is a dark complexion and emaciation, a purple tongue, or purple spots on the borders, and a choppy, deep, wiry or tight pulse.

Principle of treatment

Circulate Blood, eliminate Blood stasis, harmonise the collateral and arrest the pain.

HERBAL TREATMENT

Prescription

TAO HONG SI WU TANG
Four-Substance Decoction with Safflower and Peach Pit
Tao Ren *Semen Persicae* 10 g
Hong Hua *Flos Carthami* 10 g
Dang Gui *Radix Angelicae Sinensis* 10 g
Chi Shao *Radix Paeoniae Rubra* 10 g
Chai Hu *Radix Bupleuri* 10 g
Zhi Qiao *Fructus Aurantii* 10 g
Jie Geng *Radix Platycodi* 10 g
Xuan Shen *Radix Scrophulariae* 10 g

Explanations

- Tao Ren, Hong Hua, Chi Shao and Dang Gui promote circulation of Blood and eliminate Blood stasis.
- Chai Hu and Zhi Qiao promote Qi circulation and smooth Blood circulation.
- Jie Geng and Xuan Shen disperse the Lung-Qi, resolve Phlegm, benefit the throat and relieve pain.

Modifications

1. If there is profuse phlegm, add Chuan Bei Mu *Bulbus Fritillariae Cirrhosae* 10 g and Gua Lou Pi *Fructus Trichosanthis* 10 g to eliminate Phlegm.
2. If there is chest pain at night, add Yan Hu Suo *Rhizoma Corydalis* 10 g and Dan Shen *Radix Salviae Miltiorrhizae* 10 g to promote the Blood circulation, remove Blood stagnation and relieve pain.
3. If there is difficulty in swallowing, add Niu Bang Zi *Fructus Arctii* 10 g and Wei Ling Xian *Radix Clematidis* 10 g to regulate the Qi circulation and improve swallowing.
4. If there is a history of surgery, add Shui Zhi *Hirudo* 10 g and Xian He Cao *Herba Agrimoniae* 10 g to promote the Blood circulation and remove Blood stasis.
5. In cancer patients, add Ban Zhi Lian *Herba Scutellariae Barbatae* 15 g and Bai Hua She She Cao *Herba Hedyotis Diffusae* 20 g to eliminate Toxin and relieve the pain.

Patent remedy

Yan Hu Suo Zhi Tong Pian *Corydalis Stop Pain Tablet*

ACUPUNCTURE TREATMENT

CV-21 Xuanji, CV-22 Tiantu, LU-7 Lieque, BL-17 Geshu, SP-6 Sanyinjiao, LI-4 Hegu, PC-6 Neiguan and LR-3 Taichong. Reducing method is used on these points.

Explanations

- Long-standing persistence of pathogenic factors in the body may cause stagnation of the Blood, leading to blockage of the collateral and slowing down of circulation in the channels in the throat, and causing a throat pain with a stabbing feeling and swelling.
- BL-17, the Gathering point for the Blood, and SP-6, the crossing point of the three Yin channels of the foot, promote the Blood circulation and eliminate its stasis.
- LI-4, the Source point, promotes circulation of the Qi and Blood in the upper body and relieves the pain.
- LU-7, the Connecting point, induces the treatment into the throat and disperses the Lung-Qi so as to improve the voice.
- PC-6, the Connecting point and Confluence point of the Yin Linking Vessel, regulates the Mind and calms pain. Also, it promotes the Qi circulation in the throat so as to promote the Blood circulation.
- CV-21 and CV-22 are very important points here to regulate the circulation of Qi in the channels and eliminate stagnation and blockage in the throat so as to relieve the throat pain.

Modifications

1. If there is a severe throat pain with aggravation at night, add ST-9 and ST-10 to circulate the Blood, eliminate Blood stasis and stop the pain.
2. In case of difficulty in swallowing and drinking, vomiting, add SP-4, the Confluence point of the Penetrating Vessel, and KI-27 to cause the Stomach-Qi to descend and relieve the blockage in the throat.
3. If there is swelling in the throat due to stagnation of Blood, add ST-40, the Connecting point, to reduce the swelling and eliminate blockage of the collateral in the throat.
4. If there is restlessness due to severe throat pain, add HT-3, the Sea point, to calm the Heart and tranquillise the Mind.
5. If there is expectoration of profuse phlegm, add SP-9, the Sea point of the Spleen channel, and CV-12, the Gathering point of the Fu organs, to activate the Spleen and Stomach and resolve Phlegm.

DEFICIENCY OF YIN OF LUNG, HEART AND KIDNEY

Symptoms and signs

Prolonged persistence of a slight throat pain, dryness in the throat, thirst especially at night, but a lack of much desire to drink, and sometimes a burning feeling in the throat. If due to deficiency of Kidney-Yin, the throat symptoms are often accompanied by night sweating, heat in the palms and soles of the feet, dry stools, scanty urine, and other symptoms such as tiredness, dizziness, tinnitus, poor memory, weakness in the knees and lower back pain. If due to deficiency of Lung-Yin, there is hoarseness, a dry cough, or cough with scanty Phlegm, or even blood breaks in the Phlegm. If due to deficiency of Heart-Yin, there may be insomnia, restlessness and palpitation. There is also a red tongue with a thin peeled coating and a rapid, thready and weak pulse.

Principle of treatment

Nourish Yin and clear Deficient-Fire, moisten the throat and relieve the pain.

HERBAL TREATMENT

Prescription

SHA SHEN MAI MEN DONG TANG
Glehnia and Ophiopogonis Decoction
Sha Shen *Radix Adenophorae* 10 g
Mai Dong *Radix Ophiopogonis* 10 g
Yu Zhu *Rhizoma Polygonati Odorati* 10 g
Gan Cao *Radix Glycyrrhizae* 6 g
Sang Ye *Folium Moris* 10 g
Bai Bian Dou *Semen Dolichoris Album* 10 g
Tian Hua Fen *Radix Trichosanthis* 10 g
Zhi Qiao *Fructus Aurantii* 10 g

Explanations

- Sha Shen and Mai Dong nourish the Kidney-Yin and clear Deficient-Fire.
- Tian Hua Fen and Sang Ye nourish the Lung-Yin and reduce Deficient-Fire.
- Yu Zhu and Bai Bian Dou nourish the Stomach-Yin.
- Zhi Qiao regulates the Qi circulation and relieves pain.
- Gan Cao may tonify the Spleen-Qi and harmonise the actions of the other herbs.

Modifications

1. If there is night sweating, add Wu Wei Zi *Fructus Schisandrae* 10 g and Mu Li *Concha Ostreae* 10 g to arrest the sweating.
2. If there is insomnia, add Suan Zao Ren *Semen Ziziphi Spinosae* 10 g and Bai Zi Ren *Semen Biotae* 10 g to nourish the Heart-Yin and calm the Mind.

3. If there are dry stools, add Xuan Shen *Radix Scrophulariae* 10 g and Shou Wu *Radix Polygoni Multiflori* 10 g to nourish the Yin and promote defecation.
4. If there is heat in the palms and the soles of the feet, add Hu Huang Lian *Rhizoma Picrorhizae* 10 g and Qing Hao *Herba Artemisiae Chinghao* 10 g to clear Deficient-Fire.
5. If there is lower back pain and weakness in the knees, add Sang Ji Sheng *Ramulus Loranthi* 10 g and Bai Shao *Radix Paeoniae Alba* 10 g to strengthen the Kidney and relieve the pain.
6. If there is a dry mouth, add Sheng Di Huang *Radix Rehmanniae Recens* 10 g and Xuan Shen *Radix Scrophulariae* 10 g to nourish the Kidney-Yin and relieve the thirst.

Patent remedy

Qi Ju Di Huang Wan *Lycium Fruit, Chrysanthemum and Rehmannia Pill*

ACUPUNCTURE TREATMENT

LU-5 Chize, LU-7 Lieque, LU-8 Jingqu, KI-6 Zhaohai, KI-7 Fului, SP-6 Sanyinjiao, HT-3 Shaohai and CV-23 Lianquan. Reinforcing method is used on these points.

Explanations

- The Kidney rules water and the Yin in the body. Chronic throat pain due to deficiency of Yin is mostly related to the Kidney. Thus nourishing the Kidney-Yin should be the root treatment for such cases.
- KI-7 and LU-8, the Metal points, have the function of nourishing the Yin and promoting the secretion of Body Fluids so as to benefit and moisten the throat.
- SP-6, the crossing point of the three Yin channels of the foot, helps the above two points tonify the Yin and relieve dryness in the throat. This is the root treatment.
- LU-5, the Water point of the Lung channel, directly promotes the secretion of Body Fluids in the Lung system and moistens the throat.
- Application of LU-7 and KI-16 simultaneously is a special combination to open the Directing Vessel, moisten the throat and sedate the throat pain.
- CV-23 benefits the throat and relieves the throat pain.
- HT-3, the Water point of the Heart channel, nourishes the Yin and calms the Mind.

Modifications

1. If there is dizziness, poor memory, lower back pain, and weakness of knees, add KI-3, the Source point, and KI-10, the Sea point, to tonify the Kidney-Essence and strengthen the back.
2. If there is night sweating, heat in the palms and soles of the feet and thirst due to deficiency of Yin, add HT-6, the Accumulation point, and KI-2, the Spring point, to nourish the Yin and clear Deficient-Heat.
3. If there is a dry cough, hoarseness or blood breaks in the phlegm, add BL-13, the Back Transporting point of the Lung, and LU-6, the Accumulation point, to nourish the Lung-Yin and relieve the cough and bleeding.
4. If there is insomnia, restlessness and palpitations, add BL-15, the Back Transporting point of the Heart, and CV-14, the Front Collecting point of the Heart, to nourish the Heart-Yin and calm the Mind.
5. If there is nervousness, headache and irritability due to deficiency of Liver-Yin with hyperactivity of Deficient-Fire, add LR-3, the Source point of the Liver, and GB-20 to calm the Liver and reduce Deficient-Fire.

DEFICIENCY OF QI OF LUNG, SPLEEN AND KIDNEY

Symptoms and signs

A chronic history, slight throat pain, a feeling of cold in the throat, hoarseness, a low and weak voice, aggravation of the pain with tiredness, no swelling in the throat, sometimes a slight white phlegm in the throat, also a pale and swollen tongue with tooth marks and a wet and watery coating, and a thready, deep and slow pulse.

If this kind of throat complaint is accompanied by a pale complexion, spontaneous sweating, aversion to cold, cold hands and feet and other symptoms, such as listlessness when speaking, tiredness, a tendency to catch colds easily and a slight cough with expectoration of white phlegm, it results from deficiency of Lung-Qi. If there is a poor appetite, loose stools, abdominal distension, nausea and weakness of the muscles, it results from deficiency of Spleen-Qi. If there is general tiredness, lower back pain, weakness in the knees, nocturia, impotence and profuse and clean urine, it results from deficiency of Kidney-Qi.

Principle of treatment

Reinforce Qi, tonify Yang, dispel Cold and relieve the throat pain.

HERBAL TREATMENT

Prescription

JIN GUI SHEN QI WAN
Kidney Qi Pill from the Golden Cabinet
Shu Di Huang *Radix Rehmanniae Praeparata* 12 g
Shan Yao *Rhizoma Dioscoreae* 15 g
Shan Zhu Yu *Fructus Corni* 10 g
Ze Xie *Rhizoma Alismatis* 10 g
Fu Ling *Poria* 10 g
Rou Gui *Cortex Cinnamomi* 5 g
Zhi Fu Zi *Radix Aconiti Praeparata* 10 g
Chen Pi *Pericarpium Citri Reticulatae* 10 g

Explanations

- Shu Di Huang nourishes the Kidney-Yin.
- Shan Yao and Shan Zhu Yu strengthen the Liver and Spleen and help Shu Di Huang to nourish the Kidney.
- Rou Gui and Zhi Fu Zi warm the Kidney-Yang.
- Ze Xie and Fu Ling remove Damp and promote digestion of above greasy herbs.
- Chen Pi regulates Qi circulation.

Modifications

1. If there is shortness of breath, lassitude, a lowered voice, a poor appetite and diarrhoea due to deficiency of the Spleen-Qi, add Dang Shen *Radix Codonopsis* 10 g and Huang Qi *Radix Astragali seu Hedysari* 12 g to tonify the Spleen-Qi.
2. If there is diarrhoea before dawn with a cold lower abdomen due to deficiency of the Kidney-Yang, add Bu Gu Zhi *Fructus Psoraleae* 10 g and Wu Wei Zi *Fructus Schisandrae* 10 g to tonify the Kidney-Yang and relieve diarrhoea.
3. If there is spontaneous sweating due to deficiency of Lung-Qi, add Yi Zhi Ren *Fructus Alpiniae Oxyphyllae* 6 g and Mu Li *Concha Ostreae* 10 g to stop sweating.
4. If there is a poor appetite, add Bai Zhu *Rhizoma Atractylodis Macrocephalae* 10 g and Sha Ren *Fructus Amomi* 10 g to tonify Spleen-Qi and promote circulation.
5. If there is a chronic cough, add Dang Gui *Radix Angelicae Sinensis* 10 g and Chuan Bei Mu *Bulbus Fritillariae Cirrhosae* 10 g to regulate Blood and eliminate Phlegm.
6. If there is lower back pain or soreness of knees, add Sang Ji Sheng *Ramulus Loranthi* 10 g and Huang Jing *Rhizoma Polygonati* 15 g to tonify Kidney and relieve the pain.

Patent remedy

Jin Gui Shen Qi Wan *Kidney Qi Pill from the Golden Cabinet*

ACUPUNCTURE TREATMENT

CV-4 Guanyuan, CV-6 Qihai, ST-36 Zusanli, SP-3 Taibai, KI-3 Taixi, BL-23 Shenshu and CV-23 Lianquan. Reinforcing method is used on these points. Moxibustion should also be employed on these needles.

Explanations

- The Kidney-Qi and Yang are the root of Qi and Yang in the general body. Deficiency of Qi and Yang in other organs will sooner or later affect the Kidney, and vice versa. Deficiency of Qi or Yang in the body will cause formation of Deficient-Cold, leading to blockage of the throat by Cold. Thus to reinforce the Qi and Yang of the Kidney and dispel Cold in the throat will be the root treatment.
- KI-3, the Source point, and BL-23, the Back Transporting point of the Kidney, tonify the Kidney-Qi and warm the Kidney-Yang.
- ST-36, the Sea point, and SP-3, the Source point, activate the Spleen and Stomach and tonify the Qi.
- CV-4 and CV-6 reinforce the Qi and Yang of the body and dispel Cold.
- CV-23 relieves the blockage in the throat and sedates the pain.
- Moxibustion strongly warms the body, reinforces the Yang and dispels Cold.

Modifications

1. If there is lower back pain and weakness in the knees, add SP-6, the crossing point of the three Yin channels of the foot, and BL-58, the Connecting point, to tonify the Kidney and strengthen the back.
2. If there is nycturia and impotence, add GV-4 with moxibustion to tonify the Kidney-Yang and improve potency.
3. If there is general tiredness and coldness of hands and feet due to deficiency of Kidney-Yang add KI-10, the Sea point, to tonify the Yang and warm the Interior. Moxibustion on the needle should be employed.
4. If there are loose stools, or diarrhoea, a poor appetite and nausea, add SP-4, the Confluence point of Penetrating Vessel, and SP-9, the Sea point, to activate the Spleen and cause the Stomach-Qi to descend.
5. If there is a tendency to catch colds, cough, easily with expectoration of some white phlegm, a low voice and spontaneous sweating, add LU-9, the Source point, and BL-13, the Back Transporting point of the Lung, to tonify the Lung-Qi and strengthen the Lung.

Painful swallowing 21

吞咽疼痛

Painful swallowing is a condition characterised by pain and difficulty in swallowing of hard food, a feeling of blockage in the throat, and nausea. In some cases, there may gradually develop an inability to swallow soft food or drink, with vomiting immediately after eating. This complaint may be of either an acute or a chronic type, caused by disorder of the throat, oesophagus or stomach. Acute cases are usually caused by Excessive pathogenic factors, and in chronic cases, it may be caused by Deficient pathogenic factors or mixture of Excess and Deficiency. A clear diagnosis should be made in order to exclude cancer of the throat, oesophagus or stomach, for which a combination of treatment with Western medicine and TCM should be applied simultaneously.

In physiology, swallowing needs the cooperation between the throat and oesophagus as well as the opening of the stomach (cardia). The throat includes pharynx and larynx; the former is the musculomembranous sac comprising the nasopharynx and the oropharynx, through which the nasal cavity connects with the larynx and the oral cavity with the oesophagus, while the latter is the organ of voice, and also forms one of the upper parts of the air passages. The oesophagus is the tube that conveys food and drink from the throat down to the stomach. It begins at the level of the sixth cervical vertebra, lying close against the left side and front of the spinal column, passes downward through the neck and chest to pierce the diaphragm, and then opens into the stomach. The cardia refers to the upper opening of the stomach, which lies immediately behind the heart. Any disorders of these three organs may lead to painful swallowing.

TCM also stresses the link between the throat, oesophagus and Stomach and the interior Zang-Fu organs, especially the Lung, Spleen, Stomach and Liver, and holds that disorders of Qi, Blood, Body Fluids, Yin and Yang, channels and collaterals may all cause dysfunction of the throat, oesophagus and Stomach that results in painful swallowing. Painful swallowing in TCM is usually subsumed within the context of throat pain, stomach pain, or vomiting; if it is severe it is often considered under dysphagia. According to TCM, it can be caused either by invasion of External pathogenic factors or by Internal disorders, such stagnation of Liver-Qi, stagnation of Blood, blockage of Phlegm and Qi, hyperactivity of Fire of the Lung and Stomach or deficiency of Yin of Stomach. It may be attributed to any of the following diseases in Western medicine: acute laryngitis, chronic laryngitis, acute pharyngitis, chronic pharyngitis, acute tonsillitis, chronic tonsillitis, laryngeal polyp, fibroma of larynx, perilaryngitis, laryngeal oedema, laryngovestibulitis, laryngoxerosis, pharyngospasm, laryngopharyngitis, diphtheria, oesophageal achalasia, cardiospasm, benign oesophageal carcinoma of oesophagus, burns of oesophagus and oesophagitis.

Aetiology and pathology

The throat is connected with the oral cavity and the nose, as well as with the stomach and lung. The oesophagus connects with the throat and the cardia, and is very important as the passage for food. Invasion of the throat by external factors, or a bad diet and disorders of the interior organs can all cause painful swallowing.

Invasion of External factors

The Lung dominates the skin, and opens into the nose, and the throat connects it to the nose. Thus External invasion may directly attack the throat. Wind usually attacks the throat in combination with Heat, Cold and Dryness. Heat burns and damages the throat, Cold blocks the channels in the throat, and Dryness consumes and dries the Body Fluids in the throat and causes dryness there. All these cause dysfunction of the throat, which is followed by the development of painful swallowing.

Hyperactivity of Fire of Stomach and Lung

External invasion may also invade the Lung and Stomach through the skin, nose and throat. If these pathogenic factors are not eliminated completely, they may lead to the accumulation and stagnation of pathogenic factors in the Lung and Stomach, and then to blockage of the oesophagus and cardia, causing painful swallowing. Moreover, if there is prolonged persistence of these pathogenic factors here, then Excessive-Fire usually forms as a consequence, which may cause a burning of the throat if there is an uprising of Fire from the Lung or Stomach to the throat, and so swallowing becomes painful.

Bad diet

Overeating of pungent, sweet or fatty food, as well as drinking too much alcohol, may cause Damp-Heat to form, which may burn the throat, oesophagus and stomach. Overeating of food that is too hard, or too hot, or of too much fast food, may damage the throat and oesophagus, causing painful swallowing. Some cases of painful swallowing may be caused by the intake of toxic drugs, or liquids, that burn and damage the throat and oesophagus. Overeating of food that is too cold, and drinking of too many cold drinks may damage the Yang of the Spleen and Stomach, leading to the formation of Cold and Damp.

Irregular food intake, whether in quantity or in time, may disturb the transportation and transformation of the Stomach and Spleen, causing Damp-Phlegm to appear. When Damp accumulates in the throat, oesophagus and Stomach then the Qi and Blood circulation in the throat is blocked, food will have difficulty in passing through the throat and down the oesophagus, and swallowing is painful.

Emotional disturbance

Prolonged persistence of stress and frustration and excessive anger may cause stagnation of the Liver-Qi, and if this invades the Stomach then the Stomach fails to control its opening, and this leads to painful swallowing.

Prolonged stagnation of Qi may also cause generation of Fire, which flares up and attacks the Lung and Stomach, affecting the throat, oesophagus and cardia so painful swallowing follows. Prolonged stagnation of Qi may alternatively lead to stagnation of Blood in the throat, oesophagus and Stomach, causing painful swallowing. Finally, Liver-Qi stagnation may invade the Spleen, damaging the Qi in the Spleen. Excessive worrying and thinking also causes stagnation of Qi in the Spleen, impeding the transporting and transforming function of the Spleen so Damp forms. A mixture of Phlegm and stagnant Qi may block the food passage, resulting in painful swallowing.

Weakness of constitution

Congenital weakness, impairment of the Defensive Qi due to prolonged sickness, overstrain over a long period or senility may cause consumption of Qi and Blood, and as a consequence the throat, oesophagus and Stomach fail to be properly nourished, the passage of food becomes difficult, and painful swallowing follows.

A weak constitution may also result in disturbance of the water metabolism in the body, so Damp-Phlegm forms. The Damp-Phlegm may then ascend and and block the throat, oesophagus and Stomach, causing painful swallowing.

Excessive sexual activity, prolonged febrile diseases, too much singing and excessive intake of traditional medicines and drugs may all cause consumption of the Yin in the Lung, Liver and Kidney, so that the throat is not properly nourished, leading to pain when swallowing.

Treatment based on differentiation

Differentiation

Before giving treatment, the practitioner should first distinguish whether the painful swallowing is caused by External invasion or by Internal disorders, and whether it is due to Excess or Deficiency.

Differentiation of External invasion and Internal disorder

— External invasion is characterised by acute onset, a short duration of the pain and a relatively severe throat pain, accompanied by External symptoms such as an aversion to cold, fever, generalised body pain, stiffness in the neck, coughing, a thin tongue coating and a superficial pulse.
— Internal disorders are characterised by a chronic onset, long duration, pain that is not so severe and accompanied by symptoms related to the disorder of Interior Zang-Fu organs, with an absence of External symptoms, or much change in the tongue and pulse.

Differentiation of Excess and Deficiency

— In Excessive conditions the pain is relatively severe, aggravated by a bad diet and excessive emotion, and there is constipation, a red tongue with a greasy coating and a wiry and forceful pulse. This type often occurs in young and strong persons.
— The Deficient types are characterised by a milder pain that moves up and down, is aggravated by tiredness and exertion, with a low voice, poor appetite, night sweating, lower back pain, a thin tongue coating, or lack of coating, and a thready and weak pulse. This type is often seen in more elderly persons.

Treatment

INVASION OF WIND-COLD

Symptoms and signs

Acute onset of painful swallowing, a constant spasm and cold feeling in the throat, aggravation of the pain with cold, and a light red colour and slight swelling in the throat. Other symptoms include coughing with expectoration of white phlegm, an aversion to cold and wind, a slight fever, a runny nose with a white discharge, headache, absence of sweat, generalised body pain, a thin and white tongue coating and a superficial and tight pulse.

Principle of treatment

Dispel Wind, eliminate Cold, disperse Lung-Qi and relieve the pain.

HERBAL TREATMENT

Prescription

JING FANG BAI DU SAN
Schizonepeta and Ledebouriella Powder to Overcome Pathogenic Influences
Jing Jie *Herba Schizonepetae* 6 g
Fang Feng *Radix Ledebouriellae* 6 g
Qiang Huo *Rhizoma seu Radix Notopterygii* 6 g
Chen Pi *Pericarpium Citri Reticulatae* 10 g
Qian Hu *Radix Peucedani* 6 g
Chai Hu *Radix Bupleuri* 6 g
Jie Geng *Radix Platycodi* 5 g
Zhi Qiao *Fructus Aurantii* 6 g
Chuan Xiong *Rhizoma Ligustici Chuanxiong* 5 g
Gan Cao *Radix Glycyrrhizae* 5 g

Explanations

- Jing Jie, Fang Feng and Qiang Huo are pungent and Warm herbs, that promote sweating and dispel pathogenic Wind-Cold.
- Chai Hu and Chuan Xiong invigorate the Qi and Blood circulation and stop the pain.
- Jie Geng and Qian Hu promote the circulation of Lung-Qi and stop the cough.
- Zhi Qiao and Chen Pi promote the Qi to ease the chest.
- Gan Cao harmonises the other herbs in the prescription.

Modifications

1. If there is swelling of the throat, add Bai Bu *Radix Stemmonae* 10 g and Jiang Can *Bombys Batryticatus* 10 g to regulate the Qi and reduce the swelling.
2. If there is an aversion to cold, add Ma Huang *Herba Ephedrae* 10 g and Xi Xin *Herba Asari* 3 g to promote the Lung-Qi and dispel Wind-Cold.
3. If there is a fever, add Chai Hu *Radix Bupleuri* 5 g and Ma Huang *Herba Ephedrae* 10 g to dispel Cold and reduce the fever.
4. If there is headache, add Bai Zhi *Radix Angelicae Dahuricae* 10 g and Man Jing Zi *Fructus Viticis* 10 g to dispel Wind-Cold-Heat and sedate the headache.
5. If there is a cough and expectoration of white phlegm due to invasion of the Lung by Wind-Cold, add Zi Wan *Radix Asteris* 10 g and Xing Ren *Semen Armeniacae Amarum* 10 g to disperse the Lung-Qi and dispel the Wind-Cold.

Patent remedy

Jing Fang Bai Du Pian *Schizonepeta and Ledebouriella Tablet to Overcome Pathogenic Influences*

ACUPUNCTURE TREATMENT

TE-5 Waiguan, LI-4 Hegu, BL-12 Fengmen, BL-17 Geshu, CV-17 Tanzhong and CV-18 Yutang. Reducing method is used on these points. Moxibustion should be used on the first three points.

Explanations

- LI-4, the Source point, and TE-5, the Connecting point, promote sweating so as to relieve External symptoms due to the invasion of Wind-Cold.
- BL-12 opens the skin pores and promotes sweating so as to relieve blockage of the Lung system resulting from invasion of External factors.
- BL-17, the Back Transporting point of the diaphragm, relaxes the diaphragm, promotes descent of the Stomach-Qi and relieves painful swallowing. It also promotes the circulation of Blood and eliminates Blood stasis.
- CV-17, the Gathering point for Qi, promotes the circulation of Qi and relieves its stagnation in the chest so as to relieve blockage in the throat, oesophagus and Stomach.
- CV-18 promotes swallowing and relieves painful swallowing.

Modifications

1. If there is swelling in the throat, and much pain on swallowing, add CV-22 and CV-23 in order to reduce the swelling and relieve the pain.
2. If there is nausea or vomiting, add PC-6, the Confluent point of the Yin Linking Vessel to harmonise the Stomach, cause the Stomach-Qi to descend and relieve the vomiting.
3. If there is a cough with much white phlegm, add LU-7, the Connecting point, to disperse the Lung-Qi and relieve the cough.
4. If there is generalised body pain with a cold feeling, add BL-58, the Connecting point, and BL-63, the Accumulation point, to dispel Wind-Cold and relieve the body pain.
5. If there is hoarseness, add LU-11, the Well point, to open the collateral of the Lung and improve the voice.
6. If there is headache, add Extra Yintang and GV-16 to dispel Wind-Cold and stop the headache.

INVASION OF WIND-HEAT

Symptoms and signs

Acute onset of painful swallowing, a burning feeling, swelling and redness in the throat, with formation of pus, accompanied by a slight fever, an aversion to cold and wind, a runny nose with a yellow discharge, headache, sweating, thirst, restlessness, generalised body pain, a thin and yellow tongue coating and a superficial and rapid pulse.

Principle of treatment

Dispel Wind, clear Heat, reduce swelling and relieve the pain.

HERBAL TREATMENT

Prescription

PU JI XIAO DU YIN
Universal Benefit Decoction to Eliminate Toxin
Huang Qin *Radix Scutellariae Baicalensis* 10 g
Huang Lian *Rhizoma Coptidis* 10 g
Xuan Shen *Radix Scrophulariae* 15 g
Chai Hu *Radix Bupleuri* 6 g
Ban Lan Gen *Radix Isatidis* 15 g
Jie Geng *Radix Platycodi* 6 g
Lian Qiao *Fructus Forsythiae* 3 g
Ma Bo *Lasiosphaera seu Calvatia* 3 g
Niu Bang Zi *Fructus Arctii* 3 g
Bo He *Herba Menthae* 3 g
Jiang Can *Bombyx Batryticatus* 3 g
Sheng Ma *Rhizoma Cimicifugae* 3 g
Gan Cao *Radix Glycyrrhizae* 6 g
Chen Pi *Pericarpium Citri Reticulatae* 6 g

Explanations

- Huang Qin, Huang Lian, Ma Bo and Ban Lan Gen dispel Wind-Heat and remove Toxin.
- Chai Hu, Sheng Ma and Bo He regulate the Lung-Qi circulation and relieve throat pain.
- Xuan Shen, Jie Geng and Gan Cao nourish the Yin and reduce swelling.
- Lian Qiao, Niu Bang Zi and Jiang Can dispel Wind-Heat and smooth the throat.
- Chen Pi promotes Qi circulation, relieves the swelling and eliminates Phlegm.

Modifications

1. If there is a high fever, add Shi Gao *Gypsum Fibrosum* 20 g, Da Qing Ye *Folium Isatidis* 15 g and Zhi Mu *Rhizoma Anemarrhenae* 10 g to clear Fire and reduce the fever.
2. If there is severe swelling and pain, add Pu Gong Ying *Herba Taraxaci* 10 g and Ye Ju Hua *Flos Chrysanthemi Indici* 10 g to remove Toxin and reduce the swelling.

3. If there is headache, add Gou Teng *Ramulus Uncariae cum Uncis* 10 g and Shi Jue Ming *Concha Haliotidis* 15 g to eliminate Wind-Heat and relieve the headache.
4. If there is constipation, add Mang Xiao *Natrii Sulfas* 10 g and Da Huang *Radix et Rhizoma Rhei* 6 g to clear Excess-Fire and eliminate Toxin by means of defecation.
5. If there is thirst, add Sha Shen *Radix Adenophorae* 10 g and Sheng Di Huang *Radix Rehmanniae Recens* 15 g to nourish the Yin and clear Heat.

Patent remedy

Yin Qiao Jie Du Pian *Honeysuckle and Forsythia Tablet to Overcome Toxins*

ACUPUNCTURE TREATMENT

LI-4 Hegu, LI-11 Quchi, BL-12 Fengman, GV-14 Dazhui, CV-18 Yutang and CV-22 Tiantu. Reducing method is used on these points.

Explanations

- LI-4, the Source point, LI-11, the Sea point, and GV-14 dispel Wind, clear Heat and reduce fever so as to relieve External symptoms due to the invasion of Wind-Heat.
- BI-12 helps the above-mentioned points to clear Wind-Heat and relieve External symptoms.
- CV-18 and CV-22 promote swallowing and reduce swelling in the throat so as to relieve painful swallowing.

Modifications

1. If there is a high fever and severe painful swallowing due to swelling in the throat, use bleeding method at LI-1 and LU-11 to clear Heat, reduce the fever and relieve the throat pain.
2. If there is pain behind the chest on swallowing, add CV-21 to reduce the swelling strongly and promote swallowing.
3. If there is nausea or vomiting, add PC6, the Confluence point of the Yin Linking Vessel, and CV-12, the Gathering point for the Fu organs and the Front Collecting point of the Stomach, to harmonise the Stomach and cause the Stomach-Qi to descend so as to relieve the vomiting.
4. If there is a cough with yellow phlegm, add BL-13, the Back Transporting point, and LU-1, the Front Collecting point of the Lung, to disperse the Lung-Qi and relieve the cough.

5. If there is chest pain due to cough, add LU-6, the Accumulation point, to disperse the Lung-Qi and sedate the pain.
6. If there is thirst and a dry mouth, add ST-44 and LI-2, the Spring points, to clear Heat and preserve the Body Fluids.
7. If there is constipation, add ST-25, the Front Collecting point of the Large Intestine, and ST-37, the Lower Sea point of the Large Intestine, to promote defecation and relieve the constipation.

Case history

A 14-year-old boy had been suffering from painful swallowing for 1 week. He had fallen ill with acute pharyngitis 10 days previously and had been given antibiotics. The swelling in his throat had improved, but his throat was painful when he swallowed food. When he arrived at the clinic, he had a slightly swollen throat. He also had a thirst, a bitter taste in his mouth, constipation, a red tongue with a dry yellow coating and a pulse.

Diagnosis
Invasion of External Wind-Heat.

Principle of treatment
Promote Qi circulation, dispel Wind and clear Heat.

Herbal treatment
PU JI XIAO DU YIN
Universal Benefit Decoction to Eliminate Toxin
Huang Qin *Radix Scutellariae* 15 g
Xuan Shen *Radix Scrophulariae* 6 g
Chai Hu *Radix Bupleuri* 6 g
Ban Lan Gen *Radix Isatidis seu Baphicacanthi* 6 g
Jie Geng *Radix Platycodi Grandiflori* 6 g
Lian Qiao *Fructus Forsythiae* 3 g
Ma Bo *Lasiosphaerae seu Calvatiae* 3 g
Niu Bang Zi *Fructus Arctii* 3 g
Jiang Can *Bombyx Batryticatus* 3 g
Sheng Ma *Rhizoma Cimicifugae* 3 g
Gan Cao *Radix Glycyrrhizae* 6 g
Zhi Qiao *Fructus Aurantii* 10 g

Explanations
- Huang Qin, Ma Bo and Ban Lan Gen clear Heat and remove Fire.
- Chai Hu and Sheng Ma regulate the Qi circulation, dispel Wind-Heat and relieve the pain.
- Xuan Shen, Jie Geng and Gan Cao nourish the Yin and reduce the swelling in the throat.
- Lian Qiao, Niu Bang Zi and Jiang Can dispel Wind, clear Lung-Heat and relieve the pain.
- Zhi Qiao regulates the Qi circulation and relieves pain.

The boy had a daily treatment with this herbal decoction. His painful swallowing was relieved after 1 week of treatment. His father was followed up by letter a year later. He stated that his son had experienced no painful swallowing since the herbal treatment.

INVASION OF WIND-DRYNESS

Symptoms and signs

Acute onset of painful swallowing, dryness in the mouth and throat and on the lips, with no obvious swelling in the throat, accompanied by a slight aversion to cold, a low-grade fever, thirst, dry skin, a dry cough, scanty phlegm expectoration, a slight headache, a thin and dry tongue coating and a superficial pulse.

If the cause is Wind-Heat-Dryness, there will be expectoration of yellow phlegm, possibly with blood in the phlegm, a red tongue with a thin, yellow and dry coating and a superficial and rapid pulse. If the cause is Wind-Cold-Dryness, there will be expectoration of white phlegm, itching in the throat, a runny nose with a white discharge, a thin, white and dry tongue coating and a superficial and slow pulse.

Principle of treatment

Dispel Wind, moisten Dryness, reduce swelling and relieve the pain.

HERBAL TREATMENT

a. Prescription for Wind-Cold-Dryness

XING SU SAN
Apricot Kernel and Perilla Leaf Powder
Su Ye *Folium Perillae* 6 g
Ban Xia *Rhizoma Pinelliae* 10 g
Gan Cao *Radix Glycyrrhizae* 5 g
Qian Hu *Radix Peucedani* 10 g
Jie Geng *Radix Platycodi* 6 g
Zhi Qiao *Fructus Aurantii* 10 g
Ju Pi *Exocarpium Citri Reticulatae* 10 g
Xing Ren *Semen Armeniacae* 10 g
Fu Ling *Poria* 10 g

Explanations

- Su Ye and Qian Hu dispel Wind-Cold-Dryness and promote the Qi circulation.
- Ban Xia and Fu Ling disperse the Qi and remove Phlegm.
- Jie Geng and Xing Ren promote the circulation of Qi and resolve Phlegm.
- Zhi Qiao and Ju Pi promote the circulation of Qi and relieve the pain.
- Gan Cao harmonises the herbs in the formula.

b. Prescription for Wind-Heat-Dryness

SANG XING TANG
Mulberry Leaf and Apricot Kernel Decoction

Sang Ye *Folium Mori* 6 g
Xing Ren *Semen Armeniacae Amarum* 10 g
Sha Shen *Radix Adenophorae* 10 g
Zhe Bei Mu *Bulbus Fritillariae Thunbergii* 10 g
Dan Dou Chi *Semen Sojae Praeparatum* 10 g
Zhi Zi Pi *Pericarpium Gardeniae* 10 g
Li Pi *Exocarpium Pyrus* 10 g

Explanations

- Sang Ye and Zhi Zi Pi clear Dryness-Heat.
- Dan Dou Chi dispels Wind and relieves Exterior symptoms.
- Sha Shen and Li Pi nourish the Lung-Yin and relieve Dryness.
- Xing Ren and Zhe Bei Mu disperse the Lung-Qi and relieve the pain.

Modifications

1. If there is a swollen throat due to the invasion of Wind-Heat, add Pu Gong Ying *Herba Taraxaci* 10 g and Zhu Ye *Herba Lophatheri* 10 g to clear Heat and reduce the swelling.
2. If there is a thirst due to the invasion of Dry-Heat, add Mai Dong *Radix Ophiopogonis* 10 g and Xuan Shen *Radix Scrophulariae* 10 g to nourish the Yin of the Lung and the Stomach and relieve the thirst.
3. If there is a fever due to the predominance of Dry-Heat invasion, add Chai Hu *Radix Bupleuri* 10 g and Sheng Ma *Rhizoma Cimicifugae* 10 g to clear the Heat and reduce the fever.
4. If there is a headache due to the disturbance of the clear Yang in the head by Wind-Heat, add Chuan Xiong *Rhizoma Ligustici Chuanxiong* 10 g and Man Jing Zi *Fructus Viticis* 10 g to dispel the Wind-Heat and sedate the headache.
5. If there is a dry cough with itching in the throat, add Tian Hua Fen *Radix Trichosanthis* 10 g and Chuan Bei Mu *Bulbus Fritillariae Cirrhosae* 10 g to disperse the Lung-Qi, nourish the Yin and dispel Dryness.

Patent remedy

Qing Fei Yi Huo Pian *Clear Lungs Restrain Fire Tablet*

ACUPUNCTURE TREATMENT

LI-4 Hegu, BL-12 Fengmen, BL-13 Feishu, LU-7 Lieque, LU-8 Jingqu and ST-45 Lidui. Reducing method is used on these points, except for LU-8 and LU-5 on which a tonifying method is used.

Explanations

- LI-4, the Source point, and BL-12 dispel External pathogenic factors in order to relieve External symptoms.
- LU-7, the Connecting point, and BL-13, the Back Transporting point of the Lung, dispel External factors from the Lung system, and harmonise the collateral of the Lung in order to clear away pathogenic factors in the throat, which is the food passage.
- LU-8 and ST-45, the Metal points, are used here to promote secretion of Body Fluids in the Lung and Stomach so as to moisten the throat, oesophagus and stomach and relieve Dryness.

Modifications

1. If there is a fever and painful swallowing due to a swollen throat resulting from the invasion of Wind-Heat-Dryness, add LU-10 and LI-2, the Spring points, to clear Heat and reduce the fever and swelling.
2. If there is nausea or vomiting, add PC-6, the Confluence point of the Yin Linking Vessel, to cause the Stomach-Qi to descend and relieve vomiting,
3. If there is difficulty in swallowing due to swelling, add CV-21 and CV-22 to reduce the swelling strongly and promote swallowing.
4. If there is a severe thirst, add SP-6, the crossing point of the three Yin channels of the foot, to promote the secretion of Body Fluids and relieve the thirst.
5. If there is painful swallowing with a feeling of spasm or blockage in the throat due to invasion of Wind-Cold-Dryness, add moxibustion on LU-7 and BL-13 to disperse the Wind-Cold and Dryness and warm the collateral so as to relieve the painful swallowing.

INVASION OF TOXIN

Symptoms and signs

This condition is usually caused by ingestion of Toxic drugs or liquids that burn and damage the throat, oesophagus and stomach, leading to occurrence of painful swallowing and throat, with a severe pain also behind the chest, and in the stomach. There is an obvious burning sensation, swelling and redness in the throat, or ulceration in the throat, accompanied by fever, severe headache, restlessness, sweating, palpitations, even profuse sweating, or a fainting, rapid pulse.

Note: TCM treatment for this case will usually need to follow the necessary emergency Western medical treatment.

Principle of treatment

Clear Heat, remove Toxin, reduce swelling and relieve the pain.

HERBAL TREATMENT

Prescription

HUANG LIAN JIE DU TANG
Coptis Decoction to Relieve Toxicity
Huang Lian *Rhizoma Coptidis* 10 g
Huang Qin *Radix Scutellariae* 10 g
Huang Bai *Cortex Phellodendri* 10 g
Zhi Zi *Fructus Gardeniae* 10 g
Su Ye *Folium Perilliae* 10 g
Bai Ji *Rhizoma Bletillae* 15 g
Gan Cao *Radix Glycyrrhizae* 20 g

Explanations

- Huang Lian, Huang Qin and Huang Bai clear Fire, eliminate Toxin and relieve the pain.
- Zhi Zi clears Heat and Fire and relieves the pain.
- Su Ye dispels Wind and eliminates toxin.
- Bai Ji stops bleeding, repairs a wound and relieves the pain.
- Gan Cao in heavy dosage resolves Toxin, protects the Stomach-Qi and relieves pain.

Modifications

1. If the throat is red and swollen, add Pu Gong Ying *Herba Taraxaci* 15 g and Hu Zhang *Rhizoma Polygoni Cuspidati* 15 g to clear Fire, remove Toxin and reduce the swelling.
2. If there is a fever due to Fire and Toxin invasion, add Chai Hu *Radix Bupleuri* 15 g and Sheng Ma *Rhizoma Cimicifugae* 15 g to clear the Fire and Toxin and reduce the fever.
3. If there is a cough due to the invasion of Fire and toxin, add Qian Hu *Radix Peucedani* 10 g, Ban Lan Gen *Radix Isatidis* 20 g and Zhe Bei Mu *Bulbus Fritillariae Thunbergii* 10 g to disperse the Lung-Qi and eliminate the Toxin.
4. If there is a chest pain with a burning sensation, add Yin Hua *Flos Lonicerae* 10 g and Yu Xing Cao *Herba Houttuyniae* 20 g to clear Fire in the Upper Burner and relieve the pain.
5. If there is a stomach ache, add Shi Gao *Gypsum Fibrosum* 30 g and Zhi Mu *Rhizoma Anemarrhenae* 10 g to clear Heat and relieve the pain.
6. If there is constipation, add Da Huang *Radix et Rhizoma Rhei* 10 g and Mang Xiao *Natrii Sulfas* 10 g to eliminate Toxin through promoting defecation.

Patent remedy

Niu Huang Jie Du Pian *Cattle Gallstone Tablet to Resolve Toxin*

ACUPUNCTURE TREATMENT

LI-2 Erjian, LI-4 Hegu, LI-11 Quchi, LU-10 Yuji, ST-44 Neiting, CV-22 Tiantu and CV-23 Lianquan. Reducing method is used on these points.

Explanations

- LI-4, the Source point, and LI-11, the Sea point, clear Heat and reduce fever. They also promote defecation so as to eliminate the Toxin with the faeces.
- LI-2, ST-44 and LU-10, the Spring points from the Large Intestine, Stomach and Lung channels respectively, strongly clear Heat and remove toxin. Moreover, they can also reduce swelling in the throat and oesophagus.
- CV-22 and CV-23 reduce swelling, relieve the pain and eliminate blockage in the throat so as to alleviate painful swallowing.

Modifications

1. If there is a high fever, add GV-14, the meeting point of all the Yang channels, to clear Heat and reduce the fever.
2. If there is severe pain and swelling in the throat, add LI-1 and LU-11, the Well points, to clear Heat and relieve the throat pain.
3. If there is nausea and vomiting, add PC-6, the Confluence point of the Yin Linking Vessel, and SP-4, the Confluence point of the Penetrating Vessel, which is a special combination to harmonise the Stomach, cause the Stomach-Qi to descend and relieve the vomiting.
4. If there is constipation, add ST-25, the Front Collecting point, and ST-40, the Connecting point, to promote bowel movement and ease defecation.
5. If there is pus in the throat, use bleeding method at LU-11 and LI-1 to clear Heat and remove Toxin.

HYPERACTIVITY OF FIRE IN THE LUNG AND STOMACH

Symptoms and signs

Gradual onset of painful swallowing with an up-and-down movement, a red throat with a burning feeling, aggravation by smoke, on drinking alcohol, and on eating sweet, fatty on highly flavoured food. Other accompanying symptoms include coughing with expectoration of yellow phlegm, thirst, constipation, a foul smell in the mouth, bleeding and swollen gums, sometimes pus in the throat, and red tongue with a yellow and dry coating.

Principle of treatment

Clear Heat, promote defecation, reduce the swelling and relieve the pain.

HERBAL TREATMENT

Prescription

LIANG GE SAN plus **YU NU JIAN**
Cool the Diaphragm Powder plus *Jade Woman Decoction*
Zhi Zi *Fructus Gardeniae* 10 g
Huang Qin *Radix Scutellariae* 10 g
Yin Hua *Flos Lonicerae* 10 g
Jing Jie Sui *Spica Schizonepetae* 6 g
Bo He *Herba Menthae* 6 g
Lian Qiao *Fructus Forsythiae* 10 g
Zhu Ye *Herba Lophatheri* 10 g
Lu Gen *Rhizoma Phragmitis* 10 g
Sheng Di Huang *Radix Rehmanniae Recens* 18 g
Sha Shen *Radix Adenopherae* 12 g
Mang Xiao *Natrii Sulfas* 10 g
Da Huang *Radix et Rhizoma Rhei* 6 g
Gan Cao *Radix Glycyrrhizae* 6 g

Explanations

- Yin Hua and Lian Qiao clear Lung-Heat and release Toxin.
- Bo He and Jing Jie Sui promote the Qi circulation and dispel Heat.
- Zhu Ye, Lu Gen, Sheng Di Huang and Sha Shen clear Heat and promote the production of Body Fluids so as to relieve the thirst.
- Zhi Zi, Huang Qin and Gan Cao clear Fire in the Upper Burner.
- Da Huang and Mang Xiao clear Stomach-Fire and promote defecation.

Modifications

1. If the throat is swollen and painful, add Pu Gong Ying *Herba Taraxaci* 10 g and Zhe Bei Mu *Bulbus Fritillariae Thunbergii* 10 g to clear Heat, remove Toxin and reduce the swelling.
2. If there is thirst, add Xuan Shen *Radix Scrophulariae* 10 g to nourish the Yin and relieve the thirst.

3. If the pain is severe, add Chai Hu *Radix Bupleuri* 10 g and Bai Shao *Radix Paeoniae Alba* 10 g to moderate the Liver-Qi and relieve the pain.
4. If the gums are painful, add Ju Hua *Flos Chrysanthemi* 6 g and Gou Teng *Ramulus Uncariae cum Uncis* 10 g to reduce Fire and relieve the pain.
5. If there is constipation, increase the dosage of Da Huang *Radix et Rhizoma Rhei* to 15 g to clear Heat and promote bowel movements.
6. If the gums are bleeding, add Bai Mao Gen *Rhizoma Imperatae* 20 g and Ce Bai Ye *Cacumen Biotae* 10 g to cool the Blood and stop the bleeding.

Patent remedies

Qing Qi Hua Tan Wan *Clear the Qi and Transform Pill*
Wei Te Ling *Stomach Especially Effective Remedy*

ACUPUNCTURE TREATMENT

LU-5 Chize, LU-10 Yuji, BL-13 Feishu, ST-9 Renying, ST-42 Chongyang, ST-44 Neiting, LI-4 Hegu and CV-23 Lianquan. Reducing method is used on these points.

Explanations

- LU-5, the Water point and Sea point of the Lung channel, and LU-10, the Spring point, clear Heat and cause the Lung-Qi to descend, which is the root treatment for reducing Fire in the Lung.
- BL-13, the Back Transporting point of the Lung, clears Heat in the Lung and regulates its physiological function so as to eliminate pathogenic factors in the throat.
- ST-9, the local point, ST-42, the Source point, and ST-44, the Spring point of the Stomach channel, clear Heat from the Stomach and reduce Fire.
- LI-4, the Source point of the Large Intestine channel, clears Heat, reduces Fire and promotes defecation so as to eliminate Excessive-Fire in the Bright Yang Fu organs.
- CV-23 clears Heat in the throat and reduces swelling to relieve painful swallowing.

Modifications

1. If there is difficulty in swallowing, add CV-22 to reduce swelling and ease swallowing.
2. If there is a cough with profuse expectoration of yellow phlegm, add ST-40, the Connecting point, and CV-17, the Gathering point for the Qi, to resolve Phlegm and cause the Lung-Qi to descend so as to stop the cough.

3. If there is severe constipation, add ST-25, the Front Collecting point of the Large Intestine, to promote defecation and relieve the constipation.
4. If there is a severe thirst, add LU-8 and LI-1, the Metal points, to promote secretion of Body Fluids and relieve the thirst.

STAGNATION OF QI

Symptoms and signs

Gradual onset of painful swallowing, spasm and a feeling of tension in the throat with an up-and-down movement, painful swallowing related to the emotional state, a feeling as if a plum stone were stuck in the throat, depression, stress, a feeling of oppression over the chest, headache, a bitter taste in the mouth, insomnia, a poor appetite, slight purplish tongue with a thin coating and a wiry pulse.

Principle of treatment

Smooth Liver, circulate Qi, harmonise the emotions and relieve the pain.

HERBAL TREATMENT

Prescription

XIAO YAO SAN
Honeysuckle and Forsythia Powder
Chai Hu *Radix Bupleuri* 10 g
Dang Gui *Radix Angelicae Sinensis* 10 g
Bai Shao *Radix Paeoniae Alba* 20 g
Bai Zhu *Rhizoma Atractylodis Macrocephalae* 10 g
Fu Ling *Poria* 15 g
Gan Cao *Radix Glycyrrhizae* 5 g
Bo He *Herba Menthae* 3 g
Sheng Jiang *Rhizoma Zingiberis Recens* 5 g
Yan Hu Suo *Rhizoma Corydalis* 12 g

Explanations

- Chai Hu and Bo He regulate and promote the Liver-Qi circulation so as to remove Qi stagnation in the Liver.
- Bai Shao and Dang Gui nourish the Blood and strengthen the Liver. These two herbs can also relieve the pain directly.
- Bai Zhu, Fu Ling and Sheng Jiang tonify the Spleen and Stomach.
- Yan Hu Suo regulates the Blood circulation and relieves the pain.
- Gan Cao harmonises the actions of the other herbs in the prescription.

Modifications

1. If there is a headache or dizziness, add Chuan Xiong *Radix Ligustici Chuanxiong* 10 g and Qiang Huo *Rhizoma seu Radix Notopterygii* 10 g to regulate the Qi circulation and relieve the headache or dizziness.
2. If the emotions are unstable, add Xiang Fu *Rhizoma Cyperi* 10 g and Yu Jin *Radix Curcumae* 10 g to promote the Liver-Qi circulation and remove Qi stagnation.
3. If there is a plum-stone feeling in the throat, add Ban Xia *Rhizoma Pinelliae* 10 g and Su Ye *Folium Perillae* 10 g to disperse the Qi, resolve Phlegm and remove Qi stagnation.
4. If there is irritability, add Huang Lian *Rhizoma Coptidis* 10 g and Gou Teng *Ramulus Uncariae cum Uncis* 10 g to clear Liver-Fire and calm the Mind.

Patent remedies

Xiao Yao Wan *Honeysuckle and Forsythia Pill*
Shu Gan Wan *Soothe Liver Pill*

ACUPUNCTURE TREATMENT

LR-3 Taichong, LR-14 Qimen, ST-40 Fenglong, PC-6 Neiguan, CV-12 Zhongwan and CV-23 Lianquan. Reducing method is used on these points.

Explanations

- Stagnation of the Liver-Qi is generally the root cause of this condition. LR-3, the Source point of the Liver, and LR-14, the Front Collecting point of the Liver, smooth the Liver, promote Qi circulation and relieve depression so as to eliminate the blockage in the throat.
- Because of the stagnation of Liver-Qi, there could also be some Phlegm formation in the throat resulting from stagnation of Qi in the Spleen impeding its function of transportation and transformation.
- PC-6, the Connecting point of the Pericardium and the Confluence point of the Yin Linking Vessel, helps LR-3 and GB-20 to circulate the Liver-Qi and regulate the emotions.
- CV-12, the Gathering point for the Fu organs, and PC-6, the Confluence point of the Yin Linking Vessel, promote the physiological function of the Fu organs, cause the Stomach-Qi to descend and eliminate blockage in the oesophagus and stomach.
- CV-23, the local point, relieves the blockage in the throat and promotes swallowing.

Modifications

1. If there is nausea or vomiting, add SP-4, the Confluence point of the Penetrating Vessel, to cause the Stomach-Qi to descend and regulate the Penetrating Vessel so as to relieve the vomiting.
2. If there is depression, a feeling of fullness and pain in the chest due to stagnation of Liver-Qi, add CV-17, the Gathering point for the Qi, to smooth the Liver, circulate the Liver-Qi and relieve blockage in the chest.
3. If there is irritability, add LR-2, the Spring point, and GV-20 to clear Heat from the Liver and suppress the Liver-Yang.
4. If there is a poor appetite, abdominal fullness, flatulence and belching due to stagnation of Spleen-Qi, add LR-13, the Front Collecting point of the Spleen, and SP-6, the crossing point of the three Yin channels of the foot, to activate the Spleen and relieve the stagnation.
5. If there is insomnia, dream-disturbed sleep and sighing due to stagnation of Heart-Qi, add HT-3, the Sea point of the Heart channel, and Extra Sishencong to regulate the Heart and calm the Mind.
6. If there is a bitter taste in the mouth and constipation due to stagnation of Qi in the Lesser Yang, add GB-40, the Source point, to regulate the Lesser Yang and relieve the stagnation.

Case history

A 45-year-old woman had been suffering from pain when swallowing for 6 months. She complained of painful swallowing with a 'plum-stone sensation' in her throat. When she was under stress, or was nervous for some reason, she felt more pain in her throat. She had many diagnostic investigations, but no organic disease was found. As well as painful swallowing, she suffered headache, heat in her palms and the soles of her feet, irregular menstruation and a poor appetite. Her tongue was red with white coating and her pulse was deep and wiry.

Diagnosis
Stagnation of Liver-Qi.

Principle of treatment
Regulate Liver-Qi, remove Qi stagnation and relieve the pain.

Acupuncture treatment
PC-6, KI-6, HT-7, LR-3, SP-6, GV-20 and CV-23 were selected. Even method was used for these points. Treatment was given every other day for 1 month.

Explanations

- PC-6, the Connecting point of the Pericardium channel, and KI-6, the Confluence point of the Yin Heel Vessel, regulate the Qi circulation and relieve the pain.

- HT-7, the Stream and Source point of the Heart channel, calms the Mind, regulates the Qi circulation and removes Qi stagnation.
- LR-3, the Stream and Source point of the Liver channel, SP-6, the crossing point of the three Yin channels of the foot, and GV-20 promote the Qi circulation and calm the Mind.
- CV-23 is the patent point for regulating the Qi circulation and relieving pain.

After 30 days of treatment, her pain had been relieved. She was followed up by telephone a year later and she said she had experienced no pain when swallowing food.

ACCUMULATION OF DAMP-PHLEGM

Symptoms and signs

Gradual onset of a slight pain when swallowing, an absence of redness in the throat, slight swelling and phlegm in the throat, aggravation of the pain after eating fatty or sweet food, accompanied by a cough, occasional expectoration of phlegm from the throat, a feeling of fullness in the chest and abdomen, a poor appetite, loose stools, a thick, white and greasy tongue coating and a slippery pulse.

Principle of treatment

Descend Qi, activate the Spleen and Stomach, eliminate Damp and relieve the pain.

HERBAL TREATMENT

Prescription

DAO TAN TANG
Guide Out Phlegm Decoction
Zhi Ban Xia *Rhizoma Pinelliae Praeparata* 10 g
Chen Pi *Pericarpium Citri Reticulatae* 10 g
Fu Ling *Poria* 10 g
Gan Cao *Radix Glycyrrhizae* 5 g
Zhi Shi *Fructus Aurantii Immaturus* 10 g
Zhi Nan Xing *Rhizoma Arisaematis Praeparata* 10 g

Explanations

- Zhi Ban Xia and Zhi Nan Xing dry Damp and resolve Phlegm.
- Fu Ling promotes urination and eliminates Damp.
- Chen Pi and Zhi Shi promote the Qi circulation and eliminate Damp and Phlegm.
- Gan Cao may harmonise the actions of the other herbs in the prescription.

Modifications

1. If there is a feeling of fullness in the Stomach, add Mu Xiang *Radix Aucklandiae* 10 g and Bin Lang *Semen Arecae* 10 g to promote the Qi circulation and eliminate Phlegm.
2. If there is thick phlegm in the throat, add Yuan Zhi *Radix Polygalae* 10 g and Jie Geng *Radix Platycodi* 10 g to promote the Qi circulation and eliminate Phlegm.
3. If there is a poor appetite, add Cang Zhu *Rhizoma Atractylodis* 10 g and Sha Ren *Fructus Amomi* 10 g to dry Damp and improve the appetite.
4. If there is a cough with phlegm, add Bai Jie Zi *Semen Sinapis Albae* 10 g and Lai Fu Zi *Semen Raphani* 10 g to resolve Phlegm and disperse the Lung-Qi.

Patent remedy

Xiang Sha Liu Jun Wan *Six-Gentleman Pill with Aucklandia and Amomum*

ACUPUNCTURE TREATMENT

ST-40 Fenglong, SP-6 Sanyinjiao, SP-9 Yinlingquan, SP-4 Gongsun, PC-6 Neiguan, CV-12 Zhongwan and CV-23 Lianquan. Reducing method is used on these points.

Explanations

- This kind of painful swallowing is caused by blockage in the throat, oesophagus and Stomach by Damp-Phlegm. Since the pathogenic factors are formed because of disorder of the Spleen and Stomach, the chief treatment would be to activate the Spleen and resolve the Damp.
- ST-40, the Connecting point on the Stomach channel, SP-6, the crossing point of the three Yin channels of the foot, and SP-9, the Sea point of the Spleen channel, are prescribed here together to activate the Spleen and Stomach strongly, eliminate Damp and resolve Phlegm. This is the root treatment.
- CV-12, the Gathering point for the Fu organs, helps the above points to harmonise the Fu organs and resolve Damp-Phlegm in the body.
- SP-4, the Confluence point of the Penetrating Vessel, opens the vessel and causes the Stomach-Qi to descend so as to ease the passage of food through the oesophagus smoothly.
- PC-6, the Confluence point of the Yin Linking Vessel, opens the Vessel, harmonises the chest, and

regulates the Stomach so as to relieve the blockage in the oesophagus and Stomach.

● CV-23 resolves the blockage in the throat and relieves the throat pain.

Modifications

1. If the throat is red and swollen, add LI-2, the Spring point, and LU-11, the Well point, to clear Heat and reduce the swelling.
2. If there is a sensation of fullness in the abdomen, a poor appetite and loose stools due to weakness of the Spleen and Stomach, add SP-3, the Source point, to activate the Spleen and improve the digestion.
3. If there is an accumulation of Phlegm-Heat, manifested as a yellow and greasy tongue coating, a slippery and rapid pulse, expectoration and nasal discharge of yellow phlegm, add LU-10, the Spring point of the Lung, and BL-13, the Back Transporting point of the Lung, to clear the Heat and resolve the Phlegm.

STAGNATION OF BLOOD

Symptoms and signs

Prolonged persistence of a stabbing pain in the throat or behind the chest, difficulty in speaking or swallowing, aggravation of the chest pain at night or when emotionally upset, a slight swelling in the throat with a purplish colour, hoarseness, expectoration of phlegm containing blood and shortness of breath. Some patients might have had surgical operations on the throat, or a history of throat, oesophageal or stomach cancer. In some cases, there is a dark complexion and emaciation, a purple tongue or purple spots on the borders and a choppy, deep, wiry or tight pulse.

Principle of treatment

Circulate Blood, eliminate Blood stasis, harmonise the collateral and arrest the pain.

HERBAL TREATMENT

Prescription

TAO HONG SI WU TANG
Four-Substance Decoction with Safflower and Peach Pit
Tao Ren *Semen Persicae* 10 g
Hong Hua *Flos Carthami* 10 g
Dang Gui *Radix Angelicae Sinensis* 10 g
Chi Shao *Radix Paeoniae Rubra* 10 g
Chai Hu *Radix Bupleuri* 10 g

Zhi Qiao *Fructus Aurantii* 10 g
Jie Geng *Radix Platycodi* 10 g
Xuan Shen *Radix Scrophulariae* 10 g

Explanations

● Tao Ren, Hong Hua, Chi Shao and Dang Gui promote the circulation of Blood and eliminate Blood stasis.
● Chai Hu and Zhi Qiao promote the Qi circulation and help the Blood circulation.
● Jie Geng and Xuan Shen disperse the Lung-Qi, resolve Phlegm and benefit the throat.

Modifications

1. If there is profuse phlegm, add Chuan Bei Mu *Bulbus Fritillariae Cirrhosae* 10 g and Gua Luo Pi *Fructus Trichosanthis* 10 g to eliminate Phlegm.
2. If there is a chest pain at night, add Yan Hu Suo *Rhizoma Corydalis* 10 g and Dan Shen *Radix Salviae Miltiorrhizae* 10 g to promote the Blood circulation, remove Blood stagnation and relieve the pain.
3. If swallowing is difficult, add Niu Bang Zi *Fructus Arctii* 10 g and Wei Ling Xian *Radix Clematidis* 10 g to regulate the Qi circulation and improve the ease of swallowing.
4. If there is a history of surgery, add Shui Zhi *Hirudo* 10 g and Xian He Cao *Herba Agrimoniae* 10 g to promote the Blood circulation and remove Blood stasis.
5. If it is a cancer patient, add Ban Zhi Lian *Herba Scutellariae Barbatae* 15 g and Bai Hua She She Cao *Herba Hedyotis Diffusae* 20 g to eliminate Toxin and relieve the pain.

Patent remedies

Fu Fang Dan Shen Pian *Compound Salvia Tablet*
Mao Dong Qing *Ilex Root Tablet*

ACUPUNCTURE TREATMENT

CV-21 Xuanji, CV-22 Tiantu, BL-17 Geshu, LU-7 Lieque, SP-6 Sanyinjiao, LI-4 Hegu, PC-6 Neiguan and LR-3 Taichong. Reducing method is used on these points.

Explanations

● Stagnation of Blood may cause blockage of the channels and collateral in the throat, oesophagus and Stomach, so painful swallowing occurs.

- BL-17, the Gathering point for the Blood, and SP-6, the crossing point of the three Yin channels of the foot, promote the Blood circulation and eliminate Blood stasis.
- LI-4, the Source point, promotes the Qi and Blood circulation in the upper body and relieves pain.
- LU-7, the Connecting point, induces the treatment into the throat, disperses the Lung-Qi and harmonises the collateral in the throat.
- PC-6, the Confluence point of the Yin Linking Vessel, regulates the Mind to relieve the pain. It also increases the Qi circulation in the Stomach so as to promote the Blood circulation.
- CV-21 and CV-22 are very important points here to regulate the circulation of Qi in the channels and eliminate stagnation and blockage in the throat and oesophagus, so as to relieve painful swallowing.

Modifications

1. If there is difficulty in swallowing and drinking, or vomiting, add SP-4, the Confluence point of the Penetrating Vessel, and KI-27 to cause the Stomach-Qi to descend and relieve the blockage in the throat.
2. If the throat is swollen owing to stagnation of Blood, add ST-40, the Connecting point, to subside swelling and eliminate blockage in the collateral in the throat.
3. If there is restlessness due to severe pain, add HT-3, the Sea point, to calm the Heart and tranquillise the Mind.
4. If there is expectoration of profuse phlegm, add SP-9, the Sea point of the Spleen channel, and CV-12, the Gathering point of the Fu organs, to activate the Spleen and Stomach and resolve Phlegm.

DEFICIENCY OF YIN OF LUNG, STOMACH AND KIDNEY

Symptoms and signs

Prolonged persistence of a slight pain when swallowing, especially swallowing of hard food, a dry throat, thirst, especially at night, but not much desire to drink, sometimes a burning feeling in the throat, night sweating, heat in the palms and soles of the feet, dry stools, scanty urine, a red tongue with a thin or peeled coating and a rapid and thready and weak pulse are the general signs of Yin deficiency.

Symptoms such as hoarseness, a dry cough, a slight chest pain or cough with scanty phlegm, or even blood in the phlegm, are due to deficiency of Lung-Yin.

Symptoms such as a slight burning sensation in the stomach, thirst, dry stools and a poor appetite are due to deficiency of Stomach-Yin. Tiredness, dizziness, tinnitus, a poor memory, weakness in the knees and lower back pain are caused by deficiency of Kidney-Yin.

Principle of treatment

Nourish Yin, clear Deficient-Fire, moisten the throat and relieve the pain.

HERBAL TREATMENT

Prescription

SHA SHEN MAI MEN DONG TANG
Glehnia and Ophiopogonis Decoction
Sha Shen *Radix Adenophorae* 10 g
Mai Dong *Radix Ophiopogonis* 10 g
Yu Zhu *Rhizoma Polgonati Odorati* 10 g
Gan Cao *Radix Glycyrrhizae* 6 g
Sang Ye *Folium Mori* 10 g
Bai Bian Dou *Semen Dolichoris Album* 10 g
Tian Hua Fen *Radix Trichosanthis* 10 g
Zhi Qiao *Fructus Aurantii* 10 g

Explanations

- Sha Shen and Mai Dong nourish the Kidney-Yin and clear Fire.
- Tian Hua Fen and Sang Ye nourish the Lung-Yin and clear Fire.
- Yu Zhu and Bai Bian Dou nourish the Stomach-Yin.
- Gan Cao tonifies the Spleen-Qi and harmonises the actions of the other herbs in the prescription.
- Zhi Qiao regulates the Qi circulation and relieves the pain.

Modifications

1. If there is night sweating, add Wu Wei Zi *Fructus Schisandrae* 10 g and Mu Li *Concha Ostreae* 10 g to arrest the sweating.
2. If there is insomnia, add Suan Zao Ren *Semen Ziziphi Spinosae* 10 g and Bai Zi Ren *Semen Biotae* 10 g to nourish the Heart-Yin and calm the Mind.
3. If there are dry stools, add Xuan Shen *Radix Scrophulariae* 10 g and Shou Wu *Radix Polygoni Multiflori* 10 g to nourish the Yin and to soften the stools.
4. If the palms and soles of the feet are hot, add Hu Huang Lian *Rhizoma Picrorhizae* 10 g and Qing

Hao *Herba Artemisiae Chinghao* 10 g to clear Deficient-Fire.
5. If there is lower back pain and weakness in the knees, add Sang Ji Sheng *Ramulus Loranthi* 10 g and Bai Shao *Radix Paeoniae Alba* 10 g to strengthen the Kidney and relieve the pain.
6. If the mouth is dry, add Sheng Di Huang *Radix Rehmanniae Recens* 10 g and Xuan Shen *Radix Scrophulariae* 10 g to nourish the Kidney-Yin and relieve the thirst.

Patent remedy

Zhi Bai Di Huang Wan *Anemarrhena, Phellodendron and Rehmannia Pill*

ACUPUNCTURE TREATMENT

LU-5 Chiz, LU-7 Lieque, LU-8 Jingqu, KI-6 Zhaohai, KI-7 Fuliu, SP-6 Sanyinjiao, ST-44 Neiting and CV-23 Lianquan. Reinforcing method is used on these points.

Explanations

- Failure of the throat and oesophagus to be nourished by Yin due to deficiency of Yin of Lung, Stomach and Kidney may cause painful swallowing. The Kidney rules the Water and Yin in the body. Thus nourishing the Yin and moistening the Dryness should be the root treatment for this condition.
- KI-7 and LU-8, the Metal points, have function of nourishing the Yin and promoting the secretion of Body Fluids so as to benefit and moisten the throat.
- SP-6, the crossing point of the three Yin channels of foot, helps the above two points tonify the Yin

and relieve the Dryness in the throat. This is the root treatment.
- LU-5, the Water point of the Lung channel, directly promotes the secretion of Body Fluids in the Lung system and moistens the throat.
- LU-7 together with KI-6 is a special combination, capable of opening the Directing Vessel, moistening the throat and sedating throat pain.
- CV-23 benefits the throat and relieves throat pain.
- ST-44, the Water point and Spring point of the Stomach channel, clears Deficient-Heat.

Modifications

1. If there is dizziness, a poor memory, lower back pain, and weakness in the knees, add KI-3, the Source point, and KI-10, the Sea point, to tonify the Kidney-Essence and strengthen the back.
2. If there is night sweating, heat in the palms and soles of the feet and thirst due to deficiency of Yin, add HT-6, the Accumulation point, and KI-2, the Spring point, to nourish the Yin and clear Deficient-Heat.
3. If there is a dry cough, hoarseness or blood in the phlegm, add BL-13, the Back Transporting point of the Lung, and LU-6, the Accumulation point, to nourish the Lung-Yin and relieve the cough and bleeding.
4. If there is insomnia, restlessness and palpitations, add BL-15, the Back Transporting point of the Heart, and CV-14, the Front Collecting point of the Heart, to nourish the Heart-Yin and calm the Mind.
5. If there is nervousness, headache and irritability due to deficiency of Liver-Yin with hyperactivity of Deficient-Fire, add LR-3, the Source point of the Liver, and GB-20 to calm the Liver and reduce Deficient-Fire.

Part 5

Pain in the front of the trunk 胸腹疼痛

Chest pain 22

胸
痛

Chest pain includes both pain and a sensation of compression in the chest. It may have a variety of causes, and be attributed to any of the following diseases in Western medicine:

1. heart diseases, such as coronary artery disease, angina pectoris, myocardial infarction, myocarditis, pericarditis, pulmonary embolism and heart failure
2. lung diseases, such as pneumonia, acute bronchitis, pulmonary tuberculosis and lung cancer
3. other disorders and diseases, such as hypertension, pleurisy, Tietze's syndrome, intercostal neuralgia, herpes zoster, dermatomyositis, trauma and neurosis.

Aetiology and pathology

According to TCM, chest pain may be the result of invasion of External pathogenic factors or internal conditions of the patient, or a combination of the two. Any factor that causes obstruction of the channels and the corresponding organs in the chest may cause chest pain. Common causes are stagnation of Qi and Blood, obstruction of Phlegm, contraction of Cold and obstruction of chest Yang.

Obstruction of Qi in the chest

Emotional disturbances, such as anger, resentment, frustration and anxiety, may cause stagnation of Liver-Qi, and because the Liver promotes Qi circulation in the body as a whole this Liver-Qi stagnation may cause obstruction of Qi in the Upper Burner. If the Heart-Qi is obstructed, the chest pain occurs on the left side of the chest. If the stagnant Liver-Qi blocks the descent of the Lung-Qi, there may be a sensation of compression in the chest. This condition can be seen in cardiophrenia, hyperventilation, depression, Tietze's syndrome and intercostal neuralgia.

External Wind-Heat or Wind-Cold can directly invade the Lung, causing blockage of the Lung-Qi, generation of Heat and formation of Phlegm, injuring the Lung and causing chest pain. This condition can be seen in pneumonia, pulmonary tuberculosis and pleurisy.

Chronic Heart or Lung diseases may directly cause stagnation of Qi in the chest, such as in chronic bronchitis, emphysema, rheumatic heart disease and heart failure in different pathological conditions.

Stagnation of Blood in the Heart

Long-term stagnation of Liver-Qi in conditions of emotional disturbance and stress may cause stagnation of Blood in the chest. Invasion of Cold in the chest may cause contraction of the channels, which blocks the Blood circulation, again causing Blood stagnation. Eating of too much greasy food may cause Phlegm-Damp to accumulate in the body, which also slows down the circulation of Blood, leading to stagnation of Blood. Trauma can directly cause obstruction of the Blood circulation in the chest. Once the channels are obstructed from any of these causes, the Heart becomes blocked and is not properly nourished by Blood, and this triggers chest pain. This condition can be seen in coronary artery disease, angina pectoris, myocardial infarction, hyperlipidaemia, myocarditis and pericarditis.

In chronic disease, or in elderly people as well as those with weak constitutions, there may be a deficiency of Qi, Blood, Yin or Yang. This situation may cause the circulation of Qi and Blood to slow down, leading to obstruction of the chest by Qi, Blood, Phlegm and Fire, which causes chest pain.

Phlegm obstruction in the Heart and Lung

Excessive consumption of greasy, raw or cold food, or of alcohol, may impede the Spleen in its physiological function of transportation and transformation, which results in Phlegm formation and changes the quality of the Blood. Phlegm accumulation can cause Heat to be generated, or it may combine with Damp-Cold from the Middle Burner, obstructing the Heart and Lung in the chest and causing chest pain. This condition can be seen in hyperlipidaemia, coronary artery disease, bronchitis and asthma.

Excessive thinking and habitual working under stressful or emotional circumstances may directly injure the Spleen and generate Phlegm. When there is concurrent stagnation of Liver-Qi and uprising of Liver-Yang, this Phlegm can obstruct the Heart and cause chest pain. This condition is seen in hypertension, coronary artery disease, Tietze's syndrome and herpes zoster.

Exogenous pathogenic factors can directly invade the Lung disturbing its dispersing and descending function, which causes Phlegm-Heat to be generated, injuring the Blood and causing chest pain. This condition is seen in pneumonia, tuberculosis and pleurisy.

Obstruction of Yang in the chest

In elderly people, or those suffering from chronic diseases or with a weak constitution, the Kidney-Yang is usually weak. This deficiency will in turn cause weakness of the Spleen-Yang and Heart-Yang. This condition, compounded by carelessness in daily habits such as wearing too few clothes or overconsumption of cold, raw food and cold drinks, leaves the person vulnerable to the invasion of Exogenous pathogenic Cold

to the Upper and Middle Burners. When the Heart-Yang is very weak and blocked by Cold, the channels in the chest contract, causing chest pain. Alternatively if the Yang of the Lung, Spleen and Kidney is weak then it is the water metabolism that is disturbed; the water passage becomes blocked and cold water accumulates in the body, the Heart and Lung are attacked, causing chest pain. This condition is seen in angina pectoris, myocardial infarction, pericarditis, hydrothorax, pulmonary heart disease and heart failure in Heart and Kidney disease.

Treatment based on differentiation

Differentiation

Differentiation of location

The first step in differentiating chest pain is to identify the location of the disorder.

— If the obstruction is in the Heart (whether in the terminology of TCM or that of Western medicine) the pain is mainly on the left side of the chest, radiating to the upper back, the left shoulder and the inner side of the left arm. Other symptoms such as palpitations and restlessness may accompany the pain.
— If the obstruction is in the Lung, the breathing is not smooth and symptoms such as cough with sputum and fever accompany the chest pain.
— If the muscles and nerves of the chest are involved, the pain changes with breathing (e.g. intercostal neuralgia and trauma).
— If the costal cartilage, muscles and skin are involved, the affected areas are tender and there may be skin lesions (e.g. Tietze's syndrome and herpes zoster).

Differentiation of severity

— A severe pain or pressing pain is usually caused by obstruction of Yang or stagnation of Blood in the Heart.
— A mild pain indicates a mild obstruction or deficiency syndrome in a chronic stage.

Treatment

In the treatment of chest pain, it is important to follow the principle of treating the manifestation in an acute stage and treating the root cause in the remission. Use of a combination of TCM and Western medicine is strongly advised when there is an acute chest pain caused by severe Heart or Lung disease. If a chest pain is caused by tumour or systemic diseases, treatment should also be given to treat the underlying disease.

In acute conditions, the medication must be given promptly. As well as acupuncture treatment, use of patent herbal medicines is recommended. Some commonly used patent herbal medicines, their functions and indications are as follows:

Guan Xin Su He Wan Styrax Pill for Coronary Heart Disease. This can invigorate the Blood, promote Qi movement, disperse the Yang in the chest and stop pain. It is used for severe chest pain, such as angina pectoris, or myocardial infarction of any TCM type.

Su He Xiang Wan Styrax Pill. This can disperse Cold, promote Qi movement, warm and disperse the Yang in the chest, aromatically open the orifices and stop pain. It is used for chest pain due to obstruction of Yang in the Heart.

Sheng Mai San Generating the Pulse Powder (administered via intravenous drip). This can nourish the Yin and strengthen the Heart-Qi. It is often used in cardiogenic shock. It can decrease the oxygen consumption of the Heart, but increase its contraction, and raise the blood pressure.

Zhi Bao Dan Greatest Treasure Special Pill. This can clear Heat, open the orifices, clear turbidity and relieve toxicity. It is used for obstruction of the Heart by Phlegm-Heat.

Qi Li San Seven-Thousandths of a Tael Powder or **Yun Nan Bai Yao** Yunnan White Medicine. These two patent medicines promote circulation of the Blood, reduce swelling and stop pain. They are often used for chest pain due to trauma.

These patent herbs can be used in combination with the following treatment methods according to the differentiation of the syndromes.

EXCESS SYNDROMES OF THE HEART

OBSTRUCTION OF QI IN THE UPPER BURNER

Symptoms and signs

Chest pain of a compressing or cramping nature, which may occur under situations of emotional disturbance or stress, a sense of fullness in the chest and hypochondriac region, irritability, a bitter taste in the mouth, dream-disturbed sleep, a white, dry and thin tongue coating and a wiry pulse. This syndrome can be seen in coronary artery disease, angina pectoris, hypertension, psychosis, menopausal syndrome or premenstrual tension.

Principle of treatment

Promote Qi circulation in the chest and stop the pain.

HERBAL TREATMENT

Prescription

JIN LING ZI SAN and **DAN SHEN YIN**
Melia Toosendan Powder and *Salvia Decoction*
Chuan Lian Zi *Fructus Meliae Toosendan* 6 g
Yan Hu Suo *Rhizoma Corydalis* 6 g
Tan Xiang *Lignum Santali Albi* 3 g
Sha Ren *Fructus Amomi* 3 g
Dan Shen *Radix Salviae* 9 g

Add:

Chuan Xiong *Rhizoma Ligustici Chuanxiong* 6 g
Dai Dai Hua *Flos Citri Aurantii* 6 g
Zhi Qiao *Fructus Aurantii* 6 g
Xiang Fu *Rhizoma Cyperi* 6 g
Bai Shao *Radix Paeoniae Alba* 9 g
Dang Gui *Radix Angelicae Sinensis* 9 g

Explanations

- Emotional disturbance and stress may cause stagnation of Liver-Qi and disturbance of Qi movement in the chest. If the Qi is obstructed in the Upper Burner, the pain may start in the chest. A normal tongue coating shows there is no obvious stagnation of Blood or weakness of the internal organs. The pulse shows stagnation of Qi, especially the Liver-Qi.
- Since the Qi guides the Blood, stagnation of Qi always causes stagnation of Blood, the difference being only one of degree. This is why the formula contains both Qi-moving and also Blood-moving herbs.
- Jin Ling Zi is a very bitter and Cold herb. It is able to break up Liver-Qi obstruction and drain Heat.
- Yuan Hu Suo is a pungent and warm herb. It is able to invigorate the Qi and Blood circulation, unblock obstruction and stop the pain.
- This small formula is effective for treating pain that is due mainly to stagnation of Qi as well as to stagnation of Blood.
- In the formula Dan Shen Yin, Tan Xiang and Sha Ren, the aromatic herbs, disperse the Qi obstruction and open the orifice.

- Dan Shen is able to promote the Blood circulation, dissolve the stagnant Blood together with the other herbs that promote the Qi and Blood circulation and stop pain. It can also clear Heat in the Heart, calm the Mind, and treat restlessness and irritability.
- Chuan Xiong and Dai Dai Hua can promote the Qi and Blood circulation, especially Blood circulation, enhancing the action of Dan Shen and Yan Hu Suo.
- Xiang Fu and Zhi Qiao can strengthen the function of the Qi-moving herbs.
- Dan Gui and Bai Shao regulate and tonify the Blood so as to moderate the dispersing herbs.

Modifications

1. If there is severe pain, add Qing Pi *Pericarpium Citri Reticulatae Viride* 9 g to break up Qi stagnation in the Liver and stop the pain.
2. If there is irritability, add Xia Ku Cao *Spica Prunella* 10 g and Huang Qin *Radix Scutellariae* 12 g to clear Heat in the Liver and calm the Mind.
3. If there is a bitter taste in the mouth or insomnia, add Mu Dan Pi *Cortex Moutan Radici* 9 g and Zhi Zi *Fructus Gardeniae* 9 g to clear Liver-Heat directly.

Patent remedies

Shu Gan Wan *Soothe Liver Pill*
Xiao Yao Wan *Honeysuckle and Forsythia Pill*

ACUPUNCTURE TREATMENT

PC-6 Neiguan, LU-7 Lieque, CV-17 Tanzhong, LR-3 Taichong, LR-14 Qimen, BL-18 Ganshu, GB-34 Yanglingquan and SP-6 Sanyinjiao. Reducing method is used on these points.

Explanations

- PC-6 is a Connecting point of the Pericardium channel and a Confluence point of the Yin Linking Vessel. It specifically treats the chest pain by promoting Blood circulation and dispersing the Qi in the chest. It is also very effective for calming the Mind and treating emotional disturbance.
- LU-7 is also a Connecting point, which can open the chest and help the Lung to disperse the Qi and cause it to descend, together with CV-17 the Gathering point for the Qi, to remove the stagnation of Qi in the chest.
- LR-3, the Source point, promotes Liver-Qi circulation and regulates the function of the Liver.
- LR-14 and BL-18, the combination of Front Collecting point and Back Transporting point of the Liver, together with GB-34, the Lower Sea point, regulate the Liver-Qi and Qi in Lesser Yang channels so as to resolve the Qi obstruction in the chest.
- SP-6 promotes the Blood circulation and enhances the function of PC-6 in stopping the pain.

Modifications

1. If there is insomnia, add HT-3, the Sea point, to calm the Mind and improve the sleep.
2. If there is shortness of breath and a sensation of oppression over the chest, add SP-4 in combination with PC-6 to regulate the breath and cause the Qi to descend.
3. If the pain is radiating to the arm, add HT-5, the Connecting point, to harmonise the collateral and stop the pain.
4. If there is an extremely purplish tongue, add BL-17 to promote the Blood circulation and eliminate Blood stasis.

STAGNATION OF QI AND BLOOD IN THE HEART

Symptoms and signs

Pain on the left side of the chest with a sharp or pressing feature, which may occur in circumstances of fatigue, overwork, stress, immoderate eating or emotional disturbance. In severe cases, there is radiation to the left scapula and arm, palpitations, stiffness of the chest, distension in the hypochondriac region, irritability, a purplish tongue, or purplish spots on the sides of the tongue, with a white and dry tongue coating and a wiry or choppy pulse.

This syndrome is a development of the previous syndrome of the obstruction of Qi in the Heart. It can be seen in coronary artery disease, angina pectoris, myocarditis, pericarditis, pleurisy and intercostal neuralgia.

Principle of treatment

Spread Qi, promote Blood circulation in the Heart and stop the pain.

HERBAL TREATMENT

Prescription

DAN SHEN YIN and **TAO HONG SI WU TANG**
Salvia Decoction and *Four-Substance Decoction with Safflower and Peach Pit*
Dan Shen *Radix Salviae Miltiorrhizae* 15 g
Tan Xiang *Lignum Santali Albi* 3 g

Sha Ren *Fructus Amomi* 3 g
Qing Pi *Pericarpium Citri Reticulatae Viride* 6 g
Wu Yao *Radix Linderae* 6 g
Dang Gui *Radix Angelicae Sinensis* 9 g
Chi Shao *Radix Paeoniae Rubra* 9 g
Chuan Xiong *Rhizoma Ligustici Chuanxiong* 6 g
Tao Ren *Semen Persicae* 9 g
Hong Hua *Flos Carthami* 9 g

Explanations

- When stagnation of Qi persists for a long time, the Blood circulation also slows and stagnates. If the channel and the collateral of the Heart are blocked by stagnant Qi and Blood, chest pain follows. Any factors that worsen stagnation of Blood, such as extreme fatigue, overwork, immoderate eating, stress and emotional disturbance, may lead to chest pain.
- Dan Shen, Tao Ren, Hong Hua, Chuan Xiong and Dang Gui can promote the Blood circulation, unblock the Heart channel and stop the pain.
- Since stagnation of Qi and Blood can generate Heat, Dan Shen and Chi Shao promote the Blood circulation, clear the Heat in the Blood and dissolve the stagnant Blood.
- Tan Xiang, Sha Ren, Qing Pi and Wu Yao regulate the Qi movement in the Heart and Liver, so assisting the other herbs to stop the pain.
- When Qi and Blood circulate smoothly, chest pain disappears.

Modifications

1. If there are palpitations, add Fu Shen *Sclerotium Poria Pararadicis* 15 g and Ye Jiao Tang *Caulis Polygoni Multiflori* 12 g to calm the Mind and relieve the palpitations.
2. If there is arm pain, add Bai Zhi *Radix Angelicae Dahuricae* 6 g and Qiang Huo *Rhizoma seu Radix Notopterygii* 9 g to regulate the Qi circulation and relieve the pain.
3. If there is depression, add Chai Hu *Radix Bupleuri* 6 g and Yu Jin *Radix Curcumae* 12 g to smooth the Liver and promote the Blood circulation.
4. If there is insomnia, add Suan Zao Ren *Semen Ziziphi Spinosae* 9 g and Yu Li Ren *Semen Pruni* 9 g to calm the Mind and improve the sleep.

Patent remedies

Fu Fang Dan Shen Pian *Compound Salvia Tablet*
Guan Xin Su He Wan *Styrax Pill for Coronary Heart Disease*

ACUPUNCTURE TREATMENT

PC-6 Neiguan, HT-6 Yinxi, CV-14 Juque, BL-15 Xinshu, CV-17 Tanzhong, BL-17 Geshu, LR-3 Taichong and LU-7 Lieque. Reducing method is used on these points.

Explanations

- PC-6, the Connecting point and Confluent point, can spread the Qi and invigorate the Blood circulation in the chest, calm the Mind and stop the chest pain.
- HT-6, an Accumulation point, is particularly used in acute conditions. It can clear Heat due to stagnation of Qi and Blood and stop the acute pain.
- CV-14 and BL-15, the Front Collecting point and Back Transporting point of the Heart, are able to regulate the Qi and Blood circulation of the Heart so as to stop the pain.
- CV-17 and BL-17 are the Gathering points for the Qi and Blood. They can disperse and dissolve stagnation so as to reduce the pain.
- LR-3, the Source point, promotes circulation of the Liver-Qi. LU-7, the Connecting point, promotes the Lung-Qi. These two points move the Qi in the body so as to assist the Blood circulation.

Modifications

1. If there is nervousness, add LR-2, the Spring point, to clear Heat and calm the Liver.
2. If there is headache, add GB-20 to calm the Mind and relieve the headache.
3. If there is aggravation of the pain at night, add HT-5 to harmonise the collateral and relieve the pain.
4. If there is an extremely purplish tongue, add SP-6 to promote the Blood circulation and eliminate Blood stasis.

STAGNATION OF THE BLOOD IN THE HEART

Symptoms and signs

Fixed, compressing or stabbing pain in the chest, worse at night, with palpitations, restlessness, a purple tongue or purple spots on the sides of the tongue and a choppy and wiry pulse. In a very severe case, the chest pain is very heavy, the pain radiates to the left scapula and arm and the patient has breathlessness and cold sweating.

This syndrome can be seen in angina pectoris, myocardial infarction and cardiomyopathy.

Principle of treatment

Drive out the stagnant Blood and stop the pain.

HERBAL TREATMENT

Prescription

XUE FU ZHU YU TANG
Drive Out Stasis in the Mansion of Blood Decoction
Tao Ren *Semen Persicae* 12 g
Chai Hu *Radix Bupleuri* 6 g
Jie Geng *Radix Platycodi* 6 g
Sheng Di Huang *Radix Rehmanniae* 9 g
Gan Cao *Radix Glycyrrhizae* 6 g
Chi Shao *Radix Paeoniae Rubrae* 9 g
Chuan Xiong *Radix Ligustici Chuanxiong* 9 g
Dang Gui *Radix Angelicae Sinensis* 9 g
Hong Hua *Flos Carthami* 9 g
Zhi Qiao *Fructus Citri Aurantii* 6 g
Chuan Niu Xi *Radix Cyathulae* 9 g

Add:

Yan Hu Suo *Rhizoma Corydalis* 9 g
Wu Ling Zhi *Faeces Trogopterorum* 9 g
Ru Xiang *Resina Olibani* 6 g
Mo Yao *Resina Myrrhae* 6 g
San Qi *Radix Notoginseng* powder 3 g

Explanations

- This syndrome develops from stagnation of Qi and Blood in the Heart. In fact, stagnation of Blood is the main cause of the chest pain and stagnation of Qi is secondary. Since chest pain is caused by obstruction of the stagnant Blood in the Heart channel, there are many herbs to invigorate the Blood and dissolve the stagnant Blood in this formula.
- Tao Ren, Hong Hua, Chuan Xiong, Chuan Niu Xi, Dang Gui and Chi Shao invigorate the Blood and stop pain.
- Yan Hu Suo and Wu Ling Zhi dissolve the stagnant Blood and stop pain.
- Ru Xiang, Mo Yao and San Qi can break up the stagnant Blood, promote the Blood circulation and stop pain.
- Sheng Di Huang cools Blood Heat produced by Blood stagnation.
- Gan Cao harmonises the herbs in the formula.
- Chai Hu and Jie Geng can cause the Qi to ascend in the chest, together with Zhi Qiao, which opens the chest, and Chuan Niu Xi, which causes the Blood to descend, and activates Qi movement so as to assist the herbs which move the Blood and

unblock the obstruction of Qi and Blood in the chest. When the stagnant Blood has been dissolved, the Qi and Blood move properly, the chest pain can disappear.

Modifications

1. If there is sharp pain, add Xiang Fu *Rhizoma Cyperi* 9 g and Xue Jie *Resina Draconis* 6 g to remove the Blood stasis and relieve the pain.
2. If there is restlessness, add Yu Jin *Radix Curcumae* 9 g and Ji Xue Teng *Caulis Spatholobi* 15 g to regulate the Blood circulation and calm the Mind.
3. If there is severe pain at night, add Dan Shen *Radix Salviae Miltiorrhizae* 18 g and Bing Pian *Borneolum Syntheticum* 1 g to remove the Blood stasis and relieve the pain.

Patent remedy

Guan Xin Su He Wan *Styrax Pill for Coronary Heart Disease*

ACUPUNCTURE TREATMENT

Extra Huatuojiaji points on T4–T5, SP-6 Sanyinjiao, PC-6 Neiguan, CV-17 Tanzhong, LR-3 Taichong and LU-9 Taiyuan. Reducing method is used on these points, except for LR-3 and LU-9, on which even method is employed.

Explanations

- The Extra Huatuojiaji points on T4–T5 can harmonise the collateral, stimulate the Blood circulation in the Heart and stop the pain.
- SP-6 and PC-6 promote the Blood circulation and stop the pain.
- CV-17, a Gathering point for the Qi, together with LR-3 and LU-9, the Source points of the Liver and Lung channels, promote the Qi circulation in the Heart and chest so as to strengthen the function of the other points that invigorate Blood circulation.

Modifications

1. If there is pain with palpitations, add PC-3 and HT-3 to strengthen the Heart, calm the Mind and stop the pain.
2. If the lips and nails are purplish, add PC-9 and HT-9, the Well points, to promote the Blood circulation and revive the Heart.
3. If there is severe chest pain, add HT-5 to harmonise the collateral and relieve the pain.

OBSTRUCTION OF THE HEART BY PHLEGM-HEAT

Symptoms and signs

Chest pain with a sense of fullness in the chest, palpitations, cough with expectoration of yellow phlegm, dizziness, constipation, a yellow and greasy tongue coating and a slippery and rapid pulse. This syndrome can be seen in coronary artery disease, hyperlipaemia and pleurisy.

Principle of treatment

Transform Phlegm, clear Heat, promote Qi and Blood circulation and stop the pain.

HERBAL TREATMENT

Prescription

XIAO XIAN XIONG TANG and **GUN TAN WAN**
Minor Sinking into the Chest Decoction and Vaporise Phlegm Pill
Huang Lian *Rhizoma Coptidis* 6 g
Ban Xia *Rhizoma Pinelliae* 6 g
Gua Lou *Fructus Trichosanthis* 12 g
Huang Qin *Radix Scutellariae* 9 g
Da Huang *Radix et Rhizoma Rhei* 6 g
Meng Shi *Lapis Chloriti Usta* 15 g
Chen Xiang *Lignum Aquilariae Resinatum* 3 g

Add:

Dan Shen *Radix Salviae Miltiorrhizae* 9 g
Yu Jin *Radix Curcumae* 9 g
Zhu Ru *Caulis Bambusae in Taeniam* 9 g

Explanations

- Habitual eating of greasy food may injure the Spleen and Stomach, causing Phlegm-Heat to form in the Middle Burner. When the Qi and Blood circulation in the chest and Heart is obstructed by Phlegm-Heat, chest pain occurs.
- Huang Lian is very bitter and Cold, entering the Heart and Stomach channels. It can powerfully clear Heat from the Heart and dry Damp. Ban Xia is pungent and warm, entering the Lung, Spleen and Stomach Channels. It causes the Stomach-Qi to descend and clears Phlegm in the Upper and Middle Burners. When Huang Lian and Ban Xia are used together, they are very effective for removing Phlegm-Heat from the chest.
- Gua Lou can eliminate Phlegm-Heat from the chest directly, unblock the chest and stop the pain.

It can also promote bowel movement so as to treat constipation.
- Huang Qin clears Damp-Heat from the Upper Burner, enhancing the function of Huang Lian.
- Da Huang and Meng Shi are Cold herbs, draining Heat, directing Qi and Phlegm downwards, and promoting bowel movement so as to clear the Qi obstruction in the chest and Heat in the Upper Burner.
- Chen Xiang can cause the Qi to descend and also relieve the pain.
- Dan Shen and Yu Jin can promote the Blood circulation in the Heart.
- Yu Jin and Zhu Ru can remove Phlegm-Heat from the Heart. When Phlegm-Heat is removed, the Qi and Blood can circulate properly and chest pain disappears.

Modifications

1. If there is severe pain, add Dan Xing *Arisaema cum Bile* 9 g, Zhe Bei Mu *Bulbus Fritillariae Thunbergii* 9 g and Zhi Shi *Fructus Aurantii Immaturus* 12 g to eliminate Phlegm-Heat, break up Phlegm and unblock the chest.
2. If there is mental confusion, add Yuan Zhi *Radix Polygale* 6 g and Shi Chang Pu *Rhizoma Acori Graminei* 6 g to transform Phlegm and unblock the Heart Orifice.
3. If there is an acute obstruction of Phlegm-Heat in the Heart, there is mental confusion or loss of consciousness; use Zhi Bao Dan (patent formula, 1 pill a day) to transform the Phlegm-Heat and unblock the Orifice.
4. If there is shortness of breath, add Sang Bai Pi *Cortex Mori Radicis* 12 g and Ting Li Zi *Semen Lepidii seu Descurainiae* 9 g to cause the Lung-Qi to descend and relieve the shortness of breath.

Patent remedy

Qing Fei Yi Huo Pian *Clear Lungs Restrain Fire Tablet*

ACUPUNCTURE TREATMENT

PC-6 Neiguan, HT-5 Tongli, ST-40 Fenglong, CV-12 Zhongwan, LU-7 Lieque, SP-10 Xuehai, BL-15 Xinshu and CV-14 Juque. Reducing method is used on these points.

Explanations

- PC-6 is a Confluence point, connecting with the Yin Linking Vessel. It can promote Blood circulation, stop pain and treat mental disorders caused by obstruction of the Heart by Blood. It is also able to cause the Stomach-Qi to descend, together with ST-40, the Connecting point, to remove Phlegm from the Stomach; together with HT-5 these remove Phlegm obstruction in the Heart.

- CV-12 is a Gathering point for all the Fu organs. Together with ST-40 and PC-6, it can clear Phlegm.
- LU-7, the Connecting point, and LR-3, the Source point, can promote Qi movement in the Upper and Middle Burners so as to strengthen the function of the points that remove Phlegm.
- SP-10 is able to promote the Blood circulation and clear Blood-Heat.
- BL-15 and CV-14, the combination of the Back Transporting point and Front Collecting points of the Heart, regulate the function of the Heart and stop the pain.

Modifications

1. If there is severe pain, add BL-14 and BL-17 to promote the Blood circulation and stop the pain.
2. If there is shortness of breath, add CV-17 to disperse the Qi and relieve the shortness of breath.
3. If there is anxiety and restlessness, add PC-7 and PC-8 to clear Heat in the Heart and calm the Mind.

OBSTRUCTION OF THE HEART BY DAMP-PHLEGM

Symptoms and signs

Chest pain with a sensation of fullness in the chest and abdomen, obesity, a feeling of oppression over the chest, and heaviness in the body, tiredness, poor memory and concentration, a purplish and pale tongue with a white, sticky and thick coating and a slippery pulse.

This syndrome can be seen in coronary artery disease with hyperlipaemia, and hypertension with hyperlipaemia.

Principle of treatment

Transform Damp, promote Qi movement and stop the pain.

HERBAL TREATMENT

Prescription

WEN DAN TANG and **SU HE XIANG WAN**
Warm the Gall Bladder Decoction and *Styrax Pill*
Ban Xia *Rhizoma Pinelliae* 9 g

Ju Pi *Exocarpium Citri Reticulatae* 9 g
Fu Ling *Poria* 15 g
Zhi Shi *Fructus Aurantii Immaturus* 6 g
Zhu Ru *Caulis Bambusae in Taeniam* 6 g
Gan Cao *Radix Glycyrrhizae* 3 g

Add:

Hou Po *Cortex Magnoliae Officinalis* 6 g
Yuan Zhi *Radix Polgalae* 6 g
Chang Pu *Rhizoma Acori Graminei* 6 g
Bai Zhu *Rhizoma Atractylodis Macrocephalae* 9 g

Explanations

- Habitual eating of greasy food injures the function of the Spleen and Stomach, causing greasy Phlegm to accumulate. If this obstructs the Qi and Blood in the chest this causes pain, and obesity too. When the Qi movement is obstructed, a sensation of oppression is experienced over the chest. Damp-Phlegm is a Yin pathogenic factor, so can cause heaviness of the body. When Phlegm obstructs the Heart and the Spleen, the patient is not able to concentrate when thinking, and the memory deteriorates.
- Ban Xia, pungent and warm in nature, causes the Stomach-Qi to descend and dissolves Damp-Phlegm.
- Chen Pi is a pungent and warm herb. Its aromatic smell can clear Turbidity of the Damp-Phlegm and revive the Spleen.
- Fu Ling can strengthen the Spleen, increase urination and eliminate Damp.
- Zhi Shi can break up and drain Phlegm.
- Zhu Ru is able to transform Phlegm and cause Stomach-Qi to descend.
- Hou Po promotes Qi movement, transforms Phlegm and enhances the action of the other herbs that eliminate Phlegm.
- Yuan Zhi and Chang Pu specifically remove Phlegm from the Heart.
- Bai Zhu and Gan Cao strengthen the function of the Spleen so less Phlegm is formed.

Modifications

1. If there is a deficiency of Yang in the chest, add Gui Zhi *Ramulus Cinnamomi* 9 g and Xie Bai *Bulbus Allii Macrostemi* 9 g to disperse the Yang and promote the Qi and Blood circulation.
2. If there is a deficiency of the Spleen-Yang, add Bai Zhu *Rhizoma Atractylodis Macrocephalae* 12 g and Dang Shen *Radix Codonopsis Pilosulae* 9 g to tonify the Qi in the Middle Burner.

3. If there is oedema, add Ze Xie *Rhizoma Alismatis* 9 g, Wu Yao *Radix Linderae* 9 g and Da Fu Pi *Pericarpium Arecae* 9 g to eliminate Damp and promote the Qi movement.

Patent remedy

Su He Xiang Wan *Styrax Pill*

ACUPUNCTURE TREATMENT

PC-4 Ximen, CV-14 Juque, PC-5 Jianshi, CV-17 Tanzhong, ST-36 Zusanli, ST-40 Fenglong and HT-5 Tongli. Reducing method is used on these points, except for ST-36, on which even method is employed.

Explanations

- PC-4, the Accumulation point, is specifically used in acute conditions. It can unblock the Heart orifice and activate the function of the Heart-Qi.
- CV-14, the Front Collecting point of the Heart, regulates its function, and together with PC-4 restores the function of the Heart.
- PC-6, the Confluence point, is used specifically to treat disorders of the Stomach, Heart and chest.
- CV-17, the Front Collecting point of the Pericardium, is used to regulate the Blood and Qi in the Heart and stop the pain.
- ST-40, the Connecting point, and HT-5 are used to clear Phlegm and unblock the Heart orifice.
- ST-36, the Sea point, is used to tonify the Spleen-Qi, dissolve Phlegm and prevent Phlegm being formed.

Modifications

1. If there is severe pain in the chest and the extremities are cold, apply moxibustion on CV-4 and CV-6 to warm the Qi, dispel Cold and promote the movement Yang-Qi in the chest.
2. If there is a deficiency of Spleen-Qi, add BL-20 and BL-21 to tonify the Middle Burner and reinforce the Qi.

Case history

A 52-year-old man had been suffering from chest pain for a year. The pain often started when he walked too fast or under stress. He also suffered from headache, a feeling of distension in the head, palpitations and obesity. This was diagnosed by Western medicine as arteriosclerosis, coronary heart disease, angina pectoris, hypertension and hyperlipaemia. He received Western medical treatment. The chest pain could be relieved for a short time, but was not under control. He also had a flabby and purple tongue with purple spots on the border and white and greasy coating, and a choppy and slow pulse.

Diagnosis
Accumulation of Damp-Phlegm and deficiency of Heart-Yang.

Principle of treatment
Eliminate Phlegm, transform Damp, disperse Yang in the chest and stop the pain.

Herbal treatment
ER CHEN TANG and **GUA LOU XIE BAI GUI ZHI TANG**
Two-Cured Decoction and *Trichosanthes Fruit, Chinese Chive and Cinnamon Twig Decoction*
Ban Xia *Rhizoma Pinelliae* 9 g
Fu Ling *Poria* 9 g
Chen Pi *Pericarpium Citri Reticulatae* 6 g
Zhi Gan Cao *Radix Glycyrrhizae Praeparata* 3 g
Xie Bai *Bulbus Allii* 9 g
Gui Zhi *Ramulus Cinnamomi* 9 g
Chuan Xiong *Radix Ligustici Chuanxiong* 9 g
Shan Zha *Fructus Crataegi* 15 g
San Qi *Radix Notoginseng* powder 3 g
Dang Shen *Radix Codonopsis* 15 g

Explanations

- Ban Xia, Fu Ling, Chen Pi and Zhi Gan Cao form the formula called Er Chen Tang *Citrus and Pinellia Decoction*, which is commonly used to harmonise the Stomach-Qi, remove Damp from the Spleen and eliminate Phlegm.
- Xie Bai and Gui Zhi are able to move the Yang and Qi in the chest so as to disperse and transform Damp in the chest and stop the pain.
- Chuan Xiong and San Qi invigorate the Blood circulation, dissolve stagnant Blood and stop the pain in the chest.
- Shan Zha can promote the Blood circulation as well as remove Damp in the body.
- Dang Shen can strengthen the Qi in the Middle and Upper Burners, assisting the actions of the other herbs.

After the patient had used this formula for a month, the chest pain had disappeared and the electrocardiogram (ECG) had much improved. The patient used the formula for another 2 months in order to increase the therapeutic effect. Half a year later, the patient returned for a consultation. The ECG was normal and he had experienced no more chest pain in the intervening months.

CONTRACTION OF THE HEART CHANNEL DUE TO COLD

Symptoms and signs

Severe chest pain, with the pain radiating to the upper back and scapula, and starting or worsening after exposure to cold, shortness of breath, a feeling of stifling in the chest, fear of cold, cold hands and feet, a bluish-purple tongue with a white and greasy coating and a deep, wiry and slippery pulse.

This syndrome can be seen in angina pectoris, myocardial infarction, pulmonary heart disease and heart failure during the course of different diseases.

Principle of treatment

Expel Cold, disperse the Yang-Qi, promote Qi circulation, transform Damp-Phlegm and stop the pain.

HERBAL TREATMENT

Prescription

GUA LOU XIE BAI GUI ZHI TANG
Trichosanthis–Allium–Cinnamon Twig Decoction
Gua Lou *Fructus Trichosanthis* 12 g
Xie Bai *Bulbus Allii Macrostemi* 9 g
Gui Zhi *Ramulus Cinnamomi* 6 g

Add:

Ban Xia *Rhizoma Pinelliae* 9 g
Chen Pi *Pericarpium Citri Reticulatae* 6 g
Hou Po *Cortex Magnoliae Officinalis* 6 g
Zhi Qiao *Fructus Aurantii* 9 g
Fu Ling *Poria* 12 g

Explanations

- When Cold invades and blocks the chest, the Heart-Yang will not be able to disperse to warm the chest, so chest pain occurs.
- Gua Lou is able to eliminate Phlegm and clear the Qi obstruction in the chest so as to promote the distribution of Yang-Qi in the chest.
- Xie Bai and Gui Zhi are pungent and warm, enter the Heart channel, clear the Cold obstruction and disperse the Yang-Qi.
- Ban Xia, Chen Pi and Hou Po can transform and eliminate Damp-Phlegm, and direct the Qi downwards in the chest so as to relieve shortness of breath and a feeling of stifling in the chest.
- Zhi Qiao can unblock the chest, enhance the function of Gua Lou and clear the Qi and Phlegm obstruction in the chest. Meanwhile, Zhi Qiao enhances the function of Ban Xia, Chen Pi and Hou Po in regulating the Qi in the Upper Burner.
- Fu Ling can strengthen the Spleen, dissolve Damp, increase urination and leach out Damp. When Cold, Damp and Phlegm are removed, Yang-Qi can disperse in the chest, and chest pain stops.

Modifications

1. If the chest is very cold, with severe pain and cold extremities, add Fu Zi *Radix Aconiti Praeparata* 6 g and Gan Jiang *Rhizoma Zingiberis* 9 g to warm the Kidney-Yang and Spleen-Yang so as to warm the Heart-Yang in turn and dispel the Cold in the chest.
2. If external Cold symptoms are present, add Gui Zhi *Ramulus Cinnamomi* 6 g, Jing Jie *Herba Schizonepetae* 6 g and Qiang Huo *Rhizoma seu Radix Notopterygii* 6 g to expel the External Cold and relieve the External symptoms.
3. If there is severe Blood stagnation, add Chuan Xiong *Rhizoma Ligustici Chuanxiong* 9 g, Hong Hua *Flos Carthami* 9 g, Dang Gui *Radix Angelicae Sinensis* 9 g and Ji Xue Teng *Caulis Spatholobi* 9 g to promote the Blood circulation and stop pain.

Patent remedy

Liang Fu Wan *Galangal and Cyperus Pill*

ACUPUNCTURE TREATMENT

PC-6 Neiguan, CV-17 Tanzhong, HT-5 Tongli, BL-15 Xinshu, BL-14 Jueyinshu and BL-17 Geshu with even method. Moxibustion is used on CV-4, CV-6 or BL-20, BL-23 and BL-25.

Explanations

- PC-6, the Connecting point, promotes the Qi and Blood circulation, together with CV-17, the Gathering point of the Qi, opens Qi obstruction in the chest and stops the pain.
- Moxibustion on CV-4 and CV-6 may warm the Lower Burner and support the Heart-Yang.
- Moxibustion on BL-20, BL-23 and BL-25 can strengthen the Spleen-Yang and Kidney-Yang so as to strengthen the Heart-Yang in turn.
- HT-5, the Connecting point of the Heart, clears Phlegm, opens the collateral, promotes Qi movement and stops the pain.
- BL-15, BL-14 and BL-17 promote the Blood circulation and stop the pain.

Modifications

1. If external Cold symptoms are present, add BL-12 and BL-13 to expel the Cold and relieve the External symptoms.
2. If there is severe chest pain, add HT-6, the Accumulation point, to open the collateral and stop the pain.

3. If there is a cough, add LU-7 to dispel Cold and disperse the Lung-Qi.

DEFICIENCY SYNDROMES OF THE HEART

DEFICIENCY OF YIN AND QI OF THE HEART

Symptoms and signs

Chest pain, palpitations, shortness of breath, frequent sweating, anxiety, restlessness, a dry mouth, thirst, a red tongue with a thin coating, and a thready, wiry and irregular pulse.

This syndrome can be seen in angina pectoris, myocardial infarction, myocarditis, cardiogenic shock and pulmonary tuberculosis.

Principle of treatment

Nourish the Yin and tonify the Qi of the Heart, promote Blood circulation in the Heart and stop the pain.

HERBAL TREATMENT

Prescription

SHENG MAI SAN
Generate the Pulse Powder
Dang Shen *Radix Codonopsis Pilosulae* 12 g
Mai Dong *Radix Ophiopogonis* 12 g
Wu Wei Zi *Fructus Schisandrae* 3 g

Add:

Sheng Di Huang *Radix Rehmanniae Recens* 15 g
Zhi Gan Cao *Radix Glycyrrhizae Praeparata* 12 g
Gui Zhi *Ramulus Cinnamomi* 6 g
Bai Shao *Radix Paeoniae Alba* 9 g

Explanations

● There are several common causes of deficiency of Yin and Qi in this syndrome. Some chronic diseases such as pulmonary tuberculosis and diabetes may cause deficiency of Yin and Qi; in a febrile disease, Yin and Qi can be weakened by Excessive-Heat; overeating of spicy food or drinking too much coffee may cause Heat to be generated and consume the Yin, leading to deficiency of Yin—all these can bring about disorders of the Heart. When Yin and Qi are not sufficient to support and nourish the Heart, the patient may have chest pain and palpitations. As soon as the Heart-Qi becomes weak, the Lung-Qi

will also become insufficient, causing quick and shallow breathing. If the Lung-Qi cannot control the skin pores then Deficient-Fire due to deficiency of Heart-Yin may cause the Body Fluids to move to the body surface, so the patient sweats easily. Deficiency of Yin with formation of Deficient-Heart may also disturb the Mind, causing anxiety and restlessness.

● Dang Sheng tonifies the Qi of the Heart, Spleen and Lung. Mai Dong nourishes the Yin of the Heart and Lung. When these two sweet herbs are used with the sour herb Wu Wei Zi, which has a stabilising ability, the Heart-Qi and Heart-Yin are nourished and stabilised. This relieves sweating and thirst, calms the Mind and reduces anxiety.

● When the Yin and Qi are sufficient, the Blood can circulate smoothly, and this corrects the chest pain and palpitations.

● Sheng Di Huang can effectively nourish the Heart-Yin and reduce Deficient-Fire so as to enhance the action of Mai Dong and Wu Wei Zi in nourishing the Yin.

● Zhi Gan Cao can tonify the Heart-Qi and enhance the action of Dang Shen to treat restlessness and anxiety.

● Gui Zhi can disperse the Qi and Yang of the Heart and accelerate the Blood circulation. Bai Shao can nourish the Blood and moderate the speed of its circulation. Gui Zhi and Bai Shao are used together to regulate the Blood.

● When the Qi and Yin are sufficient, the Yin and Yang, Qi and Blood are rebalanced, and chest pain disappears.

Modifications

1. If there is severe pain, add Dan Shen *Radix Salviae Miltiorrhizae* 9 g, Yu Jin *Radix Curcumae* 9 g, Chen Xiang *Lignum Aquilariae Resinatum* 6 g and Zhi Qiao *Fructus Aurantii* 9 g to promote the Blood circulation and Qi movement so as to stop the pain.
2. If there is deficiency of the Liver-Yin with hyperactivity of Liver-Yang, manifesting as dizziness, tinnitus and irritability, add Shi Jue Ming *Concha Haliotidis* 15 g, Gou Teng *Ramulus Uncariae cum Uncis* 9 g, Zhi Zi *Fructus Gardeniae* 9 g and Mu Dan Pi *Cortex Moutan Radici* 9 g to calm the Liver and subdue the Liver-Yang.
3. If there are palpitations with insomnia, add Suan Zao Ren *Semen Ziziphi Spinosae* 9 g and He Huan Pi *Cortex Albiziae* 9 g to calm the Mind.
4. If there is frequent sweating, add Sheng Long Gu *Os Draconis* 15 g and Sheng Mu Li *Concha Ostreae* 15 g to stabilise the Body Fluids and stop the sweating.

Patent remedy

Sheng Mai Pian *Generate the Pulse Pill*

ACUPUNCTURE TREATMENT

BL-15 Xinshu, CV-14 Juque, PC-5 Jianshi, HT-7 Shenmen, PC-6 Neiguan and CV-17 Tanzhong. Even method is used.

Explanations

- BL-15 and CV-14 are the Back Transporting point and Front Collecting point of the Heart. They can regulate and tonify the Heart-Qi.
- PC-5, the River point, and HT-7, the Stream point, calm the Mind and treat restlessness and palpitations.
- PC-6, the Connecting point and Confluence point, promotes Blood circulation, and together with CV-17, the Gathering point for the Qi, regulates the Qi and stops the chest pain.

Modifications

1. If there are palpitations, restlessness and a warm feeling in the chest, add PC-8 to reduce Heat in the chest, and PC-7 to calm the Mind.
2. If there is frequent sweating, add KI-6 to reduce the sweating.

Case history

A 54-year-old man was admitted to the hospital with severe chest pain as the chief complaint. He was also suffering from palpitations, sweating, tiredness, restlessness and shortness of breath at that time. The ECG showed a myocardial infarction. The patient had suffered from angina pectoris several times in the previous 3 years. He also had a red tongue with purple spots on the border and without a tongue coating. His pulse was thready and rapid.

Diagnosis
Deficiency of the Qi and Yin of the Heart and stagnation of Qi and Blood.

Principle of the treatment
Nourish Qi and Yin of the Heart, promote the Qi and Blood circulation and stop the pain.

Herbal treatment
SHENG MAI SAN and **SHI XIAO SAN**
Generate the Pulse Powder and *Sudden Smile Powder*
Dang Shen *Radix Codonopsis Pilosulae* 20 g
Mai Dong *Radix Ophiopogonis* 15 g
Wu Wei Zi *Fructus Schisandrae* 6 g

Pu Huang *Pollen Typhae* 10 g
Wu Ling Zhi *Faeces Trogopterorum* 10 g
Sheng Di Huang *Radix Rehmanniae Recens* 15 g
Bai He *Bulbus Lilii* 30 g
Bai Zi Ren *Semen Biotae* 15 g

Explanations

- Dang Shen, Mai Dong and Wu Wei Zi form the formula called Sheng Mai San, which is able to nourish the Yin and tonify the Qi of the Heart.
- Shi Xiao San contains two substances, Pu Huang and Wu Ling Zhi. They can promote the Blood circulation, dissolve stagnant Blood and stop the pain.
- Sheng Di Huang, Bai He and Bai Zi Ren can nourish the Heart-Yin and calm the Mind.

Thirty minutes after the formula was given, the pain was much relieved. After the second dose of the herbs 4 hours later, the pain disappeared completely. This formula was continued for another 10 days, after which the ECG had much improved. The patient recovered and was discharged from the hospital after a further 2 weeks. He continued to take this formula but without Pu Hu and Wu Ling Zhi once a day for 2 months. At a follow-up consultation 6 months later, he said he had experienced no further chest pain.

DEFICIENCY OF YIN OF HEART AND KIDNEY

Symptoms and signs

Chest pain with a stabbing sensation, palpitations, night sweating, irritability, insomnia, weakness of the back and knees, dizziness, tinnitus, dry eyes, a red tongue with purple spots and a thready, choppy and irregular pulse.

This syndrome can be seen in coronary artery disease, angina pectoris, menopausal syndrome, myocarditis and pulmonary tuberculosis.

Principle of treatment

Nourish Yin, clear Deficient-Heat, promote Blood circulation and stop the pain.

HERBAL TREATMENT

Prescription

YI GUAN JIAN and **ER ZHI WAN**
Linking Decoction and *Two-Ultimate Pill*
Sheng Di Huang *Radix Rehmanniae Recens* 18 g
Sha Shen *Radix Adenopherae* 12 g
Mai Dong *Radix Ophiopogonis* 12 g
Dang Gui *Radix Angelicae Sinensis* 9 g
Gou Qi Zi *Fructus Lycii* 15 g
Chuan Lian Zi *Fructus Meliae Toosendan* 3 g

Nu Zhen Zi *Fructus Ligustri Lucidi* 12 g
Han Lian Cao *Herba Ecliptae* 12 g

Add:

Dan Shen *Radix Salviae Miltiorrhizae* 12 g
Dan Pi *Cortex Moutan Radicis* 9 g
Yi Mu Cao *Herba Leonuri* 9 g
Chuan Niu Xi *Radix Cyathulae* 9 g
Mu Li *Concha Ostreae* 15 g

Explanations

- Sheng Di Huang is sweet and Cold in nature, entering the Heart and Kidney channels. It can nourish the Yin, clear Heat and cool the Blood.
- Gou Qi Zi and Dang Gui are able to tonify the Blood and moisten Dryness.
- Sha Shen and Mai Dong both can nourish the Yin in the Upper Burner so as to provide a better condition of Qi and Blood circulation.
- Chuan Lian Zi is bitter and Cold in nature, and can drain Liver-Fire and unblock the obstruction of Qi.
- Nu Zhen Zi and Han Lian Cao nourish the Kidney-Yin and reduce Deficient-Fire, but do not have the greasy nature of many Yin-tonifying herbs.
- Dan Shen, Dan Pi and Yi Mu Cao clear Heat and promote the Blood circulation so as to stop pain.
- Chuan Niu Xi can cause the Blood to descend.
- Mu Li can descend Liver-Yang, stabilise the Body Fluids and stop night sweating.

Modifications

1. If there is severe pain, add Chen Xiang *Lignum Aquilariae Resinatum* 6 g and Chuan Xiong *Rhizoma Ligustici Chuanxiong* 9 g to regulate the Qi and Blood so as to relieve the pain.
2. If there is severe night sweating, add Zhi Mu *Rhizoma Anemarrhenae* 9 g, Huang Bai *Cortex Phellodendri* 9 g and Di Gu Pi *Cortex Lycii Radicis* 9 g to nourish the Yin and reduce Deficient-Fire.
3. If there are severe palpitations and insomnia, add Suan Zao Ren *Semen Ziziphi Spinosae* 9 g and Bai Zi Ren *Semen Biotae* 9 g to calm the Mind and improve the sleep.
4. If there is tinnitus with a high-toned noise, add Shi Jue Ming *Concha Haliotidis* 15 g and Gou Teng *Ramulus Uncariae cum Uncis* 9 g to cause the Liver-Yang to descend and reduce Liver-Fire.
5. If there is Qi deficiency, add Dang Shen *Radix Codonopsis Pilosulae* 9 g and Zhi Gan Cao *Radix Glycyrrhizae Praeparata* 6 g to activate the Spleen and tonify the Qi.

Patent remedy

Qi Ju Di Huang Wan *Lycuim Fruit, Chrysanthemum and Rehmannia Pill*

ACUPUNCTURE TREATMENT

PC-6 Neiguan, PC-7 Daling, PC-8 Laogong, KI-3 Taixi, HT-7 Shenmen, LR-3 Taichong, CV-14 Juque, CV-17 Tanzhong, BL-15 Xinshu and SP-6 Sanyinjiao. Even method is used.

Explanations

- PC-7, the Stream point, reduces Heart-Fire.
- KI-3, the Source point, tonifies the Kidney-Yin so as to nourish the Heart-Yin.
- HT-7, the Stream point, clears Heart-Heat, calms the Mind and treats restlessness and palpitations.
- PC-8, the Spring point, clears Deficient-Heat from the Heart and treats a warm sensation in the chest.
- LR-3, the Source point, regulates the Liver-Qi.
- PC-6 and CV-17 promote the Qi circulation so as to regulate the Blood circulation in the chest and stop the pain.
- BL-15 and CV-14, the Back Transporting point and Front Collecting point of the Heart, regulate the Heart-Qi and stop chest pain.
- SP-6 promotes the Blood circulation and tonifies the Yin and Blood.

Modifications

1. If there is dizziness and irritability due to hyperactivity of the Liver-Yang, add GB-20 and LR-2 to calm the Liver and suppress the Liver-Yang.
2. If there is night sweating, add SI-3 and HT-6 to reduce the sweating.
3. If there is insomnia, palpitations and restlessness, add BL-44, BL-47 and BL-49 to harmonise and tonify the Heart, Liver and Spleen.

Case history

A 52-year-old woman complained of chest pain and pressure in the chest. The pain was triggered or worsened by stressful situations. She suffered also from dry eyes, reduced vision and general tiredness. Her menstruation had been irregular for a year, and she often had migraine after menstruation. She had a purple-red tongue with a thin coating and a deep, thready and choppy pulse.

Diagnosis
Deficiency of Yin and Blood and stagnation of Liver-Qi.

Principle of treatment
Nourish the Yin and Blood, smooth the Liver and stop the pain.

Herbal treatment
XIAO YAO SAN
Free and Relaxed Powder
Chai Hu *Radix Bupleuri* 6 g
Dang Gui *Radix Angelicae Sinensis* 9 g
Bai Shao *Radix Paeoniae Alba* 12 g
Bai Zhu *Rhizoma Atractylodis Macrocephalae* 9 g
Gan Cao *Radix Glycyrrhizae* 6 g
Bo He *Herba Menthae* 3 g
Sheng Jiang *Rhizoma Zingiberis Recens* 3 g
Yan Hu Suo *Rhizoma Corydalis* 9 g
Sheng Di Huang *Radix Rehmanniae Recens* 12 g
Dan Shen *Radix Salviae Miltiorrhizae* 9 g
Gou Qi Zi *Fructus Lycii* 9 g
Ju Hua *Flos Chrysanthemi* 6 g
Xiang Fu *Rhizoma Cyperi* 9 g

Explanations

- The formula Xiao Yao San can smooth the Liver, promote the Liver-Qi circulation, nourish the Blood and strengthen the Spleen.
- Sheng Di Huang and Dan Shen can clear the Heat in the chest, nourish the Yin, promote the Blood circulation and stop the pain.
- Gou Qi Zi nourishes the Blood and Yin, and together with Ju Hua benefits the eyes.
- Xiang Fu can circulate the Qi in the Triple Burner channel so as to regulate the Qi circulation in the chest and stop the pain.
- Yan Hu Sho arrests the pain.

After herbal treatment for 20 days, the pain had gone. She used the herbs continuously for another 6 months and the other symptoms disappeared too.

DEFICIENCY OF YANG OF THE KIDNEY AND HEART

Symptoms and signs

Chest pain, purple lips and nails, shortness of breath, palpitations, tiredness, an aversion to cold, weakness of the back and cold of the limbs, oedema, a purplish-pale tongue and a deep, weak and irregular pulse.

This syndrome can be seen in angina pectoris, myocardial infarction, heart failure, rheumatic heart diseases, pulmonary heart disease and chronic bronchitis.

Principle of treatment

Tonify the Yang, warm the interior, promote the Blood circulation and stop the pain.

HERBAL TREATMENT

Prescription

JIN GUI SHEN QI WAN
Kidney Qi Pill
Rou Gui *Ramulus Cinnamomi* 6 g
Fu Zi *Radix Aconiti Carmichaeli Praeparata* 9 g
Shu Di Huang *Radix Rehmanniae Praeparata* 24 g
Shan Zhu Yu *Fructus Corni* 12 g
Shan Yao *Rhizoma Dioscoreae Oppositae* 12 g
Fu Ling *Poria* 9 g
Mu Dan Pi *Cortex Moutan Radicis* 9 g
Ze Xie *Rhizoma Alismatis* 9 g

Add:

Gan Jiang *Rhizoma Zingiberis* 9 g
Ren Shen *Radix Ginseng* 9 g
Bai Zhu *Rhizoma Atractylodis Macrocephalae* 9 g
Chen Xiang *Lignum Aquilariae Resinatum* 3 g
Che Qian Zi *Semen Plantagini* 12 g

Explanations

- Rou Gui and Fu Zi are very pungent and warm, strengthening the Yang and warming the interior. Shu Di Huang can tonify the Kidney-Essence so as to provide a substantial foundation for the Kidney-Yang.
- Shan Zhu Yu and Shan Yao tonify and stabilise the Essence of the Liver and Spleen respectively.
- Ze Xie can eliminate turbid Damp from the Lower Burner so as to assist Shu Di Huang to tonify the Kidney-Essence.
- Mu Dan Pi can disperse and clear the restrained Heat from the Liver so as to assist Shan Zhu Yu to stabilise the Liver-Yin.
- Fu Ling dissolves Damp in the Middle Burner and assists Shan Yao to strengthen the Spleen-Qi.
- Gan Jiang warms the Middle Burner, and assists Rou Gui and Fu Zi to strengthen the Kidney-Yang and Heart-Yang.
- Ren Shen and Bai Zhu tonify the Spleen-Qi so as to control the Water ascending from the Lower Burner.
- Chen Xiang can cause the Qi to descend and stop the pain.
- Che Qian Zi can increase urination and leach out Damp.
- When the Heart-Yang becomes stronger, it can disperse the Warmth in the chest and improve the Blood circulation, so chest pain is reduced. When the Kidney-Yang becomes stronger, it can accelerate the water metabolism and also support the Heart-Yang so as to maintain the balance

between Yin and Yang, and between the Upper and the Lower Burners.

Modifications

1. If there is severe pain and sweating, use Su He Xiang Wan *Styrax Pill* (1 pill a day) in the mean time to promote the Qi circulation in the chest and stop the pain; use Sheng Long Gu *Os Draconis* 15 g, Sheng Mu Li *Concha Ostreae* 15 g, Zhi Gan Cao *Radix Glycyrrhizae Praeparata* 6 g and Wu Wei Zi *Fructus Schisandrae* 6 g to stop the sweating.
2. If there is restlessness and insomnia, add Yuan Zhi *Radix Polygalae* 6 g and Suan Zao Ren *Semen Ziziphi Spinosae* 9 g to calm the Mind and improve sleep.
3. If there is severe Blood stagnation, add Chuan Xiong *Rhizoma Ligustici Chuanxiong* 9 g, Hong Hua *Flos Carthami* 9 g and Tao Ren *Semen Persicae* 9 g to invigorate the Blood circulation and eliminate Blood stasis.
4. If there is severe oedema, add Huang Qi *Radix Astragali seu Hedysari* 12 g, Gui Zhi *Ramulus Cinnamomi* 9 g, together with Bai Zhu *Rhizoma Atractylodis Macrocephalae* 12 g and Fu Ling *Poria* 15 g to strengthen the Spleen and promote Water metabolism.

Patent remedy

Jin Gui Shen Qi Wan *Kidney Qi Pill*

ACUPUNCTURE TREATMENT

PC-6 Neiguan, CV-17 Tanzhong, BL-14 Jueyinshu, BL-15 Xinghu, BL-17 Geshu, BL-23 Shenshu, CV-4 Guanyuan and CV-6 Qihai. Even method is used on these points.

Explanations

- PC-6, the Connecting point and the Confluence point, regulates the Qi and Blood of the Heart and stops the pain in the chest.
- CV-17, the Gathering point for the Qi, disperses the Qi and unblocks the chest so as to stop pain.
- BL-14, BL-15 and BL-17 tonify and regulate the Blood of the Heart, calm the Mind and treat the chest pain.
- BL-23, CV-4 and CV-6 can tonify the Kidney and strengthen the Qi and Blood so as to strengthen the Yang in the chest.

Modifications

1. If there is deficiency of Spleen-Qi, add ST-36 and SP-6 to activate the Spleen and tonify the Qi and Blood.
2. If there is restlessness and palpitations, add BL-44 and HT-7 to calm the Mind.
3. If there is oedema, add BL-20, ST-36 and CV-9 together with BL-23, CV-6 to reduce the oedema.

OTHER SYNDROMES

ACCUMULATION OF PHLEGM-HEAT IN THE LUNG

Symptoms and signs

High fever, thirst, cough with expectorate of ferruginous sputum, chest pain, shortness of breath, scanty urine, a red tongue with a dry and yellow coating and slippery, rapid and forceful pulse.

This syndrome can be seen in pneumonia and acute bronchitis.

Principle of treatment

Clear Heat, relieve Toxicity, regulate the Lung-Qi and transform Phlegm.

HERBAL TREATMENT

Prescription

MA XING SHI GAN TANG and **WEI JING TANG**
Ephedra, Apricot Kernel, Gypsum and Licorice Decoction and *Reed Decoction*
Ma Huang *Herba Ephedrae* 6 g
Shi Gao *Gypsum Fibrosum* 30 g
Xing Ren *Semen Armeniacae Amarum* 9 g
Zhi Gan Cao *Radix Glycyrrhizae Praeparata* 6 g
Wei Jing *Rhizoma Phragmitis* 30 g
Tao Ren *Semen Persicae* 9 g
Yi Yi Ren *Semen Coicis* 15 g
Dong Gua Ren *Semen Benincasae* 12 g

Add:

Chi Shao *Radix Paeoniae Rubra* 9 g
Gua Lou *Fructus Trichosanthis* 15 g
Yu Jin *Radix Curcumae* 12 g

Explanations

- When pathogenic Heat invades the Lung and disturbs the dispersing and descending function of the Lung-Qi, the Lung-Qi is obstructed, and symptoms such as high fever, quick and shallow breathing, cough with sputum and chest pain appear.

- Ma Huang is pungent and Hot in nature, entering the Lung channel and dispersing the Lung-Qi. Shi Gao is very pungent and Cold in nature, entering the Lung and Stomach channel; it powerfully clears Heat and relieves Toxicity so as to reduce high fever. It can cause the Lung-Qi to descend and calm the breath and, together with Ma Huang, regulate the Lung-Qi, unblock Qi obstruction in the chest and so stop the pain.
- Shi Gao clears Heat and reduces fever.
- Xing Ren causes the Lung-Qi to descend as well as transforming Phlegm so as to treat cough.
- Zhi Gan Cao moderates the Hot and Cold herbs in the formula.
- Wei Jing, Yi Yi Ren and Dong Gua Ren clear Heat from the Lung, transform Damp, and reduce cough and Phlegm.
- Tao Ren is able to promote the Blood circulation. Gua Lou clears Phlegm-Heat obstruction in the chest, Chi Shao and Yu Jin regulate the Blood circulation and cool the Blood so as to stop bleeding. These four herbs are also used to stop the chest pain.

Modifications

1. If there is a high fever and semi-consciousness, add An Gong Niu Huang Wan *Calm the Palace Pill with Cattle Gallstone* (patent formula, 1 pill a day) to clear Heat, relieve Toxicity and unblock the Orifices.
2. If there is a lot of blood in the sputum, add Ce Bai Ye *Cacumen Biotae* 12 g, Bai Mao Gen *Rhizoma Imperatae* 15 g to cool the Blood and stop the bleeding.
3. If there is constipation, add Da Huang *Radix et Rhizoma Rhei* 6 g to clear Heat and promote bowel movement.
4. If there is deficiency of Qi and Yin, add Sha Shen *Radix Glehniae* 12 g and Mai Dong *Radix Ophiopogonis* 15 g to tonify the Qi and the Yin.

Patent remedy

Qing Qi Hua Tan Wan *Clear the Qi and Transform Phlegm Pill*

ACUPUNCTURE TREATMENT

LU-5 Chize, LU-7 Lieque, LU-8 Jingqu, BL-13 Feishu, LT-11 Quchi and GV-14 Dazhui. Reducing method is used on these points.

Explanations

- LU-7, the Connecting point, disperses the Lung-Qi and unblocks the chest.
- BL-13, the Back Transporting point of the Lung, regulates and strengthens the function of the Lung.
- LU-5, the Sea point, reduces Heat from the Lung, assists BL-13 to cause the Lung-Qi to descend, transforms Phlegm and stops the chest pain.
- LU-8, the River point, clears Heat, transforms Phlegm and stops cough and chest pain.
- GV-14 reduces fever and expels external pathogenic Heat.

Modifications

1. If there is bloody sputum, add LU-6, the Accumulation point, and PC-8, the Spring point, to clear Heat in the Blood and stop the bleeding.
2. If there is itching and irritation in the throat, add KI-6, in combination with LU-7, to reduce Deficient-Heat and benefit the throat.
3. If there is constipation, add ST-25, the Front Collecting point of the Large Intestine, and CV-12, the Gathering point for the Fu organs, to promote the bowel movement.
4. If there is a feeling of oppression in the chest, add PC-6 and LR-3 to regulate the Qi in the chest and relieve the feeling of oppression.

STAGNATION OF BLOOD IN THE CHEST DUE TO TRAUMA

Symptoms and signs

Chest pain usually occurs after physical trauma on the chest, with aggravation of the pain by deep breathing or palpation; there is a normal tongue and a wiry pulse. In a chronic case, there may be tingling and numbness in the affected area, a purple tongue and a wiry and choppy pulse.

Principle of treatment

Promote the Qi and Blood circulation and stop the pain.

HERBAL TREATMENT

Prescription

HUO LUO XIAO LING DAN
Fantastically Effective Pill to Invigorate the Collaterals
Dang Gui *Radix Angelicae Sinensis* 9 g
Dan Shen *Radix Salviae Miltiorrhizae* 9 g

Ru Xiang *Resina Olibani* 6 g
Mo Yao *Resina Myrrhae* 9 g

Add:

San Qi *Radix Notoginseng* powder 3 g
Chai Hu *Radix Bupleuri* 6 g
Zhi Qiao *Fructus Aurantii* 6 g

Explanations

- Trauma or chronic strain may directly obstruct the channels, so the Qi and Blood cannot circulate properly, leading to chest pain. In a chronic case, Blood stagnation exists not only in the channel but also in the collateral and sensations of tingling and numbness may appear.
- Dang Gui and Dan Shen invigorate the Blood circulation and stop the pain.
- Ru Xing and Mo Yao break up stagnant Blood, reduce swelling and stop the pain.
- San Qi is an important herb for treating trauma because it not only invigorates Blood but also stops bleeding. It can also reduce swelling and stop the pain.
- Chai Hu disperses the Liver-Qi and promotes Qi movement in the Triple Burner passage. Zhi Qiao unblocks Qi obstruction in the chest. These two herbs regulate the Qi circulation so as to assist the herbs that regulate the Blood.

Modifications

1. If there is severe pain, add Qi Li San (patent formula, 0.5 g each time, three times a day) to invigorate the Blood circulation, reduce swelling and stop the pain.
2. If there is Blood deficiency in the chronic stage, add Huang Qi *Radix Astragali seu Hedysari* 12 g, Gui Zhi *Ramulus Cinnamomi* 9 g, Shu Di Huang *Radix Rehmanniae Praeparata* 12 g and Bai Shao *Radix Paeoniae Alba* 12 g to tonify the Qi and Blood.
3. If there is obstruction of the collateral by stagnant Blood, add Wang Bu Liu Xin *Semen Vaccariae* 9 g, Jiang Can *Bombyx Batryticatus* 9 g and Di Long *Lumbricus* 9 g to open the collateral and eliminate Blood stasis.

4. In the subacute and chronic stages, some herbal lotions, plasters and tinctures can be applied to invigorate the Qi and Blood.

Patent remedies

Jin Gu Die Shang Wan *Muscle and Bone Traumatic Injury Pill*
Sheng Tian Qi Fen *Raw Pseudoginseng*

ACUPUNCTURE TREATMENT

PC-6 Neiguan, CV-17 Tanzhong, BL-17 Geshu, BL-18 Ganshu, LR-3 Taichong, LR-14 Qimen, SP-6 Sanyinjiao, SP-10 Xuehai and TE-6 Zhigou. Reducing method is used on these points.

Explanations

- PC-6, the Connecting point and Confluent point, regulates the Qi and Blood in the chest and stops pain.
- CV-17, the Gathering point for the Qi, promotes the Qi circulation in the chest and stops the pain.
- BL-18 and LR-14, the Back Transporting point and the Front Collecting point of the Liver, regulate the Blood circulation and unblock obstruction in the Heart channel.
- BL-17, SP-10 and SP-6 are all able to invigorate the Blood circulation and stop the pain.
- TE-6 and LR-3 regulate the Liver-Qi and the Gall Bladder to stop the chest pain.

Modifications

1. If there is severe pain, add PC-8 and CV-4 to reduce Heat in the Blood and strengthen the Qi so as to stop the pain.
2. If there is Blood deficiency, add BL-20 and ST-36 to strengthen the Spleen and tonify the Blood.
3. If there is an aggravation of the chest pain at night, add HT-6 and HT-5, the Accumulation points and Connecting points of the Heart channel, to invigorate the Blood circulation and eliminate Blood stasis.

Breast pain 23

乳
房
疼
痛

Breast pain is a disorder characterised by distension and pain in one or both breasts, or on the nipple, or even aggravation of breast pain by touching the clothing. In some cases, the breast pain may refer to the chest or axillary regions. It occurs in both men and women, but mostly women, especially those between the ages of 20 and 40 years. The pain varies in nature, and may be distending, stabbing, contracting, burning, slight, severe, or bearing-down. Distending pain is the most frequently encountered, and it is generally accompanied by disorders of menstruation such as dysmenorrhoea or irregular menstruation, or of lactation or the emotions.

Breast pain may be attributed to any of the following diseases in Western medicine: acute or chronic mastitis, perimastitis, hyperplasia of the mammary glands, galactoschesis, stagnation mastitis, and fibrosclerosis of breast and lobule of mammary gland.

Aetiology and pathology

Invasion of External factors

Bad lifestyle habits with lack of attention to wearing proper clothing, especially during the breast-feeding period, and lack of personal hygiene, may leave the individual vulnerable to the invasion of External Cold or Toxic Heat, leading to stagnation of Qi in the collateral and blockage in the breast, or retention of milk, causing breast pain.

Emotional disorders

There is a saying in TCM that the Liver is in charge of the nipples, because the Liver channel penetrates the diaphragm, covers the hypochondriac regions and chest, and contacts the nipples. Excessive anger, stress, frustration and unhappiness may impair the physiological function of Liver, slowing down the flow of Qi and causing stagnation of the Liver-Qi, and blockage of the collateral in the breast, and distending breast pain follows. Since the circulation of Qi brings about the circulation of Blood, the Qi stagnation results in Blood stagnation. Long-standing stagnation of the Liver-Qi may cause stagnation of the Blood in the breast, resulting in a severe stabbing breast pain. Prolonged persistence of Liver-Qi stagnation may also generate Liver-Fire, leading to burning and damage of the collateral in the breast, and a burning breast pain.

Excessive meditation and thinking, or invasion of the Spleen by Liver-Qi, may impair the Spleen's physiological function of transportation and transformation, causing Damp-Phlegm to form. If this blocks the collateral in the breast then breast pain is triggered.

Bad diet

Eating of too much raw or cold food may cause impairment of the Yang in the Spleen and Stomach, leading to the formation of Cold and Damp in the body. Eating of too much fatty, sweet and some highly flavoured food may also impair the Spleen and Stomach and cause Damp-Heat or Excessive-Heat to form. The Stomach channel passes through the breast, so if Damp-Phlegm, Damp-Heat or Excessive-Heat accumulates in the Stomach and Spleen it may travel along the Stomach channel to the breast, blocking the collateral in the breast and causing breast pain.

Accumulation of milk in the breast

Excessive production of milk beyond the needs of the infant may cause a constant fullness in the breast and impede the Qi and milk circulation, so breast pain follows. Extreme emotional upsets and excessive thinking, or eating of too much sweet, fatty or highly flavoured food during the breast-feeding period, may cause the Qi to stagnate and Heat to form in the breast, so breast pain follows.

Senility and weakness of the body

Decline of the Kidney-Qi after middle age, constitutional weakness, excessive bleeding in menstruation or after labour, prolonged sickness, excessive strain, or lack of sufficient and nutritious food, can all cause deficiency of the Qi and Blood, or even of the Kidney-Essence. When the Penetrating and Directing Vessels are empty, the breast is not nourished, and breast pain occurs.

Treatment based on differentiation

Differentiation

Differentiation of Excess and Deficiency

Breast pain, generally speaking, can be caused either by Excessive factors or Deficient factors. However, it is mostly caused by Excessive factors. Even if it is caused by Deficient factors, there is often a mixture of Excess and Deficiency. The key method to differentiate Excess and Deficiency is to see if the breast is hard or soft. If the breast pain is accompanied by a hard breast, it is usually caused by Excessive factors, whereas breast pain accompanied by a soft breast is usually caused by Deficient factors.

— Generally speaking, Excessive causes include: invasion of External Cold, stagnation of Liver-Qi, accumulation of Damp-Phlegm, stagnation of Blood, accumulation of milk, hyperactivity of Toxic Fire, etc.
— Deficient causes include deficiency of Qi and Blood, and deficiency of Yin of Liver and Kidney.

Differentiation of character of the pain

— Acute onset of breast pain with a contracting feeling, aggravation of the pain by exposure to cold, or aversion to cold, is usually caused by invasion of cold.
— Acute sharp breast pain, or chronic pain with acute aggravation after emotional upset, or breast pain with a moving nature, with distension of the breast, depression, headache or dysmenorrhoea, is usually caused by stagnation of Liver-Qi.
— Chronic breast pain with a stabbing nature and fixed location, aggravation of the breast pain at night, a purplish colour of the tongue and menstrual flow, is usually caused by stagnation of Blood.
— Breast pain with formation of nodules, soft in nature, heaviness of the body, nausea, loose stool, a poor appetite and a greasy tongue coating, is usually caused by accumulation of Damp-Phlegm.
— Acute onset of breast pain with a burning feeling, redness and swelling of the breast, thirst, fever, constipation, formation of carbuncles or furuncles with pus on the breast, or a red tongue, is usually caused by hyperactivity of Toxic Fire.
— Chronic and slight breast pain with intermittent aggravation, or aggravation of the breast pain by exertion and during the day, with tiredness, or an aversion to cold, is usually caused by deficiency of Qi and Blood.
— Chronic and slight breast pain with intermittent aggravation, or aggravation of the breast pain during the menstruation period, with poor vision and memory, hair loss, lower back pain, or weakness of knees, is usually caused by deficiency of the Liver and Kidney.

Treatment

EXCESSIVE TYPES OF BREAST PAIN

INVASION OF COLD

Symptoms and signs

Acute occurrence of breast pain, aggravation of pain on exposure to cold, a feeling of contraction in the breast, an aversion to cold, a runny nose with a white discharge, headache, generalised body pain, a thin and white tongue coating and a superficial and wiry pulse.

Principle of treatment

Dispel Cold, warm the channel and sedate the pain.

HERBAL TREATMENT

Prescription

GUI ZHI TANG and **ZHENG QI TIAN XIANG SAN**
Cinnamon Twig Decoction and *Correct Qi Heaven Fragrant Powder*
Gui Zhi *Ramulus Cinnamomi* 12 g
Bai Shao *Radix Paeoniae Alba* 6 g
Sheng Jiang *Rhizoma Zingiberis Recens* 6 g
Wu Yao *Radix Linderae* 10 g
Chen Pi *Pericarpium Citri Reticulatae* 10 g
Zi Su Ye *Folium Perillae* 6 g
Xiang Fu *Rhizoma Cyperi* 10 g

Explanations

- Gui Zhi and Bai Shao used concurrently can dispel Wind and Cold so as to relieve External symptoms.
- Sheng Jiang and Zi Su Ye, pungent and Warm herbs, help Gui Zhi to dispel External Wind and Cold. They also warm the channels and relieve the breast pain.
- Wu Yao, a pungent and Hot herb entering the Liver channel, expels Cold and promotes Qi movement in the breast so as to relieve the breast pain.
- Chen Pi and Xiang Fu promote circulation of the Liver-Qi so as to relieve breast pain.

Modifications

1. If there is severe breast pain, add Yan Hu Suo *Rhizoma Corydalis* 10 g to invigorate the Qi and Blood circulation and stop the pain.
2. If there is severe cramp in the breast, increase the dosage of Bai Shao *Radix Paeoniae Alba* to 15 g and add Zhi Gan Cao *Radix Glycyrrhizae Praeparata* 6 g to moderate the speed of Qi circulation and harmonise the collateral so as to stop the pain.
3. If there is a severe aversion to cold, add Zhi Fu Zi *Radix Aconiti Praeparata* 9 g to expel Cold and warm the channels.
4. If there is lower abdominal pain, add Xiao Hui Xiang *Fructus Foeniculi* 6 g and Rou Gui *Cortex Cinnamomi* 6 g to warm the Lower Burner and Kidney and disperse Cold.

Patent remedy

Jing Fang Bai Du Pian Schizonepeta and Ledebouriella Tablet to Overcome Pathogenic Influences

ACUPUNCTURE TREATMENT

LI-4 Hegu, TE-5 Waiguan, BL-12 Fengmen, LU-7 Lieque, PC-6 Neiguan and CV-17 Tanzhong. Reducing method is used on these points. Moxibustion is employed on the first four points.

Explanations

- Invasion of external Cold causing breast pain usually has an acute onset. LI-4, TE-5 and LU-7 are used here to promote sweating in order to dispel the External Cold.
- BL-12 dispels Wind and relieves External symptoms.
- CV-17 and PC-6 regulate the Qi circulation in the chest and breast, and harmonise the collateral and channels in order to eliminate blockage in the breast.
- Moxibustion dispels Cold and warms the channels.

Modifications

1. If there is severe breast pain, add PC-4, the Accumulation point, and ST-40, the Connecting point, to harmonise the collateral and sedate the pain.
2. If there is generalised body pain, add BL-63, the Accumulation point, and BL-64, the Source point, to eliminate pathogenic factors at the Greater Yang level of the body.
3. If there is distension of the breast, add LR-14, the Front Collecting point of the Liver, to promote the Qi circulation and relieve the distension.
4. If there is nausea and vomiting, add CV-12, the Front Collecting point of the Stomach, to harmonise the Stomach and cause the Stomach-Qi to descend.

STAGNATION OF LIVER-QI

Symptoms and signs

Distension and pain in the breast, with aggravation before menstruation and alleviation after menstruation, pain related to the emotional situation and formation of soft nodules in the breast, accompanied by irritability, hypochondriac pain and distension, depression, a feeling of oppression across the chest, insomnia, a normal-coloured tongue with a white coating, and a wiry and tight pulse.

Principle of treatment

Smooth the Liver and circulate the Qi, relieve stagnation and sedate the pain.

HERBAL TREATMENT

Prescription

XIAO YAO SAN
Free and Relaxed Powder
Chai Hu *Radix Bupleuri* 10 g
Bai Shao *Radix Paeoniae Alba* 12 g
Dang Gui *Radix Angelicae Sinensis* 10 g
Chuan Xiong *Rhizoma Ligustici Chuanxiong* 6 g
Dai Dai Hua *Flos Citri Aurantii* 6 g
Zhi Qiao *Fructus Aurantii* 10 g
Xiang Fu *Rhizoma Cyperi* 10 g
Zhi Gan Cao *Radix Glycyrrhizae Praeparata* 5 g

Explanations

- Emotional disturbance and stress may cause stagnation of the Liver-Qi and disturbance of the Qi movement in the breast, leading to breast pain. A normal tongue coating and colour show there is no obvious stagnation of Blood or weakness of the internal organs. The pulse shows stagnation of Qi, especially the Liver-Qi.
- Chai Hu and Bai Shao smooth the Liver, promote its physiological function and relieve breast pain.
- Dan Gui, in combination with Bai Shao, regulates and tonifies the Blood in the Liver and also moderates the Qi-circulating herbs.
- Xiang Fu and Zhi Qiao can strengthen the function of the Qi-circulating herbs.
- Since Qi is the guide of Blood, stagnation of Qi leads to stagnation of Blood, the difference being only in degree. That is why this prescription contains both Qi-moving herbs and Blood-moving herbs.
- Chuan Xiong and Dai Dai Hua can promote the Qi and Blood circulation, especially the Blood circulation.
- Zhi Gan Cao and Bai Shao harmonise the Liver and relieve breast pain.

Modifications

1. If there is severe breast pain, or severe distension of the breast, add Chuan Lian Zi *Fructus Meliae* *Toosendan* 10 g and Qing Pi *Pericarpium Citri Reticulatae Viride* 10 g to break up Qi stagnation in the Liver and stop the pain.
2. If there is an occasional stabbing pain in the breast, add Yan Hu Suo *Rhizoma Corydalis* 10 g to promote the Blood circulation and relieve the pain.
3. If there are nodules in the breast, add Yu Jin *Radix Curcumae* 10 g and Gua Lou *Fructus Trichosanthis* 10 g to promote the Qi circulation, soften the hard lumps and relieve the pain.
4. If there are red spots on the breast or nipples, add Mu Dan Pi *Cortex Moutan Radici* 10 g to clear Heat in the Blood, remove Toxin and eliminate the red spots.
5. If there is irritability and headache, add Xia Ku Cao *Spica Prunella* 10 g and Huang Qin *Radix Scutellariae* 12 g to clear Heat in the Liver, calm the Mind and relieve the headache.
6. If there is a bitter taste in the mouth, add Zhi Zi *Fructus Gardeniae* 9 g to clear Heat in the Liver and Gall Bladder and remove the bitter taste.
7. If there is pain radiating to the arm, add Tan Xiang *Lignum Santali* 3 g and Dan Shen *Radix Salviae* 10 g to promote the Blood circulation in the Heart and relieve the pain.
8. If there is insomnia and restlessness, add Duan Long Gu *Os Draconis* 15 g and Huang Lian *Rhizoma Coptidis* 5 g to clear Heat in the Heart, calm the Mind and improve the sleep.
9. If there is nausea and a poor appetite, add Sha Ren *Radix Aenophorae* 5 g to harmonise the Stomach and improve the appetite.
10. If there is irregular menstruation or dysmenorrhoea, add Shu Di *Radix Rehmanniae Praeparata* 10 g and Yi Mu Cao *Herba Leonuri* 10 g to regulate the menstruation and relieve the dysmenorrhoea.
11. If there is constipation, add Da Huang *Radix en Rhizoma Rhei* 10 g to promote defecation and relieve the constipation.

Patent remedies

Shu Gan Wan *Soothe Liver Pill*
Xiao Yao Wan *Free and Relaxed Pill*

ACUPUNCTURE TREATMENT

LR-3 Taichong, LR-5 Ligou, LR-14 Qimen, LI-4 Hegu, PC-6 Neiguan, CV-17 Tanzhong and BL-18 Ganshu. Reducing method is used on these points.

Explanations

- The Liver channel belongs to the Liver and connects to the Gall Bladder, penetrating the diaphragm and covering the hypochondriac regions and the chest. Stagnation of the Liver-Qi would cause breast pain, so the key treatment should be to smooth the Liver and circulate the Qi.
- LR-3, the Source point of the Liver, LR-14, the Front Collecting point, and BL-18, the Back Transporting point of the Liver, are used to smooth the Liver and promote the Qi circulation.
- LR-5, the Connecting point, harmonises the collateral and sedates pain in the breast.
- PC-6 and CV-17 promote the Qi circulation in the chest and sedate the breast pain.
- LI-4 is used to promote the Qi circulation and relieve pain.

Modifications

1. If there is a feeling of fullness and oppression across the chest, add LU-7 and KI-6 to clear the blockage in the chest and sedate the chest pain.
2. If there is severe breast pain, or severe distension, add LR-6, the Accumulation point, to break up Qi stagnation of the Liver and stop the pain.
3. If there is an occasional stabbing pain in the breast, add BL-17, the Gathering point for the Blood, to promote the Blood circulation and relieve the pain.
4. If there are nodules in the breast, add ST-40, the Connecting point, to promote the Qi circulation, soften the hard lumps and relieve the pain.
5. If there are red spots on the breast, add ST-44 and LR-2, the Spring points, to clear Heat in the Blood, remove Toxin and eliminate the red spots.
6. If there is irritability, add GV-20 to clear Heat in the Liver, calm the Mind and relieve the irritability.
7. If there is a headache, add GV-20 to suppress the Liver-Yang and relieve the headache.
8. If there is a bitter taste in the mouth, add GB-40, the Source point, and GB-43, the Spring point, to clear Heat in the Liver and Gall Bladder and remove the bitter taste.
9. If there is chest pain radiating to the arm, add HT-3, the Sea point, and HT-6, the Accumulation point, to promote the Blood circulation in the Heart and relieve the pain.
10. If there is insomnia and restlessness, add HT-8, the Spring point, to clear Heat in the Heart, calm the Mind and improve the sleep.
11. If there is nausea and a poor appetite, add CV-12, the Front Collecting point of the Stomach, to harmonise the Stomach and improve the appetite.
12. If there is irregular menstruation or dysmenorrhoea, add KI-3 and CV-6 to regulate the menstruation and relieve the dysmenorrhoea.
13. If there is constipation, add ST-25, the Front Collecting point of the Large Intestine, to promote defecation and relieve the constipation.

Case history

A 35-year-old woman had complained of breast pain for 6 months. In the previous year, her relationship with her husband had been difficult and they often had quarrels. She became depressed and was given medication. Then she developed breast pain, which was worse before menstruation and also in stressful situations. Her gynaecologist and her doctor told her the breast pain was caused by the stress and asked her to continue her antidepressive medications. Besides breast pain, she had been suffering from other symptoms such as chest pain with a sense of pressure over the chest, insomnia, headaches in the occipital region and sometimes eye pain, irritability, nervousness, tiredness and irregular menstruation for one year. Her tongue had a thin and slight yellow coating, a red tip and edges and a slight purple colour at the edges, and a deep, thready, wiry and slightly rapid pulse.

Diagnosis
Breast pain due to stagnation of the Liver-Qi with generation of Liver-Fire.

Principle of treatment
Smooth the Liver, promote the Liver-Qi circulation, harmonise the collateral, reduce the Liver-Fire and relieve the pain.

Herbal treatment
XIAO YAO SAN
Free and Relaxed Powder
Chai Hu *Radix Bupleuri* 6 g
Dang Gui *Radix Angelicae Sinensis* 10 g
Bai Shao *Radix Paeoniae Alba* 12 g
Yan Hu Suo *Rhizoma Corydalis* 10 g
Sheng Di Huang *Radix Rehmanniae Recens* 12 g
Xia Ku Cao *Spica Prunella* 10 g
Huang Qin *Radix Scutellariae* 12 g
Ju Hua *Flos Chrysanthemi* 5 g
Xiang Fu *Rhizoma Cyperi* 10 g
Gan Cao *Radix Glycyrrhizae* 5 g

Explanations

- Chai Hu and Bai Shao smooth the Liver, promote the Liver-Qi circulation and relieve the breast pain.
- Xiang Fu helps Chai Hu to promote the Liver-Qi circulation and relieve the breast pain.
- Yan Hu Suo promotes the Qi and Blood circulation and relieves the breast pain.
- Sheng Di Huang, Huang Qin, Ju Hua and Xiao Ku Cao clear Heat in the Liver, reduce Liver-Fire, sedate the headache and relieve nervousness.

- Dang Gui nourishes the Liver-Blood and smoothes the Liver.
- Gan Cao, in combination with Bai Shao, harmonises the Liver and relieves the breast pain.

Acupuncture treatment

LR-2, LR-3, LR-5, LR-14, LI-4, PC-6, CV-17, HT-8 and GB-20. Reducing method was used on these points. Treatment was given once every other day.

Explanations

- LR-3, the Source point of the Liver, and LR-14, the Front Collecting point of the Liver, are used to smooth the Liver, promote the Qi circulation and relieve breast pain.
- LR-2, the Spring point, is used to reduce Liver-Fire and calm the Liver.
- LR-5, the Connecting point, harmonises the collateral and sedates pain in the breast.
- PC-6 and CV-17 promote the Qi circulation in the chest and sedate the breast pain.
- LI-4 promotes Qi circulation, clears Heat in the Liver and relieves the pain.
- HT-8, the Spring point, clears Heat in the Heart, calms the Mind and improves the sleep.

After treatment for 3 weeks, she was much calmer, her breast pain had begun to diminish, and her sleep pattern and irritability had also improved. Treatment frequency was reduced to once every 3 days, and after another 3 weeks her breast pain had disappeared. She continued with the herbal treatment for another 6 months, during which the other symptoms also resolved.

ACCUMULATION OF DAMP-PHLEGM

Symptoms and signs

Gradual onset of breast pain with feelings of fullness, distension and heaviness, and the formation of soft nodules in the breast, accompanied by tiredness, nausea, phlegm in the throat, coughing with expectoration of white phlegm, a feeling of fullness in the stomach region, a poor appetite, loose stools, obesity, somnolence, a white and greasy tongue coating and a slippery pulse.

Principle of treatment

Resolve Damp, eliminate Phlegm, circulate the collateral and sedate the pain.

HERBAL TREATMENT

Prescription

DAO TAN TANG
Guide Out Phlegm Decoction
Ban Xia *Rhizoma Pinelliae* 10 g

Tian Nan Xing *Rhizoma Arisaematis* 10 g
Chen Pi *Pericarpium Citri Reticulatae* 5 g
Fu Ling *Poria* 10 g
Gua Lou *Fructus Tricosanthis* 10 g
Chang Pu *Rhizoma Acori Graminei* 10 g
Hou Po *Cortex Magnoliae Officinalis* 10 g
Zhi Shi *Fructus Citri Aurantii Immaturus* 10 g
Xie Bai *Bulbus Allii* 10 g
Gui Zhi *Ramulus Cinnamomi* 6 g
Sha Ren *Fructus seu Semen Amomi* 5 g

Explanations

- Ban Xia and Tian Nan Xing resolve Damp and eliminate Phlegm.
- Chen Pi and Sha Ren promote the Qi circulation and harmonise the Stomach so as to eliminate Damp-Phlegm.
- Fu Ling and Gua Lou resolve Damp-Phlegm.
- Hou Po and Zhi Shi break Qi stagnation and eliminate Damp. Also, Zhi Shi is a good herb for relieving the breast pain.
- Gui Zhi warms the Yang of the body and eliminates blockage of the channels by Damp-Phlegm.
- Xie Bai is a special herb that eliminates Damp-Phlegm in the breast and relaxes the chest.
- Chang Pu eliminates Damp in the chest and clarifies the Mind.

Modifications

1. If there is distension of the breast, add Zhi Qiao *Fructus Aurantii* 10 g and Xiang Fu *Rhizoma Cyperi* 10 g to promote the Qi circulation in the chest and relieve the distension.
2. If there are nodules in the breast, add Yu Jin *Radix Curcumae* 10 g and Zhe Bei Mu *Bulbus Fritillariae Thunbergii* 10 g to eliminate Damp-Phlegm in the breast and soften the nodules.
3. If there is an occasional stabbing pain in the breast, add Yan Hu Suo *Rhizoma Corydalis* 10 g to promote the Blood circulation and relieve the pain.
4. If there is a burning feeling in the breast, add Xia Ku Cao *Spica Prunella* 10 g and Huang Qin *Radix Scutellariae* 12 g to clear Heat in the breast and remove Toxin.
5. If there is a yellow and greasy tongue coating and a slippery and rapid pulse due to the accumulation of Damp-Heat, remove Tian Nan Xing, Gui Zhi and Xie Bai from the prescription and add Huang Lian *Rhizoma Coptidis* 5 g, Cang Zhu *Rhizoma Atractylodis* 10 g and Zhu Ru *Caulis Bambusae in Taeniam* 10 g to clear the Heat and resolve the Damp.

6. If there is depression, irritability and headache, add Gou Teng *Ramulus Uncariae cum Uncis* 10 g to calm the Liver and relieve the headache.

7. If there is a bitter taste in the mouth, add Zhi Zi *Fructus Gardeniae* 9 g to clear Heat in the Liver and Gall Bladder and remove the bitter taste.

8. If there is diarrhoea or loose stools, add Bai Zhu *Rhizoma Atractylodis Macrocephalae* 10 g and Ge Gen *Radix Puerariae* 10 g to activate the Spleen, eliminate Damp and relieve the diarrhoea.

9. If there is nausea and a poor appetite, add Sha Ren *Radix Aenophorae* 5 g to harmonise the Stomach and improve the appetite.

10. If there is insomnia and restlessness, add Duan Long Gu *Os Draconis* 15 g and Huang Lian *Rhizoma Coptidis* 5 g to clear Heat in the Heart, calm the Mind and improve the sleep.

11. If there is irregular menstruation, add Dang Gui *Radix Angelicae Sinensis* 10 g and Yi Mu Cao *Herba Leonuri* 10 g to relieve blockage in the Penetrating and Directing Vessels and regulate the menstruation.

12. If there is amenorrhoea, add Chuan Xiong *Rhizoma Ligustici Chuanxiong* 6 g and Chuan Niu Xi *Radix Cyathulae* 10 g to eliminate Blood stagnation and regulate the menstruation.

Patent remedy

Xiao Luo Wan *Reduce Scrofula Pill*

ACUPUNCTURE TREATMENT

LI-4 Hegu, SP-6 Sanyinjiao, SP-9 Yinlingquan, ST-36 Zusanli, ST-40 Fenglong, CV-12 Zhongwan, LR-3 Taichong, LR-14 Qimen and PC-6 Neiguan. Reducing method is used on these points.

Explanations

- Formation of Damp-Phlegm is usually caused by bad diet or weakness of the Spleen and Stomach, or of Kidney, leading to disorder of Water metabolism in the body. Weakness of Spleen and Stomach together with a bad diet is often seen.
- LI-4 and LR-3, the Source points, promote the Qi and Blood circulation and relieve breast pain.
- SP-6 and ST-36, the crossing points of the three Yin channels of the foot and the Sea point of the Stomach channel respectively, activate the Spleen and Stomach and eliminate Damp.
- SP-9, the Sea point, and ST-40, the Connecting point, resolve Damp and eliminate Phlegm. ST-40

also harmonises the collateral in the breast and sedates the pain.
- CV-12, the Gathering point for the Fu organs and the Front Collecting point of the Stomach, activates the Stomach and resolves Damp in the body.
- Accumulation of Damp-Phlegm in the body and breast blocks the Qi circulation and causes Qi stagnation. PC-6 and LR-14 promote the Qi circulation and relieves the blockage in the breast caused by the Damp-Phlegm.

Modifications

1. If there is severe pain in the breast, add PC-4 and ST-34, the Accumulation points of the Pericardium and Stomach channels respectively, to harmonise the collateral and sedate the pain.

2. If there is distension of the breast, add PC-3, the Sea point, to promote the Qi circulation in the chest and relieve the distension.

3. If there are nodules in the breast, add Ah Shi points around the nodules to eliminate Damp-Phlegm in the breast and soften the nodules.

4. If there is an occasional stabbing pain in the breast, add SP-6 and BL-17 to promote the Blood circulation and relieve the pain.

5. If there is a burning feeling in the breast, add PC-8 and LR-2, the Spring points, to clear Heat in the breast and remove Toxin.

6. If there is depression, irritability and a headache, add GB-20 and LR-8 to calm the Liver and relieve the headache.

7. If there is a bitter taste in the mouth, add GB-40 and GB-43 to clear Heat in the Liver and Gall Bladder and remove the bitter taste.

8. If there is a poor appetite and loose stools, add SP-3, the Source point, to activate the Spleen and Stomach, eliminate Damp and improve the appetite.

9. If there is nausea, add SP-4 in combination with PC-6 to cause the Stomach-Qi to descend and relieve the nausea.

10. If there is insomnia and restlessness, add HT-3, the Sea point, and HT-8, the Spring point, to clear Heat in the Heart, calm the Mind and improve the sleep.

11. If there is amenorrhoea, add ST-28 and ST-29 to promote the Qi and Blood circulation and regulate menstruation.

12. If there is abdominal distension, add ST-30 to regulate the Qi circulation in the abdomen and relieve the distension.

13. If there is profuse leucorrhoea, add BL-22 and BL-32 to eliminate Damp in the Lower Burner and relieve the leucorrhoea.

STAGNATION OF BLOOD

Symptoms and signs

Prolonged persistence of stabbing breast pain with a fixed location, and aggravation at night, accompanied by scar formation after operation or trauma, amenorrhoea, dysmenorrhoea or discharge of purplish blood during menstruation, restlessness, insomnia, a purplish tongue, with a thin coating or ecchymoses and a wiry and choppy pulse.

Principle of treatment

Promote Blood circulation, eliminate stagnant Blood and sedate the pain.

HERBAL TREATMENT

Prescription

XUE FU ZHU YU TANG
Drive Out Stasis in the Mansion of Blood Decoction
Chi Shao *Radix Paeoniae Rubra* 6 g
Chuan Xiong *Rhizoma Ligustici Chuanxiong* 9 g
Dang Gui *Radix Angelicae Sinensis* 9 g
Hong Hua *Flos Carthami* 9 g
Yan Hu Suo *Rhizoma Corydalis* 6 g
Yu Jin *Radix Curcumae* 10 g
Xiang Fu *Rhizoma Cyperi* 10 g
Zhi Qiao *Fructus Aurantii* 10 g
Gan Cao *Radix Glycyrrhizae* 6 g

Explanations

- Xiang Fu, Zhi Qiao and Yu Jin regulate the Liver-Qi and relieve the breast pain.
- Chuan Xiong, Hong Hua and Yan Hu Suo promote the Blood circulation, eliminate Blood stasis and relieve breast pain.
- Dang Gui tonifies the Liver-Blood and harmonises the Liver.
- Chi Shao promotes the Blood circulation and clears Heat in the Blood.
- Gan Cao harmonises the herbs in the prescription and relieves the pain.

Modifications

1. If there is depression, add Chai Hu *Radix Bupleuri* 6 g to regulate the Liver-Qi and relieve the depression.
2. If there is severe breast pain with cramp, add Bai Shao *Radix Paeoniae Alba* 12 g to smooth the muscles and tendons so as to stop the breast pain and relieve the cramp.
3. If there are palpable and immobile nodules, add Mu Li *Concha Ostreae* 18 g and Wang Bu Liu Xing *Semen Vaccariae* 10 g to promote the Blood circulation and remove the nodules.
4. If there is breast cancer, add Bai Hua She Shi Cao *Herba Oldenlandiae* 20 g and Zi Hua Di Ding *Herba Violae* 20 g to clear Heat, remove Toxin and reduce the swelling.
5. If there is night sweating and hot flushes due to deficiency of Liver-Yin, add Huang Bai *Cortex Phellodendri* 12 g and Sheng Di Huang *Radix Rehmanniae Recens* 12 g to nourish the Liver-Yin and clear Deficient-Heat.
6. If there are Heart palpitations, add Dan Shen *Radix Salviae Miltiorrhizae* 20 g to clear Heat in the Heart and calm the palpitations.
7. If there is insomnia, add Huang Lian *Rhizoma Coptidis* 5 g to clear Heat in the Heart and improve the sleep.
8. If there is lower abdominal pain, add Wu Yao *Radix Linderae* 6 g to promote the Qi circulation and relieve the pain.
9. If there is amenorrhoea, add E Zhu *Rhizoma Zedoariae* 10 g and Pu Huang *Pollen Typhoo* 12 g to eliminate Blood stagnation and promote menstruation.
10. If there is irregular menstruation or dysmenorrhoea, add Shu Di *Radix Rehmanniae Praeparata* 10 g and Yi Mu Cao *Herba Leonuri* 10 g to regulate the menstruation and relieve the dysmenorrhoea.
11. If there is scar formation on the breast or poor wound healing after a breast operation, add Mo Yao, *Resina Myrrhae* 6 g and San Qi *Radix Notoginseng* 10 g to reduce the scar and promote healing of the wound.
12. If there is generalised tiredness, add Huang Qi *Radix Astragali seu Hedysari* 10 g and Dang Shen *Radix Codonopsis Pilosulae* 10 g to tonify the Qi and relieve the tiredness.
13. If there is constipation, add Da Huang *Radix en Rhizoma Rhei* 10 g to promote defecation and relieve the constipation.

Patent remedy

Yan Hu Suo Zhi Tong Pian *Corydalis Stop Pain Tablet*

ACUPUNCTURE TREATMENT

SP-6 Sanyinjiao, SP-10 Xuchai, BL-17 Geshu, LI-4 Hegu, ST-40 Fenglong, CV-17 Tanzhong, LR-3 Taichong and LR-14 Qimen. Reducing method is used on these points.

Explanations

- Stagnation of Blood causing breast pain is usually due to persistent Liver-Qi stagnation, accumulation of Damp-Phlegm or hyperactivity of toxic Fire, which lead to severe blockage of the collateral and channels in the breast. The root treatment is to promote the Blood circulation and eliminate the Blood stasis.
- SP-6, the crossing point of the three Yin channels of the foot, SP-10, the point called Sea of Blood, and BL-17, the Gathering point for the Blood, promote the Blood circulation, eliminate Blood stasis and relieve the breast pain.
- LI-4 and LR-3, the Source points, promote the Qi circulation so as to promote Blood circulation. They can also sedate the breast pain.
- CV-17, the Gathering point for Qi in the body generally, relaxes the chest and smoothes the Qi circulation in the chest and breast so as to help the above points promote the Blood circulation.
- ST-40, the Connecting point, harmonises the collateral and relieves the blockage in the breast.
- LR-14, the Front Collecting point of the Liver, smoothes the Liver, promotes the Liver-Qi circulation, relaxes the chest and relieves the pain.

Modifications

1. If there is severe breast pain, add PC-4 and KI-9, the Accumulation points of the Pericardium channel and the Yin Linking Vessel respectively, to sedate the breast pain.
2. If there are palpable and immobile nodules, add LR-5, the Connecting point, to promote the Blood circulation and resolve the nodules.
3. If there is depression, add LR-8, the Sea point, and LR-12 to regulate the Liver-Qi and relieve the depression.
4. If there is a feeling of oppression over the chest, add CV-16, the Connecting point of the Directing Vessel, to unblock the chest and relieve the feeling of oppression.
5. If there is restlessness, palpitation and insomnia due to extreme pain, add HT-7 and HT-3 to tranquillise the Mind and calm the Heart.
6. If there is night sweating and hot flushes due to deficiency of the Liver-Yin, add HT-6, the Accumulation point, and KI-7, the Metal point, to nourish the Liver-Yin and clear Deficient-Heat.
7. If there is lower abdominal pain, add SP-8, the Accumulation point, and ST-28 to promote the Qi and Blood circulation in the abdomen and relieve the pain.

8. If there is amenorrhoea or dysmenorrhoea, add CV-3 and ST-29 to promote the Qi and Blood circulation in the Lower Burner, eliminate Blood stasis and regulate the menstruation.
9. If there is irregular menstruation, add KI-3 and CV-6 to tonify the Kidney and regulate the menstruation.
10. If there is scar formation with poor wound healing after a breast operation, add some surrounding points around the wound to promote healing.
11. If there is generalised tiredness, add ST-36 and CV-4 to tonify the Qi and relieve the tiredness.
12. If there is constipation, add ST-25, the Front Collecting point of the Large Intestine, to promote defecation and relieve the constipation.

HYPERACTIVITY OF TOXIC FIRE

Symptoms and signs

Redness, swelling, heat and a burning pain in the breast, especially around the nipple, aggravation of the pain on touching the breast, accompanied by fever, a slight aversion to cold, thirst, constipation, restlessness, a red tongue with a yellow and dry coating and a rapid and slippery pulse.

Principle of treatment

Clear Heat and remove Toxin, reduce swelling and sedate the pain.

HERBAL TREATMENT

Prescription

WU WEI XIAO DU YIN
Five-Ingredient Decoction to Eliminate Toxin
Jin Yin Hua *Flos Lonicerae* 20 g
Ye Ju Hua *Flos Chrysanthemi Indici* 15 g
Pu Gong Ying *Herba Taraxaci* 30 g
Zi Hua Di Ding *Herba Violae* 30 g
Zi Bei Tian Kui *Herba Begonia Fibristipulatae* 15 g

Explanations

- Jin Yin Hua and Pu Gong Ying clear Heat and eliminate Toxin so as to stop the pain.
- Ye Ju Hua, Zi Hua Di Ding and Zi Bei Tian Kui eliminate Toxin, cool the Blood and reduce swelling.

Modifications

1. If there is obvious redness and swelling of the breast due to severe Toxin, add Huang Lian

Rhizoma Coptidis 10 g and Da Qing Ye *Folium Isatidis* 10 g to clear Heat, remove the Toxin and reduce the swelling.

2. If there is a fever, add Shi Gao *Gypsum Fibrosum* 20 g and Sheng Ma *Rhizoma Cimicifugae* 5 g to clear Heat and reduce the fever.

3. If there is a headache, add Man Jing Zi *Fructus Viticis* 10 g to sedate the headache.

4. If there is pus or ulceration in the breast, add Zhe Bei Mu *Bulbus Fritillariae Thunbergii* 10 g and Zao Jiao Ci *Spina Gledisiae* 10 g to clear Heat, eliminate the pus and reduce the ulceration.

5. If there is a burning feeling in the breast, add Xia Ku Cao *Spica Prunella* 10 g and Huang Qin *Radix Scutellariae* 12 g to clear Heat in the breast and remove Toxin.

6. If there are nodules in the breast, add Yu Jin *Radix Curcumae* 10 g to eliminate Damp-Phlegm in the breast and soften the nodules.

7. If there is an occasional stabbing pain in the breast, add Yan Hu Suo *Rhizoma Corydalis* 10 g to promote Blood circulation and relieve the pain.

8. If there is a yellow and greasy tongue coating and a slippery and rapid pulse due to the accumulation of Toxic Damp-Heat, add Huang Lian *Rhizoma Coptidis* 5 g and Cang Zhu *Rhizoma Atractylodis* 10 g to clear the Heat and resolve the Damp.

9. If there is nausea or vomiting, add Zhu Ru *Caulis Bambusae in Taeniam* 10 g and Xuan Fu Hua *Flos Inulae* 10 g to cause the Stomach-Qi to descend and relieve the vomiting.

10. If there is restlessness and insomnia, add Huang Lian *Rhizoma Coptidis* 10 g and Zhu Ye *Herba Lophatheri* 10 g to clear Heat and calm the Mind.

11. If there is severe thirst, add Zhi Mu *Rhizoma Anemarrhenae* 10 g and Tian Hua Fen *Radix Trichosanthis* 10 g to clear the Heat, promote secretion of Body Fluids and relieve the thirst.

12. If there is constipation, add Da Huang *Radix et Rhizoma Rhei* 10 g and Mang Xiao *Natrii Sulfas* 10 g to clear Heat, reduce Fire and promote defecation.

Patent remedy

Niu Huang Jie Du Wan *Cattle Gallstone Pill to Resolve Toxin*

ACUPUNCTURE TREATMENT

LI-2 Erjian, LI-4 Hegu, LI-11 Quchi, ST-40 Fenglong, ST-44 Neiting, SP-6 Sanyinjiao, BL-17 Geshu and GV-10 Lingtai. Reducing method is used on these points.

Explanations

- Invasion of Toxic Heat, generation of Toxin due to prolonged persistence of Qi stagnation, and accumulation of Damp-Phlegm may all cause hyperactivity of Toxic Fire, leading to damage and burning of the collateral and muscle in the breast, causing breast pain.
- LI-2, the Spring point, LI-4, the Source point, and LI-11, the Sea point, are used to clear Heat, remove Toxin and promote defecation in order to eliminate Toxic Fire.
- ST-44, the Spring point, cools Heat, reduces fever and removes Toxin.
- ST-40, the Connecting point, harmonises the collateral and reduces swelling.
- SP-6 and BL-17 cool the Blood and remove Toxin.
- GV-10 clears Heat, removes Toxin and reduces the swelling.

Modifications

1. If there is a high fever, add GV-14, the meeting point of all the Yang channels, to clear Heat and reduce the fever.

2. If there is pus or ulceration in the breast, add ST-16 and ST-18 to clear Heat, eliminate the pus and reduce the ulceration.

3. If there is restlessness and insomnia, add HT-3 and HT-7 to clear Heat in the Heart and tranquillise the Mind.

4. If there is distension and pain in the breast and chest, add PC-6, the Connecting point, and CV-17, the Gathering point for the Qi, to promote the Qi circulation in the chest and sedate the pain.

5. If there is a stabbing pain in the breast or bleeding from the breast, add SP-10 and BL-17 to clear Heat in the Blood and remove Toxin.

6. If there is restlessness due to pain, add Extra Sishencong and HT-3 to calm the Heart and tranquillise the Mind.

7. If there is insomnia, add HT-8 to clear Heat in the Heart and improve the sleep.

8. If the appetite is poor, add SP-3, the Source point, to activate the Spleen and improve the appetite.

9. If there is nausea, add SP-4 to cause the Stomach-Qi to descend and relieve the nausea.

10. If there is constipation, add ST-25, the Front Collecting point of the Large Intestine, and ST-37, the Lower Sea point, to promote defecation, remove Toxin and relieve the constipation.

11. If there is a yellow and greasy tongue coating, add CV-12, the Gathering point for the Fu organs, and SP-2, the Spring point, to clear Heat and eliminate Damp.

12. If there is diarrhoea, add SP-9, the Sea point of the Spleen channel, to eliminate Damp-Phlegm, activate the Spleen and relieve the diarrhoea.

XU TYPE OF BREAST PAIN

DEFICIENCY OF QI AND BLOOD

Symptoms and signs

Gradual onset of a slight breast pain that moves up and down with breast softness and a bearing-down sensation, and aggravation of the pain after menstruation, accompanied by scanty menstruation with a light red colour of the blood, a pale complexion, hair loss, a poor appetite, generalised tiredness, palpitations, shortness of breath, an aversion to cold, coldness in the limbs, nycturia, lower back pain, a pale and swollen tongue with tooth marks and a deep, weak and thready pulse.

Principle of treatment

Reinforce Yang Qi and tonify Blood, harmonise the collateral and sedate the pain.

HERBAL TREATMENT

Prescription

REN SHEN TANG plus **YOU GUI WAN**
Ginseng Decoction plus *Restore the Right-Kidney Pill*
Ren Shen *Radix Ginseng* 6 g
Zhi Gan Cao *Radix Glycyrrhizae Praeparata* 10 g
Zhi Fu Zi *Radix Aconiti Carmichaeli Praeparata* 6 g
Shu Di Huang *Radix Rehmanniae Praeparata* 10 g
Shan Zhu Yu *Fructus Corni* 10 g
Du Zhong *Cortex Eucommiae* 10 g
Xian Ling Pi *Herba Epimedii* 10 g
Huang Qi *Radix Astragali* 10 g
Ba Ji Tian *Radix Morindae Officinalis* 10 g
Lu Jiao Jiao *Colla Cervi Cornu* 10 g

Explanations

- Ren Shen greatly tonifies the Qi and strengthens the body.
- Huang Qi and Zhi Gan Cao tonify the Qi, activate the Spleen and raise the Qi to the breast.
- Shu Di Huang and Shan Zhu Yu tonify the Kidney-Essence so as to tonify the Blood.
- Du Zhong, Ba Ji Tian and Lu Jiao Jiao strengthen the bones, tonify the Kidney-Essence and benefit the Blood.
- Zhi Fu Zi and Xian Ling Pi warm the body and channels and dispel Interior Cold.

Modifications

1. If there is obvious hair loss and scanty menstruation due to Blood deficiency, add Dang Gui *Radix Angelicae Sinensis* 10 g to tonify the Blood and nourish the hair.
2. If there is an obvious shortness of breath, pale complexion and tiredness due to Qi deficiency, add Shan Yao *Rhizoma Dioscorea* 10 g to activate the Spleen and tonify the Qi.
3. If there is distension of the breast, add Yan Hu Suo *Rhizoma Corydalis* 12 g and Xiang Fu *Rhizoma Cyperi* 10 g to promote the Qi circulation and relieve the distension.
4. If there is cramp in the breast, add Bai Shao *Radix Paeoniae Alba* 12 g together with Gan Cao *Radix Glycyrrhizae Praeparata* 6 g to relieve the cramp.
5. If there is coldness in the abdomen, hands and feet, add Rou Gui *Cortex Cinnamomi* 5 g and Gan Jiang *Rhizoma Zingiberis* 5 g to warm the Interior and dispel Cold.
6. If there is insomnia, add Bai Zi Ren *Semen Biotae* 10 g and Ye Jiao Teng *Caulis Polygoni Multiflori* 15 g to nourish the Heart-Blood and tranquillise the Mind.
7. If the appetite is poor, add Gu Ya *Fructus Oryzae Germinatus* 12 g and Mai Ya *Fructus Hordei Germinatus* 12 g to promote digestion and improve the appetite.
8. If there is nausea and belching, add Sha Ren *Fructus Amomi* 5 g and Ban Xia *Rhizoma Pinelliae Praeparata* 5 g to harmonise the Stomach, cause the Stomach-Qi to descend and relieve the uprising of Stomach-Qi.
9. If there are loose stools or diarrhoea, add Bai Zhu *Rhizoma Atractylodis Macrocephalae* 10 g and Fu Ling *Poria* 12 g to activate the Spleen and Stomach, eliminate Damp and relieve the diarrhoea.
10. If there is scanty or irregular menstruation, add Chuan Xiong *Rhizoma Ligustici Chuanxiong* 10 g and Yi Mu Cao *Herba Leonuri* 10 g to regulate the Blood circulation and promote menstruation.

Patent remedies

Dang Gui Bu Xue Pian *Angelica Decoction to Tonify the Blood*
Shi Quan Da Bu Wan *All-Inclusive Great Tonifying Pill*

ACUPUNCTURE TREATMENT

SP-3 Taibai, SP-6 Sanyinjiao, KI-3 Taixi, ST-36 Zusanli, CV-4 Guanyuan, CV-6 Qihai, PC-6 Neiguan and LR-3 Taichong. Reinforcing method is used on the first six points; even method is used on PC-6 and LR-3.

Explanations

- Prolonged sickness, excessive bleeding during menstruation, a bad diet and overstrain may all cause a deficiency of Qi and Blood, so the breast is not properly nourished, causing breast pain.
- SP-3, the Source point, and SP-6 activate the Spleen and promote Qi and Blood production.
- ST-36 activates the Spleen and Stomach and reinforces Qi and Blood production.
- KI-3, the Source point, tonifies the Kidney and benefits the Kidney-Essence so as to promote the production of Qi and Blood.
- CV-4 and CV-6 reinforce the Qi and Yang generally in the body, and strengthen the constitution.
- LR-3, the Source point, and PC-6, the Confluence point of the Yin Linking Vessel, promote the Qi circulation in the chest and harmonise the collateral in the breast so as to sedate the pain.

Modifications

1. If there is distension or cramp of the breast, add CV-17, the Gathering point for the Qi, and LR-14, the Front Collecting point of the Liver, to promote the Qi circulation and relieve the distension and cramp.
2. If there is occasional severe breast pain, add PC-4, the Accumulation point, to harmonise the collateral and relieve the breast pain.
3. If there is depression, add GB-8 and LR-8 to promote the Qi circulation and relieve the depression.
4. If there is generalised tiredness, add GV-20 to raise the Qi and Yang and relieve the tiredness.
5. If the appetite is poor, add CV-12 to activate the Spleen and Stomach and eliminate Damp.
6. If there is nausea, add SP-4 to cause the Stomach-Qi to descend and relieve the nausea.
7. If there are loose stools or diarrhoea, add SP-9 and ST-25 to activate the Spleen and relieve the diarrhoea.
8. If the hands and feet are cold, or there is aversion to cold, add moxibustion on CV-4, CV-6 and ST-36 to warm the Yang and Qi and dispel Cold.
9. If there is lower back pain, add BL-23 and BL-58 to reinforce the Kidney and strengthen the back.
10. If there is insomnia and palpitations, add HT-7 to tonify the Heart and tranquillise the Mind.
11. If there is irregular menstruation, add LR-12 and ST-29 to smooth the Blood circulation and regulate the menstruation.
12. If there is a headache, add GB-20 to harmonise the collateral and sedate the headache.

DEFICIENCY OF YIN OF THE LIVER AND KIDNEY

Symptoms and signs

A slight breast pain with a soft or sometimes swollen breast, and aggravation of the pain during or after menstruation, accompanied by irregular or scanty menstruation, tiredness, dizziness, vertigo, tinnitus, thirst, heat in the body or hot flushes, restlessness, night sweating, lower back pain, a red tongue with cracks and a scanty or peeled coating and a deep, thready and rapid pulse.

Principle of treatment

Nourish the Yin of Liver and Kidney and harmonise the collateral.

HERBAL TREATMENT

Prescription

ZUO GUI YIN
Restore Left-Kidney Decoction
Sheng Di Huang *Radix Rehmanniae Recens* 12 g
Shu Di Huang *Radix Rehmanniae Praeparata* 12 g
He Shou Wu *Polygoni Multiflori* 15 g
Gou Qi Zi *Fructus Lycii* 10 g
Shan Zhu Yu *Fructus Corni* 10 g
Nu Zhen Zi *Fructus Ligustri Lucidi* 10 g
Dang Gui *Radix Angelicae Sinensis* 10 g
Dan Shen *Radix Salviae Miltiorrhizae* 10 g
Bai Shao *Radix Paeoniae Alba* 10 g
Suan Zao Ren *Semen Ziziphi Spinosae* 10 g

Explanations

- Shu Di Huang and Shan Zhu Yu tonify the Kidney and benefit the Essence.
- Dang Gui and He Shou Wu tonify the Blood and nourish the Essence.
- Gou Qi Zi and Nu Zhen Zi nourish the Yin of the Liver and Kidney and benefit the Kidney-Essence.
- Sheng Di clears Deficient-Heat and cools the Blood.
- Bai Shao harmonises the Liver and relieves the pain in the breast.
- Dan Shen and Suan Zao Ren calm the Mind, clear Heat in the Heart and relieve restlessness.

Modifications

1. If there is underdevelopment of the breast owing to deficiency of Kidney-Essence, add Zi He Che

Placenta Hominis 10 g, Lu Jiao Jiao *Colla Cervi Cornu* 10 g and Du Zhong *Cortex Eucommiae* 10 g to tonify the Kidney and reinforce the Essence.

2. If there is irregular menstruation and hot flushes due to menopause, add Xian Ling Pi *Herba Epimedii* 10 g and Huang Bai *Cortex Phellodendri* 10 g to tonify the Yin and Yang of the Kidney and relieve the hot flushes.

3. If there is nervousness and headache, add Ju Hua *Flos Chrysanthemi* 10 g and Gou Teng *Ramulus Uncariae cum Uncis* 10 g to calm the Liver and clear Heat in the Liver.

4. If there is generalised tiredness, add Huang Qi *Radix Astragali seu Hedysari* 10 g and Zhi Gan Cao *Radix Glycyrrhizae Praeparata* 10 g to tonify the Qi and relieve the tiredness.

5. If there is a severe thirst, add Mai Men Dong *Radix Ophiopogonis* 10 g to promote the secretion of Body Fluids and relieve the thirst.

6. If there is night sweating, add Ma Huang Gen *Radix Ephedrae* 10 g and Wu Wei Zi *Fructus Schizandrae* 10 g to arrest the sweating.

7. If there is lower back pain, add Ba Ji Tian *Radix Morindae Officinalis* 10 g to reinforce the Kidney, strengthen the back and relieve the lower back pain.

Patent remedy

Qi Ju Di Huang Wan *Lycuim Fruit, Chrysanthemum and Rehmannia Pill*

ACUPUNCTURE TREATMENT

SP-6 Sanyinjiao, KI-3 Taixi, KI-6 Zhaohai, KI-7 Fuliu, LR-3 Taichong, LR-8 Ququan, LU-7 Lieque and PC-6 Neiguan. Reinforcing method is used on the first six points; even method is used on LU-7 and PC-6.

Explanations

- Constitutional weakness, giving birth to many children and overstrain may all cause weakness of the Liver and Kidney, leading to Yin deficiency in the Liver and Kidney.
- KI-3, the Source point, and KI-7, the Metal point, nourish the Kidney-Yin and promote secretion of Body Fluids so as to tonify the root Yin of the body.
- LR-3, the Source point, and LR-8, the Sea point and Water point, tonify the Liver-Yin and calm the Liver.
- SP-6, the crossing point of the three Yin channels of the foot, nourishes the Yin and clears Deficient-Heat.

- KI-6 and LU-7, a special combination, open the Directing Vessel, nourish the Yin and regulate the Qi circulation in the breast.
- PC-6 harmonises the collateral in the breast and sedates the pain.

Modifications

1. If there is underdevelopment of the breast owing to Kidney-Essence deficiency, add CV-4 and CV-6 to tonify the Kidney and reinforce the Essence.

2. If there is irregular menstruation and hot flushes due to menopause, add KI-2 and KI-10 to tonify the Yin and Yang of the Kidney and relieve the hot flushes.

3. If there is dysmenorrhoea, add SP-8, the Accumulation point, and LR-12 to harmonise the menstruation and relieve the pain.

4. If there is nervousness and headache, add CV-20 and LR-2 to calm the Liver, clear Heat in the Liver and relieve the nervousness.

5. If there is headache, add GB-20 to suppress the Liver-Yang and relieve the headache.

6. If there is generalised tiredness, add ST-36 and CV-6 to tonify the Qi and Yin of the body and relieve the tiredness.

7. If there is a severe thirst, add LU-8, the Metal point, to promote the secretion of Body Fluids and relieve the thirst.

8. If there is night sweating, add HT-6 to stop the sweating.

9. If there is insomnia and restlessness, add HT-3, the Sea point, and HT-8, the Spring point, to clear Heat in the Heart, calm the Mind and improve the sleep.

10. If there is lower back pain, add BL-23 and BL-58 to reinforce the Kidney and strengthen the back.

Case history

A 49-year-old woman had been experiencing menopausal syndrome for 2 years, and was treated by hormone replacement therapy. Prior to starting this therapy, she had experienced breast pain, especially on the left side. After receiving the therapy, her hot flushes improved slightly, but she suffered much more breast pain on both sides and she gained 15 kg in weight. During the previous 2 months, the breast pain became a stabbing pain and worsened at night. Her breasts were sometimes hard to the touch. Because of the severe breast pain, she was afraid she had breast cancer, so had visited different gynaecologists but her treatment remained almost the same. As well as the breast pain, she had hot flushes, night sweating, heat in the palms and soles of the feet, always felt too warm, and had restlessness, lower back pain, generalised tiredness, headache, a thin and slight yellow tongue coating, with one peeled spot on the right edge, and a thready and wiry pulse.

Diagnosis
Breast pain due to deficiency of Yin of Liver and Kidney with stagnation of Blood.

Principle of the treatment
Nourish Yin, promote Blood circulation and stop the pain.

Herbal treatment
ZUO GUI YIN plus **ER ZHI WAN**
Restore Left-Kidney Decoction plus *Two-Ultimate Pill*
Shu Di Huang *Radix Rehmanniae Praeparata* 12 g
Shan Zhu Yu *Fructus Corni* 10 g
Chuan Lian Zi *Fructus Meliae Toosendan* 3 g
Pu Huang *Pollen Typhae* 10 g
Wu Ling Zhi *Faeces Trogopterorum* 10 g
Bai Shao *Radix Paeoniae Alba* 10 g
Nu Zhen Zi *Fructus Ligustri Lucidi* 12 g
Han Lian Cao *Herba Ecliptae* 12 g
Dang Shen *Radix Codonopsis Pilosulae* 20 g
Huang Bai *Cortex Phellodendri* 10 g
Sheng Di Huang *Radix Rehmanniae Recens* 12 g
Suan Zao Ren *Semen Ziziphi Spinosae* 10 g

Explanations

- Shu Di Huang and Shan Zhu Yu tonify the Kidney and benefit the Essence.
- Nu Zhen Zi and Han Lian Cao nourish the Yin of the Liver and Kidney and benefit the Kidney-Essence.
- Sheng Di and Huang Bai clear Deficient-Heat and cool the Blood.
- Dang Shen tonifies the Qi and relieves tiredness.
- Bai Shao and Chuan Lian Zi harmonise the Liver and relieve pain in the breast.
- Pu Huang and Wu Ling Zhi promote the Blood circulation and eliminate Blood stasis so as to relieve breast pain.

- Suan Zao Ren calms the Mind, clears Heat in the Heart and relieves the restlessness.

Acupuncture treatment
SP-6, KI-2, KI-3, KI-6, KI-7, LR-3, LR-8, LU-7 and PC-6. Reinforcing method is used on the first six points; even method is used on LU-7 and PC-6. Treatment was given once every 2 days.

Explanations

- KI-3, the Source point, and KI-7, the Metal point, nourish the Kidney-Yin and promote the secretion of Body Fluids so as to tonify the root Yin of the body.
- LR-3, the Source point, and LR-8, the Sea point and Water point, tonify the Liver-Yin and calm the Liver.
- KI-2, the Spring point, clears Deficient-Heat, reduces Fire and relieves hot flushes.
- SP-6, the crossing point of the three Yin channels of the foot, nourishes the Yin, clears Deficient-Heat and promotes the Blood circulation so as to eliminate Blood stasis.
- KI-6 and LU-7, a special combination, open the Directing Vessel, nourish the Yin and regulate the Qi circulation in the breast.
- PC-6 harmonises the collateral in the breast and sedates the pain.

After treatment for 1 month, her hot flushes had resolved and the breast pain was also much better; she only had the pain from time to time, and the stabbing pain in the breast had gone. After this, the herbal treatment remained the same, but acupuncture was given only once every 4 days. Two months later, she was completely free of the breast pain, and her general condition had also improved greatly. The acupuncture treatment was stopped while the herbal treatment was continued for another 4 months. A year later, she had a consultation for some other complaint, and she said she had experienced no more breast pain. She had also stopped the hormone replacement therapy and had lost 10 kg over the course of a year which she felt happy about.

Axillary pain 24

腋
部
疼
痛

Pain in the axillary fossa may occur on one side or both sides of the body. There are several channels passing through the axillary fossa, including the three Yin channels of the hand and the Gall Bladder channel of foot Lesser Yang. Any factor that obstructs these channels, may cause pain in the axillary fossa. Axillary pain may be attributed to any of the following disorders in Western medicine: intercostal neuralgia from the third to the eighth intercostal nerve, herpes zoster, injury or trauma of pectoralis muscle, serratus anterior muscle and latissimus dorsi muscle, axillary lymphadenitis from lymphangitis, mastitis, axillary furuncle and folliculitis.

Aetiology and pathology

Stagnation of Qi and Blood

Trauma or injury of the arm and trunk in an accident may directly cause stagnation of Qi and Blood with blockage of the channels, and so axillary pain follows.

Invasion of Toxic Heat to the channels

Invasion of Toxic Heat to the axillary fossa may be caused by a wound in the arm or in the axillary fossa. Local infection, such as eczema or folliculitis, is a common cause of such pain. Lymphangitis and mastitis can also develop into and influence the axillary glands. Herpes zoster may cause Toxic Heat to accumulate in this region. When it obstructs the Qi and Blood circulation, the pain starts with redness, swelling and tenderness in the area.

Accumulation of Damp-Heat in the locality

Pathogenic factor Damp-Heat can invade the axillary fossa through a wound. Some skin diseases, such as eczema and tinea in the axillary fossa, can cause secondary pain owing to accumulation of Damp-Heat in the area, leading to stagnation of Qi and Blood and obstruction of the channels and collateral, and so pain follows.

Treatment based on differentiation

Differentiation

Differentiation of character of the pain

— Acute and severe pain is usually caused by Excessive pathogenic factors. Mild lingering pain is often caused by deficiency of Qi and Blood.
— Pain with red, swelling, tenderness and warmth in the local region is usually caused by Heat or Toxic Heat.
— Pain with a burning sensation, swelling and deep red colour of skin indicates the presence of toxic Heat, particularly when fever and chills accompany the pain.
— Pain in the axillary fossa with a swollen arm is usually caused by accumulation of Damp and stagnation of Qi.
— Stabbing and sharp pain suggests Blood stagnation.
— Distending pain is usually caused by Qi stagnation.
— Pain in the axillary fossa, worsened by abduction of the arm and emotional upset, indicates Qi and Blood stagnation.

Differentiation of the skin lesions

— Pain, swelling and a bluish colour in the axillary fossa indicate stagnation of Qi and Blood. This is often seen in trauma.
— Red, painful and tender carbuncles or folliculitis in the axillary fossa are caused by Heat or Toxic Heat.
— If pus is formed and the skin lesion is not so red and the pain is also less heavy, this indicates accumulation of Damp-Heat.
— A very painful, red, serpiginous, vesicular eruption of skin along the intercostal nerve of the affected axillary fossa indicates Damp-Heat in the Liver channel. This is seen in herpes zoster.
— Reddish and oozing skin lesions with a burning and itchy sensation are caused by Damp-Heat, such as in eczema.
— Red, itchy, circular skin lesions, which worsen with warmth or after sweating, are caused by Wind-Damp-Heat, such as in tinea.

Treatment

STAGNATION OF QI AND BLOOD

Symptoms and signs

Pain in the axillary fossa that is worsened by abduction of the arm and emotional upset, and is sometimes stabbing, accompanied by a normal or purplish tongue with a white coating and a deep and wiry pulse.

This syndrome can be found in trauma and the remote consequences of herpes zoster.

Principle of treatment

Invigorate Qi and Blood circulation, open the channels and relieve the pain.

HERBAL TREATMENT

Prescription

FU YUAN HUO XUE TANG
Revive Health by Invigorating the Blood Decoction
Tao Ren *Semen Persicae* 9 g
Hong Hua *Flos Carthami* 9 g
Dang Gui *Radix Angelicae Sinensis* 9 g
Chuan Shan Jia *Squama Manitis* 6 g
Chai Hu *Radix Bupleuri* 6 g
Tian Hua Fen *Radix Trichosanthis* 9 g
Jiu Da Huang *Radix et Rhizoma Rhei* 6 g
Gan Cao *Radix Glycyrrhizae* 3 g
Rice wine 10–20 ml

Explanations

- Tao Ren and Hong Hua promote the Blood circulation, reduce the stagnant Blood and stop the pain.
- Dang Gui promotes the Blood circulation and tonifies the Blood.
- Chuan Shan Jia is able to open the channels and the collateral, and promote Qi movement so as to stop the pain.
- Chai Hu can disperse constrained Qi and remove stagnation of Blood; Tian Hua Fen can clear Heat produced by stagnation of Qi; Da Huang can promote the Qi and Blood circulation and remove stagnant Blood. These three herbs are specifically used to remove and dissolve stagnant Blood due to trauma.
- Gan Cao can harmonise the other herbs in the formula and protect the Stomach from the Blood-moving herbs.

- Rice wine is pungent and warm in nature and has dispersing action. It can promote the Qi and Blood circulation and enhance the function of the other herbs.

Modifications

1. If there is severe Qi stagnation, add Mu Xiang *Radix Aucklandiae* 6 g and Qing Pi *Pericarpium Citri Reticulatae Viride* 6 g to regulate the Qi and relieve the stagnation.
2. If there is severe stagnation of Blood, add Yan Hu Suo *Rhizoma Corydalis* 9 g, Ru Xiang *Resina Olibani* 9 g and Mo Yao *Resina Myrrhae* 9 g to regulate the Blood and eliminate the stasis.
3. If there is deficiency of Qi, add Huang Qi *Radix Astragali seu Hedysari* 12 g to strengthen the Qi so as to assist the Blood circulation.
4. If the pain is influenced by Cold and Wind, add Qiang Huo *Rhizoma seu Radix Notopterygii* 9 g and Gui Zhi *Ramulus Cinnamomi* 6 g to expel Wind-Cold and warm the channels.
5. If there is numbness, add Di Long *Lumbricus* 9 g and Jiang Can *Bombyx Batryticatus* 9 g to open the channels and collaterals.

Patent remedy

Yan Hu Suo Zhi Tong Pian *Corydalis Stop Pain Tablet*

ACUPUNCTURE TREATMENT

GB-22 Yuanye, GB-23 Zhejin, TE-5 Waiguan, LR-3 Taichong, LR-14 Qimen, SP-6 Sanyinjiao and SP-10 Xuehai. Reducing method is used on these points.

Explanations

- GB-22 and GB-23 open the Gall Bladder channel and stop the pain.
- TE-5, the Connecting point, LR-14, the Front Collecting point of the Liver, and LR-3, the Source point, regulate the Qi and relieve the pain.
- SP-6 and SP-10 regulate the Blood and stop the pain.

Modifications

1. If there is aggravation of pain on exposure to wind and cold, add BL-12, BL-13, BL-20 and ST-36 to strengthen the Interior and expel Wind-Cold.
2. If there is severe pain, add local Ah Shi points and PC-6 to harmonise the collateral and relieve the pain.
3. If there is pain as a consequence of herpes zoster, add PC-4 and GB-38 to relieve the pain.

INVASION OF TOXIC HEAT TO THE CHANNELS

Symptoms and signs

Pain with redness, swelling, tenderness and warmth in the locality, accompanied by chills, fever, headache, thirst, a red tongue with dry, yellow coating and a rapid and slippery pulse. This syndrome can be seen in acute lymphangitis, lymphadenitis, furuncle and folliculitis.

Principle of treatment

Reduce Fire, remove Heat Toxin and relieve the pain.

HERBAL TREATMENT

Prescription

WU WEI XIAO DU YIN
Five-Ingredient Decoction to Eliminate Toxin
Jin Yin Hua *Flos Lonicerae* 15 g
Ye Ju Hua *Flos Chrysanthemi* 15 g
Pu Gong Ying *Herba Taraxaci* 15 g
Zi Hua Di Ding *Herba Violae* 15 g
Zi Bei Tian Kui *Herba Begonia Fibristipulatae* 9 g

Explanations

These five herbs all reduce Fire and remove Toxic Heat. When the Toxic Heat is cleared and there is no disturbance of the Qi and Blood circulation, the pain disappears.

Modifications

1. If there are severe chills, fever and headache, add Huang Lian *Rhizoma Coptidis* 6 g, Huang Qin *Radix Scutellariae* 12 g, Zhi Zi *Fructus Gardeniae* 9 g and Da Qing Ye *Folium Isatidis* 12 g to clear Heat and reduce the fever.
2. If the skin is red with a burning feeling owing to disturbance of the Blood by Toxic Heat, add Zi Cao *Radix Arnebiae seu Lithospermi* 9 g, Sheng Di Huang *Radix Rehmanniae Recens* 9 g, Chi Shao *Radix Paeoniae Rubra* 9 g and Xuan Shen *Radix Scrophulariae* 9 g to cool the Blood and reduce the pain.
3. If there is severe pain, add Qing Pi *Pericarpium Citri Reticulatae Viride* 9 g and Yan Hu Suo *Rhizoma Corydalis* 9 g to regulate the Qi and Blood circulation and reduce the pain.
4. If there are hard glands and tenderness under the arm, add Xuan Shen *Radix Scrophulariae* 9 g, Mu Li *Concha Ostreae* 15 g and Zhe Bei Mu *Bulbus Fritillariae Thunbergii* 15 g to soften the hardness.

5. If there is deficiency of the Qi and Blood, add Dang Shen *Radix Codonopsis Pilosulae* 9 g, Huang Qi *Radix Astragali seu Hedysari* 12 g, Bai Shao *Radix Paeoniae Alba* 9 g and Dang Gui *Radix Angelicae Sinensis* 9 g to tonify the Qi and Blood and strengthen the body resistance.

Patent remedy

Niu Huang Jie Du Pian *Cattle Gallstone Tablet to Resolve Toxin*

ACUPUNCTURE TREATMENT

GB-22 Yuanye, GB-23 Zhejin, GB-43 Xiaxi, LR-2 Xingjian, LR-14 Qimen, ST-44 Neiting, TE-3 Zhongzhu and LI-11 Quchi. Reducing method is used in these points.

Explanations

- GB-22 and GB-23, the local points, clear obstruction in the channels and reduce the pain.
- LR-14 regulates the Liver-Qi.
- GB-43, LR-2 and SP-44, the Spring points, reduce Excess-Heat.
- TE-3 and LI-11 disperse constrained Heat so as to assist the action of other herbs in reducing Toxic Heat.

Modifications

1. If the pain is severe and the Blood is disturbed, use the Blood-letting technique on the Ah Shi points and BL-40 to reduce Heat in the Blood.
2. If there is acute mastitis, add points from the Bright Yang channels such as ST-16, ST-37, ST-40 and LI-7 to reduce the Heat and swelling.

ACCUMULATION OF DAMP-HEAT

Symptoms and signs

Pain in the axillary fossa with redness and burning feeling in the area, accompanied by oozing skin lesions, thirst, a bitter taste in the mouth, irritability, constipation, scanty urine, a red tongue with a yellow and greasy coating and a rapid and slippery pulse.

This syndrome can be seen in herpes zoster, acute eczema and furuncle with pus formation.

Principle of treatment

Clear Heat, transform Damp and relieve the pain.

HERBAL TREATMENT

Prescription

LONG DAN XIE GAN TANG
Gentianae Decoction to Drain the Liver
Long Dan Cao *Radix Gentianae* 9 g
Huang Qin *Radix Scutellariae* 9 g
Zhi Zi *Fructus Gardeniae* 9 g
Ze Xie *Rhizoma Alismatis* 9 g
Mu Tong *Caulis Akebiae* 5 g
Che Qian Zi *Semen Plantaginis* 6 g
Dang Gui *Radix Angelicae Sinensis* 6 g
Sheng Di Huang *Radix Rehmanniae Recens* 12 g
Chai Hu *Radix Bupleuri* 6 g
Gan Cao *Radix Glycyrrhizae* 6 g

Explanations

- Long Dan Cao is very bitter and Cold in nature, entering the Liver channel. It can clear Heat from the Liver as well as transform Damp so as to reduce the pain.
- Zhi Zi and Mu Tong are also bitter and Cold in nature. They enter the Heart channel, clear Heat and reduce fever directly. They can increase urination and leach out Damp-Heat so as to enhance the function of Long Dan Cao.
- Che Qian Zi and Ze Xie transform and leach out Damp. Huang Qin clears Heat from the Upper and Middle Burners. These three herbs assist Long Dan Cao in different ways.
- Chai Hu disperses constrained Fire and Qi, and prevents side-effects caused by the downward-draining herbs.
- Dang Gui and Sheng Di Huang tonify the Blood and Yin so as to reduce side-effects caused by the very bitter and Cold herbs.
- Gan Cao moderates the harsh herbs and harmonises the herbs in the formula.

Modifications

1. If there is a viral infection, add Ban Lan Gen *Radix Isatidis* 12 g and Da Qing Ye *Folium Isatidis* 12 g to clear Heat and remove Toxin.
2. If there is pain as a consequence of herpes zoster, add Bai Shao *Radix Paeoniae Alba* 9 g, Shu Di Huang *Radix Rehmanniae Praeparata* 9 g, Chuan Xiong *Rhizoma Ligustici Chuanxiong* 9 g and Mu Li Concha Ostreae 15 g to tonify the Blood, invigorate the Blood circulation and clear the obstruction.
3. If there is itching of skin lesions, add Bai Xian Pi *Cortex Dictamni Radicis* 9 g, Jing Jie *Herba Schizonepetae* 9 g and Di Fu Zi *Fructus Kochiae* 9 g to reduce the itching.

Patent remedy

Long Dan Xie Gan Wan *Gentianae Pill to Drain the Liver*

ACUPUNCTURE TREATMENT

GB-22 Yuanye, GB-23 Zhejin, GB-43 Xiaxi, LR-3 Taichong, LR-14 Qimen, TE-2 Yemen, ST-44 Neiting, SP-4 Gongsun, SP-9 Yinlingquan and SP-10 Xuehai. Reducing method is used on these points.

Explanations

- GB-22 and GB-23, the local points, open the channels.
- LR-3 and LR-14 spread Liver-Qi so as to relieve stagnation of Qi.
- TE-2, GB-43 and ST-44, the Spring points, clear Heat and reduce fever.
- SP-9, the Sea point, and SP-4, the Connecting point, remove Damp-Heat.
- SP-6 regulates the Blood circulation and stops the pain.

Modifications

1. If there is severe pain, add Ah Shi points and BL-40 to promote the Blood circulation and stop the pain.
2. If there is a bitter taste in the mouth and acid regurgitation, add GB-40 and GB-34 to spread Qi from the Lesser Yang channel and reduce constrained Heat.

Case history

A 29-year-old woman had been suffering from chronic furunculosis for 10 years under the armpits and in the groins. The big furuncles were 6 cm × 6 cm in size and the small ones were 0.5 cm × 0.5 cm. They were, in the beginning, very painful, swollen and red in colour. Sometimes she had a fever. There was hardly any time when furuncles were absent in those regions. She was often treated with antibiotics, but sometimes had to be treated by incision and drainage. She had a quite busy and stressful job, and often felt tired and sleepy, but still had a normal appetite and bowel movements. She had a red tip to her tongue, and a white, greasy and uneven coating. Her pulse was slightly soft. Under the armpits and groins, there were several tender furuncles of a dark-red colour, and the skin there was thick, dark and full of scars.

Diagnosis
Restrained Damp-Heat.

Principle of treatment
Transform Damp-Heat, disperse the restrained Qi and Heat and stop the pain.

Herbal treatment
WU WEI XIAO DU YIN
Five-Ingredient Decoction to Eliminate Toxin
Yin Hua *Flos Lonicerae* 15 g
Lian Qiao *Fructus Forsythiae* 12 g
Huang Qin *Radix Scutellariae* 12 g
Huang Bai *Cortex Phellodendri* 12 g
Pu Gong Ying *Herba Taraxaci* 15 g
Zi Hua Di Ding *Herba cum Radice Violae Yedoensitis* 12 g
Bai Zhi *Radix Angelicae Dahuricae* 6 g
Lu Gen *Rhizoma Phragmitis* 15 g
Yi Yi Ren *Semen Coicis* 15 g
Chi Shao *Radix Paeoniae Rubrae* 12 g
Bai Zhu *Rhizoma Atractylodis Macrocephalae* 15 g
Xiang Fu *Rhizoma Cyperi* 12 g

Explanations

- In the 'Yellow Emperor's Classic of Internal Medicine', it indicates that 'almost all painful and swelling skin disorders were linked with Heart-Fire'. This syndrome started with excess Toxic Heat; after many courses of antibiotics it became more complicated. Since antibiotics are considered in TCM to be very bitter and Cold, they can powerfully reduce Heat in the body. However, since the pathogenic Heat is also very powerful, it should be eliminated instead of being simply restrained by antibiotics. If antibiotics are used for too long, they may injure the Spleen and Stomach, causing Damp to form, and when this accumulates in the body and mixes with Heat, the antibiotics fail to eliminate the pathogens completely.
- In this formula, the many pungent and Cold herbs, such as Yin Hua, Lian Qiao, Bai Zhi and Chi Shao, disperse and clear the restrained Qi and Heat.
- Huang Qin and Huang Bai clear Heat and dry Damp.
- Pu Gong Ying and Zi Hua Di Ding specifically clear Toxic Heat.
- Bai Zhi, Lu Gen and Yi Yi Ren transform Damp and eliminate the pus.
- Chi Shao regulates Blood circulation, clears Heat in the Blood, reduces the swelling and stops the pain.
- Bai Zhu tonifies the Spleen-Qi and dries Damp in the Middle Burner.
- Xiang Fu regulates the Qi circulation in the Triple Burner channel.

After using the herbs for 14 days, no new furuncles had formed in the area. The skin colour had also improved. The patient continued with herbs for another 6 weeks in order to enhance the effect of dispersing the restrained Qi and Heat; the formula was changed slightly to include Chai Hu *Radix Bupleuri* 6 g and Shi Gao *Gypsum* 15 g, and omit Bai Zhi and Yi Yi Ren, as there was no more pus and no new furuncles. The patient was followed up 6 months later and she said she had experienced no new furuncles or pain in those regions since the treatment.

Epigastric pain 25

胃
脘
疼
痛

Epigastric pain includes pain occurring under the xiphoid and between the costal arches. According to TCM, epigastric pain is mostly classified as a disorder of Stomach, often caused by invasion of External factors such as Cold, Damp and Heat. Internal factors include weakness of the Internal organs, mental disorders and stress. Other causative factors include bad diet and eating habits, and trauma.

Epigastric pain may be attributed to any of the following diseases in Western medicine: acute or chronic gastritis, gastrospasm, gastrointestinal dyspepsia, gastroneurosis, hyperchlorhydria, gastric ulcer, duodenal ulcer, hepatitis and carcinoma of the stomach. (Epigastric pain caused by acute perforation of gastroduodenal ulcer, gastric bleeding and carcinoma of the stomach is not discussed here.)

Aetiology and pathology

The Stomach is one of the Fu organs. Since, according to TCM theory, it receives and ripens the food, it should be full of Qi and Blood to perform this function, so it is regarded as a Yang organ, the source of Qi and Blood generation in the body. The Stomach and Spleen have an external–internal relationship; the Stomach-Qi descends and transports the ripe food to the Spleen, and the Spleen transforms it into Nutritive Essence, Qi and Blood. When the Spleen-Qi ascends, the Nutritive Essence is transported to the whole body to support the functions of different organs. Because the function of Spleen and Stomach determines the health of a person, they are called the 'foundation of life after birth'.

In pathological conditions, because the Stomach is the first stop of food and drinks in the body and it opens to the external environment, it is easily injured by External pathogenic factors and unhealthy diets and drink. It is also easily influenced by the Liver; stress and emotional disturbance can cause stagnation of the Liver-Qi, which can influence the Stomach. Any factor that disturbs the movement of Qi in the Stomach, the Middle Burner, and disturbs the balance of Yin and Yang of the Stomach, can cause epigastric pain.

Invasion of Exogenous pathogenic factors

The Exogenous pathogenic Cold, Heat and Damp-Heat are common causes of epigastric pain. The Stomach channel and organ are mainly involved in these conditions.

Cold can invade the Stomach if cold drinks or raw and cold food are eaten frequently (see next section). It can also invade the Stomach if there is improper breathing. Since it can contract the muscles, tendons, channels, and obstruct the Qi and Blood, the pain may start in the epigastric region. Some medicine or herbs of a Cold nature can also injure the Stomach if they are used improperly.

Heat can invade the Stomach if there is over-consumption of spicy food, or heating drinks (see next section). Heat can also disturb the Stomach in certain stages of febrile diseases. Some medicines of a hot nature can also act as a Heat factor, disturbing the Stomach if the dosage is too large or they are used for too long. Because Heat can consume the Body Fluids and the Yin, the channels and organs will fail to be properly nourished, the movement of Qi and Blood will be slower than normal, and epigastric pain follows.

Damp-Heat can also invade the Stomach because of a bad diet. Greasy food, milk products and alcohol can directly generate Damp-Heat. Eating of unhygienic or rotten food may cause Damp-Heat to form in the Middle Burner, which is seen in cases of acute gastritis, dysentery and influenza.

Improper diet and eating habits

Different tastes and quality of the food may influence the Qi and Blood in the Middle Burner. A good meal should be balanced, being moderate in terms of its taste, nature, quality and quantity. This is the basic principle of Chinese diet. If the food and drink that is consumed is in some way unbalanced, it may cause epigastric pain.

Most spicy food, such as of hot pepper, spices, onion and garlic, may produce Heat, and further consume Yin and Body Fluid. Coffee and alcohol have the same action. When the Stomach is not properly nourished, the Qi and Blood move more slowly, which can cause pain in the epigastrium.

Cold drinks and food, such as raw vegetables and fruits, may injure the Qi and Yang if they are consumed habitually. Cold obstructs the Qi, blocks the Blood circulation and also causes pain. Milk products and sweet and greasy food may easily generate Damp, and often Damp-Heat. Damp-Heat also obstructs the Qi movement in the Middle Burner and causes epigastric pain.

Sour, salty and bitter foods can injure the Yin of the body if they are eaten habitually. Food like glutinous rice, maize, sorghum and millet as well as brown bread, although containing essential nutrients and good for constipation, are not easy to digest, especially for people who have a weak Stomach or Spleen. They may injure the Qi and cause Qi stagnation and epigastric pain.

Eating habits also directly influence the function of the Stomach. For instance, eating hot food followed by cold food or drinks, or eating several kinds of food with different tastes or qualities either together or within in a short time, may burden the Stomach and Spleen, which may injure the Stomach-Qi and also cause Qi stagnation, and in the long run the Yang of Stomach and Spleen will be injured, causing epigastric pain.

Eating too much at one time, such as when on holiday or attending a party, may cause food stagnation, which may generate Damp-Heat and obstruct the movement of Qi and Blood. Similarly, eating too little, such as on extreme weight-loss diets, may first generate Heat then over a longer period may weaken the Qi and Yang in the Middle Burner, so the Stomach is not supported by the Qi, Yin and Yang. Eating a large amount of food that is not very nutritious, for instance when on some vegetarian diets or slimming diet, may weaken the Spleen-Qi causing Damp to accumulate. In the long run, this weakens the Yang of the Spleen and Stomach. All these conditions can cause epigastric pain.

Moreover, eating food irregularly instead of three meals a day may over a long period of time weaken the Stomach-Qi. Skipping breakfast may weaken the Spleen-Qi, causing deficiency of Qi and Blood, while skipping lunch may over time generate Stomach-Heat, causing deficiency of Yin and Qi, and skipping dinner or eating too late in the day may over time consume the Yin of the Stomach, leading to deficiency of Stomach-Yin. Constant nibbling may disturb the normal functions of the Stomach and intestine, causing Qi stagnation and Damp accumulation, resulting in deficiency of Stomach-Qi. Changing one's diet too quickly or too frequently—for instance, going to boarding school, living alone, going on frequent trips whether on business or vacation to other countries, or trying different diets to lose weight—may also weaken the Qi of the Stomach and Spleen. These conditions can also all cause epigastric pain.

Eating too quickly may cause extra work for the Stomach, and lead to stagnation of Qi, weakening the Qi of Stomach and Spleen. Eating while working, reading, studying, watching TV or engaged in discussion may cause stagnation of the Qi of Spleen and Liver. Eating under stress or emotional disturbance, such as when fearful, angry, sad, anxious or pondering over problems, may also cause the same type of stagnation. These habits all lead to poor digestion and eventually can cause epigastric pain as the Liver-Qi eventually overcontrols the Stomach, triggering pain.

Emotional disturbance

Of the seven emotions, anger and worry directly influent the function of Stomach and Spleen and can cause epigastric pain. Prolonged anger, frustration, indignation, animosity, a sense of being insulted and resentment may cause stagnation of Liver-Qi, which then overcontrols the Stomach and Spleen according to the Five Element theory. As soon as the Stomach-Qi is obstructed, and is not able to descend, epigastric pain starts together with a sensation of fullness and nausea. Pensiveness, worry and inability to make up one's mind may also cause stagnation of Liver-Qi, weakening the transportation and transformation functions of the Spleen and Stomach, causing accumulation of food and consequently epigastric pain.

Stagnation of Blood

Trauma, operation, adhesions or a chronic disorder of the Stomach may lead to stagnation of Qi and Blood; when the channels are obstructed, epigastric pain appears.

Weakness of Qi of Spleen and Stomach

A weak constitution, acute or chronic disease, a bad diet or dietary habits, or taking the wrong medicines may cause deficiency and stagnation of Qi in the Middle Burner, and trigger epigastric pain.

Weakness of Qi and Blood

Poor constitution, eating irregularly for a long time, or following a diet with a low nutritional value may cause deficiency of the Qi and Blood, and weakness of the muscles and the body in general. When the Stomach is too weak to digest heavy food, epigastric pain may follow.

Weakness of Stomach-Yin

The Stomach is a Yang organ, being full of Qi and Blood. It tends to generate Heat during the process of ripening food, and this Heat can consume the Body Fluids and cause deficiency of Yin. Prolonged overindulgence in spicy food, alcohol or coffee may also cause deficiency of Stomach-Yin. When the channel is not properly nourished, epigastric pain may occur.

Weakness of Stomach-Yang

Deficiency of the Stomach-Yang develops from the above stages of deficiency of the Qi and Blood, and deficiency of the Stomach-Yin. A weak constitution, chronic digestive disease, a bad diet over a long term, taking the wrong medicines, overdosage or long-term use of herbs or medicines of a Cold nature also cause deficiency of the Stomach-Yang. When the Yang is not able to warm the Stomach, the function of the organ is greatly impeded, the Qi stagnates, the food accumulates, the channel is contracted, the Blood circulation is obstructed, and epigastric pain follows.

Treatment based on differentiation

Differentiation

Differentiation of location

Before giving treatment, it is important to differentiate epigastric pain clearly from the pain accompanying other similar syndromes, such as true Heart pain, hypochondriac pain and abdominal pain. It is particularly important to ensure that the epigastric pain is not caused by a disorder of the liver, gall bladder or heart.

— Epigastric pain is located in the epigastric region, and starts in this region, though it may radiate to or influence the hypochondriac region, chest or abdomen.
— 'True heart pain' includes angina pectoris and myocardial infarction. This pain can radiate to the stomach region, neck, or upper back, but it is mainly in the chest, is pressing in nature, accompanied by breathlessness, cold extremities and a heavy cold sweat.
— Hypochondriac pain results from disorders of the Liver and Gall Bladder (in both Western and TCM terminology). These include hepatitis, early stages of cirrhosis of the liver, cholecystitis, cholelithiasis and angiocholitis. The pain is largely in the hypochondrium. If the Liver-Qi attacks the Stomach, the pain is in both the epigastric and hypochondriac regions, but the hypochondriac pain, which is influenced by emotions, is the chief location, while the epigastric pain is secondary.
— Abdominal pain is centred over the abdomen and, in most cases, is caused by a disorder of the Spleen, Small and Large Intestine or Liver. Since the Stomach, Small and Large Intestine and Spleen work together in the process of digestion, disorders of the abdomen often influence the Stomach as well. In this case, there may be both a pain in the abdomen and a disorder of bowel movement.

Differentiation of Excess and Deficiency

— Before the treatment is applied, it is also important to differentiate between Excess and Deficiency syndromes.
— Excess syndrome is characterised by acute, severe pain and a short history of the disorder.
— Deficiency syndrome is characterised by milder, lingering pain, with a long history of the disorder and a recurrent nature.

Treatment

In some acute conditions, such as gastric bleeding and acute perforation of gastroduodenal ulcer, TCM treatment of epigastric pain should be combined with Western medical treatment. The general principle of treatment is to regulate the Qi and harmonise the Stomach so as to relieve the pain, reducing the Excess or tonifying the weakness to treat the root, and stopping pain to treat the manifestations. Since the Stomach is the first stop of the herbs in the treatment, a proper treatment often brings an effective result in a short time. However, patients may also have to modify any bad diets or dietary habits and reduce stress so as to maintain the condition. Moreover, it is also important to select herbs that will not place any extra burden or irritation on the stomach.

EXCESS SYNDROMES

INVASION OF COLD TO THE STOMACH

Symptoms and signs

Sudden epigastric pain of a cramping nature, with a sensation of pressure and heaviness, accompanied by a preference for warm drinks, a white tongue coating and a wiry and forceful pulse.

This syndrome can be seen in acute gastritis or after excessive consumption of cold food and drinks.

Principle of treatment

Expel the Cold, regulate the Qi in the Stomach and stop the pain.

HERBAL TREATMENT

Prescription

LIANG FU WAN
Galangal and Cyperus Pill
Gao Liang Jiang *Rhizoma Alpiniae Officinarum* 9 g
Xiang Fu *Rhizoma Cyperi* 9 g

Explanations

● This is a syndrome in which External Cold invades the Stomach, causing contraction of the Stomach channel and obstruction of Qi and the Blood, so epigastric pain follows.
● Gao Liang Jiang, very pungent and warm in nature, specifically enters the Stomach channel. It can effectively expel the Cold in the Stomach and relieve cramp.
● Xiang Fu can promote the Qi circulation in the Stomach and Liver channels so as to stop the pain. It also relieves the anxiety caused by the pain.
● This simple but effective formula is particularly useful after excessive consumption of cold food and drink.

Modifications

1. If the pain is not severe and is caused by excessive consumption of cold drinks, use Sheng Jiang *Rhizoma Zingiberis* 6 g, brown sugar 6 g with 200 ml water. Cook them together for 10 minutes, then drink the liquid slowly.
2. If there is External Wind-Cold syndrome, add Zi Su Ye *Folium Perillae* 9 g to expel the Wind-Cold, Chen Pi *Pericarpium Citri Reticulatae* 9 g and Zhi Gan Cao *Radix Glycyrrhizae Praeparata* 6 g to harmonise the Stomach-Qi.
3. If there is vomiting, add Ban Xia *Radix Pinelliae* 9 g to cause the Stomach-Qi to descend and relieve the vomiting.
4. If the pain is fixed and heavy, add Yan Hu Suo *Rhizoma Corydalis* 9 g to promote the Qi and Blood circulation and stop the pain.
5. If the Cold in the Stomach is severe and the cramp is obvious, add Wu Zhu Yu *Fructus Evodiae* 6 g to expel the Cold and warm the Stomach.
6. If the pain is caused by emotional disturbance, add Chai Hu *Radix Bupleuri* 6 g and Mu Xiang *Radix Aucklandiae* 6 g to regulate the Liver-Qi.

ACUPUNCTURE TREATMENT

CV-12 Zhongwan, ST-36 Zusanli, SP-4 Gongsun and PC-6 Neiguan. Even method is used on these points.

Explanations

● CV-12 is the Front Collecting point of the Stomach and ST-36 is the Lower Sea point of the Stomach. These two points are used in combination to clear obstruction in the Stomach channel, expel the Cold and stop the pain.

- PC-6 and SP-4 are the Confluence points, being able to clear Qi obstruction in the chest and Stomach and stop the pain.

Modifications

1. If the Cold is severe, apply moxibustion on CV-12 and PC-6 to expel the Cold and warm the Interior.
2. If the pain is severe and leading to restlessness, add LR-3, the Source point, and GB-20, to disperse the Liver-Qi so as to relieve the pain and calm the Mind.

INVASION OF COLD-DAMP

Symptoms and signs

Acute onset of stomach pain with nausea and vomiting, a feeling of fullness in the epigastric region, fever, chills, generalised pain, a white and sticky tongue coating and a soft pulse.

This syndrome can be seen in acute gastritis, influenza, incorrect use or side-effects of some medicines, and excessive consumption of cold food and drinks.

Principle of treatment

Expel the Cold, transform the Damp, regulate the Qi in the Middle Burner and stop the pain.

HERBAL TREATMENT

Prescription

HUO XIANG ZHENG QI SAN
Agastache Upright Qi Powder
Huo Xiang *Herba Agastachis* 9 g
Zi Su Ye *Folium Perillae* 6 g
Bai Zhi *Radix Angelicae Dahuricae* 6 g
Jie Geng *Radix Platycodi* 6 g
Chen Pi *Pericarpium Citri Reticulatae* 9 g
Ban Xia *Rhizoma Pinelliae* 6 g
Hou Po *Cortex Magnoliae Officinalis* 6 g
Da Fu Pi *Pericarpium Arecae* 9 g
Fu Ling *Poria* 12 g
Gan Cao *Radix Glycyrrhizae* 6 g
Da Zao *Fructus Ziziphi Jujubae* 6 g
Sheng Jiang *Rhizoma Zingiberis Recens* 6 g

Explanations

- This is a syndrome in which External Cold-Damp invades the Exterior of the body and the Middle Burner, disturbing the descent of the Stomach-Qi and the ascent of the Spleen-Qi. Huo Xiang and Zi Su Ye are warm and aromatic herbs, expelling the Wind-Cold and releasing the Exterior. They can smooth the Stomach-Qi and also eliminate the Cold-Damp from the Middle Burner.
- Bai Zhi and Jie Geng enhance the action of above two herbs to expel the Wind-Cold.
- Chen Pi and Ban Xia smooth the Stomach-Qi, transform the Phlegm and stop vomiting.
- Hou Po and Da Fu Pi regulate the Qi in the Stomach and abdomen, treating fullness of the Stomach and distension in the abdomen.
- Fu Ling tonifies the Spleen and transforms the Damp, treating the source of the Damp-Cold.
- Sheng Jiang, Da Zao and Gan Cao are able to strengthen the Middle Burner.
- As soon as the Exterior syndrome is treated, Cold-Damp is transformed from the Middle Burner and the epigastric pain disappears.

Modifications

1. If there is severe epigastric pain due to the Cold invasion, add Gao Liang Jiang *Rhizoma Alpiniae Officinarum* 9 g and Xiang Fu *Rhizoma Cyperi* 9 g to warm the Stomach and spread the Qi so as to relieve the pain.
2. If there is diarrhoea, add Gan Jiang *Rhizoma Zingiberis* 9 g to warm the Spleen and stop the diarrhoea.
3. If there is severe vomiting, add Wu Zhu Yu *Fructus Evodiae* 6 g to cause the Stomach-Qi to descend and relieve the vomiting.

ACUPUNCTURE TREATMENT

CV-12 Zhongwan, LI-4 Hegu, TE-5 Waiguan, ST-36 Zusanli and SP-3 Taibai. Reducing method is used on the first three points; even method is used on the last two points.

Explanations

- CV-12, the Front Collecting point of the Stomach, and ST-36, the Lower Sea point of the Stomach, can regulate the Stomach-Qi, expel the Cold and stop the pain.
- LI-4, the Source point of Large Intestine, TE-5, the Connecting point of the Triple Burner, can expel the Cold from Exterior and treat the Exterior symptoms.
- SP-3, the Source point, can strengthen the Spleen and transform the Damp in the Middle Burner so as to harmonise the Stomach.

Modifications

1. If there is vomiting, apply indirect moxibustion with ginger on CV-8, to transform the Damp and warm the Middle Burner.
2. If there is diarrhoea, add SP-9 to activate the Spleen and relieve the diarrhoea.
3. If there is severe epigastric pain add ST-34, the Accumulation point, to harmonise the collateral and stop the pain.

Case history

A 41-year-old woman complained of epigastric pain after consuming too much cold food and drink the day before. The pain was constant, with a cramping nature and distension. She also had diarrhoea about five times a day. Her tongue coating was white and her pulse was soft and slightly superficial.

Diagnosis
Invasion of Cold-Damp to the Stomach.

Principle of treatment
Eliminate Damp, harmonise the Middle Burner and stop the pain.

Herbal treatment
HUO XIANG ZHENG QI SAN
Agastache Upright Qi Powder
Huo Xiang *Herba Agastachis* 9 g
Zi Su Ye *Folium Perillae* 6 g
Bai Zhi *Radix Angelicae Dahuricae* 6 g
Gan Jiang *Rhizoma Zingiberis* 6 g
Chen Pi *Pericarpium Citri Reticulatae* 9 g
Ban Xia *Rhizoma Pinelliae* 6 g
Hou Po *Cortex Magnoliae Officinalis* 6 g
Da Fu Pi *Pericarpium Arecae* 9 g
Fu Ling *Poria* 12 g
Gan Cao *Radix Glycyrrhizae* 6 g

Explanations
This formula can expel the Wind-Cold from the Exterior and transform the Cold-Damp from the Middle Burner so as to restore the function of the Stomach and Spleen, and stop the pain.

After taking the herbs for only 1 day, the patient found the pain and diarrhoea had disappeared. She was followed up 6 months later and she said she had experienced no pain after the herbal treatment.

STAGNATION OF FOOD

Symptoms and signs

Epigastric pain with full and distending sensation, belching with a foul smell, vomiting, which can reduce the pain, a normal or slightly red tongue with a sticky coating and a wiry, slippery pulse.

This syndrome often happens after overeating, a change of diet or poor digestion when under stress.

Principle of treatment

Promote digestion, regulate the Qi of the Stomach and Liver and stop the pain.

HERBAL TREATMENT

Prescription

BAO HE WAN
Preserving and Harmonising Pill
Jiao Mai Ya *Fructus Hordei Germinatus* 9 g
Jiao Shen Qu *Massa Fermentata Medicinalis* 9 g
Jiao Shan Zha *Fructus Crataegi* 9 g
Ban Xia *Rhizoma Pinelliae* 9 g
Chen Pi *Pericarpium Citri Reticulatae* 9 g
Fu Ling *Poria* 12 g
Lai Fu Zi *Semen Raphani* 6 g
Lian Qiao *Fructus Forsythiae* 6 g

Explanations

- Epigastric pain in this syndrome is caused by overeating with retention of food in the Stomach, leading to obstruction of Qi movement in the Middle Burner.
- Jiao Mai Ya, Jiao Shen Qu and Jiao Shan Zha promote the digestion of wheat, alcohol and meat respectively.
- Ban Xia and Chen Pi cause the Stomach-Qi to descend and relieve nausea and vomiting. These two herbs also regulate the Qi in the Stomach so as to promote digestion.
- Fu Ling tonifies the Spleen, and together with Chen Pi and Ban Xia removes the Phlegm in the Middle Burner that is produced by food stagnation.
- Lai Fu Zi enters the Large Intestine channel, promotes the transportation of the Fu organs, causes the Qi to descend, reduces fullness in the Stomach and abdomen and treats constipation.
- Lian Qiao, a Cold and aromatic herb, can clear the Heat generated by food stagnation. When the undigested food is removed and the Qi moves freely in the Middle Burner, the epigastric pain disappears.

Modifications

1. If there are external symptoms, add Zi Su Ye *Folium Perillae* 9 g and Huo Xiang *Herba Agastachis* 9 g to expel the Wind-Cold and also cause the Stomach-Qi to descend.

2. If there is vomiting, add Zhu Ru *Caulis Bambusae in Taeniam* 9 g and Huang Qin *Radix Scutellariae* 12 g together with Ban Xia *Rhizoma Pinelliae* 9 g to cause the Stomach-Qi to descend and transform the Phlegm in the Stomach.

3. If there is constipation, add Zhi Shi *Fructus Aurantii Immaturus* 12 g to promote bowel movement.

4. If there is abdominal pain and distension, add Mu Xiang *Radix Aucklandiae* 6 g together with Hou Po *Cortex Magnoliae Officinalis* 6 g to regulate the Qi in the intestine and stop the pain.

5. If there is food stagnation due to anger, stress or frustration, add Xiang Fu *Rhizoma Cyperi* 12 g, Chai Hu *Radix Bupleuri* 9 g and Huang Qin *Radix Scutellariae* 12 g to disperse the Liver-Qi and harmonise the Stomach so as to assist the digestion.

6. If there is food stagnation due to emotional distress, such as fear, sorrow or loneliness, add Zi Su Ye *Folium Perillae* 9 g and Zhi Qiao *Fructus Aurantii* 9 g to disperse the stagnation. Also Zhu Ru *Caulis Bambusae in Taeniam* 12 g to smooth the Stomach-Qi; add Dang Shen *Radix Codonopsis Pilosulae* 9 g, Mai Dong *Radix Ophiopogonis* 12 g and Bai He *Bulbus Lilii* 15 g to strengthen the Qi in the Heart and Lung so as to treat depression.

ACUPUNCTURE TREATMENT

CV-12 Zhongwan, ST-36 Zusanli, BL-21 Weishu, ST-25 Tianshu and PC-6 Neiguan. Reducing method is used on these points.

Explanations

- CV-12, the Front Collecting point of the Stomach and the Gathering point for the Fu organs, can transport the food and promote digestion. ST-36, the Lower Sea point of the Stomach, can strengthen the function of the Spleen and Stomach, promote digestion and reduce food stagnation. These two points can regulate the Stomach-Qi and stop epigastric pain.
- BL-21, the Back Transporting point of the Stomach, is used together with CV-12 to regulate the Stomach-Qi.
- ST-25, the Front Collecting point of the Large Intestine, regulates the Qi in the Large Intestine and reduces food stagnation.
- PC-6, the Confluence point of the Yin Linking Vessel and the Connecting point, can smooth the Stomach-Qi and relieve pain. It can also disperse the Qi in the chest and release emotional distress.

Modifications

1. If there are Exterior symptoms, add LI-4 and TE-5 to expel the Wind and release the Exterior symptoms.
2. If stress is involved, add LR-3, the Source point, and GB-34, the Lower Sea point of the Gall Bladder, to disperse the Liver-Qi and promote digestion.
3. If there is depression, add CV-17, the Gathering point for the Qi, LU-7, the Connecting point of the Lung, and LI-4, the Source point of the Large Intestine, to regulate the Lung-Qi, disperse the restrained Qi and promote digestion.

DISHARMONY BETWEEN THE LIVER AND STOMACH

Symptoms and signs

Epigastric pain with a distending sensation and belching, which starts or gets worse in times of stress or emotional disturbance, distension and pain in the hypochondriac region, irregular bowel movement, a white, thin tongue coating and a wiry pulse.

This syndrome can be seen in chronic gastritis, gastroduodenal ulcer, gastroneurosis and Stomach cancer.

Principle of treatment

Disperse the Liver-Qi and harmonise the Liver and the Stomach.

HERBAL TREATMENT

Prescription

CHAI HU SHU GAN SAN
Bupleurum Soothing the Liver Powder
Chai Hu *Radix Bupleuri* 6 g
Xiang Fu *Rhizoma Cyperi* 9 g
Zhi Qiao *Fructus Aurantii* 6 g
Chuan Xiong *Rhizoma Ligustici Chuanxiong* 6 g
Bai Shao *Radix Paeoniae Alba* 9 g
Zhi Gan Cao *Radix Glycyrrhizae Praeparata* 3 g

Explanations

- Chai Hu and Xiang Fu spread the Liver-Qi.
- Zhi Ke unblocks the chest and regulates the Stomach-Qi.
- Chuan Xiong invigorates the Blood. It can also regulate the Qi circulation together with Chai Hu and Xiang Fu.
- Bai Shao can nourish the Yin and Blood of the Liver. It can also harmonise the Liver together with Zhi Gan Cao so as to stop the pain.

Modifications

1. If there is obvious stagnation of the Liver-Qi add Qing Pi *Pericarpium Citri Reticulatae Viride* 9 g and Chuan Lian Zi *Fructus Meliae Toosendan* 9 g to promote circulation of the Liver-Qi, clear the obstruction and stop the pain.
2. If there is occasional stabbing pain due to Blood stagnation, add Yan Hu Suo *Rhizoma Corydalis* 9 g and Dan Shen *Radix Salviae Miltiorrhizae* 9 g to regulate the Blood circulation and stop the pain.
3. If there is belching, add Chen Xiang *Lignum Aquilariae Resinatum* 3 g and Zhu Ru *Caulis Bambusae in Taeniam* 9 g to cause the Stomach-Qi to descend and relieve the belching.
4. If there is vomiting due to accumulation of Phlegm and ascent of Stomach-Qi, add Zhu Ru *Caulis Bambusae in Taeniam* 9 g and Ban Xia *Rhizoma Pinelliae* 9 g to eliminate the Phlegm and cause the Stomach-Qi to descend.
5. If the appetite is poor, add Bai Zhu *Rhizoma Atractylodis* 12 g and Fu Ling *Poria* 12 g to strengthen the Stomach and Spleen and promote digestion.
6. If there is overeating when under stress, add Fu Ling *Poria* 15 g and Bai Zhu *Rhizoma Atractylodis* 12 g to strengthen the Middle Burner; increase the dosage of Xiang Fu *Rhizoma Cyperi* 12 g, Bai Shao *Radix Paeoniae Alba* 12 g and Zhi Gan Cao *Radix Glycyrrhizae Praeparata* 9 g to moderate the Liver-Qi.
7. If there is abdominal pain with distension, add Mu Xiang *Radix Aucklandiae* 6 g and Hou Po *Cortex Magnoliae Officinalis* 6 g to regulate the Qi in the intestine and relieve the abdominal distension.

ACUPUNCTURE TREATMENT

ST-36 Zusanli, CV-12 Zhongwan, PC-6 Neiguan, BL-18 Ganshu, LR-14 Qimen, LR-3 Taichong and GB-34 Yanglingquan. Even method is applied on ST-36; reducing method is used on the rest of the points.

Explanations

- ST-36 and CV-12 are able to strengthen the Spleen, regulate the Stomach and promote digestion.
- PC-6, the Confluence point, is used to regulate the Qi in the chest and epigastric region, and treat the pain and emotional disturbance.
- BL-18 and LR-14, the Back Transporting point and the Front Collecting point of the Liver, are used to regulate the Liver-Qi and harmonise the function of the Liver and Stomach.
- LR-3, the Source point, and GB-34, the Lower Sea point, can disperse the Liver-Qi and reduce Qi stagnation so as to harmonise the Liver and Stomach.

Modifications

1. If there is a sensation of fullness in the Stomach, add BL-21, the Back Transporting point of the Stomach, and SP-4, the Confluence point of the Penetrating Vessel, to promote digestion and reduce the pain and distension.
2. If there is severe acid regurgitation and belching, add BL-19, the Back Transporting point of the Gall Bladder, and GB-40, the Source point, to regulate the Qi and reduce Heat in the Lesser Yang Fu organs.

Case history

A 29-year-old woman had been suffering from epigastric pain for 2 months. The pain radiated to the hypochondriac region, and worsened under stress. She also had a sensation of fullness in the chest, irritability and a poor appetite. Her tongue colour was normal with a white coating, and her pulse was wiry and slippery.

Diagnosis
Disharmony between the Liver and Stomach.

Principle of treatment
Smooth the Liver, promote the Liver-Qi circulation and harmonise the Stomach.

Acupuncture treatment
CV-12, PC-6, ST-36, LI-4 and LR-3. Reducing method was used on these points.

Explanations

- CV-12, the Front Collecting point of the Stomach, harmonises the Stomach-Qi and regulates the Qi in the Middle Burner. PC-6, the Connecting point, regulates the Qi in the Stomach and calms the Mind. ST-36 is the Lower Sea point and LI-4 is the Source point. They can strengthen the transportation and transformation function of the Spleen and the Stomach. When these four points are used together, the Qi in the Middle Burner is regulated and the pain can be reduced.
- LR-3 can regulate the Liver-Qi so as to rebuild the balance between the Liver and the Stomach.

After four treatments, the pain was under control. She was followed up by letter a year later. She replied that she had experienced no pain since the treatment.

LIVER-FIRE ATTACKING THE STOMACH

Symptoms and signs

A pressing epigastric pain with a burning sensation, accompanied by irritability, a bitter taste in the mouth, acid regurgitation, a preference for cold drinks, constipation and scanty urine, a red tongue with yellow coating and a wiry, rapid pulse.

This syndrome is often seen in acute and chronic gastric ulcer or duodenal ulcer.

Principle of treatment

Smooth the Liver, reduce Liver-Fire and harmonise the Stomach.

HERBAL TREATMENT

Prescription

ZUO JIN WAN and **HUA GAN JIAN**
Restoring the Left Pill and *Canopy Pill*
Huang Lian *Rhizoma Coptidis* 6 g
Wu Zhu Yu *Fructus Evodiae* 1 g
Qing Pi *Pericarpium Citri Reticulatae Viride* 6 g
Chen Pi *Pericarpium Citri Reticulatae* 9 g
Chi Shao Yao *Radix Paeoniae Rubrae* 9 g
Mu Dan Pi *Cortex Moutan Radicis* 9 g
Zhi Zi *Fructus Gardeniae* 9 g
Zhe Bei Mu *Bulbus Fritillariae Thunbergii* 9 g
Ze Xie *Rhizoma Alismatis* 9 g

Explanations

- This is a syndrome in which Liver-Fire attacks the Stomach, obstructing the Stomach-Qi. Huang Lian, very bitter and Cold in nature, can directly reduce the Liver-Fire. Since it also enters the Heart and Stomach channel, it can also clear the Heat in the Heart and Stomach, treating stomach pain, acid regurgitation, irritability, thirst and a desire for cold drinks.
- Wu Zhu Yu is a very pungent and Hot herb, but is used in a very small dosage for Excessive-Heat syndrome as it enters the Liver channel, disperses the restrained Fire and promotes the circulation of Liver-Qi. It can also cause the Stomach-Qi to descend and assist Huang Lian to treat nausea and vomiting.
- Qing Pi disperses the Liver-Qi and Chen Pi regulates the Stomach-Qi.
- Chi Shao and Dan Pi cool the Blood and invigorate the Blood circulation so as to avoid Blood stagnation caused by Excessive-Heat.

- Zhi Zi clears Heat in the Triple Burner, and together with Ze Xie regulates the water passage and leaches out Heat by increasing urination.
- Zhe Bei Mu can disperse restrained Heat and clear obstruction.
- As soon as the Fire is removed and Liver-Qi and the Stomach-Qi are harmonised, the pain will disappear.

Modifications

1. If there is obvious irritability, add Dan Shen *Radix Salviae Miltiorrhizae* 12 g to clear Heat in the chest and relieve the irritability.
2. If there is acid regurgitation, add Wa Leng Zi *Concha Arcae* 15 g to reduce the acid.
3. If there is an obvious thirst, dry and bitter in the mouth, add Shi Gao *Gypsum Fibrosum* 15 g to clear Stomach-Heat, and Chuan Lian Zi *Fructus Meliae Toosendan* 9 g to clear and drain Liver-Heat.
4. If there is constipation, add Da Huang *Radix et Rhizoma Rhei* 6 g and Zhi Shi *Fructus Aurantii Immaturus* 12 g to promote bowel movement and clear Heat.
5. If there is vomiting, add Zhu Ru *Caulis Bambusae in Taeniam* 9 g to cause the Stomach-Qi to descend and clear Stomach-Heat.
6. If there is food stagnation, add Jiao Mai Ya *Fructus Hordei Germinatus* 9 g, Jiao Shen Qu *Massa Fermentata* 9 g and Jiao Shan Zha *Fructus Crataegi* 9 g to promote digestion and relieve the food stagnation.
7. If there is obvious depression or stress, add Xiang Yuan *Fructus Citri* 9 g and Fo Shou *Fructus Citri Sarcodactylis* 9 g to gently disperse the Liver-Qi without injuring the Yin and Qi of the Liver.
8. If there is obvious restrained Heat in the Liver, add Chuan Lian Zi *Fructus Meliae Toosendan* 9 g to drain the Heat and disperse the Liver-Qi.
9. If the pain refers to the hypochondriac region, add Yu Jin *Radix Curcumae* 12 g and Qing Pi *Pericarpium Citri Reticulatae Viride* 9 g to regulate the Blood and Qi in the Liver.
10. If there is gastric bleeding, add Da Huang *Radix et Rhizoma Rhei* 9 g, Huang Lian *Rhizoma Coptidis* 9 g and Huang Qin *Radix Scutellariae* 12 g to clear Heat, and San Qi *Radix Notoginseng* 12 g and Bai Ji *Rhizoma Bletillae* 12 g to stop the bleeding.

ACUPUNCTURE TREATMENT

PC-6 Neiguan, ST-36 Zusanli, CV-12 Zhongwan, LI-4 Hegu, GB-34 Yanglingquan, GB-43 Xiaxi, LR-2 Xingjian and ST-44 Neiting. Reducing method is used on these points.

Explanations

- PC-6, the Connecting point and Confluence point, can regulate the Qi, clear Heat in the chest and epigastric region and stop the pain there. It can also calm the Mind and treat emotional disturbance.
- ST-36, CV-12 and LI-4 are able to strengthen the Stomach and the Spleen, promote digestion, relieve Qi stagnation and stop the pain.
- GB-34 can promote circulation of the Liver-Qi so as to reduce Liver-Fire.
- LR-2, GB-43 and ST-44, the Spring points, can directly reduce Fire in the Liver and Stomach, treat acid regurgitation, irritability, bitter taste in the mouth and thirst.

Modifications

1. If there is severe pain, add ST-34, the Accumulation point, to harmonise the collateral and reduce the pain.
2. If there is obvious acid regurgitation, add GB-40 to regulate the Qi in the Lesser Yang channel and relieve the acid regurgitation.
3. If there is obvious irritability, restlessness and anxiety, add PC-7, the Source point, to calm the Mind.
4. If there is gastric bleeding, add PC-4, the Accumulation point, and SP-6 to cool the Blood and stop the bleeding.

STAGNATION OF BLOOD IN THE STOMACH

Symptoms and signs

Epigastric pain that is sharp and fixed in one place, and worsens after meals, accompanied by vomiting of blood, haemafecia, a purple tongue and a choppy pulse.

This syndrome can be seen in gastroduodenal ulcers, chronic gastritis and stomach cancer.

Principle of treatment

Invigorate Blood and stop the pain.

HERBAL TREATMENT

Prescription

SHI XIAO SAN and **DAN SHEN YIN**
Sudden Smile Powder and Salvia Decoction
Pu Huang *Pollen Typhae* 9 g
Wu Ling Zhi *Faeces Trogopterorum* 9 g
Dan Shen *Radix Salviae Miltiorrhizae* 9 g
Tan Xiang *Lignum Santali* 3 g
Sha Ren *Fructus Amomi* 3 g
Da Huang *Radix et Rhizoma Rhei* 3 g
Zhi Gan Cao *Radix Glycyrrhizae Praeparata* 3 g

Explanations

- This syndrome can be caused by trauma and chronic disorder of the Stomach. When there is stagnation of Qi and Blood, the channel will be obstructed, causing pain that starts in the epigastric region.
- Wu Ling Zhi is pungent, Warm and sweet in nature. It stops pain by effectively removing the stagnant Blood without injuring it.
- Pu Huang is able to either invigorate the Blood circulation or stop bleeding. It is particularly suitable for treating bleeding conditions caused by stagnation of Blood.
- Dan Shen can cool the Blood and promote its circulation, effectively relieving epigastric pain.
- Tan Xiang and Sha Ren regulate the Qi circulation and cause the Stomach-Qi to descend so as to assist Dan Shen, Wu Ling Zhi and Pu Huang in moving the Blood and stopping the pain.
- Da Huang promotes bowel movement and promotes the Qi and Blood circulation in the Small and Large Intestine.
- Zhi Gan Cao can moderate the actions of the other herbs in the formula as well as the speed of development of the disease.

Modifications

1. If there is gastric bleeding, add San Qi *Radix Notoginseng* 9 g and Bai Ji *Rhizoma Bletillae* 9 g to stop the bleeding.
2. If the digestion is poor, add Jiao Mai Ya *Fructus Hordei Germinatus* 9 g, Jiao Shen Qu *Massa Fermentata* 9 g and Jiao Shan Zha *Fructus Crataegi* 9 g, to promote the digestion.
3. If there is deficiency of the Spleen-Qi, add Dang Shen *Radix Codonopsis Pilosulae* 9 g, Bai Zhu *Rhizoma Atractylodis* 9 g and Fu Ling *Poria* 12 g to activate the Spleen and tonify the Spleen-Qi.

ACUPUNCTURE TREATMENT

CV-12 Zhongwan, ST-34 Liangqiu, LR-3 Taichong, ST-36 Zusanli, SP-6 Sanyinjiao, SP-10 Xuehai, BL-17 Geshu and BL-18 Ganshu. Even method is used on these points.

Explanations

- CV-12, together with ST-34, the Accumulation point, causes the Stomach-Qi to descend, regulates the Qi and Blood of the Stomach and relieves the pain.
- LR-13, the Gathering point of the Zang organs, regulates the Qi and Blood of the Liver. It can harmonise the Spleen and the Liver, and promote the Qi and Blood circulation together with BL-18.
- SP-10, SP-6 and BL-17 specifically regulate the Blood circulation and stop the pain.

Modifications

1. If there is bleeding in the Stomach, add ST-44 and SP-10 to stop the bleeding.
2. If there is severe pain, add SP-4 and PC-6, the Confluence points of the Penetrating and Yin Linking Vessels, to relieve the pain.

MIXTURE OF HEAT AND COLD IN THE STOMACH

Symptoms and signs

Epigastric pain with fullness, vomiting, irregular bowel movement or diarrhoea, a thin and yellow tongue coating and a wiry pulse.

This syndrome is often seen in acute and chronic gastritis, hyperchlorhydria, gastrostenosis, acute or chronic gastroduodenal ulcers, anorexia and taking of medicines incorrectly.

Principle of treatment

Harmonise and strengthen the Stomach, clear the obstruction, and regulate Cold and Heat in the Stomach.

HERBAL TREATMENT

Prescription

BAN XIA XIE XIN TANG
Pinellia Decoction
Ban Xia *Rhizoma Pinelliae* 9 g
Huang Qin *Radix Scutellariae* 9 g
Huang Lian *Rhizoma Coptidis* 3 g
Gan Jiang *Rhizoma Zingiberis* 6 g
Dang Shen *Radix Codonopsis Pilosulae* 9 g
Gan Cao *Radix Glycyrrhizae* 6 g
Da Zao *Fructus Ziziphi Jujubae* 6 g

Explanations

- This syndrome happens after eating the wrong food or taking the wrong medication, or in conditions of stress; these injure the Stomach-Qi, and develop the Cold and Heat in the Middle Burner, so the Qi becomes blocked in the Stomach.
- Ban Xia, pungent and Warm in nature, enters the Stomach. It can disperse the Qi obstruction and reduce sensations of fullness in the Stomach. It also causes the Stomach-Qi to descend, reduces the Qi obstruction and relieves nausea and vomiting.
- Gan Jiang, pungent and Hot in nature, expels Cold in the Stomach. Together with Ban Xia it also unblocks the Qi obstruction.
- Huang Lian and Huan Qin, bitter and Cold in nature, clear Heat in the Stomach. These four herbs are used together to disperse the Qi and cause it to descend, and regulate Cold and Heat so that epigastric pain and distension can be reduced.
- Dang Shen, Gan Cao and Da Zao tonify the Spleen, strengthen the Qi in the Middle Burner, which has been injured.
- When these herbs are used in combination, the Qi obstruction disappears, the Stomach-Qi becomes stronger and moves properly, the Heat and Cold becomes balanced, and the epigastric pain then disappears.

Modifications

1. If there is obvious nausea, use Sheng Jiang *Rhizoma Zingiberis Recens* 9 g instead of Gan Jiang *Rhizoma Zingiberis* 6 g to cause the Stomach-Qi to descend and relieve the vomiting.
2. If the appetite and digestion are poor, add Bai Zhu *Rhizoma Atractylodis Macrocephalae* 12 g and Fu Ling *Poria* 12 g to strengthen the Spleen and promote the digestion.

ACUPUNCTURE TREATMENT

CV-12 Zhongwan, PC-6 Neiguan, SP-4 Gongsun, ST-36 Zusanli and GB-40 Qiuxu. Even method is used on these points.

Explanations

- CV-12 causes the Stomach-Qi to descend and reduces nausea and vomiting.
- PC-6 and SP-4 can regulate the Qi in the chest and epigastric region and stop the pain.

- ST-36 strengthens the Spleen and Stomach and harmonises the Middle Burner.
- GB-40, the Source point of the foot Lesser Yang channel, regulates the Qi and harmonises the Qi in the epigastric region.

Modifications

1. If there is diarrhoea, add ST-25, the Front Collecting point of the Large Intestine, and SP-9, the Sea point of the Spleen channel, to transform Damp and relieve the diarrhoea.
2. If there is a sensation of fullness in the epigastrium, add ST-21 to regulate the Stomach-Qi and relieve the fullness.

DEFICIENT SYNDROMES

WEAKNESS OF THE SPLEEN AND STOMACH

Symptoms and signs

Slight and lingering epigastric pain that occurs or is worsened after eating cold or heavy food, with a preference for soft, warm and light food, a poor appetite, a sensation of fullness in the stomach, irregular bowel movements, a pale, white tongue coating and a soft, weak pulse.

This syndrome can be seen in chronic gastritis, gastroduodenal ulcer and chronic hepatitis.

Principle of treatment

Strengthen the Spleen, harmonise the Stomach and stop the pain.

HERBAL TREATMENT

Prescription

LIU JUN ZI TANG
Six Gentlemen Decoction
Dang Shen *Radix Codonopsis Pilosulae* 12 g
Bai Zhu *Rhizoma Atractylodis Macrocephalae* 9 g
Fu Ling *Poria* 9 g
Zhi Gan Cao *Radix Glycyrrhizae Praeparata* 6 g
Ban Xia *Rhizoma Pinelliae* 6 g
Chen Pi *Pericarpium Citri Reticulatae* 6 g

Explanations

- This is a syndrome in which the Spleen and Stomach are too weak to carry out their functions, so the channels are obstructed, causing epigastric pain.

- Dang Shen, Bai Zhu, Fu Ling and Zhi Gan Cao form a basic formula called Si Jun Zi Tang *Four Gentlemen Decoction* to tonify the Spleen-Qi. The herb with the strongest function in this formula is Dang Shen. Bai Zhu can dry Damp in the Middle Burner. Fu Ling can transform Damp in the Middle Burner by increasing urination. Zhi Gan Cao can harmonise the actions of the other herbs in the formula. These four herbs can tonify the Spleen-Qi but are not harsh, are Warm but not too Hot, and nourish the body but are not sticky, so they have been given the name 'four gentlemen'.
- Ban Xia can cause the Stomach-Qi to descend and Chen Pi can regulate the Stomach-Qi, so they can relieve the sensation of fullness in the Stomach and improve the appetite.
- When the six herbs are used together, the Spleen-Qi is strengthened and its functions of transportation and transformation will be improved, so the epigastric pain disappears.

Modifications

1. If there is severe pain, add Mu Xiang *Radix Aucklandiae* 6 g and Sha Ren *Fructus Amomi* 6 g to regulate the Qi in the Stomach and Middle Burner.
2. If there is stagnation of food, add Jiao Mai Ya *Fructus Hordei Germinatus* 9 g, Jiao Shen Qu *Massa Fermentata Medicinalis* 9 g and Jiao Shan Zha *Fructus Crataegi* 9 g to promote digestion and relieve the food stagnation.
3. If there is obvious Cold, add Gao Liang Jiao *Rhizoma Alpiniae Officinarum* 9 g to warm the Stomach and dispel the Cold.
4. If there is a mixture of Heat and Cold in the Middle Burner, add Huang Qin *Radix Scutellariae* 9 g and Huang Lian *Rhizoma Coptidis* 3 g, together with Ban Xia *Rhizoma Pinelliae* 9 g, to regulate the Heat and Cold and harmonise the Middle Burner.

ACUPUNCTURE TREATMENT

CV-12 Zhongwan, BL-21 Weishu, LR-13 Zhangmen, BL-20 Pishu, ST-36 Zusanli and PC-6 Neiguan. Even method is used on these points.

Explanations

- CV-12 and BL-21, LR-13 and BL-20 are the Front Collecting points and Back Transporting points of the Stomach and Spleen respectively. They can tonify the Spleen and Stomach so as to strengthen their physiological functions.

- ST-36, the Lower Sea point, can tonify the Stomach. Together with PC-6, it can also regulate the Qi in the epigastrium and stop the pain.

Modifications

1. If there is severe pain, add ST-34, the Accumulation point, to harmonise the collateral and reduce the pain.
2. If there is food stagnation, add SP-6 and ST-40 to promote digestion and relieve the food stagnation.
3. If there is obvious Cold in the Middle Burner, add SP-3 and CV-6 with moxibustion to tonify the Qi and warm the Yang of the Spleen and Stomach.

DEFICIENCY OF QI AND BLOOD

Symptoms and signs

Intermittent epigastric pain alleviated by warmth and pressure, and aggravated by tiredness, accompanied by a pale complexion, generalised tiredness, a dry mouth, warm palms, a poor appetite, loose stools, a pale tongue with a white coating and a thready and weak pulse.

This syndrome can be found in gastroduodenal ulcer, chronic hepatitis and neurasthenia.

Principle of treatment

Warm the Stomach, tonify the weakness, harmonise the Stomach and stop the pain.

HERBAL TREATMENT

Prescription

XIAO JIAN ZHONG TANG
Minor Strengthening the Middle Decoction
Yi Tang *Saccharum Granorum* 15 g
Bai Shao *Radix Paeoniae Alba* 12 g
Gui Zhi *Ramulus Cinnamomi* 6 g
Zhi Gan Cao *Radix Glycyrrhizae Praeparata* 3 g
Sheng Jiang *Rhizoma Zingiberis Recens* 6 g
Da Zao *Fructus Ziziphi Jujubae* 9 g

Explanations

- This syndrome is caused by deficiency of Qi and Blood in the Middle Burner. Deficiency of Qi may generate Cold, and deficiency of Blood may generate Heat. In this case, the warm herbs, which tonify the Qi and warm the Yang, may injure the Yin and Blood; the herbs that nourish the Blood and Yin may weaken the Yang and Qi. The Spleen and Stomach are too weak to digest greasy and tonifying herbs. So this is a very difficult condition to treat, but it is seen quite often in many chronic diseases.
- In this formula, the sweet and slightly warm Yi Tang is used with a big dosage to tonify the weakness of the Spleen-Qi, nourish the Blood, relieve cramp and stop the pain in the epigastrium. It does not have a sticky nature and is easily accepted by the Stomach.
- Bai Shao, sour in nature, together with the sweet Yi Tang, can generate the Yin, tonify the Blood, moisten the tendons and relieve the pain.
- Gui Zhi and Sheng Jiang, pungent in nature, together with the sweet Yi Tang, can generate the Yang and tonify the Qi.
- Gui Zhi and Bai Shao can harmonise the Blood so as to stop the pain.
- Da Zao and Zhi Gan Cao are also sweet herbs, and assist Yi Tang to strengthen the Middle Burner and relieve the pain.
- When these herbs are used together, they can tonify either Qi or Blood without the side-effect of increasing the Cold or Warmth in the Middle Burner. When the Stomach is strong and harmonised, the pain disappears.

Modifications

1. If there is severe pain, add Yan Hu Suo *Rhizoma Corydalis* 9 g to relieve the pain.
2. If there is severe deficiency of Qi, add Huang Qi *Radix Astragali seu Hedysari* 12 g to tonify the Qi.
3. If there is severe deficiency of Blood, add Dang Gui *Radix Angelicae Sinensis* 12 g to tonify the Blood.
4. If there is acid regurgitation, add Duan Wa Leng Zi *Concha Arcae* 15 g to reduce the acid regurgitation.

ACUPUNCTURE TREATMENT

SP-6 Sanyinjiao, ST-36 Zusanli, BL-17 Geshu, BL-20 Pishu, BL-21 Weishu, BL-23 Shenshu, GB-34 Yanglingquan and PC-6 Neiguan. Even method is used on these points.

Explanations

- SP-6, the crossing point of the three Yin channels of the foot, together with BL-17, the Gathering point for Blood, tonify the Blood and promote its circulation.

- ST-36, BL-20, BL-21 and BL-23 tonify the Spleen, Stomach and Kidney so as to generate the Qi and Blood.
- ST-36 and GB-34, the Lower Sea points, and PC-6, the Confluence point, regulate the Qi in the Middle Burner and stop the pain.

Modifications

1. If the pain is severe, add ST-34, the Accumulation point, to reduce the pain.
2. If there is acid regurgitation, add GB-40, the Source point, to regulate the Qi in the Lesser Yang Fu organs and relieve the acid regurgitation.

Case history

A 40-year-old man had suffered from epigastric pain for 4 years. The pain became worse at night after eating a heavy meal or in stressful situations. It had a lingering, distending nature and occasionally referred to the hypochondriac region. The patient also had a poor appetite, loose stools, an aversion to cold, and was tired and very stressed. He had a pale tongue with a thin and white coating and a wiry, thready and deep pulse.

Diagnosis
Deficiency of Qi, Blood and Yang in the Middle Burner with stagnation of Liver-Qi.

Principle of treatment
Tonify the Qi and Yang of the Spleen, nourish the Blood, disperse the Liver-Qi and stop the pain.

Herbal treatment
HUANG QI JIAN ZHONG TANG and **XIAO YAO SAN**
Astragalus Decoction to Construct the Middle and Free and Relaxed Powder
Huang Qi *Radix Astragali seu Hedysari* 12 g
Yi Tang *Saccharum Granorum* 15 g
Bai Shao *Radix Paeoniae Alba* 12 g
Gui Zhi *Ramulus Cinnamomi* 6 g
Zhi Gan Cao *Radix Glycyrrhizae Praeparata* 3 g
Sheng Jiang *Rhizoma Zingiberis Recens* 6 g
Da Zao *Fructus Ziziphi Jujubae* 9 g
Chai Hu *Radix Bupleuri* 6 g
Xiang Fu *Rhizoma Cyperi* 9 g
Bai Zhu *Rhizoma Atractylodis Macrocephalae* 9 g
Fu Ling *Poria* 12 g

Explanations

- Yi Tang, as well as all the sweet-tasting herbs, nourishes the Qi and Blood in the Middle Burner, and also the Yin and Yang.
- Huang Qi, Bai Zhu, Fu Ling and Zhi Gan Cao tonify the Spleen-Qi and dry Damp.
- Huang Qi, Gui Zhi and Sheng Jiang warm the Stomach-Yang and stimulate the Spleen-Qi.
- Bai Shao and Da Zao nourish the Blood.
- Chai Hu and Xiang Fu disperse the Liver-Qi so as to harmonise the Liver and Spleen.

After 3 months of treatment, the pain as well as the other symptoms were under control. He was followed up a year later and he said he had experienced no pain since the herbal treatment.

DEFICIENCY OF SPLEEN-QI AND STAGNATION OF LIVER-QI

Symptoms and signs

Slight epigastric pain, occurring or worsening with stressful or emotional disturbance, accompanied by a poor appetite, belching, hypochondriac distension, tiredness, depression, a pale tongue with thin and white coating and a thready and wiry pulse.

This syndrome can be seen in hepatitis, chronic gastritis and gastroduodenal ulcer.

Principle of treatment

Promote Liver-Qi circulation and tonify the Spleen.

HERBAL TREATMENT

Prescription

XIAO YAO SAN
Free and Relaxed Powder
Chai Hu *Radix Bupleuri* 9 g
Dang Gui *Radix Angelicae Sinensis* 9 g
Bai Shao *Radix Paeoniae Alba* 12 g
Bai Zhu *Rhizoma Atractylodis Macrocephalae* 9 g
Fu Ling *Poria* 15 g
Gan Cao *Radix Glycyrrhizae* 6 g
Bo He *Herba Menthae* 3 g
Sheng Jiang *Rhizoma Zingiberis Recens* 3 g
Yan Hu Suo *Rhizoma Corydalis* 9 g
Xiang Fu *Rhizoma Cyperi* 9 g

Explanations

- When the Spleen-Qi is deficient, it fails to generate Qi and Blood. When the Blood is insufficient to nourish the Liver, the Liver-Qi stagnates. Alternatively, long-term persistence of stressful or emotional disturbance causes Liver-Qi stagnation, so the Liver overcontrols the Spleen causing deficiency of the Spleen-Qi and of the Blood.
- In this formula, the pungent and Warm herb Dang Gui and the sour and Cold herb Bai Shao are used together to tonify and harmonise the Blood and soften the Liver so as to assist the circulation of Liver-Qi. Chai Hu can promote the Liver-Qi

circulation so as to relieve its stagnation. These three herbs are particularly used to regulate the Liver.

- Bai Zhu and Fu Ling can tonify the Spleen-Qi and transform Damp in the Middle Burner.
- Sheng Jiang causes the Stomach-Qi to descend and improves the appetite.
- Bo He disperses the constrained Heat due to stagnation of Qi.
- Gan Cao harmonises the function of the other herbs in the formula.
- There are two herbs added to this standard formula. Xiang Fu regulates the Qi and Yan Hu Suo regulates the Blood. They are added specifically to reduce the pain. As soon as the Liver-Qi moves properly, the functions of the Spleen and Stomach become normal, and the epigastric pain disappears.

Modifications

1. If there is pain of a cramping nature, increase the dosage of Bai Shao to 15 g and Zhi Gan Cao to 10 g to moderate the cramp and relieve the pain.
2. If there is obvious stagnation of Qi and Blood, add Yu Jin *Radix Curcumae* 9 g and Chuan Xiong *Radix Ligustici Chuanxiong* 9 g to regulate the Qi and Blood and relieve the stagnation.
3. If there is severe weakness of the Spleen, add Dang Shen *Radix Codonopsis Pilosulae* 9 g and Huang Qi *Radix Astragali seu Hedysari* 9 g to tonify the Spleen-Qi, and Chen Pi *Pericarpium Citri Reticulatae* 9 g to promote Qi movement in the Middle Burner.
4. If there is food stagnation, add Jiao Mai Ya *Fructus Hordei Germinatus* 9 g, Jiao Shen Qu *Massa Fermentata Medicinalis* 9 g and Jiao Shan Zha *Fructus Crataegi* 9 g to promote digestion and relieve the stagnation.
5. If there is formation of Liver-Heat due to Qi stagnation, manifested as irritability, nervousness, headache and a red tongue and rapid pulse, add Mu Dan Pi *Cortex Moutan Radicis* 9 g and Zhi Zi *Fructus Gardeniae* 9 g to reduce the Heat and relieve the irritability.

ACUPUNCTURE TREATMENT

LR-3 Taichong, LR-13 Zhangmen, LR-14 Qimen, GB-34 Yanglingquan, BL-18 Ganshu, BL-20 Pishu, BL-21 Weishu, CV-12 Zhongwan, ST-36 Zusanli and SP-6 Sanyinjiao. Even method is used on these points.

Explanations

- LR-3, the Source point, and GB-34, the Lower Sea point, can promote the circulation of Liver-Qi and regulate the physiological function of the Liver.
- LR-14 and BL-18, the Front Collecting point and the Back Transporting point of the Liver, can regulate the Liver-Qi and tonify the Liver-Blood.
- LR-13 and BL-20, CV-12 and BL-21 are the Front Collecting points and Back Transporting points of the Spleen and Stomach respectively, together with ST-36 and SP-6, strengthen the Spleen and Stomach, generate Qi and Blood, against overcontrol by the Liver.

Modifications

1. If there is severe pain, add ST-34, the Accumulation point, to reduce the pain.
2. If there is food stagnation, add ST-25 and LI-4 to promote digestion and relieve the stagnation.
3. If there is obvious emotional disturbance, add PC-6 to calm the Mind, LR-2 to reduce Liver-Heat, and CV-17 to unblock the chest.

DEFICIENCY OF STOMACH-YIN

Symptoms and signs

Mild epigastric pain with a slight burning feeling in the stomach, accompanied by thirst, a dry and bitter taste in the mouth and throat, acid regurgitation, constipation, a red tongue with a dry, thin and peeled coating, and a thready and rapid pulse.

This syndrome can be seen in gastric ulcer and chronic gastritis.

Principle of treatment

Nourish Stomach-Yin and stop the pain.

HERBAL TREATMENT

Prescription

YI GUAN JIAN and **SHAO YAO GAN CAO TANG**
Linking Decoction and *Peony and Licorice Decoction*
Sheng Di Huang *Radix Rehmanniae* 18 g
Sha Shen *Radix Adenopherae* 12 g
Mai Dong *Radix Ophiopogonis* 12 g
Dang Gui *Radix Angelicae Sinensis* 9 g
Gou Qi Zi *Fructus Lycii* 15 g
Chuan Lian Zi *Fructus Meliae Toosendan* 3 g
Bai Shao *Radix Paeoniae Alba* 12 g
Zhi Gan Cao *Radix Glycyrrhizae Praeparata* 6 g

Explanations

- Sha Shen, Mai Dong and Sheng Di Huang are able to nourish the Yin and clear Deficient-Heat in the Stomach.
- Gou Qi Zi and Dang Gui tonify the Liver-Blood amd smooth the Liver.
- Chuan Lian Zi promotes the circulation of Liver-Qi and drains Liver-Fire. Since it is very bitter and cold, it is used in only small amounts.
- Bai Shao and Zhi Gan Cao nourish the Yin and smooth the Liver so as to stop the pain. If the Stomach-Yin is sufficient, the epigastric pain will be relieved.

Modifications

1. If there is severe pain, add Xiang Yuan *Fructus Citri* 9 g and Fo Shou *Fructus Citri Sarcodactylis* 9 g to promote the circulation of Liver-Qi without consuming the Yin.
2. If there is severe acid regurgitation, add Huang Lian *Rhizoma Coptidis* 6 g, Wu Zhu Yu *Fructus Evodiae* 1 g and Wa Leng Zi *Concha Arcia* 12 g to clear Heat in the Liver and Stomach and relieve the acid regurgitation.
3. If there is constipation, add Gua Lou Ren *Semen Trichosanthis* 12 g and Huo Ma Ren *Fructus Cannabis* 12 g to moisten the intestines and promote bowel movement.

ACUPUNCTURE TREATMENT

CV-12 Zhongwan, LR-13 Zhangmen, BL-20 Pishu, BL-21 Weishu, CV-6 Qihai, ST-36 Zusanli, SP-6 Sanyinjiao and KI-3 Taixi. Even method is used on these points.

Explanations

- LR-13 and BL-20, CV-12 and BL-21 are the Front Collecting and Back Transporting points of the Spleen and Stomach respectively. They can strengthen and harmonise the physiological functions of the Spleen and Stomach.
- CV-6, and ST-36, the Lower Sea point, tonify the Qi of the Kidney and Spleen. SP-6, the crossing point of the three Yin channels of the foot, tonifies the Yin and Blood.
- KI-3, the Source point, tonifies the Kidney-Yin.

Modifications

1. If there is constipation, add ST-37, ST-25 and ST-44

to regulate the intestine, clear Heat and promote defecation.
2. If there is a dry mouth and thirst, add KI-6 to clear Deficient-Heat and nourish the Yin generally.
3. If there is acid regurgitation, add GB-34 and GB-40 to clear Heat in the Fu organs and relieve the acid regurgitation.
4. If there is gastric bleeding, add SP-10, ST-44 and PC-4 to clear Stomach-Heat and stop the bleeding.

DEFICIENCY OF SPLEEN-YANG

Symptoms and signs

Slight epigastric pain that becomes worse with hunger, and is alleviated after eating, which is of a lingering nature, and is better with warmth and pressure in the locality accompanied by a poor appetite, tiredness, an aversion to cold, cold limbs, soft stools, a pale tongue with a white coating and a deep, weak and slow pulse.

Principle of treatment

Warm the Spleen and Stomach and stop the pain.

HERBAL TREATMENT

Prescription

LI ZHONG WAN
Regulating the Middle Decoction
Dang Shen *Radix Codonopsis Pilosulae* 9 g
Bai Zhu *Rhizoma Atractylodis Macrocephalae* 9 g
Gan Jiang *Rhizoma Zingiberis* 6 g
Zhi Gan Cao *Radix Glycyrrhizae Praeparata* 6 g

Explanations

- When the Spleen-Yang is too weak to warm the Middle Burner, then interior Cold forms, causing the channels and interior organs to contract, obstructing the Qi and Blood circulation, and triggering epigastric pain.
- In this formula, Dang Shen and Bai Zhu strengthen the Spleen-Qi.
- Gan Jiang warms and disperses the Spleen-Yang and expels Cold in the Middle Burner.
- Zhi Gan Cao moderates pain and harmonises the actions of the other herbs in the formula.
- When the Spleen-Qi and Spleen-Yang become stronger, the interior Cold is relieved and the epigastric pain disappears.

Modifications

1. If there is obvious Qi deficiency, add Huang Qi *Radix Astragali seu Hedysari* 12 g to tonify the Qi.
2. If there are obvious Cold symptoms, add Rou Gui *Cortex Cinnamomi* 6 g to warm the Spleen-Yang and dispel the Interior Cold.
3. If there is nausea and vomiting, add Ban Xia *Rhizoma Pinelliae* 9 g and Sheng Jiang *Rhizoma Zingiberis Recens* 6 g to cause the Stomach-Qi to descend and relieve the vomiting.
4. If the digestion is poor, add Jiao Mai Ya *Fructus Hordei Germinatus* 9 g, Jiao Shen Qu *Massa Fermentata Medicinalis* 9 g and Jiao Shan Zha *Fructus Crataegi* 9 g to promote the digestion.

ACUPUNCTURE TREATMENT

BL-20 Pishu, BL-21 Weishu, BL-23 Shenshu, ST-36 Zusanli, PC-6 Neiguan, CV-4 Guangyuan, CV-6 Qihai, CV-12 Zhongwan and LR-3 Taichong. Even method is used. It is also advisable to apply moxibustion.

Explanations

- BL-20, BL-21 and BL-23, the Back Transporting points of the Spleen, Stomach and Kidney respectively, tonify these organs and regulate their physiological functions.
- CV-12, ST-36 and PC-6 regulate the Stomach-Qi and stop epigastric pain.
- CV-4 and CV-6 warm and strengthen the Original Qi and tonify the Blood.
- LR-3, the Source point, smoothes the Liver, regulates circulation of the Liver-Qi, promotes digestion and stops the pain.

Modifications

1. If there is severe pain, add ST-34, the Accumulation point, to harmonise the collateral and reduce the pain.
2. If there is distension in the abdomen and diarrhoea, add SP-4 together with ST-36 to activate the Spleen and regulate the Middle Burner.

Hypochondriac pain 26

胁
部
疼
痛

Hypochondriac pain is pain occurring in an area level with the seventh rib down to a level slightly below the costal arch. It can be either a subjective feeling or an objective symptom. Hypochondriac pain may be attributed to any of the following diseases in Western medicine: acute and chronic hepatitis, early stages of cirrhosis of the liver, liver cancer, acute and chronic cholecystitis, cholelithiasis, angiocholitis, acute and chronic pancreatitis, gastric ulcer, duodenal ulcer, pleuritis, Tietze's disease, intercostal neuralgia and herpes zoster. Hypochondriac pain can also accompany heart diseases, such as angina pectoris and myocardial infarction, and neurosis as well as some mental–physical disorders such as depression and hyperventilation.

Aetiology and pathology

Stagnation of the Liver-Qi and disturbance of the Liver-Fire

Anger, rage, resentment may cause the Qi to ascend; frustration, depression and excessive work stress may cause Liver-Qi stagnation; anxiety and fear may cause the Qi to descend. If the emotional strain is greater than normal, the movement of the Liver-Qi is disturbed, and the Liver and Gall Bladder channels as well as their collateral are obstructed, causing pain. Stagnation of Qi may also generate Heat and injure the channels and collateral, also causing hypochondriac pain.

Stagnation of Blood

If stagnation of Liver-Qi persists over a long period because of emotional disturbance, it may in turn cause stagnation of Blood. Physical overexertion may also injure the Liver and Gall Bladder channels and cause Blood stagnation. Finally, trauma, operation and chronic infection in the hypochondriac region can directly cause Blood stagnation. All these factors obstruct the Qi movement and Blood circulation in this area, triggering hypochondriac pain.

Accumulation of Damp-Heat

Living in a region with warm weather and a high humidity, or habitual indulgence in spicy or greasy food or milk products, may cause Damp-Heat to accumulate in the Middle Burner. This disturbs the function not only of the Spleen and Stomach, but also of the Liver and Gall Bladder. When the Damp-Heat covers and clogs up the Liver and Gall Bladder, the Liver-Qi is not able to move freely, and hypochondriac pain follows. When the Damp-Heat also obstructs the bile secretion and excretion, there may be jaundice as well.

Deficiency of Qi and Blood

Deficiency of Qi and Blood can be caused by many different chronic diseases. Overwork in stressful circumstances over a long period, giving birth to many children and heavy bleeding during menstruation can all also cause deficiency of Qi and Blood. When the Qi is too weak to move, it may stagnate. If the Blood is not sufficient to nourish the Liver, the latter becomes rigid and the Qi cannot move properly. Both of these situations may precipitate hypochondriac pain. Moreover, these factors may weaken the Spleen, the source of Qi and Blood production, causing further Blood deficiency and stagnation of the Liver-Qi.

Deficiency of Liver-Yin

Long-term mental or physical overwork or emotional strain, or excessive sexual activity, may weaken the Kidney-Essence and the Liver-Blood and cause Liver-Yin deficiency. Chronic disease and ageing also weaken the Liver-Yin. If the Liver-Yin is not sufficient to nourish the Liver, it can lead to Liver-Qi stagnation, Liver-Fire disturbance and Liver-Blood stagnation. All these conditions can be the cause of hypochondriac pain.

Treatment based on differentiation

Differentiation

Differentiation of character of the pain

Hypochondriac pain is directly caused by the disorders of the Liver and Gall Bladder, the channels and the organs.

— Pain with a distending and moving nature, and associated with emotions, is caused by Qi stagnation.
— Sharp and fixed pain in the hypochondriac region, which gets worse in the night, is caused by Blood stagnation.
— Severe pain, sometimes with jaundice, fever and chills, is often caused by Damp-Heat.
— Hypochondriac pain with irritability, a bitter taste in the mouth, scanty urine, insomnia and dream-disturbed sleep, is usually caused by Excessive-Heat in the Liver.
— Hypochondriac pain, with irritability, scanty and irregular menstruation, a red tongue and a thready, wiry pulse indicate deficiency of Liver-Yin with Deficient-Heat.

Differentiation according to the signs of tongue and pulse

— A wiry pulse is the typical sign in hypochondriac pain. A normal tongue body with thin white coating and a wiry pulse is often seen in Liver-Qi stagnation.
— A thick, yellow coating of the tongue and a wiry, slippery or moderate pulse show the accumulation of Damp-Heat.
— A red tongue, and a wiry and rapid pulse indicate Liver-Heat disturbance.
— A purple tongue body, or purple spots on the border of the tongue, together with a wiry and irregular pulse indicate Blood stagnation.
— A pale tongue and a thready, wiry pulse indicate Blood deficiency.
— A thin, red tongue body and a thready, wiry pulse suggest deficiency of Yin.

Differentiation of the location of the pain according to Western medical diagnosis

The diagnosis according to Western medicine is helpful in the differentiation of the syndrome as it provides information on the location of the pain.

— Cholecystitis, cholelithiasis and angiocholitis may cause right hypochondriac pain; sometimes it radiates to the right side of the back and scapula.
— Hepatitis causes hypochondriac pain too; however, the pain is not heavy, but with distension in the hypochondriac region and upper abdomen. Nausea, vomiting, an aversion to greasy food and tiredness accompany this.
— Early stages of cirrhosis of liver and liver cancer can cause right hypochondriac pain. A hard mass or the edge of the enlarged liver can be found on palpation.
— Gastric ulcer or duodenal ulcer may also cause the hypochondriac pain. Gastric ulcer causes pain under the xiphoid and is associated with the left side of the hypochondrium. Duodenal ulcer causes pain under the xiphoid and is associated with the right side of the hypochondrium.
— Pancreatitis may cause hypochondriac pain. Depending on the involved part of the pancreas, the pain can be in the left or the right hypochondrium. In most cases, the pain radiates to the back.
— The pain in angina pectoris and myocardial infarction can be associated with the hypochondria in some special cases. The pain is more severe than in the other types; sometimes the pain radiates to the left shoulder and arm.

— The pain in pleurisy may be associated with the hypochondria, but the pain is worse in deep breath.
— Tietze's disease causes pain in the involved costal cartilage too. The pain is getting worse in deep breathing, or by palpation and percussion.
— Intercostal neuralgia may cause pain along the intercostal nerve and the pain is very sharp.
— Herpes zoster shows skin lesions along the involved nerve.
— Hypochondriac pain caused by mental disorders or emotional strain has distending and moving features, and often happens under stress or emotional disturbance.

Treatment

EXCESS SYNDROMES

STAGNATION OF LIVER-QI AND RESTRAINT OF THE LIVER-FIRE

Symptoms and signs

Hypochondriac pain with distending and moving features, which starts or worsens in stressful situations, with distension in the sides of abdomen, and a sensation of fullness in the gastric region and stifling in the chest, accompanied by shortness of breath, a reduced appetite, belching, a thin, white tongue coating and a wiry pulse. If the stagnant Liver-Qi produces Liver-Fire, there will also be irritability, heartburn, a bitter taste in the mouth, scanty urine and constipation, a tongue that is red, or red at the edges, with a yellow coating and a wiry, forceful and rapid pulse.

The syndrome of Qi stagnation can be seen in chronic hepatitis, chronic cholecystitis, cholelithiasis, intercostal neuralgia, depression and hyperventilation. The syndrome of restraint of the Liver-Fire can be found in the acute and subacute stages of these diseases.

Principle of treatment

Disperse the Liver-Qi and stop the pain.

HERBAL TREATMENT

Prescription a

CHAI HU SHU GAN SAN
Bupleurum Soothing the Liver Powder
Chai Hu *Radix Bupleuri* 6 g

Xiang Fu *Fructus Aurantii* 9 g
Zhi Qiao *Rhizoma Cyperi* 9 g
Chuan Xiong *Rhizoma Ligustici Chuangxiong* 6 g
Bai Shao *Radix Paeoniae Alba* 9 g
Zhi Gan Cao *Radix Glycyrrhizae Praeparata* 6 g

Explanations

- Chai Hu is pungent and neutral, and enters the Gall Bladder and Liver channels. It is effective for dispersing and causing the Liver-Qi to ascend so as to promote its free flow.
- Xiang Fu is pungent, slightly bitter and sweet, and enters the Liver and Triple Burner channels. It is the most commonly used herb to induce movement of the Liver-Qi, as it is both moderate and effective.
- Zhi Qiao specifically unblocks the chest and treats the feeling of stiffness in the chest and shortness of breath.
- Chuan Xiong promotes the Blood circulation so as to assist the movement of Qi.
- Bai Shao is sour and cold, and enters the Liver channel, softens the Liver and assists the movement of Liver-Qi; together with Zhi Gan Cao, it can slow down the pathological process and relieve acute pain.
- This formula is a very well designed one for regulating and dispersing the Liver-Qi. It improves the balance among the Liver, Gall Bladder, Triple Burner, Stomach and Lung, and between Qi and Blood as well. It is particularly effective for treating hypochondriac pain due to stress and emotional disturbance. Usually, after taking this formula for 3 days, both pain and stress improve.

Prescription b

DA CHAI HU TANG
Major Bupleurum Decoction
Chai Hu *Radix Bupleuri* 9 g
Huang Qin *Radix Scutellariae* 12 g
Ban Xia *Rhizoma Pinelliae* 9 g
Bai Shao *Radix Paeoniae Alba* 12 g
Zhi Shi *Fructus Aurantii Immaturus* 9 g
Da Huang *Radix et Rhizoma Rhei* 3 g
Sheng Jiang *Rhizoma Zingiberis Recens* 6 g
Da Zao *Fructus Ziziphi Jujubae* 6 g

Explanations

- This formula can harmonise the Liver and remove obstructions. It is particularly useful for treating hypochondriac pain due to Liver-Qi stagnation that has affected the transportation functions of the Stomach and Large Intestine. Besides the hypochondriac pain, there are other symptoms such as nausea, vomiting, irritability, a sensation of fullness in the chest, distension in the abdomen and constipation.

- Chai Hu disperses and causes the Liver-Qi to ascend. Bai Shao softens the Liver. These two herbs together regulate the Liver and treat hypochondriac pain.
- Ban Xia smoothes the Stomach-Qi, together with Huang Qin, which clears Heat, and relieves nausea, irritability and distension in the hypochondriac region and the Stomach.
- Zhi Shi and Da Huang regulate the Qi in the intestines, promote bowel movement and treat abdominal distension and constipation. Da Huang is also able to drain Heat, regulate the Blood and remove obstruction.
- This formula can be used to treat acute pancreatitis, acute cholecystitis, cholelithiasis and irritable bowel syndrome.

Prescription c

ZUO JIN WAN
Left Metal Pill
Huang Lian *Rhizoma Coptidis* 6 g
Wu Zhu Yu *Fructus Evodiae* 1 g

Explanations

This small formula is very effective to treat hypochondriac pain with belching and Heartburn due to the Liver-Fire attacking the Stomach. Huang Lian, bitter and Cold in nature, enters the Heart, Liver and Stomach channel, being able directly and indirectly to clear the Liver-Heat. Wu Zhu Yu, pungent and very hot in nature, can smooth the Stomach-Qi, treat belching, and together with Huang Lian, treat Heartburn. Wu Zhu Yu can also reduce the side-effects of Huang Lian. Because Huang Lian is very cold, it reduces the Fire, but may cause restrained Heat. Wu Zhu Yu is able to disperse the restrained Heat so as to assist Huang Lian to clear the Heat. Since Wu Zhu Yu is used with very small dosage, only one sixth of Huang Lian, the main action of this formula is still to clear the Liver-Heat, harmonise the Liver and Stomach.

Modifications

1. If the distending pain is severe, add Qing Pi *Pericarpium Citri Reticulatae Viride* 9 g and Chuan

Lian Zi *Fructus Meliae Toosendan* 9 g to break up the Qi stagnation in the Liver and stop the pain.

2. If there is a fixed pain in the hypochondriac region, add Yu Jin *Radix Curcumae* 9 g and Yan Hu Suo *Rhizoma Corydalis* 9 g to promote the Qi movement and Blood circulation so as to stop the pain.

3. If the pain is associated with the sides of the lower abdomen, and there is Cold in the Liver channel, add Wu Yao *Radix Linderae* 9 g to expel the Cold from the channel, disperse the Liver-Qi and relieve the pain. If there is Heat in the Liver channel, add Chuan Lian Zi *Fructus Meliae Toosendan* 9 g to drain the Heat from the channel, disperse the Liver-Qi and stop the pain.

4. If there is a digestive disorder, add Chen Pi *Pericarpium Citri Reticulatae* 9 g to regulate the Stomach-Qi, and Mu Xiang *Radix Aucklandiae* 6 g to regulate the Qi of the Liver and Large Intestine, and promote digestion.

5. If the Liver-Qi partially turns to Liver-Heat, there is slight irritability and warm sensation in the chest, add Ban Xia *Rhizoma Pinelliae* 9 g and Huang Qin *Radix Scutellariae* 12 g to regulate the Lesser Yang channel, or Zhi Zi *Fructus Gardeniae* 9 g and Dan Dou Chi *Semen Sojae Praeparatum* 9 g to disperse Heat in the chest.

6. If the Liver-Qi turns into Liver-Fire, which is manifested as thirst, a bitter taste in the mouth, irritability, insomnia, a red tongue with a dry yellow coating and a wiry, rapid pulse, add Mu Dan Pi *Cortex Moutan Radicis* 9 g and Zhi Zi *Fructus Gardeniae* 9 g to clear Liver-Heat directly. According to the Five Element theory, to treat an Excess syndrome, you need to reduce the Son organ. Huang Lian *Rhizoma Coptidis* 6 g and Dan Shen *Radix Salviae Miltiorrhizae* 12 g can be added to clear the Fire of the Heart, which is the Son organ of the Liver. It is an effective method for reducing Fire from the Liver indirectly.

Patent remedies

Xiao Yao Wan *Free and Relaxed Pill*
Shu Gan Wan *Soothe Liver Pill*
Long Dan Xie Gan Wan *Gentiana Draining the Liver Pill*

ACUPUNCTURE TREATMENT

TE-6 Zhigou, GB-34 Yanglingquan, LR-3 Taichong, PC-6 Neiguan, LU-7 Lieque and SP-6 Sanyinjiao. Reducing method is used on the first five points; even method is used on SP-6.

Explanations

- TE-6, a River point, is able to regulate the Qi in the Lesser Yang channel. It is very effective for treating hypochondriac pain, both the root and manifestations in different types.
- GB-34, a Lower Sea point, regulates the Liver-Qi, specifically treating disorder of Fu organs and stopping hypochondriac pain.
- LR-3, a Source point, is able to regulate the Liver-Qi and stop the pain.
- PC-6 can calm the Mind, and smooth the Qi in the chest and hypochondriac region, because it is a Confluence point for the Yin Linking Vessel, which passes through the hypochondria.
- LU-7, a Connecting point and Confluence point of the Directing Vessel, is used to disperse and cause the Qi to descend in the body generally so as to assist the free flow of the Liver-Qi. It is particularly effective for treating hypochondriac pain accompanied by distension in depression, premenstrual tension and hyperventilation.
- SP-6, where the three Yin channels of foot meet, regulates the Blood so as to assist the movement of the Qi.

Modifications

1. If there is constipation and abdominal distension, add ST-25, the Front Collecting point of the Large Intestine, and CV-12, the Gathering point for the Fu organs, to regulate the Qi in the Stomach and intestines, and LR-14, the Front Collecting point of the Liver, to regulate the Liver-Qi.
2. If there is a fixed pain with distending sensation, add BL-18 and LR-14, the Back Transporting point and the Front Collecting point of the Liver respectively, to regulate the movement of the Liver-Qi. Add BL-17 and LR-13, the Gathering point for the Blood and the Zang organs respectively, to invigorate the Blood and regulate the function of the Liver.
3. If there is Liver-Heat, add LR-2 and GB-43, the Spring points, to reduce the Heat, and LR-14 to regulate the Liver-Qi.
4. If there is pain in the sides of lower abdomen, add LR-12 to unblock the obstruction and stop the pain.

Case history

A 55-year-old woman had been suffering from hypochondriac pain following an emotional disturbance for 10 days. The pain was moving, and accompanied by a distending sensation, belching throughout the day, acid regurgitation, a reduced appetite and dream-disturbed sleep. She had a red tongue with a dry, yellow coating and a wing pulse.

Diagnosis
Stagnation of Liver-Qi. This was an acute Excess syndrome due to stagnation of Liver-Qi resulting from emotional disturbance.

Principle of treatment
Disperse the Liver-Qi, clear the Liver-Heat, harmonise the Stomach and Liver and stop the pain.

Herbal treatment
CHAI HU SHU GAN SAN
Bupleurun Soothing the Liver Powder
Chai Hu *Radix Bupleuri* 6 g
Xiang Fu *Rhizoma Cyperi* 4.5 g
Zhi Qiao *Fructus Aurantii* 4.5 g
Chen Pi *Pericarpium Citri Reticulatae* 6 g
Chuan Xiong *Rhizoma Ligustici Chuanxiong* 4.5 g
Shao Yao *Radix Paeoniae Alba* 4.5 g
Zhi Gan Cao *Radix Glycyrrhizae Praeparata* 1.5 g

And:

ZUO JIN WAN
Left Metal Pill
Huang Lian *Rhizoma Coptidis* 6 g
Wu Zhu Yu *Fructus Evodiae* 1 g

(Both are patent formulae.)

Explanations

- Chai Hu Shu Gan San disperses the Liver-Qi, softens the Liver, stops the pain and reduces distension in the hypochondriac region.
- Zuo Jin Wan contains Huang Lian and Wu Zhu Yu. Huang Lian can directly reduce Liver-Heat. Wu Zhu Yu can dispel restrained Liver-Qi and Heat as well as soothing the Stomach-Qi.

After using the herbs for 3 days, the hypochondriac pain and belching were much reduced. After another 3 days' treatment, all the symptoms had disappeared. The patient was followed up years later and she stated she had experienced no pain since the herbal treatment.

STAGNATION OF BLOOD

Symptoms and signs

Hypochondriac pain with a sharp and fixed nature that becomes worse at night, with a palpable mass in the area, accompanied by a purple tongue, or one with purple spots on the sides, and a white tongue coating, and a deep, wiry or unsmooth pulse.

This syndrome can be seen in patients with prolonged Liver-Qi stagnation, trauma, adhesions after an operation, tumour, or chronic infection in the locality.

Principle of treatment

Invigorate the Blood, eliminate the stagnant Blood, open the channels and collateral and stop the pain.

HERBAL TREATMENT

Prescription a

JIN LING ZI SAN and **SHI XIAO SAN**
Melia Toosendan Powder and *Sudden Smile Powder*
Jin Ling Zi *Fructus Meliae Toosendan* 9 g
Yan Hu Suo *Rhizoma Corydalis* 9 g
Pu Huang *Pollen Typhae* 9 g
Wu Ling Zhi *Faeces Trogopterorum* 9 g

Explanations

- When the Liver-Qi stagnates, it can cause Blood stagnation in turn as the Qi can no longer promote the circulation of the Blood. Trauma, operation, tumour and chronic infection in the locality can also directly cause Qi and Blood stagnation. The combination of the two formulae is particularly useful for treating hypochondriac pain due to Qi and Blood stagnation. The characteristic symptoms of this are a fixed and distending pain in the hypochondriac region and a palpable mass that is not very hard.
- Jin Ling Zi, also called Chuan Lian Zi, disperses the Liver-Qi and drains Liver-Fire.
- Yan Hu Suo, which can promote Qi movement and Blood circulation, is very effective in stopping the pain.
- Pu Huang and Wu Ling Zhi are able to dissolve stagnant Blood and stop pain. When the Qi and Blood move freely, the pain will disappear.
- This formula is often used in cholecystitis, cholelithiasis, intercostal neuralgia, duodenal ulcer, pancreatitis, hypochondriac pain in premenstrual tension and hypochondriac pain due to anger or depression.

Prescription b

YAN HU SUO SAN
Corydalis Powder
Dang Gui *Radix Angelicae Sinensis* 9 g
Yan Hu Suo *Rhizoma Corydalis* 9 g
Pu Huang *Pollen Typhae* 9 g
Jiang Huang *Rhizoma Curcumae Longae* 9 g
Chi Shao *Radix Paeoniae Rubra* 9 g
Ru Xiang *Resina Olibani* 9 g
Mo Yao *Resina Myrrhae* 9 g
Mu Xiang *Radix Aucklandiae* 6 g
Rou Gui *Cortex Cinnamomi* 6 g
Sheng Jiang *Rhizoma Zingiberis Recens* 3 g
Gan Cao *Radix Glycyrrhizae* 3 g

Explanations

- This formula particularly treats fixed hypochondriac pain that has a distending sensation and is associated to the lateral sides of the lower abdomen. It is caused by Cold invasion in the Liver channel, and Qi and Blood stagnation that is more severe than in the previous case. So, compared with the first formula, there are more herbs to break up stagnant Blood and relieve pain, such as Ru Xiang, Mo Yao, Rou Gui and Jiang Huang. These herbs warm the Liver channel and dispel the stagnation.
- Mu Xiang and Dang Gui regulate the Qi and Blood respectively.
- Yan Hu Suo and Mu Xiang invigorate the Blood and Qi, and are effective in stopping pain. Sheng Jiang and Gan Cao strengthen the Spleen so as to rebuild the balance between the Liver and Spleen.
- Chi Shao is Cold, and can promote the circulation of Blood, so it moderates the harsh properties of the Hot herbs without causing Blood stagnation.
- In clinical practice, this formula is used to treat the same diseases or disorders as in the first formula but where the pain is more severe.

Prescription c

GE XIA ZHU YU TANG
Drive Out Blood Stasis Below the Diaphragm Decoction
Tao Ren *Semen Persicae* 9 g
Hong Hua *Flos Carthami* 9 g
Yan Hu Suo *Rhizoma Corydalis* 6 g
Wu Ling Zhi *Faeces Trogopterorum* 9 g
Chuan Xiong *Rhizoma Ligustici Chuanxiong* 9 g
Dang Gui *Radix Angelicae Sinensis* 9 g
Dan Pi *Cortex Moutan Radicis* 6 g
Chi Shao *Radix Paeoniae Rubra* 6 g
Xiang Fu *Rhizoma Cyperi* 9 g
Zhi Qiao *Fructus Aurantii* 6 g
Wu Yao *Radix Linderae* 6 g
Gan Cao *Radix Glycyrrhizae* 6 g

Explanations

- This formula particularly treats severe Blood stagnation, where a mass can be felt in the hypochondriac region and the pain is not so severe. The first five herbs are able to invigorate the Blood circulation, dispel stagnant Blood and stop the pain.
- Chi Shao and Dan Pi clear Heat in the Blood as the stagnation may in turn generate Heat.
- Xiang Fu and Wu Yao specifically promote the movement of Qi in the Liver channel.

- Zhi Qiao unblocks the chest, and dispels the Qi stagnation in the Stomach and Spleen so as to assist the movement of Liver-Qi.
- Dang Gui tonifies the Blood and promotes its circulation as the herbs that dispel stagnant Blood may injure the Blood too.
- Gan Cao harmonises the herbs in the different channels, organs and levels in the formula.
- This formula can be used for chronic hepatitis, early stages of liver cirrhosis, tumour and trauma.

Prescription d

FU YUAN HUO XUE TANG
Revive Health by Invigorating the Blood Decoction
Da Huang *Radix et Rhizoma Rhei* 12 g
Chai Hu *Radix Bupleuri* 9 g
Dang Gui *Radix Angelicae Sinensis* 12 g
Tao Ren *Semen Persicae* 6 g
Hong Hua *Flos Carthami* 6 g
Chuan Shan Jia *Squama Manitis* 6 g
Gua Lou Ren *Semen Trichosanthis* 9 g
Gan Cao *Radix Glycyrrhizae* 6 g

Add:

Yan Hu Suo *Rhizoma Corydalis* 9 g
Chuan Xiong *Rhizoma Ligustici Chuanxiong* 9 g
Mu Xiang *Radix Aucklandiae* 6 g
Qing Pi *Pericarpium Citri Reticulatae Viride* 6 g

Explanations

- This formula particularly treats acute pain due to stagnation of Blood after trauma. The Blood stagnates not only in the channels but also in the collateral. The symptoms are characterised by severe pain in the hypochondriac region.
- In this formula, a high dosage of Da Huang is used for draining out the stagnant Blood, breaking up the stagnation, together with Chai Hu, which disperses and causes the Liver-Qi to ascend and dispels stagnant Blood in the hypochondriac region.
- Tao Ren, Hong Hua and Dang Gui invigorate the Blood, dissolve stagnant Blood, reduce the swelling and stop the pain.
- Chuan Shan Jia characteristically breaks up stagnant Blood in the collateral.
- Gua Lou Ren clears Heat from the stagnation and dispels stagnant Blood.
- Gan Cao harmonises the actions of the other herbs in the formula.
- The pain-relieving action is stronger if Yan Hu Suo and Chuan Xiong are added to invigorate the Blood, and Mu Xiang and Qing Pi are added to promote the movement of Qi in the Liver channel.

Prescription e

TAO HONG SI WU TANG
Four-Substance Decoction with Safflower and Peach Pit
Bai Shao *Radix Paeoniae Alba* 9 g
Dang Gui *Radix Angelicae Sinensis* 12 g
Shu Di Huang *Radix Rehmanniae Praeparata* 9 g
Chuan Xiong *Rhizoma Ligustici Chuanxiong* 9 g
Tao Ren *Semen Persicae* 9 g
Hong Hua *Flos Carthami* 9 g

Add:

Yu Jin *Radix Curcumae* 9 g
Yan Hu Suo *Rhizoma Corydalis* 9 g

Explanations

- This formula is able to tonify Blood and promote Blood circulation. It is especially suitable for Blood stagnation combined with deficiency of Blood. When a patient complains of tiredness or only temporary pain relief after using herbs or acupuncture to invigorate the Blood and remove stagnation, this indicates that the Blood is insufficient and cannot cope with the moving herbs, which both stimulate and consume the Blood.
- In this formula Tao Ren, Hong Hua, Chuan Xiong, Dang Gui, Yu Jin and Yan Hu Suo are able to invigorate the Blood, remove stagnant Blood and stop the pain.
- Dan Gui, Bai Shao and Shu Di Huang can tonify the Blood so as to assist the herbs that promote Blood circulation.

Patent remedies

Bie Jia Jian Wan *Turtle Shell Pill*
Yan Hu Suo Zhi Tong Pian *Corydalis Stop Pain Tablet*

ACUPUNCTURE TREATMENT

TE-6 Zhigou, GB-34 Yanglingquan, LR-13 Zhangmen, LR-14 Qimen, BL-13 Feishu, LR-3 Taichong, GB-40 Qiuxu, SP-6 Sanyinjiao, SP-10 Xuehai, BL-18 Ganshu and BL-17 Geshu. Reducing method is used on these points.

Explanations

- TE-6, a River point, is also a Fire point. GB-34 is a Lower Sea point. They are the commonly used points for treating hypochondriac pain of different types as they can regulate the Qi in the Lesser Yang channels.

- LR-13, the Gathering point for the Zang organs, is able to regulate the Qi and Blood, and treats most of the chronic disorders when the Zang organs are involved.
- LR-14 and BL-18, the Front Collecting point and the Back Transporting point of the Liver respectively, are able to regulate the function of the Liver and promote the Blood circulation. They are also local points for treating hypochondriac pain.
- LR-3 and GB-40 are the Source points, which can regulate the Liver-Qi and reduce stagnation.
- SP-6, SP-10 and BL-17 are able to invigorate the Blood and stop pain.

Modifications

1. If there is hypochondriac pain due to the diseases of the Lung and pleura, add CV-22, CV-17, LU-5 and LU-6 to regulate the Lung-Qi.
2. If the pain is due to angina pectoris, add PC-6, the Confluence point, to promote the Blood circulation in the Heart and stop the pain. Add HT-6, the Accumulation point, to treat the acute pain. Add BL-15, the Back Transporting point of the Heart, to regulate the function of the Heart. Add CV-17, the Gathering point for the Qi, to disperse the Qi in the chest so as to assist the Blood circulation, or Extra Huatuojiaji points between T4 and T6, to regulate the Qi and Blood in the chest and Heart.
3. If the pain is due to Stomach disorder, add CV-12, the Gathering point for the Fu organs, to harmonise the Qi movement. Add ST-36, the Lower Sea point, to regulate the Stomach and strengthen the Spleen. Add BL-20 and BL-21, the Back Transporting point of the Spleen and Stomach respectively, to regulate the Spleen and Stomach.
4. If the pain is caused by diseases of Liver and Gall Bladder, add BL-19, the Back Transporting point of the Gall Bladder, together with BL-18 to regulate the Liver and Gall Bladder.
5. If the pain is caused by trauma, add KI-6, with GB-40 to regulate the Qi and Blood and stop the pain.
6. If there is intercostal neuralgia, add the Huatuojiaji points in the affected region to regulate the function of the nerves.
7. If the pain is caused by stagnation of Qi and Blood from excessive thinking and overwork, add ST-36 to strengthen the Spleen, and PC-6 to calm the Mind, reduce the tension and stop the pain. Use reinforcing method on SP-6 to regulate the Blood and tonify the Blood.

Case history

A 60-year-old woman had been suffering from hypochondriac pain on her left side for 3 days after a car accident. The pain got worse if she took a deep breath or cough. Her tongue was normal, with a white coating and her pulse was wiry and deep.

Diagnosis
Stagnation of Qi and Blood in the Liver and Gall Bladder channels.

Principle of treatment
Open the channels, invigorate the Qi and Blood and stop the pain.

Acupuncture treatment
TE-6, GB-34, GB-40, KI-6 and PC-6. Reducing method was used on these points.

Explanations

- TE-6, the River point, and GB-34, the Lower Sea point and the Gathering point for the tendons, are able to promote the Qi movement in the Lesser Yang channels.
- GB-40, the Source point, and KI-6, the Confluence point of the Yin Heel Vessel, can regulate the Qi and Blood and stop pain.
- PC-6, the Connecting point, can also regulate the Qi and Blood, and calm the Mind, reducing anxiety caused by the pain.

After the first treatment, the pain had lessened. After another four treatments, it had disappeared. She was followed up 2 years later and she stated she had experienced no pain since the acupuncture treatment.

ACCUMULATION OF DAMP-HEAT IN THE LIVER AND GALL BLADDER

Symptoms and signs

Hypochondriac pain, accompanied by a bitter taste in the mouth, a poor appetite, nausea, vomiting, jaundice, scanty urine, a yellow and sticky tongue coating and a wiry and slippery pulse.

This syndrome can be seen in acute hepatitis, cholecystitis, cholelithiasis, herpes zoster and malaria.

Principle of treatment

Clear the Heat, transform the Damp, disperse the Liver-Qi and stop the pain.

HERBAL TREATMENT

Prescription a

LONG DAN XIE GAN TANG
Gentiana Draining the Liver Decoction
Long Dan Cao *Radix Gentianae* 9 g

Huang Qin *Radix Scutellariae* 9 g
Zhi Zi *Fructus Gardeniae* 9 g
Ze Xie *Rhizoma Alismatis* 9 g
Mu Tong *Caulis Akebiae* 9 g
Che Qian Zi *Semen Plantaginis* 9 g
Dang Gui *Radix Angelicae Sinensis* 9 g
Sheng Di Huang *Radix Rehmanniae Recens* 9 g
Chai Hu *Radix Bupleuri* 6 g
Gan Cao *Radix Glycyrrhizae* 6 g

Explanations

- When Damp-Heat accumulates in the Liver and Gall Bladder, the channels and collateral are obstructed, the Liver-Qi cannot move freely and hypochondriac pain appears. Damp-Heat blocks the Qi movement of the Spleen and Stomach, which may cause symptoms such as poor appetite, nausea and vomiting.
- Long Dan Cao is bitter and Cold in nature, entering the Liver channel. It is able to clear Excessive-Heat, and treat thirst and a bitter taste in the mouth. It can eliminate Damp and treat jaundice and turbid urine. Since it can powerfully clear Damp-Heat, it is the chief herb in the formula.
- Huang Qin and Zhi Zi are both bitter and Cold in nature, and reduce Fire.
- Ze Xie, Mu Tong and Che Qian Zi can eliminate Damp-Heat by promoting urination.
- Heat may injure the Blood and the Yin, and Damp may block the Qi. Dang Gui tonifies the Blood, Sheng Di Huang nourishes the Yin and Chai Hu disperses the Liver-Qi. These three herbs are used to reduce the side-effects of the bitter and cold herbs.
- Gan Cao can clear Heat and remove Toxin.
- When Heat is reduced, and Damp is eliminated, the Qi can move freely and the pain and the other symptoms disappear. This formula can be used for herpes zoster, intercostal neuralgia, cholelithiasis and cholecystitis.

Modifications

1. If there is severe pain, add Chuan Lian Zi *Fructus Meliae Toosendan* 9 g and Yan Hu Suo *Rhizoma Corydalis* 9 g to regulate the Qi and Blood and stop the pain.
2. If there is a sensation of fullness in the abdomen and hypochondria, add Yu Jin *Radix Curcumae* 9 g, Ho Po *Herba Menthae* 6 g and Zhu Ru *Caulis Bambusae in Taeniam* 9 g to transform the Phlegm and regulate the Qi movement in the Middle Burner.

3. If there is cholelithiasis, add Da Huang *Radix et Rhizoma Rhei* 9 g, Jin Qian Cao *Herba Lysimachiae* 18 g and Hai Jin Sha *Spora Lygodii* 15 g to remove the stone and promote the bile secretion and excretion.

Prescription b

YIN CHEN HAO TANG
Artemisia Yinchenhao Decoction
Yin Chen Hao *Herba Artemisiae Capillaris* 15 g
Zhi Zi *Fructus Gardeniae* 9 g
Da Huang *Radix et Rhizoma Rhei* 6 g

Explanations

- This formula is designed for jaundice due to accumulation of Damp-Heat in the Middle Burner. If bile secretion and excretion are obstructed by the Damp-Heat, jaundice may follow. A bitter taste with a sticky sensation in the mouth and turbid, strong smelling urine indicate that Damp-Heat has accumulated in the body. As well as hypochondriac pain and distension, symptoms include nausea, abdominal distension and scanty urine.
- Yin Chen Hao, an aromatic herb, can disperse and clear Damp-Heat.
- Zhi Zi, bitter and cold, enters the Triple Burner channel and clears Damp-Heat from the Triple Burner passage. It can promote urination and also drain Damp-Heat.
- Da Huang drains Heat, promotes the Blood circulation and reduces the pain. It also promotes bowel movement so as to eliminate Damp-Heat.
- These three herbs all have the function of accelerating bile secretion and excretion, which can reduce pain, inflammation and jaundice. This formula is particularly useful in acute hepatitis, and jaundice due to cholecystitis or leptospirosis.

Modifications

1. In the early stages of hepatitis, add Yin Hua *Flos Lonicerae* 12 g, Lian Qiao *Fructus Forsythiae* 12 g, Da Qing Ye *Folium Isatidis* 12 g and Ban Lan Gen *Radix Isatidis* 12 g to clear Heat and eliminate Toxin.
2. If there is severe hypochondriac pain, add Yu Jin *Radix Curcumae* 12 g, Chuan Lian Zi *Fructus Meliae Toosendan* 9 g and Chai Hu *Radix Bupleuri* 9 g to regulate the Qi and Blood and eliminate Damp-Heat.
3. If there is nausea and vomiting, add Chen Pi *Pericarpium Citri Reticulatae* 9 g and Zhu Ru *Caulis Bambusae in Taeniam* 12 g to smooth the Stomach and cause the Stomach-Qi to descend.

4. If there is fever, add Zhi Bao Dan *Greatest Treasure Special Pill* (patent formula, 1 pill a day) to remove Damp-Heat Toxin.

Patent remedies

Li Dan Pai Shi Pian *Benefit Gall Bladder Discharge Stone Tablet*

Long Dan Xie Gan Wan *Gentiana Draining the Liver Pill*

ACUPUNCTURE TREATMENT

TE-6 Zhigou, GB-34 Yanglingquan, LR-3 Taichong, GB-24 Riyue, LR-14 Qimen, BL-18 Ganshu, LI-11 Quchi, and SP-9 Yinlingquan. Reducing method is used on these points.

Explanations

- TE-6 and GB-34 regulate the Qi, and disperse and reduce Damp-Heat, in the Lesser Yang channels and stop the pain.
- LR-3, the Source point, disperses the Liver-Qi so as to eliminate Damp-Heat.
- BL-19 and GB-24, the Back Transporting point and Front Collecting point respectively of the Gall Bladder, can regulate the Qi of Gall Bladder, transform Damp-Heat and stop the pain.
- LR-14 and BL-18, the Back Transporting point and Front Collecting point respectively of the Liver, can regulate the Liver, promote the Qi movement and stop the pain.
- LI-11 and SP-9, the Sea points, can clear Heat and eliminate Damp from the Fu organs.

Modifications

1. If the Heat is pronounced, add LR-2, the Spring point, to reduce Fire.
2. If there is fever with chills, add LI-4 and GV-14 to expel the Exogenous pathogenic factors from the Exterior and reduce the fever.
3. If there is nausea and vomiting due to obstruction of the Stomach-Qi by Damp-Heat, add CV-12, PC-6 and ST-40 to smooth the Stomach-Qi, and remove Phlegm-Heat.

Case history

A 47-year-old woman had been suffering from hypochondriac pain and a burning sensation in the stomach for 8 years. The symptoms worsened if she was stressed or emotionally disturbed or ate heavy food. The condition was diagnosed as chronic chole-cystitis and she was given medication by her general practitioner, but the pain and the burning sensation were not getting better. The muscles on her back and shoulders were very stiff, also her concentration was poor and she often felt sad and tired. She had a purple tongue with a yellow and greasy coating. Her right pulse was soft and her left pulse was thready and wiry.

Diagnosis
Accumulation of Damp-Heat in the Middle Burner and stagnation of Liver-Qi.

Principle of treatment
Eliminate Damp-Heat, open the channel, disperse the Liver-Qi and strengthen the Spleen-Qi.

Herbal treatment
WEN DAN TANG and **XIAO YAO SAN**
Warming the Gall Bladder Decoction and *Free and Relaxed Powder*
Ban Xia *Rhizoma Pinelliae* 6 g
Ju Pi *Exocarpium Citri Grandis* 6 g
Fu Ling *Poria* 9 g
Gan Cao *Radix Glycyrrhizae* 3 g
Zhu Ru *Caulis Bambusae in Taeniam* 9 g
Zhi Shi *Fructus Aurantii Immaturus* 9 g

Add:

Dang Gui *Radix Angelicae Sinensis* 6 g
Bai Shao *Radix Paeoniae Alba* 6 g
Chai Hu *Radix Bupleuri* 6 g
Bai Zhu *Rhizoma Atractylodis Macrocephalae* 9 g
Bo He *Herba Menthae* 1 g
Sheng Jiang *Rhizoma Zingiberis Recens* 3 g

Add:

Xiang Fu *Rhizoma Cyperi* 9 g
Yu Jin *Radix Curcumae* 6 g
Dan Shen *Radix Salviae Miltiorrhizae* 6 g

Explanations
- Wen Dan Tang eliminates Damp-Heat in the Middle Burner and opens the channels.
- Xiao Yao San tonifies the Blood, softens the Liver and strengthens the Spleen-Qi.
- Xiang Fu disperses the Liver-Qi.
- Yu Jin promotes the Blood circulation and transforms the Damp.
- Dan Shen and Xiang Fu stop pain and reduce the burning sensation in the Stomach.

After 1 month of treatment, the symptoms were under control. She took the herbs for another 3 months to maintain the result. She was followed up 2 years later and she said she had experienced almost no pain after the herbal treatment.

DEFICIENCY SYNDROMES

DEFICIENCY OF QI AND BLOOD AND STAGNATION OF THE LIVER-QI

Symptoms and signs

Chronic, mild and lingering hypochondriac pain, which worsens when stressed, angry or anxious, accompanied by headache, dizziness, a dry mouth and throat, tired, a poor appetite, irregular menstruation, a pale or pink tongue with white coating and a thready and wiry pulse.

This syndrome is often seen in chronic hepatitis, cholecystitis, chronic gastroduodenal ulcer, depression and premenstrual tension.

Principle of treatment

Tonify the Blood, promote the free flow of the Liver-Qi and strengthen the Spleen.

HERBAL TREATMENT

Prescription

XIAO YAO SAN
Free and Relaxed Powder
Chai Hu *Radix Bupleuri* 9 g
Dang Gui *Radix Angeliace Sinensis* 12 g
Bai Shao *Radix Paeoniae Alba* 15 g
Bai Zhu *Rhizoma Atractylodis Macrocephalae* 9 g
Fu Ling *Poria* 15 g
Gan Cao *Radix Glycyrrhizae* 6 g
Bo He *Herba Menthae* 3 g
Sheng Jiang *Rhizoma Zingiberis Recens* 3 g

Explanations

- This is a syndrome of Blood deficiency, stagnation of the Liver-Qi and weakness of the Spleen. The hypochondriac pain has a chronic process. The patient has a Blood deficiency condition, which may be caused by weak constitution, chronic disease, too many operations, giving birth to many children, long-term overwork or excessive thinking. When the Blood fails to nourish the Liver, the Liver becomes rigid and the Qi of the Liver stagnates. It easily influences or overcontrols the Spleen, which is the source of the Qi and the Blood. That is the reason the root and manifestations of the syndrome are not very clear in the chronic stage.
- In this formula, Dang Gui and Bai Shao are able to tonify the Blood, smooth the Liver and promote the Liver-Qi movement, which is the treatment for the cause of this disorder.

- Chai Hu promotes the free flow of the Liver-Qi together with Dang Gui and Bai Shao, in order to treat the hypochondriac pain.
- Bai Zhu and Fu Ling can strengthen the Spleen-Qi, dry the Damp and provide more Qi and Blood to support the Liver.
- Meanwhile, since the Liver-Qi very easily attacks the Spleen in a pathogenic condition, it is necessary to treat the Liver and Spleen together. Sheng Jiang smoothes the Stomach-Qi, improves the appetite. Gan Cao tonifies the Spleen-Qi. Both of them assist Bai Zhu and Fu Ling to strengthen the Middle Burner.
- Bo He, in very small dosage, slightly disperses the Heat produced by Qi stagnation. Meanwhile, it assists Chai Hu to promote the Liver-Qi movement.
- This formula is often used in treating hypochondriac pain in hepatitis, chronic gastritis, gastroduodenal ulcer, premenstrual tension syndrome and depression.

Modifications

1. If there are obvious symptoms due to Liver-Heat, add Zhi Zi *Fructus Gardeniae* 9 g and Mu Dan Pi *Cortex Moutan Radicis* 9 g to clear the Heat and cool the Blood.
2. If there is deficiency of Blood, add Shu Di Huang *Radix Rehmanniae Praeparata* 9 g and Sheng Di Huang *Radix Rehmanniae Recens* 9 g to tonify the Blood and reduce the Empty-Heat resulting from deficiency of Blood.
3. If the Liver-Qi stagnation is pronounced, add Xiang Fu *Rhizoma Cyperi* 9 g and Yu Jin *Radix Curcumae* 9 g to disperse the Liver-Qi and stop the pain.
4. If there is obvious dizziness, blurred vision and the eyes easily get tired, add Ju Hua *Flos Chrysanthemi* 6 g and Gou Qi Zi *Fructus Lycii* 9 g to expel Liver Heat and nourish the Yin and the Blood.
5. If there is irregular menstruation, add Huai Niu Xi *Radix Achyranthis Bidentatae* 9 g and Yi Mu Cao *Herba Leonuri* 9 g to regulate the menstruation.

Patent remedy

Xiao Yao Wan *Free and Relaxed Pill*

ACUPUNCTURE TREATMENT

SP-6 Sanyinjiao, CV-4 Guanyuan, ST-36 Zusanli, BL-20 Pishu, LR-3 Taichong, LR-14 Qimen, GB-34 Yanglingquan, TE-6 Zhigou, PC-6 Neiguan, and GB-40 Qiuxu. Even method is used on these points.

Explanations

- SP-6, the crossing point of three Yin channels of the foot, can tonify the Blood and promote the Blood circulation. CV-4 is able to generate the Blood and invigorate the Blood. These two points are used to treat Blood deficiency and stagnation.
- ST-36, the Lower Sea point, and BL-20, the Back Transporting point of the Spleen, are able to tonify the Spleen, generate the Blood and Qi so as to treat the Spleen and Blood deficiency.
- LR-3, the Source point, LR-14, the Front Collecting point of the Liver, and BL-18, the Back Transporting point of the Liver, can regulate and promote the movement of Liver-Qi and treat its stagnation.
- GB-34 and TE-6 particularly treat the hypochondriac pain.
- PC-6, a Connecting point as well as the Confluence point for the Yin Linking Vessel, is very effective for calming the Mind, smoothing the Qi in the chest, reducing stress and treating irritability, restlessness, depression and other symptoms of emotional disturbance.
- GB-40, the Source point, treats distension in the hypochondriac region and distension in the breasts in premenstrual tension.

Modifications

1. If the Liver-Heat is obvious, add LR-2 and GB-43, the Spring points, to reduce Fire, and LR-8, the Sea point, to nourish the Yin so as to reduce the Fire.
2. If the Blood deficiency is obvious, add KI-3 and BL-23, the Source point and the Back Transporting point of the Kidney, to tonify the Kidney Essence and generate the Blood.
3. If the Liver-Qi stagnation is pronounced, add LU-7 to unblock the Lung-Qi, so as to accelerate the action of dispersing it.

STAGNATION OF THE LIVER-QI AND WEAKNESS OF THE SPLEEN-QI

Symptoms and signs

Hypochondriac pain and distension, with depression, a sensation of fullness in the chest, a poor appetite, irritability, a bitter taste in the mouth and dry throat. The tongue coating is white and thin. The pulse is wiry in the Liver position and moderate in the Spleen position.

This syndrome can be seen in hepatitis and cholecystitis.

Principle of treatment

Spread the Liver-Qi, strengthen the Spleen and harmonise the Liver and Spleen.

HERBAL TREATMENT

Prescription

XIAO CHAI HU TANG
Small Bupleurum Decoction
Chai Hu *Radix Bupleuri* 6 g
Huang Qin *Radix Scutellariae* 12 g
Ban Xia *Rhizoma Pinelliae* 9 g
Ren Shen *Radix Ginseng* 9 g
Gan Cao *Radix Glycyrrhizae* 6 g
Sheng Jiang *Rhizoma Zingiberis Recens* 6 g
Da Zao *Fructus Ziziphi Jujubae* 6 g

Explanations

- This syndrome is characterised by stagnation of the Liver-Qi and weakness of the Spleen-Qi. The Liver-Qi disturbs the function of the Spleen and Stomach.
- Chai Hu disperses the Liver-Qi and causes it to ascend, directly treating the Liver-Qi stagnation. Huang Qin, bitter and Cold in nature, causes Qi to descend, clears the Heat, relieves irritability, the warm sensation in the chest, the bitter taste in the mouth and dry mouth.
- Ban Xia, pungent and warm in nature, disperses Qi stagnation in the Upper and Middle Burners. It can also smooth the Stomach-Qi and together with Huang Qin, regulate the Qi in the Upper Burner and Middle Burner. Since Huang Qin and Ban Xia regulate the Qi, they can also assist Chai Hu to regulate the Qi movement of the Liver.
- Ren Shen, Gan Cao, Sheng Jiang and Da Zao tonify the Spleen and strengthen the Middle Burner against the influence of the Liver.
- This formula can be used in treating the hypochondriac pain in hepatitis, cholecystitis, pyelonephritis, influenza, gastritis, premenstrual tension and depression.

Modifications

1. If there is obvious Qi stagnation, add Zhi Qiao *Fructus Aurantii* 9 g to unblock the chest, Chen Pi *Pericarpium Citri Reticulatae* 9 g to regulate the Qi in the Middle Burner and Jie Geng *Radix Platycodi* 6 g to lift the Qi.

2. If the pain is obvious, add Mu Xiang *Radix Aucklandiae* 6 g to regulate the Liver and Spleen-Qi, and Bai Shao *Radix Paeoniae Alba* 12 g to soften the Liver.

3. If the Heat is obvious, add Bo He *Herba Menthae* 3 g, Qing Hao *Herba Artemisiae Chinghao* 9 g and Zhi Zi *Fructus Gardeniae* 9 g to dispel and clear the Heat.

Patent remedy

Xiao Yao Wan plus Shen Ling Bai Zhu Wan
Free and Relaxed Pill plus *Panax–Poria–Atractylodis Pill*

ACUPUNCTURE TREATMENT

TE-6 Zhigou, GB-34 Yanglingquan, TE-5 Waiguan, GB-40 Quixu, LR-3 Taichong, LU-7 Lieque, PC-6 Neiguan, LI-4 Hegu, ST-25 Tianshu and ST-36 Zusanli. Even method is used on these points.

Explanations

- TE-6 and GB-34 disperse the Qi in the hypochondriac region and stop the pain.
- TE-5, the Connecting point, and GB-40, the Source point, disperse the Qi in the Lesser Yang channels, together with LR-3, the Source point, and LU-7, the Connecting point, to strengthen the effect of the first two points, and treat the hypochondriac pain, depression and fullness in the chest.
- PC-6 can smooth the Qi in the chest and Stomach, clear Heat, and relieve irritability, nausea and poor appetite.
- LI-4, the Source point, ST-25, the Front Collecting point, and ST-36, the Lower Sea point, can tonify the Spleen and strengthen the Qi in the Middle Burner.
- When the Liver-Qi is dispersed, the Spleen-Qi is strengthened and the balance between the two organs will be rebuilt.

Modifications

1. If there is fever with chills, add LI-11 and CV-14 to reduce the fever.
2. If the nausea is obvious and the tongue coating is yellow and sticky, add CV-12 and ST-40 to eliminate Damp-Heat and smooth the Stomach-Qi.
3. If there is abdominal pain, add SP-6 to nourish the Liver and stop the pain.
4. If there is thirst, add TE-2 and LR-8 to increase the Body Fluids and reduce the thirst.

DEFICIENCY OF THE LIVER-YIN AND STAGNATION OF THE LIVER-QI

Symptoms and signs

Mild, but lingering hypochondriac pain, which worsens after physical exertion or in stressful situations, accompanied by a sensation of warmth in the chest, heartburn, irritability, headache, dizziness, a dry mouth and throat, a red tongue with no coating and a wiry, thready and rapid pulse.

This syndrome can be seen in chronic hepatitis, chronic gastritis, intercostal neuralgia, neurosis, premenstrual tension and menopausal syndrome.

Principle of treatment

Nourish the Liver-Yin, soften the Liver, reduce the Heat and disperse the Liver-Qi.

HERBAL TREATMENT

Prescription

YI GUAN JIAN
Linking Decoction
Sheng Di Huang *Radix Rehmanniae Recens* 18 g
Sha Shen *Radix Adenopherae* 12 g
Mai Dong *Radix Ophiopogonis* 12 g
Dang Gui *Radix Angelicae Sinensis* 9 g
Gou Qi Zi *Fructus Lycii* 12 g
Chuan Lian Zi *Fructus Meliae Toosendan* 3 g

Explanations

- If the Liver-Yin is not sufficient to nourish the Liver, the Liver-Qi may stagnate and cause hypochondriac pain. Prolonged persistence of stagnation of Qi may generate Heat, which may also injure the Liver-Yin. This formula is designed for deficiency of Liver-Yin and stagnation of Liver-Qi with restrained Liver-Heat.
- Sheng Di Huang, sweet and Cold in nature, enters the Heart, Liver and Kidney channels. It can nourish the Yin and clear the Heat.
- Sha Shen and Mai Dong both are sweet and Cold, having a similar function to Sheng Di Huang. Since the Blood belongs to the Yin, deficiency of the Liver-Yin accompanies deficiency of Liver-Blood in most cases. Dang Gui and Gou Qi Zi tonify the Blood and moisten Dryness so as to nourish the Liver-Yin. These five herbs can smooth the Liver, thus the Liver-Qi can move properly and the hypochondriac pain will be reduced.

• Chuan Lian Zi, bitter and Cold in nature, enters the Liver channel, drains down the Heat, breaks up the Qi stagnation and restraint of Heat, promotes the Liver-Qi movement and directly treats hypochondriac pain, distension and irritability. Although Chuan Lian Zi is bitter and Cold and has the action tendency of consuming the Yin, its dosage is low and there are enough herbs in this formula to correct its possible side-effects.

Modifications

1. If the pain is pronounced, add Xiang Fu *Rhizoma Cyperi* 9 g and Chai Hu *Radix Bupleuri* 6 g to regulate the Liver-Qi. Add Bai Shao *Radix Paeoniae Alba* 12 g and Zhi Gan Cao *Radix Glycyrrhizae Praeparata* 6 g to moderate the Liver-Qi, and Yu Jin *Radix Curcumae* 9 g and Mu Dan Pi *Cortex Moutan Radicis* 9 g to regulate the Blood and stop the pain.
2. If there is insomnia, add Suan Zao Ren *Semen Ziziphi Spinosae* 9 g and Bai Zi Ren *Semen Biotae* 9 g to calm the Mind.
3. If there is dizziness, and the eyes are obviously dry, add Ju Hua *Flos Chrysanthemi* 6 g, Nu Zhen Zi *Fructus Ligustri Lucidi* 9 g and Han Lian Cao *Herba Ecliptae* 9 g to nourish the Yin and reduce Heat.
4. If there is constipation, add Gua Lou Ren *Semen Trichosanthis* 12 g and Huo Ma Ren *Fructus Cannabis* 12 g to moisten the Intestines and promote bowel movement.

Patent remedy

Xiao Yao Wan plus Liu Wei Di Huang Wan
Free and Relaxed Pill plus *Six-Flavour Rehmanniae Pill*

ACUPUNCTURE TREATMENT

KI-3 Taixi, KI-6 Zhaohai, LR-8 Ququan, BL-23 Shenshu, BL-18 Ganshu, BL-15 Xinshu and SP-6 Sanyinjiao. Reinforcing method is used on these points. Also add PC-6 Neiguan, TE-6 Zhigou, LR-3 Taichong, GB-40 Qiuxu and LU-9 Taiyuan. Even or reducing method is used on these points.

Explanations

• KI-3, the Source point, is able to tonify the Kidney, KI-6 nourishes the Kidney-Yin and reduces Empty-Heat. LR-8, the Sea point, nourishes the Liver-Yin and also reduces Deficient-Heat. SP-6 is able to tonify the Blood and promote the Blood circulation. These four points are especially used for nourishing the Liver-Yin and Kidney-Yin, and softening the Liver so as to disperse the Liver-Qi.
• BL-23, BL-18 and BL-15 are the Back Transporting points of the Kidney, Liver and Heart respectively. They can tonify and harmonise the function of these three organs so as to treat emotional disturbance.
• PC-6 smoothes the Qi in the chest and reduces tension and calms the Mind, together with the other points that treat emotional disturbance.
• TE-6 and GB-34 disperse the Qi in the Lesser Yang channels and stop the hypochondriac pain.
• GB-40, LR-3 and LU-9, the Source points, disperse the Liver-Qi and the Qi in the chest.
• When the Yin of the Liver is sufficient, the Liver becomes soft, the Qi can move freely, and pain and emotional and digestive disorders disappear.

Modifications

1. If there is restlessness, insomnia and dream-disturbed sleep, add HT-7 to calm the Mind and spirit.
2. If there are night sweats, add SI-3 and HT-6 to reduce the sweating.

Abdominal pain 27

腹
痛

Abdominal pain is pain occurring in the area between the epigastrium and the top of the pubis. Generally speaking, either External or Internal causative factors may result in abdominal pain. External factors include invasion of Wind, Cold, Heat and Damp. Internal factors include weakness of the Internal organs due to constitution, age, emotional state and character. Abdominal pain can also be caused by other factors such as trauma and bad diet. The main involved organs are the Spleen, Liver, Kidney and their correspondent channels. Abdominal pain may be attributed to any of the following diseases in Western medicine: enteritis, duodenal ulcer, ulcerative colitis, irritable bowel syndrome (IBS), subacute appendicitis, dysentery, hepatitis, hepatocirrhosis, adhesions in the abdomen after operation or chronic infection, tumour and ascariasis. Abdominal pain caused by urogenital diseases and lumbar disorders is not discussed here. It is strongly advised that acute abdominal pain accompanying the following diseases should be diagnosed and treated in combination with Western medicine: acute cholecystitis, acute intestinal haemorrhagia, perforation, obstruction of the Large Intestine, intussusception, volvulus, acute pancreatitis, appendicitis, peritonitis, intoxication and allergy.

Aetiology and pathology

Invasion of Exogenous pathogenic factors

Exogenous pathogenic Cold, Heat, Damp-Cold or Damp-Heat are the most common factors causing abdominal pain. Cold has a contracting nature and obstructs the channels, collateral, muscles and the Zang-Fu organs, slows down the Qi and Blood circulation, and so causes pain. Heat has a burning and consuming nature, and has an upward-moving tendency. It can consume and concentrate the Blood and Yin, so it slows the circulation of Blood, resulting in its stagnation and the accumulation of water or Phlegm. Heat or Fire may disturb the normal movement of both Qi and Blood, causing stagnation of Qi and Blood. Once this occurs, it may cause pain due to channel obstruction. Damp is a substantial pathogenic factor of the Yin type, and has a heavy and sticky nature. It may combine with Cold or Heat to obstruct the Qi and Blood circulation, causing pain.

Generally speaking, all these pathogenic factors invade the superficial parts of the body, for instance because of abrupt changes of season. When the weather changes too quickly, people who do not take proper care to wear the correct clothing, or who have a weak constitution or are chronically sick, stressed or fatigued, are particularly vulnerable to attack by these Exogenous pathogenic factors. Invasion of Exogenous pathogenic factors may also be caused by bad eating habits (see below).

Bad diet and eating habits

Habitual consumption of cold drinks, or cold or raw food, such as salad or fruit, may cause Cold to invade the Stomach directly. This disturbs the Qi and Blood in the Middle Burner and can cause acute pain. In the long run, it also injures the Spleen-Yang and weakens its function, causing chronic abdominal pain.

Consumption of too much spicy food, coffee or alcohol may cause Excessive-Heat to form in the Bright Yang Fu organs and channels. In the long run, they also consume the Yin of the Bright Yang Fu organs, causing stagnation of the Qi and Blood, and abdominal pain follows. Overindulgence in fatty or sweet food or milk products may generate Damp-Heat in the Middle Burner. Since these kinds of food are rich in energy and nutrition, they are relatively much more difficult to digest and they place an extra burden on the Spleen, Stomach and Small and Large Intestines. If these food and drinks are not transported and transformed properly, they accumulate in the Middle Burner, and easily generate Damp-Heat, which causes abdominal pain.

Overeating directly causes food to accumulate in the Middle Burner and obstruct the Qi and Blood, resulting in acute abdominal pain. On the other hand, eating too little or following a strict weight-loss diet may weaken the Qi in the Middle Burner, leading to disharmony of the Qi and Blood. If the channels and organs in the abdomen fail to be properly supported by Qi and Blood, abdominal pain follows. An irregular food intake or bad eating habits, such as frequent nibbling or a restricted food choice may weaken the Spleen-Qi and bring about abdominal pain.

Intake of dirty or unfresh food may cause toxins to invade the Middle Burner directly, injuring the transportation and transformation of the Spleen, disturbing circulation of the Qi, Blood and Body Fluids, and generating toxic Heat, which causes abdominal pain. Food allergies can also cause abdominal pain. Where there is disharmony and weakness in the Spleen, Kidney and Large and Small Intestines, certain foods may injure the Spleen and cause Heat or Damp-Heat to accumulate in the Middle Burner, triggering abdominal pain.

Physical trauma

Trauma, wounds or adhesions after an operation or from long-lasting infection in the abdomen may cause the Qi and Blood to stagnate and block the channels in the abdomen, and abdominal pain follows.

Emotional disturbance

Habitual pensiveness and pondering over problems, procrastination over decisions and worrying can all directly weaken and block the Spleen-Qi, causing abdominal pain. Excessive stress and frustration may cause stagnation of the Liver-Qi. Furthermore, prolonged anger, indignation, animosity, a sense of being insulted and a tendency to become enraged may cause the Liver-Qi and Liver-Yang to ascend and attack the Spleen. In the Five Element theory this is called the Wood overcontrolling the Earth. When the functions of the Spleen, Stomach and the Small and Large Intestines are disturbed, abdominal pain may be triggered. Also, stagnant Liver-Qi eventually turns to Liver-Fire, which consumes the Blood and Body Fluids in the Middle Burner, causing stagnation of Blood, and abdominal pain.

Depression, sorrow, grief and sadness may weaken and block the Lung-Qi. The Lung is where the Qi from the whole body congregates. If the Lung-Qi stagnates, this in turn may cause the Qi circulation to slow down in the Liver, Spleen and Large and Small Intestines, causing abdominal pain. Fear as well as nervousness, worry and anxiety may cause the Qi to descend, depleting the Kidney-Qi and Spleen-Qi and blocking the free flow of Liver-Qi. Any of these emotions can cause disharmony of the Qi and Blood circulation in the abdomen, and trigger abdominal pain.

Weakness of Spleen-Qi and Spleen-Yang

A weak constitution, chronic sickness, unhealthy diet and bad eating habit, may all cause deficiency of the Spleen-Qi and Yang. When the Qi and Yang fail to warm the organs and channels in the abdomen, interior Cold may form, blocking the Middle Burner and channels, and causing abdominal pain.

Deficiency of Blood

A weak constitution, chronic disease and bad diet may alternatively cause deficiency of Blood. When the channels, tendons, muscles and Internal Zang-Fu organs are not properly nourished by Blood, they go into spasm, causing abdominal pain.

Weakness of Body Fluid in the Intestines

Constitutional Yang Excess, long-lasting febrile disease or habitual eating of spicy food may cause Excessive-Heat to form in the Intestines, which may consume the Yin and Body Fluids, leading to deficiency of Yin and Body Fluid. When the Small and Large Intestines and the other Zang-Fu organs are not properly nourished then abdominal pain, constipation and thirst may follow.

Treatment based on differentiation

Differentiation

In everyday practice, it is very important to differentiate the symptoms clearly in order to get an overall view of the abdominal pain. Special attention should be paid to the following characteristics of the pain: its quality, timing, location, duration, factors that trigger, worsen or alleviate it, and accompanying symptoms.

Differentiation of pain quality

— Distending and migrating pain that is not palpable, is usually caused by stagnation of Qi.
— Sharp, fixed pain that is palpable is usually caused by stagnation of Blood.
— Cramping, severe pain of sudden onset is usually caused by stagnation of the Blood, invasion of Cold or severe stagnation of Qi.
— Pain with a burning sensation is usually caused by Heat.
— Lingering pain, mild pain of long duration, is usually caused by deficiency.

Differentiation of timing

— Pain that occurs or is aggravated at night is usually caused by stagnation of Blood.
— Pain that starts at around 5 a.m. is usually caused by deficiency of Kidney-Yang.
— Pain that begins on waking up in the morning is usually caused by disharmony between the Liver and Spleen.
— Pain that starts after eating certain foods is usually caused by a food intolerance or allergy, or food poisoning.

Differentiation of location

In accordance with TCM

— Pain under the gastrium and above the navel is usually caused by disorder of the Stomach, Heart or Spleen.
— Pain below the navel is usually caused by disorder of the Spleen, Large Intestine or Kidney.
— Pain on the sides of the lower abdomen is usually caused by Liver disorder, for instance accumulation of Cold in the Liver channel, deficiency of Liver-Blood or deficiency of Kidney-Essence.

— Pain in the lower abdomen is usually caused by urogenital disorders.
— Pain around the navel is usually caused by ascariasis.
— Generalised pain over the whole abdomen is usually caused by disorder of the Spleen and Liver.

In accordance with Western medicine

— Pain located in the right upper abdomen is usually caused by disorder of the Liver and Gall Bladder. If this radiates to the back it is usually caused by a disorder of the Gall Bladder.
— Pain slightly on the right of the upper abdomen is usually caused by duodenal disorder.
— Pain in the left upper abdomen is usually caused by a disorder of the stomach. If this radiates to the back it is usually caused by a disorder of the pancreas.
— Pain around the waist and towards the back is usually caused by a disorder of the kidney or a renal stone.
— Pain around the navel is usually a sign of early-stage appendicitis.
— Pain in the right lower abdomen is usually caused by appendicitis or IBS.
— Pain in the lower abdomen generally is usually caused by a disorder of bladder or uterus.

Differentiation of duration

— Acute pain is usually an Excess syndrome.
— Chronic pain is usually a Deficiency syndrome, or mixture of Excess and Deficiency.

Differentiation of factors that trigger, aggravate and relieve the pain

— Pain that starts or is aggravated after consuming cold food or cold drinks is usually caused by Excessive-Cold invasion or deficiency of the Spleen-Yang.
— Pain that starts after overeating is usually caused by accumulation of food.
— Pain after consuming food that has begun to decay or has not been cleaned is usually caused by Damp-Heat or Heat Toxin in the Intestine, or dysentery.
— Pain that starts or is aggravated after eating fatty or greasy food is usually caused by deficiency of Spleen-Qi.
— If the pain is aggravated after eating it is an Excessive syndrome; if it is alleviated after eating it is a Deficient syndrome.

— Pain that starts or is aggravated by stress or emotional disturbance is usually caused by disharmony between the Liver and Spleen.
— Pain that starts after trauma or an operation is usually caused by stagnation of Qi and Blood.
— Pain in someone with a weak constitution or after prolonged disease is usually caused by Deficiency.
— If the pain is alleviated by pressure it is a Deficiency syndrome; if it worsens on pressure it is an Excessive syndrome.

Differentiation of accompanying symptoms

— Constipation is usually caused by Excessive-Heat in the Intestine.
— Difficult bowel movements and abdominal distension are usually caused by stagnation of Qi.
— Soft and sticky stools with blood, mucus and tenesmus are usually caused by Damp-Heat in the Intestine.
— Defecation with a strong bad smell is usually caused by food stagnation, or Damp-Heat in the Intestine.
— Alternating diarrhoea and constipation is usually caused by stagnation of the Liver-Qi.

Treatment

EXCESSIVE SYNDROMES

INVASION OF EXOGENOUS PATHOGENIC COLD

Symptoms and signs

Sudden onset of severe abdominal pain with a cramping nature, accompanied by a preference for warmth, lack of thirst, clear urine, normal or soft stools, a white and sticky tongue coating and deep, wiry and slow pulse.

This syndrome is often seen in acute enteritis, influenza and after excessive consumption of cold drinks, raw and cold food.

Principle of treatment

Warm the Interior and disperse the Cold.

HERBAL TREATMENT

Prescription

LIANG FU WAN and **ZHENG QI TIAN XIANG SAN**
Galangal and Cyperus Pill and *Correct Qi Heaven Fragrant Powder*
Gao Liang Jiang *Rhizoma Alpiniae Officinarum* 6 g

Gan Jiang *Rhizoma Zingiberis* 6 g
Wu Yao *Radix Linderae* 10 g
Chen Pi *Pericarpium Citri Reticulatae* 10 g
Zi Su Ye *Folium Perillae* 6 g
Xiang Fu *Rhizoma Cyperi* 10 g

Explanations

● The combination of these two formulae is especially useful for treating invasion of Cold in the abdomen, which obstructs the Qi movement in the Spleen, Liver, Stomach and Kidney channels.
● Gao Liang Jiang is a pungent and hot herb, entering the Stomach channel. It is able to warm the Stomach and expel Cold. This herb is particularly effective for treating upper abdominal pain.
● Gan Jiang is a pungent and hot herb, entering the Spleen channel. It specifically expels Cold from the Middle Burner and warms the Spleen. This herb is particularly effective for treating pain around the umbilicus.
● Wu Yao is a pungent and hot herb, entering the Liver and Kidney channels. It expels Cold and promotes movement of the Qi in these channels. It is particularly effective for alleviating pain in the centre or at the sides of the lower abdomen.
● Zi Su Ye can smooth the Stomach-Qi and Chen Pi can promote its movement; Xiang Fu can disperse the Liver-Qi. These three herbs used together regulate the Qi and relieve pain; they are three Hot herbs that warm different channels, disperse Cold and promote the movement of Qi in the abdomen.
● When Cold is eliminated and the Qi can flow fluently, abdominal pain disappears.

Modifications

1. If there is severe pain, add Yan Hu Suo *Rhizoma Corydalis* 10 g to invigorate the Qi and Blood circulation so as to stop the pain.
2. If there is severe cramp, add Bai Shao *Radix Paeoniae Alba* 15 g and Zhi Gan Cao *Radix Glycyrrhizae Praeparata* 6 g to regulate the Qi movement and harmonise the tendons so as to stop the pain.
3. If there is severe Cold, add Gui Zhi *Ramulus Cinnamomi* 9 g and Fu Zi *Radix Aconiti Praeparata* 9 g to expel the Cold and warm the channels.
4. If there is lower abdominal pain, add Xiao Hui Xiang *Fructus Foeniculi* 6 g and Rou Gui *Cortex Cinnamomi* 9 g to warm the Lower Burner and Kidney, and disperse Cold.

Patent remedy

Liang Fu Wan *Galangal and Cyperus Pill*

ACUPUNCTURE TREATMENT

CV-6 Qihai, ST-36 Zusanli, SP-4 Gongsun, CV-12 Zhongwan, SP-15 Daheng, GB-34 Yanglingquan and LI-4 Hegu. Reinforcing method is used on the first three points, and reducing method on the last four.

Explanations

- CV-6, the Sea of Qi, can strengthen and disperse the Qi so as to expel Cold.
- ST-36, the Sea point, strengthens the function of the Spleen, warms the Middle Burner and treats the disorder of the Fu organs.
- CV-12 is the Gathering point for all the Fu organs. It can regulate the Qi in the Fu organs so as to stop pain.
- SP-4, the Connecting point, and SP-15 promote the transportation in the Small and Large Intestines and strengthen the function of the Spleen.
- GB-34, the Lower Sea point, regulates the Liver-Qi and relieves cramp.
- LI-4, the Source point, promotes the movement of Qi in the Large Intestine.

Modifications

1. If there is pain above the navel, add CV-10 and ST-24 in order to relieve the pain.
2. If there is pain below the navel, add ST-27 to relieve the pain.
3. If the pain is associated with the sides of the abdomen, add LR-13 to regulate the Liver-Qi and relieve the pain.
4. If there is pain around the navel, add ST-25, CV-9 and CV-7 to relieve the pain.
5. If there is pain in the lower abdomen, add CV-14 to regulate the Qi circulation there.
6. If there is severe pain, add SP-6 and moxibustion on CV-6 to promote the Qi and Blood circulation.
7. If there is abdominal distension, add SP-4 to strengthen the Spleen and cause the Qi to descend in the Penetrating Vessel.

INVASION OF DAMP-COLD

Symptoms and signs

Sudden onset of abdominal pain of a distending nature and alleviated by warmth, accompanied by urgent diarrhoea with gurgling sound, a poor appetite, nausea and vomiting. There may also be a fever, chills, a blocked nose and headache, a white and greasy tongue coating and a soft pulse. This syndrome may be seen following excessive consumption of cold food and drinks, or in influenza and acute gastroenteritis.

Principle of treatment

Expel the Cold and transform Damp from both the Exterior and the Middle Burner.

HERBAL TREATMENT

Prescription

HUO XIANG ZHENG QI SAN
Agastache Upright Qi Powder
Huo Xiang *Herba Agastachis* 6 g
Zi Su Ye *Folium Perillae* 6 g
Chen Pi *Pericarpium Citri Reticulatae* 9 g
Hou Po *Cortex Magnoliae Officinalis* 6 g
Da Fu Pi *Pericarpium Arecae* 9 g
Bai Zhu *Rhizoma Atractylodis Macrocephalae* 9 g
Fu Ling *Poria* 12 g
Ban Xia *Rhizoma Pinelliae* 6 g
Bai Zhi *Radix Angelicae Dahuricae* 6 g

Explanations

- Huo Xiang and Zi Su Ye are warm and aromatic herbs. They are able to expel Cold, transform Damp from the Middle Burner and superficial portions of the body and harmonise the function of Spleen, Stomach and Bladder channels and organs.
- Chen Pi specifically regulates the Qi, dries Damp in the region above the navel. Da Fu Pi regulates the Qi and transforms Damp below the navel and Hou Po has the same function but works on the whole abdomen. These three herbs are very effective for relieving abdominal pain and distension.
- Bai Zhu and Fu Ling can tonify the Spleen and strengthen its function so as to cause the Spleen-Qi to ascend, and dissolve Damp in the Middle Burner. Ban Xia and Zi Su Ye can smooth the Stomach-Qi, stop vomiting and improve the appetite. These four herbs used together restore the proper Qi movement in the Middle Burner.
- Bai Zhi can treat a headache that has a heavy sensation, which is an accompanying symptom in this syndrome. It is able to expel Cold and transform Damp, and also releases the Exterior syndrome.
- When all these herbs are used together, Damp-Cold can be eliminated and dissolved, the Qi can move freely, and then the abdominal pain stops.

Modifications

1. If there is severe pain, add Gui Zhi *Ramulus Cinnamomi* 9 g to disperse the Yang-Qi, expel Cold and relieve the pain.

2. If there is severe abdominal distension, add Mu Xiang *Radix Aucklandiae* 6 g to regulate the Qi in the Liver and Large Intestine channel.

Patent remedy

Huo Xiang Zheng Qi Wan (Pian) *Agastache Upright Qian Pill (Tablet)*

ACUPUNCTURE TREATMENT

ST-25 Tianshu, LI-4 Hegu, ST-37 Shangjuxu, ST-38 Tiaokou and SP-9 Yinlingquan. Even method is used on these points.

Explanations

- ST-25 is the Front Collecting point of the Large Intestine channel, ST-37 is the Low Sea point and LI-4 is the Source point. These three points used together regulate the Qi movement in the Large Intestine and promote its function.
- ST-38 is the Lower Sea point of the Small Intestine; SP-9 is the Sea point of the Spleen channel. These two points can transform Damp, stop diarrhoea and relieve the abdominal pain.

Modifications

1. If there is severe Cold in the Middle Burner, apply moxibustion on CV-8 to strengthen the Spleen-Yang and expel the Cold.
2. If there is severe pain above the navel, add CV-12 and ST-36 to regulate the Fu organs.
3. If there is pain in the sides of the abdomen, add LR-13, the Front Collecting point of the Spleen and the Confluence point for the Zang organs, to regulate the Liver-Qi and harmonise the Spleen.
4. If there is pain in the lower abdomen, apply moxibustion on CV-4 to strengthen the Yang in the Lower Burner.

Case history

A 55-year-old-woman was suffering from abdominal pain and diarrhoea. Three months previously, she had developed dysentery. After treatment with Western medicine, this cleared up, but she continued to suffer from abdominal pain with a cold sensation around the navel, and had diarrhoea four to six times a day. These became worse after eating cold or raw food. She also had abdominal distension, a poor appetite, belching, was generally tired, and had cold limbs, a pale tongue with a white coating and a deep, slow and slightly wiry pulse.

Diagnosis
Accumulation of Cold-Damp in the Middle Burner and deficiency of Spleen-Yang.

Principle of treatment
Expel Cold, transform Damp, warm the Yang and strengthen the Spleen.

Acupuncture treatment
ST-25, SP-9, ST-36, CV-8 and CV-12. Reducing method was used on the first two points, reinforcing method is applied on ST-36, and moxibustion is applied on CV-8 and CV-12.

Explanations
- ST-25, the Front Collecting point of the Large Intestine, can promote the transportation function of the Large Intestine and reduce the accumulation of Cold-Damp.
- SP-9, the Sea point, can transform Damp in the Middle Burner and reduce the diarrhoea.
- ST-36, the Lower Sea point, can strengthen the Spleen, Stomach and Small and Large Intestines.
- Moxibustion on CV-8 and CV-12 can expel Cold in the Middle Burner and warm the Spleen-Yang.

After 1 month of treatment, the patient had recovered.

ACCUMULATION OF EXCESSIVE-HEAT IN THE LARGE INTESTINE

Symptoms and signs

Abdominal pain and distension that is worsened by compression, accompanied by constipation, a sensation of fullness in the chest and upper abdomen, thirst, irritability, scanty urine, a red tongue with a yellow, dry coating and a forceful, rapid and slippery pulse.

This syndrome is often seen in people who habitually indulge in spicy food, those with a Yang constitution, or during a febrile disease. It can also be seen in IBS, intestinal obstruction and adhesions after abdominal operation and constipation.

Principle of treatment

Drain Heat, promote the bowel movement, clear the obstruction and stop the pain.

HERBAL TREATMENT

Prescription

DA CHENG QI TANG
Major Order the Qi Decoction
Da Huang *Radix et Rhizoma Rhei* 10 g
Mang Xiao *Natrii Sulfas* 10 g
Zhi Shi *Fructus Aurantii Immaturus* 6 g
Hou Po *Cortex Magnoliae Officinalis* 6 g

Explanations

- Da Huang is a bitter and cold herb, powerfully draining Heat and purging the bowel. Mang Xiao is salty and cold, clearing Heat, softening the faeces and moistening the Intestine. Both of these substances focus on removing obstruction and clearing Heat in the Large Intestine.
- Zhi Shi and Hou Po specifically promote the movement of Qi in the Large Intestine, relieve the obstruction and assist Da Huang and Mang Xiao to relieve constipation.
- When the four substances are used together, Heat is reduced and the faeces are eliminated, so the Qi obstruction is removed and the abdominal pain disappears.

Modifications

1. If there is fever, add Shi Gao *Gypsum Fibrosum* 15 g to clear Heat and reduce the fever.
2. If there is severe pain, add Mu Xiang *Radix Aucklandiae* 9 g and Qing Pi *Pericarpium Citri Reticulatae Viride* 9 g to regulate the Qi in the Large Intestine and Liver channels.
3. If there is constipation, add Huo Ma Ren *Fructus Cannabis* 12 g and Xing Ren *Semen Armeniacae Amarum* 9 g to promote bowel movement and relieve the constipation.
4. If there is severe abdominal cramp, add Yan Hu Suo *Rhizoma Corydalis* 9 g, Bai Shao *Radix Paeoniae Alba* 12 g and Zhi Gan Cao *Radix Glycyrrhizae* 6 g to relieve the cramp.
5. If there is a thirst, add Xuan Shen *Radix Scrophulariae* 12 g and Mai Men Dong *Radix Ophiopogonis* 12 g to nourish the Body Fluids and relieve the thirst.
6. If there is Deficiency of Yin, add Sheng Di Huang *Radix Rehmanniae Recens* 12 g and Shi Hu *Herba Dendrobii* 12 g to nourish the Yin and clear Deficient-Heat.

Patent remedy

Fang Feng Tong Sheng Wan *Ledebouriella Pill That Sagely Unblocks*

ACUPUNCTURE TREATMENT

LI-4 Hegu, LI-11 Quchi, SP-14 Fujie, ST-37 Shangjuxu, LR-2 Xingjian, CV-12 Zhongwan and CV-6 Qihai. Reducing method is used on these points.

Explanations

- LI-4 is the Source point of the Large Intestine channel, and LI-11 is the Sea point. Both can clear Heat from the Large Intestine.
- ST-37 is the Lower Sea point of the Large Intestine. Together with SP-14 it can promote the movement of Qi and clear obstruction in the Large Intestine.
- LR-2, the Spring point, reduces Liver-Fire and regulates the Liver so as to regulate the Stomach and Large Intestine in turn.
- CV-12 and CV-6 clear obstruction in the Fu organs and stop the pain.

Modifications

1. If there is a fever, add ST-44, the Spring point, to clear Fire and reduce the fever.
2. If there is Yin deficiency, add KI-6 to nourish the Yin and reduce Deficient-Heat.
3. If there is constipation, add ST-25, the Front Collecting point of the Large Intestine, and TE-6 to remove the obstruction in the Large Intestine and promote bowel movement.

ACCUMULATION OF DAMP-HEAT TOXIN

Symptoms and signs

Acute or subacute onset of abdominal pain, which is of fixed location in most cases, but can be spread throughout the abdomen, accompanied by abdominal distension, soft stools or diarrhoea containing blood and mucus, urgent and frequent bowel movement, tenesmus, scanty urine, a red tongue with yellow and greasy coating and a slippery and rapid pulse.

This syndrome is often seen in dysentery, and the acute or active stage of colitis.

Principle of treatment

Clear Heat Toxin, transform Damp, clear the obstruction and stop the abdominal pain.

HERBAL TREATMENT

Prescription

BAI TOU WENG TANG
Pulsatilla Decoction
Bai Tou Weng *Radix Pulsatillae* 9 g
Huang Lian *Rhizoma Coptidis* 6 g
Huang Bai *Cortex Phellodendri* 6 g

Qin Pi *Cortex Fraxini* 6 g
Dang Gui *Radix Angelicae Sinensis* 9 g
Bai Shao *Radix Paeoniae Alba* 9 g
Mu Xiang *Radix Aucklandiae* 6 g
Yan Hu Suo *Rhizoma Corydalis* 6 g

Explanations

- Since there is accumulation of Damp and Heat Toxin in the Spleen and Large Intestine, this could in turn invade the Middle and Lower Burners.
- Bai Tou Weng, Huang Lian and Huang Bai are very bitter and cold herbs, and have a descending action. They are able to clear Heat, and dry Damp in the Middle and Lower Burners. Qin Pi is a bitter, Cold and astringent herb; it can clear Heat and bind up the intestine, and is especially used for prolonged diarrhoea and urgent bowel movement. Since Damp and Heat Toxin must be eliminated, the astringent Qin Pi should not be used too early or in large dosage. These four herbs combined treat the root of the disorder.
- Since the chief complaint is abdominal pain, it is better to use some herbs to treat the pain directly. Dang Gui and Bai Shao enter the Liver and Spleen channels; the first promoting Blood circulation and tonifying the Blood, and the second nourishing the Yin and relaxing the tendons. Together they can regulate the Blood, harmonise the Qi circulation, relieve cramp and stop the pain.
- Mu Xiang can regulate the Qi in the Liver and Large Intestine. Yan Hu Suo can invigorate the Qi and Blood. They can directly stop the pain.

Modifications

1. If there is fever, add Jin Yin Hua *Flos Lonicerae* 12 g, Ma Chi Xian *Herba Portulacae* 18 g and Da Huang *Radix et Rhizoma Rhei* 6 g to clear Heat and remove the Toxicity.
2. If there is a discharge of more blood than mucus in the stool, add Zi Cao *Radix Arnebiae seu Lithospermi* 12 g, Huai Hua *Flos Sophorae* 9 g and Di Yu *Radix Sanguisorbae* 9 g to cool the Blood and stop the bleeding.
3. If there is a discharge of more mucus than blood in the stool, add Fu Ling *Poria* 12 g and Yi Yi Ren *Semen Coicis* 12 g to transform Damp.
4. If there is pronounced tenesmus, add Bai Shao *Radix Paeoniae Alba* 12 g to moderate the Qi in the Large Intestine.
5. If there is Spleen weakness manifesting as tiredness and a poor appetite, add Dang Shen *Radix Codonopsis Pilosulae* 12 g and Bai Zhu

Rhizoma Atractylodis Macrocephalae 9 g to tonify the Spleen and transform Damp.

6. If there is stagnation of the Liver-Qi, add Xiang Fu *Rhizoma Cyperi* 9 g and Chai Hu *Radix Bupleuri* 9 g to disperse the Liver-Qi.

Patent remedy

Huang Lian Su Pian *Coptis Extract Tablet*

ACUPUNCTURE TREATMENT

ST-25 Tianshu, ST-37 Shangjuxu, SP-15 Daheng, SP-9 Yinlingquan, SP-10 Xuehai, LI-4 Hegu, LI-11 Quchi and LR-2 Xingjian. In the acute stage, reducing method is used. Deep needling is essential, with the needle left in place generally for 30 minutes. After the acute stage, even method is used, and shallow needling is required. During the recovery stage, add ST-36 Zusanli.

Explanations

- ST-25 is the Front Collecting point of the Large Intestine, LI-4 is the Source point and ST-37 is the Lower Sea point. These three points together regulate the Qi and Blood in the Large Intestine.
- SP-15 is able to promote the transportation function of the Large Intestine and stop the pain. SP-9, the Sea point, can reduce Damp-Heat in the intestine and reduce mucus and pus in the stool.
- SP-10 can cool the Blood and regulate it so as to stop bleeding and reduce blood in the stool.
- LI-4 and LI-11, the Source point and Sea point respectively of the Large Intestine channel, are used to clear Heat from the Large Intestine.
- LR-3, the Source Point, harmonises the Liver, and reduces Qi stagnation of the Liver so as to regulate in turn the Qi of the Large Intestine.
- ST-36, the Lower Sea point of the Stomach, is an important point for tonification, strengthens the Spleen-Qi and regulates the function of the Spleen, Stomach and Large Intestine.

Modifications

1. If there is severe pain, add CV-6 to regulate the Qi and stop the pain.
2. If there is fever, add ST-44, the Spring point, and LI-1 and SI-1, the Well points, to clear Heat Toxin and reduce the fever.
3. If there is a discharge of more blood than mucus in the stool, add KI-6 and SP-1 to reduce Heat, cool the Blood and regulate it.

4. If there is a discharge of more mucus than blood in the stool, add SP-3 to transform Damp.

5. If there is tenesmus, add BL-29 to regulate the movement of Qi in the intestines.

6. If there is an aggravation of abdominal pain by stress, add GB-20, and BL-18, the Back Transporting point of the Liver, to smooth the Liver and promote the Liver-Qi circulation.

Case history

A 23-year-old woman had been complaining of severe abdominal pain after suffering from colitis for 1 year. The colitis started suddenly with very heavy abdominal pain, and loss of a lot of blood and mucus in the stool. Her bowel movement was irregular and sometimes she also suffered from constipation. She was treated for more than 6 months with Western medicines, and the blood and mucus had improved, but the abdominal pain and constipation remained. The abdominal pain was on the right side, and was constant and heavy in nature with cramp in the lower abdomen. She felt tired and could not sleep well because of the pain. She had no appetite, and felt better from warmth applied to the back and lower abdomen. She had a dark red tongue with a red tip and white and thick coating. Her pulse was weak, soft and deep.

Diagnosis
Accumulation of Damp-Heat Toxin in the Middle Burner with formation of internal Cold, disturbance of Qi and Blood in the Large Intestine.

Principle of treatment
Clear Heat toxin, transform Damp, warm and strengthen the Spleen, promote the Qi movement, regulate the Blood and stop the pain.

Herbal treatment
BAI TOU WENG TANG
Pulsatilla Decoction
Bai Tou Weng *Radix Pulsatillae* 9 g
Huang Lian *Rhizoma Coptidis* 6 g
Huang Bai *Cortex Phellodendri* 6 g
Qin Pi *Cortex Fraxini* 6 g
Bai Shao *Radix Paeoniae Alba* 9 g
Yan Hu Suo *Rhizoma Corydalis* 6 g
Dang Gui *Radix Angelicae Sinensis* 9 g
Bai Zhu *Rhizoma Atractylodis Macrocephalae* 9 g
Hou Po *Cortex Magnoliae Officinalis* 6 g
Wu Yao *Radix Linderae* 6 g
Xiao Hui Xiang *Fructus Foeniculi* 6 g
Rou Gui *Cortex Cinnamomi* 2 g
Zhi Gan Cao *Radix Glycyrrhizae Praeparata* 6 g

Explanations
- Bai Tou Weng Tang is a formula that is very effective in eliminating Damp-Heat Toxin from the intestines.
- Bai Shao and Zhi Gan Cao can nourish the Liver and relax the muscles so as to relieve the abdominal pain.
- Dang Gui and Bai Shao can regulate the circulation of Blood to stop the bleeding in the stool.

- Huo Po and Wu Yao regulate the Qi in the Middle and Lower Burners so as to stop pain and reduce tenesmus.
- Xiao Hui Xiang and Rou Gui are effective for warming the Lower Burner, Kidney-Yang and Spleen-Yang.
- Bai Zhu directly tonifies the Spleen-Qi and strengthens the physiological function of Spleen. Also, together with Hou Po, Xiao Hui Xiang and Wu Yao dry Damp and reduce mucus in the stool.
- Yan Hu Suo is very effective for regulating the Qi and Blood so as to stop the pain.

After taking this formula for 2 weeks, the patient said there was much less pain in her abdomen than before, but she still had no appetite; the white and thick tongue coating had become thinner, and her pulse was not so deep. The formula was then varied a bit; Wu Yao, Rou Gui and Xiao Hui Xiang were omitted because there was not so much Cold in the Lower and Middle Burners. Huang Qin *Radix Scutellariae* 4 g, Mu Xiang *Radix Aucklandiae* 3 g, Ban Xia *Rhizoma Pinelliae* 3 g and Chen Pi *Pericarpium Citri Reticulatae* 3 g were added to promote digestion, regulate the Stomach-Qi and Spleen-Qi and improve the appetite. Huo Ma Ren *Fructus Cannabis* 4 g was added to moisten the Large Intestine and treat the constipation.

After 2 weeks, her appetite had obviously improved. After another month's treatment, there was no more abdominal pain, blood and mucus in the stool or constipation, so she could return to working normally.

ACCUMULATION OF DAMP-HEAT

Symptoms and signs

Acute abdominal pain with distension and diarrhoea, and alleviation of the pain after defecation, accompanied by a burning sensation in the anus, thirst, a red tongue with a yellow and greasy coating and a rapid and moderate pulse.

This syndrome is often seen in acute enteritis, influenza, sunstroke, after excessive consumption of spicy or fatty food, and food allergy.

Principle of treatment

Clear Heat, transform Damp, promote urination and stop the diarrhoea.

HERBAL TREATMENT

Prescription

GE GEN HUANG QIN HUANG LIAN TANG
Kudzu, Coptis and Scutellaria Decoction
Huang Qin *Radix Scutellariae* 12 g
Huang Lian *Rhizoma Coptidis* 6 g

Ge Gen *Radix Puerariae* 6 g
Jin Yin Hua *Flos Lonicerae* 12 g
Mu Tong *Caulis Akebiae* 6 g
Fu Ling *Poria* 12 g
Che Qian Zi *Semen Plantaginis* 9 g

Explanations

- Huang Qin and Huang Lian are cold and bitter, entering the Large Intestine channel. They are effective for clearing Heat and drying Damp in the channel.
- Ge Gen is pungent and cold, entering the Bright Yang channels. It can not only clear Heat, but can also cause the clear Spleen-Qi to ascend so as to stop the diarrhoea.
- Yin Hua can enhance the action of Huang Qin and Huang Lian to reduce Heat.
- Mu Tong, Fu Ling and Che Qian Zi promote urination and eliminate Damp.

Modifications

1. If there is a predominance of Damp, add Fu Ling *Poria* 15 g and Xiang Ru *Herba Elsholtziae seu Moslae* 9 g to transform the Damp.
2. If there is a sensation of burning in the anus, add Huang Bai *Cortex Phellodendri* 9 g to clear the Heat in the Lower Burner.
3. If there is a fever caused by the heat of the sun, add Shi Gao *Gypsum Fibrosum* 18 g and Chai Hu *Radix Bupleuri* 9 g to clear Heat and reduce the fever.

Patent remedy

Ge Gen Qin Lian Pian *Kudzu, Coptis and Scutellaria Tablet*

ACUPUNCTURE TREATMENT

LI-4 Hegu, LI-11 Quchi, ST-39 Xiajuxu, SP-6 Sanyinjiao, ST-25 Tianshu and CV-6 Qihai. Reducing method is used on these points.

Explanations

- LI-4, the Source point, and LI-11, the Sea point, are used to clear Heat in the Large Intestine. They can also expel Wind-Heat and reduce fever if there is an Exterior syndrome.
- ST-39, the Lower Sea point of the Small Intestine, and SP-9, the Sea point of the Spleen channel, are able to reduce Heat, transform Damp in the

Middle and Lower Burners and stop the abdominal pain.
- SP-6 is an important point to resolve Damp and stop pain in the lower abdomen.
- ST-25, the Front Collecting point of the Large Intestine, is used to regulate the function of the Large Intestine.
- CV-6 regulates the Qi and relieves the obstruction so as to stop abdominal pain.
- When all these points are used together, diarrhoea stops and the abdominal pain disappears.

Modifications

1. If there are Exterior symptoms, add TE-5, the Connecting point, to expel the External pathogenic factors.
2. If there is a high fever, add GV-14, the meeting point of all the Yang channels, and ST-44, the Spring point, to clear Heat and reduce the fever.
3. If there is indigestion, add CV-12, the Gathering point for the Fu organs, to regulate the Stomach and promote the digestion.

Case history

One summer, a 35-year-old woman arrived at the clinic complaining of acute abdominal pain that became worse before bowel movement. She also had diarrhoea over ten times a day, a chill, fever, distension in her abdomen, nausea, thirst, scanty urine, a yellow and greasy tongue coating and soft and a rapid pulse.

Diagnosis
Invasion of Damp-Heat to the Intestines.

Principle of treatment
Clear Heat, transform Damp, strengthen the Spleen and stop the abdominal pain.

Acupuncture treatment
LI-4, LI-11, ST-25, SP-9 and ST-44. Reducing method was used on these points.

Explanations

- LI-4, the Source point, and LI-11, the Sea point, are used to clear Heat, promote digestion and relieve Exterior symptoms.
- ST-25, the Front Collecting point of the Large Intestine, regulates Qi, promotes digestion and relieves the obstruction in the Large Intestine.
- SP-9, the Sea point, transforms Damp and clears Heat.
- ST-44, the Spring point, clears Heat and reduces Fire from the Large Intestine.

After the first treatment, she immediately sweated and the abdominal pain and distension diminished. The fever that night also lessened. After 2 weeks of treatment she had recovered from the abdominal pain.

ACCUMULATION OF FOOD

Symptoms and signs

Abdominal pain and distension after overeating, or eating fatty or greasy food, alleviated after defecation, diarrhoea or constipation with a very strong foul smell, thirst, irritability, nausea or a reduced appetite, a thick and greasy tongue coating and a slippery pulse.

Principle of treatment

Promote digestion, remove accumulation and stop abdominal pain.

HERBAL TREATMENT

Prescription

BAO HE WAN
Preserve Harmony Pill
Mai Ya *Fructus Hordei Germinatus* 9 g
Shen Qu *Massa Fermentata Medicinalis* 9 g
Shan Zha *Fructus Crataegi* 9 g
Zhi Ban Xia *Rhizoma Pinelliae Praeparatae* 9 g
Chen Pi *Pericarpium Citri Reticulatae* 9 g
Lai Fu Zi *Semen Raphani* 6 g
Fu Ling *Poria* 12 g
Lian Qiao *Fructus Forsythiae* 3 g
Mu Xiang *Radix Aucklandiae* 6 g
Sha Ren *Fructus Amomi* 6 g
Zhi Shi *Fructus Aurantii Immaturus* 6 g

Explanations

- This syndrome is caused by accumulation of undigested food in the Bright Yang Fu organs, obstructing the Qi circulation.
- The first three herbs when combined promote digestion. Mai Ya particularly promotes the digestion of wheat, rice and fruits, Shen Qu particularly promotes the digestion of grains and alcohol, and Shan Zha particularly promotes the digestion of meat, fat and milk. All these three herbs are deep-fried so as to work in the Middle Burner directly.
- Zhi Ban Xia and Chen Pi can smooth the Stomach-Qi; Lai Fu Zi can cause the Qi in the intestines to descend and promote bowel movement. These three herbs can regulate the Qi, eliminate food stagnation and relieve the abdominal pain.
- Fu Ling, with Zhi Ban Xia and Chen Pi, can transform Damp in the Middle Burner.
- Lian Qiao can break up the accumulation of food and clear Heat caused by food stagnation.

- Mu Xiang and Sha Ren can relieve Qi obstruction in the Large Intestine.
- Zhi Shi can assist Bing Lang to cause Qi to descend and break up food accumulation.
- These are all effective for stopping abdominal pain and distension. When the food is digested, the accumulated food will be eliminated and transformed, and the abdominal pain will disappear.

Modifications

1. If there is a strong foul smell in the stool, add Huang Lian *Rhizoma Coptidis* 6 g to clear Fire in the Large Intestine and relieve the foul smell.
2. If there is a poor appetite, add Hou Po *Cortex Magnoliae Officinalis* 9 g and Jiang Huang *Rhizoma Curcumae Longae* 9 g to regulate the Qi circulation in the Middle Burner and improve the appetite.
3. If there is constipation, add Da Huang *Radix et Rhizoma Rhei* 6 g to disperse the Qi stagnation and promote defecation.
4. If there is nausea, add Zi Su Geng *Caulis Perillae* 9 g to cause the Stomach-Qi to descend and relieve the nausea.

Patent remedy

Bao He Wan *Preserve Harmony Pill*

ACUPUNCTURE TREATMENT

ST-21 Liangmen, ST-25 Tianshu, CV-10 Xiawan, LI-14 Binao and LI-11 Quchi. Reducing method is used on these points.

Explanations

- ST-21 and CV-10 are able to promote digestion and reduce a distending pain in the abdomen.
- ST-25, the Front Collecting point, and LI-11, the Sea point, can clear Heat from the Bright Yang channels and Fu organs and promote transportation in the Large Intestine.
- LI-4, the Source point, can clear Heat and regulate the function of the Large Intestine.

Modifications

1. If there is thirst, add ST-44, the Spring point, to clear Heat and relieve the thirst.
2. If there is belching, add PC-6 and SP-4 to cause the Stomach-Qi to descend and relieve the belching.

STAGNATION OF THE LIVER-QI

Symptoms and signs

Abdominal pain, especially in stressful situations radiating to the sides, with distension in the abdomen, irregular bowel movements, diarrhoea alternating with sometimes constipation, irritability, a sensation of fullness in the chest and hypochondriac region, a poor appetite, a white tongue coating and a wiry pulse.

This syndrome is often seen after prolonged stress caused by overwork or excessive thinking, as well as in emotional disturbance such as anxiety, habitual worrying, anger or frustration. It can also be seen in IBS and chronic colitis.

Principle of treatment

Disperse the Liver-Qi, promote the transportation of the Fu organs, eliminate the obstruction and stop the pain.

HERBAL TREATMENT

Prescription

LIU MO TANG and **CHAI HU SHU GAN SAN**
Six Milled-Herb Decoction and *Bupleurum Soothing the Liver Powder*
Mu Xiang *Radix Aucklandiae* 6 g
Wu Yao *Radix Linderae* 9 g
Chen Xiang *Lignum Aquilariae Resinatum* 3 g
Da Huang *Radix et Rhizoma Rhei* 6 g
Bing Lang *Semen Arecae* 6 g
Zhi Shi *Fructus Aurantii Immaturus* 6 g
Chai Hu *Radix Bupleuri* 6 g
Xiang Fu *Rhizoma Cyperi* 9 g
Chuan Xiong *Rhizoma Ligustici Chuanxiong* 9 g
Zhi Qiao *Fructus Aurantii* 9 g
Bai Shao *Radix Paeoniae Alba* 12 g
Zhi Gan Cao *Radix Glycyrrhizae* 6 g

Explanations

- This is a syndrome caused by stagnation of Liver-Qi. The free flow of Liver-Qi promotes the physiological function of the Spleen, Stomach and Small and Large Intestines. When the Liver-Qi stagnates, the digestion, transformation and transportation function of these organs becomes disturbed. When the circulation of the Qi is obstructed, the stool is not moved along the Large Intestine properly, causing abdominal pain and distension over the whole area. A stressful and depressive situation may aggravate the stagnation of Liver-Qi, leading to difficult defecation or constipation, and causing abdominal pain. In contrast, when the Liver-Qi attacks the Spleen and Large Intestine, there may be diarrhoea or frequent bowel movements.

- Mu Xiang enters the Liver, Spleen and Large Intestine channel. It is a pungent and bitter herb, which can relieve Qi stagnation in these channels and organs, and cause the Qi to descend in the Large Intestine. It is an important herb for regulating Qi and stopping abdominal pain.

- Wu Yao and Chen Xiang are also pungent and bitter. They enter the Spleen and Kidney channels, and are especially effective for regulating the Qi, removing obstruction and stopping the pain in the lower and lateral sides of the abdomen.

- Bing Lang, Zhi Shi and Da Huang specifically cause Qi to descend in the Large Intestine and reduce distension. They are very useful herbs for constipation when the distending pain is pronounced.

- Chai Hu and Xiang Fu are two of the most commonly used herbs for dispersing and regulating the Liver-Qi.

- Chuan Xiong invigorates the Blood circulation and relieves the pain. Zhi Ke unblocks the chest. These two herbs enhance the action of the herbs that remove the obstruction and stop the pain.

- Bai Shao and Zhi Gan Cao smooth and harmonise the Liver so as to benefit the proper movement of the Liver-Qi.

- When the Qi moves freely in the Middle Burner, Liver and Triple Burner channels, then abdominal pain and other symptoms will disappear.

Modifications

1. If the emotions are unstable, add Yu Jin *Radix Curcumae* 9 g to regulate the Qi and remove its stagnation.
2. If the appetite is poor, add Jiang Huang *Rhizoma Curcumae Longae* 9 g and Mai Ya *Fructus Hordei Germinatus* 9 g to regulate the Qi and improve the appetite.
3. If there is distension of the abdomen, add Qing Pi *Pericarpium Citri Reticulatae Viride* 9 g to promote the circulation of Qi.
4. If there is a sensation of fullness in the chest and hypochondriac region, add Chuan Lian Zi *Fructus Meliae Toosendan* 9 g to regulate the circulation of Qi and relieve the fullness.

Patent remedies

Mu Xiang Shun Qi Wan *Saussurea Smooth Qi Pill*
Shu Gan Wan *Soothe Liver Pill*
Xiao Yao Wan *Free and Relaxed Pill*

ACUPUNCTURE TREATMENT

LR-3 Taichong, LR-13 Zhangmen, LR-14 Qimen, CV-12 Zhongwan, CV-17 Tanzhong, PC-6 Neiguan, ST-35 Dubi and ST-36 Zusanli. Reducing method is used on these points.

Explanations

- LR-3, LR-13 and LR-14 are used to regulate the Liver-Qi. LR-13, the Gathering point for the Zang organs, is particularly suitable for treating chronic pain. LR-14, the Front Collecting point of the Liver, is effective for treating pain in the sides of the abdomen as well as the hypochondriac region. LR-3, the Source point, is particularly useful for dispersing and harmonising the Liver-Qi, and together with CV-17, the Gathering point for the Qi, it smoothes the Liver and promotes the circulation of Qi.
- PC-6, the Connecting point, clears Heat and relieves irritability.
- ST-25, ST-36 and CV-12 regulate the Qi in the Middle Burner and stop the pain in the abdomen.

Modifications

1. If the pain is above the navel, add CV-10 to relieve the pain.
2. If the pain is below the navel, add CV-6 to regulate the Qi circulation and relieve the pain.

DISHARMONY BETWEEN THE LIVER AND SPLEEN

Symptoms and signs

Sudden onset of abdominal pain in stressful situations, together with borborygmus, cramp, diarrhoea with the abdominal pain, which starts with the urge to defecate and subsides after completion, a thin and white tongue coating and a wiry pulse in the Liver position and a moderate pulse in the Spleen position.

This syndrome can be seen in IBS, colitis and hyperthyroidism.

Principle of treatment

Smooth the Liver, strengthen the Spleen and stop the pain.

HERBAL TREATMENT

Prescription

TONG XIE YAO FANG
Important Formula for Painful Diarrhoea
Bai Zhu *Rhizoma Atractylodis Macrocephalae* 9 g
Bai Shao *Radix Paeoniae Alba* 9 g
Chen Pi *Pericarpium Citri Reticulatae* 9 g
Fang Feng *Radix Ledebouriellae* 6 g

Explanations

- Bai Zhu is a bitter and warm herb, entering the Spleen channel, drying Damp and strengthening the Spleen. Bai Shao is a sour, bitter and cold herb, entering the Liver channel, smoothing the Liver and relieving stagnation of the Liver-Qi. These two herbs are able to regulate the function of the Liver and Spleen and rebuild the balance between them.
- When the Liver-Qi overcontrols the Spleen, the movement of the Qi and water transformation in the Middle Burner become disturbed. Chen Pi regulates the Qi in the Middle Burner and dries Damp, and together with Bai Zhu stops diarrhoea.
- Fang Feng disperses Qi stagnation in the Spleen and the Liver and together with Bai Shao treats acute and severe abdominal pain.
- When the Liver and Spleen are back in harmony, the abdominal pain disappears.

Modifications

1. If there is vomiting, add Ban Xia *Rhizoma Pinelliae* 6 g and Huang Lian *Rhizoma Coptidis* 6 g to smooth the Stomach-Qi and relieve the vomiting.
2. If there is irritability, add Chai Hu *Radix Bupleuri* 9 g and Xiang Fu *Rhizoma Cyperi* 9 g to disperse the Liver-Qi.
3. If there is severe abdominal pain, add Chuan Lian Zi *Fructus Meliae Toosendan* 6 g and Yan Hu Suo *Rhizoma Corydalis* 9 g to regulate the Liver-Qi and stop the pain.
4. If there is weakness of the Spleen, add Dang Shen *Radix Codonopsis Pilosulae* 12 g and Fu Ling *Poria* 15 g to activate the Spleen and tonify the Spleen-Qi.

Patent remedy

Chai Hu Shu Gan Wan *Bupleurum Soothing the Liver Pill*

ACUPUNCTURE TREATMENT

LR-3 Taichong, LR-14 Qimen, PC-6 Neiguan, ST-36 Zusanli, SP-6 Sanyinjiao and SP-3 Taibai. Reducing method is used on the first three points, and reinforcing method on the last three.

Explanations

- LR-3, the Source point, together with LR-14, the Front Collecting point, and PC-6, the Connecting point, promote circulation of the Liver-Qi and sedate the abdominal pain.
- ST-36, the Lower Sea point, and SP-6, the crossing point of the three Yin channels of the foot, regulate the movement of Qi and the Blood circulation in the abdomen and stop the pain.
- SP-3, the Source point, and ST-36, the Sea point, strengthen the Spleen and harmonise the Spleen and Liver.

Modifications

1. If there is vomiting, add CV-12, the Gathering point for the Fu organs and the Front Collecting point of the Stomach, to regulate the Stomach and relieve the vomiting.
2. If there is irritability, add LR-2 to reduce Liver-Heat and calm the Liver.
3. If there is severe diarrhoea, add SP-9 and ST-25 to transform Damp and regulate the Large Intestine.

STAGNATION OF BLOOD

Symptoms and signs

Stabbing pain in the abdomen with a fixed location, aggravation of the pain at night and, in some cases, a palpable mass in the abdomen, accompanied by a purple colour to the lips and nails, a dark complexion, a purple tongue, or purple spots on its borders and a choppy, deep, wiry or tight pulse.

This syndrome can be seen in chronic cases of abdominal pain, tumour, trauma, adhesions and the early stage of liver cirrhosis.

Principle of treatment

Promote the Qi and Blood circulation, eliminate Blood stasis and stop the pain.

HERBAL TREATMENT

Prescription a

GE XIA ZHU YU TANG
Drive Out Blood Stasis Below the Diaphragm Decoction
Tao Ren *Semen Persicae* 9 g

Hong Hua *Flos Carthami* 9 g
Yan Hu Suo *Rhizoma Corydalis* 6 g
Wu Ling Zhi *Faeces Trogopterorum* 9 g
Chuan Xiong *Rhizoma Ligustici Chuanxiong* 9 g
Dang Gui *Radix Angelicae Sinensis* 9 g
Dan Pi *Cortex Moutan Radicis* 6 g
Chi Shao *Radix Paeoniae Rubra* 6 g
Xiang Fu *Rhizoma Cyperi* 9 g
Zhi Qiao *Fructus Aurantii* 6 g
Wu Yao *Radix Linderae* 6 g
Gan Cao *Radix Glycyrrhizae* 6 g
Chen Pi *Pericardium Citri Reticulatae* 9 g
Sha Ren *Fructus Amomi* 6 g

Explanation

- This is a formula that is suitable for upper abdominal pain radiating to the hypochondriac region. The herbs in this formula can be divided into two groups. One group is to invigorate the Blood circulation and eliminate Blood stasis. Another group is to regulate the Qi circulation. Tao Ren, Hong Hua, Yan Hu Suo, Wu Ling Zhi, Chuan Xiong, Dang Gui, Chi Shao and Dan Pi are the most commonly used herbs to invigorate the Blood circulation and relieve pain, but there are some differences among these.
- Tao Ren and Hong Hua, pungent and warm herbs, break up and disperse stagnant Blood. These two herbs are indicated where there is stagnation of Blood in particular regions of the body, and especially for pain or swelling in the abdomen, and pain of the limbs after trauma or operation.
- Yan Hu Suo regulates both the Qi and Blood circulation and is very effective for stopping pain.
- Wu Ling Zhi breaks up Blood stasis, but does not consume the Blood or disturb the normal Blood circulation. Dang Gui can tonify and move the Blood. Both of them are especially suitable for Blood stagnation in a Deficient syndrome.
- Chuan Xiong strongly activates the Blood circulation, reaching all parts of the body and stopping the pain effectively.
- Chi Shao and Dan Pi clear Heat in the Blood generated by its stagnation.
- Xiang Fu, Zhi Qiao and Wu Yao particularly regulate the Liver-Qi, treating the pain in the sides of the abdomen.
- Sha Ren regulates the Spleen-Qi, treating pain in the middle or lower abdomen.
- Chen Pi regulates the Stomach-Qi as well as the Spleen-Qi, treating pain in the upper and middle area of the abdomen.
- Gan Cao harmonises the actions of the other herbs in the formula.

Modifications

1. If there is irritability and restlessness, add Chai Hu *Radix Bupleuri* 9 g to regulate the Liver-Qi.
2. If there is severe abdominal pain and cramp, add Bai Shao *Radix Paeoniae Alba* 12 g to smooth the muscles and tendons so as to stop the pain and relieve the cramp.
3. If there are palpable and immobile masses, add Mu Li *Concha Ostreae* 18 g and E Zhu *Rhizoma Curcumae* 9 g to reduce the masses.
4. If the Liver-Yin is deficient, add Bai Shao *Radix Paeoniae Alba* 12 g and Sheng Di Huang *Radix Rehmanniae Recens* 12 g to nourish the Liver-Yin.

Prescription b

SHAO FU ZHU YU TANG
Drive Out Blood Stasis in the Lower Abdomen Decoction
Xiao Hui Xiang *Fructus Foeniculi* 6 g
Gan Jiang *Rhizoma Zingiberis* 6 g
Yan Hu Suo *Rhizoma Corydalis* 9 g
Mo Yao *Resina Myrrhae* 6 g
Dang Gui *Radix Angelicae Sinensis* 12 g
Rou Gui *Cortex Cinnamomi* 6 g
Chuan Xiong *Radix Ligustici Chuanxiong* 6 g
Chi Shao *Radix Paeoniae Rubra* 9 g
Pu Huang *Pollen Typhae* 12 g
Wu Ling Zhi *Faeces Trogopterorum* 9 g

Explanations

- This is a formula that is effective for treating lower abdominal pain due to stagnation of Blood in the Lower Burner that is partially caused by deficiency of the Kidney-Yang. All the herbs in this formula are warm herbs, especially Xiao Hui Xiang, Gan Jiang and Rou Gui, which can warm the Lower Burner so as to promote the circulation of the Blood. The remaining herbs in the formula are used to regulate the Blood.
- Pu Huang, Wu Ling Zhi, Yan Hu Suo and Chuan Xiong are very effective for stopping the pain. Mo Yao can break up the stasis.
- Chi Shao can clear Heat in the Blood and reduce the side-effects of the hot herbs.
- Dang Gui regulates and tonifies the Blood.

Modifications

1. If there is obvious Liver-Qi stagnation, add Chai Hu *Radix Bupleuri* 9 g and Xiang Fu *Rhizoma Cyperi* 9 g to promote the Liver-Qi circulation.
2. If there is distension in the abdomen, add Qing Pi *Pericarpium Citri Reticulatae Viride* 9 g and Wu Yao *Radix Linderae* 3 g to regulate the Spleen-Qi and relieve the distension.

Patent remedy

Yan Hu Suo Zhi Tong Pian *Corydalis Stop Pain Tablet*

ACUPUNCTURE TREATMENT

LR-3 Taichong, LR-14 Qimen, PC-6 Neiguan, CV-6 Qihai, SP-6 Sanyinjiao, BL-17 Geshu and Ah Shi points. Reducing method is used on these points. For acute Blood stagnation, such as trauma, the distant points are selected. For chronic cases with stagnation of Blood, the local points are selected. For pain due to adhesions or a scar, the local points are also very important.

Explanations

- The Ah Shi points are used to clear obstruction in the Blood circulation and stop the pain directly.
- PC-6, LR-3 and CV-6 promote the circulation of Qi and stop pain.
- SP-6, the crossing point of the three Yin channels of the foot, and BL-17, the Gathering point for the Blood, invigorate the Blood circulation, eliminate its stasis and stop the pain.
- LR-14, the Front Collecting point as well as the point where the Liver, Spleen and Yin Linking Vessel meet, smoothes the Liver, promotes the Liver-Qi circulation and reduces the pain.

DEFICIENCY SYNDROMES

DEFICIENCY OF SPLEEN-QI

SYMPTOMS AND SIGNS

Slight, lingering abdominal pain that begins or worsens after eating a heavy meal or unusual foods and improves after rest or warm, light food, accompanied by loose stools, a poor appetite, belching and abdominal distension, a pale tongue with white coating and a weak pulse.

This syndrome can be seen in many chronic diseases, such as chronic colitis, enteritis, cholecystitis, hepatitis, pancreatitis, duodenal ulcer, IBS and food allergy.

Principle of treatment

Strengthen the Spleen and relieve the abdominal pain.

HERBAL TREATMENT

Prescription

XIAO JIAN ZHONG TANG
Minor Strengthening the Middle Decoction
Yi Tang *Saccharum Granorum* 15 g
Gui Zhi *Ramulus Cinnamomi* 6 g
Bai Shao *Radix Paeoniae Alba* 12 g
Zhi Gan Cao *Radix Glycyrrhizae Praeparata* 6 g
Sheng Jiang *Rhizoma Zingiberis Recens* 3 g
Da Zao *Fructus Ziziphi Jujubae* 6 g

Explanations

● This is a formula that is especially suitable for abdominal pain with slight cramping due to deficiency of the Spleen-Qi. Since there is deficiency of the Yang-Qi, interior Cold forms, leading to weakness of the Spleen and Stomach and undernourishment of the interior organs and channels, which causes abdominal pain.

● Yi Tang, sweet and slightly warm, enters the Spleen channel, tonifies the Spleen, and generates the Qi and Blood without the side-effects of consuming the Yin or weakening the Yang. Gui Zhi, a pungent and warm herb, promotes the Yang and Qi circulation. Bai Shao, a sour and cold herb, nourishes the Yin and relieves the cramp. The two herbs, together with Yi Tang, are used to harmonise, strengthen and nourish the Spleen so as to stop the pain.

● Zhi Gan Cao, together with Gui Zhi, warms the Yang, and with Bai Shao nourishes the Yin Zhi. Gan Cao by itself can tonify the Spleen-Qi.

● Sheng Jiang, a pungent and warm herb, regulates the Stomach-Qi and promotes digestion, assisting Gui Zhi to disperse the Yang-Qi.

● Da Zao promotes the transformation of Blood in the Middle Burner so as to assist Bai Shao in tonifying Blood.

● When these five herbs are used together, the Spleen is strengthened, the Qi, Blood, Yin and Yang are harmonised and the pain disappears.

Modifications

1. If there is obvious Blood deficiency, add Dang Gui *Radix Angelicae Sinensis* 9 g to tonify the Blood.
2. If there is obvious Qi deficiency, add Huang Qi *Radix Astragali seu Hedysari* 15 g to strengthen the Qi.

Prescription b

XIANG SHA LIU JUN ZI TANG
Six-Gentlemen Decoction with Aucklandia and Amomum
Dang Shen *Radix Codonopsis Pilosulae* 9 g
Bai Zhu *Rhizoma Atractylodis Macrocephalae* 9 g
Fu Ling *Poria* 12 g
Zhi Gan Cao *Radix Glycyrrhizae Praeparata* 6 g
Chen Pi *Pericarpium Citri Reticulatae* 6 g
Zhi Ban Xia *Rhizoma Pinelliae Praeparata* 6 g
Mu Xiang *Radix Aucklandiae* 9 g
Sha Ren *Fructus Amomi* 6 g

Explanations

● This is a formula that is particularly suitable for abdominal pain with distending sensation, belching, a poor appetite and loose stools after eating a heavy meal.

● Dang Shen, Bai Zhu, Fu Ling and Zhi Gan Cao, known as Si Jun Zi Tang—Four-Gentlemen Decoction—can tonify the Spleen-Qi.

● Zhi Ban Xia and Chen Pi harmonise the Stomach-Qi, transform Phlegm and treat a poor appetite, belching and upper abdominal distension.

● Mu Xiang and Sha Ren promote the movement of Qi and treat the pain and distension in the abdomen and loose stools.

● When the above herbs are used together, they can strengthen the Spleen and relieve the abdominal pain as well as other symptoms.

Modifications

1. If there is severe pain, add Yan Hu Suo *Rhizoma Corydalis* 15 g and Xiang Fu *Rhizoma Cyperi* 9 g to promote the circulation of Qi and Blood and relieve the pain.
2. If the appetite is poor, add Gu Ya *Fructus Oryzae Germinatus* 9 g and Mai Ya *Fructus Hordei Germinatus* 9 g to promote digestion and improve the appetite.

Patent remedies

Si Jun Zi Pian *Four-Gentlemen Tablet*
Shen Ling Bai Zhu Wan (Pian) *Panax–Poria–Atractylodis Pill (Tablet)*

ACUPUNCTURE TREATMENT

BL-20 Pishu, BL-21 Weishu, ST-36 Zusanli, SP-6 Sanyinjiao and SP-3 Taibai. Reinforcing method and moxibustion are used on these points.

Explanations

● BL-20 and BL-21, the Back Transporting points of the Spleen and Stomach, tonify the Spleen and Stomach and regulate their physiological functions.

- ST-36, the Lower Sea point, together with SP-3, the Source point, strengthen the Spleen-Qi, transform Damp and promote digestion.
- SP-6 strengthens the Spleen, regulates the Qi and Blood and stops the pain.

Modifications

1. If there is chronic pain with food stagnation, add BL-25 to regulate the intestine and promote digestion.
2. If there is aggravation of the pain with stress, add BL-18 and LR-3 to smooth the Liver and regulate the Liver-Qi.
3. If there is chronic diarrhoea, add SP-9 to transform Damp and relieve the diarrhoea.

Case history

A 60-year-old-woman had been suffering from colitis for more than 5 years. The chief complaint was a lingering abdominal pain, which always worsened with stress or after eating cold or raw food, or a heavy meal. When the abdominal pain worsened, there was also diarrhoea. Accompanying symptoms were blood and mucus in the stool, nausea and tiredness. She had a purple and pale tongue with a thin white coating and a wiry and thready pulse.

Diagnosis
Deficiency of Spleen-Qi, stagnation of Liver-Qi and accumulation of Damp in the Middle Burner.

Principle of treatment
Strengthen the Spleen-Qi, transform Damp, regulate the Liver-Qi and stop the pain.

Herbal treatment
SI JUN ZI TANG
Four-Gentlemen Decoction
Dang Shen *Radix Codonopsis Pilosulae* 12 g
Bai Zhu *Rhizoma Atractylodis Macrocephalae* 12 g
Fu Ling *Poria* 15 g
Gan Cao *Radix Glycyrrhizae* 6 g
Bai Shao *Radix Paeoniae Alba* 12 g
Chai Hu *Radix Bupleuri* 6 g
Mu Xiang *Rhizoma Cyperi* 6 g

Explanations

- The first four herbs form the basic formula, known as Si Jun Zi Tang—Four-Gentleman Decoction—which activates the Spleen and Stomach and tonifies the Spleen-Qi.
- Chai Hu regulates the Liver-Qi.
- Bai Shao nourishes Liver-Yin and Blood. When it is combined with Zhi Gan Cao, it can smooth the Liver and relieve the cramping pain.
- Mu Xiang, entering the Liver and Large Intestine channels, regulates the Qi circulation and stops pain.

Acupuncture treatment
ST-25, ST-36, SP-3, SP-6, SP-9, LR-3 and LI-4. Even method was used on these points.

Explanations

- ST-36, the Lower Sea point, strengthens the Middle Burner.
- SP-3, the Source point, together with SP-6 and SP-9, can strengthen the Spleen, transform Damp and stop the abdominal pain.
- LR-3, the Source point, promotes the circulation of Liver-Qi so as to reduce the tension in the abdomen.
- ST-25, the Front Collecting point of the Large Intestine, and LI-4, the Source point, relieve stagnant food, promote digestion and stop the abdominal pain.

After 3 months of treatment with Chinese herbs and acupuncture, the complaint was under control.

DEFICIENCY OF SPLEEN-YANG

Symptoms and signs

Abdominal pain with a cold and cramping nature, which worsens after eating cold food, accompanied by loose stools, cold limbs, a preference for warm drinks and food, a poor appetite, a pale tongue with a white and moist coating and a deep, slow and weak pulse.

This syndrome can be seen in chronic colitis, IBS and chronic dysentery.

Principle of treatment

Tonify the Spleen-Yang, warm the interior and relieve the pain.

HERBAL TREATMENT

Prescription

LI ZHONG WAN
Regulating the Middle Decoction
Ren Shen *Radix Ginseng* 9 g
Gan Jiang *Rhizoma Zingiberis* 6 g
Bai Zhu *Rhizoma Atractylodis Macrocephalae* 12 g
Zhi Gan Cao *Radix Glycyrrhizae Praeparata* 6 g

Explanations

- Ren Shen, a sweet, slightly warm herb, can powerfully tonify the Spleen-Qi and the Qi of the whole body.
- Gan Jiang, a pungent and hot herb, warms the Spleen and expels Cold.
- Bai Zhu, a bitter and warm herb, enhances the function of Ren Shen to tonify the Spleen-Qi as well as dry Damp in the Middle Burner.

- Zhi Gan Cao harmonises the actions of the other herbs in the formula.
- When the Spleen-Qi is sufficient, Cold is eliminated from the Middle Burner and the abdominal pain stops.

Modifications

1. If the pain is severe, add Gui Zhi *Ramulus Cinnamomi* 9 g and Bai Shao *Radix Paeoniae Alba* 15 g to harmonise the Qi and Blood and relieve the pain.
2. If there is diarrhoea, add Fu Ling *Poria* 12 g to eliminate Damp, and Huang Qi *Radix Astragali seu Hedysari* 12 g and Sheng Ma *Rhizoma Cimicifugae* 6 g to cause the Spleen-Qi to ascend.

Patent remedy

Fu Zi Li Zhong Wan *Prepared Aconite Pill to Regulate the Middle*

ACUPUNCTURE TREATMENT

BL-20 Pishu, BL-23 Shenshu, BL-25 Dachangshu, BL-26 Guanyuanshu, GV-4 Mingmen, SP-3 Taibai, SP-6 Sanyinjiao, SP-9 Yinlingquan and KI-3 Taixi.

Reinforcing method is used on these points. Moxibustion can be applied too.

Explanations

- BL-20 and BL-23, BL-25 and BL-26, the Back Transporting points, strengthen the Kidney and Spleen, and promote their physiological functions.
- BL-25 and BL-26 relieve the pain.
- GV-4 tonifies the Kidney-Yang and expels internal Cold so as to warm the Spleen-Yang. It is especially effective when moxibustion is applied on this point.
- SP-6 regulates the Blood, transforms Damp and stops the pain.
- SP-9 strengthens the Spleen, transforms Damp and treats abdominal distension and loose stools.
- KI-3 and SP-3, the Source points, specifically regulate the function of the Kidney and Spleen.
- Moxibustion is very effective to warm the Yang and expel Cold.

Modifications

1. If there is severe abdominal pain, apply moxibustion on CV-6 to warm the Interior and relieve the pain.
2. If there is diarrhoea in an elderly person, apply moxibustion on CV-8 and CV-4 to stop diarrhoea.

Dysmenorrhoea 28

痛
经

Dysmenorrhoea is severe pain appearing in the lower abdomen or sacral region during, before or after menstruation. It may greatly influence the daily life and work.

Dysmenorrhoea is divided into primary and secondary dysmenorrhoea in the Western medical classification. Dysmenorrhoea occurring after the menarche without the existence of organic disease is considered to be primary dysmenorrhoea, or functional dysmenorrhoea. Dysmenorrhoea caused by a distinct organic disease, such as pelvic inflammation or endometriosis, is called secondary dysmenorrhoea.

Aetiology and pathology

Generally speaking, the aetiology of dysmenorrhoea includes the invasion of External pathogenic factors, abnormal emotions, dysfunction of the internal Zang-Fu organs, bad diet and excessive sexual activity. The pathogenic factors may cause either stagnation of the Qi and Blood in the Penetrating and Directing Vessels and blockage in the Uterus or failure of regulation of these Vessels, or insufficient nourishment of the Uterus by the Qi and Blood.

Qi and Blood should circulate freely in the body, particularly in the Penetrating and Directing Vessels. Emotional disturbances may cause the Qi and Blood to stagnate, causing blockage in the above Vessels and the Uterus, and resulting in dysmenorrhoea.

Constitutional weakness may cause weakness of the above Vessels. Weakness of the Spleen and Stomach may cause deficiency of Qi and Blood. Prolonged sickness may lead to consumption of the Qi, Blood and Kidney-Essence. The normal blood loss during menstruation will aggravate any deficiency of the Qi and Blood, leading to undernourishment of the Penetrating and Directing Vessels and Uterus. Constitutional Yang deficiency may cause Interior Cold to form, whereas constitutional Yin deficiency may cause Deficient-Heat to form. During menstruation, blood in the Penetrating and Directing Vessels and Uterus may meet this Cold or Heat, causing blockage in these Vessels and the Uterus. All of these can precipitate dysmenorrhoea.

Accumulation of Cold-Damp or Damp-Heat in the Lower Burner may slow down the circulation of Qi and Blood, causing a blockage in the above Vessels and the Uterus, leading to dysmenorrhoea.

Stagnation of Liver-Qi

Emotional stimulation is a very important causative factor in dysmenorrhoea. Emotional disturbances include frequent anger, frustration, resentment, stress and insult. There should be a free and smooth circulation of Qi in the Liver; prolonged or habitual emotional disturbance, especially excessive anger and stress during menstruation, pregnancy or shortly after delivery, may cause the Liver-Qi and the Qi in the Penetrating and Directing Vessels and the Uterus to stagnate, causing dysmenorrhoea. Furthermore, Qi circulation leads to Blood circulation, and Qi stagnation leads to Blood stagnation. So if the stagnation of Liver-Qi persists over a long period, it may in turn cause stagnation of Blood, which aggravates the dysmenorrhoea.

Accumulation of Cold-Damp

Women belong to the category of Yin, especially during their monthly periods or soon after the period as well as after giving birth. Also, excessive environmental exposure to Cold and Damp, such as living, working or walking in a humid place, may allow these pathogenic factors to invade the Lower Burner, and affect the Penetrating and Directing Vessels as well as the Uterus. Cold is characterised by contraction and stagnation, and Damp is characterised by viscosity, heaviness and stagnation. When these two pathogenic factors in combination attack women, they usually invade the Lower Burner, leading to Qi and Blood stagnation and accumulation of Cold-Damp in the Uterus. Finally, drinking too many cold beverages, eating too much cold and raw food, swimming, taking a cold shower or excessive sexual intercourse during the menstrual period or soon after, as well as after giving birth, may also easily allow Cold-Damp to invade the Uterus, leading to stagnation of Qi and Blood. All of these factors can lead to dysmenorrhoea.

Downward flow of Damp-Heat

Overeating of sweet food, fatty or greasy food, meat or milk products, as well as drinking too much alcohol, may impair the Spleen and Stomach, leading to the formation of Damp-Heat. Damp is characterised by stagnation, viscosity and heaviness; Heat is characterised by burning. When Damp-Heat forms in the body, it may flow downward to the Lower Burner, disturbing the Penetrating and Directing Vessels and damaging the Uterus. This downward flow may also cause the Qi and Blood to stagnate, precipitating dysmenorrhoea.

In fact, this downward flow of Damp-Heat may also be caused by incomplete elimination of an invasion of External Damp-Heat, or overlong persistence of Cold-Damp in the body. A further cause is lack of personal hygiene, which can cause Damp-Heat to invade the Lower Burner, leading to dysmenorrhoea.

Deficiency of Qi and Blood

Prolonged illness, dysfunction of the Internal Zang-Fu organs, a bad diet, as well as excessive physical or mental work may cause deficiency of Qi and Blood, leading to failure of the Penetrating and Directing Vessels to fill with Blood, and undernourishment of the Uterus, leading to dysmenorrhoea.

The normal circulation of Blood is promoted by the Qi, so if the Qi is deficient, this may cause the Blood circulation to slow, resulting in stagnation of the Blood in the Penetrating and Directing Vessels and Uterus, and causing dysmenorrhoea. This kind of dysmenorrhoea is due to a mixture of Deficiency and Excess, and is difficult to treat.

Deficiency of Essence of Liver and Kidney

A weakness of the constitution, excessive bleeding during menstruation, giving birth to several children, multiple curettage, excessive sexual activity or masturbation, prolonged weakness of the Spleen and Stomach, and prolonged deficiency of the Qi and Blood, as well as chronic sickness may cause a deficiency of the Essence of Liver and Kidney, leading to Emptiness in the Penetrating and Directing Vessels and undernourishment of the Uterus, and causing dysmenorrhoea. The Kidney-Yin is the root Yin of the body, and if this is deficient then the body as a whole, as well as the above Vessels and the Uterus, will be undernourished. A deficiency of the Yin of the Liver and Kidney may also cause Deficient-Heat to form, leading to hyperactivity of Deficient-Fire. When this Deficient-Fire burns the Uterus and channels and collateral, it causes dysmenorrhoea. The Kidney-Yang is the root Yang of the body generally, and if it becomes deficient this will cause Deficient-Cold to form in the body, leading to insufficient warming of the Penetrating and Directing Vessels and Uterus, to contraction and stagnation in these Vessels and organs and finally to stagnation of the Qi and Blood, causing dysmenorrhoea.

Why does dysmenorrhoea occur only around the period of menstruation and not between the periods or when periods have ceased? This is because at the latter times, even if pathogenic factors are present, the circulation of Qi and Blood in the Penetrating and Directing Vessels is not much disturbed, the Uterus is able to maintain its physiological function, so there is no dysmenorrhoea. During or around menstruation, however, the Directing Vessel transmits an abundance of Blood to the Penetrating Vessel, and this vessel in turn discharges much more Blood to the Uterus. At this time, pathogenic factors may more easily influence these two vessels to cause either blockage or undernourishment of these vessels and the Uterus, leading to dysmenorrhoea. After the menstrual period, the Qi and Blood in these Vessels is again properly regulated, as the Penetrating Vessel doesn't need to transmit so much Blood to the Uterus, so these Vessels and the Uterus will not be easily influenced by these pathogenic factors, thus there is no dysmenorrhoea.

In summary, the chief location for dysmenorrhoea is the Penetrating and Directing Vessels and the Uterus, the chief disorder is of Qi and Blood, and the chief complaint is pain.

Treatment based on differentiation

Differentiation

Before giving the treatment, a clear differentiation should be made.

Differentiation of Excess and Deficiency

It can be seen from the above description that dysmenorrhoea can be subdivided into two groups: dysmenorrhoea due to Excess and dysmenorrhoea due to Deficiency. The first group includes stagnation of Qi and Blood, accumulation of Cold-Damp and downward flow of Damp-Heat; the second includes deficiency of Qi and Blood, deficiency of the Yin of the Liver and Kidney and deficiency of the Kidney-Yang. In practice, dysmenorrhoea that is due to a mixture of Excess and Deficiency is also commonly seen. It is necessary to find out which causative factor is the most important, and which cause is less important. Proper treatment can be given only when this differentiation is clearly made.

— Severe pain and constant pain are usually caused by Excessive factors.
— Slight pain and intermittent pain are usually caused by Deficiency.
— Pain occurring before and during the period is usually of the Excessive type.
— Pain occurring after the period is of the Deficient type.
— Pain occurring before and during the period with scanty and sticky or purplish-coloured blood is usually of the Excessive type.
— Pain occurring after the period with light-red-coloured blood loss and diluted blood discharge is usually of the Deficient type.

— If the pain is aggravated by pressure it is of the Excessive type.
— Pain that is alleviated by pressure indicates Deficiency.

Differentiation of Qi stagnation or Blood stagnation

— If there is a distending or wandering pain, a pain with a feeling of swelling, and the pain is closely associated with the emotional state, it is usually caused by stagnation of Qi.
— If the pain is stabbing in nature with a fixed location and associated abdominal masses, and is worse at night, it is usually caused by stagnation of Blood.

Differentiation of Heat and Cold

— If the pain is alleviated on contact with heat, and aggravated by cold, this indicates it is a Cold type. This type can be caused by invasion of external cold, accumulation of Cold-Damp, deficiency of Qi or deficiency of Kidney-Yang.
— If it is accompanied by an aversion to cold, a slight fever, generalised body pain, a runny nose, a cough with white phlegm, a thin tongue coating and a superficial and tight pulse, it is caused by invasion of External Cold.
— If it is accompanied by white leucorrhoea with no smell, no itching, a sensation of heaviness in the lower abdomen, a poor appetite, a white and greasy tongue coating and a slippery pulse, it is caused by accumulation of Cold-Damp.
— If it is accompanied by scanty blood loss of a light red colour, with tiredness, a pale complexion, cold hands and feet, shortness of the breath, a poor appetite, a thin and white tongue coating and a threthy and weak pulse, it is caused by deficiency of Qi.
— If it is accompanied by scanty or irregular menstruation, cold hands and feet, a lower back pain with a cold sensation, profuse clear urine, oedema, a pale tongue with a wet coating and a deep and slow pulse, it is caused by deficiency of Kidney-Yang.
— If the pain is alleviated by contact with cold and aggravated by heat, this indicates it is of the Hot type. This type of dysmenorrhoea can be caused by downward flow of Damp-Heat and deficiency of the Yin of Liver and Kidney.
— If it is accompanied by a feeling of heaviness in the lower abdomen, leucorrhoea with a smelly yellow discharge, genital itching, loose stools, a

fever or feverish feeling, deep and yellow urine, a yellow and greasy tongue coating and a slippery and rapid pulse, it is caused by downward flow of Damp-Heat.

— If it is accompanied by scanty and sticky menstruation, a burning feeling in the lower abdomen, night sweating, heat in the palms and soles of the feet, thirst, dry stools, a red tongue with a scanty coating and a thready and rapid pulse, it is caused by deficiency of the Yin of Liver and Kidney.

Differentiation of the character of the pain

— Pain with a distending feeling, or with a wandering nature is usually caused by stagnation of Qi.
— Pain with a stabbing feeling, or with a fixed location, or with a pulling sensation is usually caused by stagnation of Blood.
— Pain with a burning feeling is usually caused by downward flow of Damp-Heat or deficiency of the Yin of Liver and Kidney.
— Pain with a cold feeling is usually caused by accumulation of Cold-Damp, deficiency of Qi or deficiency of Kidney-Yang.
— A cramping pain is usually caused by Cold in the Uterus.
— Pain with a bearing-down sensation is usually caused by deficiency of Qi.

Differentiation of location

— Pain on one or both sides of the lower abdomen is usually caused by stagnation of Qi, and a related disorder of the Liver.
— Pain in the centre line of the abdomen is usually caused by stagnation of Blood.
— Pain at the lower abdomen that moves up and down and refers to the sacrum is usually caused by a disorder of the Kidney, and is related to the Kidney and Bladder channels.

Differentiation of the menstrual cycle

— If the cycle is prolonged and the menstrual blood is dark and clotted, this indicates stagnation of Blood.
— If the cycle is prolonged and the menstrual blood is light red, this indicates deficiency of Qi.
— If the cycle is irregular and the blood is scanty, this indicates Deficient type.
— If the cycle is short and the blood loss is scanty, this also indicates Deficient type.

Treatment

The general principle of treatment is to regulate the Qi and Blood in the Penetrating and Directing Vessels. Since the pathogenic factors for dysmenorrhoea vary according to whether it is caused by Excess or Deficiency, other principles, such as whether to promote the Qi circulation, to promote the Blood circulation, to eliminate Blood stasis, to eliminate Damp, to disperse Cold, to clear Heat, to tonify the Qi and Blood, or to tonify the Liver and Kidney, etc. will vary according to the causation. Moreover, treatment for dysmenorrhoea differs depending on whether the treatment is given during menstruation or after it. During menstruation, treatment is given only to treat the symptoms by regulating the Blood and stopping the pain. At other times of the cycle, treatment can also be given to treat the root causes by regulating the Penetrating and Directing Vessels and eliminating pathogenic factors.

When using herbal prescriptions to treat dysmenorrhoea, some herbs can be applied for symptomatic treatment in order to strengthen the therapeutic effect, so if Cold is predominant, Ai Ye *Folium Artemisiae Argyi*, Xiao Hui Xiang *Fructus Foeniculi*, Gan Jiang *Rhizoma Zingiberis*, Wu Yao *Radix Linderae* or Wu Zhu Yu *Fructus Evodiae* can be added to dispel the Cold and relieve the pain. If Heat is predominant, Chuan Lian Zhi *Fructus Meliae Toosendan*, Dan Pi *Cortex Moutan Radicis* or Chi Shao *Radix Paeoniae Rubra* can be added to clear the Heat and relieve the pain.

If stagnation of Qi is predominant, Xiang Fu *Rhizoma Cyperi*, Chuan Lian Zi *Fructus Meliae Toosendan*, Yan Hu Suo *Rhizoma Corydalis*, Mu Xiang *Radix Aucklandiae*, Zhi Qiao *Fructus Aurantii* or Bin Lang *Semen Arecae* can be added to invigorate the flow of Qi and relieve the pain. If stagnation of Blood is predominant, San Qi *Radix Notoginseng*, Mo Yao *Resina Myrrhae*, Pu Huang *Pollen Typhae* or Wu Ling Zhi *Faeces Trogopterorum* can be added to promote the circulation of the Blood and relieve the pain.

STAGNATION OF QI

Symptoms and signs

Distending pain in the lower abdomen, especially on one or both sides of the abdomen, a dislike of pressure, accompanied by a feeling of fullness and distension in the chest and hypochondriac region, depression, headache, irritability, a poor appetite, insomnia, a slightly purplish colour to the menstrual blood, a purplish tongue and a wiry pulse.

Principle of treatment

Smooth the Liver, promote the Qi circulation, remove Blood stasis and relieve the pain.

HERBAL TREATMENT

Prescription

XIAO YAO SAN
Free and Relaxed Powder
Chai Hu *Radix Bupleuri* 10 g
Dang Gui *Radix Angelicae Sinensis* 10 g
Bai Shao *Radix Paeoniae Alba* 10 g
Zhi Xiang Fu *Rhizoma Cyperi Praeparata* 10 g
Yan Hu Suo *Rhizoma Corydalis* 10 g
Chuan Xiong *Rhizoma Ligustici Chuanxiong* 6 g
Gan Cao *Radix Glycyrrhizae* 5 g
Bo He *Herba Menthae* 3 g

Explanations

- Chai Hu and Zhi Xiang Fu regulate and promote the circulation of Liver-Qi so as to remove Qi stagnation in the Liver channel.
- Bai Shao and Gan Cao smooth and harmonise the Liver and relieve spasm so as to relieve the pain.
- Dang Gui nourishes the Blood and strengthens the Liver.
- Yan Hu Suo and Chuan Xiong promote the circulation of Qi and Blood and eliminate Blood stagnation so as to relieve the pain.
- Bo He clears Heat in the Liver resulting from stagnation of the Liver-Qi.

Modifications

1. If there is stagnation of Qi due to the accumulation of Cold, and abdominal pain with a dull sensation, add Wu Yao *Radix Linderae* 5 g to regulate the Qi circulation and relieve the pain.
2. If there is stagnation of Qi due to its deficiency, add Huang Qi *Radix Astragali seu Hedysari* 10 g to activate the Spleen and tonify the Qi.
3. If there is distension of the breast, or formation of cysts in the breast, add Ju He *Semen Citri Reticulatae* 10 g to promote the circulation of Qi, harmonise the collateral and reduce the cysts.
4. If there is a sharp pain, add Yu Jin *Radix Curcumae* 10 g to regulate the Qi and Blood circulation and relieve the pain.
5. If the menstruation is irregular, add Yi Mu Cao *Herba Leonuri* 15 g to regulate the menstruation.

6. If there are many purplish clots in the menstrual blood, add Mo Yao *Resina Myrrhae* 10 g to eliminate Blood stasis and relieve the pain.
7. If there is restlessness and insomnia due to severe pain, add Xue Jie *Resina Draconis* 5 g and Dan Shen *Radix Salviae Miltiorrhizae* 10 g to promote the circulation of Blood, calm the Mind and relieve the pain.
8. If there is nervousness and irritability, add Xia Ku Cao *Spica Prunellae* 10 g and Ju Hua *Flos Chrysanthemi* 10 g to clear Heat in the Liver and calm the Liver.
9. If there is a headache, add Jue Ming Zi *Semen Cassiae* 10 g to relieve the headache.
10. If there is nausea and vomiting due to severe pain, add Wu Zhu Yu *Fructus Evodiae* 3 g and Zhu Ru *Caulis Bambusae in Taeniam* 10 g to regulate the Stomach-Qi and stop the vomiting.
11. If the appetite is poor, add Mai Ya *Fructus Hordei Germinatus* 15 g to promote the appetite and improve digestion.

Patent remedies

Yan Hu Suo Zhi Tong Pian *Corydalis Stop Pain Tablet*
Yi Mu Cao Gao *Leonurus Syrup*

ACUPUNCTURE TREATMENT

PC-6 Neiguan, LI-4 Hegu, LR-13 Zhangmen, LR-5 Ligou, ST-28 Shuidao, ST-29 Guilai and SP-6 Sanyinjiao. Reducing method is used on these points.

Explanations

- PC-6, the Connecting point of the Pericardium channel, is used to unblock the chest and calm the Mind.
- LI-4 and LR-3, 'the four gate points', are used to promote the circulation of Qi and relieve pain.
- LR-5, the Connecting point, is used to harmonise the collateral, promote the circulation of Qi and relieve the pain.
- ST-28 and ST-29, the local points, and SP-6, the crossing points of the three Yin channels of the foot, are used together to promote the circulation of Qi and Blood and relieve stagnation so as to relieve the pain.

Modifications

1. If there is severe abdominal pain, add LR-6 and SP-8, the Accumulation points, to harmonise the collateral, promote the circulation of Qi and Blood and relieve the pain.

2. If the menstruation is irregular, add CV-6 and KI-3 to regulate the menstruation.
3. If the menstrual blood is dark with clots, add SP-10 to promote the circulation of Qi and Blood and eliminate Blood stasis.
4. If there is hypochondriac pain, add LR-14, the Front Collecting point, and GB-40, the Source point, to harmonise the Liver and relieve the pain.
5. If there is a sensation of fullness and oppression in the chest, add CV-17, the Gathering point for the Qi, to promote the circulation of Qi and relax the chest.
6. If there is nervousness and headache, add GB-20 to calm the Liver and clear Heat there.
7. If there is restlessness and insomnia due to severe pain, add HT-3 and Extra Anmian to calm the Mind and improve the sleep.
8. If there is a poor appetite or nausea and vomiting, add CV-12 and SP-4 to regulate the Stomach-Qi and improve the appetite.

Precautions

1. Try to relax as much as possible, especially during the menstrual period.
2. Avoid negative emotions so far as is possible.
3. Do exercise such as Taijiquan so as to release negative Qi in the body.
4. Try to maintain a regular lifestyle and avoid stress.

STAGNATION OF BLOOD

Symptoms and signs

Stabbing pain in the lower abdomen 1 or 2 days before or during the menstrual period, which worsens at night, with a discharge of big purplish blood clots in the menstruation and alleviation of pain after the blood clot discharge, accompanied by cyst formation in the ovary and uterus, a purplish tongue or purplish spots on the tongue and a wiry and choppy pulse.

Principle of treatment

Promote the Qi and Blood circulation, eliminate Blood stasis and relieve the pain.

HERBAL TREATMENT

Prescription

GE XIA ZHU YU TANG

Drive Out Blood Stasis Below the Diaphragm Decoction
Zhi Qiao *Fructus Aurantii* 10 g

Wu Yao *Radix Linderae* 10 g
Zhi Xiang Fu *Rhizoma Cyperi Praeparata* 10 g
Yan Hu Suo *Rhizoma Corydalis* 10 g
Dang Gui *Radix Angelicae Sinensis* 10 g
Chuan Xiong *Rhizoma Ligustici Chuanxiong* 6 g
Chi Shao *Radix Paeoniae Rubra* 10 g
Tao Ren *Semen Persicae* 10 g
Hong Hua *Flos Carthami* 10 g
Dan Pi *Cortex Moutan Radicis* 10 g
Wu Ling Zhi *Faeces Trogopterorum* 10 g
Gan Cao *Radix Glycyrrhizae* 5 g

Explanations

- Since the Qi circulation promotes the circulation of Blood, many herbs to promote the circulation of Qi are prescribed. Zhi Qiao, Wu Yao, Zhi Xiang Fu and Yan Hu Suo all promote the flow of Qi, coordinate the function of the Liver and relieve the pain.
- Dang Gui tonifies the Blood and promotes its circulation.
- Chuan Xiong, Chi Shao, Hong Hua, Tao Ren, Dan Pi and Wu Ling Zhi promote the circulation and eliminate stasis of the Blood and relieve the pain.
- Gan Cao relieves spasm and pain. It can also moderate the action of other herbs in the formula.

Modifications

1. If there is severe pain, add Xue Jie *Resina Draconis* 5 g to promote the circulation of Blood and relieve the pain.
2. If the menstruation is irregular, add Yi Mu Cao *Herba Leonuri* 15 g to regulate the menstruation.
3. If there is abdominal pain with a distending sensation and constipation, add Bing Lang *Semen Arecae* 10 g to promote the circulation of Qi and relieve the abdominal distension.
4. If cysts or masses form in the ovaries or Uterus, add Ju He *Semen Citri Reticulatae* 10 g and Kun Bu *Thallus Laminariae* 10 g to regulate the circulation of Qi and reduce the swelling.
5. If there is profuse bleeding with purplish blood loss during menstruation, or lingering bleeding with purplish blood, add San Qi *Radix Notoginseng* 10 g and Bai Ji *Rhizoma Bletillae* 10 g to promote circulation and eliminate stasis of the Blood and stop the excessive bleeding.
6. If there is distending pain in the breast, add Yu Jin *Radix Curcumae* 10 g to regulate the circulation of Qi and Blood and relieve the distension.
7. If there is restlessness and insomnia due to pain, add Dan Shen *Radix Salviae Miltiorrhizae* 10 g to calm the Mind and relieve the restlessness.

8. If there is nausea and vomiting due to pain, add Wu Zhu Yu *Fructus Evodiae* 3 g, Zhu Ru *Caulis Bambusae in Taeniam* 10 g to regulate the Stomach-Qi and stop the vomiting.

Patent remedies

Tong Jing Wan *Regulate Menses Pill*
If there is profuse bleeding, add Yun Nan Bai Yao *Yunnan White Medicine*

ACUPUNCTURE TREATMENT

ST-28 Shuidao, ST-29 Guilai, SP-6 Sanyinjiao, SP-8 Diji, BL-17 Geshu, BL-18 Ganshu, LI-4 Hegu, LR-3 Taichong and LR-5 Ligou. Reducing method is used on these points.

Explanations

- ST-28 and ST-29, the local points on the abdomen, are used to promote the circulation of Qi and Blood and relieve the pain.
- SP-6, the crossing point of the three Yin channels of the foot, and BL-17, the Gathering point for the Blood, are used to promote the circulation and eliminate stasis of the Blood and stop the pain.
- SP-8, the Accumulation point, and LR-5, the Connecting point, are used to harmonise the collateral, promote the circulation of Qi and Blood and relieve the pain.
- LI-4, LR-3 and BL-18 are used to promote the circulation of Qi in order to promote the circulation of Blood.

Modifications

1. If there is hypochondriac or breast pain, add PC-6 and LR-14 to promote the circulation of Qi and relieve the pain.
2. If the menstruation is irregular, add CV-4 and KI-3 to regulate the menstruation.
3. If there is severe dysmenorrhoea, add LR-6, the Accumulation point, to promote the circulation of Qi and Blood, remove Blood stasis and relieve the pain.
4. If there is nausea and vomiting, add SP-4 and CV-12 to harmonise the Stomach, cause the Stomach-Qi to descend and relieve the vomiting.
5. If the appetite is poor, add ST-36, the Sea point, and SP-3, the Source point, to activate the Spleen and Stomach and improve the appetite.

Precautions

1. Try to calm the emotions.
2. When there is stagnation of Liver-Qi, a method of promoting the circulation of Blood should also be used together with a method of promoting the circulation of Qi in order to prevent Blood stagnation.
3. When treating stagnation of Blood, one should also use a method for promoting the circulation of Qi.
4. If there is excessive blood loss during menstruation, both a method of promoting Blood circulation and a method of stopping bleeding should be used simultaneously.
5. If a cyst or mass has formed that is more than 5 cm in diameter, and conservative methods have already been used but still there is much bleeding, an operation should be considered.

Case history

A 35-year-old woman had been suffering mainly from severe abdominal pain during menstruation for 3 years. She was the mother of one child and, 3 years previously, she had for the first time had an abortion. She was mildly depressed after this, but was given no treatment. Three months after the abortion, she started to have a slight distending pain in the abdomen during menstruation. At the beginning, the pain was not very severe and was tolerable with the aid of normal painkillers. However, it became worse and worse until she had to take very strong painkillers in order to stop the stabbing pain during menstruation. Her cycle and duration of menstruation were normal.

When she arrived at the practice, she still had a feeling of depression, insomnia, hypochondriac pain, a feeling of oppression over her chest, generalised tiredness, dark and purplish-coloured blood loss during menstruation with big clots, a purplish tongue with a thin and white coating, and a wiry pulse.

Diagnosis
Dysmenorrhoea due to stagnation of Qi and Blood.

Principle of treatment
Smooth the Liver, promote the Qi and Blood circulation, eliminate Blood stasis and relieve the pain.

Herbal treatment
XIAO YAO SAN and **GE XIA ZHU YU TANG**
Free and Relaxed Powder and *Drive Out Blood Stasis Below the Diaphragm Decoction*
Chai Hu *Radix Bupleari* 10 g
Bai Shao *Radix Paeoniae Alba* 10 g
Zhi Qiao *Fructus Aurantii* 10 g
Zhi Xiang Fu *Rhizoma Cyperi Praeparata* 10 g
Yan Hu Suo *Rhizoma Corydalis* 10 g
Dang Gui *Radix Angelicae Sinensis* 10 g
Chuan Xiong *Rhizoma Ligustici Chuanxiong* 6 g
Chi Shao *Radix Paeoniae Rubra* 10 g
Wu Ling Zhi *Faeces Trogopterorum* 10 g
Huang Qi *Radix Astragali seu Hedysari* 10 g
Gan Cao *Radix Glycyrrhizae* 5 g

Explanations

- Chai Hu and Bai Shao smooth and harmonise the Liver.
- Zhi Qiao and Xiang Fu harmonise the Liver and promote the circulation of Liver-Qi.
- Yan Hu Suo, Chuan Xiong, Chi Shao and Wu Ling Zhi promote the circulation and eliminate stasis of Blood and relieve the pain.
- Huang Qi tonifies the Qi and Dang Gui tonifies the Blood to relieve tiredness. Dang Gui can also prevent damage to the Blood from the strong Blood circulation herbs.
- Gan Cao relieves spasm and pain. It can also moderate the actions of the other herbs in the formula.

Acupuncture treatment

ST-28 Shuidao, ST-29 Guilai, SP-6 Sanyinjiao, SP-8 Diji, PC-6 Neiguan, LR-3 Taichong, LR-5 Ligou and LR-14 Qimen. Reducing method is used on these points. For the first 3 weeks, treatment was given twice a week; after this, it was given once a week.

Explanations

- ST-28 and ST-29, the local points on the abdomen, were used to promote the circulation of Qi and Blood and relieve abdominal pain.
- SP-6, the crossing point of the three Yin channels of the foot, promotes the circulation of Blood, eliminates Blood stasis and stops the pain.
- SP-8, the Accumulation point, and LR-5, the Connecting point, harmonise the collateral, promote the circulation of Qi and Blood and relieve the abdominal pain.
- PC-6, the Connecting point, LR-3, the Source point, and LR-14, the Front Collecting point, smooth the Liver and promote the circulation of Liver-Qi in order to promote the circulation of Blood.

After a month of treatment, her dysmenorrhoea had decreased. After 3 months of treatment, her pain had disappeared completely. One year later, she was followed up by telephone and she stated she had not suffered from any further dysmenorrhoea since the treatment.

ACCUMULATION OF COLD-DAMP

Symptoms and signs

Pain in the lower abdomen with a cold sensation before or during menstruation, which is alleviated by contact with warmth and aggravated by pressure on the lower abdomen, accompanied by scanty and dark menses with blood clots, white-coloured leucorrhoea with no smell, and no vaginal itching. Other symptoms include an aversion to cold, diarrhoea with loose stools, lower back pain with a cold or bearing-down sensation, cold limbs, a white and greasy tongue coating and a deep, slow and slippery pulse.

Principle of treatment

Warm the channels, eliminate Cold and Damp, promote the Blood circulation and relieve the pain.

HERBAL TREATMENT

Prescription

SHAO FU ZHU YU TANG
Drive Out Blood Stasis in the Lower Abdomen Decoction
Dang Gui *Radix Angelicae Sinensis* 10 g
Chuan Xiong *Rhizoma Ligustici Chuanxiong* 10 g
Chi Shao *Radix Paeoniae Rubra* 10 g
Yan Hu Suo *Rhizoma Corydalis* 10 g
Wu Ling Zhi *Faeces Trogopterorum* 5 g
Pu Huang *Pollen Typhae* 10 g
Mo Yao *Resina Myrrhae* 5 g
Rou Gui *Cortex Cinnamomi* 10 g
Xiao Hui Xiang *Fructus Foeniculi* 5 g
Gan Jiang *Rhizoma Zingiberis* 10 g
Cang Zhu *Rhizoma Atractylodis* 10 g
Fu Ling *Poria* 10 g

Explanations

- Dang Gui, Chuan Xiong and Chi Shao nourish and promote the Blood, and dissipate Blood stasis.
- Yan Hu Suo, Wu Ling Zhi, Pu Huang and Mo Yao remove Blood stasis and relieve pain.
- Rou Gui, Xiao Hui Xiang and Gan Jiang warm the channels and Interior and dispel Cold.
- Cang Zhu and Fu Ling activate the Spleen and dry Damp.
- This prescription warms the channels, dispels Cold, dries Damp, removes Blood stasis and alleviates the pain.

Modifications

1. If there is severe pain and a cold sensation in the abdomen, cold limbs and profuse cold perspiration, add Fu Zi *Radix Aconiti Praeparata* 6 g and Ai Ye *Folium Artemisiae Argyi* 10 g to warm the channels and interior, dispel Cold and relieve the pain.
2. If there is lower back pain and white leucorrhoea, add Huai Niu Xi *Radix Achyranthis Bidentatae* 10 g and Du Zhong *Cortex Eucommiae* 10 g to tonify the Kidney and relieve the pain.
3. If there is diarrhoea with loose stools, add Bu Gu Zhi *Fructus Psoraleae* 10 g to tonify the Kidney-Yang and stop the diarrhoea.
4. If the appetite is poor, add Bai Zhu *Rhizoma Atractylodis Macrocephalae* 9 g to activate the Spleen and improve the appetite.

5. If there is nausea, add Zhi Ban Xia *Rhizoma Pinelliae Praeparata* 10 g to harmonise the Stomach, eliminate Cold-Damp, cause the Stomach-Qi to descend and relieve the nausea.

Patent remedy

Ai Fu Nuan Gong Wan *Mugwort and Prepared Aconite Pill for Warming the Uterus*

ACUPUNCTURE TREATMENT

ST-29 Guilai, ST-36 Zusanli, ST-40 Fenglong, SP-6 Sanyinjiao, SP-9 Yinlingquan, CV-4 Guanyuon and CV-6 Qihai. Reducing method is used on all these points except for the last two, on which reinforcing method is used. Moxibustion is also used on ST-29, ST-36, ST-40, CV-4 and CV-6.

Explanations

- ST-29, the local point on the abdomen, is used to eliminate Damp, promote the circulation of Blood in the Uterus and stop the pain.
- ST-36, the Sea point, and SP-6, the crossing point of the three Yin channels of the foot, tonify the Spleen and Stomach and reinforce the Qi.
- ST-40, the Connecting point, and SP-9, the Sea point, activate the Spleen and dry Damp.
- CV-4 and CV-6 warm the Uterus and dispel Cold in the body.
- Moxibustion warms the channels and interior and dispels Cold. It can also promote the circulation of Blood and stop the pain.

Modifications

1. If there is a cold sensation in the lower abdomen, add a moxa box on the abdomen instead of moxibustion on CV-4 and CV-6, to warm the Interior and dispel Cold.
2. If there is an aversion to cold, add L1-4 with moxibustion to dispel External Cold, warm the channels and promote the circulation of Qi.
3. If the pain is severe, add SP-8, the Accumulation point, to harmonise the collateral and sedate the pain.
4. If the menstrual blood is dark with clots, add SP-10 and LR-3 to promote the circulation of Qi and Blood and remove Blood stagnation.
5. If there is white leucorrhoea, add CV-2 to eliminate Damp and stop the leucorrhoea.
6. If there is diarrhoea with loose faeces, add SP-3 to activate the Spleen, tonify the Spleen-Qi and stop the diarrhoea.

7. If there is lower back pain, add BL-23 to warm the Kidney and relieve the pain.

Precautions

1. The patient should not eat too much cold or raw food or drink too much during menstruation, because this can cause an attack of Cold-Damp, leading to aggravation of the dysmenorrhoea.
2. The patient should wear sufficient clothing and avoid standing and working in a cold place during menstruation.

Case history

A 20-year-old woman had been suffering from pain in the lower abdomen during menstruation for 1 year. She remembered that once she had taken a cold shower when she was sweating heavily after sport, and the dysmenorrhoea had started a month later. Since then she had never got rid of the abdominal pain during menstruation. The pain usually began at the first day of menstruation and lasted until her menstruation was finished. Her menstruation lasted for 4 days and the cycle was normal. She had visited a few gynaecologists, but they could not help her, since all the examinations showed nothing wrong. She had also taken different painkillers, but they did not help the pain.

She felt strongly that the abdominal pain during the menstruation worsened if she ate too much cold food during this time. Her pain was accompanied by cold extremities, a lower back pain with a sensation of coldness, white-coloured leucorrhoea, dark menses with some small clots, a poor appetite, a sensation of fullness in her stomach, loose stools twice a day, a white and greasy tongue coating and a deep and slippery pulse.

Diagnosis
Accumulation of Cold-Damp in the Penetrating and Directing Vessels.

Principle of treatment
Warm the channels, dispel Cold, eliminate Damp, remove Blood stasis and relieve the pain.

Herbal treatment
SHAO FU ZHU YU WAN
Drive Out Blood Stasis in the Lower Abdomen Decoction
Dang Gui *Radix Angelicae Sinensis* 10 g
Chuan Xiong *Rhizoma Ligustici Chuanxiong* 10 g
Chi Shao *Radix Paeoniae Rubra* 10 g
Yan Hu Suo *Rhizoma Corydalis* 10 g
Pu Huang *Pollen Typhae* 10 g
Rou Gui *Cortex Cinnamomi* 10 g
Xiao Hui Xiang *Fructus Foeniculi* 5 g
Gan Jiang *Rhizoma Zingiberis* 10 g
Cang Zhu *Rhizoma Atractylodis* 10 g
Fu Ling *Poria* 10 g
Bai Zhu *Rhizoma Atractylodis Macrocephalae* 9 g
Zhi Ban Xia *Rhizoma Pinelliae Praeparata* 10 g

Explanations

- Dang Gui, Chuan Xiong and Chi Shao promote the circulation and dissipate stasis of Blood.
- Yan Hu Suo and Ru Xiang remove Blood stasis and relieve the pain.
- Rou Gui, Xiao Hui Xiang and Gan Jiang warm the channels and interior and dispel Cold.
- Bai Zhu and Fu Ling activate the Spleen and tonify the Spleen-Qi.
- Cang Zhu and Zhi Ban Xia activate the Spleen and dry Damp.

Acupuncture treatment

ST-28, ST-29, ST-36, ST-40, SP-6, SP-8, SP-9 and CV-4. Reducing method was used on all these points except for the last point, on which reinforcing method was used. Moxibustion was also used on ST-28, ST-29, ST-36, ST-40 and CV-4.

Explanations

- ST-28 and ST-29, the local points on the abdomen, eliminate Damp, promote the circulation of Blood in the Uterus and stop the pain.
- ST-36, the Sea point, and SP-6, the crossing points of the three Yin Channels of the foot, tonify the Spleen and Stomach and reinforce the Qi.
- ST-40, the Connecting point, and SP-9, the Sea point, activate the Spleen and dry Damp.
- SP-8, the Accumulation point, harmonises the collateral and relieves the pain.
- CV-4 warms the Uterus and dispels Cold in the body.
- Moxibustion warms the channels and Interior and dispels Cold. It can also promote the circulation of Blood and stop the pain.

After treatment for a month, the pain during her next menstruation had diminished, especially in its intensity. After treatment for 2 months, the pain during menstruation was almost gone, so the herbal treatment was stopped, and acupuncture was continued alone for a further month. She has not suffered from dysmenorrhoea since; 6 months later she was followed up and she reported that the dysmenorrhoea had disappeared completely.

DOWNWARD FLOW OF DAMP-HEAT

Symptoms and signs

Dark and sticky menstruation with small clots, abdominal pain with a sensation of heat in the lower abdomen before menstruation, a dislike of pressure, a slight fever or feverish feeling, deep yellow urine and painful urination, yellow leucorrhoea with a foul smell, genital itching, lower back pain with a bearing-down sensation, a red tongue with a greasy coating and a wiry and rapid pulse.

Principle of treatment

Clear Heat and eliminate Damp, remove Blood stasis and relieve the pain.

HERBAL TREATMENT

Prescription

QING RE TIAO XUE TANG
Clear Heat and Regulate Blood Decoction
Huang Lian *Rhizoma Coptidis* 10 g
Huang Bai *Cortex Phellodendri* 10 g
Sheng Di Huang *Radix Rehmanniae* 15 g
Mu Dan Pi *Cortex Moutan Radicis* 10 g
Dang Gui *Radix Angelicae Sinensis* 10 g
Bai Shao *Radix Paeoniae Alba* 10 g
Xiang Fu *Rhizoma Cyperi* 10 g
Yan Hu Suo *Rhizoma Corydalis* 10 g
Chuan Xiong *Rhizoma Ligustici Chuanxiong* 10 g
Hong Hua *Flos Carthami* 10 g
Tao Ren *Semen Persicae* 10 g
E Zhu *Rhizoma Curcumae* 10 g

Explanations

- Huang Lian, in high dosage, and Huang Bai strongly clear Heat and dry Damp in the Lower Burner.
- Sheng Di Huang and Mu Dan Pi clear Heat in the Blood.
- Dang Gui and Bai Shao nourish the Liver-Blood and relieve the pain.
- Xiang Fu and Yan Hu Suo invigorate the flow of Qi and relieve the pain.
- Chuan Xiong, Hong Hua, Tao Ren and E Zhu promote the circulation of Blood and eliminate Blood stasis.

Modifications

1. If there is severe pain or pelvic inflammation, add Pu Gong Ying *Herba Taraxaci* 30 g and Bai Jang Cao *Herba Patriniae* 30 g to clear Heat and remove Toxin.
2. If there is profuse bleeding, add Zhi Zi *Fructus Gardeniae* 6 g and Di Yu *Radix Sanguisorbae* 10 g to clear Heat in the Blood and stop the bleeding.
3. If there is lower back pain, add Chuan Niu Xi *Radix Cyathulae* 10 g to strengthen the back and relieve the pain.
4. If there is genital itching, add Bai Xian Pi *Cortex Dictamni Radicis* 10 g and Ku Shen *Radix Sophorae Flavescentis* 10 g to clear Damp-Heat and relieve the itching.
5. If there is profuse yellow leucorrhoea, add Chun Bai Pi *Cortex Ailanthi* 10 g and Cang Zhu *Rhizoma Atractylodes* 10 g to clear Heat, dry Damp and relieve the leucorrhoea.

6. If there is scanty urination, add Ze Xie *Rhizoma Alismatis* 10 g to promote urination and clear Damp-Heat in the Lower Burner.

Patent remedy

San Miao Wan *Three-Marvel Pill*

ACUPUNCTURE TREATMENT

ST-28 Shuidao, ST-29 Guilai, CV-2 Qugu, SP-6 Sanyinjiao, SP-8 Diji, SP-9 Yinlingquan, LR-5 Ligou and BL-32 Ciliao. Reducing method is used on these points.

Explanations

- St-28 and ST-29, the local points, promote the circulation of Qi and Blood, eliminate Damp-Heat and relieve the pain.
- CV-2, BL-32 and SP-9 eliminate Damp-Heat.
- SP-8, the Accumulation point, harmonises the collateral and sedates the pain.
- SP-6, the crossing point of the three Yin channels of the foot, and LR-5, the Connecting point, eliminate Damp-Heat in the Lower Burner, promote the circulation of Qi and Blood, harmonise the collateral and sedate the pain.

Modifications

1. If the blood loss in menstruation is dark with clots, add SP-10 to promote the circulation of Qi and Blood and remove Blood stasis.
2. If there is a sensation of heat in the lower abdomen, add SP-2 and ST-44 to clear Heat in the Lower Burner.
3. If there is yellow urine or leucorrhoea, add KI-2 to clear Heat, promote urination and eliminate Damp.
4. If there is genital itching, add LR-12 to eliminate Damp-Heat and stop the itching.
5. If there is irregular menstruation, add KI-10 and LR-8, the Sea points, to regulate the menstruation and strengthen the Liver and Kidney.
6. If there is a slight fever, add LI-11 and GV-14 to clear Heat and reduce the fever.
7. If there is lower back pain, add BL-58 and GB-30 to eliminate Damp-Heat, regulate the circulation of Qi and relieve the pain.
8. If there is diarrhoea, add ST-40 and SP-3 to activate the Spleen and stop the diarrhoea.

Precautions

1. The patient should avoid eating too much pungent, sweet or fatty food or drinking too much alcohol, which will impair the Spleen and Stomach aggravating the Damp-Heat.
2. Herbal treatment is usually essential as well as acupuncture in order to achieve a good therapeutic result.
3. Attention needs to be paid to personal hygiene in order to prevent infection and avoid invasion of Damp-Heat.

Case history

A 31-year-old woman had been suffering from pain in the lumbosacral region during menstruation for 5 months. As well as the dysmenorrhoea, she had yellow and sticky leucorrhoea with itching, a dry mouth but not much desire to drink, yellow urine with a sensation of heat, a bearing-down sensation in the lower back and abdomen, sometimes a mild fever, generalised tiredness, infertility, a yellow and greasy coating and a slippery and rapid pulse. Her menstruation was irregular and scanty with some small clots. She had been diagnosed with chronic pelvic inflammation 2 years previously, but after treatment with antibiotics, her dysmenorrhoea had not improved.

Diagnosis
Dysmenorrhoea due to downward flow of Damp-Heat.

Principle of treatment
Eliminate Damp, clear Heat, promote the Qi and Blood circulation and relieve the pain.

Herbal treatment
QING RE TIAO XUE TANG
Clear Heat and Regulate Blood Decoction
Huang Lian *Rhizoma Coptidis* 5 g
Huang Bai *Cortex Phellodendri* 10 g
Bai Jang Cao *Herba Patriniae* 20 g
Sheng Di Huang *Radix Rehmanniae Recens* 15 g
Bai Xian Pi *Cortex Dictamni Radicis* 10 g
Dang Gui *Radix Angelicae Sinensis* 10 g
Xiang Fu *Rhizoma Cyperi* 10 g
Yan Hu Suo *Rhizoma Corydalis* 10 g
Chuan Xiong *Rhizoma Ligustici Chuanxiong* 10 g
Hong Hua *Flos Carthami* 10 g
Tao Ren *Semen Persicae* 10 g

Explanations

- Huang Lian and Huang Bai clear Heat strongly and dry Damp in the Lower Burner.
- Bai Jiang Cao and Sheng Di Huang clear Heat in the Blood and remove Toxin.
- Dang Gui regulates the menstruation, nourishes the Liver-Blood and relieves the pain.
- Xiang Fu and Yan Hu Suo invigorate the circulation of Qi and relieve the pain.

- Chuan Xiong, Hong Hua and Tao Ren promote the circulation of Blood and eliminate Blood stasis.
- Bai Xian Pi eliminates Damp-Heat and relieves vaginal itching.

Acupuncture treatment
ST-28, ST-29, CV-2, SP-6, SP-8, SP-9, LR-5 and LR-12. Reducing method was used on these points.

Explanations

- ST-28, ST-29 and CV-2, the local points, promote the circulation of Qi and Blood, eliminate Damp-Heat and relieve the pain.
- SP-8, the Accumulation point, harmonises the collateral and sedates pain. SP-6, the crossing point of the three Yin channels of the foot, and SP-9, the Sea point, activate the Spleen and eliminate Damp-Heat in the Lower Burner.
- LR-5, the Connecting point, and LR-12 promote the circulation of Qi and Blood, harmonise the collateral, eliminate Damp-Heat and sedate the pain.

After treatment over a 3-week period, her menstruation came and the pain was slightly improved. She did not have purplish clots in the menstrual blood. After 2 months of treatment, the yellow leucorrhoea was under control and the vaginal itching disappeared.

During the second menstruation after the treatment, she no longer suffered from dysmenorrhoea. The same treatment was continued for a further month in order to maintain the effect. A year later she was followed up by letter and she said she had experienced no further pain since the treatment.

DEFICIENCY OF QI AND BLOOD

Symptoms and signs

Slight pain in the lower abdomen during or after menstruation, with either scanty blood loss with a light red colour or profuse or lingering blood loss, accompanied by alleviation of the pain with pressure, a bearing-down sensation in the lower abdomen, a sallow complexion, dizziness, generalised tiredness, palpitations, insomnia and dream-disturbed sleep, a loss of appetite, constipation, a pale tongue and a thin and weak pulse.

Principle of treatment

Activate the Spleen, tonify the Qi and Blood and relieve the pain.

HERBAL TREATMENT

Prescription

BU ZHONG YI QI TANG and **GUI PI TANG**
Tonifying the Middle and Benefiting Qi Decoction and Tonifying the Spleen Decoction

Ren Shen *Radix Ginseng* 5 g
Huang Qi *Radix Astragali seu Hedysari* 10 g
Bai Zhu *Rhizoma Atractylodis Macrocephalae* 10 g
Dang Gui *Radix Angelicae Sinensis* 10 g
Chuan Xiong *Rhizoma Ligustici Chuanxiong* 6 g
Shu Di Huang *Radix Rehmanniae Praeparata* 15 g
Bai Shao *Radix Paeoniae Alba* 15 g
Mu Xiang *Radix Saussureae* 6 g

Explanations

- Ren Shen, Huang Qi and Bai Zhu activate the Spleen and tonify the Qi.
- Dang Gui and Shu Di Huang harmonise and regulate the menstruation and tonify the Blood.
- Chuan Xiong promotes the circulation and eliminates stasis of the Blood and relieves the pain.
- Mu Xiang and Bai Shao harmonise the circulation of Qi, smooth the Liver and stop the pain.
- As a whole, this decoction can tonify the Blood and Qi, promote the circulation of Blood, and relieve the pain.

Modifications

1. If there is profuse bleeding during menstruation or lingering, add Xue Yu Tan *Carbonisatus Crinis* 10 g and Bai Ji *Rhizoma Bletillae* 10 g to stop the bleeding.
2. If there is a distending pain, add Xiang Fu *Rhizoma Cyperi* 5 g to promote the circulation of Qi and relieve the pain.
3. If there is severe pain, add Yan Hu Suo *Rhizoma Corydalis* 10 g to regulate the circulation of Qi and Blood and relieve the pain.
4. If there is scanty menstruation, add Lu Jiao Jiao *Colla Cervi Cornu* 15 g to tonify the Blood and benefit the Kidney-Essence.
5. If there is a bearing-down sensation in the abdomen, add Sheng Ma *Rhizoma Cimicifugae* 5 g and Chai Hu *Radix Bupleuri* 5 g to lift up the Qi and relieve the bearing-down sensation.
6. If there is dizziness, add Tian Ma *Rhizoma Gastrodiae* 10 g and Ji Xue Teng *Caulis Spatholobi* 20 g to tonify the Blood and subdue Interior Wind.
7. If there are palpitations and insomnia, add Bai Zi Ren *Semen Biotae* 10 g, Suan Zao Ren *Semen Ziziphi Spinosae* 15 g to tonify the Heart and calm the Mind.
8. If there is anorexia and lose stools, add Fu Ling *Poria* 10 g and Shen Qu *Medicinalis Massa Fermentata* 15 g to activate the Spleen and Stomach and improve the appetite.

9. If there is an aversion to cold and cold hands and feet, add Zhi Fu Zi *Radix Aconiti Carmichaeli Praeparata* 10 g and Rou Gui *Cortex Cinnamomi* 5 g to warm the interior and dispel Cold.

10. If there is oedema and scanty urination, add Yi Mu Cao *Herba Leonuri* 10 g and Ze Xie *Rhizoma Alisma* 10 g to promote urination and reduce the oedema.

Patent remedy

Ba Zhen Yi Mu Wan *Women's Precious Pill*

ACUPUNCTURE TREATMENT

ST-28 Shuidao, CV-6 Qihai, ST-36 Zusanli, SP-3 Taibai, SP-6 Sanyinjiao, SP-9 Yinlingquan and KI-3 Taixi. Tonifying method is used on these points. Moxibustion should be used on CV-6, ST-36 and SP-9.

Explanations

- ST-28, the local point, regulates menstruation and relieves the pain.
- CV-6 and KI-3 tonify the Kidney and Original Qi so as to benefit the Essence in order to reinforce the Blood.
- ST-36 and SP-9, the Sea points, and SP-3, the Source point, activate the Spleen and Stomach and tonify the Qi so as to reinforce the Blood.
- SP-6, the crossing point of the three Yin channels of the foot, activates the Spleen and tonifies the Blood.
- Moxibustion could warm the body and Yang-Qi and dispel Cold.

Modifications

1. If there is scanty menstruation, add KI-10 to reinforce the Qi and Blood and regulate the menstruation.
2. If there is profuse bleeding during menstruation, add SP-1 to stop the bleeding.
3. If there is severe pain during menstruation, add SP-8, the Accumulation point, to harmonise the collateral and relieve the pain.
4. If there are cold hands and feet and an aversion to cold, add CV-4 with moxibustion to warm the Interior and dispel Cold.
5. If there is dizziness, add CV-20 to lift up the Qi and relieve the dizziness.

6. If there is a headache, add GB-20 to regulate the circulation of Qi and Blood in the head and relieve the headache.
7. If there are palpitations, add PC-6 and HT-7 to nourish the Blood and calm the Mind.
8. If there is a poor appetite, add CV-12, the Front Collecting point of the Stomach, and LR-13, the Front Collecting point of the Spleen, to tonify the Spleen and Stomach and improve the appetite.
9. If there is diarrhoea, add SP-3 to activate the Spleen and relieve the diarrhoea.
10. If there is oedema, add TE-6 and KI-6 to promote urination and relieve the oedema.

Precautions

The patient should be given the following advice:

1. Try to maintain a regular daily life.
2. Eat sufficient nutritious food.
3. It is important to eat adequate meat, especially red meat.
4. Any mild chronic sickness should be treated adequately.

Case history

A 45-year-old woman had been suffering from pain in the lower abdomen 2 days after menstruation for more than a year. She also had scanty blood loss during menstruation, a delayed cycle, which was between 40 and 50 days, and when the menstrual period came it usually lasted for 2 days. The blood was a light red colour. This was accompanied by a poor appetite, generalised tiredness, dizziness, palpitations, a tendency to catch colds easily, a pale complexion, a pale tongue with tooth marks and a thin and white coating and thin and weak pulse.

Diagnosis
Dysmenorrhoea due to deficiency of Qi and Blood.

Principle of treatment
Activate the Spleen, tonify the Qi and Blood and relieve the pain.

Herbal treatment
BU ZHONG YI QI TANG and **GUI PI TANG**
Tonifying the Middle and Benefiting Qi Decoction and *Tonifying the Spleen Decoction*
Ren Shen *Radix Ginseng* 10 g
Huang Qi *Radix Astragali seu Hedysari* 10 g
Bai Zhu *Rhizoma Atractylodis Macrocephalae* 10 g
Dang Gui *Radix Angelicae Sinensis* 10 g
Lu Jiao Jiao *Colla Cervi Cornu* 15 g
Shu Di Huang *Radix Rehmanniae Praeparata* 15 g
Chuan Xiong *Rhizoma Ligustici Chuanxiong* 6 g
Mu Xiang *Radix Saussureae* 6 g
Rou Gui *Cortex Cinnamomi* 5 g
Shen Qu *Medicinalis Massa Fermentata* 15 g

Explanations

- Ren Shen, Huang Qi and Bai Zhu activate the Spleen and tonify the Qi generally.
- Lu Jiao Jiao, Dang Gui and Shu Di Huang harmonise and regulate the menstruation and tonify the Blood.
- Chuan Xiong and Mu Xiang promote the circulation of Qi and Blood, eliminate Blood stasis and relieve the pain.
- Rou Gui warms the Interior and dispels Cold.
- Shen Qu promotes digestion and improves the appetite.

Acupuncture treatment
ST-28, CV-4, CV-6, ST-36, SP-3, SP-6, GB-39 and KI-3. Tonifying method was used on these points. Moxibustion was used on CV-4, CV-6, ST-36 and SP-3.

Explanations

- ST-28, the local point, regulates menstruation and relieves the pain.
- CV-4, CV-6 and KI-3 tonify the Kidney and Source Qi so as to benefit the Essence in order to reinforce the Blood.
- ST-36, the Sea point, and SP-3, the Source point, activate the Spleen and Stomach and tonify the Qi so as to reinforce the Blood.
- SP-6, the crossing point of the three Yin channels of the foot, and GB-39, the Gathering point for the Marrow, activate the Spleen and tonify the Blood.
- Moxibustion can warm the body and Yang-Qi and dispel Cold.

After treatment for 1 week, she started to feel that she had more energy and she was not so tired as before. Three weeks later her menstrual period arrived and the pain had greatly improved. The cycle was 35 days, which was shorter that it used to be, and blood loss was more extensive, and lasted for 3 days.

After treatment for another 4 weeks, her next menstrual period was almost on time, and the blood loss lasted for 4 days. The abdominal pain during her menstruation was again much improved. After 4 months of treatment her dysmenorrhoea had disappeared. Also, she did not get tired so easily, and complexion and appetite were back to normal. A year later she was followed up and she reported she had experienced no further dysmenorrhoea since the treatment.

DEFICIENCY OF YIN OF LIVER AND KIDNEY

Symptoms and signs

Slight pain in the lower abdomen 1 or 2 days after menstruation, scanty and sticky menstruation, with a sensation of heat in the palms and soles of the feet, hot flushes, night sweating, tinnitus, dizziness, irritability, insomnia, palpitation, constipation, a red tongue with a scanty or peeled coating and a thin and rapid pulse.

Principle of treatment

Tonify the Yin of the Liver and Kidney and relieve the pain.

HERBAL TREATMENT

Prescription

TIAO GAN TANG
Regulate Liver Decoction
Dang Gui *Radix Angelicae Sinensis* 10 g
Bai Shao *Radix Paeoniae Alba* 10 g
E Jiao *Colla Corii Asini* 12 g
Yan Hu Suo *Rhizoma Corydalis* 10 g
Shan Zhu Yu *Fructus Corni* 12 g
Ba Ji Tian *Radix Morindae Officinalis* 10 g
Shan Yao *Rhizoma Dioscoreae* 10 g
Gan Cao *Radix Glycyrrhizae* 5 g
Huang Bai *Cortex Phellodendri* 10 g
Mu Dan Pi *Cortex Moutan Radicis* 10 g

Explanations

- Dang Gui, Bai Shao and E Jiao nourish the Liver-Blood and regulate the menstruation.
- Yan Hu Suo promotes the circulation of Qi and Blood and relieves the pain.
- Shan Zhu Yu and Ba Ji Tian nourish the Yin of the Liver and Kidney and regulate the Penetrating and Directing Vessels.
- Shan Yao and Gan Cao activate the Spleen and tonify the Qi.
- Huang Bai and Mu Dan Pi nourish the Yin and clear Deficient-Heat.

Modifications

1. If there is scanty menstruation, add Lu Jiao Jiao *Colla Cervi Cornu* 15 g to tonify the Kidney, benefit the Essence and regulate the menstruation.
2. If there is severe pain, add Chuan Xiong *Rhizoma Ligustici Chuanxiong* 6 g to promote the circulation of Qi and Blood and relieve the pain.
3. If there are hot flushes and night sweating, add Qin Jiao *Radix Gentianae Macrophyllae* 10 g to clear Deficient-Heat and stop the sweating.
4. If there is a dry cough due to Deficient-Heat in the Lung, add Di Gu Pi *Cortex Lycii Radicis* 12 g to clear the Deficient-Heat and relieve the cough.
5. If there is lower back pain, add Du Zhong *Cortex Eucommiae* 10 g and Xu Duan *Radix Dipsaci* 10 g to tonify the Kidney and strengthen the lower back.

6. If there is irritability, add Shi Jue Ming *Concha Haliotidis* 20 g to calm the Liver and relieve the irritability.
7. If there is insomnia, add Suan Zhao Ren *Semen Ziziphi Spinosae* 15 g to calm the Heart and tranquillise the Mind.
8. If there is hypochondriac pain, add Chuan Lian Zi *Fructus Meliae Toosendan* 10 g to harmonise the collateral and promote the Liver-Qi circulation.

Patent remedies

Liu Wei Di Huang Wan *Six-Flavour Rehmanniae Pill*
Qi Ju Di Huang Wan *Lycuim Fruit, Chrysanthemum and Rehmannia Pill*

ACUPUNCTURE TREATMENT

KI-3 Taixi, KI-4 Dazhong, KI-5 Shuiquan, KI-6 Zhaohai, KI-7 Fuliu, KI-10 Yingu, SP-6 Sanyinjiao and CV-6 Qihai. Tonifying method is used on these points.

Explanations

- KI-3, the Source point and Stream point of the Kidney channel, and CV-6 tonify the Kidney, reinforce the Kidney-Qi and regulate the menstruation.
- KI-4, the Connecting point, and KI-5, the Accumulation point, harmonise the collateral and relieve the pain.
- SP-6, the crossing point of the three Yin channels of the foot, KI-6 and KI-7 nourish the Yin and clear Deficient-Heat.
- KI-10, the Sea point and the Water point, nourishes the Yin of the Liver and Kidney, regulates the menstruation and clears Deficient-Heat.

Modifications

1. If there is scanty and sticky menstruation, add LR-8, the Sea point, to tonify the Liver-Blood and regulate the menstruation.
2. If there is severe abdominal pain, add ST-28 and SP-8 to regulate the Qi and Blood and relieve the pain.
3. If there is dizziness, add GB-8 to relieve the dizziness.
4. If there is nervousness, add GB-20 to calm the Liver and relieve the nervousness.
5. If there are hot flushes, add KI-2 to clear Deficient-Heat and reduce Fire.
6. If there is tinnitus, add GB-2 and TE-21 to regulate the circulation of Qi in the ear and improve the hearing.

7. If there is night sweating, add HT-6 to stop the sweating.
8. If there is lower back pain, add BL-58 to harmonise the collateral and relieve the pain.
9. If there is weakness of the lower back and knees, add GB-34 and GB-39 to tonify the Qi and Blood and strengthen the back and knees.
10. If there is constipation, add ST-25 and ST-37 to nourish the Yin and regulate the circulation of Qi in the Large Intestine so as to relieve the constipation.

Precautions

The patient should be given the following advice:

1. Try to maintain a regular daily life.
2. Don't eat too much pungent food and don't drink too much alcohol.
3. Limit sexual intercourse.

DEFICIENCY OF KIDNEY-YANG

Symptoms and signs

Pain in the lower abdomen with a cold sensation during or after menstruation, alleviation of the pain by warmth and aggravation by pressure or contact with cold, with a scanty and dark menstruation, an aversion to cold, cold limbs, a pale complexion, a poor appetite, generalised tiredness, loose stools, or diarrhoea with undigested food, a pale tongue with a wet coating and a deep, weak and slow pulse.

Principle of treatment

Warm the channels and Uterus, dispel Cold and relieve the pain.

HERBAL TREATMENT

Prescription

WEN JING TANG
Warm the Menses Decoction
Gui Zhi *Ramulus Cinnamomi* 10 g
Wu Zhu Yu *Fructus Evodiae* 10 g
Dang Gui *Radix Angelicae Sinensis* 10 g
Chuan Xiong *Rhizoma Ligustici Chuanxiong* 10 g
E Jiao *Colla Corii Asini* 10 g
Mai Men Dong *Radix Ophiopogonis* 10 g
Bai Shao *Radix Paeoniae Alba* 10 g
Ren Shen *Radix Ginseng* 5 g
Ban Xia *Rhizoma Pinelliae* 10 g
Sheng Jiang *Rhizoma Zingiberis Recens* 10 g
Gan Cao *Radix Glycyrrhizae* 5 g

Explanations

- Gui Zhi and Wu Zhu Yu warm the channels and Uterus, dispel Cold and relieve the pain.
- Dang Gui and Chuan Xiong tonify the Blood, promote its circulation and relieve pain.
- E Jiao together with Dang Gui and Mai Men Dong nourish the Blood and the Yin.
- Bai Shao and Gan Cao relieve the spasm and pain.
- Ren Shen tonifies the Qi and benefits the Kidney-Essence.
- Sheng Jiang and Ban Xia moderate the Stomach and resolve Damp.

Modifications

1. If the limbs are cold, add Zhi Fu Zi *Radix Aconiti Praeparata* 6 g and Ai Ye *Folium Artemisiae Argyi* 10 g to warm the Yang and dispel Cold.
2. If there is lower back pain, add Ba Ji Tian *Radix Morindae Officinalis* 10 g to tonify the Kidney and strengthen the lower back.
3. If there is frequent nycturia, add Yi Zhi Ren *Fructus Alpiniae Oxyphyllae* 10 g and Rou Gui *Cortex Cinnamomi* 3 g to tonify the Kidney and relieve the nycturia.
4. If there is scanty menstruation, add Lu Jiao Jiao *Colla Cervi Cornu* 15 g to tonify the Kidney and regulate the menstruation.
5. If there is diarrhoea with undigested food, add Bu Gu Zhi *Fructus Psoraleae* 10 g and Rou Dou Kou *Semen Myristicae* 10 g to warm the Kidney-Yang and stop the diarrhoea.

Patent remedy

Jin Gui Shen Qi Wan *Kidney Qi Pill*

ACUPUNCTURE TREATMENT

CV-4 Guanyuan, CV-6 Qihai, KI-3 Taixi, KI-4 Dazhong, KI-5 Shuiquan, KI-10 Yingu and SP-8 Diji. Tonifying method is used on these points. Moxibustion is used on CV-4, CV-6 and KI-3.

Explanations

- CV-4 and CV-6 tonify the Kidney-Essence and regulate the menstruation.
- KI-3, the Source point and Stream point of the Kidney channel, and KI-10, the Sea point, tonify the Kidney, reinforce the Kidney-Qi and regulate the menstruation.
- KI-4, the Connecting point, and KI-5, the Accumulation point, harmonise the collateral and relieve the pain.
- SP-8, the Accumulation point, regulates the menstruation and relieves the pain.
- Moxibustion is applied to dispel Cold.

Modifications

1. If there is scanty and sticky menstruation, add LR-8, the Sea point, to tonify the Liver-Blood and regulate the menstruation.
2. If there is difficulty in passing the menstrual Blood, add SP-6, the crossing point of the three Yin channels of the foot, to promote the circulation of Blood and regulate the menstruation.
3. If there is severe abdominal pain, add ST-28 and SP-8 to regulate the Qi and Blood and relieve the pain.
4. If there is dizziness, add GB-8 to relieve the dizziness.
5. If there is tinnitus, add GB-2 and TE-21 to regulate the circulation of Qi in the ear and improve the hearing.
6. If there is lower back pain, add BL-58 to harmonise the collateral and relieve the pain.
7. If there is weakness of the lower back and knees, add GB-34 and GB-39 to tonify the Qi and Blood and strengthen the back and knees.
8. If there is diarrhoea, add SP-3 and ST-25 to tonify the Spleen and Stomach and relieve the diarrhoea.

Precautions

The patient should be given the following advice:

1. Try to maintain a regular daily life.
2. Avoid overeating of cold and raw food.
3. Limit sexual intercourse.
4. Eat sufficient red meat every day.
5. Keep the lower abdomen and lower back warm.

Case history

A 46-year-old woman was suffering from pain in the lower abdomen during menstruation, which was alleviated by warmth and pressure. It was accompanied by irregular and dark menses, an aversion to cold, generalised tiredness, cold extremities, hot flushes, occasional night sweating, restlessness, insomnia, a poor appetite, diarrhoea, oedema in the legs, a pale and swollen tongue with a scanty and peeled coating and a deep, weak and thready pulse.

Diagnosis
Dysmenorrhoea due to deficiency of both Kidney-Yin and Kidney-Yang.

Principle of treatment
Tonify the Kidney and benefit the Yin and Yang of the Kidney.

Herbal treatment
ER XIAN TANG
Two-Immortal Decoction
Xian Mao *Rhizoma Curculiginis* 10 g
Xian Ling Pi *Herba Epimedium* 10 g
Dang Gui *Radix Angelicae Sinensis* 10 g
Chuan Xiong *Rhizoma Ligustici Chuanxiong* 10 g
Ba Ji Tian *Radix Morindae Officinalis* 10 g
Huang Bai *Cortex Phellodendri* 10 g
Zhi Mu *Rhizoma Anemarrhenae* 10 g
Huang Lian *Rhizoma Coptidis* 5 g

Explanations

- Xian Mao, Ba Ji Tian and Xian Ling Pi tonify the Kidney-Yang and dispel Cold.
- Huang Bai and Zhi Mu tonify the Kidney-Yin and clear Deficient-Heat.
- Dang Gui and Chuan Xiong regulate the menstruation and relieve the pain.
- Huang Lian clears Heat and calms the Mind.

Acupuncture treatment
CV-4, CV-6, KI-3, KI-7, KI-10, LR-3, LR-8, ST-28, ST-29, GB-20 and HT-8. Reinforcing method was used on these points. Acupuncture treatment was given once every week for the first 2 months, and then once every 2 weeks.

Explanations

- CV-4 and CV-6 tonify the Kidney-Essence and regulate the menstruation.
- KI-3, the Source point and Stream point of the Kidney channel, and KI-10, the Sea point, tonify the Kidney, reinforce the Kidney-Qi and regulate the menstruation.
- K17, the Metal point, nourishes the Kidney-Yin and relieves hot flushing.
- LR-3, the Source point, and LR-8, the Sea point, tonify the Liver-Blood and promote the circulation of Liver-Qi so as to relieve the pain.
- ST-28 and ST-29, the local points, regulate the circulation of Qi and Blood and relieve dysmenorrhoea.
- GB-20 and HT-8 clear Heat, calm the Mind and regulate the emotions.

After treatment for 2 months, the patient no longer had much dysmenorrhoea, although the menstruation was still irregular, but the colour of the blood loss was less dark. The same treatment was continued for another 3 months, and the dysmenorrhoea disappeared and the other general symptoms also improved. One year later, she had amenorrhoea.

Part 6

Back pain 腰背疼痛

Pain in the entire back 29

腰
背
疼
痛

Pain occurring over the entire back may be attributed to any of the following disorders in Western medicine: influenza, fever due to infectious disease, lung disease, heart diseases, renal disease, muscle strain or traumatic injury of the back, rheumatism, rheumatoid arthritis, hyperplastic spondylosis, deformation or injury of spinal column. If the pain is related to a disorder of the Internal organs, the TCM treatment should be combined with Western medical treatment.

Aetiology and pathology

Invasion of External factors

Invasion of External pathogenic factors such as Wind, Cold, Heat and Damp may cause acute back pain, chronic back pain or scapular pain with acute exacerbation. Exposure to Wind, Cold, Heat or Damp for too long may cause some of these factors to invade of the back generally, blocking the channels and causing stagnation of Qi and Blood in the whole of the back, so pain follows.

Wind tends to rise and attack the upper body, usually in combination with one or more of the other pathogenic factors. If the Wind is predominant, there is a predominance of pain in the upper back.

Cold characteristically causes contraction of the muscles, tendons and channels and stagnation of the Qi and Blood in the channels. Because of this pathogenic feature, invasion of Wind-Cold to the back may cause sudden and severe pain with a cold sensation that is aggravated by contact with cold and alleviated by contact with warmth.

Heat characteristically has an ascending movement and a burning nature. If Wind-Heat invades the back, there is a pain with a burning or hot sensation, which is aggravated by contact with warmth and alleviated by contact with cold.

Damp is characterised by viscosity, heaviness and stagnation. It is a Yin pathogenic factor that tends to obstruct the functions of the Qi and impair the Yang-Qi. It usually attacks the body in combination with Wind, Cold or Heat. If Wind-Damp with Cold or Heat invades the back, the circulation of Qi and Blood in the channels is disturbed, leading to accumulation of Damp and stagnation of Qi and Blood on the back, so a pain with swelling and heaviness occurs and, generally speaking, it tends to be located more in the lower back.

Invasion of these pathogenic factors may take place through the skin pores, or eating of the wrong foods, or the wrong lifestyle habits. When the weather changes too quickly, people who do not take proper care of themselves, or with a weak constitution, or acute or chronic disease, or under stress or in a tired state, may be more vulnerable to these pathogenic factors than other

349

people. Also if these External pathogenic factors are not quickly eliminated from the body and channels then the person is vulnerable to further invasion of these factors, leading to aggravation of the back pain.

Emotional disturbance

The Liver is in charge of maintaining free flow of Qi in the body generally. Excessive stress, frustration or anger may cause dysfunction of the Liver, leading to stagnation of Qi in the channels, and causing generalised back pain. This type of back pain is usually associated with symptoms such as unstable emotions, irritability, depression, headache or nervousness. If the Liver-Qi stagnation lasts for a long time, it may in turn cause stagnation of Blood, which aggravates the back pain.

Physical trauma

Physical traumas such as falling over, a car accident, wounds or inappropriate surgery on the back may directly damage the local muscles, tendons and channels, leading to stagnation of the Qi and Blood, and causing back pain.

Sleeping on a hard bed or too soft a mattress, or in bad conditions, may also cause Qi and Blood to stagnate in the channels passing through the back and an imbalance in the strength of the muscles along the spine, causing back pain.

Inadequate exercise

Apart from the above specific causes, generalised back pain can also be a consequence of inadequate physical exercise, especially by people whose work is sedentary. Lack of proper daily exercise may lead the tendons, muscles and joints around the back to become weak, causing the circulation of Qi and Blood to slow, and generalised back pain follows.

It is clear, however, that those with a weak constitution should avoid lifting heavy weights or undertaking excessive exercise. They should, in contrast, engage in sensible, regular exercises to strengthen their back gradually so as to keep the tendons, muscles and channels supple. Taijiquan is an excellent example of exercise that helps to strengthen the back and calms the Mind at the same time.

Bad diet

Bad diets include eating too little, eating irregularly and eating food of poor quality; these may cause deficiency of the Qi and Blood due to poor functioning of the Spleen and Stomach in digesting, transporting and transforming the food. When the muscles, tendons, bones and channels are not properly nourished, generalised back pain follows.

Unhealthy diets, such as eating too much fatty, greasy, sweet, cold or raw food, or drinking too much alcohol, may block the Spleen and Stomach, leading to the formation of Damp-Phlegm. When this pathogenic factor blocks the channels passing through the back, generalised back pain is seen to be caused by the stagnation of Qi and Blood in the channels.

Overstrain and weak constitution

Overstrain, a poor constitution, excessive bleeding during menstruation and prolonged sickness may all cause consumption of the Qi, Blood, Yin and Yang, leading to deficiency conditions in the body. When the Qi, Blood, Yin and Yang fail to warm the channels, and tonify the muscles, tendons and bones in the back, then generalised back pain occurs.

This syndrome can often be seen in those with a weak constitution who have pain in the entire back. Excessive physical work also refers to working for too many hours without adequate rest for many years.

Treatment based on differentiation

Differentiation

Differentiation of External or Internal origin

Entire back pain can be caused either by invasion of External pathogenic factors or by Internal disorders.

— If it is caused by invasion of External pathogenic factors, it is usually acute, and accompanied by External symptoms such as headache, fever, an aversion to cold, runny nose, or coughing.
— If it is caused by disorders of Internal organs, it is chronic and has no External symptoms.

Differentiation of the character of the pain

— Acute onset of back pain with a burning or pricking sensation or sharp pain, aggravation of the pain by exposure to warmth and wind, alleviation by cold, with fever, or an aversion to cold, is usually caused by invasion of Wind-Heat.
— Sharp pain over the whole back with a cold sensation, aggravation of the pain by exposure to

cold, and alleviation of pain by warmth, with an aversion to cold, or a slight fever, is usually caused by invasion of Wind-Cold.

— Whole back pain after exposure to cold and damp weather, aggravation of the pain in rainy or cold weather, with heaviness and stiffness of the muscles on the back with a cold sensation, or limitation of extension and flexion of the back, is usually caused by invasion of Cold-Damp.

— Persistent entire back pain, which is aggravated by tiredness and exertion, and alleviated back pain by rest, with fatigue, a pale complexion, or a poor appetite, is often caused by deficiency of Qi.

— Stabbing pain in the back, with aggravation of the pain by pressure, emotions, and at night, a history of sprain of the back, or rigidity in the whole back, is usually caused by stagnation of Qi and Blood.

Treatment

INVASION OF WIND-HEAT

Symptoms and signs

Back pain with a burning or pricking sensation or a sharp pain, aggravated by exposure to warmth and wind, and alleviated by cold, accompanied by a thirst, sore throat, fever, sweating, a cough with yellow sputum, constipation, dark and scanty urine, a thin and yellow tongue coating and a superficial and rapid pulse.

Principle of treatment

Dispel Wind, clear Heat and relieve the pain.

HERBAL TREATMENT

Prescription

YIN QIAO SAN
Honeysuckle and Forsythia Powder
Yin Hua *Flos Lonicerae* 10 g
Lian Qiao *Fructus Forsythiae* 10 g
Dou Chi *Semen Sojae Praeparatum* 6 g
Niu Bang Zi *Fructus Arctii* 10 g
Bo He *Herba Menthae* 6 g, decocted later
Jing Jie Sui *Spica Schizonepetae* 6 g
Jie Geng *Radix Platycodi* 10 g
Gan Cao *Radix Glycyrrhizae* 6 g
Lu Gen *Rhizoma Phragmitis* 10 g
Yu Xing Cao *Herba Houttuyniae* 30 g
Pu Gong Ying *Herba Taraxaci* 15 g
Zhu Ye *Herba Lophatheri* 10 g

Explanations

- Yin Hua and Lian Qiao, pungent in flavour and cool in property, are used to dispel Wind and clear pathogenic Heat so as to relieve the Exterior symptoms.
- Bo He, Jing Jie and Dou Chi induce sweating and dispel External pathogenic factors. Niu Bang Zi, Jie Geng and Gan Cao remove toxin, clear Heat, treat sore throat and eliminate Phlegm. Furthermore, Niu Bang Zi, pungent and cool in nature, is a good herb to dispel External Heat.
- Lu Gen removes pathogenic Heat, promotes the production of Body Fluids and relieves thirst and restlessness.
- Zhu Ye can specifically promote urination, which helps to drive out pathogenic factors by passing water.
- Yu Xing Cao and Pu Gong Ying are used to clear Heat and eliminate Toxin.
- When Wind-Heat is dispelled, the back pain will disappear.

Modifications

1. If there is entire back pain with burning sensation, add Zhi Mu *Rhizoma Anemarrhenae* 10 g and Xi Qian Cao *Herba Siegesbeckiae* 10 g to clear Heat in the channel and relieve the pain.

2. If the back pain is worse at night and there is waking at night owing to severe pain, add Dan Shen *Radix Salviae Miltiorrhizae* 10 g to promote the circulation of Blood, calm the Mind and relieve the pain.

3. If there is a feeling of heaviness in the back, add Cang Zhu *Rhizoma Atractylodis* 10 g to activate the Spleen, eliminate Damp and relieve the feeling of heaviness.

4. If there is a high fever, add Chai Hu *Radix Bupleuri* 15 g and Shi Gao *Gypsum Fibrosum* 30 g to clear Heat and reduce the fever.

5. If there is constipation, add Da Huang *Radix et Rhizoma Rhei* 10 g and Mang Xiao *Natrii Sulfas* 10 g to eliminate Heat, promote defecation and relieve the constipation.

6. If there is a thirst, add Mai Men Dong *Radix Ophiopogonis* 12 g and Sha Shen *Radix Glehniae* 12 g to nourish the Yin, promote the secretion of Body Fluids and relieve the thirst.

7. If there is a sore or swollen throat, add Xuan Shen *Radix Scrophulariae* 12 g to clear Heat, reduce the swelling and relieve the sore throat.

8. If there is a cough and expectoration of much sputum, add Bei Mu *Bulbus Fritillariae* 10 g and

Wei Jing *Rhizoma Phragmitis* 20 g to clear Heat, eliminate Phlegm and stop the cough.
9. If there is chest pain and expectoration of yellow sputum, add Huang Qin *Radix Scutellariae* 15 g and Dong Gua Ren *Semen Benincasae* 30 g to clear Heat in the Lung and relieve the chest pain.

Patent remedies

Yin Qiao Pian *Honeysuckle and Forsythia Tablet*
Huang Lian Shang Qing Wan *Coptis Pill to Clear Heat of Upper Burner*

ACUPUNCTURE TREATMENT

LI-4 Hegu, TE-5 Waiguan, GB-20 Fengchi, GB-35 Yangjiao, GV-14 Dazhui, BL-40 Weizhong, BL-58 Feiyang and BL-63 Jinmen. Reducing method is used on these points.

Explanations

- LI-4, the Source point of the Large Intestine channel, dispels Wind, clears Heat and promotes the circulation of Qi. This is an important point in the body to sedate body pain due to the invasion of External factors.
- TE-5, the Connecting point of the Triple Burner channel and also the Confluence point communicating with the Yang Linking Vessel, disperses pathogenic factors on the body surface and relieves the back pain.
- GB-20 is the meeting point of the Gall Bladder channel and the Yang Linking Vessel. This vessel connects with all the Yang channels and dominates the superficial portion of the body. Needling at GB-20 eliminates Wind, clears Heat, relieves External symptoms and stops the back pain.
- GB-35, the Accumulation point of the Yang Linking Vessel, harmonises the collateral and relieves the back pain.
- GV-14, the meeting point of all the Yang channels, invigorates the Yang-Qi and clears Heat. It also can be needled with a three-edged needle to cause bleeding so as to obtain quick results.
- BL-40, the Sea point, and BL-58, the Connecting point, dispel Wind-Heat in the Bladder channel, harmonise the collateral and treat the back pain.
- BL-63, the Accumulation point, harmonises the collateral, relieves stagnation of Qi and Blood and sedates the back pain.

Modifications

1. If there is generalised back pain with a burning sensation, add BL-66, the Spring point, to clear Heat in the channel and relieve the pain.
2. If the pain worsens at night and there is waking at night owing to the severe back pain, add SP-6, the crossing point of the three Yin channels of the foot, to promote the circulation of Blood and relieve the pain.
3. If there is a feeling of heaviness in the back, add SP-9 to activate the Spleen, eliminate Damp and relieve the heaviness.
4. If there is a fever, add LI-11, the Sea point of the Large Intestine channel, to clear Heat, reduce fever and regulate the Qi and Blood so as to relieve the back pain.
5. If there is a common cold infection, add BL-12 to dispel Wind and relieve the external symptoms.
6. If there is a cough, add LU-5, the Sea point of the Lung channel, and BL-13, the Back Transporting point of the Lung, to disperse the Lung-Qi and relieve the cough.
7. If there is chest pain, add PC-4, the Accumulation point, to harmonise the collateral and relieve the pain.
8. If there is a thirst, add LU-8, the Metal point, to clear Heat, promote the secretion of Body Fluids and relieve the thirst.
9. If there is constipation, add ST-25, the Front Collecting point of the Large Intestine, and ST-37, the Lower Sea point of the Large Intestine, to clear Heat, regulate the Large Intestine and promote defecation.
10. If there is a sore throat, add LU-10, the Spring point, and CV-23 to clear Heat in the Lung system and relieve the throat pain.

Case history

A 21-year-old woman had been suffering from pain over the whole back and a high fever for 4 days. One week previously she had been swimming and when she returned home she felt a bit tension in the whole back, together with a slight aversion to cold. The same evening, her menstrual period started. The next day, her back pain became much worse. She went to her local doctor and received aspirin tablets for her cold. After taking this medicine for 1 day, her back pain failed to improve. She then developed high fever 4 days before visiting the accupuncture clinic. Her temperature was 39.5°C. She also had a headache, throat pain and swelling, a lack of sweating, thirst, restlessness, and coughing with expectoration of yellow sticky phlegm. The day before she came to the clinic, her doctor wanted to give her antibiotics, but she did not want these. She continued with the aspirin till she came to the clinic with her mother. She complained that her whole back was burning, it was difficult to lie down on her back, her temperature was then 39.3°C, she was not sweating but her skin was hot, her tongue had a red tip, and a yellow and dry coating, and her pulse was superficial and rapid.

Diagnosis
Entire back pain due to invasion of Wind-Heat.

Principle of treatment
Dispel Wind, clear Heat, reduce fever and relieve the back pain.

Acupuncture treatment
LI-4, TE-5, GB-20, GB-35, GV-14, LU-5, LU-7, BL-58 and BL-63. Reducing method was used on these points. Treatment was given once every day.

Explanations

- LI-4, the Source point, and TE-5, the Connecting point and the Confluence point communicating with the Yang Linking Vessel, were used to dispel Wind, clear Heat and promote the circulation of Qi so as to relieve the back pain due to invasion of External factors.
- Needling on GB-20 eliminates Wind, clears Heat, relieves External symptoms and stops entire back pain.
- GB-35, the Accumulation point of the Yang Linking Vessel, harmonises the collateral and relieves back pain.
- GV-14, the meeting point of all the Yang channels, invigorates the Yang-Qi and clears Heat.
- LU-5, the Sea point, and LU-10, the Spring point, disperse the Lung-Qi, clear Heat in the Lung and relieve coughing and throat swelling.
- BL-58, the Connecting point, and BL-63, the Accumulation point, dispel Wind-Heat in the Bladder channels, harmonise the collateral, relieve stagnation of Qi and Blood and sedate generalised back pain.

During the first acupuncture treatment, she experienced some sweating, her body temperature started to fall within 2 hours and her back pain felt better. The same evening her body temperature dropped to 38.5°C and she could lie down to sleep. After the second treatment, her temperature was 37.8°C, and her back pain was much improved. A total of another four treatments were given, after which her back pain and fever had disappeared.

INVASION OF WIND-COLD

Symptoms and signs

Sharp pain in the whole back with a cold sensation, which is aggravated by exposure to cold, and alleviated by exposure to warmth. Accompanying symptoms include a stiff neck and back, an aversion to cold, a slight fever, a cough with white phlegm, a lack of thirst, a thin and white tongue coating and a superficial and tight pulse.

Principle of treatment

Dispel Wind, eliminate Cold, harmonise the collateral and relieve the pain.

HERBAL TREATMENT

Prescription

GUI ZHI JIA GE GEN TANG
Cinnamon Twig Decoction plus Kudzu
Gui Zhi *Ramulus Cinnamomi* 10 g
Bai Shao *Radix Paeoniae Alba* 6 g
Sheng Jiang *Rhizoma Zingiberis* 5 g
Zhi Gan Cao *Radix Glycyrrhizae Praeparata* 6 g
Ge Gen *Radix Puerariae* 12 g
Qiang Huo *Rhizoma seu Radix Notopterygii* 12 g

Explanations

- Qiang Huo and Gui Zhi dispel pathogenic Wind and Cold from the muscles and skin, relieve External symptoms and stop the back pain.
- Bai Shao is an assistant herb to nourish the Yin and harmonise the Nutritive system.
- Ge Gen dispels Wind, harmonises the collateral, relieves tension at the back and stops back pain.
- Sheng Jiang not only aids Gui Zhi to dispel pathogenic factors from the muscles and skin but also warms the Stomach.
- Zhi Gan Cao tonifies the Qi.

Modifications

1. If there is generalised pain in body, add Du Huo *Radix Angelicae Pubescentis* 10 g to dispel Wind-Cold and relieve the pain.
2. If there is a feeling of heaviness in the back, add Cang Zhu *Rhizoma Atractylodis* 10 g to eliminate Damp and relieve the feeling of heaviness.
3. If the back pain worsens at night and there is waking at night owing to severe back pain, add Dan Shen *Radix Salviae Miltiorrhizae* 10 g to promote the circulation of Blood, calm the Mind and relieve the pain.
4. If there is an absence of sweating, add Ma Huang *Herba Ephedrae* 10 g to open the skin pores, promote sweating and relieve External symptoms.
5. If there is an aversion to cold or wind on the back, add Jing Jie *Herba Schizonepetae* 10 g and Fang Feng *Radix Ledebouriellae* 10 g to dispel Wind and eliminate Cold.

6. If there is a headache, add Chuan Xiong *Rhizoma Ligustici Chuanxiong* 10 g and Gao Ben *Rhizoma et Radix Ligustici* 10 g to promote the circulation of Qi and relieve the headache.

7. If there is a cough, add Jie Geng *Radix Platycodi* 10 g and Ju Hong *Exocarpium Citri Grandis* 5 g to disperse the Lung-Qi, eliminate Phlegm and relieve the cough.

Patent remedy

San She Dan Zhui Feng Wan *Three Snake Gall Bladder Dispel Wind Pill*

ACUPUNCTURE TREATMENT

GB-20 Fengchi, BL-12 Fengmen, BL-14 Jueyinshu, BL-58 Feiyang, LU-7 Lieque and LI-4 Hegu. Reducing method is used on these points.

Explanations

- GB-20 is the meeting point of the Gall Bladder and Yang Linking Vessel. This Vessel connects with all the Yang channels and dominates the superficial level of the body. Needling at GB-20 dispels Wind, eliminates Cold and stops the back pain.
- BL-12, the Meeting point of the Governing Vessel and Bladder channel, and BL-14, the Back Transporting point of the Pericardium, eliminate pathogenic Wind, warm the channel and stop the pain.
- BL-58, the Connecting point of the Bladder channel, harmonises the collateral, dispels Wind-Cold and relieves the pain.
- LU-7, the Connecting point of the Lung channel, and LI-4, the Source point of the Large Intestine channel, are a pair of points from externally and internally related channels. They dispel Wind, eliminate Cold and stop pain. LI-4 is also a very good point for sedating the back pain.

Modifications

1. If there is pain of the general body, add TE-5, the Connecting point, to dispel Wind-Cold, harmonise the collateral and relieve the pain.
2. If the back is stiff, add a few Extra Huatuojiaji points and cupping on the local area to promote the circulation of Qi and Blood and relieve the stiffness.
3. If there is a sharp pain at night, add Ah Shi points and SP-6 to promote the circulation of Blood, eliminate Blood stasis and relieve the pain.

4. If there is a feeling of heaviness in the back, add SP-9 to eliminate Damp and relieve the feeling of heaviness.
5. If there is a limitation of movement in the back, add BL-60 and BL-62, with strong stimulation, to promote the circulation of Qi in the Bladder channel and Yang Heel Vessel so as to improve the movement.
6. If there is an absence of sweating, add to SI-3 and BL-10 to open the skin pores, promote sweating and relieve External symptoms.
7. If there is an aversion to cold or wind at the back, add moxibustion on BL-12 and BL-58 to dispel Wind and eliminate Cold.
8. If there is a headache, add Extra Yintang to promote the circulation of Qi in the head and relieve the headache.
9. If there is a cough, add BL-13, the Back Transporting point of the Lung, to disperse the Lung-Qi, eliminate Phlegm and relieve the cough.

INVASION OF COLD-DAMP

Symptoms and signs

Pain over the whole back usually after exposure to cold and damp conditions, which is aggravated in rainy or cold weather, accompanied by heaviness and stiffness of the back muscles together with a sensation of coldness, limitation of extension and flexion of the back, a poor appetite, sensation of fullness in the stomach, a white and sticky tongue coating, and a deep and slow pulse.

Principle of treatment

Dispel Cold, eliminate Damp and relieve the pain.

HERBAL TREATMENT

Prescription

QIANG HUO SHENG SHI TANG
Notopterygium Dispelling Dampness Decoction
Qiang Huo *Rhizoma seu Radix Notopterygii* 10 g
Du Huo *Radix Angelicae Pubescentis* 10 g
Chuan Xiong *Rhizoma Ligustici Chuanxiong* 10 g
Man Jing Zi *Fructus Viticis* 10 g
Gan Cao *Radix Glycyrrhizae* 6 g
Fang Feng *Radix Ledebouriellae* 6 g
Gao Ben *Rhizoma et Radix Ligustici* 10 g

Explanations

- Qiang Huo dispels Wind, Cold and Damp from the upper body and Du Huo dispels Wind, Cold and

Damp from the lower body. These two herbs in combination dispel Wind, Cold and Damp from the whole back and the joints in order to treat back pain.
- Fang Feng, Man Jing Zi and Gao Ben dispel Wind, eliminate Cold and relieve the headache.
- Chuan Xiong promotes the circulation of Qi and Blood and dispels Wind so as to relieve back pain.
- Gan Cao coordinates the effects of the other herbs in the formula.

Modifications

1. If there is a feeling of severe heaviness in the back, add Cang Zhu *Rhizoma Atractylodis* 10 g and Bai Zhi *Radix Angelicae Dahuricae* 10 g to dispel Wind, eliminate Damp and relieve the feeling of heaviness.
2. If there is back pain with an obvious cold sensation, add Gui Zhi *Ramulus Cinnamomi* 10 g to warm the channels, dispel Cold and relieve the cold sensation.
3. If the back pain worsens at night and there is waking at night owing to severe pain, add Dan Shen *Radix Salviae Miltiorrhizae* 10 g to promote the circulation of Blood, calm the Mind and relieve the pain.
4. If there is an absence of sweating, add Ma Huang *Herba Ephedrae* 10 g to open the skin pores, promote sweating and relieve Eternal symptoms.
5. If there is nausea with a feeling of heaviness in the Stomach, add Huo Xiang *Herba Agastachis* 5 g and Chen Pi *Exocarpium Citri Grandis* 5 g to harmonise the Stomach, cause the Stomach-Qi to descend, resolve Damp and relieve the nausea.
6. If there is a poor appetite and feeling of fullness in the Stomach, add Bai Kou Ren *Semen Amoni Rotundus* 5 g and Sha Ren *Fructus Amomi* 5 g to dry Damp, improve the appetite and relieve the feeling of fullness.
7. If there is diarrhoea, add Fu Ling *Poria* 10 g and Cang Zhu *Rhizoma Atractylodis* 10 g to dry Damp, activate the Spleen and relieve the diarrhoea.

Patent remedy

Tian Ma Qu Feng Bu Pian *Gastrodia Dispel Wind Formula Tablet*

ACUPUNCTURE TREATMENT

GB-20 Fengchi, BL-12 Fengman, BL-20 Pishu, BL-58 Feiyang, BL-62 Shenmai, SI-3 Houxi, TE-6 Zhigou, LU-7 Lieque and LI-4 Hegu. Reducing method is used on these points.

Explanations

- GB-20, the meeting point of the Gall Bladder channel and the Yang Linking Vessel, and BL-12, the meeting point of the Governing Vessel and the Bladder channel, dispel Wind, Cold and Damp in the Bladder channel, Yang Linking Vessel and Governing Vessel, and relieve the back pain.
- LU-7, the Connecting point of the Lung channel, and LI-4, the Source point of the Large Intestine channel, are a pair of points from externally and internally related channels. Together with TE-6 they dispel Wind, eliminate Cold, relieve External symptoms and stop generalised body pain. LI-4 is also a very good point for sedating the back pain.
- BL-20, the Back Transporting point of the Spleen, activates the Spleen and Stomach, eliminates Damp and relieves the diarrhoea.
- BL-58, the Connecting point, harmonises the collateral, dispels Wind-Cold and relieves the pain.
- BL-62 and SI-3 in combination dispel Wind, Cold and Damp, remove blockage in the Governing Vessel and relieve the back pain.

Modifications

1. If there is a feeling of severe heaviness in the back, add SP-9 to eliminate Damp and relieve the feeling of heaviness.
2. If there is back pain with an obvious cold sensation, add moxibustion on BL-12, BL-58 and LI-4 to warm the channels, dispel Cold and relieve the cold sensation.
3. If the back pain worsens at night and there is waking at night owing to severe back pain, add SP-6 and HT-7 to promote the circulation of Blood, calm the Mind and relieve the pain.
4. If there is an absence of sweating, add KI-6 and BL-10 to open the skin pores, promote sweating and relieve External symptoms.
5. If there is nausea with a feeling of heaviness in the Stomach, add BL-21, the Back Transporting point of the Stomach, to harmonise the Stomach, cause the Stomach-Qi to descend, resolve Damp and relieve the nausea.
6. If there is a poor appetite and a feeling of fullness in the Stomach, add SP-4 to cause the Stomach-Qi to descend, dry Damp, improve the appetite and relieve the feeling of fullness.
7. If there is diarrhoea, add SP-3, the Source point, to dry Damp, activate the Spleen and relieve the diarrhoea.

DEFICIENCY OF SPLEEN-QI

Symptoms and signs

Persistent pain in the entire back, which worsens with tiredness and exertion and is alleviated by rest, accompanied by fatigue, a pale complexion, a poor appetite, loose stools, a shortness of breath, palpitations, cold limbs, spontaneous sweating, a low voice, a pale tongue with tooth marks and a deep, thready and weak pulse.

Principle of treatment

Tonify the Spleen-Qi and sedate the pain.

HERBAL TREATMENT

Prescription

BU ZHONG YI QI TANG
Tonifying the Middle and Benefiting Qi Decoction
Dang Shen *Radix Codonopsis Pilosulae* 9 g
Bai Zhu *Rhizoma Atractylodis Macrocephalae* 9 g
Fu Ling *Poria* 12 g
Huang Qi *Radix Astragali seu Hedysari* 10 g
Chuan Xiong *Rhizoma Ligustici Chuanxiong* 10 g
Bai Shao *Radix Paeoniae Alba* 10 g
Qin Jiao *Radix Gentianae Macrophyllae* 12 g
Gui Zhi *Ramulus Cinnamomi* 10 g
Zhi Gan Cao *Radix Glycyrrhizae Praeparata* 6 g

Explanations

- Dang Shen, Bai Zhu, Fu Ling and Zhi Gan Cao, known as Si Jun Zi Tang—Four-Gentlemen Decoction, activate the Spleen and tonify the Spleen-Qi.
- Huang Qi tonifies the Spleen-Qi and lifts up Qi to the back.
- Chuan Xiong promotes the circulation of Blood and relieves the back pain.
- Bai Shao nourishes the Blood, harmonises the Liver and relieves the back pain.
- Qin Jiao and Gui Zhi promote the circulation of Qi and Blood in the channels, harmonise the collateral and relieve the back pain.

Modifications

1. If the back pain is related to changes in the weather, add Qiang Huo *Rhizoma seu Radix Notopterygii* 10 g to dispel External pathogenic factors, harmonise the collateral and relieve the back pain.

2. If there is an occasional stabbing pain, add Tao Ren *Semen Persicae* 10 g and Hong Hua *Flos Carthami* 5 g to promote the circulation of Blood, eliminate Blood stasis and relieve the pain.
3. If there is a sensation of heaviness in the back, add Huai Niu Xi *Radix Achyranthis Bidentatae* 6 g and Di Long *Lumbricus* 10 g to eliminate Damp in the channels and relieve the feeling of heaviness.
4. If the hands and feet are cold, with an aversion to cold and a slow pulse, add Gan Jiang *Rhizoma Zingiberis* 10 g and Rou Gui *Cortex Cinnamomi* 3 g to warm the body and dispel Interior Cold.
5. If there is shortness of breath and lassitude, add Ren Shen *Radix Ginseng* 10 g to tonify the Qi and relieve the shortness of breath.
6. If there is dizziness, vertigo, hair loss, a dry skin and scanty menstruation due to deficiency of Blood, add Dang Gui *Radix Angelicae Sinensis* 10 g and Shu Di Huang *Radix Rehmanniae Praeparata* 10 g to tonify the Blood and regulate the menstruation.
7. If there is a cough with expectoration of white phlegm, add Zhi Ban Xia *Rhizoma Pinelliae Praeparata* 6 g and Chen Pi *Pericarpium Citri Reticulatae* 5 g to resolve Damp and stop the cough.
8. If there is a poor appetite, add Gu Ya *Fructus Oryzae Germinatus* 10 g and Mai Ya *Fructus Hordei Germinatus* 10 g to promote digestion and improve the appetite.
9. If there is diarrhoea, add Ge Gen *Radix Puerariae* 10 g to lift the Spleen-Qi and relieve the diarrhoea.

Patent remedy

Bu Zhong Yi Qi Wan *Tonifying the Middle and Benefiting Qi Pill*

ACUPUNCTURE TREATMENT

BL-11 Dashu, BL-20 Pishu, BL-23 Shenshu, BL-58 Feiyang, BL-62 Shenmai, SI-3 Houxi and GB-39 Xuanzhong. Reinforcing method is used on these points.

Explanations

- BL-11, the Gathering point of the Bones, and GB-39, the Gathering point for the Marrow, tonify the Marrow and strengthen the bones in the back.
- BL-20, the Back Transporting point of the Spleen, and BL-23, the Back Transporting point of the

Kidney, activate the Spleen, tonify the Kidney-Qi and benefit the back.

- BL-62 and SI-3 open the Governing Vessel and relieve the pain in the back.
- BL-58, the Connecting point, harmonises the collateral and relieves the back pain.

Modifications

1. If there is severe pain in a fixed location, add some local Ah Shi points, to harmonise the collateral, promote the circulation of Qi and Blood and relieve the pain.
2. If there is tension and cramping in the back, add GB-34, the Gathering point for the tendons, to relax the tendons, smooth the collateral and sedate the pain.
3. If there is a feeling of tiredness in the back, add moxibustion to warm the channels and promote the circulation of Qi to the local area.
4. If there is an aversion to cold on the back, add cupping on the back to dispel Cold and relieve the pain.
5. If there is dizziness, add GV-20 and GB-20 to raise the energy to the head and relieve the dizziness.
6. If the appetite is poor, add SP-3, the Source point, to activate the Spleen and improve the appetite.
7. If there is lower back pain, hair loss and a poor memory, add KI-3, the Source point, to tonify the Kidney and benefit the Essence.
8. If there is insomnia, add HT-3 and HT-7 to calm the Mind and Heart and improve the sleep.

Case history

A 32-year-old woman had been suffering from pain over the whole back for 2 years. The woman had undergone an abortion 2 years previously. She didn't stay at home afterwards to rest and went back to work immediately. She felt very tired and, a month after the abortion, she started to feel pain over her whole back that moved up and down, closely related to her energetic level. If she was very tired, she would feel more back pain, and if she had enough rest and sleeping, she would feel better. Painkillers did not help the pain. She had several physical check-ups, but each time nothing abnormal was found. Two months previously, she had moved her house and her back pain became much worse.

When she arrived at the clinic, she had a pale complexion, a constant feeling of tiredness, cold hands and feet, shortness of breath and sweating on exertion, a low voice, a poor appetite, loose stools, one to two instances of nycturia and tiredness in the legs. The muscles in the back were soft with slight tenderness everywhere, a pale tongue with some tooth marks and a thin and white coating, and a thready and weak pulse.

Diagnosis
Entire back pain due to deficiency of the Qi of the Spleen and Kidney.

Principle of treatment
Activate the Spleen, tonify the Kidney-Qi and strengthen the back.

Herbal treatment
SI JUN ZI TANG
Four-Gentlemen Decoction
Ren Shen *Radix Ginseng* 5 g
Bai Zhu *Rhizoma Atractylodis Macrocephalae* 10 g
Fu Ling *Poria* 10 g
Huang Qi *Radix Astragali seu Hedysari* 10 g
Du Zhong *Cortex Eucommiae* 10 g
Sang Ji Sheng *Ramus Loranthi* 10 g
Dang Gui *Radix Angelicae Sinensis* 10 g
Chuan Xiong *Rhizoma Ligustici Chuanxiong* 10 g
Ge Gen *Radix Puerariae* 10 g
Zhi Gan Cao *Radix Glycyrrhizae Praeparata* 3 g

This prescription was given every day.

Explanations

- Ren Shen and Huang Qi invigorate the Original Qi and strengthen the Spleen so as to lift the Qi to the back.
- Bai Zhu and Fu Ling strengthen the Spleen, tonify the Spleen-Qi and eliminate Damp.
- Du Zhong and Sang Ji Sheng tonify the Kidney-Qi, strengthen the back and relieve the back pain.
- Dang Gui and Chuan Xiong nourish the Blood, promote its circulation and relieve the pain.
- Ge Gen helps Huang Qi to lift the Qi to the back and relieves the back pain.
- Zhi Gan Cao harmonises the effect of the other herbs in the prescription.

Acupuncture treatment
BL-11, BL-20, BL-23, BL-58, BL-62, SI-3, KI-3, SP-3 and SP-6. Reinforcing method was applied on these points. Treatment was given once every 3 days.

Explanations

- BL-11, the Gathering point for the Bones, and GB-39, the Gathering point for the Marrow, tonify the Marrow and strengthen the bones in the back.
- BL-20, the Back Transporting point of the Spleen, and SP-3, the Source point, activate the Spleen and tonify the Spleen-Qi.
- BL-23, the Back Transporting point of the Kidney, and KI-3, the Source point, tonify Kidney-Qi and benefit the back.
- BL-62 and SL-3 open the Governing Vessel and relieve the pain in the back.
- BL-58, the Connecting point, harmonises the collateral and relieves the back pain.
- SP-6, the crossing point of the three Yin channels of the foot, activates the Spleen, tonifies the Qi of the Spleen and Kidney and relieves the back pain.

After 2 weeks of treatment, her back pain was much relieved. Meanwhile, she was advised to have adequate rest. After another 2 weeks of treatment, her back pain had almost completely disappeared. In addition, her energy levels were much better, and her appetite, stools and nycturia had also improved. Acupuncture was then given once every week, and one package of the same herbs was used for 3 days. Two months later, her back pain was under control. She was followed up 6 months later and she stated she had experienced no back pain since the treatment.

STAGNATION OF QI AND BLOOD

Symptoms and signs

History of sprain in the back, rigidity and pain over the whole back that is characteristically a stabbing pain, aggravated by pressure or by emotional upset and worsening during the night, with waking at night due to the pain. Accompanying symptoms include depression, headache, neck pain, generalised body stiffness, a dark and purplish tongue with a thin and white coating and a thready and wiry pulse.

Principle of treatment

Promote circulation of Qi and Blood, eliminate Blood stasis and relieve the pain.

HERBAL TREATMENT

Prescription

SHEN TONG ZHU YU TANG
Meridian Passage
Dang Gui *Radix Angelicae Sinensis* 12 g
Chuan Xiong *Rhizoma Ligustici Chuanxiong* 12 g
Tao Ren *Semen Persicae* 10 g
Hong Hua *Flos Carthami* 6 g
Xiang Fu *Rhizoma Cyperi* 10 g
Qiang Huo *Rhizoma seu Radix Notopterygii* 10 g
Qin Jiao *Radix Gentianae* 10 g
Mo Yao *Resina Myrrhae* 6 g
Wu Ling Zhi *Faeces Trogopterorum* 6 g
Di Long *Lumbricus* 10 g
Gan Cao *Radix Glycyrrhizae* 6 g

Explanations

- Dang Gui, Chuan Xiong, Tao Ren and Hong Hua promote the circulation of Blood and eliminate Blood stasis.
- Mo Yao and Wu Ling Zhi eliminate Blood stasis to sedate the pain.
- Xiang Fu promotes the circulation of Qi to reinforce the effect of the herbs for Blood circulation.

- Qiang Huo and Qin Jiao harmonise the collateral, eliminate Damp and relieve the back pain.
- Di Long eliminates Blood stasis and Damp in the collateral.
- Gan Cao harmonises the effect of the other herbs in the prescription.

Modifications

1. If there is restlessness and insomnia, add Dan Shen *Radix Salviae Miltiorrhizae* 15 g to calm the Mind, promote the circulation of Blood and improve the sleep.
2. If the limbs are cold, add Gui Zhi *Ramulus Cinnamomi* 10 g to warm the channels and dispel Cold.
3. If there is depression, add Chai Hu *Radix Bupleuri* 10 g and Bai Shao *Radix Paeoniae Alba* 10 g to harmonise the Liver, promote the circulation of Liver-Qi and relieve the depression.
4. If there is dysmenorrhoea or scanty menstruation, add Yi Mu Cao *Herba Leonuri* 15 g and Huai Niu Xi *Radix Achyranthis Bidentatae* 10 g to promote the circulation of Blood and regulate the menstruation.
5. If there is a pale complexion, hair loss and a dry skin due to deficiency of Blood, add E Jiao *Colla Corii Asini* 10 g to tonify the Blood and nourish the hair and skin.
6. If there is a sensation of fullness in the abdomen, add Mu Xiang *Radix Aucklandiae* 12 g and Chen Pi *Pericarpium Citri Reticulatae* 10 g to promote the circulation of Qi and relieve the feeling of fullness.
7. If there is a slight fever at night, add Qing Hao *Herba Artemisiae Chinghao* 12 g to clear Heat in the Blood and reduce the fever.
8. If there is constipation, add Da Huang *Radix et Rhizoma Rhei* 10 g to promote defecation and relieve the constipation.

Patent remedies

Te Xiao Yao Tong Ling *Special Efficacy Lower Back Pain Pill*
Yu Xue Bi Chong Ji *Stagnant Blood Bi Syndrome Infusion*
Yun Nan Bai Yao *Yunnan White Medicine*

ACUPUNCTURE TREATMENT

BL-15 Xinshu, BL-17 Geshu, BL-18 Ganshu, GB-35 Yangjiao, BL-58 Feiyang, BL-59 Fuyang, BL-62 Shenmai and SI-3 Houxi. Reducing method is used on these points.

Explanations

- BL-15, the Back Transporting point of the Heart, which is the king of the five organs, invigorates the circulation of Blood, calms the Mind and relieves the back pain.
- BL-17, the Gathering point for the Blood, promotes its circulation, eliminates Blood stasis and relieves the pain.
- BL-18, the Back Transporting point of the Liver, smoothes the Liver, promotes the circulation of Liver-Qi and relieves depression.
- GB-35, the Accumulation point of the Yang Linking Vessel, and BL-59, the Accumulation point of the Yang Heel Vessel, harmonise the collateral, promote the circulation of Qi and Blood and relieve the pain.
- BL-58, the Connecting point, harmonises the collateral, promotes the circulation of Qi and Blood and relieves the back pain.
- BL-62 and SI-3 in combination open the Governing Vessel and relieve the back pain.

Modifications

1. If there is a severe stabbing back pain, add SP-6 to regulate the circulation of Blood and relieve the pain.
2. If there is intolerance of cold, add BL-20 and GV-4 to invigorate the Yang-Qi and dispel Cold.
3. If there is general tiredness, add KI-3 to tonify the Kidney and reinforce the Qi so as to relieve the tiredness.
4. If there is chest pain, add PC-4, the Accumulation point, and PC-6, the Connecting point, to regulate the circulation of Qi and Blood in the chest and relieve the pain.
5. If there is depression, add LR-3 to smooth the Liver, promote the circulation of Liver-Qi and relieve the depression.
6. If there is a headache and nervousness, add GB-20 to calm the Liver and relieve the headache.
7. If there is restlessness and insomnia, add HT-3 and HT-7 to calm the Mind and improve the sleep.
8. If there is constipation, add BL-25, the Back Transporting point of the Large Intestine, to promote defecation and relieve the constipation.

Case history

A 30-year-old man had been suffering from back pain over the whole back for 2 years which had been much worse for the previous 6 days. He had sprained his lower back 2 years previously whilst lifting a heavy object. Investigations by hospital staff had revealed nothing wrong with his vertebrae, and he was given painkillers and physiotherapy. His back pain was almost under control after 2 weeks of medication and physiotherapy; however, it had never completely gone. Six days before coming to the clinic, he suddenly got a severe back pain when he got out of his car after driving for 5 hours. He took some painkillers and stayed in bed, but this did not help. He could not sleep because of the severe pain. The hospital team had always suspected there might be herniation, but nothing was revealed on the tests.

He came to the clinic assisted by his wife. He had the following symptoms: rigidity and pain in the whole back, which was mainly fixed at the level of T7 and L4–L5, but with tenderness on pressure over the whole back, severe muscle tension, limitation of movement, radiation of the back pain to the right leg along the Gall Bladder channel, aggravation of the back pain by coughing, sneezing and defecation, accompanied by insomnia, restlessness, a poor appetite, a purplish tongue with a thin and white coating and a thready and wiry pulse.

Diagnosis
Entire back pain due to stagnation of Qi and Blood.

Principle of treatment
Promote circulation of Qi and Blood, eliminate Blood stasis and relieve the pain.

Herbal treatment
SHEN TONG ZHU YU TANG
Meridian Passage
Dang Gui *Radix Angelicae Sinensis* 12 g
Chuan Xiong *Rhizoma Ligustici Chuanxiong* 12 g
Tao Ren *Semen Persicae* 10 g
Hong Hua *Flos Carthami* 6 g
Xiang Fu *Rhizoma Cyperi* 10 g
Mo Yao *Resina Myrrhae* 6 g
Wu Ling Zhi *Faeces Trogopterorum* 6 g
Huai Niu Xi *Radix Achyranthis Bidentatae* 10 g
Di Long *Lumbricus* 10 g
Gan Cao *Radix Glycyrrhizae* 6 g

Explanations

- Dang Gui, Chuan Xiong, Tao Ren and Hong Hua promote the circulation of Blood, eliminate Blood stasis and relieve the back pain.
- Mo Yao and Wu Ling Zhi eliminate Blood stasis and sedate the back pain.
- Xiang Fu promotes the circulation of Qi to reinforce the effect of the herbs for Blood circulation.
- Huai Niu Xi and Di Long eliminate Blood stasis and Damp in the collateral.
- Gan Cao harmonises the effect of the other herbs in the prescription.

Acupuncture treatment
BL-17, BL-58, BL-62, GB-35, GB-36, SP-6, HT-3 and SI-3. Reducing method was used on these points. Moxibustion was used on BL-17 and GB-58. Treatment was given once a day.

Explanations

- BL-17, the Gathering point for the Blood, promotes its circulation, eliminates Blood stasis and relieves the pain.
- BL-58, the Connecting point, harmonises the collateral, promotes the circulation of Qi and Blood and relieves the back pain.
- BL-62 and SI-3 in combination open the Governing Vessel and relieve the back pain.
- GB-35, the Accumulation point of the Yang Linking Vessel, harmonises the collateral, promotes the circulation of Qi and Blood and relieves the pain.
- GB-36, the Accumulation point of the Gall Bladder channel, harmonises the collateral, eliminates Blood stagnation in this channel and relieves the pain.
- SP-6, the crossing point of the three Yin channels of the foot, helps BL-17 promote the circulation and eliminate stasis of the Blood.
- HT-3 calms the Mind and improves sleep.

After two sessions of acupuncture treatment, his back pain was a bit better, he could turn his back slightly more easily and he slept slightly better. The same acupuncture and herbal treatment was continued for 2 more weeks and his back pain much improved, and was no longer aggravated by coughing, sneezing and defecation. The acupuncture was given once every 3 days and the herbal treatment remained the same. Three weeks later, his back pain was completely under control. He continued to take the same herbs for one more month, after which he reported he was free of back pain.

Upper back pain 30

上背疼痛

Upper back pain may occur either on one side or over the entire upper back, that is from the level of C7 down to that of T7. Mostly it occurs on one side. According to TCM theory, upper back pain can be caused by invasion of External pathological factors, stagnation of Qi, deficiency of the Yin or Yang of the Heart, stagnation of Phlegm and Blood in the Heart, or flaring-up of Liver-Fire. Upper back pain may be attributed to any of the following conditions in Western medicine: rachiopathy, injury to the soft tissue of the upper back, deformation or injury of the spinal column, spondylopathy, herpes zoster or its sequelae, angina pectoris or acute myocardial infarction, pleuritis or pleural tumour.

Aetiology and pathology

Invasion of External factors

Overlong exposure to Wind, Cold, Heat or Damp may cause invasion of these pathogenic factors into the upper back, Lung and Heart.

Wind tends to rise and invade the human body in combination with other pathogenic factors; contraction and stagnation are the characteristics of Cold. If there is an invasion of Wind-Cold, therefore, the channels and muscles on the upper back contract, leading to stagnation of Qi and Blood, and pain follows. Invasion of Wind-Cold to the Lung or Heart may also impede the Lung's functions of dispersing the Lung-Qi and the Heart's function of promoting the circulation of Blood, so causing chest pain and upper body pain.

The characteristics of Heat are ascending and burning. It can also consume the Blood and Yin, slowing down the circulation of Blood, which causes the Blood to stagnate. Heat also disturbs the normal movement of the Qi and Blood, which will also lead to stagnation. If Wind-Heat invades the body, the Qi and Blood in the channel will be disturbed, leading to a slowing down or even stagnation of the circulation of Qi and Blood in the locality, which manifests as swelling, redness and pain. Furthermore, if Wind-Heat invades the Lung or Heart it may cause dysfunction of these organs, and trigger off chest pain along with the upper back pain.

Damp is a Yin pathogenic factor with a heavy and sticky nature that tends to obstruct the physiological activities of the Qi and specifically impair the Yang-Qi. If Wind-Damp invades the body, the circulation of Qi and Blood in the channels is disturbed, again leading to a slowing down or stagnation of the circulation of Qi and Blood in the locality, and causing upper back pain together with a feeling of heaviness and lassitude. When Wind-Damp blocks the Lung and Heart, it causes chest pain with upper back pain.

These pathogenic factors may invade the body through its superficial layers, through the nose and mouth, or through eating foods that are inappropriate for the season. Sudden changes in the weather, with a lack of proper self-care, or a weak constitution, or if suffering from an acute or a chronic disease, or excessive stress or overexertion, may all lead to invasion of external factors into the body, and cause upper back pain.

Deficiency of Qi

Overstrain, a poor constitution, an unhealthy diet and eating habits or a prolonged sickness may cause consumption of the Qi, leading to its deficiency. If the Qi is too weak to promote the circulation of Blood, they may lead to stagnation of Qi and Blood. When Qi and Blood stagnate in the channels the upper back is undernourished, causing upper back pain.

Stagnation of Qi and Blood

Qi and Blood should circulate freely in the channels; if they stagnate then upper back pain will occur. The stagnation of Qi and Blood can be due to various causes, including emotional disturbance and trauma to the body.

Emotional disturbance

Excessive stress and frustration may impede the Liver's function of promoting the free flow of Qi; this leads to stagnation of the Liver-Qi, and upper back pain follows. Qi is the leader for Blood, so stagnation of the Liver-Qi will in turn cause stagnation of Blood, which aggravates the upper back pain. If there is Qi stagnation, there is a distending pain and feeling of oppression in the chest and upper back, and the onset of the pain is related to the emotional state.

If Liver-Qi stagnation persists for a long time it will gradually lead to the formation of Liver-Fire, which manifests as sudden severe anger, or habitual indignation, animosity, a feeling of being insulted or rage that causes the Liver-Fire to rise up. When Liver-Fire burns the channels in the upper back, then upper back pain occurs. The Liver-Fire will also consume the Blood and Body Fluids, leading to deficiency of the Blood and Yin, so the upper back is not properly nourished, again causing upper back pain.

Depression, sorrow, grief and sadness may weaken and block the Lung-Qi, where the Qi of the whole body meets. Fear with nervousness, worry and anxiety may also direct the Qi downward, and block its free flow. Both these situations may cause the Qi to stagnate and precipitate upper back pain.

All such emotional disturbances cause the circulation of Qi and Blood in the upper back to become unharmonious, leading to blockage of the channels and muscles and causing upper back pain.

Trauma

Physical trauma, wounds or adhesions after an operation or chronic infection on the upper back may directly damage the channels and muscles, leading to stagnation of the Qi and Blood, and causing upper back pain.

Obstruction of the Heart Vessels

Obstruction in the Heart often occurs in old age, prolonged disease and deficiency of the Qi or Yang, attack by Cold, emotional distress and stagnation of Phlegm.

A poor constitution, chronic disease, or an unhealthy diet and eating habits may cause the Qi or Yang to become deficient. If there is insufficient Qi or Yang, the flow of Blood will be less strong, and the circulation easily becomes impeded. The accumulation and stagnation of Cold and accumulation of Phlegm also hinder the function of the Qi, adversely affecting the Heart Vessels and the circulation of Blood and Qi. Consequently, there will be obstruction in the Heart Vessels, and this manifests as a feeling of oppression and pain in the chest that radiates to the shoulder and upper back.

Emotional disturbance may cause the Qi to stagnate. A deficiency of the Qi, Yang or Blood will cause the Blood circulation to slow, so Blood blocks the Heart Vessels; this manifests as localised twinges of pain that worsen at night.

Consumption of too many cold drinks or cold and raw food, such as salad and fruit, may cause Cold to invade the Spleen directly, leading to dysfunction of its function of transporting and transforming, and the formation of Cold-Phlegm in the body. Upper back pain due to the accumulation of Cold manifests as sudden onset of serious pain in the chest and upper back that is relieved by warmth, and an intolerance of cold.

Overconsumption of fatty or sweet food or milk products may generate Damp-Heat in the Middle Burner. Since these kinds of food are rich in energy and nutritious, they are more difficult to digest than other food and drinks, and place an extra burden on the Spleen and Stomach. The symptoms of Phlegm accumulation are a sensation of stifling and oppression, and pain in the chest and upper back.

Treatment based on differentiation

Differentiation

Differentiation of External or Internal origin

Upper back pain can be caused either by invasion of External pathogenic factors or by Internal disorders.

— If it is caused by invasion of External pathogenic factors, it is usually acute, and accompanied by External symptoms such as headache, fever, an aversion to cold, runny nose, or coughing.
— If it is caused by disorder of the Internal organs, it is chronic and has no External symptoms.

Differentiation of character of the pain

— Acute onset of upper back pain with a burning or pricking sensation, or sharp pain, aggravation of the pain by exposure to warmth and wind, and alleviation by cold, with fever, or an aversion to cold, is usually caused by invasion of Wind-Heat.
— Sharp and sudden pain in the upper back, a cold sensation in the upper back, aggravation of the pain by exposure to cold, and alleviation by warmth, an aversion to cold, or slight fever, is usually caused by invasion of Wind-Cold.
— Fixed upper back pain with a heavy sensation, an aversion to wind, a heavy sensation in body or limbs, poor appetite, dull stomach, or a greasy tongue coating, is often caused by invasion of Wind-Damp.
— Intermittent upper back pain, aggravation of the pain when tired, with a pale complexion, poor appetite, loose stool, shortness of breath, or aversion to cold, is often caused by deficiency of Qi.
— Long-lasting upper back pain with a fixed location, intermittent stabbing pain, or aggravation of the pain by emotional upset and at night, is usually caused by stagnation of Qi and Blood.
— Oppression and pain in the chest, which radiate to the shoulder and upper back, with the pain often located at the left, aggravation of pain at night, or palpitations, is often caused by obstruction of the Heart Vessels.

Treatment

INVASION OF WIND-HEAT

Symptoms and signs

Sudden upper back pain with a burning or pricking sensation, or a sharp pain, or constant pain, which worsens on aggravation of pain by exposure to warmth and alleviated by cold, accompanied by sweating, thirst, fever, a cough with expectoration of yellow phlegm, dark and scanty urine, accompanied by sweating, a thin and yellow tongue coating and a superficial and rapid pulse.

Principle of treatment

Dispel Wind, clear Heat and arrest the pain.

HERBAL TREATMENT

Prescription

YIN QIAO SAN
Honeysuckle and Forsythia Powder
Jin Yin Hua *Flos Lonicerae* 10 g
Lian Qiao *Fructus Forsythiae* 10 g
Dan Dou Chi *Semen Sojae Praeparatum* 6 g
Niu Bang Zi *Fructus Arctii* 10 g
Bo He *Herba Menthae* 6 g, decocted later
Jing Jie *Spica Schizonepetae* 6 g
Jie Geng *Radix Platycodi* 10 g
Gan Cao *Radix Glycyrrhizae* 6 g
Zhu Ye *Herba Lophatheri* 10 g
Lu Gen *Rhizoma Phragmitis* 10 g

Explanations

- In the formula, Jin Yin Hua and Lian Qiao, pungent in flavour and cool in property, relieve the Exterior syndrome and clear pathogenic Heat and Toxin.
- Bo He, Jing Jie and Dan Dou Chi expel Exogenous pathogens and induce sweating so as to relieve chill, fever, sweating and headache.
- Niu Bang Zi, Jie Geng and Gan Cao clear toxin and remove Phlegm so as to relieve a sore throat and cough. Also, Niu Bang Zi, pungent and cool in nature, is good at dispelling Exterior Heat.
- Zhu Ye and Lu Gen remove pathogenic Heat and promote the production of Body Fluids so as to relieve thirst and restlessness. In particular, Zhu Ye can promote urination, which helps to drive pathogenic factors out of the body.

Modifications

1. If there is a high fever, add Chai Hu *Radix Bupleuri* 9 g and Shi Gao *Gypsum Fibrosum* 30 g to clear Heat and reduce the fever.
2. If there is constipation, add Da Huang *Radix et Rhizoma Rhei* 10 g to clear Heat and promote defecation.
3. If there is a thirst, add Mai Dong *Radix Ophiopogonis* 12 g and Sha Shen *Radix Glehniae* 12 g to promote secretion of Body Fluids and relieve the thirst.
4. If there is a sore throat, add Xuan Shen *Radix Scrophulariae* 12 g to benefit the throat and relieve the soreness.

Patent remedies

Yin Qiao Pian *Honeysuckle and Forsythia Tablet*
Huang Lian Shang Qing Pian *Coptis Tablet to Clear Heat of Upper Burner*

ACUPUNCTURE TREATMENT

GV-14 Dazhui, GB-20 Fengchi, LI-4 Hegu, TE-5 Waiguan, SI-11 Tianzong, BL-58 Feiyang, BL-60 Kunlun and some local Ah Shi points. Reducing method is used on these points.

Explanations

- GV-14, the meeting point of all the Yang channels, invigorates the Yang-Qi and clears Heat. It also can be needled with a three-edged needle to cause bleeding, which gives a better result in clearing Heat.
- GB-20 is the meeting point of the Gall Bladder channel and the Yang Linking Vessel. This Vessel connects with all the Yang channels and dominates the superficial level of the body. Needling at GB-20 can eliminate Wind so as to stop pain.
- LI-4, the Source point of the Large Intestine channel, dispels Wind-Heat. It is also an important point for promoting the circulation of Qi in the superficial layers of the body so as to relieve the upper back pain.
- TE-5, the Connecting point of the Triple Burner channel and also the Confluence point communicating with the Yang Linking Vessel, disperses pathogenic factors on the body surface.
- SI-11 dispels Wind-Heat in the upper back and stops the pain.

- BL-58, the Connecting point, harmonises the collateral and sedates the pain.
- BL-60 dispels Wind-Heat in the upper back and relieves the pain.
- Local Ah Shi points promote the circulation of Qi and Blood, eliminate stagnation in the channels and stop the pain.

Modifications

1. If there is a fever, add LI-11, the Sea point of the Large Intestine channel, to clear Heat and reduce the fever.
2. If there is a cough, add LU-5, the Sea point of the Lung channel, and BL-13, the Back Transporting point of the Lung, to stop the cough and clear Heat.
3. If there is chest pain, add LU-6, the Accumulation point, to harmonise the collateral and sedate the pain.
4. If there is a burning feeling in the upper back, add BL-66, the Spring point, to clear Heat and relieve the burning feeling.

Case history

A 32-year-old man had been suffering from upper back pain with an aversion to wind for 1 day. To begin with, he had sneezing, a cough with sticky sputum and a runny nose with little discharge. When he arrived at the clinic, all these symptoms were still present, together with generalised body pain, a sore throat, a slight thirst, sweating, a thin and yellow tongue coating and a superficial and rapid pulse.

Diagnosis
Invasion of Wind-Heat.

Principle of treatment
Dispel Wind, clear Heat, circulate the collateral and sedate the pain.

Herbal treatment
YIN QIAO SAN
Honeysuckle and Forsythia Powder
Jin Yin Hua *Flos Lonicerae* 10 g
Lian Qiao *Fructus Forsythiae* 10 g
Niu Bang Zi *Fructus Arctii* 10 g
Bo He *Herba Menthae* 6 g, decocted later
Jing Jie *Spica Schizonepetae* 6 g
Jie Geng *Radix Platycodi* 10 g
Gan Cao *Radix Glycyrrhizae* 6 g
Yan Hu Suo *Rhizoma Corydalis* 15 g
Chuan Lian Zi *Fructus Meliae Toosendan* 10 g

Explanations

- Jin Yin Hua and Lian Qiao, pungent in flavour and cool in nature, relieve the Exterior symptoms and clear pathogenic Heat and Toxin.

- Bo He and Jing Jie expel Exogenous Heat and induce sweating.
- Niu Bang Zi, Jie Geng and Gan Cao dispel Wind-Heat in the Upper Burner, open the nasal orifice and relieve cough.
- Yan Hu Suo and Chuan Lian Zi regulate the circulation of Qi and relieve the pain.

The patient was treated with a herbal decoction daily. The upper back pain had disappeared after 10 days. Three months later he was followed up and he reported that he had experienced no further pain.

INVASION OF WIND-COLD

Symptoms and signs

Sharp and sudden pain in the upper back, with a cold sensation in the upper back, which is aggravated by exposure to cold and alleviated by warmth, accompanied by a purplish or slight blue colour to the face, a thin and white tongue coating and a superficial and tight pulse.

Principle of treatment

Dispel Wind, eliminate Cold, and circulate the collateral and sedate the pain.

HERBAL TREATMENT

Prescription

GUI ZHI JIA GE GEN TANG
Cinnamon Twig Decoction plus Kudzu
Gui Zhi *Ramulus Cinnamomi* 10 g
Bai Shao *Radix Paeoniae Alba* 6 g
Sheng Jiang *Rhizoma Zingiberis Recens* 5 g
Zhi Gan Cao *Radix Glycyrrhizae Praeparata* 6 g
Da Zao *Fructus Ziziphi Jujubae* 5 g
Ge Gen *Radix Puerariae* 12 g

Explanations

- Gui Zhi expels pathogenic Wind-Cold and warms the channels and collateral so as to relieve Exterior symptoms.
- Bai Shao is an assistant herb to harmonise the Nutritive and Defensive Qi systems so as to relieve External symptoms and pain.
- Sheng Jiang can not only aid Gui Zhi in expelling pathogenic factors but also warm the Stomach and arrest vomiting.
- Da Zao is a tonic for the Stomach and Blood.
- Zhi Gan Cao tonifies the Middle Burner and the Qi.

Modifications

1. If there is severe upper back pain, add Qiang Huo *Rhizoma seu Radix Notopterygii* 10 g and Du Huo *Radix Angelicae Pubescentis* 10 g to dispel Cold and relieve the pain.
2. If there is a high fever with no sweating, add Jing Jie *Herba Schizonepetae* 10 g, Fang Feng *Radix Ledebouriellae* 10 g and Chi Shao *Radix Paeoniae Rubra* 12 g to dispel Wind and reduce the fever.
3. If there is a headache, add Gao Ben *Rhizoma et Radix Ligustici* 10 g to relieve the headache.

Patent remedy

San She Dan Zhui Feng Wan *Three Snake Gall Bladder Dispel Wind Pill*

ACUPUNCTURE TREATMENT

GB-20 Fengchi, BL-12 Fengmen, LU-7 Lieque, BL-58 Feiyang, BL-60 Kunlun, LI-4 Hegu and some local Ah Shi points. Reducing method is used on these points.

Explanations

- GB-20 is the meeting point of the Gall Bladder channel and the Yang Linking Vessel. This Vessel connects with all the Yang channels and dominates the superficial levels of the body. Needling at GB-20 eliminates Wind so as to stop the pain.
- BL-12, the Meeting point of the Governing Vessel and the Bladder channel, and BL-13, the Back Transporting point of the Lung, are the gateways through which pathogenic Wind invades the body. Application of acupuncture and cupping to these two points disperses Wind-Cold and promotes the Lung's function of dispersing the Lung-Qi.
- LU-7, the Connecting point of the Lung channel, and LI-4, the Source point of the Large Intestine channel, are a pair of points from externally and internally related channels. Use of these two points in combination eliminates Wind and stops the pain. LU-7 is used for pain in the head and neck; LI-4 is important for sedating body pain due to External invasion.
- BL-58, the Connecting point, harmonises the collateral and sedates the pain.
- BL-60 dispels Wind-Cold in the upper back and relieves the pain.
- Local Ah Shi points promote the circulation of Qi and Blood, eliminate stagnation in the channels and stop the pain.

Modifications

1. If the muscles are stiff, add Extra Huatuojiaji around C5–T3 and cupping on the local area to promote the circulation of Qi and Blood and relieve the stiffness.
2. If there is a severe aversion to cold on the upper back, add moxibustion at the upper back to dispel Cold and warm the channels.
3. If the pain worsens at night, add BL-17, the Gathering point for the Blood, to promote its circulation and relieve the pain.
4. If there is a fever, add GV-14, the meeting point of all the Yang channels, to clear Heat and reduce the fever.
5. If there is a headache, add Extra Taiyang and Extra Yintang, to sedate the headache.

Case history

A 19-year-old boy had been suffering from upper back pain for 1 day. He also had sneezing, a cough with thin and clear sputum and a runny nose with a white discharge. When he arrived at the clinic, all these symptoms were still present, together with generalised body pain, a lack of thirst, a thin and white tongue coating and a superficial pulse.

Diagnosis
Invasion of Wind-Cold.
   The key symptoms are acute-onset upper back pain with an aversion to cold, a thin and white discharge from the nose, the tongue conditions and the pulse.

Principle of treatment
Dispel Wind, eliminate Cold, circulate the collateral and sedate the pain.

Acupuncture treatment
GB-20, BL-13, LU-7, BL-58, BL-60 and LI-4 together with some local Ah Shi points. Reducing method was used on all these points once a day.

Explanations

- GB-20 is the meeting point of the Gall Bladder channel and the Yang Linking Vessel. Needling at GB-20 can eliminate Wind and stop the upper back pain.
- BL-12, the Meeting point of the Governing Vessel and the Bladder channel, and BL-13, the Back Transporting point of the Lung, are the gateways for dispersing Wind-Cold and promoting the Lung's function in dispersing the Lung-Qi.
- LU-7, the Connecting of the Lung channel, and LI-4, the Source point of the Large Intestine channel, are a pair of points from externally and internally related channels. They eliminate Wind and stop the pain.
- BL-58, the Connecting point, harmonises the collateral and sedates the pain.

- BL-60 dispels Wind-Cold in the upper back and relieves the pain.
- Local Ah Shi points promote the circulation of Qi and Blood, eliminate stagnation in the channels and stop the pain.

Due to the short duration of the problem, the upper back pain was under control in 2 days. One year later he was followed up and he said that he had experienced no further pain after the acupuncture treatment.

INVASION OF WIND-DAMP

Symptoms and signs

Fixed upper back pain with a heavy sensation, and an aversion to wind, together with a heavy sensation in the body or limbs, a poor appetite, a feeling of dullness in the stomach, a greasy tongue coating and a rolling pulse.

Principle of treatment

Dispel Wind, dry Damp and sedate the pain.

HERBAL TREATMENT

Prescription

QIANG HUO SHENG SHI TANG
Notopterygium Dispelling Dampness Decoction
Qiang Huo *Rhizoma seu Radix Notopterygii* 10 g
Du Huo *Radix Angelicae Pubescentis* 10 g
Chuan Xiong *Rhizoma Ligustici Chuanxiong* 10 g
Man Jing Zi *Fructus Viticis* 10 g
Gan Cao *Radix Glycyrrhizae* 6 g
Fang Feng *Radix Ledebouriellae* 6 g
Gao Ben *Rhizoma et Radix Ligustici* 10 g

Explanations

- In the Qiang Huo Sheng Shi Tang, Qiang Huo can dispel Wind-Damp from the upper body and Du Huo tends to dispel Wind-Damp from the lower body. The combination of these two herbs can expel Wind-Damp from the whole body and the joints so as to treat the upper back pain.
- Fang Feng and Gao Ben can dispel Wind-Cold and relieve the headache.
- Chuang Xiong promotes the circulation of Blood and expels Wind so as to arrest the pain.
- Man Jing Zi dispels Wind and relieves the upper back pain.
- Gan Cao coordinates the effects of the other herbs in the formula.

Modifications

1. If there is a nasal discharge and sneezing, add Huo Xiang *Herba Agastachis* 12 g (decocted later) to dispel Damp and relieve the sneezing.
2. If there is diarrhoea, add Fu Ling *Poria* 10 g to relieve the diarrhoea.
3. If the appetite is poor, add Ji Nei Jin *Endothelium Corneum Gigeriae Galli* 15 g and Mai Ya *Fructus Hordei Germinatus* 30 g to improve the appetite and promote digestion.

Patent remedy

Tian Ma Qu Feng Bu Pian *Gastrodia Dispel Wind Formula Tablet*

ACUPUNCTURE TREATMENT

GB-20 Fengchi, SI-13 Quyuan, TE-5 Waiguan, SP-9 Yinlingquan, BL-58 Feiyang, BL-60 Kunlun and some local Ah Shi points. Reducing method is used on all these points.

Explanations

- GB-20 disperses Wind from the Lesser Yang channel and stops the upper back pain.
- SI-13 is a local point for upper back pain. Cupping is applied to this point.
- TE-5, the Connecting point of the Triple Burner channel, is suitable for eliminating Damp, and clearing and regulating the water passage.
- SP-9 is the Sea point of the Spleen channel, which can regulate and strengthen the Spleen so as to eliminate Damp.
- BL-58, the Connecting point, harmonises the collateral and sedates the pain.
- BL-60 dispels Wind-Damp in the upper back and relieves pain.
- Local Ah Shi points promote the circulation of Qi and Blood, eliminate stagnation in the channels and stop the pain.

Modifications

1. If there is pain at the scapular region, add SI-9 and TE-14 to relieve the pain in the locality.
2. If there is a headache and heavy sensation in the head, add ST-8 to eliminate Damp in the head and relieve the headache.
3. If there is vomiting, add PC-6, the Connecting point of the Pericardium channel, to regulate the Stomach and cause the Stomach-Qi to descend.

Case history

A 33-year-old man had been suffering from upper back pain with aversion to cold for 2 days. At the same time, he had a runny nose with a white discharge, a slight fever (37.3°C), generalised body pain with a feeling of heaviness and a poor appetite. When he arrived at the clinic, all these symptoms were still in existence; he also had a greasy and white tongue coating and a soft pulse.

Diagnosis
Invasion of Wind-Damp.

Principle of treatment
Dispel Wind, dry Damp and sedate the pain.

Acupuncture treatment
GB-20, SI-13, TE-5, SP-9, BL-58 and BL-60. Reducing method is used on all these points and some local points. Treatment was given once every day.

Explanations

- GB-20 disperses Wind and stops the upper back pain.
- SI-13 is a local point for back pain in the corresponding areas.
- TE-5, the Connecting point of the Triple Burner channel, eliminates Damp and dispels Wind.
- SP-9, the Sea point of the Spleen channel, regulates and strengthens the Spleen and eliminates Damp.
- BL-58, the Connecting point, harmonises the collateral and sedates the pain.
- BL-60 dispels Wind-Damp in the upper back and relieves the pain.
- Local Ah Shi points promote the circulation of Qi and Blood, eliminate stagnation in the channels and stop pain.

After 5 days of treatment, his upper back pain had disappeared. He was followed up by letter 2 years later, and replied he had experienced no further pain since the acupuncture treatment.

DEFICIENCY OF QI

Symptoms and signs

Intermittent occurrence of upper back pain, which worsens when feeling tired, accompanied by a pale complexion, a poor appetite, loose stools, shortness of breath, an aversion to cold, a tendency to catch cold, spontaneous sweating, a low voice, a pale tongue and a thready and weak pulse.

Principle of treatment

Tonify Qi and circulate the collateral.

HERBAL TREATMENT

Prescription

YU PING FENG SAN plus **BU ZHONG YI QI TANG**
Jade Windscreen Powder plus *Tonifying the Middle and Benefiting Qi Decoction*
Huang Qi *Radix Astragali seu Hedysari* 15 g
Bai Zhu *Rhizoma Atractylodis Macrocephalae* 10 g
Dang Shen *Radix Codonopsis Pilosulae* 9 g
Fu Ling *Poria* 12 g
Chuan Xiong *Rhizoma Ligustici Chuanxiong* 10 g
Bai Shao *Radix Paeoniae Alba* 10 g
Fang Feng *Radix Ledebouriellae* 10 g
Zhi Gan Cao *Radix Glycyrrhizae Praeparata* 6 g

Explanations

- Dang Shen, Bai Zhu, Fu Ling and Zhi Gan Cao, known as Si Jun Zi Tang—Four-Gentlemen Decoction, activate the Spleen and tonify the Spleen-Qi.
- Huang Qi is used to tonify the Spleen-Qi, strengthen the Defensive Qi and lift up the Qi to the back.
- Chuan Xiong activates the circulation of Blood and relieves the upper back pain.
- Bai Shao nourishes the Blood, harmonises the Liver and relieves the pain.
- Fang Feng dispels External pathogenic invasion.

Modifications

1. If there is an aversion to cold and cold limbs, add Gui Zhi *Ramulus Cinnamomi* 10 g to warm the channels and dispel Cold.
2. If the upper back pain is related to weather changes, add Qin Jiao *Radix Gentianae Macrophyllae* 10 g and Qiang Huo *Rhizoma seu Radix Notopterygii* 10 g to dispel External pathogenic factors, harmonise the collateral and relieve the pain.
3. If there is a cold abdomen and slow pulse, add Gan Jiang *Rhizoma Zingiberis* 10 g to warm the Interior and dispel Cold.
4. If the appetite is poor, add Gu Ya *Fructus Oryzae Germinatus* 10 g and Mai Ya *Fructus Hordei Germinatus* 10 g to promote digestion and improve appetite.
5. If there is diarrhoea, add Zhi Ban Xia *Rhizoma Pinelliae Praeparatae* 6 g to resolve Damp in the body and stop the diarrhoea.
6. If there is a stabbing pain in the upper back, add Tao Ren *Semen Persicae* 10 g and Hong Hua *Flos Carthami* 5 g to promote the circulation and eliminate stasis of the Blood.

7. If there is a feeling of heaviness in the upper back, add Huai Niu Xi *Radix Achyranthis Bidentatae* 6 g and Di Long *Lumbricus* 10 g to eliminate Damp in the channels and relieve the heaviness.

Patent remedy

Bu Zhong Yi Qi Wan *Tonifying the Middle and Benefiting Qi Pill*

ACUPUNCTURE TREATMENT

BL-11 Dashu, BL-13 Feishu, BL-15 Xinshu, BL-20 Pishu and ST-36 Zusanli. Reinforcing method is used on these points. Moxibustion is used on BL-13 and BL-20.

Explanations

- BL-11, the Gathering point for the Bones, strengthens the upper back and relieves the pain in the neck and back.
- BL-13, the Back Transporting point of the Lung, regulates and tonifies the Qi of the Lung.
- BL-15, the Back Transporting point of the Heart, tonifies the Heart-Qi and relieves the upper back pain.
- BL-20, the Back Transporting point of the Spleen, activates the Spleen and tonifies the Qi.
- ST-36, the Sea point, restores the normal conversion of Food Essence into Qi and Blood so as to tonify the Qi in the body generally.

Modifications

1. If there is numbness in the upper back, use Plum Blossom needling to promote the circulation of Qi and Blood and relieve the numbness.
2. If there is an intolerance to cold in the upper back, add GV-12, and GV-14, the meeting point of all the Yang channels, to invigorate the Yang-Qi and resist the pathogenic factors.
3. If there is a stabbing pain in the upper back, add BL-17, the Gathering point of the Blood, to promote circulation and eliminate stasis of the Blood and relieve the pain.
4. If there is a feeling of heaviness in the upper back, add TE-6 to eliminate Damp in the channels and relieve the heaviness.
5. If there is generalised tiredness, add SP-6 and KI-3 to tonify the Original Qi and relieve the tiredness.
6. If there is diarrhoea, add SP-9 to activate the Spleen, eliminate Damp and relieve the diarrhoea.

Case history

A 26-year-old woman had been suffering from upper back pain for 1 month. During the first two days, she had felt very tired because of stress in her job. Afterwards, she had upper back pain as well as tiredness. If she rested, the pain would improve. When she came to the clinic, she also had a pale complexion, shortness of breath, a tendency to catch colds, an aversion to wind, generalised extreme tiredness, a pale tongue and a thready pulse.

Diagnosis
Upper back pain due to deficiency of Qi.

Principle of treatment
Tonify the Qi and circulate the collateral.

Acupuncture treatment
BL-11, BL-13, BL-15, LR-3 and ST-36. Reinforcing method was used on all these points except for LR-3, on which reducing method was used. Treatment was given once every other day.

Explanations

- BL-11, the Gathering point for the Bones, relieves the pain in the neck and back.
- BL-13, the Back Transporting point of the Lung, regulates and tonifies the Lung-Qi.
- BL-15, the Back Transporting point of the Heart, regulates the Heart and tonifies the Heart-Qi.
- SP-36, the Sea point, restores the normal conversion of Food Essence into Qi and Blood so as to tonify the Qi in the body generally.
- LR-3, the Source point, harmonises the Liver and relieves stress.

The woman also took Yu Ping Feng San (6 g) three times a day together with the acupuncture. After 2 weeks of treatment, her upper back pain had disappeared. She was followed up a year later, and she said the pain had disappeared after the treatment.

STAGNATION OF QI AND BLOOD

Symptoms and signs

Long duration of stabbing upper back pain with a fixed location and intermittent occurrence, which is aggravated by emotional upset and at night, accompanied by purplish colour of the face, a purplish tongue with a thin coating and a wiry and choppy pulse.

Principle of treatment

Circulate Qi and Blood, smooth the collateral and sedate the pain.

HERBAL TREATMENT

Prescription

SHEN TONG ZHU YU TANG
Meridian Passage

Qin Jiao *Radix Gentianae Macrophyllae* 10 g
Chuan Xiong *Rhizoma Ligustici Chuanxiong* 12 g
Tao Ren *Semen Persicae* 10 g
Hong Hua *Flos Carthami* 6 g
Gan Cao *Radix Glycyrrhizae* 6 g
Qiang Huo *Rhizoma seu Radix Notopterygii* 10 g
Mo Yao *Resina Myrrhae* 6 g
Xiang Fu *Rhizoma Cyperi* 10 g
Wu Ling Zhi *Faeces Trogopterorum* 6 g
Huai Niu Xi *Radix Achyranthis Bidentatae* 6 g
Di Long *Lumbricus* 10 g
Dang Gui *Radix Angelicae Sinensis* 12 g

Explanations

- Dang Gui, Chuan Xiong, Tao Ren and Hong Hua promote the circulation of Blood and eliminate Blood stasis.
- Mo Yao and Wu Ling Zhi eliminate Blood stasis and sedate the pain.
- Xiang Fu promotes the circulation of Qi so as to reinforce the effect on Blood circulation.
- Huai Niu Xi guides Blood stasis down and tonifies the loins and knees.
- Qinjiao, Qiang Huo and Di Long harmonise the collateral and sedate the pain.
- Gan Cao harmonises the herbs in the formula.

Modifications

1. If there is abnormal menstruation, add Yi Mu Cao *Herba Leonuri* 15 g to regulate the menstruation.
2. If there is a feeling of fullness in the abdomen, add Mu Xiang *Radix Aucklandiae* 12 g to promote the circulation of Qi and relieve the fullness.
3. If the limbs are cold, add Gui Zhi *Ramulus Cinnamomi* 6 g to warm the body and dispel Cold from the body.
4. If there is constipation, add Da Huang *Radix et Rhizoma Rhei* 10 g to promote defecation.

Patent remedies

Yun Nan Bai Yao *Yunnan White Medicine*
Xiao Huo Luo Dan *Minor Invigorate the Collaterals Special Pill*

ACUPUNCTURE TREATMENT

BL-10 Tianzhu, BL-17 Geshu, BL-42 Pohu, SI-6 Yanglao, SI-12 Bingfeng and BL-63 Jinmen. Reducing method is used on these points.

Explanations

- BL-10 promotes the smooth circulation of Qi and Blood. Needling at this point can relieve the upper back pain.
- BL-17, the Gathering point for the Blood, promotes its circulation and eliminates Blood stasis so as to sedate the upper back pain.
- BL-42 activates the circulation and removes obstruction of Blood, remove obstruction from the channels and collateral and relieve the pain.
- SI-12 treats pain in the neck and back.
- SI-6 and BL-63, the Accumulation points, harmonise the collateral and relieve the pain.

Modifications

1. If there is numbness in the upper back, add TE-5 and Plum Blossom needles to regulate the circulation of Qi and Blood and relieve the numbness.
2. If the upper back is intolerant of cold, add ST-36 and GV-14 to invigorate the Yang-Qi and dispel Cold.
3. If there is chest pain, add PC-6, the Connecting point of the Pericardium channel, to regulate the circulation of Qi in the Upper Burner and relieve the chest pain.
4. If the pain is aggravated by emotional upset, add LR-3 and GB-20 to calm the Liver and sedate the pain.
5. If the pain worsens at night, add SP-6 and SI-3 to promote the circulation of Blood and relieve the pain.

OBSTRUCTION OF THE HEART VESSELS

Symptoms and signs

Oppression and pain in the chest, often located on the left side, which radiates to the shoulder and upper back, and worsens at night, accompanied by a dark purple tongue with ecchymoses, and a thready and uneven or knotted and intermittent pulse. There could also be a feeling of oppression in the chest, a greasy tongue coating and a slippery pulse due to obstruction of Phlegm in the Heart. Or there may be sudden attacks of severe pain in the chest, referring to the upper back, and alleviated by warmth, with a deep and slow pulse due to obstruction of the Heart by Cold. Or there could be a distending pain radiating to the upper back, with a feeling of oppression in the chest, and aggravation of the pain by stress and emotional upset, together with a reddish tongue with a thin white coating and a wiry pulse due to stagnation of Liver-Qi.

Principle of treatment

Promote the circulation of Qi and Blood, tonify the Qi or Yang and resolve Phlegm.

HERBAL TREATMENT

Prescription

GUA LOU XIE BAI BAN XIA TANG
Trichosanthis–Allium–Pinellia Decoction
Gua Lou *Fructus Trichosanthis* 12 g
Xie Bai *Bulbus Allii Macrostemi* 30 g
Bai Jiu (liquor) 30 to 60 ml
Ban Xia *Rhizoma Pinelliae* 10 g

Explanations

- Gua Lou unblocks the chest and eliminates Phlegm.
- Ban Xia removes Phlegm, causing uprising Qi to descend.
- Xie Bai and Bai Jiu move the Yang and eliminate Phlegm.
- All these herbs together treat chest pain referring to the upper back due to obstruction of the Heart Vessels.

Modifications

1. If there is shortness of breath due to deficiency of Qi, add Dang Shen *Radix Codonopsis* 15 g to tonify the Qi and activate the Spleen.
2. If there is shortness of breath due to hyperventilation resulting from stagnation of Liver-Qi, add Yu Jin *Radix Curcumae* 10 g and Zhi Ke *Fructus Aurantii* 10 g to promote the circulation of Liver-Qi and relieve the shortness of breath.
3. If there are palpitations, add Wu Wei Zi *Fructus Schisandrae* 10 g to calm the Mind and stop the palpitations.
4. If there is insomnia, add Suan Zao Ren *Semen Ziziphi Spinosae* 12 g to tranquillise the Mind and improve the sleep.
5. If there is chest pain, add San Qi *Radix Notoginseng* 10 g to promote the circulation of Blood and relieve the pain.

Patent remedies

Guan Xin Su He Wan *Styrax Pill for Coronary Heart Disease*
Fu Fang Dan Shen Pian *Compound Salvia Tablet*

ACUPUNCTURE TREATMENT

BL-15 Xinshu, BL-17 Geshu, SP-6 Sanyinjiao and HT-5 Tongli. Reducing method is used on these points.

Explanations

- BL-15, the Back Transporting point of the Heart, which is the king of the five organs, invigorates the Qi of the Zang-Fu organs and dispels the stagnation.
- BL-17, the Gathering point for the Blood, improves its circulation and relieves the pain.
- HT-5, the Connecting point of the Heart channel, harmonises the collateral, eliminates Blood stagnation and relieves the chest pain.
- SP-6 promotes the circulation of Blood and eliminates Blood stasis so as to sedate the pain.

Modifications

1. If there is numbness in the upper back, add Plum Blossom needles to regulate the circulation of Qi and Blood and relieve the numbness.
2. If there is a headache, add Extra Taiyang and Extra Yintang to relieve the headache.
3. If there is severe chest pain, add HT-6 and PC-4, the Accumulation points, to harmonise the collateral and sedate the pain.
4. If there are palpitations, add HT-3, the Sea point, to calm the Heart and relieve the palpitations.

Case history

A 62-year-old man had been suffering from upper back pain with stuffiness in the chest for 3 years. In the beginning, he just had stuffiness of the chest and shortness of breath, then two years previously, he had oppression and pain in the chest radiating to the shoulder and upper back, often localised in the left side of the chest and worsening at night. The Western medical diagnosis made 3 years previously was myocardial infarction. At the time of presentation the main complaint was upper back pain with stuffiness in the chest that becomes severe during the night or after when tired, with shortness of breath, a dark purple tongue with spots and a thready and choppy or knotted and intermittent pulse.

Diagnosis
Obstruction of the Heart Vessels.
The key symptoms of obstruction of the Heart Vessels are: 3 years of the same case history, a chronic and prolonged attack of upper back pain with oppression of the chest, and sometimes chest pain, shortness of breath, a dark purple tongue with spots and a thready and choppy or knotted and intermittent pulse.

Principle of treatment
Promote the circulation of Qi and Blood and sedate the pain.

Acupuncture treatment
BL-15, BL-17, SP-6, PC-4, HT-6 and HT-5. Reducing method was used on these points. Treatment was given every other day.

Explanations

- BL-15, the Back Transporting point of the Heart, which is the king of the five organs, invigorates the circulation of Qi and Blood and dispels the stagnation.
- BL-17, the Gathering point for the Blood, promotes its circulation, eliminates obstruction and relieves the pain.
- HT-5, the Connecting point of the Heart channel, harmonises the collateral and relieves the chest pain.
- SP-6 promotes the circulation of Blood.
- HT-6 and PC-4, the Accumulation points, sedate the chest pain.

Gua Lou Xie Bai Ban Xia Tang *Trichosanthis-Allium-Pinellia Decoction* and Dan Shen Yin *Salvia Decoction* were prescribed at the same time. Alcohol and smoking were forbidden. If there were attacks of upper back pain, Guan Xin Su He Wan *Styrax Pill for Coronary Heart Disease* was given at once to sedate the pain.

Because of the prolonged duration of the disease, the upper back pain took 2 weeks to disappear. One year later he was followed up and he said his back pain was well controlled after this treatment.

Scapular pain 31

肩
肿
疼
痛

Scapular pain may occur on one side of the body or on both, but it is mostly confined to one scapula. Scapular pain may be attributed to any of the following conditions in Western medicine: injury to the soft tissue of the scapular, herpes zoster and its sequelae, angina pectoris or acute myocardial infarction, etc.

Aetiology and pathology

Invasion of External factors

Invasion of External factors such as Wind, Cold, Heat and Damp is one of the most common causes of both acute scapular pain and chronic scapular pain with acute exacerbations. Overexposure to Wind, Cold, Heat or Damp may allow these factors to invade the scapula, blocking the channels and causing stagnation of the Qi and Blood around the scapular region.

Wind tends to rise and attack the upper body. It usually attacks the body in combination with other pathogenic factors, such as Cold, Heat or Damp.

Cold characteristically causes contraction of the muscles, tendons and channels, and subsequently stagnation of the Qi and Blood in the channels. Because of these pathogenic features, when Wind-Cold invades the scapular regions it may cause sudden and severe scapular pain accompanied by a cold sensation, and External symptoms such as an aversion to cold, a slight fever, headache, and a runny nose with a white-coloured discharge.

Heat characteristically rises and is burning in nature. If Wind-Heat invades the scapular region, it causes scapular pain accompanied by a burning or hot sensation, together with swelling in the area and limitation of shoulder movement. Heat can also consume the Body Fluids, Blood and Yin, which leads to concentration of the Blood, so the circulation of the Blood slows, and the Qi and Blood stagnate in the hand Greater Yang or Lesser Yang channels or the foot Greater Yang channel, which may aggravate the scapular pain.

Damp is characterised by viscosity, heaviness and stagnation. It is a Yin pathogenic factor that tends to impede the functions of the Qi and impair the Yang-Qi. It usually attacks the body in combination with Wind, Cold or Heat. If there is invasion of Wind-Damp with Cold or Heat, it disturbs the circulation of the Qi and Blood in the hand Greater Yang or Lesser Yang channels or the foot Greater Yang channel, leading to accumulation of Damp and stagnation of Qi and Blood in the locality, so causing scapular pain with swelling and heaviness.

Emotional disturbance

The Liver is in charge of maintaining the free flow of Qi of the general body. If there is excessive stress, frustration, or prolonged anger, this may cause dysfunction of the Liver, leading to stagnation of the Liver-Qi. If the Liver-Qi stagnates, it may in turn cause stagnation of the Qi in the channels around the scapular regions, and this precipitates scapular pain accompanied by unstable emotions, irritability, depression, headache or nervousness. If the Liver-Qi stagnation lasts for a long time, it may then cause the Blood to stagnate, which aggravates the scapular pain.

In additional to stagnation of the Liver-Qi, excessive thinking may cause stagnation of the Qi and Blood in the Heart, leading to disharmony of the collateral—the Small Intestine channel, so causing scapular pain with pain in the chest, palpitations, restlessness or insomnia.

Excessive grief and sadness disturb the Lung, leading to stagnation of the Lung-Qi, and causing scapular pain accompanied by pain along the Lung channel, a feeling of oppression over the chest, prolonged cough or shortness of breath.

Excessive meditation may cause dysfunction of the Spleen, so that Damp-Phlegm forms in the body. When the channels around the scapular regions are blocked by this pathogenic factor, there is scapular pain with a sensation of heaviness and local swelling, nausea, a poor appetite or loose stools.

Physical trauma

All kinds of physical trauma may cause scapular pain, including falling down, wounds and insect bites, inappropriate operations on the shoulder and the formation of adhesions after an operation. Physical trauma may directly damage the local muscles, tendons and channels, leading to stagnation of the Qi and Blood, and causing scapular pain. If there is acute scapular pain due to above factors, Chinese herbal treatment and acupuncture treatment can have relatively good results. However, if the pain is chronic, the result can be poor.

Bad diet and eating habits

Bad eating habits include eating too little, eating irregularly and eating food of poor quality. These may cause the Qi and Blood to become deficient owing to poor functioning of the Spleen and Stomach in digesting, transporting and transforming food, leading to undernourishment of the muscles, tendons, bones and channels which results in scapular pain. Bad diet includes overconsumption of fatty, greasy or sweet food, or cold or raw food as well as drinking too much alcohol, which may cause the Spleen and Stomach to become blocked, so Damp-Phlegm forms. When this pathogenic factor blocks the channels around the scapular regions, scapular pain appears due to the stagnation of Qi and Blood in the channels.

Overstrain and weak constitution

Overstrain, a poor constitution, excessive menstrual bleeding, and prolonged sickness can all cause the Qi, Blood, Yin or Yang to be consumed, leading to deficiency of the Qi, Blood, Yin or Yang in the body. When the Qi, Blood, Yin or Yang fail to warm the channels and tonify the muscles and tendons around the scapular regions, scapular pain occurs.

This syndrome can often be seen in those with a weak constitution who have scapular pain. Excessive physical work, or working for long hours without adequate rest over many years, can also cause this syndrome.

Treatment based on differentiation

Differentiation

Differentiation of External or Internal origin

Scapular back pain can be caused either by invasion of External pathogenic factors or by Internal disorders.

— If it is caused by invasion of External pathogenic factors, it is usually acute, and accompanied by External symptoms such as headache, fever, an aversion to cold, runny nose, or coughing.
— If it is caused by disorder of the Internal organs, it is chronic and has no External symptoms.

Differentiation of character of the pain

— Acute onset of sharp pain at the scapula, aggravation of the pain by exposure to wind and cold, or rainy weather, alleviation of the pain by warmth and dryness, or sometimes a swollen shoulder with difficult shoulder movement, is usually caused by invasion of Wind-Cold-Damp.
— Sudden scapular pain with a burning sensation, or pricking pain, or sharp and constant pain, with sticky sweating, aggravation of the pain by exposure to warmth and damp, or alleviation of pain with cold, is usually caused by Wind-Damp-Heat.

— Long-lasting scapular pain with intermittent occurrence, aggravation of the pain by emotional upset and stress, and alleviation by relaxation, with tension in the scapular regions and whole back, chest pain, insomnia, depression or headache, is usually caused by stagnation of Qi.

— Long-lasting scapular pain with a fixed location, stabbing pain, worsening of the pain at night, and alleviation by movement and during the day-time, with a history of trauma or operation, is often caused by stagnation of Blood.

— Chronic scapular pain with a diffused location, mostly scapular pain in both shoulders, with tiredness in the shoulder and scapular regions, aggravation of the pain by tiredness and exertion, and alleviation by rest and relaxation, a pale complexion, hair loss, or a poor appetite, is often caused by deficiency of Qi and Blood.

Treatment

INVASION OF WIND-COLD-DAMP

Symptoms and signs

Acute onset of sharp pain at the scapula, which is aggravated by exposure to Wind and Cold or rainy weather and alleviated by contact with warmth and dryness, and occasionally with a swollen shoulder and difficult shoulder movement, accompanied by external symptoms such as an aversion to cold, generalised body pain, headache, a runny nose with a white-coloured discharge, a slightly purplish tongue with a thin and white coating and a superficial and tight pulse.

Principle of treatment

Dispel Wind, eliminate Cold, dry Damp, circulate the collateral and sedate the pain.

HERBAL TREATMENT

Prescription

JUAN BI TANG
Remove Painful Obstruction Decoction
Qiang Huo *Rhizoma seu Radix Notopterygii* 10 g
Du Huo *Radix Angelicae Pubescentis* 10 g
Rou Gui *Cortex Cinnamomi* 6 g
Qin Jiao *Radix Gentianae Macrophyllae* 15 g
Dang Gui *Radix Angelicae Sinensis* 12 g
Chuan Xiong *Rhizoma Ligustici Chuanxiong* 10 g
Zhi Gan Cao *Radix Glycyrrhizae Praeparata* 6 g

Hai Feng Teng *Caulis Piperis Futokadsurae* 30 g
Sang Zhi *Fructus Gardeniae* 30 g
Ru Xiang *Resina Olibani* 6 g
Mu Xiang *Radix Aucklandiae* 6 g

Explanations

- Qiang Huo, Du Huo and Qin Jiao dispel Wind and dry Damp. These three herbs also relieve External symptoms and relieve generalised body pain.
- Hai Feng Teng and Sang Zhi harmonise the collateral in the upper limbs and relieve the scapular pain.
- Chuan Xiong, Dang Gui and Ru Xiang promote the circulation and eliminate the stasis of Blood in the collateral. Chuan Xiong is also a very good herb for dispelling Wind-Cold in the upper limbs and scapular regions and sedating the pain.
- Rou Gui warms the body and channels, dispels Cold and relieves the pain.
- Mu Xiang promotes the circulation of Qi in the channels and sedates the pain.
- Zhi Gan Cao harmonises the herbs in the formula.
- When Wind-Cold and Damp are eliminated, the circulation of Blood is regulated and the collateral harmonised and the scapular pain will disappear gradually.

Modifications

1. If there is a fever, add Chai Hu *Radix Bupleuri* 15 g to dispel Wind and relieve the fever.
2. If there is extreme aversion to cold in the shoulder and scapular region, add Zhi Fu Zi *Radix Aconiti Lateralis Praeparata* 6 g and Gan Jiang *Rhizoma Zingiberis* 10 g to warm the channels and dispel Cold.
3. If there is swelling in the scapular region, add Han Fang Ji *Radix Stephania Tetrandrae* 10 g to dispel Damp and reduce the swelling.
4. If there is severe limitation of shoulder movement, add Lu Lu Tong *Fructus Liquidambaris* 10 g and Luo Shi Teng *Caulis Trachelospermi* 15 g to harmonise the collateral and improve the shoulder movement.
5. If there is severe scapular pain or aggravation of the pain at night, add Jiang Huang *Rhizoma Curcumae* 10 g to promote the circulation of Blood and relieve the pain.
6. If there is a very runny nose and cough, add Ma Huang *Herba Ephedrae* 10 g and Zi Su Ye *Folium Perillae* 10 g to dispel Wind-Cold and disperse the Lung-Qi.

Patent remedy

Han Shi Bi Chong Ji *Cold-Damp Bi Syndrome Infusion*

ACUPUNCTURE TREATMENT

GB-20 Fengchi, LI-4 Hegu, TE-5 Waiguan, SI-4 Wangu, SI-10 Naoshu, SI-11 Tianzong and BL-58 Feiyang. Reducing method is used on these points.

Explanations

- GB-20 is the meeting point of the Gall Bladder channel and the Yang Linking Vessel; TE-5 is the Connecting point of the Triple Burner channel and the point that connects with the Yang Linking Vessel. This vessel connects with all the Yang channels and dominates the superficial level of the body. Needling at GB-20 and TE-5 dispel Wind, eliminate Cold, promote the function of the Triple Burner and eliminate Damp.
- LI-4, the Source point of the Large Intestine channel, dispels Wind and Cold, promotes sweating and eliminates Damp. LI-4 is also a very good point for promoting the circulation of Qi and Blood and relieving the pain.
- SI-4, the Source point, and SI-7, the Connecting point, harmonise the collateral around the scapular regions and relieve the pain.
- SI-10 and SI-11, the local points, promote the circulation of Qi and Blood in the locality and relieve the pain.
- BL-58, the Connecting point of the Bladder channel, harmonises the collateral and dispels Wind, Cold and Damp. This point is also very good for relieving the pain on the back.

Modifications

1. If there is shoulder pain along the Large Intestine channel, add LI-15, the meeting point of the Bright Yang channel of hand and the Yang Heel Vessel, LI-6, Connecting point, and LI-7, the Accumulation point, to promote the circulation of Qi in the channel, dispel Wind-Cold and eliminate Damp.
2. If there is shoulder pain along the Triple Burner channel, add TE-14 and TE-4, the Source point, also TE-7, the Accumulation point, to harmonise the collateral, promote the circulation of Qi, dispel External factors and relieve the pain.
3. If there is pain between the scapular regions, add BL-59, the Accumulation point of the Yang Heel Vessel, BL-40, the Sea point of the Bladder channel, and some local Ah Shi points, to harmonise the collateral, promote the circulation of Qi and Blood and relieve the pain.
4. If the neck is stiff, add SI-3 and LU-7 to dispel External pathogenic factors and relieve the stiffness.
5. If there is tension and cramp in the scapular region, add Huahuojiaji points on C5–C7 to relax the muscles and sedate the pain.
6. If the pain worsens at night, add SP-6 and BL-17 to promote the circulation of Blood and alleviate the pain.
7. If there is neck pain, add GB-21 to relieve the pain.
8. If there is a headache, add Extra Taiyang and Extra Yintang to harmonise the collateral and relieve the headache.
9. If there is a fever, add GV-14, the meeting point of all the Yang channels, to dispel Heat and reduce the fever.
10. If there is a cough, add BL-13, the Back Transporting point of the Lung, to dispel Wind-Cold and relieve the cough.

Case history

A 58-year-old woman had been suffering from scapular pain for 3 weeks. At first she had a cold, infection, and was mainly suffering from throat pain, headache and generalised body pain together with a runny nose, a slight cough and a mild scapular pain on both sides of the body. She was given some herbs for her cold. Two days later, the general cold symptoms improved, but her scapular pain remained. Gradually this worsened over the next 2 weeks, and she often woke up at night.

When she arrived at the clinic, she had scapular pain mainly on the right side, which radiated along the Triple Burner channel with limitation of shoulder movement and was sensitive to cold and humidity, accompanied by a slight aversion to cold, headache in the occipital region, a stiff neck, a feeling of heaviness in the body generally, a thin, white and slightly greasy tongue coating and a superficial and tight pulse.

Diagnosis
Scapular pain due to invasion of Wind-Cold-Damp.

Principle of treatment
Dispel Wind, eliminate Cold, dry Damp and circulate the collateral and sedate the pain.

Acupuncture treatment
GB-20, LI-4, TE-4, TE-5, TE-7, TE-14, SI-4, SI-7, SI-11 and SP-6. Reducing method was used on these points. The acupuncture treatment was given once every other day in order to achieve a quick result.

Explanations
- Needling at GB-20 and TE-5 dispels Wind, eliminate Cold and promotes the Triple Burner's function of eliminating Damp.
- LI-4, the Source, dispels Wind and Cold, promotes sweating and eliminates Damp. It is also a very good point for promoting the circulation of Qi and Blood and relieving pain.

- SI-4, the Source point, SI-7, the Connecting point, and TE-14 harmonise the collateral around the scapular regions and relieve the shoulder pain.
- SI-11, the local point, promotes the circulation of Qi and Blood in the locality and relieves the pain.
- SP-6, the crossing point of the three Yin channels of the foot, promotes the circulation of Blood and relieves the pain.

After two sessions of treatment, her scapular pain had much improved and she could sleep without waking up at night. Her general cold symptoms were also under control. After 2 weeks of treatment, the scapular pain had disappeared completely. During the treatment, she was advised to wear enough warm clothes. She did not take any painkillers during the treatment. Six months later, she was followed up by a letter and she replied that she had experienced no more pain since the acupuncture treatment.

INVASION OF WIND-DAMP-HEAT

Symptoms and signs

Sudden scapular pain with a burning sensation, or a pricking pain, or a sharp and constant pain, which is aggravated by exposure to warmth and damp, and alleviated by cold. Accompanying symptoms included sticky sweating, an aversion to cold, thirst, fever, a generalised feeling of heaviness in the body, a cough with expectoration of slightly yellow phlegm, dark and scanty urine, a red tip to the tongue and a thin and yellow coating, and a superficial and rapid pulse.

Principle of treatment

Dispel Wind, dry Damp, clear Heat and arrest the pain.

HERBAL TREATMENT

Prescription

JIA WEI XUAN BI TANG
Modified Disband Painful Obstruction Decoction
Han Fang Ji *Radix Stephaniae Tetrandrae* 15 g
Xing Ren *Semen Armeniacae* 10 g
Hua Shi *Talcum* 15 g
Zhi Zi *Fructus Gardeniae* 10 g
Chi Xiao Dou *Semen Phaseoli Calcarati* 10 g
Yi Yi Ren *Semen Coicis* 15 g
Zhi Ban Xia *Rhizoma Pinelliae Praeparata* 10 g
Can Sha *Excrementum Bombycis Mori* 10 g
Lian Qiao *Fructus Forsythiae* 10 g
Jiang Huang *Rhizoma Curcumae Longae* 15 g
Hai Tong Pi *Cortex Erythrinae* 15 g
Sang Zhi *Ramulus Mori* 15 g

Explanations

- Han Fang Ji and Sang Zhi dispel Wind, Heat and Damp and relieve External symptoms.
- Zhi Zi and Lian Qiao clear Heat and reduce fever.
- Chi Xiao Dou, Hua Shi, Can Sha and Yi Yi Ren dispel Wind and Damp and promote urination so as to eliminate Damp.
- Xing Ren and Ban Xia resolve Damp-Phlegm and relieve the cough.
- Jiang Huang and Hai Tong Pi harmonise the collateral, promote the circulation of Qi and Blood and relieve the scapular pain.

Modifications

1. If there is an aversion to cold in the scapular region, add Fang Feng *Radix Ledebouriellae* 6 g to dispel Wind and relieve External symptoms.
2. If there is severe scapular pain, add Chuan Xiong *Rhizoma Ligustici Chuanxiong* 10 g to promote the circulation of Qi and Blood and relieve the pain.
3. If there is a fever, add Huang Qin *Radix Scutellariae* 10 g to clear Heat and reduce the fever.
4. If there is a burning feeling and swelling with formation of red spots or blisters in the scapular region, add Long Dan Cao *Radix Gentianae* 10 g and Sheng Di Huang *Radix Rehmanniae Recens* 10 g to dispel Heat, remove Toxin and reduce the swelling.
5. If there is coughing with profuse phlegm, add Jie Geng *Radix Platycodi* 10 g to eliminate Phlegm and relieve the cough.
6. If there is expectoration of yellow and thick phlegm, add Gua Lou *Fructus Trichosanthis* 12 g to clear Heat and resolve Phlegm.
7. If there is a sore throat, add Da Qing Ye *Folium Isatidis* 10 g to clear Heat and relieve the throat pain.
8. If there is a thirst, add Mai Men Dong *Radix Ophiopogonis* 12 g to promote the secretion of Body Fluids and relieve the thirst.

Patent remedies

Shi Re Bi Chong Ji *Damp-Heat Bi Syndrome Infusion*
Feng Shi Xiao Tong Wan *Wind-Damp Dispel Pain Pill*

ACUPUNCTURE TREATMENT

GB-20 Fengchi, LI-4 Hegu, TE-6 Zhigou, SI-4 Wangu, SI-7 Zhizheng, SI-10 Naoshu, SI-11 Tianzong, ST-40 Fenglong and SP-9 Yinlingquan. Reducing method is used on these points.

Explanations

- GB-20, the meeting point of the Gall Bladder channel and the Yang Linking Vessel, dispels Wind, clears Heat and relieves External symptoms.
- LI-4, the Source point, and TE-6 dispel Wind and clear Heat. They can also promote sweating so as to eliminate Damp. LI-4 is also a very good point for promoting the circulation of Qi and Blood and relieving the pain.
- SI-4, the Source point, and SI-7, the Connecting point, harmonise the collateral in the scapular region and relieve the pain.
- SI-10 and SI-11, the local points, promote the circulation of Qi and Blood in the locality and relieve the pain.
- ST-40 and SP-9 dispel Damp in the channels and in the body generally.

Modifications

1. If there is shoulder pain along the Large Intestine channel, add LI-15, the meeting point of the Bright Yang channel of the hand and the Yang Heel Vessel, and LI-6, the Connecting point, LI-2, the Spring point, and LI-7, the Accumulation point, to promote the circulation of Qi in the channel, dispel Wind, clear Heat and eliminate Damp.
2. If there is shoulder pain along the Triple Burner channel, add TE-14, TE-4, the Source point, TE-2, the Spring point, and TE-7, the Accumulation point, to harmonise the collateral, promote the circulation of Qi, dispel External factors and relieve the pain.
3. If there is pain between the scapular regions, add BL-58, the Connecting point of the Bladder channel, BL-59, the Accumulation point of the Yang Heel Vessel, and GB-35, the Accumulation point of the Yang Linking Vessel, to harmonise the collateral and relieve the pain.
4. If there are red spots or blisters in the scapular region, add local surrounding points around the red spots or blisters to clear Heat, reduce swelling and relieve the pain.
5. If there is scapular pain at a fixed location, add some local Ah Shi points to harmonise the collateral, promote the circulation of Qi and Blood and relieve the pain.
6. If there is tension and cramp in the scapular region, add Huatuojiaji points on C5–C7 to relax the muscles and sedate the pain.
7. If the pain worsens at night, add SP-6 and BL-17 to promote the circulation of Blood and alleviate the pain.
8. If there is pain in the neck, add GB-21 and BL-11 to dispel External factors and relieve the neck pain.
9. If the neck is stiff, add SI-3 and LU-7 to dispel Wind and Damp and relieve the stiffness.
10. If there is occipital pain, add BL-10 and GV-16 to dispel Wind and relieve the headache.
11. If there is difficulty in urination, add BL-40, the Sea point of the Bladder channel, to promote urination and eliminate Damp.
12. If there is a fever, add GV-14, the meeting point of all the Yang channels, to dispel Heat and reduce the fever.
13. If there is a cough, add BL-13, the Back Transporting point of the Lung, to dispel Wind and relieve the cough.

STAGNATION OF QI

Symptoms and signs

Long duration of scapular pain of intermittent occurrence that is aggravated by emotional upset and stress and alleviated by relaxation, accompanied by tension in the scapular region and over the whole back, chest pain, insomnia, depression, headache, nervousness, a thin and white tongue coating and a wiry and forceful pulse.

Principle of treatment

Smooth the Liver, promote Qi circulation, harmonise the collateral and relieve the pain.

HERBAL TREATMENT

Prescription

CHAI HU SHU GAN SAN
Bupleurum Soothing the Liver Powder
Chai Hu *Radix Bupleuri* 6 g
Xiang Fu *Rhizoma Cyperi* 9 g
Zhi Qiao *Fructus Aurantii* 6 g
Chuan Xiong *Rhizoma Ligustici Chuanxiong* 6 g
Chuan Lian Zi *Fructus Meliae Toosendan* 9 g
Bai Shao *Radix Paeoniae Alba* 9 g
Zhi Gan Cao *Radix Glycyrrhizae Praeparata* 3 g

Explanations

- Chai Hu and Xiang Fu smooth the Liver and promote the circulation of Liver-Qi.
- Zhi Qiao relaxes the chest and regulates the circulation of Qi.

- Chuan Lian Zi promotes the circulation of Qi and relieves the pain.
- Chuan Xiong invigorates the circulation of Blood and sedates pain. Together with Chai Hu and Xiang Fu it can also regulate the circulation of Qi.
- Bai Shao can nourish the Yin and Blood of the Liver. It can also harmonise the Liver together with Zhi Gan Cao so as to stop the pain.

Modifications

1. If the stagnation of Liver-Qi is obvious, add Qing Pi *Pericarpium Citri Reticulatae Viride* 9 g to promote the circulation of Liver-Qi, remove the obstruction and stop the pain.
2. If there is nervousness, add Xia Ku Cao *Spica Prunellae* 10 g and Gou Teng *Ramulus Uncariae cum Uncis* 10 g to calm the Liver and subdue the Liver-Yang.
3. If there is a headache, add Man Jing Zi *Fructus Viticis* 10 g and Chuan Niu Xi *Radix Cyathulae* 10 g to relieve the headache.
4. If there is chest pain, add Yu Jin *Tuber Curcumae* 10 g to promote the circulation of Qi in the chest and relieve the chest pain.
5. If there is an occasional stabbing scapular pain due to Blood stagnation, or worsening of the pain and waking at night due to the pain, add Yan Hu Suo *Rhizoma Corydalis* 9 g to promote the circulation of Blood and relieve the pain.
6. If there is Chest pain and insomnia, add Dan Shen *Radix Salviae Miltiorrhizae* 10 g and Huang Lian *Rhizoma Coptidis* 5 g to regulate the circulation of Blood, clear Heat in the Heart and stop the pain.
7. If the appetite is poor, add Bai Zhu *Rhizoma Atractylodis* 10 g and Fu Ling *Poria* 12 g to strengthen the Stomach and Spleen and promote digestion.
8. If there is abdominal pain with distension, add Mu Xiang *Radix Aucklandiae* 5 g and Hou Po *Cortex Magnoliae Officinalis* 5 g to regulate the Qi in the Large Intestine and relieve the distension.

Patent remedies

Shu Gan Wan *Soothe Liver Pill*
Xiao Yao Wan *Free and Relaxed Pill*

ACUPUNCTURE TREATMENT

LR-3 Taichong, BL-15 Xinshu, BL-18 Ganshu, PC-6 Neiguan, SI-4 Wangu, SI-7 Zhizheng, SI-10 Naoshu, SI-11 Tianzong and LI-4 Hegu. Reducing method is used on these points.

Explanations

- LR-13, the Source point of the Liver channel, and LI-4, the Source point of the Large Intestine channel, smooth the Liver, promote the circulation of Qi and relieve the pain.
- BL-15, the Back Transporting point of the Heart, and BL-18, the Back Transporting point of the Liver, together with PC-6, regulate the Mind, smooth the Liver and promote the circulation of Qi so as to relieve the pain.
- SI-4, the Source point, and SI-7, the Connecting point, harmonise the collateral around the scapula and relieve the pain.
- SI-10 and SI-11, the local points, promote the circulation of Qi and Blood in the locality and relieve the pain.

Modifications

1. If there is pain between the scapular regions, add BL-59, the Accumulation point of the Yang Heel Vessel, GB-35, the Accumulation point of the Yang Linking Vessel, BL-40, the Sea point of the Bladder channel, and some local Ah Shi points, to harmonise the collateral, promote the circulation of Qi and Blood and relieve the pain.
2. If there is tension and cramp in the scapular region, add GB-34, the Gathering point for the tendons, to relax the tendons, smooth the collateral and sedate the pain.
3. If the pain worsens at night owing to stagnation of Blood, add SP-6 and BL-17 to promote the circulation of Blood and alleviate the scapular pain.
4. If the neck is stiff, add SI-3 and LU-7 to relieve the stiffness.
5. If there is neck pain, add GB-21 to relieve the pain.
6. If there is a headache, add GB-20 to calm the Liver and relieve the headache.
7. If there is nervousness, add GV-20 to calm the Mind, subdue the Liver-Yang and regulate the emotions.
8. If there is restlessness and insomnia, add HT-3, the Sea point, and HT-8, the Spring point, to calm the Mind and Heart and improve sleep.
9. If there is shoulder pain along the Large Intestine channel, add LI-15, the meeting point of the Bright Yang channel of the hand and the Yang Heel Vessel, and LI-6, the Connecting point, and LI-7, the Accumulation point, to promote the circulation of Qi in the channel, dispel Wind-Cold and eliminate Damp.

10. If there is shoulder pain along the Triple Burner channel, add TE-14, and TE-4, the Source point, and TE-7, the Accumulation point, to harmonise the collateral, promote the circulation of Qi, dispel external factors and relieve the pain.

STAGNATION OF BLOOD

Symptoms and signs

History of trauma or operation, scapular pain of long duration and with a fixed location, a stabbing pain, which worsens at night and is alleviated by movement and better during the daytime, accompanied by a purplish colour to the face, a purplish tongue with a thin and white coating and a wiry and choppy pulse.

Principle of treatment

Promote Qi and Blood circulation, smooth the collateral and sedate the pain.

HERBAL TREATMENT

Prescription

SHEN TONG ZHU YU TANG
Meridian Passage
Qin Jiao *Radix Gentianae* 10 g
Chuan Xiong *Rhizoma Ligustici Chuanxiong* 12 g
Tao Ren *Semen Persicae* 10 g
Hong Hua *Flos Carthami* 6 g
Qiang Huo *Rhizoma seu Radix Notopterygii* 10 g
Mo Yao *Resina Myrrhae* 6 g
Xiang Fu *Rhizoma Cyperi* 10 g
Wu Ling Zhi *Faeces Trogopterorum* 6 g
Huai Niu Xi *Radix Achyranthis Bidentatae* 6 g
Di Long *Lumbricus* 10 g
Dang Gui *Radix Angelicae Sinensis* 12 g
Gan Cao *Radix Glycyrrhizae* 6 g

Explanations

- Dang Gui, Chuang Xiong, Tao Ren, and Hong Hua promote the circulation and eliminate the stasis of Blood.
- Di Long, Mo Yao and Wu Ling Zhi eliminate Blood stasis, smooth the collateral and sedate pain.
- Xiang Fu promotes the circulation of Qi so as to reinforce the effect of the Blood circulation.
- Qin Jiao and Qiang Huo harmonise the collateral and relieve the pain.
- Huai Niu Xi guides Blood stasis downward and eliminates it.

- Gan Cao harmonises the actions of the other herbs in the prescription.

Modifications

1. If there is trauma, add Xue Jie *Sanguis Draconis* 3 g and San Qi *Radix Notoginseng* 10 g to promote the circulation of Blood, eliminate its stasis and promote wound healing.
2. If there is depression, add Chai Hu *Radix Bupleuri* 5 g and Bai Shao *Radix Paeoniae Alba* 10 g to smooth the Liver and promote the circulation of Qi.
3. If there is tiredness, add Bai Zhu *Rhizoma Atractylodis* 10 g and Fu Ling *Poria* 12 g to strengthen the Stomach and Spleen and promote the production of Qi.
4. If there is chest pain or angina pectoris, palpitations and shortness of breath due to stagnation of Blood in the Heart, add Dan Shen *Radix Salviae Miltiorrhizae* 10 g to regulate the circulation of Blood in the Heart, calm the Mind and stop the pain.

Patent remedy

Xiao Huo Luo Dan *Minor Invigorate the Collaterals Special Pill*

ACUPUNCTURE TREATMENT

LR-3 Taichong, LI-4 Hegu, BL-17 Geshu, BL-18 Ganshu, SI-4 Wangu, SI-6 Yanglao, SI-7 Zhizheng, SI-10 Naoshu, SI-11 Tianzong and GB-35 Yangjiao. Reducing method is used on these points.

Explanations

- LR-3 and LI-4, the Source points, smooth the Liver and promote the circulation of Qi so as to promote the circulation of Blood and relieve the pain.
- BI-17, the Gathering point for the Blood, and BL-18, the Back Transporting point of the Liver, regulate the circulation of Blood and eliminate its stasis so as to relieve the pain.
- SI-4, the Source point, SI-6, the Accumulation point, and SI-7, the Connecting point, harmonise the collateral around the scapula, eliminate Blood stasis and relieve the pain.
- SI-10 and SI-11, the local points, promote the circulation of Qi and Blood in the locality and relieve the pain.
- GB-35, the Accumulation point of the Yang Linking Vessel, promotes the circulation of Qi and Blood in this Vessel and relieves the scapular pain.

Modifications

1. If there is pain between the scapular regions, add BL-58, the Connecting point, BL-59, the Accumulation point of the Yang Heel Vessel, and BL-63, the Accumulation point, to promote the circulation of Blood in the channels, eliminate Blood stasis and relieve the pain.
2. If there is severe pain of fixed location, add some local Ah Shi points, to harmonise the collateral, promote the circulation of Qi and Blood and relieve the pain.
3. If there is tension and cramp in the scapular region, add GB-34, the Gathering point for the tendons, to relax the tendons, smooth the collateral and sedate the pain.
4. If the pain worsens at night owing to stagnation of Blood, add SP-6 to promote the circulation of Blood and alleviate the pain.
5. If the neck is stiff, add SI-3 and LU-7 to relieve the stiffness.
6. If there is neck pain, add GB-21 to relieve the pain.
7. If there is a headache, add BL-62, the Confluence point of the Yang Heel Vessel, to calm the Mind and relieve the headache.
8. If there is insomnia due to worsening of the pain at night, add HT-3 and HT-7 to calm the Mind and Heart and improve the sleep.
9. If there is shoulder pain along the Large Intestine channel, add LI-15, the meeting point of the Bright Yang channel of the hand and the Yang Heel Vessel, LI-6, the Connecting point, and LI-7, the Accumulation point, to promote the circulation of Qi in the channel, dispel Wind-Cold and eliminate Damp.
10. If there is shoulder pain along the Triple Burner channel, add TE-14, and TE-4, the Source point, and TE-7, the Accumulation point, to harmonise the collateral, promote the circulation of Qi, dispel external factors and relieve the pain.

Case history

A 45-year-old man had been suffering from scapular pain on the left side for 6 years. This pain came and went in close relation to his emotional state. Over the past 10 years, he had also been suffering from heart disease. About 6 years previously, he had experienced a cardiac infarction, after which he felt a stabbing pain in the left scapular region. Occasionally, he also experienced left chest pain referring to the scapular region. He sometimes took some painkillers for the scapular pain, and received physiotherapy when the pain was severe. However, the various investigative tests could find nothing wrong in the scapular region. He even went to see a psychiatrist for his scapular pain, but the psychiatrist could not help him. In the previous 10 days, due to a lot of stress at home, his scapular pain became worse and worse, and painkillers did not help. He went to his cardiologist to have a general check-up, but his heart situation was stable.

When he arrived at the clinic, he had chest pain and scapular pain on the left side, with tenderness in SI-11 and SI-12, accompanied by shortness of breath, a feeling of fullness in the chest, insomnia and frequent waking from the scapular pain, a thin and white tongue coating and a wiry and forceful pulse.

Diagnosis
Scapular pain due to stagnation of Qi and Blood.

Principle of treatment
Smooth the Liver, promote the circulation of Qi and Blood, remove Blood stasis and relieve the pain.

Herbal treatment
SHEN TONG ZHU YU TANG
Meridian Passage
Chuan Xiong *Rhizoma Ligustici Chuanxiong* 12 g
Dang Gui *Radix Angelicae Sinensis* 12 g
Tao Ren *Semen Persicae* 10 g
Hong Hua *Flos Carthami* 6 g
Dan Shen *Radix Salviae Miltiorrhizae* 10 g
Xiang Fu *Rhizoma Cyperi* 10 g
Jiang Huang *Rhizoma Curcumae Longae* 10 g
Yan Hu Suo *Rhizoma Corydalis* 15 g
Di Long *Lumbricus* 10 g
Mo Yao *Resina Myrrhae* 6 g
Wu Ling Zhi *Faeces Trogopterorum* 6 g
Gan Cao *Radix Glycyrrhizae* 6 g

Explanations

- Dang Gui, Chuang Xiong, Tao Ren and Hong Hua promote the circulation of Blood and eliminate Blood stasis.
- Dan Shen promotes the circulation of Blood in the Heart and calms the Mind.
- Di Long, Mo Yao and Wu Ling Zhi eliminate Blood stasis, smooth the collateral and sedate the pain.
- Xiang Fu and Yan Hu Suo promote the circulation of Qi so as to reinforce the effect of the Blood circulation.
- Jiang Huang promotes the circulation of Qi and Blood in the collateral and relieves the pain.
- Gan Cao harmonises the actions of the other herbs in the formula and relieves the muscle tension in the back.

Acupuncture treatment
LR-3, LI-4, BL-15, BL-17, BL-18, SI-4, SI-6, SI-7, SI-11, SI-12 and HT-6. Reducing method was used on these points. Acupuncture was given once every 3 days.

Explanations

- LR-3 and LI-4, the Source points, smooth the Liver and promote the circulation of Qi so as to promote the Blood circulation and relieve the pain.

- BL-15, the Back Transporting point of the Heart, BL-17, the Gathering point for the Blood, and BL-18, the Back Transporting point of the Liver, regulate the circulation of Qi and Blood, smooth the emotions and eliminate Blood stasis so as to relieve the pain.
- HT-6, the Accumulation point, regulates the Heart and sedates the pain in the chest.
- SI-4, the Source point, SI-6, the Accumulation point, and SI-7, the Connecting point, harmonise the collateral around the scapular regions, eliminate Blood stasis and relieve the pain.
- SI-11 and SI-12, the local points, promote the circulation of Qi and Blood in the locality and relieve the pain.

After 1 month of treatment, his scapular pain was much better. He also felt his emotions were much more stable than before the treatment, and his chest pain was under control. He continued with the same treatment for another month, by which time he had got rid of the scapular pain. He was followed up 2 years later and he reported that he had experienced no further pain in the scapular area.

DEFICIENCY OF QI AND BLOOD

Symptoms and signs

Chronic scapular pain of diffuse location, mostly on both sides and with a sensation of tiredness in the shoulder and scapular regions, which is aggravated by tiredness and exertion and alleviated by rest and relaxation, and accompanied by a pale complexion, dizziness, a poor memory, hair loss, lower back pain, a poor appetite, loose stools, a pale tongue with a thin and white coating and a thin and weak pulse.

Principle of treatment

Tonify Qi and Blood, nourish the channels and relieve the pain.

HERBAL TREATMENT

Prescription

BU ZHONG YI QI TANG plus **SI WU TANG**
Tonifying the Middle and Benefiting Qi Decoction plus *Four Substance Decoction*
Dang Shen *Radix Codonopsis Pilosulae* 9 g
Bai Zhu *Rhizoma Atractylodis Macrocephalae* 9 g
Fu Ling *Poria* 12 g
Huang Qi *Radix Astragali seu Hedysari* 10 g
Dang Gui *Radix Angelicae Sinensis* 10 g
Shu Di Huang *Radix Rehmanniae Praeparata* 15 g
Chuan Xiong *Rhizoma Ligustici Chuanxiong* 10 g
Bai Shao *Radix Paeoniae Alba* 10 g
Zhi Gan Cao *Radix Glycyrrhizae Praeparata* 6 g

Explanations

- Dang Shen, Bai Zhu, Fu Ling and Zhi Gan Cao, known as Si Jun Zi Tang—Four-Gentlemen Decoction, can activate the Spleen and tonify the Spleen-Qi.
- Huang Qi tonifies the Spleen-Qi and lifts up Qi to the back.
- Dang Gui and Chuan Xiong nourish the Blood and relieve the scapular pain.
- Shu Di Huang tonifies the Kidney-Essence so as to promote the production of Blood.
- Bai Shao nourishes the Blood, harmonises the Liver and relieves the scapular pain.

Modifications

1. If the scapular pain is related to weather changes, add Qin Jiao *Radix Gentianae Macrophyllae* 10 g and Qiang Huo *Rhizoma seu Radix Notopterygii* 10 g to dispel external pathogenic factors, harmonise the collateral and relieve the pain.
2. If the hands and feet are cold, with an aversion to cold and a slow pulse, add Gan Jiang *Rhizoma Zingiberis* 10 g to warm the body and dispel Interior Cold.
3. If the appetite is poor, add Gu Ya *Fructus Oryzae Germinatus* 10 g and Mai Ya *Fructus Hordei Germinatus* 10 g to promote digestion and improve the appetite.
4. If there is diarrhoea, add Zhi Ban Xia *Rhizoma Pinelliae Praeparata* 6 g to resolve Damp in the body and stop the diarrhoea.
5. If there is a stabbing pain, add Tao Ren *Semen Persicae* 10 g and Hong Hua *Flos Carthami* 5 g to promote the circulation of Blood and eliminate Blood stasis.
6. If there is a sensation of heaviness in the scapular region, add Huai Niu Xi *Radix Achyranthis Bidentatae* 6 g and Di Long *Lumbricus* 10 g to eliminate Damp in the channels and relieve the heaviness.

Patent remedies

Ba Zheng Tang *Eight-Herb Decoction for Rectification*
Bu Zhong Yi Qi Wan *Tonifying the Middle and Benefiting Qi Pill*

ACUPUNCTURE TREATMENT

ST-36 Zusanli, CV-4 Guanyuan, SP-6 Sanyinjiao, BL-17 Geshu, BL-18 Ganshu, SI-4 Wangu, SI-6 Yanglao, SI-7 Zhizheng, SI-11 Tianzong and GB-39 Xuanzhong. Reinforcing method is used on these points.

Explanations

- ST-36, the Sea point, and SP-6, the crossing point of the three Yin channels of the foot, and GB-39, the Gathering point for the Marrow, tonify the Qi and Blood so as to nourish the body and relieve the pain.
- CV-4 tonifies the Original Qi and strengthens the body.
- BL-17 and BL-18 tonify the Blood and promote easy circulation of the Blood.
- SI-4, the Source point, SI-6, the Accumulation point, and SI-7, the Connecting point, harmonise the collateral around the scapular, promote the circulation of Qi and Blood and relieve the pain.
- SI-11, the local point, promotes the circulation of Qi and Blood in the locality and relieves the pain.

Modifications

1. If there is pain between the scapular regions, add BL-58, the Connecting point, BL-59, the Accumulation point of the Yang Heel Vessel, and BL-63, the Accumulation point, to harmonise the collateral, promote the circulation of Blood in the channels and relieve the pain.
2. If there is severe pain of fixed location, add some local Ah Shi points to harmonise the collateral, promote the circulation of Qi and Blood and relieve the pain.
3. If there is tension and cramp in the scapular regions, add GB-34, the Gathering point for the tendons, to relax the tendons, smooth the collateral and sedate the pain.
4. If there is a feeling of tiredness in the scapular regions, add moxibustion to warm the channels and bring the Qi to the locality.
5. If there is an aversion to cold in the scapular region, add cupping in the area to dispel Cold and relieve the pain.
6. If there is dizziness, add GV-20 and GB-20 to raise the Qi to the head and relieve the dizziness.
7. If the appetite is poor, add SP-3, the Source point, to activate the Spleen and improve the appetite.
8. If there is lower back pain, hair loss and a poor memory, add KI-3, the Source point, to tonify the Kidney and benefit the Essence.
9. If there is insomnia, add HT-3 and HT-7 to calm the Mind and Heart and improve the sleep.
10. If there is shoulder pain along the Large Intestine channel, add LI-15, LI-6 and LI-7 to promote the circulation of Qi in the channel and relieve the pain.
11. If there is shoulder pain along the Triple Burner channel, add TE-4, TE-27 and TE-14 to harmonise the collateral, promote the circulation of Qi and relieve the pain.

Middle back pain 32

中
背
疼
痛

Middle back pain may occur on one side or over the entire middle back, in the area between vertebrae T8 and T12. According to TCM theory, middle back pain is often caused by invasion of External factors, accumulation of Damp-Heat in the Gall Bladder, deficiency of the Qi, Blood, Yin or Yang of the Heart, or stagnation of Qi and Blood. Middle back pain may be attributed to any of the following disorders in Western medicine: cholecystitis and cholelithiasis, rheumatism, rheumatoid arthritis (RA), hyperplastic spondylitis, muscle strain or traumatic injury of the middle region, deformation or injury of spinal column. Also, it may sometimes be caused by heart disease—for instance, myocardial infarction or angina pectoris—and in these cases Western medical treatment should be combined with the TCM treatment.

Aetiology and pathology

Invasion of External factors

Overexposure to Wind, Cold or Damp-Heat may cause them to invade the middle back.

Wind tends to invade the upper body, such as the head and the sense organs, and often in combination with other pathogenic factors. When Wind-Cold invades, the channels, tendons and muscles in the middle back contract, leading to stagnation of Qi and Blood, and so causing middle back pain.

Cold is characterised by contraction. When it invades the body, it may obstruct the channels, slowing the circulation of Qi and Blood, and causing pain.

Heat rises up and burns by nature. It can consume the Blood and Yin. In spring or early summer, Wind and Heat often combine, disturbing the Qi and Blood circulation. If the foot Greater Yang channel and Governing Vessel are invaded by Wind-Heat, the Qi and Blood in the locality stagnate, causing swelling, redness and pain.

Damp is a Yin pathogenic factor that tends to obstruct the functions of the Qi of the Spleen and impair the Yang-Qi. It has a heavy and sticky nature. When Damp invades the body, it may cause Damp to accumulate in the channels and collaterals, leading to stagnation of Qi and Blood; when Damp accumulates in the Bladder channel then middle back pain occurs.

Bad diet

The Spleen and Stomach are very important for the digestion, transportation and transformation of food. Overconsumption of alcohol, and of meat or pungent, hot, sweet, or highly flavoured food, causes dysfunction of the Spleen and Stomach, leading to the formation of Damp-Heat. Furthermore, habitual eating of raw and cold food impairs the Spleen and Stomach, leading to the formation of Cold-Damp. When Damp-Heat or Cold-Damp block the channels and collateral, they disturb the circulation of Qi and Blood resulting in middle back pain and other symptoms.

Deficiency of Qi

Overwork, both physical and mental, may gradually consume the Qi and Blood. A weak constitution, giving birth to several children, bad diet and poor eating habits, and prolonged sickness may all damage the Qi and Blood, leading to their deficiency. Qi is the energy that circulates the Blood and distributes it to all parts of the body, and when there is insufficient Qi to circulate the Blood freely, then both the Qi and Blood stagnate, the channels, tendons and muscles on the middle back fail to be nourished, and middle back pain follows.

Stagnation of Qi and Blood

Excessive emotional disturbance, such as excessive stress and frustration, may in turn disturb the Liver's function of maintaining the free flow of Liver-Qi, directly causing the Liver-Qi to stagnate. Furthermore, habitual anger, indignation, a feeling of being insulted and enraged may cause both stagnation of Liver-Qi and flaring-up of Liver-Fire. Since Qi is the guide for Blood circulation, if Liver-Qi stagnation persists over a long period this may result in Blood stagnation. When there is stagnation of Qi and Blood, the circulation of the channels and collateral also becomes blocked, causing pain. Sometimes, the stagnant Liver-Qi turns into Liver-Fire, which consumes the Blood and Body Fluids, slowing down the Blood flow, leading to Blood stagnation and again causing pain.

As well as these emotions that cause the disharmony of Qi and Blood circulation in the middle back, inappropriate physical movement, especially of the trunk, may easily cause Qi and Blood stagnation in this area. When the Qi and Blood are blocked in the channels, tendons and muscles of the middle back, pain follows as a consequence. Physical trauma, operation scars and chronic infection on the middle back may all directly damage the channels, tendons and muscles, inducing stagnation of Qi and Blood, and causing middle back pain.

Treatment based on differentiation

Differentiation

Differentiation of External or Internal origin

Middle back pain can be caused either by invasion of External pathogenic factors or by Internal disorders.

— If it is caused by invasion of External pathogenic factors, it is usually acute, and accompanied by External symptoms such as headache, fever, an aversion to cold, runny nose, or coughing.
— If it is caused by disorder of the Internal organs, it is chronic and has no External symptoms.

Differentiation of character of the pain

— Acute onset of sudden middle back pain with a burning or pricking sensation, or sharp or constant pain, with sweating, aggravation of the pain by exposure to warmth, and alleviation by cold, thirst or fever, an aversion to cold, or cough, is often caused by invasion of Wind-Heat.
— Acute onset of sharp and sudden pain in the middle back, aggravation of the pain by exposure to cold, with limitation of back movement, alleviation by warmth, slight fever, or an aversion to cold, is often caused by invasion of Wind-Cold.
— Acute onset of middle back pain with a heavy sensation, heaviness of the limbs, lassitude, an aversion to cold and damp, slight fever, or a poor appetite, is often caused by invasion of Wind-Damp.
— Middle back pain with a burning sensation and heaviness, aggravation of the back pain after exposure to humid and hot weather, lassitude, low fever, a slight aversion to cold, or sticky sweating, is usually caused by invasion of Damp-Heat.
— Slight middle back pain, which may be aggravated by tiredness and alleviated by rest, with a pale complexion, poor appetite, loose stool, shortness of breath, an aversion to cold, cold hands and feet, or spontaneous sweating, is usually caused by deficiency of Qi.
— Long-lasting middle back pain with a fixed location, intermittent occurrence of a stabbing pain, aggravation of the pain at night and with emotional upset, with a purplish colour of face, is often caused by stagnation of Qi and Blood.

Treatment

INVASION OF WIND-HEAT

Symptoms and signs

Sudden middle back pain with a burning or pricking sensation, or a sharp or constant pain, which is aggravated by exposure to warmth and alleviated by cold, accompanied by sweating, thirst or fever, an aversion to cold, a cough with yellow phlegm, dark and scanty urine, a thin and yellow tongue coating and a superficial and rapid pulse.

Principle of treatment

Dispel Wind, clear Heat and arrest the pain.

HERBAL TREATMENT

Prescription

YIN QIAO SAN
Honeysuckle and Forsythia Powder
Jin Yin Hua *Flos Lonicerae* 10 g
Lian Qiao *Fructus Forsythiae* 10 g
Dan Dou Chi *Semen Sojae Praeparatum* 6 g
Niu Bang Zi *Fructus Arctii* 10 g
Bo He *Herba Menthae* 6 g, decocted later
Jing Jie *Spica Schizonepetae* 6 g
Jie Geng *Radix Platycodi* 10 g
Gan Cao *Radix Glycyrrhizae* 6 g
Zhu Ye *Herba Lophatheri* 10 g
Lu Gen *Rhizoma Phragmitis* 10 g

Explanations

- Yin Hua and Lian Qiao, pungent in flavour and cool in property, relieve the Exterior symptoms and clear pathogenic Heat.
- Bo He, Jing Jie and Dan Dou Chi expel Exogenous pathogenic factors and induce diaphoresis so as to relieve External symptoms.
- Niu Bang Zi, Jie Geng and Gan Cao relieve sore throat and cough by clearing away Toxin and removing Phlegm.
- Niu Bang Zi, pungent and cool in properties, is good for dispelling Exterior Heat.
- Zhu Ye and Lu Gen remove pathogenic Heat, promote the production of Body Fluids and relieve the thirst and restlessness. Zhu Ye can also induce urination, which helps to drive pathogenic factors out of the body by passing water.
- The prescription sedates the middle back pain due to invasion of Wind-Heat.

Modifications

1. If there is a high fever, add Chai Hu *Radix Bupleuri* 15 g and Shi Gao *Gypsum Fibrosum* 30 g to clear Heat and reduce the fever.
2. If there is a sore throat, add Xuan Shen *Radix Scrophulariae* 12 g to clear Heat and benefit the throat.
3. If there is a cough and expectoration of yellow phlegm, add Bei Mu *Bulbus Fritillariae* 10 g and Jie Geng *Radix Platycodi* 12 g to eliminate Phlegm and relieve the cough.
4. If there is a thirst, add Mai Dong *Radix Ophiopogonis* 12 g and Sha Shen *Radix Glehniae* 12 g to nourish Body Fluids and relieve the thirst.
5. If there is constipation, add Da Huang *Radix et Rhizoma Rhei* 10 g to clear Heat and promote defecation.

Patent remedies

Yin Qiao Pian *Honeysuckle and Forsythia Tablet*
Huang Lian Shang Qing Wan *Coptis Pill to Clear Heat of Upper Jiao*

ACUPUNCTURE TREATMENT

GV-14 Dazhui, BL-17 Geshu, BL-18 Ganshu, BL-58 Feiyang, LI-4 Hegu and TE-5 Waiguan. Reducing method is used on these points.

Explanations

- GV-14, the meeting point of all the Yang channels, dispels Heat and reduces fever. It also can be pricked with a three-edged needle to cause bleeding in order to strengthen the effect in clearing Heat and reducing fever.
- BL-17, the Gathering point for the Blood, activates the circulation of Blood in order to stop the pain.
- BL-18, the Back Transporting point of the Liver, regulates Qi and Blood in the Liver and relieves pain.
- LI-4, the Source point of the Large Intestine channel, dispels Wind-Heat at the body surface and sedates the middle back pain.
- TE-5, the Connecting point of the Triple Burner channel and also the Confluence point communicating with the Yang Linking Vessel, disperses pathogenic factors on the body surface.
- BL-58, the Connecting point of the Bladder channel, harmonises the collateral and sedates the middle back pain.

Modifications

1. If there is a fever, add LI-11, the Sea point of the Large Intestine channel, to clear Heat and reduce the fever.
2. If there is a headache, add GB-20 to dispel Wind-Heat and relieve the headache.
3. If there is a cough, add LU-7 to dispel Wind-Heat and disperse the Lung-Qi so as to stop the cough.
4. If there is expectoration of profuse yellow phlegm, add LU-5, the Sea point, to clear Heat in the Lung and eliminate Phlegm.
5. If there is constipation, add ST-25, the Front Collecting point of the Large Intestine, to clear Heat, promote the circulation of Qi in the Large Intestine and promote defecation.

Case history

A 17-year-old boy had been suffering from middle back pain for 6 days. He had got caught in heavy rain 10 days previously and caught pneumonia, for which he was hospitalised. After antibiotic treatment for 5 days, his high fever, cough with deep yellow sputum and shortness of breath were under control, but his middle back pain and chest pain on the right side remained. He also still had a lower-grade fever, thirst, a sore throat, dry coughing, a thin and yellow tongue coating and a rapid and superficial pulse.

Diagnosis
Middle back pain due to invasion of Wind-Heat.

Principle of treatment
Dispel Wind, clear Heat and arrest the pain.

Acupuncture treatment
GV-14, BL-17, BL-18, BL-58, LI-4, PC-6 and LU-7. Reducing method is used on these points. One treatment was given every day.

Explanations

- GV-14, the meeting point of all the Yang channels, dispels Wind, clears Heat and reduces fever. It was pricked with a three-edged needle to cause bleeding.
- BL-17, the Gathering point for the Blood, activates the circulation of blood in order to stop the pain.
- BL-18, the Back Transporting point of the Liver, regulates the Qi and Blood in the Liver and relieves the pain.
- LI-4, the Source point of the Large Intestine channel, and LU-7, the Connecting point, dispel Wind-Heat, disperse the Lung-Qi and sedate the middle back pain.
- BL-58, the Connecting point, harmonises the collateral and sedates middle back pain.
- PC-6, the Connecting point, harmonises the collateral over the chest and relieves the chest pain.

His middle back pain was much better after the second treatment. After one week of treatment his chest pain started to become better and the middle back pain was almost under control. Another one week of treatment was given and his complaint of middle back and chest pain were completely relieved.

INVASION OF WIND-COLD

Symptoms and signs

Sharp and sudden pain at the middle back, aggravated by exposure to cold and alleviated by warmth, accompanied by limitation of back movement, a slight fever, an aversion to cold, a purplish tongue with a thin and white coating and a superficial and tight pulse.

Principle of treatment

Dispel Wind, eliminate Cold, circulate the collateral and sedate the pain.

HERBAL TREATMENT

Prescription

GUI ZHI JIA GE GEN TANG
Cinnamon Twig Decoction plus Kudzu
Gui Zhi *Ramulus Cinnamomi* 10 g
Bai Shao *Radix Paeoniae Alba* 6 g
Sheng Jiang *Rhizoma Zingiberis Recens* 5 g
Zhi Gan Cao *Radix Glycyrrhizae Praeparata* 6 g
Da Zao *Fructus Ziziphi Jujubae* 5 g
Ge Gen *Radix Puerariae* 12 g

Explanations

- In the formula, Gui Zhi expels pathogenic Wind and Cold from the muscles and skin and relieves exterior symptoms.
- Ge Gen relieves External symptoms and stops pain.
- Bai Shao is an assistant herb to harmonise the Nutritive and Defensive Qi system and relieve External symptoms.
- Sheng Jiang not only aids Gui Zhi to expel pathogenic factors from the muscles and skin but also warms the Stomach and arrests the middle back pain.
- Da Zao is a tonic for the Stomach and Blood.
- Zhi Gan Cao tonifies the Middle Burner and Qi.
- When Wind-Cold is dispelled, the middle back pain will disappear.

Modifications

1. If there is severe pain with cold feeling, add Qiang Huo *Rhizoma seu Radix Notopterygii* 10 g and Du Huo *Radix Angelicae Pubescentis* 10 g to dispel Wind-Cold and relieve the pain.

2. If there is a high fever with no sweating, add Jing Jie *Herba Schizonepetae* 10 g, Fang Feng *Radix Ledebouriellae* 10 g to dispel Wind-Cold, promote sweating and reduce the fever.
3. If there is a headache, add Gao Ben *Rhizoma et Radix Ligustici* 10 g to dispel Wind-Cold and sedate the headache.
4. If there is a cough with white phlegm, add Jie Geng *Radix Platycodi* 12 g to eliminate Phlegm and stop the cough.

Patent remedy

San She Dan Zhui Feng Wan *Three Snake Gall Bladder Dispel Wind Pill*

ACUPUNCTURE TREATMENT

GB-20 Fengchi, BL-13 Feishu, BL-14 Jueyinshu, BL-58 Feiyang, SI-3 Houxi, LU-7 Lieque and LI-4 Hegu. Reducing method is used on these points.

Explanations

- GB-20 is the meeting point of the Gall Bladder channel and the Yang Linking Vessel. This vessel connects with all the Yang channels and dominates the superficial level of the body. Needling at GB-20 can dispel Wind-Cold and stop the middle back pain. BL-13, the Back Transporting point of the Lung, is the gateway through which pathogenic Wind invades the body. Application of acupuncture and cupping on these two points can dispel Wind-Cold and disperse the Lung-Qi.
- Needling at BL-14 can eliminate pathogenic Wind, warm the channels and arrest the pain.
- BL-58, the Connecting point, harmonises the collateral and sedates the middle back pain.
- SI-3, the Stream point and one of the eight Confluence points, communicates with the Governing Vessel. Needling at this point can open the vessel and stop the pain.
- LU-7, the Connecting point of the Lung channel, and LI-4, the Source point of the Large Intestine channel, are a pair of points on externally and internally related channels. They dispel Wind-Cold and stop the pain. LU-7 is suitable for pain in the head and neck; LI-4 is an important point for sedating pain in the body.

Modifications

1. If the neck is stiff, add GB-20 and GB-21 to promote the Qi and Blood circulation and relieve the stiffness.

2. If there is nasal obstruction, add LI-20 to open the nasal Orifice and clear the obstruction.
3. If there is stomach pain, add ST-34, the Accumulation point of the stomach channel, to stop the pain.
4. If there is diarrhoea, add ST-25, the Front Collecting point of the Large Intestine, to regulate this channel and arrest the diarrhoea.

INVASION OF WIND-DAMP

Symptoms and signs

Middle back pain with a heavy sensation, heaviness of the limbs, lassitude, an aversion to cold and damp, a slight fever, a poor appetite, diarrhoea, a sticky tongue coating and a deep and rolling pulse.

Principle of treatment

Dispel Wind, dry Damp and sedate the pain.

HERBAL TREATMENT

Prescription

QIANG HUO SHENG SHI TANG
Notopterygium Dispelling Dampness Decoction
Qiang Huo *Rhizoma seu Radix Notopterygii* 10 g
Du Huo *Radix Angelicae Pubescentis* 10 g
Chuan Xiong *Rhizoma Ligustici Chuanxiong* 10 g
Man Jing Zi *Fructus Viticis* 10 g
Gan Cao *Radix Glycyrrhizae* 6 g
Fang Feng *Radix Ledebouriellae* 6 g
Gao Ben *Rhizoma et Radix Ligustici* 10 g

Explanations

- Qiang Huo dispels Wind-Damp from the upper body and Du Huo dispels Wind-Damp from the lower body. The combination of these two herbs can expel Wind-Damp from the whole body and the joints to treat the back pain.
- Fang Feng and Gao Ben dispel Wind-Cold and relieve the headache.
- Chuan Xiong expels Wind, promotes circulation of Blood and arrests the middle back pain.
- Man Jing Zi dispels Wind and arrests the middle back pain.
- Gan Cao coordinates the effects of the other herbs in the formula.

Modifications

1. If there is a nasal discharge and sneezing, add Huo Xiang *Herba Agastachis* 12 g to dispel Wind and eliminate Damp.

2. If the appetite is poor, add Ji Nei Jin *Endothelium Corneum Gigeriae Galli* 15 g and Mai Ya *Fructus Hordei Germinatus* 30 g to improve the appetite.

3. If there is diarrhoea, add Fu Ling *Poria* 10 g and Su Ye *Folium Perillae* 10 g to eliminate Damp and stop the diarrhoea.

4. If there is a feeling of fullness in the abdomen, add Chen Pi *Pericarpium Citri Reticulatae* 5 g and Bai Zhu *Rhizoma Atractylodis* 10 g to promote the circulation of Qi and dry Damp in the Middle Burner.

Patent remedy

Tian Ma Qu Feng Bu Pian *Gastrodia Dispel Wind Formula Tablet*

ACUPUNCTURE TREATMENT

LU-7 Lieque, TE-5 Waiguan, BL-17 Geshu, BL-18 Ganshu, BL-40 Weizhong, BL-58 Feiyang, SP-6 Sanyinjiao and SP-9 Yinlingquan. Reducing method is used on these points.

Explanations

- LU-7, the Connecting point, dispels Wind-Damp and relieves External symptoms.
- TE-5, the Connecting point of the Triple Burner channel and also the Confluence point communicating with the Yang Linking Vessel, disperses pathogenic factors on the body surface.
- BL-17 promotes the circulation of Blood, removes obstruction and relieves the pain.
- BL-18, the Back Transporting point of the Liver, soothes the Liver, regulates the circulation of Qi and relieves the middle back pain.
- BL-40, the Lower Sea point of the Bladder, promotes urination and eliminates Damp.
- SP-6, the crossing point of the three Yin channels of the foot, and SP-9, the Sea point of the Spleen channel, regulate the Spleen-Qi, strengthen the Spleen and resolve Damp.
- BL-58, the Connecting point of the Bladder channel, harmonises the collateral and sedates the middle back pain.

Modifications

1. If the middle back is stiff, add Extra Huatuojiaji T7-12 points with cupping to eliminate Damp and promote the circulation of Qi and Blood so as to arrest the middle back pain.

2. If there is headache and heaviness of the head, add GB-20 to expel Wind and eliminate Damp.

3. If there is joint pain, add SI-3, the Stream point of the Small Intestine channel, to stop the joint pain.

4. If there is diarrhoea, add ST-25 and ST-36 to strengthen the Stomach and Large Intestine and stop the diarrhoea.

5. If the appetite is poor, add CV-12 and SP-3 to activate the Stomach and Spleen and improve the appetite.

Case history

A 23-year-old fisherwoman had been suffering from middle back pain for 5 days. Five days previously, she had caught a cold after washing clothes in a river. She had a severe aversion to cold, a slight fever, middle back pain and diarrhoea with a watery discharge. When she arrived at the clinic, her fever and diarrhoea were relieved but she still had the aversion to cold and middle back pain. She also had sore limbs with a heavy sensation, a poor appetite, a thick, white and greasy tongue coating and a slow and slippery pulse.

Diagnosis
Middle back pain due to invasion of Wind-Damp.

Principle of treatment
Dispel Wind, dry Damp and sedate the pain.

Herbal treatment
QIANG HUO SHENG SHI TANG
Notopterygium Dispelling Dampness Decoction
Qiang Huo *Rhizoma seu Radix Notopterygii* 10 g
Du Huo *Radix Angelicae Pubescentis* 10 g
Cang Zhu *Rhizoma Atractylodis* 10 g
Gan Cao *Radix Glycyrrhizae* 6 g
Fang Feng *Radix Ledebouriellae* 6 g
Hou Po *Cortex Magnoliae Officinalis* 10 g
Huo Xiang *Herba Agastachis* 10 g
Fu Ling *Poria* 20 g

Explanations

- Huo Xiang and Qiang Huo dispel Wind-Damp from the upper body. Du Huo dispels Wind-Damp from the lower body. These herbs together expel Wind-Damp from the whole body and the joints so as to treat the middle back pain.
- Fang Feng dispels Wind-Cold and relieves External symptoms.
- Fu Ling and Cang Zhu activate the Spleen and Stomach and eliminate Damp in the Middle Burner.
- Gan Cao coordinates the effects of the other herbs in the prescription.

She was treated with herbs daily. After 10 days of treatment, her middle back pain disappeared. She was followed up a year later and she stated she had not suffered from middle back pain any more after she had finished the herbal treatment.

INVASION OF DAMP-HEAT

Symptoms and signs

Middle back pain with a burning sensation and feeling of heaviness, which is aggravated after exposure to a humid and hot environment, accompanied by lassitude, thirst with no desire to drink, yellow urine, a low fever, a slight aversion to cold, sticky sweating or jaundice, a red tongue with a yellow and greasy coating and a soft and rapid pulse.

Principle of treatment

Clear Heat, dry Damp and harmonise the collateral.

HERBAL TREATMENT

Prescription

SAN REN TANG
Three-Nut Decoction
Xin Ren *Semen Armeniacae Amarum* 10 g
Hua Shi *Talcum* 15 g, decocted earlier
Tong Cao *Medulla Tetrapanacis* 3 g
Bai Kou Ren *Semen Amoni Cardamoni* 6 g, decocted later
Zhu Ye *Herba Lophatheri* 12 g
Hou Po *Cortex Magnoliae Officinalis* 6 g
Yi Yi Ren *Semen Coicis* 15 g
Ban Xia *Rhizoma Pinelliae* 6 g

Explanations

- Xin Ren facilitates the flow of Lung-Qi in the Upper Burner.
- Bai Kou Ren dispels Damp and promotes the circulation of Qi.
- Yi Yi Ren eliminates Damp-Heat and strengthens the Spleen.
- Hua Shi, Tong Cao and Zhu Ye strengthen the effects of expelling Damp and clearing Heat.
- Ban Xia and Hou Po can promote the circulation of Qi and dispel Damp.
- When Damp is eliminated and Heat is cleared, the middle back pain will disappear.

Modifications

1. If there is a nasal discharge and sneezing, add Huo Xiang *Herba Agastachis* 12 g and Yu Xin Cao *Herba Houttuyniae* 30 g to clear Damp-Heat and relieve External symptoms.
2. If the appetite is poor, add Pei Lan *Herba Eupatorii* 10 g and Mai Ya *Fructus Hordei Germinatus* 20 g to eliminate Damp-Heat and improve the appetite.
3. If there is diarrhoea, add Fu Ling *Poria* 10 g and Cang Zhu *Rhizoma Atractylodis* 10 g to dry Damp and stop the diarrhoea.
4. If there is a high fever, add Huang Lian *Rhizoma Coptidis* 10 g and Shi Gao *Gypsum Fibrosum* 30 g to clear Heat and reduce the fever.

Patent remedies

Shi Re Bi Chong Ji *Damp-Heat Bi Syndrome Infusion*
Feng Shi Xiao Tong Wan *Wind-Damp Dispel Pain Pill*

ACUPUNCTURE TREATMENT

BL-17 Geshu, BL-18 Ganshu, BL-20 Pishu, BL-58 Feiyang, SP-9 Yinlingquan, ST-36 Zusanli and TE-3 Zhongzhu. Even method is used on these points.

Explanations

- BL-17, the Gathering point of the Blood, activates the circulation of Blood in order to stop the pain.
- BL-18, the Back Transporting point of the Liver, regulates the Qi and Blood of the Liver and relieves the pain.
- BL-20, the Back Transporting point of the Spleen, strengthens the Spleen and eliminates Damp.
- BL-58, the Connecting point of the Bladder channel, harmonises the collateral and sedates the middle back pain.
- SP-9, the Sea point of Spleen channel, promotes urination and eliminates Damp-Heat.
- ST-36, the Sea point of Stomach channel, eliminates Damp and promotes the circulation of Qi and Blood.
- TE-3, the Stream point of the Triple Burner channel, relaxes the muscles and tendons, and activates the flow of Qi and Blood in the channels and collateral of the back so as to relieve the middle back pain.

Modifications

1. If there is diarrhoea, add ST-25, the Front Collecting point of the Large Intestine, to regulate the function of the Stomach and intestines and relieve the diarrhoea.
2. If there is a headache, add ST-8 to expel Wind and arrest the headache.
3. If there is vomiting, add CV-12 and PC-6 to eliminate Damp and stop the vomiting.
4. If there is a heavy sensation in the limbs, add SP-3 and ST-40 to promote the circulation of Qi and resolve Damp.

DEFICIENCY OF QI

Symptoms and signs

Slight middle back pain, which is aggravated by tiredness and alleviated by rest, accompanied by a pale complexion, a poor appetite, loose stool, shortness of breath, an aversion to cold, cold hands and feet, spontaneous sweating, a low voice, a pale tongue and a thready and weak pulse.

Principle of treatment

Tonify Qi and circulate the Blood to relieve the pain.

HERBAL TREATMENT

Prescription

BU ZHONG YI QI TANG
Tonifying the Middle and Benefiting Qi Decoction
Ren Shen *Radix Ginseng* 6 g
Huang Qi *Radix Astragali seu Hedysari* 15 g
Bai Zhu *Rhizoma Atractylodis Macrocephalae* 10 g
Zhi Gan Cao *Radix Glycyrrhizae Praeparata* 6 g
Dang Gui *Radix Angelicae Sinensis* 12 g
Chen Pi *Pericarpium Citri Reticulatae* 6 g
Sheng Ma *Rhizoma Cimicifugae* 3 g
Chai Hu *Radix Bupleuri* 3 g

Explanations

- Huang Qi tonifies the Qi and elevates the Yang.
- Ren Shen, Bai Zhu and Zhi Gan Cao activate the Spleen and tonify the Qi.
- Chen Pi promotes the flow of Qi in the Middle Burner so as not to cause Qi stagnation.
- Dang Gui tonifies the Blood.
- Sheng Ma and Chai Hu are used together as guiding herbs to lift the Yang-Qi to the middle back.

Modifications

1. If there is shortness of breath and lassitude, add Wu Wei Zi *Fructus Schisandrae* 10 g to tonify the Lung-Qi and relieve the shortness of breath.
2. If there is diarrhoea, add Fu Ling *Poria* 10 g to eliminate Damp and relieve the diarrhoea.
3. If there is an aversion to cold and cold limbs, add Gui Zhi *Ramulus Cinnamomi* 10 g to warm the channels and dispel Cold.

Patent remedy

Bu Zhong Yi Qi Wan *Tonifying the Middle and Benefiting Qi Pill*

ACUPUNCTURE TREATMENT

BL-13 Feishu, BL-20 Pishu, BL-21 Weishu, BL-58 Feiyang and ST-36 Zusanli. Reinforcing method with moxibustion is used on all these points.

Explanations

- BL-13, the Back Transporting point of the Lung, regulates and tonifies the Qi of the Lung.
- BL-20 and BL-21, the Back Transporting points of the Spleen and Stomach respectively, work for 'the basis of acquired energy after birth', and strengthen the Qi of the Spleen and Stomach.
- BL-58, the Connecting point of the Bladder channel, harmonises the collateral and sedates the middle back pain.
- ST-36, the Sea point, activates the Spleen and Stomach and reinforces the Qi of the Lung to arrest the pain.

Modifications

1. If there is numbness in the limbs, add LR-3 to promote the circulation of Qi.
2. If there is an intolerance of cold, add GV-14, the meeting point of all the Yang channels, to invigorate the Yang-Qi and improve the resistance to pathogenic factors.
3. If there is constipation, add ST-25, the Front Collecting point of the Large Intestine, to promote the circulation of Qi and promote defecation.
4. If there is shortness of breath, add CV-12 with moxa to warm and tonify the Lung-Qi.

STAGNATION OF QI AND BLOOD

Symptoms and signs

Long duration of middle back pain of fixed location, with intermittent stabbing pain, which worsens at night, history of operation or trauma to the middle back, accompanied by a purplish-coloured face, a purplish tongue with a thin coating and a wiry and choppy pulse.

Principle of treatment

Circulate Qi and Blood, smooth the collateral and sedate the pain.

HERBAL TREATMENT

Prescription

SHEN TONG ZHU YU TANG
Meridian Passage
Qin Jiao *Radix Gentianae Macrophyllae* 10 g

Chuan Xiong *Rhizoma Ligustici Chuanxiong* 12 g
Tao Ren *Semen Persicae* 10 g
Hong Hua *Flos Carthami* 6 g
Gan Cao *Radix Glycyrrhizae* 6 g
Qiang Huo *Rhizoma seu Radix Notopterygii* 10 g
Mo Yao *Resina Myrrhae* 6 g
Xiang Fu *Rhizoma Cyperi* 10 g
Wu Ling Zhi *Faeces Trogopterorum* 6 g
Huai Niu Xi *Radix Achyranthis Bidentatae* 6 g
Di Long *Lumbricus* 10 g
Dang Gui *Radix Angelicae Sinensis* 12 g

Explanations

- Dang Gui, Chuan Xiong, Tao Ren and Hong Hua promote the circulation of Blood and eliminate Blood stasis.
- Mo Yao and Wu Ling Zhi eliminate Blood stasis and sedate the pain.
- Xiang Fu promotes the circulation of Qi and reinforces the effect of other herbs in promoting the circulation of Blood.
- Huai Niu Xi guides Blood stasis down and tonifies the back.
- Qin Jiao, Di Long and Qiang Huo harmonise the collaterals and relieve the pain.
- Gan Cao harmonises the herbs in the formula.

Modifications

1. If there is abnormal menstruation, add Yi Mu Cao *Herba Leonuri* 15 g to improve the circulation of Blood and regulate menstruation.
2. If there is a feeling of fullness in the abdomen, add Mu Xiang *Radix Aucklandiae* 12 g to promote the circulation of Qi and relieve the fullness.
3. If the limbs are cold, add Gui Zhi *Ramulus Cinnamomi* 6 g to warm the channels and dispel Cold.
4. If there is a fever at night, add Qing Hao *Herba Artemisiae Chinghao* 15 g to clear Heat in the Blood and reduce the fever.
5. If there is constipation, add Da Huang *Radix et Rhizoma Rhei* 10 g to promote bowel movement and relieve the constipation.

Patent remedies

Yu Xue Bi Chong Ji *Stagnant Blood Bi Syndrome Infusion*
Yun Nan Bai Yao *Yunnan White Medicine*

ACUPUNCTURE TREATMENT

BL-18 Ganshu, BL-20 Pishu, BL-22 Sanjiaoshu, BL-58 Feiyang, SP-6 Sanyinjiao and SI-3 Houxi. Reducing method is used on these points.

Explanations

- BL-18, the Back Transporting point of the Liver, relieves and soothes the depressed Liver-Qi and promotes the circulation of Qi and Blood. Needling this point may relieve the pain in the middle back.
- BL-20 strengthens the Spleen and benefits the Qi.
- BL-22 activates the circulation of Qi and removes obstruction from the channels and collateral so as to relieve the pain.
- BL-58, the Connecting point of the Bladder channel, harmonises the collateral and sedates the middle back pain.
- SI-3 clears blockage in the middle back and relieves the pain.
- SP-6, the crossing point of three Yin channels of the foot, promotes the circulation of Blood, eliminates Blood stasis and sedates the middle back pain.

Modifications

1. If there is severe middle back pain, add some local Ah Shi points to harmonise the collateral and sedate the pain.
2. If there is an intolerance to cold, add ST-36 and GV-14 to invigorate the Yang-Qi and remove Blood stasis.
3. If there is abdominal pain, add PC-6 and LI-4 to regulate the Qi and Blood of the Stomach and intestines so as to relieve the abdominal pain.
4. If there is constipation, add ST-25 to promote bowel movement and relieve the constipation.

Case history

A 36-year-old man had been suffering from middle back pain of fixed location for a month. It occurred during a physical exercise. He was given painkillers by a doctor, but these could help the pain for only a very short time.

When he arrived at the clinic, his main manifestations were middle back pain, which radiated to the chest, especially the right chest, a stabbing pain, aggravated by deep breathing, and worsening at night (he woke up almost every night due to pain), a normal tongue with a thin coating and a wiry and choppy pulse.

Diagnosis
Middle back pain due to stagnation of Qi and Blood.

Principle of treatment
Promote Blood circulation, remove Blood stagnation and sedate the pain.

Acupuncture treatment
BL-17, BL-18, BL-58, BL-62, SP-6, PC-6, SI-3 and Ah Shi points. Reducing method was used on these points. Treatment was given every day.

Explanations

- BL-17, the Gathering point for the Blood, was used to promote its circulation and relieve the back pain.
- BL-18, the Back Transporting point of the Liver, relieves and soothes the depressed Liver-Qi and promotes the circulation of Qi and Blood.
- BL-58, the Connecting point of the Bladder channel, harmonises the collateral and sedates the middle back pain.
- BL-62 and SI-3, a special combination, open the middle back, harmonise the collateral and relieve the middle back pain.

- SP-6, the crossing point of the three Yin channels of the foot, and PC-6, the Connecting point of the Pericardium channel, promote the circulation of Qi and Blood, calm the Mind and relieve the middle back pain.
- The Ah Shi points were punctured with Plum-Blossom needles to promote the circulation of Blood in the locality and relieve the pain.

After 2 weeks of treatment, his middle back pain was under control. He was followed up a year later and he stated he had experienced no further pain.

Lower back pain 33

腰
痛

Lower back pain may occur on one side or over the entire lower back, but is mostly at one side. The lower back is the area between vertebrae L1 and S3. Most people have experienced lower back pain at least once in their lifetime, so it is a common complaint in everyday practice, especially in the developed countries.

Generally speaking, according to TCM lower back pain is often caused by invasion of Cold-Damp or Damp-Heat, accumulation of Cold-Damp, downward flow of Damp-Heat, deficiency of the Kidney-Essence, stagnation of Qi or stagnation of Blood. Lower back pain may be attributed to any of the following disorders in Western medicine: renal disease, rheumatism, rheumatoid arthritis, hyperplastic spondylitis, disc herniation in the lumbar area, lower back blockage, lumbar muscular strain or traumatic injury of the lower back region, or deformation or injury of spinal column.

In Western medicine, lower back pain may be encountered in many departments, including internal medicine, surgery and gynaecology. The causes can generally be subdivided into four groups:

1. disorder of the joints—for example, rheumatoid spondylitis, hypertrophic spondylitis, tuberculous spondylitis, or supportive spondylitis.
2. disorder of the intervertebral soft tissues—for instance, chronic lumbar muscular sprain or fibrofascitis.
3. pressure on the spinal nerves, for instance, spinal compression or acute myelitis.
4. local causes including disease and disorder in the deep-seated organs—for instance, kidney disease including nephritis, pyelonephritis, nephrolithiasis, nephroptosis, hydronephrosis, pyonephrosis and renal tuberculosis, or other diseases such as pancreatitis, penetrating ulcer, cholecystitis, cholelithiasis, retroversion or retroflexion of the uterus, endometriosis, chronic annexitis or chronic prostatitis.

Lower back pain often implies different causes, at different ages; for instance, in growing boys and girls there could be weakness in the lower back, whereas a feeling of extreme weariness every day may be associated with slight lateral curvature of the spine. In elderly people, the commonest cause is osteoarthrosis, which is associated with permanent rigidity of the back especially in the morning, and often with great tenderness to the touch, with or without any deformity. In young workers, lower back pain that starts suddenly while working (for instance, lifting something too heavy) is mostly due to inappropriate exertion or sudden wrong movement, and the cause is often disc herniation, which produces a severe pain in the lower back, which may refer to one or two legs, with limitation of movement. Influenza may also cause lower back pain, associated with generalised body pain, fever, headache and sneezing.

With the development of modern surgical techniques, operations for intervertebral disorder became increasingly common; in the 1940s there was a large increase in disc surgery; however, in the 1950s it became apparent that a great number of these operations were failing. Failed back surgery may cause unrelenting low back pain, sciatica and other functional impairment.

Aetiology and pathology

Invasion of Wind, Cold and Damp

In this case the lower back pain is due to blockage in the channels and collaterals by Wind, Cold and Damp resulting in obstruction of the circulation of Qi.

Damp and Cold are Yin pathogenic factors that tend to obstruct the functions of the Qi generally and specifically impair the Yang-Qi. Damp has a heavy and sticky nature; invasion of Damp, singly or in combination with Wind and Cold, may easily obstruct the circulation of Qi and Blood. The Greater Yang channel is the most superficial of all the channels in the body, and the Governing Vessel is the governor of all the Yang channels in the body, so Wind, Cold and Damp usually attack these two channels, leading to stagnation of Qi and Blood, and causing lower back pain. This kind of lower back pain is often characterised by a feeling of heaviness in the lower back with a cold sensation, lassitude, an aversion to cold and aggravation of the pain in cold and humid weather. The precipitating factors include living in cold and damp places, exposure to rain, wading through water, being drenched with sweat and consuming too much cold or uncooked food in a short period. Invasion of Cold-Damp often occurs in those with a deficiency of the Qi or Yang of the Spleen or Kidney.

Invasion of Damp-Heat

In this case the lower back pain is due to obstruction of the circulation of Qi in the channels and collaterals and impairment of the Yin and Blood by Heat. This kind of lower back pain is characterised by a burning and heavy sensation, a low-grade fever, lassitude, deep yellow urine, a yellow and greasy tongue coating and a slippery and rapid pulse. The precipitating factors include living in warm and damp places, exposure to rain, wading through water, and being drenched with sweat in summer.

Accumulation of Cold-Damp

Overconsumption of cold drinks, or cold or raw food such as salad and fruit, may cause cold to accumulate directly in the Stomach. This disturbs the circulation of Qi and Blood circulation in the channels and, in the long run, may cause lower back pain due to stagnation of Qi and Blood. These eating and drinking habits may also impair the Yang of the Spleen and Stomach, leading to poor transportation and transformation of food, and Cold-Damp may form in the body. When this blocks the Qi and Blood circulation, it causes lower back pain. Furthermore, when external Wind, Cold and Damp are incompletely eliminated from the body, Cold-Damp accumulates in the channels and internal Zang-Fu organs, causing lower back pain.

Accumulation of Cold-Damp can also be caused by a weakness of the Lung-Qi in its function of Water distribution. The Lung is the so-called 'upper source of Water', and when the Lung is weak, owing to various causes, it fails to cause Water to descend to the Lower Burner and be dispersed to the superficial levels of the body, and as a consequence Cold-Damp accumulates in the body.

A deficiency of the Kidney-Qi or Kidney-Yang can also cause poor transformation of Water in the body, so Cold-Damp once again accumulates. The Kidney-Yang is the root Yang of the body, and if it is deficient then the Yang activity in the other Zang-Fu organs is impaired, and in particular there is impairment of the water-transporting and transforming functions, so that Cold-Damp forms in the body. If Cold-Damp blocks the circulation in the channels, lower back pain occurs.

Downward flow of Damp-Heat

When Cold-Damp accumulates in the body over a long time, or in people who have a Yang excess, the Cold-Damp may turn into Damp-Heat, which impairs the channels and causes stagnation of the Qi and Blood, causing lower back pain.

Overconsumption of fatty or sweet food, or milk products, may damage the Spleen and Stomach, impairing the functions of digestion, transportation and transformation, leading to the generation of Damp-Heat in the body. Overconsumption of spicy food, coffee or alcohol may cause Excessive-Heat to form in the body, resulting in aggravation of the Damp-Heat accumulation. When the channels are blocked and the circulation of Qi and Blood slows down, then lower back pain appears. A lack of personal hygiene in the genital region, or sexual intercourse, swimming, walking or heavy work during menstruation may cause invasion of toxic Damp-Heat to the Lower Burner, which triggers lower back pain.

Stagnation of Qi and Blood

Qi and Blood should circulate freely in the channels and collaterals. If the Qi and Blood stagnate owing to various causes, the channels and collaterals become blocked, leading to lower back pain.

Excessive stress, or habitual frustration or depression may disturb the Liver-Qi. Prolonged anger, indignation, animosity, a feeling of being insulted or enraged may all cause stagnation of the Liver-Qi with hyperactivity of the Liver-Yang. In these conditions, the stagnation of Qi may in turn cause the Blood to stagnate, which greatly aggravates the blockage in the channels, and precipitates lower back pain.

Physical trauma, inappropriate or incorrect use of epidural injections, inappropriate operations on the lower back or adhesions after an operation may all directly damage the channels, muscles, tendons and bones, so the Blood stagnates and causes lower back pain.

Deficiency of Kidney-Essence

The kidneys are located on both sides of the spinal column in the loin area of the back. The Kidney-Essence is the root energy of the body, and the lower back needs to be nourished by Kidney-Essence. Congenital weakness, giving birth to several children, excessive sexual activity, prolonged sickness, excessive bleeding during menstruation, excessive strain, an irregular diet and eating too little as well as excessive mental exertion, may all weaken the Kidney. When the Kidney-Essence is deficient, the lumbar region will be undernourished, and cause lower back pain. The symptoms of deficiency of Kidney-Essence depend on whether it is deficiency of Kidney-Yin or deficiency of Kidney-Yang.

Treatment based on differentiation

Differentiation

Differentiation of External or Internal origins

Lower back pain can be caused either by invasion of External pathogenic factors or by Internal disorders.

— If it is caused by invasion of External pathogenic factors, it is usually acute, and accompanied by External symptoms such as headache, fever, an aversion to cold, runny nose or coughing.
— If it is caused by disorder of the internal organs, it is chronic and has no External symptoms.

Differentiation of character of the pain

— Acute onset of lower back pain after exposure to cold and damp weather, aggravation of the back pain on rainy days, with a heavy sensation and stiffness in the lumbar region, limitation of the movement in the lower back, a cold feeling in the lower back, upper back pain, an aversion to cold, or slight fever, is usually caused by invasion of Wind-Cold-Damp.
— Acute onset of low back pain with burning and a feeling of heaviness, a hot sensation on touching, limitation of movement, which is worsened by exposure to warmth and warm compression, and better with cold compression, local redness and swelling, dislike of pressure, accompanied by fever, thirst but disinclination to drink, or loose stools, is often caused by invasion of Wind-Damp-Heat.
— Chronic lower back pain with a heavy sensation and stiffness, aggravation of the lower back pain on rainy days, with limitation of the movement in the lower back, a cold feeling in the lower back, cold hands and feet, an aversion to cold, nausea or loose stools, is usually caused by accumulation of Cold-Damp.
— Lower back pain associated with the emotional state, pain in the hypochondriac regions, or genital region, wandering pain that comes and goes, pain with distending feeling, or aggravation of the pain by emotional upset, is usually caused by stagnation of Liver-Qi.
— Rigidity and stabbing pain in the lower back, which is generally fixed in one place or one point, aggravation of the pain by pressure and at night, with limitation of movement, or a history of lumbar sprain, is often caused by stagnation of Blood.
— Insidious onset of protracted lower back pain with soreness, accompanied by lassitude and weakness of the loins and knees, aggravated by fatigue and alleviated by bed rest, with poor hearing, dizziness, poor memory and concentration, loose teeth or tiredness, is often caused by deficiency of Kidney-Essence.

Treatment

INVASION OF WIND-COLD-DAMP

Symptoms and signs

Lower back pain usually occurring after exposure to cold and damp weather, which worsens on rainy days, accompanied by a heavy sensation and stiffness in the lumbar region, limitation of movement in the lower back, a cold feeling in the lower back, upper back pain, an aversion to cold, a slight fever, a white and greasy tongue coating and a superficial and slippery pulse.

Principle of treatment

Dispel Wind, eliminate Cold-Damp and relieve the pain.

HERBAL TREATMENT

Prescription

QIANG HUO SHENG SHI TANG
Notopterygium Dispelling Dampness Decoction
Qiang Huo *Rhizoma seu Radix Notopterygii* 10 g
Du Huo *Radix Angelicae Pubescentis* 10 g
Chuan Xiong *Rhizoma Ligustici Chuanxiong* 10 g
Gan Cao *Radix Glycyrrhizae* 6 g
Fang Feng *Radix Ledebouriellae* 6 g
Gao Ben *Rhizoma et Radix Ligustici* 10 g

Explanations

- Qiang Huo can dispel Wind-Damp from the upper body and Du Huo tends to dispel Wind-Damp from the lower body. The combination of these two herbs can expel Wind-Damp from the whole body and joints so as to treat the upper back pain.
- Fang Feng and Gao Ben can dispel Wind-Cold and relieve the pain and headache.
- Chuang Xiong promotes the circulation of Blood and expels Wind so as to arrest lower back pain.
- Gan Cao coordinates the effects of the other herbs in the formula.

Modifications

1. If there is a nasal discharge and sneezing, add Huo Xiang *Herba Agastachis* 12 g (decocted later) to dispel Damp and relieve the sneezing.
2. If there is an aversion to cold and cold limbs, add Gui Zhi *Ramulus Cinnamomi* 10 g to dispel Wind-Cold, relieve External symptoms and arrest the pain.
3. If there is lower back pain with a cold sensation, add Fu Zi *Radix Aconiti Lateralis Praeparata* 10 g and Du Huo *Radix Angelicae Pubescentis* 10 g to dispel Cold and relieve the pain.
4. If there is lower back pain with a heavy sensation, add Cang Zhu *Rhizoma Atractylodis* 10 g and Han Fang Ji *Radix Stephaniae Tetrandrae* 10 g to dry Damp and relieve the pain.

5. If there is a poor appetite and a feeling of fullness in the abdomen, add Sha Ren *Fructus Amomi* 5 g to dry Damp and regulate the circulation of Qi in the Middle Burner.
6. In case of diarrhoea, add Fu Ling *Poria* 10 g to relieve the diarrhoea.

Patent remedies

Shang Shi Zhi Tong Gao *Injury 'from' Damp Stop Pain Plaster*
Da Huo Luo Dan *Greater Invigorate the Collaterals Special Pill*

ACUPUNCTURE TREATMENT

LI-4 Hegu, TE-5 Waiguan, TE-6 Zhigou, GB-20 Fengchi, BL-40 Weizhong and BL-60 Kunlun. Reducing method is used on these points. Moxibustion is applied on LI-4, TE-5 and BL-40.

Explanations

- LI-4 and TE-5 dispel Cold, eliminate Damp and relieve External symptoms.
- GB-20 dispels Wind and relieves external invasion as well as relieving the upper back pain.
- TE-6 dispels External Wind and promotes water discharge so as to eliminate Damp.
- BL-40, a distal point, dispels Damp, warms the limbs and promotes the free flow of Qi in the channels in order to treat the lower back pain.
- BL-60 dispels Cold and Damp in the superficial parts of the body, harmonises the collateral and relieves the lower back pain.

Modifications

Lower back pain may also be caused by blockage in different channels, such as the Gall Bladder, Bladder, Liver or Stomach channels or the Governing or Girdle Vessels. Therefore different points may need to be combined with those above, as follows.

1. If there is also pain in the middle of the back, add SI-3 and BL-62, the Confluence points for the Governing Vessel, together with GV-1, the Connecting point, to promote the circulation of Qi and relieve pain in the middle of the back.
2. If there is lower back pain due to blockage of the Girdle Vessel, manifested as heaviness in the lower back, a feeling as if a belt is tightening the lower back, a cold sensation in the upper body with warmth in the lower body, or vice versa, a feeling as if sitting in the bath, or pain radiating

to the sides of the abdomen, add GB-26, GB-27 and GB-41 to harmonise the Girdle Vessel, eliminate Damp and relieve the pain.

3. If there is lower back pain radiating to the leg along the Bladder channel, add BL-36, the local point, BL-58, the Connecting point, and BL-63, the Accumulation point, to harmonise the collateral and sedate the pain.
4. If there is lower back pain radiating to the leg along the Gall Bladder channel, add GB-29, GB-30, GB-36 and GB-40 to eliminate Damp, harmonise the collateral and sedate the pain.
5. If there is lower back pain radiating to the leg along the Stomach channel, add ST-30, ST-34, ST-40 and ST-42 to promote the circulation of Qi in the Stomach channel and relieve the pain.
6. If there is lower back pain radiating to the leg along the Liver channel, add LR-3, LR-5, LR-6 and LR-12 to regulate the Liver channel, promote the circulation of Qi and relieve the pain.
7. If there is sacral pain, add BL-32 and BL-53, the local points, to harmonise the collateral and arrest the pain.
8. If there is a severe aversion to cold in the lower back, add a moxa box over the lower back to warm the lower back, dispel Cold and relieve the pain.
9. If there is a feeling of heaviness in the body, add ST-40 to resolve Damp and eliminate Phlegm.
10. If the appetite is poor, add SP-4 and ST-36 to promote the circulation of Qi in the Middle Burner to improve the appetite.
11. If there is diarrhoea, add BL-20, the Back Transporting point of the Spleen, to activate the Spleen, eliminate Damp and relieve the diarrhoea.
12. If there is scanty urination, add SP-6 to promote urination and relieve Damp accumulation.
13. If there is abdominal pain, add BL-25, the Back Transporting point of the Large Intestine, to ease the pain.

Case history

A 44-year-old male worker had been suffering from lower back pain for 3 days. He had lived in a cold and damp room for a few years. His main symptoms were lower back pain, usually occurring after exposure to cold and damp and worsening on rainy days, together with a heavy sensation and stiff muscles in the dorsolumbar region, limitation of extension and flexion of the back, heavy sensation in the lumbar area, pain radiating downwards to the buttocks and legs, a poor appetite, loose stools, a white and sticky tongue coating and a deep and slow pulse.

Diagnosis
Lower back pain due to invasion of Wind-Cold-Damp.

Principle of treatment
Dispel Cold, dry Damp and relieve the pain.

Acupuncture treatment
LI-4, TE-5, TE-6, GB-20, BL-20, BL-23 and BL-40. Reducing method is used on all these points. One treatment was given every other day.

Explanations
- LI-4 and TE-5 dispel Wind-Cold, eliminate Damp and relieve External symptoms.
- GB-20 dispels Wind and relieves external invasion as well as relieving the upper back pain.
- TE-6 dispels External Wind and promotes water discharge so as to eliminate Damp.
- BL-20, the Back Transporting point of the Spleen, and BL-23, the Back Transporting point of the Kidney, eliminate Damp.
- BL-40 eliminates Damp and strengthens the lower back as well as harmonising the collateral in the back so as to relieve the lower back pain.

After 10 days of treatment, his lower back pain was obviously relieved. He was given a further month of treatment, after which his lower back pain had disappeared completely. A year later he was followed up, and he stated there had been no more lower back pain since the acupuncture treatment.

INVASION OF WIND-DAMP-HEAT

Symptoms and signs

Lower back pain with a feeling of burning and heaviness, a hot sensation to the touch and limitation of movement, which is worsened on exposure to warmth and warm compressions, and is alleviated by cold compressions, together with local redness and swelling, and a dislike of pressure, accompanied by fever, thirst but disinclination to drink, loose stools or diarrhoea, a greasy feeling in the mouth, a sensation of fullness in the chest and abdomen, painful urination or scanty urination with deep yellow urine, a red tongue with a yellow and greasy coating and a superficial, slippery and rapid pulse.

Principle of treatment

Dispel Wind, clear Heat, eliminate Damp and relieve the pain.

HERBAL TREATMENT

Prescription

XUAN BI TANG
Disband Painful Obstruction Decoction
Han Fang Ji *Radix Stephaniae Tetrandrae* 10 g

Xing Ren *Semen Armeniacae Amarum* 10 g
Hua Shi *Talcum* 15 g
Zhi Zi *Fructus Gardeniae* 10 g
Chi Xiao Dou *Semen Phaseoli Calcarati* 10 g
Yi Yi Ren *Semen Coicis* 10 g
Zhi Ban Xia *Rhizoma Pinelliae Praeparatum* 5 g
Can Sha *Excrementum Bombycis Mori* 5 g
Lian Qiao *Fructus Forsythiae* 10 g
Jiang Huang *Rhizoma Curcumae Longae* 10 g
Hai Tong Pi *Cortex Erythrinae* 10 g
Sang Zhi *Ramulus Mori* 10 g

Explanations

- Zhi Zi and Lian Qiao clear Heat, reduce fever and dispel Wind, so as to relieve External symptoms.
- Zhi Ban Xia, Chi Xiao Dou and Can Sha eliminate Damp-Heat and harmonise the Stomach.
- Hua Shi and Yi Yi Ren promote urination and eliminate Damp in the Lower Burner.
- Xing Ren dispels Damp-Heat in the Lung and stops the cough.
- Han Fang Ji, Jiang Huang, Hai Tong Pi and Sang Zhi dispel Damp-Heat in the joints, muscles and channels so as to relieve the lower back pain.

Modifications

1. If there is extreme lower back pain, add Huai Niu Xi and Chuan Niu Xi *Radix Achyranthis Bidentatae et Radix Cyathulae* 6 g to induce the herbal treatment to enter the lower back region directly and relieve the pain.
2. If there is lower back pain with a burning sensation, add Huang Bai *Cortex Phellodendri* 12 g to clear Heat.
3. If there is a thirst, scanty urine and a red tongue, add Mu Tong *Caulis Aristolochiae* 3 g to clear Damp-Heat and promote urination.
4. If there is urethral calculus, add Jin Qian Cao *Herba Lysimachiae* 10 g and Hai Jin Sha *Spora Lygodii* 9 g to dissolve the stone and promote urination.
5. If there is diarrhoea, add Fu Ling *Poria* 15 g and Cang Zhu *Rhizoma Atractylodis* 10 g to activate the Spleen and relieve the diarrhoea.
6. If there is urinary bleeding, add Xiao Ji *Herba Cephalanoploris* 15 g to cool the Blood and stop the bleeding.
7. If there is generalised body pain, add Luo Shi Teng *Caulis Trachelospermi* 10 g to dispel External Wind, Damp and Heat and harmonise the collateral so as to relieve the pain.

Patent remedy

Shi Re Bi Chong Ji *Damp-Heat Bi Infusion*

ACUPUNCTURE TREATMENT

LI-2 Erjian, LI-4 Hegu, TE-5 Waiguan, TE-6 Zhigou, GB-20 Fengchi, BL-40 Weizhong, BL-60 Kunlun and BL-66 Zutonggu. Reducing method is used on these points.

Explanations

- LI-4 and TE-5 dispel Cold, eliminate Damp and relieve External symptoms.
- GB-20 dispels Wind, relieves external invasion and relieves the upper back pain.
- TE-6 dispels external Wind and promotes water discharge so as to eliminate Damp.
- LI-2 and BL-66, the Spring point, clear Heat, reduce fever and relieve the lower back pain.
- BL-40, a distal point, dispels Damp and promotes the free flow of Qi in the channels in order to treat the lower back pain.
- BL-60 dispels Damp-Heat in the superficial parts of the body, harmonises the collateral and relieves the lower back pain.

Modifications

1. Since lower back pain may be caused by blockage in specific channels, various points may need to be added to the above depending on the specific symptoms (see Wind-Cold-Damp invasion, p. 398).
2. If there is fever, add GV-14 to clear Heat and reduce fever.
3. If there is generalised body pain, an aversion to cold, a stiff neck and throat pain, add BL-10 and BL-12 to dispel Wind, Damp and Heat and relieve External symptoms.
4. If there is a cough with yellow phlegm, add LU-5 to clear Heat in the Lung and relieve the cough.
5. If there is sacral pain, add BL-32 and BL-53, the local points, to harmonise the collateral and arrest the pain.
6. If there is a severe burning sensation in the lower back, add BL-67 with bleeding method to clear Heat and relieve the burning sensation.
7. If there is a feeling of heaviness in the body, add SP-6 to resolve Damp and eliminate Phlegm.
8. If there is scanty and painful urination, add KI-4 and KI-5 to promote urination and relieve the pain.

9. If the appetite is poor, add CV-12, the Front Collecting point of the Stomach, to harmonise the Stomach and improve the appetite.

10. If there is diarrhoea, add BL-20, the Back Transporting point of the Spleen, to activate the Spleen, eliminate Damp and relieve the diarrhoea.

ACCUMULATION OF COLD-DAMP

Symptoms and signs

Chronic lower back pain with a heavy sensation, cold feeling and stiffness, which worsens on rainy days, together with limitation of movement in the lower back, cold hands and feet, an aversion to cold, nausea, loose stools, tiredness, a poor appetite, a white and greasy tongue coating and a slippery and slow pulse.

Principle of treatment

Warm the body, eliminate Cold, resolve Damp and relieve the pain.

HERBAL TREATMENT

Prescription

SHEN ZHAO TANG
Retention in Kidney Decoction
Gan Cao *Radix Glycyrrhizae* 10 g
Gan Jiang *Rhizoma Zingiberis* 10 g
Fu Ling *Poria* 10 g
Bai Zhu *Rhizoma Atractylodis Macrocephalae* 10 g
Gui Zhi *Ramulus Cinnamomi* 10 g
Du Huo *Radix Angelicae Pubescentis* 10 g

Explanations

- Gan Jiang eliminates Cold and warms the lower back.
- Fu Ling and Bai Zhu strengthen the Spleen and remove Damp.
- Gui Zhi dispels Cold, warms the channels and relieves the lower back pain.
- Du Huo eliminates Cold-Damp and relieves pain.
- Gan Cao nourishes the Qi and regulates the actions of the other herbs in the formula.
- When Cold-Damp is eliminated, the Qi and Blood circulate freely in the channels and collateral, and the lower back pain gradually disappears.

Modifications

1. If there is lower back pain with a cold sensation, clear urine, oedema, a pale and swollen tongue and slow pulse caused by deficiency of Kidney-Yang, add Zhi Fu Zi *Radix Aconiti Lateralis Praeparata* 10 g and Du Zhong *Cortex Eucommiae* 10 g to tonify the Kidney-Yang, dispel Cold and relieve the pain.

2. If there is a feeling of lassitude in the loins and a deep and weak pulse, add Bu Gu Zhi *Fructus Psoraleae* 10 g to tonify the Kidney and relieve the pain.

3. If there is lower back pain with a heavy sensation, add Cang Zhu *Rhizoma Atractylodis* 10 g and Fang Ji *Radix Stephaniae Tetrandrae* 10 g to dry Damp and relieve the pain.

4. If there is a poor appetite and feeling of fullness in the abdomen, add Sha Ren *Fructus Amomi* 5 g to dry Damp and regulate the circulation of Qi in the Middle Burner.

5. If there is generalised tiredness, a pale complexion, a pale tongue and weak pulse, add Huang Qi *Radix Astragali seu Hedysari* 12 g and Dang Shen *Radix Codonopsis Pilosulae* 10 g to tonify the Spleen-Qi.

Patent remedies

Han Shi Bi Chong Ji *Cold-Damp Bi Syndrome Infusion*
Mu Gua Wan *Chaenomelis Pill*
Tian Ma Wan *Gastrodia Pill*

ACUPUNCTURE TREATMENT

BL-40 Weizhong, BL-58 Feiyang, BL-60 Kunlun, BL-64 Jinggu, SP-6 Sanyinjiao, SP-9 Yinlingquan and KI-3 Taixi. Reducing method is used on these points, except for SP-6, KI-3 and BL-64, on which tonifying method is used. Moxibustion is advisable on BL-40, BL-64, SP-9 and KI-3.

Explanations

- BL-40, a commanding point for the back, and BL-60 promote urination, eliminate Damp and invigorate the free flow of Qi in the back in order to treat the lower back pain.
- BL-58, the Connecting point, and BL-64, the Source point, harmonise the collateral, promote the circulation of Qi in the Bladder channel and relieve the lower back pain.
- SP-6, SP-9 and KI-3 activate the Spleen and Kidney so as to promote urination and eliminate Damp.

Lower back pain may be caused by blockage in different channels, such as the Gall Bladder, Bladder, Liver or Stomach channels or the Governing or Girdle

Vessels. So different points may need to be combined with the above, according to the pattern of invasion of Wind-Cold-Damp, as shown in the modifications below.

Modifications

1. If there is an extreme aversion to cold at the lower back, add GV-4 and a moxa box over the lower back to warm it, dispel Cold and relieve the pain.
2. If there is a feeling of heaviness in the body, add ST-40 to resolve Damp and eliminate Phlegm in the body.
3. If the appetite is poor, add SP-3 and ST-36 to activate the Spleen and Stomach and improve the appetite.
4. If there is diarrhoea, add BL-20, the Back Transporting point of the Spleen, and BL-25, the Back Transporting point of the Large Intestine, to activate the Spleen, eliminate Damp and relieve the diarrhoea.
5. If there is generalised tiredness, add CV-4 to tonify the Original Qi and relieve the tiredness.

DOWNWARD FLOW OF DAMP-HEAT

Symptoms and signs

Chronic lower back pain, possibly with acute exacerbation, often referring to the lower abdominal region, and a burning sensation in the lower back, accompanied by painful or difficult urination, leucorrhoea, a bitter taste in the mouth, fever, nausea, vomiting, diarrhoea, a red tongue with a yellow and greasy coating at the back and a slippery and rapid pulse.

Principle of treatment

Clear Heat, eliminate Damp and relieve the pain.

HERBAL TREATMENT

Prescription

SI MIAO SAN
Four-Marvel Powder
Cang Zhu *Rhizoma Atractylodis* 10 g
Huang Bai *Cortex Phellodendri* 12 g
Chuan Niu Xi *Radix Cyathulae* 6 g
Yi Yi Ren *Semen Coicis* 15 g
Han Fang Ji *Radix Stephaniae Tetrandrae* 10 g
Fu Ling *Poria* 15 g
Luo Shi Teng *Caulis Trachelospermi* 20 g

Explanations

- Cang Zhu and Han Fang Ji clear Heat, dry Damp and relieve the lower back pain.
- Huang Bai clears Heat and removes Damp in the Lower Burner.
- Yi Yi Ren and Fu Ling clear Heat and promote urination.
- Luo Shi Teng eliminates Damp-Heat, promotes the circulation of Qi and Blood in the channels and relieves the lower back pain.
- Chuan Niu Xi guides all the herbs downward to the lower back region, invigorates the circulation of Blood, reinforces the Kidney and strengthens the tendons and bones so as to arrest the lower back pain.

Modifications

1. If there is a thirst, scanty urine and a red tongue, add Zhi Zi *Fructus Gardeniae* 12 g and Mu Tong *Caulis Aristolochiae* 3 g to clear Heat, eliminate Damp and promote urination.
2. If there is urethral calculus, add Jin Qian Cao *Herba Lysimachiae* 10 g and Hai Jin Sha *Spora Lygodii* 10 g to dissolve the stone and promote urination.
3. If there is a bitter taste in the mouth and insomnia, add Huang Lian *Rhizoma Coptidis* 5 g and to eliminate Damp-Heat, calm the Mind and improve the sleep.
4. If there is frequent, urgent and painful urination, add Che Qian Zi *Semen Plantaginis* 12 g to eliminate Damp-Heat in the Lower Burner, promote urination and relieve the pain.
5. If there is urinary bleeding, add Xiao Ji *Herba Cephalanoploris* 15 g to cool the Blood and stop the bleeding.
6. If there is genital itching and oozing or leucorrhoea, add She Chuang Zi *Fructus Cnidii* 10 g to eliminate Damp-Heat in the Lower Burner and stop the itching.

Patent remedy

San Miao Wan *Three-Marvel Pill*

ACUPUNCTURE TREATMENT

TE-2 Yemen, TE-4 Yangchi, TE-6 Zhigou, BL-40 Weizhong, BL-58 Feiyang, BL-60 Kunlun, BL-66 Zutonggu, SP-9 Yinlingquan and GB-34 Yanglingquan. Reducing method is used on these points.

Explanations

- TE-4, the Source point, and TE-6 promote the physiological function of the Triple Burner and increase water discharge to eliminate Damp-Heat.
- TE-2 and BL-66, the Spring point, clear Heat, reduce fever and relieve the lower back pain.
- BL-40, a commanding point for the back, BL-58, the Connecting point, and BL-60 promote the free flow of Qi in the channels in order to treat the lower back pain.
- SP-9 and GB-34, the Sea points, clear Heat and eliminate Damp in the Lower Burner.

Modifications

1. Since lower back pain may be caused by blockage in specific channels, various points may need to be added to the above, depending on the specific symptoms (see Wind-Cold-Damp invasion, p. 398).
2. If there is a fever, add GV-14 to clear Heat and reduce the fever.
3. If there is sacral pain, add some local Ah Shi points to harmonise the collateral and arrest the pain.
4. If there is a severe burning sensation and aversion to heat in the lower back, add BL-67 to clear Heat and relieve the burning sensation.
5. If there is scanty and painful urination, add BL-32 and KI-4 to promote urination and relieve the pain.
6. If there is a feeling of heaviness in the body, add SP-6 to resolve Damp and eliminate Phlegm.
7. If the appetite is poor, add BL-20, the Back Transporting point of the Spleen, to activate the Spleen and improve the appetite.
8. If there is diarrhoea, add SP-3, the Source point, to activate the Spleen, eliminate Damp and relieve the diarrhoea.
9. If there is profuse leucorrhoea, add GB-27 and GB-41 to eliminate Damp and relieve the leucorrhoea.

Case history

A 37-year-old man had been suffering from lumbago for 2 years. He had been drinking alcohol excessively for more than 6 years, and would feel the lower back pain when he drank too much, or if in a hot and humid environment during the summer. His pain was characterised by a heavy sensation in the lumbar region, and besides the pain he had limitation of extension and flexion in the back, deep yellow urine, painful urination with a hot sensation, genital itching, irritability, a bitter taste in his mouth, a thirst, a yellow and sticky tongue coating and a slippery and wiry pulse.

Diagnosis
Downward flow of Damp-Heat.

Principle of treatment
Clear Heat, dry Damp and relieve the pain.

Herbal treatment
SI MIAO SAN
Four-Marvel Powder
Cang Zhu *Rhizoma Atractylodis* 10 g
Huang Bai *Cortex Phellodendri* 12 g
Chuan Niu Xi *Radix Cyathulae* 6 g
Yi Yi Ren *Semen Coicis* 15 g
She Chuang Zi *Fructus Cnidii* 10 g
Bi Xie *Rhizoma Dioscoreae Septemlobae* 30 g
Fang Ji *Radix Stephaniae Tetrandrae* 10 g
Fang Feng *Radix Ledebouriellae* 12 g

Explanations

- Cang Zhu and Fang Feng dry Damp and relieve pain.
- Huang Bai clears Heat and removes Damp in the Lower Burner.
- Yi Yi Ren clears Heat and promotes urination.
- Niu Xi guides all the herbs downward to the lower back region, invigorates the circulation of Blood and arrests the lower back pain.
- She Chuang Zi, Han Fang Ji and Bi Xie eliminate Damp-Heat in the Lower Burner, stop itching and relieve the lower back pain.

He was treated daily with this herbal decoction. After treatment for 3 weeks, his lower back pain was almost under control. He continued with the treatment for more weeks, after which the pain had disappeared. When he was followed up 6 months later, he stated he had experienced no further pain since then.

STAGNATION OF LIVER-QI

Symptoms and signs

Intermittent lower back pain of a wandering nature, associated with the emotional state, and pain in the hypochondriac or genital region, with a distending feeling, which is aggravated by emotional upset, accompanied by irritability, nervousness, insomnia, headache, a poor appetite, loose stools when nervous, abdominal pain, a purplish or red tongue with a thin and yellow coating and a wiry or wiry and rapid pulse.

Principle of treatment

Smooth the Liver, promote the circulation of Qi and relieve the pain.

HERBAL TREATMENT

Prescription

CHAI HU SHU GAN SAN
Bupleurum Soothing the Liver Powder
Chai Hu *Radix Bupleuri* 6 g
Xiang Fu *Rhizoma Cyperi* 9 g
Chuan Xiong *Rhizoma Ligustici Chuanxiong* 9 g
Zhi Qiao *Fructus Aurantii* 9 g
Zhi Shi *Fructus Aurantii Immaturus* 6 g
Bai Shao *Radix Paeoniae Alba* 12 g
Zhi Gan Cao *Radix Glycyrrhizae Praeparata* 6 g

Explanations

- Chai Hu and Xiang Fu are the two most commonly used herbs to disperse and regulate the Liver-Qi.
- Chuan Xiong invigorates the circulation of Blood and relieves pain. Zhi Ke and Zhi Shi promote the circulation of Qi. These three herbs enhance the action of the herbs that remove obstruction and stop the pain.
- Bai Shao and Zhi Gan Cao smooth and harmonise the Liver so as to benefit the proper movement of Liver-Qi.
- When Qi moves fluently in the Liver channel, lower back pain and other symptoms will disappear.

Modifications

1. If there is lower back pain referring to the groin, add Chuan Lian Zi *Fructus Meliae Toosendan* 10 g to regulate the Liver-Qi and remove Qi stagnation.
2. If there is contraction of the scrotum and inguinal herniation, add Xiao Hui Xiang *Fructus Foeniculi* 10 g and Bing Lang *Semen Arecae* 5 g to harmonise the Liver and dispel Cold in the Liver channel.
3. If there is a feeling of fullness in the chest and hypochondriac region, add Yu Jin *Radix Curcumae* 9 g to regulate the circulation of Qi and relieve the fullness.
4. If there is distension of the abdomen, add Qing Pi *Pericarpium Citri Reticulatae Viride* 9 g to promote the circulation of Qi.
5. If there is a headache, irritability, nervousness and headache, add Xia Ku Cao *Spica Prunellae* 10 g and Gou Teng *Ramulus Uncariae cum Uncis* 10 g to calm the Liver and subdue the Liver-Yang.
6. If the appetite is poor, add Jiang Huang *Rhizoma Curcumae Longae* 9 g and Mai Ya *Fructus Hordei Germinatus* 9 g to regulate the Qi and improve the appetite.

Patent remedies

Shu Gan Wan *Soothe Liver Pill*
Xiao Yao Wan *Free and Relaxed Pill*

ACUPUNCTURE TREATMENT

LR-3 Taichong, LR-5 Ligou, LR-6 Zhongdu, LR-11 Yinlian, LR-12 Jimai, LR-14 Qimen, PC-6 Neiguan and SP-6 Sanyinjiao. Reducing method is used on these points.

Explanations

- LR-3, the Source point of the Liver channel, and LR-14, the Front Collecting point of the Liver, smooth the Liver, regulate the Liver-Qi circulation and arrest the pain.
- LR-5, the Connecting point, and LR-6, the Accumulation point, harmonise the collateral and relieve the lower back pain.
- LR-11 and LR-12, the local points, promote the circulation of Qi and Blood in the Liver channel and relieve the lower back and pain in the genital region.
- PC-6, the Connecting point, calms the Mind and smoothes the emotions.
- SP-6, the crossing point of the three Yin channels of the foot, regulates the Liver, promotes the circulation of Blood and relieves the abdominal and lower back pain.

Modifications

1. Since lower back pain may be caused by blockage in specific channels, various points may need to be added to the above, depending on the specific symptoms (see Wind-Cold-Damp invasion, p. 398).
2. If there is a feeling of fullness in the chest together with a feeling of oppression, add CV-17, the Gathering point for the Qi, to smooth the Liver and promote the circulation of Qi in the chest.
3. If there is emotional instability, add Extra Sishencong to calm the Mind and regulate the emotions.
4. If there is irritability and nervousness, add LR-2, the Spring point, to clear Heat in the Liver and calm it.
5. If there is a headache, add GB-20 to sedate it.
6. If there is insomnia, add HT-3 and Extra Anmian to calm the Mind and improve the sleep.
7. If there is abdominal pain, add ST-28 to promote the circulation of Qi and Blood in the abdomen and relieve the pain.

STAGNATION OF BLOOD

Symptoms and signs

History of lumbar sprain, rigidity and stabbing pain in the lower back, which is generally fixed in one place or on one point, and is aggravated by pressure and worsens at night, accompanied by limitation of movement, a dark and purplish tongue with a thin coating and a deep and wiry pulse.

Principle of treatment

Promote Qi and Blood circulation, remove Blood stagnation and relieve the pain.

HERBAL TREATMENT

Prescription

SHEN TONG ZHU YU TANG
Meridian Passage
Qin Jiao *Radix Gentianae Macrophyllae* 10 g
Chuan Xiong *Rhizoma Ligustici Chuanxiong* 12 g
Tao Ren *Semen Persicae* 10 g
Hong Hua *Flos Carthami* 6 g
Gan Cao *Radix Glycyrrhizae* 6 g
Qiang Huo *Rhizoma seu Radix Notopterygii* 10 g
Mo Yao *Resina Myrrhae* 6 g
Xiang Fu *Rhizoma Cyperi* 10 g
Wu Ling Zhi *Faeces Trogopterorum* 6 g
Huai Niu Xi *Radix Achyranthis Bidentatae* 6 g
Di Long *Lumbricus* 10 g
Dang Gui *Radix Angelicae Sinensis* 10 g

Explanations

- Dang Gui, Chuan Xiong, Tao Ren and Hong Hua promote the circulation of Blood and eliminate Blood stasis.
- Dang Gui promotes the circulation of Blood and nourishes it, so as to prevent harm to the Blood by the strong Blood-circulating herbs.
- Mo Yao and Wu Ling Zhi eliminate Blood stasis and sedate the lower back pain.
- Xiang Fu promotes the circulation of Qi to reinforce the effect of promoting the circulation of Blood.
- Huai Niu Xi guides Blood stasis down and tonifies the loins and knees.
- Qin Jiao, Qiang Huo and Di Long harmonise the collateral and relieve the pain
- Gan Cao harmonises the herbs in the formula.

Modifications

1. If there is a severe stabbing pain, add San Qi *Radix Notoginseng* 10 g to eliminate Blood stasis and relieve the pain.

2. If there is lower back pain due to prolonged persistence of External Wind-Cold-Damp, add Du Huo *Radix Angelicae Pubescentis* 10 g and Lao Guan Cao *Herba Erodii seu Ceranii* 10 g to eliminate the Wind-Cold-Damp and relieve the pain.

3. If there is lower back pain with weakness of the knees and generalised tiredness due to deficiency of Kidney-Essence, add Du Zhong *Cortex Eucommiae* 10 g and Shu Di Huang *Radix Rehmanniae Praeparata* 12 g to tonify the Kidney and relieve the pain.

4. If there is irregular menstruation due to stagnation of Blood, add Yi Mu Cao *Herba Leonuri* 10 g and Bai Shao *Radix Paeoniae Alba* 12 g to nourish the Blood and regulate the menstruation.

5. If there are cold limbs, a pale complexion, a deep and slow pulse and a pale tongue, add Gui Zhi *Ramulus Cinnamomi* 6 g or Gan Jiang *Rhizoma Zingiberis* 6 g to warm the Interior and channels and dispel Cold.

6. If there is abdominal pain, add Mu Xiang *Radix Aucklandiae* 12 g and Yu Jin *Radix Curcumae* 10 g to promote the circulation of Qi and Blood and relieve the pain.

Patent remedies

Te Xiao Yao Tong Ling *Special Efficacy Lower Back Pain Pill*
Yu Xue Bi Chong Ji *Stagnant Blood Bi Syndrome Infusion*
Yun Nan Bai Yao *Yunnan White Medicine*

ACUPUNCTURE TREATMENT

LI-4 Hegu, LR-3 Taichong, BL-17 Geshu, BL-40 Weizhong, BL-64 Jinggu, BL-67 Zhiyin and SP-6 Sanyinjiao. Reducing method is used on these points.

Explanations

- LI-4 and LR-3 promote the circulation of Qi so as to promote the circulation of Blood. Also, they have the function of sedating the pain.
- BL-17, the Gathering point for the Blood, together with BL-40, the commanding point for the back, and SP-6, the crossing point of the three Yin channels of the foot, promote the circulation of Blood, remove Blood stagnation and relieve the lower back pain.
- BL-64, the Source point, and BL-67, the Well point, promote the circulation of Qi and Blood in the Bladder channel and collateral and sedate the lower back pain.

Modifications

1. Since lower back pain may be caused by blockage in specific channels, various points may need to be added to the above, depending on the specific symptoms (see Wind-Cold-Damp invasion, p. 398).
2. If there is a severe stabbing pain, add some local Ah Shi points and bleeding method on BL-40 to activate the circulation of Blood and relieve the pain.
3. If there is limitation of movement in the lower back, add Extra Shoubeiyaotongdian to promote the circulation of Qi and Blood and relieve pain.
4. If the pain worsens at night, add KI-6 to promote the circulation of Blood at night and relieve the pain.
5. If there is restlessness and insomnia due to the pain, add HT-3 and HT-7 to calm the Mind and improve sleep.
6. If there is a headache, add GB-20 and BL-10 to promote the circulation of Qi and Blood in the head and relieve the headache.
7. If there is constipation, add BL-25, the Back Transporting point of the Large Intestine, to promote defecation and relieve the constipation.

Case history

A 52-year-old woman had been suffering from chronic lower back pain that had worsened during the past 10 days. Her lower back pain had started after she fell off a horse whilst riding 10 years previously. She was sent to the hospital immediately, and tests indicated that she did not have a bone fracture but there was some local soft tissue injury. She received 20 sessions of massage, and her lower back pain was much improved by this treatment. But shortly after the massage treatment the pain came back.

Over the past 10 years, she often took painkillers if she had severe lower back pain. On arrival at the clinic, she was suffering from a stabbing pain in the lower back, mainly on the left side, and the pain sometimes referred down the left leg to the ankle along the Gall Bladder channel. During the previous 10 days, she woke up a few times every night and had to get up to walk around in order to alleviate the pain. The pain was usually worse in the early morning. She also had a thin and white tongue coating and a thready pulse.

Diagnosis
Stagnation of Blood in the Gall Bladder channel.

Principle of treatment
Promote Qi circulation, eliminate Blood stasis and relieve the pain.

Acupuncture treatment
LI-4, BL-17, BL-40, GB-29, GB-30, GB-34, GB-36 and GB-40. Reducing method was used on these points.

Explanations

- LI-4, the Source point, and BL-17, the Gathering point for the Blood, promote the circulation of Blood and eliminate Blood stasis.
- BL-40, the commanding point for the back, removes Qi and Blood stagnation and relieves lower back pain.
- GB-29 and GB-30, the very important local points, harmonise the channel.
- GB-34, the Gathering point for the tendons, GB-36, the Accumulation point, and GB-40, the Source point, together promote the circulation of Qi and Blood and remove Blood stagnation in the Gall Bladder channel so as to relieve lower back pain and pain in the legs.

After 1 month of acupuncture treatment, her lower back pain disappeared. Two years later, she was followed up by letter, and she replied she had experienced no further pain after the acupuncture treatment.

DEFICIENCY OF KIDNEY-ESSENCE

Symptoms and signs

Insidious onset of protracted lower back pain with soreness, accompanied by lassitude and weakness of the loins and knees, which worsens with fatigue and is alleviated by bed rest, accompanied by poor hearing, dizziness, a poor memory and concentration, loose teeth and generalised tiredness.

If the deficiency is of Kidney-Yang, there is also a cold sensation in the lower back and abdomen, a pale complexion, low potency or impotency, nycturia, cold limbs, an aversion to cold, a pale tongue with tooth marks and a wet coating and a deep and thready or deep and slow pulse.

If the deficiency is of Kidney-Yin, there is also irritability, insomnia, a dry mouth and throat, a flushed face, a feverish sensation in the chest, palms and soles of the feet, constipation, a red tongue with a scanty or peeled coating and a weak or thready and rapid pulse.

Principle of treatment

Nourish the Kidney and relieve the pain.

HERBAL TREATMENT

Prescription a: for deficiency of Kidney-Yang

JIN GUI SHEN QI WAN
Kidney Qi Pill
Shu Di Huang *Radix Rehmanniae Praeparata* 12 g
Shan Yao *Rhizoma Dioscoreae* 15 g
Shan Zhu Yu *Fructus Corni* 10 g
Ze Xie *Rhizoma Alismatis* 10 g
Fu Ling *Poria* 10 g

Dan Pi *Cortex Moutan Radicis* 10 g
Gui Zhi *Ramulus Cinnamomi* 10 g
Fu Zi *Radix Aconiti Carmichaeli Praeparata* 10 g

Prescription b: for deficiency of Kidney-Yin

ZUO GUI WAN
Restoring the Left Pill
Shu Di Huang *Rhizoma Rehmanniae Praeparata* 12 g
Shan Yao *Rhizoma Dioscoreae* 15 g
Shan Zhu Yu *Fructus Corni* 6 g
Tu Si Zi *Semen Cuscutae* 10 g
Gou Qi Zi *Fructus Lycii* 12 g
Chuan Niu Xi *Radix Cyathulae* 6 g
Lu Jiao Jiao *Colla Cervi Cornus* 6 g
Gui Ban Jiao *Colla Plastri Testudinis* 10 g

Explanations

- In Jin Gui Shen Qi Wan, Shu Di Huang nourishes the Kidney-Essence.
- Shan Yao and Shan Zhu Yu strengthen the Liver and Spleen to assist Shu Di Huang to tonify the Kidney.
- Gui Zhi and Fu Zi warm the Kidney-Yang and dispel interior Cold and Cold in the channels.
- Ze Xie and Fu Ling remove Damp and promote discharge of Damp from the body.
- Dan Pi clears Liver-Fire and coordinates the functions of the other herbs in the prescription so as to control the greasy herbs.

- In Zuo Gui Wan, Shu Di Huang tonifies the Kidney and nourishes the Kidney-Yin.
- Gou Qi Zi nourishes the Yin of the Liver and Kidney and benefits the vision.
- Shan Zhu Yu tonifies the Essence of Liver and Kidney and arrests night sweating.
- Gui Ban Jiao and Lu Jiao Jiao in combination tonify the Essence. The former is good at tonifying the Kidney-Yang; the latter is good at nourishing the Kidney-Yin.
- Tu Si Zi and Chuan Niu Xi strengthen the waist and knees and reinforce the muscles and joints.
- Shan Yao tonifies the Spleen and Kidney.

Modifications

1. If there is a low voice, poor appetite and diarrhoea due to deficiency of Spleen-Qi, add Dang Shen *Radix Codonopsis Pilosulae* 10 g and Huang Qi *Radix Astragali Pilosulae* 12 g to tonify the Spleen-Qi and activate the Spleen and Stomach.
2. If there is diarrhoea before dawn with a cold lower abdomen due to failure of the Spleen to be warmed by the Kidney-Yang, add Bu Gu Zhi

Fructus Psoraleae 10 g and Wu Wei Zi *Fructus Schisandrae* 10 g to tonify the Kidney-Yang and stop the diarrhoea.
3. If there is seminal emission, enuresis and frequent nocturnal urination, add Yi Zhi Ren *Fructus Alpiniae Oxyphyllae* 6 g to tonify the Kidney and consolidate it.
4. If there is insomnia due to deficiency of Yin of the Heart and Kidney, add Huang Lian *Rhizoma Coptidis* 10 g and E Jiao *Colla Corii Asini* 10 g to nourish Yin and calm the Mind.
5. If there is a headache and vertigo due to hyperactivity of the Liver-Yang caused by deficiency of Kidney-Yin, add Tian Ma *Rhizoma Gastrodiae* 10 g and Gou Teng *Uncariae cum Uncis* 15 g to nourish the Yin and calm the Liver.
6. If there is a tidal fever or feverish sensation in the palms and soles, add Di Gu Pi *Cortex Lycii Radicis* 12 g to clear Deficient-Heat and relieve the fever.

Patent remedies

For deficiency of Kidney-Yang:
Jin Gui Shen Qi Wan *Kidney Qi Pill*
Yao Tong Pian *Waist Pain 'Lumbago' Tablet*

For deficiency of Kidney-Yin:
Liu Wei Di Huang Wan *Six-Flavour Rehmanniae Pill*

ACUPUNCTURE TREATMENT

BL-23 Shenshu, BL-40 Weizhong, GB-34 Yanglingquan, GB-39 Xuanzhong, BL-58 Feiyang, KE-3 Taixi, KI-10 Yingu and SP-6 Sanyinjiao. Reinforcing method is used on these points.

Explanations

- BL-23, the Back Transporting point of the Kidney, KI-3, the Source point, and KI-10, the Sea point, tonify the Kidney, and strengthen the back and bones so as to treat the root cause.
- BL-40, the commanding point for the back, promotes the circulation of Qi and Blood in the Bladder channel and relieves the lower back.
- BL-58, the Connecting point, harmonises the collateral and sedates the lower back pain.
- GB-34, the Gathering point for the tendons, and GB-39, the Gathering point for the Marrow, strengthen the tendons and bones so as to consolidate the back.
- SP-6, the crossing point of the three Yin channels of the foot, nourishes the Liver, Spleen and Kidney so as to promote the production of Qi and Blood.

Modifications

1. Since lower back pain may be caused by blockage in specific channels, various points may need to be added to the above, depending on the specific symptoms (see Wind-Cold-Damp invasion, p. 398).
2. If there is a cold sensation in the lower back, add GV-4 with moxibustion and a moxa box on the lower back to warm it and dispel Cold.
3. If there is weakness in the knees, add LR-8 to strengthen the knees.
4. If there is impotency, add CV-4 and CV-6 to reinforce the Kidney and improve the potency.
5. If there is insomnia, add HT-3 and PC-6 to calm the Mind and improve sleep.
6. If there is dizziness, add GB-20 to regulate the Qi and Blood in the head and relieve the dizziness.
7. If there is generalised tiredness, add ST-36 and GV-20 to lift up the energy and relieve the tiredness.
8. If there is diarrhoea, add BL-20 and BL-25 to strengthen the Spleen and stop the diarrhoea.
9. If there is constipation, add LI-4 to promote defecation.
10. If there is profuse night sweating, add HT-6 and KI-2 to clear Deficient-Heat and stop the sweating.
11. If there is nervousness and headache, add LR-2, the Spring point, to clear Heat in the Liver and calm it.

Case history

A 69-year-old woman had been suffering from lower back pain for 4 years. Four years previously, she had started to feel an uncomfortable sensation in her lumbar region. Afterwards, this turned into a lower back pain that was sore in nature and moved up and down. The pain did not radiate to the legs along the Bladder channel, was aggravated after heavy exertion and alleviated by rest, and there was weakness of the loins and knees. Accompanying symptoms included tiredness, poor hearing, hair loss, an aversion to cold, cold hands and feet, a pale complexion, a white and wet tongue coating and a deep and slow pulse.

On examination, there was tenderness both in the lower back and in the Bladder channel on each side, but especially on the right side.

Diagnosis
Deficiency of Kidney-Yang.

Principle of treatment
Tonify Kidney-Yang, warm the channels and relieve the pain.

Acupuncture treatment
BL-23, BL-40, BL-58, KI-3, GB-39, SP-6 and some local Ah Shi points. Reinforcing method was used on these points, and moxibustion was used on BL-23 and KI-3. Treatment was given once every other day.

Explanations

- BL-23, the Back Transporting point of the Kidney, and KI-3, the Source point, tonify the Kidney, and strengthen the back and bones so as to treat the root cause.
- BL-40, the commanding point for the back, promotes the circulation of Qi and Blood in the Bladder channel and relieves pain in the lower back.
- BL-58, the Connecting point, harmonises the collateral and sedates the lower back pain.
- GB-34, the Gathering point for the tendons, strengthens the tendons and bones so as to consolidate the back.
- SP-6, the crossing point of the three Yin channels of the foot, nourishes the Liver, Spleen and Kidney so as to promote the production of Qi and Blood.
- Ah Shi points harmonise the collateral and sedate the local pain.
- Moxibustion warms the channels and dispels interior Cold, as well as promoting the circulation of Qi and Blood in the channels.

After 2 months of treatment, her lower back pain had improved greatly. The acupuncture treatment was stopped but she continued with a patent remedy: Ba Wei Di Huang Wan, taking eight pills three times daily for another 2 months in order to consolidate the therapeutic effect. When she was followed up a year later, she stated she had experienced no further pain after the treatment.

Coccyx pain 34

骶
骨
疼
痛

Pain in the coccyx, according to TCM theory, is often caused by invasion of pathogenic Cold and Damp or Damp-Heat, deficiency of Kidney-Qi or stagnation of Qi and Blood. Coccyx pain may be attributed to any of the following disorders in Western medicine: rheumatism, rheumatoid arthritis, muscle strain or traumatic injury in the coccyx region, and deformation or injury to the spinal column and coccyx.

Aetiology and pathology

Invasion by Cold-Damp

In this situation coccyx pain is caused by an obstruction of the circulation of Qi in the channels and collaterals. Cold and Damp are the Yin pathogenic factors: Cold is characterised by contraction and stagnation; Damp is characterised by heaviness and stagnation. When Cold-Damp invades the coccyx, it may impede the functions of the Qi, and specifically impair the Yang-Qi, which leads to stagnation of the Qi and Blood in the locality and disturbance of the channels, causing coccyx pain with a cold sensation and feeling of heaviness to occur.

Invasion of Cold-Damp usually happens to people who live in a cold and damp place for too long, or frequently go out in the rain without waterproof clothing, or wade through or work in water, or who remain in clothes drenched from sweating, or consume too much cold or uncooked food. If in addition there is a deficiency of Qi or Yang of the Spleen or Kidney, such people will be particularly vulnerable to attack by Cold-Damp.

Invasion by Damp-Heat

Since Damp is characterised by heaviness and stagnation, and Heat is characterised by burning and consumption of Yin, if Damp-Heat invades the Lower Burner and the coccyx, it obstructs the circulation of Qi in the channels and collateral and impairs the Yin and Blood, causing coccyx pain.

Damp-Heat usually invades people who fail to maintain personal hygiene in their genital and anal regions, who walk and live in a damp and dirty place, or who remain in clothes drenched from sweating in summer or after work or sport. Moreover, if Cold-Damp persists for a long time in the body it will gradually transform into Damp-Heat.

Invasion of Damp-Heat to the coccyx can also be caused by the downward flow of Damp-Heat to the Lower Burner and coccyx, leading to coccyx pain. Internal Damp-Heat is usually caused by bad diets, such as frequent eating of pungent, sweet, or fatty or greasy food, or milk products, or drinking too much alcohol, which result in poor transportation and transformation by the Spleen and Stomach.

Deficiency of the Kidney-Essence

The Kidney dominates the Bones and produces the Marrow. Congenital weakness, excessive strain, prolonged sickness, a poor diet, excessive sexual activity or senility, may cause the Kidney to function poorly, leading to deficiency of the Kidney-Essence. When the coccyx is not properly nourished by the Kidney-Essence then coccyx pain follows.

Stagnation of Qi and Blood

The Qi and Blood should circulate freely in the body and channels. If they stagnate in the region of the coccyx because of various causes, they block the channels, causing coccyx pain. Stagnation of the Qi and Blood may be caused by emotional disturbance, trauma or congenital deformity.

Treatment based on differentiation

Differentiation

Differentiation of External or Internal origin

Coccyx pain can be caused either by invasion of External pathogenic factors or by Internal disorders.

— In case it is caused by invasion of External pathogenic factors, it is usually acute, and accompanied by External symptoms such as headache, fever, an aversion to cold, runny nose or coughing.
— If it is caused by disorders of Internal organs, it is chronic and has no External symptoms.

Differentiation of character of the pain

— Acute onset of coccyx pain after exposure to cold and damp, aggravation of the coccyx pain on rainy days, with a heavy sensation and stiffness of the muscles in the coccyx region and a cold feeling, limitation of extension and flexion of the back, lower back pain radiating to the buttocks and lower limbs, cold feeling in the lower back, an aversion to cold, or a slight fever, is usually caused by invasion of Cold-Damp.

— Acute onset of coccyx pain, lower back pain and pain in the coccyx region with a heavy and warm or hot sensation, or even swelling of the coccyx, sticky sweating, thirst but with no desire to drink, fever, or painful urination, is often caused by invasion of Damp-Heat.
— Stabbing pain in the coccyx, with rigidity at the lower back, aggravation of the coccyx pain by pressure and at night, or a history of physical trauma to the coccyx or adjacent region, is often caused by stagnation of Blood.
— Insidious onset of protracted coccyx pain with soreness, weakness of the lower back, legs and knees, aggravation of the coccyx pain by tiredness and alleviation of pain by rest, is often caused by deficiency of Kidney-Essence.

Treatment

INVASION OF COLD-DAMP

Symptoms and signs

Coccyx pain usually occurring after exposure to cold and damp, which worsens on rainy days, with a heavy sensation and stiffness of the muscles in the coccyx region, and a cold feeling, accompanied by symptoms such as limitation of extension and flexion of the back, lower back pain radiating to the buttocks and lower limbs, a cold feeling in the lower back, an aversion to cold, a slight fever, slight generalised body pain, a white and greasy tongue coating and a superficial and slippery pulse.

Principle of treatment

Dispel Cold, dry Damp and relieve the pain.

HERBAL TREATMENT

Prescription

YI YI REN TANG
Coix Decoction
Yi Yi Ren *Semen Coicis* 15 g
Chuan Xiong *Rhizoma Ligustici Chuanxiong* 10 g
Ma Huang *Herba Ephedrae* 10 g
Gui Zhi *Ramulus Cinnamomi* 6 g
Qiang Huo *Rhizoma seu Radix Notopterygii* 10 g
Du Huo *Radix Angelicae Pubescentis* 10 g
Chuan Wu *Radix Aconiti Lateralis Praeparata* 6 g, decocted for more than 2 hours
Cang Zhu *Rhizoma Atractylodis* 10 g

Gan Cao *Radix Glycyrrhizae* 6 g
Sheng Jiang *Rhizoma Zingiberis* 5 g
Chuan Niu Xi *Radix Cyathulae* 5 g

Explanations

- Yi Yi Ren and Cang Zhu eliminate Damp in the Lower Burner and coccyx.
- Qiang Huo and Du Huo dispel Wind, Cold and Damp, relieve External symptoms and stop the coccyx pain.
- Chuan Wu and Sheng Jiang warm the Yang-Qi of the body, eliminate Cold-Damp and promote the circulation of Qi and Blood.
- Ma Huang and Gui Zhi open the skin pores and promote sweating so as to dispel Wind and Cold and relieve External symptoms.
- Chuan Niu Xi and Chuan Xiong promote the circulation of Blood and relieve the coccyx pain. Chuan Niu Xi also dispels Cold-Damp and leads the treatment to the Lower Burner and coccyx.
- Gan Cao harmonises the actions of the other herbs in the prescription.

Modifications

1. If there is an aversion to cold and general body pain, add Fang Feng *Radix Ledebouriellae* 10 g and Sang Zhi *Ramulus Mori* 10 g to dispel Wind-Cold and relieve External symptoms.
2. If there is lower back pain with a feeling of heaviness, add Bu Gu Zhi *Fructus Psoraleae* 10 g and Du Zhong *Cortex Eucommiae* 10 g to tonify the Kidney, strengthen the lower back and relieve the pain.
3. If the coccyx pain worsens at night, add Pu Huang *Pollen Typhae* 10 g and San Qi *Radix Notoginseng* 10 g to promote the circulation of Blood and relieve the pain.
4. If there is a poor appetite and fullness in the abdomen, add Bai Zhu *Rhizoma Atractylodis Macrocephalae* 10 g and Sha Ren *Fructus Amomi* 5 g to activate the Spleen and dry Damp.
5. If there is generalised tiredness, shortness of breath and a pale complexion due to deficiency of Qi, add Huang Qi *Radix Astragali seu Hedysari* 12 g and Dang Shen *Radix Codonopsis Pilosulae* 10 g to activate the Spleen and Spleen-Qi.

Patent remedy

Du Huo Ji Sheng Tang *Angelica Pubescens and Loranthus Decoction*

ACUPUNCTURE TREATMENT

LU-7 Lieque, LI-4 Hegu, GB-20 Fengchi, BL-12 Fengmen, BL-35 Huiyang, BL-58 Feiyang, BL-62 Shenmai, GV-3 Yaoyangguan and SI-3 Houxi. Reducing method is used on these points.

Explanations

- LI-4, the Source point of the Large Intestine channel, and LU-7, the Connecting point of the Lung channel, are a pair of points from Externally and Internally related channels. Together they dispel Wind, eliminate Cold, relieve External symptoms and stop generalised body pain. LI-4 is also a very good point for sedating the coccyx pain.
- GB-20 and BL-12 dispel Wind, Cold and Damp in the Bladder channel and Governing Vessel, and relieve the coccyx pain.
- BL-20, the Back Transporting point of the Spleen, activates the Spleen and Stomach, eliminates Damp and relieves the diarrhoea.
- BL-58, the Connecting point, harmonises the collateral, dispels Wind-Cold and relieves the pain.
- BL-35 and GV-3, the local points, harmonise the collateral in the coccyx region and relieve the pain.
- BL-62 and SI-3 in combination dispel Wind, Cold and Damp, remove blockage in the Governing Vessel and relieve the coccyx pain.

Modifications

1. If there is severe heaviness of the back, add SP-9 to eliminate Damp and relieve the feeling of heaviness.
2. If there is lower back pain with an obvious cold sensation, add moxibustion on BL-12, BL-58 and LI-4 to warm the channels, dispel Cold and relieve the cold sensation.
3. If there is worsening of the back pain at night and waking at night due to severe pain, add SP-6 and HT-7 to promote the circulation of Blood, calm the Mind and relieve the severe pain.
4. If there is nausea with a feeling of heaviness in the Stomach, add BL-21, the Back Transporting point of the Stomach, to harmonise the Stomach, help the Stomach-Qi to descend, resolve Damp and relieve the nausea.
5. If there is a poor appetite and a feeling of fullness in the Stomach, add SP-4 to help the Stomach-Qi to descend, dry Damp, improve the appetite and relieve the fullness.
6. If there is diarrhoea, add SP-3, the Source point, to dry Damp, activate the Spleen and relieve the diarrhoea.

Case history

A 36-year-old man had been suffering from coccyx pain, with a heavy and cold sensation for 3 weeks. Three weeks previously he had caught a cold after walking in the rain, when he had an aversion to cold, a slight fever, and headache and coccyx pain. He did not take too much care over these complaints, and the coccyx pain became worse and worse.

When he arrived at the clinic, he stated that when it rained his coccyx pain usually worsened and he sometimes woke up at night. Also, he still had a slight aversion to cold and a fever (37.4°C), a sensation of heaviness in the coccyx, limitation of extension and flexion in the lower back with pain radiating to the buttocks, a white and greasy tongue coating, and a superficial and slippery pulse.

Diagnosis
Coccyx pain due to invasion of Cold-Damp.

Principle of treatment
Dispel Wind and Cold, dry Damp and relieve the pain.

Acupuncture treatment
LI-4, BL-12, BL-35, BL-58, BL-62, BL-64, SP-6, GV-3 and SI-3. Reducing method was used on these points. Treatment was given once a day.

Explanations

- LI-4, the Source point, and BL-12 dispel Wind, eliminate Cold, relieve External symptoms and stop generalised body pain. LI-4 can also sedate the coccyx pain.
- SP-6, the crossing point of the three Yin channels of the foot, activates the Spleen and Stomach, eliminates Damp, promotes the circulation of Blood and relieves the coccyx pain.
- BL-58, the Connecting point, and BL-64, the Source point, harmonise the channel and collateral, dispel Wind-Cold and relieve the coccyx pain.
- BL-35 and GV-3, the local points, harmonise the collateral in the coccyx region and relieve the pain.
- BL-62 and SI-3 in combination dispel Wind, Cold and Damp, remove blockage in the Governing Vessel and relieve the coccyx pain.

After three treatment sessions, his general symptoms were much better, and his coccyx pain had also improved somewhat. He could also sleep without waking up at night. After another week of treatment the coccyx pain was under control. He was followed up 2 months afterwards and he reported that he had experienced no coccyx pain since the treatment.

INVASION OF DAMP-HEAT

Symptoms and signs

Coccyx pain that is usually worse on rainy and hot days, or lower back pain and pain in the coccyx region with a heavy and warm or hot sensation, or even swelling at the coccyx. Other symptoms include sticky sweating, thirst with no desire to drink, fever, deep yellow urine, a red tongue with a yellow and greasy coating and a slippery and rapid pulse.

Principle of treatment

Clear Heat, eliminate Damp and relieve the pain.

HERBAL TREATMENT

Prescription

SI MIAO SAN
Four-Marvel Powder
Huang Bai *Cortex Phellodendri* 12 g
Cang Zhu *Rhizoma Atractylodis* 10 g
Chuan Niu Xi *Radix Cyathulae* 6 g
Yi Yi Ren *Semen Coicis* 15 g
Jin Qian Cao *Herba Lysimachiae* 20 g

Explanations

- Huang Bai and Cang Zhu clear Heat, reduce fever and dry Damp in the Lower Burner.
- Yi Yi Ren clears Heat and promotes urination so as to eliminate Damp in the Lower Burner.
- Chuan Niu Xi guides all herbs downward to the coccyx region, invigorates the circulation of Blood, eliminates Blood stasis and reinforces the Kidney.
- Jin Qian Cao promotes urination and eliminates Damp-Heat in the Lower Burner.

Modifications

1. If there is swelling, pain and ulceration around the coccyx, add Sheng Di Huang *Radix Rehmanniae Recens* 10 g and Pu Gong Ying *Herba Taraxaci* 15 g to clear Heat, eliminate Toxin, reduce the swelling and promote healing of the ulceration.
2. If the coccyx pain worsens at night, add Pu Huang *Pollen Typhae* 10 g and San Qi *Radix Notoginseng* 10 g to promote the circulation of Blood and relieve the pain.
3. If there is a fever and thirst, add Zhi Zi *Fructus Gardeniae* 10 g to clear Heat, reduce the fever, eliminate Damp and relieve the pain.
4. If there is lassitude in the loins, a dry throat and feverish sensations in the palms and soles of the feet, add Zhi Mu *Rhizoma Anemarrhenae* 12 g to clear Heat and nourish the Yin.

5. If there is a bitter taste in the mouth and insomnia, add Huang Lian *Rhizoma Coptidis* 5 g to clear Heat, eliminate Damp and calm the Mind.

6. If there is frequent and urgent painful urination, add Mu Tong *Caulis Aristolochiae* 6 g and Che Qian Zi *Semen Plantaginis* 12 g to eliminate Damp-Heat, promote urination and relieve the urination pain.

7. If there is bloody urine, add Xiao Ji *Herba Cephalanoploris* 12 g to cool the Blood and stop the bleeding.

8. If there is urethral calculus, add Hai Jin Sha *Spora Lygodii* 10 g to promote urination and dissolve the stone.

Patent remedy

San Miao Wan *Three-Marvel Pill*

ACUPUNCTURE TREATMENT

LI-4 Hegu, TE-6 Zhigou, BL-35 Huiyang, BL-40 Weizhong, BL-58 Feiyang, BL-62 Shenmai, BL-66 Zutonggu, GV-3 Yaoyangguan and SI-3 Houxi. Reducing method is used on these points.

Explanations

- LI-4, the Source point, and TE-6 dispel External factors, clear Heat and eliminate Damp.
- BL-40, a commanding point for the back, and BL-58, the Connecting point, promote the free flow of Qi in the channels and harmonise the collateral in order to treat the lower back pain and coccyx pain.
- BL-66, the Spring point, clears Heat and eliminates Damp in the Lower Burner.
- BL-35 and GV-3, the local points, harmonise the collateral in the coccyx region and relieve the pain.
- BL-62 and SI-3 in combination dispel Wind, Cold and Damp, remove blockage in the Governing Vessel and relieve the coccyx pain.

Modifications

1. If there is a fever, add GV-14 to clear Heat and reduce the fever.

2. If there is sacral pain, add some local Ah Shi points to harmonise the collateral and arrest the pain.

3. If there is a severe burning sensation and aversion to heat in the lower back, add BL-67 to clear Heat and relieve the burning sensation.

4. If there is scanty and painful urination, add BL-32 and KI-4 to promote urination and relieve the urination pain.

5. If there is a feeling of heaviness in the body, add SP-6 to resolve Damp and eliminate Phlegm from the body.

6. If the appetite is poor, add BL-20, the Back Transporting point of the Spleen, to activate the Spleen and improve the appetite.

7. If there is diarrhoea, add SP-3, the Source point, to activate the Spleen, eliminate Damp and relieve the diarrhoea.

8. If there is profuse leucorrhoea, add GB-27 and GB-41 to eliminate Damp and relieve the leucorrhoea.

DEFICIENCY OF KIDNEY-ESSENCE

Symptoms and signs

Insidious onset of protracted coccyx pain with soreness, which worsens when tired and is alleviated by rest, accompanied by weakness in the lower back, legs and knees.

If the deficiency is of Kidney-Yang, there is also a cold feeling in the lower back, pallor, cold limbs, a normal taste in the mouth, polyuria, a pale tongue and a deep and feeble, or faint, or deep and slow pulse.

If the deficiency is of Kidney-Yin, there is also a dry mouth and throat, a flushed face, a feverish sensation in the chest, palms and soles of the feet, irritability, insomnia, a red tongue with a scanty coating and a thready and weak or thready and rapid pulse.

Principle of treatment

Tonify the Kidney, benefit the Essence and relieve the pain.

HERBAL TREATMENT

Prescription a: for deficiency of Kidney-Yang

JIN GUI SHEN QI WAN
Kidney Qi Pill
Shu Di Huang *Radix Rehmanniae Praeparata* 12 g
Shan Yao *Rhizoma Dioscoreae* 15 g
Shan Zhu Yu *Fructus Corni* 10 g
Ze Xie *Rhizoma Alismatis* 10 g
Fu Ling *Poria* 10 g
Gui Zhi *Ramulus Cinnamomi* 6 g
Fu Zi *Radix Aconiti Carmichaeli Praeparata* 6 g, decocted first
Tu Si Zi *Semen Cuscutae* 10 g
Du Zhong *Cortex Eucommiae* 10 g

Prescription b: for deficiency of Kidney-Yin

ZUO GUI WAN
Restoring the Left Pill
Shu Di Huang *Rhizoma Rehmanniae Praeparata* 12 g
Shan Yao *Rhizoma Dioscoreae* 15 g
Shan Zhu Yu *Fructus Corni* 6 g
Tu Si Zi *Semen Cuscutae* 10 g
Gou Qi Zi *Fructus Lycii* 12 g
Chuan Niu Xi *Radix Cyathulae* 6 g
Lu Jiao Jiao *Colla Cervi Cornus* 6 g
Gui Ban Jiao *Colla Plastri Testudinis* 10 g

Explanations

- In Jin Gui Shen Qi Wan, Shu Di Huang tonifies the Kidney, benefits the Essence and consolidates the bones.
- Shan Yao and Shan Zhu Yu strengthen the Liver and Spleen to help Shu Di Huang tonify the Kidney.
- Gui Zhi and Fu Zi tonify the Kidney-Yang and dispel Cold.
- Ze Xie and Fu Ling remove Damp and promote urination.
- Tu Si Zi and Du Zhong tonify the Kidney, benefit the Essence and strengthen the back and bones.

- In Zuo Gui Wan, Shu Di Huang tonifies the Kidney and benefits the Essence.
- Shan Yao and Shan Zhu Yu strengthen the Liver and Spleen to help Shu Di Huang tonify the Kidney.
- Gou Qi Zi nourishes the Yin of the Liver and Kidney and benefits the eyes.
- Gui Ban Jiao, Tu Si Zi and Lu Jiao Jiao tonify the Kidney and strengthen the bones.
- Chuan Niu Xi has the effect of strengthening the waist and knees and reinforcing the muscles and joints.

Modifications

1. If there is shortness of breath, lassitude, a low voice, a poor appetite and diarrhoea due to deficiency of the Spleen-Qi, add Dang Shen *Radix Codonopsis Pilosulae* 10 g and Huang Qi *Radix Astragali Pilosulae* 12 g to tonify the Spleen-Qi.
2. If there is diarrhoea before dawn with cold in the lower abdomen due to deficiency of Kidney-Yang, add Bu Gu Zhi *Fructus Psoraleae* 10 g and Wu Wei Zi *Fructus Schisandrae* 10 g to tonify the Kidney-Yang and stop the diarrhoea.
3. If there is seminal emission, enuresis and frequent nocturnal urination due to deficiency of the Kidney-Qi, add Yi Zhi Ren *Fructus Alpiniae Oxyphyllae* 6 g to tonify the Kidney-Qi and arrest the seminal emission.

4. If there is insomnia due to disharmony between the Heart and Kidney, add Huang Lian *Rhizoma Coptidis* 5 g and E Jiao *Colla Corii Asini* 10 g to clear Deficient-Fire, balance the Heart and Kidney and improve sleep.
5. If there is headache and vertigo due to hyperactivity of Liver-Yang caused by deficiency of the Yin of the Liver and Kidney, add Tian Ma *Rhizoma Gastrodiae* 10 g and Gou Teng *Uncariae cum Uncis* 15 g to subdue the Liver-Yang and relieve the vertigo.
6. If there is a tidal fever or feverish sensation in the palms and soles of the feet due to deficiency of Yin, add Di Gu Pi *Cortex Lycii Radicis* 12 g to clear Deficient-Heat.

Patent remedies

Jin Gui Shen Qi Wan *Kidney Qi Pill* for deficiency of Kidney-Yang
Liu Wei Di Huang Wan *Six-Flavour Rehmanniae Pill* for deficiency of Kidney-Yin

ACUPUNCTURE TREATMENT

BL-23 Shenshu, BL-35 Huiyang, BL-40 Weizhong, BL-58 Feiyang, GB-39 Xuanzhong, KI-3 Taixi, KI-10 Yingu, GV-3 Yaoyangguan and SP-6 Sanyinjiao. Reinforcing method is used on these points.

Explanations

- BL-23, the Back Transporting point of the Kidney, KI-3, the Source point, and KI-10, the Sea point, tonify the Kidney, and strengthen the back and bones so as to treat the root cause.
- BL-40, a commanding point for the back, and BL-58, the Connecting point, promote the free flow of Qi in the channels and harmonise the collateral in order to treat pain in the lower back and coccyx.
- GB-39, the Gathering point for the Marrow, strengthens the tendons and bones so as to consolidate the back and coccyx.
- SP-6, the crossing point of the three Yin channels of the foot, nourishes the Liver, Spleen and Kidney so as to promote the production of Qi and Blood.
- BL-35 and GV-3, the local points, harmonise the collateral in the coccyx region and relieve pain.

Modifications

1. If there is a cold sensation in the lower back, add GV-4 with moxibustion and a moxa box on

the lower back to warm the lower back and dispel Cold.

2. If there is weakness in the knees, add GB-34, the Gathering point for the tendons, to strengthen the knees.
3. If there is impotency, add CV-4 and CV-6 to reinforce the Kidney and improve the potency.
4. If there is insomnia, add HT-3 and PC-6 to calm the Mind and improve the sleep.
5. If there is dizziness, add GB-20 to regulate the Qi and Blood in the head and relieve the dizziness.
6. If there is generalised tiredness, add ST-36 and GV-20 to lift up the energy and relieve the tiredness.
7. If there is diarrhoea, add BL-20 and BL-25 to strengthen the Spleen and stop the diarrhoea.
8. If there is constipation, add LI-4 to promote defecation.
9. If there is profuse night sweating, add HT-6 and KI-2 to clear Deficient-Heat and stop the sweating.
10. If there is nervousness and headache, add LR-2, the Spring point, to clear Heat in the Liver and calm it.

Case history

A 75-year-old woman had been suffering from coccyx pain for 5 years. The onset was gradual, and the pain mostly occurred when she was tired and resolved after she had rested. Sometimes she suffered from coccyx pain when she walked too much. Other symptoms were heat in the body, a thirst, a dry throat, dry stools, slight night sweating, lower back pain and soreness, weakness in the knees, a poor memory, dizziness, tinnitus in the left ear, irritability, nervousness, occasional headaches, a red tongue with a scanty coating, and one small area of peeled coating on the left edge, and a thready, weak and slightly rapid pulse.

Diagnosis
Coccyx pain due to deficiency of Yin of Liver and Kidney.

Principle of treatment
Nourish Yin, tonify the Kidney and relieve the pain.

Acupuncture treatment
BL-23, BL-35, BL-58, GB-20, GB-39, KI-3, KI-7, KI-10, GV-3 and SP-6. Reinforcing method was used on these points. Treatment was given once every 3 days.

Explanations

- BL-23, the Back Transporting point of the Kidney, KI-3, the Source point, and KI-10, the Sea point, tonify the Kidney, and strengthen the back and bones so as to treat the root cause.
- KI-7, the Metal point, and SP-6, the crossing point of the three Yin channels of the foot, nourish the Yin of the Liver and Kidney and clear Deficient-Heat.
- BL-58, the Connecting point, harmonises the collateral and relieves the coccyx pain.

- GB-39, the Gathering point for the Marrow, strengthens the tendons and bones so as to consolidate the back and coccyx.
- BL-35 and GV-3, the local points, harmonise the collateral in the coccyx region and relieve the pain.
- GB-20 calms the Mind, smoothes the Liver and tranquillises the Mind.

Herbal treatment
Liu Wei Di Huang Wan *Six-Flavour Rehmanniae Pill*, three times per day, 12 pills each time.

After treatment for 1 month, her coccyx pain was almost under control. After this, acupuncture was given once every week for another 2 months, by which time her coccyx pain had disappeared. She was followed up a year later and she replied she had experienced no further coccyx pain since the treatment.

STAGNATION OF QI AND BLOOD

Symptoms and signs

A stabbing pain in the coccyx that is aggravated by pressure and worsens at night, with a history of physical trauma to the coccyx or adjacent region, accompanied by rigidity in the lower back, restlessness or insomnia due to the coccyx pain, a dark purplish tongue and a thready or choppy pulse.

Principle of treatment

Promote Qi and Blood circulation, eliminate Blood stasis and relieve the pain.

HERBAL TREATMENT

Prescription

SHEN TONG ZHU YU TANG
Meridian Passage
Dang Gui *Radix Angelicae Sinensis* 10 g
Chuan Xiong *Rhizoma Ligustici Chuanxiong* 12 g
Tao Ren *Semen Persicae* 10 g
Hong Hua *Flos Carthami* 6 g
Mo Yao *Resina Myrrhae* 6 g
Xiang Fu *Rhizoma Cyperi* 10 g
Wu Ling Zhi *Faeces Trogopterorum* 6 g
Chuan Niu Xi *Radix Cyathulae* 6 g
Di Long *Lumbricus* 10 g
Gan Cao *Radix Glycyrrhizae* 6 g

Explanations

- Dang Gui, Chuang Xiong, Tao Ren and Hong Hua promote the circulation of Blood and eliminate Blood stasis.

- Mo Yao and Wu Ling Zhi eliminate Blood stasis and sedate coccyx pain.
- Xiang Fu promotes the circulation of Qi to reinforce the effect of the circulation of Blood.
- Chuan Niu Xi and Di Long promote the circulation of Blood in the channels and relieve coccyx pain.
- Chuan Niu Xi guides Blood stasis down and tonifies the back and coccyx.
- Gan Cao harmonises the actions of the other herbs in the prescription.

Modifications

1. If there is swelling around the coccyx, add San Qi *Radix Notoginseng* 10 g to promote the circulation of Blood, eliminate Blood stasis and reduce the swelling.
2. If there is lower back pain with an aversion to Wind-Damp, add Du Huo *Radix Angelicae Pubescentis* 10 g to dispel the Wind and relieve the pain.
3. If there is lower back pain with weakness of the lower back, add Du Zhong *Cortex Eucommiae* 10 g and Shu Di Huang *Radix Rehmanniae Praeparata* 12 g to tonify the Kidney and relieve the pain.
4. If there is irregular menstruation due to stagnant Blood, add Yi Mu Cao *Herba Leonuri* 10 g to regulate the menstruation.
5. If there are cold limbs, a pale complexion, a deep and slow pulse and a pale tongue, add Gui Zhi *Ramulus Cinnamomi* 6 g and Gan Jiang *Rhizoma Zingiberis* 6 g to warm the Kidney-Yang and relieve the pain.

Patent remedy

Te Xiao Yao Tong Ling *Special Efficacy Lower Back Pain Pill*

ACUPUNCTURE TREATMENT

BL-17 Geshu, BL-35 Huiyang, BL-40 Weizhong, BL-58 Feiyang, BL-62 Shenmai, BL-63 Jinmen, SI-3 Houxi, GV-2 Yaoshu and SP-6 Sanyinjiao. Reducing method is used on these points.

Explanations

- BL-17, the Gathering point for the Blood, and SP-6, the crossing point of the three Yin channels of the foot, promote the circulation of Blood and eliminate Blood stasis.

- BL-40, a commanding point for the back, BL-58, the Connecting point, and BL-63, the Accumulation point, promote the free flow of Qi in the channels and harmonise the collateral to relieve the pain in the lower back and coccyx.
- BL-62 and SI-3 in combination open the Governing Vessel and relieve coccyx pain.
- BL-35 and GV-2, the local points, harmonise the collateral in the coccyx region and relieve pain.

Modifications

1. If there is a severe coccyx pain, add LI-4 and LR-3 to promote the circulation of Qi and Blood and relieve the pain.
2. If there is swelling around the coccyx, add some local Ah Shi points to promote the circulation of Qi and Blood and reduce the swelling.
3. If there is restlessness due to pain, add GB-20 to calm the Mind.
4. If there is insomnia, add HT-3 and HT-7 to calm the Heart and tranquillise the Mind.
5. If there is aversion to cold in the lower back, add moxibustion to warm the channel and dispel Cold.

Case history

A 20-year-old man had been suffering from coccyx pain after falling down whilst horse riding 5 days previously. He visited his doctor and was given some painkillers; however, the pain did not improve much.

When he arrived at the clinic, he still had some swelling around the coccyx, together with a big blue spot, which was about 10 × 10 cm, worsening of the pain at night and frequent waking due to pain, restlessness, an inability to sit and lie down and, because of the coccyx pain, he could not easily defecate as usual. His appetite, tongue coating and pulse were normal.

Diagnosis
Coccyx due to stagnation of Blood.

Principle of treatment
Promote circulation of Qi and Blood, eliminate Blood stasis and relieve the pain.

Acupuncture treatment
GV-2, GV-26, BL-17, BL-40, BL-35, BL-58 and SP-6. Reinforcing method was applied for all these points. Treatment was given two times per week.

Explanations
- GV-2 and BL-35 are the local points to promote the circulation of Qi and Blood, harmonise the collateral and relieve the coccyx pain.
- Needling at GV-26 with reducing method conducts

the circulation of Qi and Blood in the Governing Vessel, which passes through the sacral region.

- BL-40, the commanding point for the back, and BL-58, the Connecting point, disperse the stagnation of Blood from the collateral and relieve the pain.
- BL-17, the Gathering point for the Blood, and SP-6, the crossing point of the three Yin channels of the foot, were used to promote the circulation of Blood, eliminate Blood stasis and relieve the pain.

After 1 month of treatment, his coccyx pain had disappeared. Two months later, he was followed up by telephone and he replied he had experienced no pain since the treatment.

Part 7

Upper limb pain 上肢疼痛

Shoulder pain 35

肩
痛

Shoulder pain may occur on one or both sides of the shoulder, and is mainly associated with the shoulder joint itself, or its attached tendons and muscles, as well as the shoulder blade. The pain may refer to the upper and back part of the thorax, upper arm or even the entire arm.

According to TCM theory, shoulder pain may be caused by a disturbance of one of the six Yang channels of the hand or of the Lung channel. Both External invasion and disorder of the internal Zang-Fu organs may cause disturbances in one or more of these channels, leading to stagnation of Qi and Blood, at which point pain occurs. More specifically shoulder pain is generally caused by invasion of External pathogenic factors, deficiency of Qi, stagnation of Qi, stagnation of Blood or accumulation of Damp-Phlegm in the channels. Shoulder pain may be attributed to any of the following disorders in Western medicine: subacromial bursitis, synovitis of the shoulder joint, periarthritis of the shoulder joint, tendinitis of the shoulder, calcification of the shoulder tendon, shoulder–hand syndrome, tendinitis of the supraspinatus muscle, calcification of the supraspinatus tendon, rheumatic arthritis of the shoulder and traumatic arthritis of the shoulder.

Aetiology and pathology

Invasion of External factors

Contraction and stagnation are the characteristics of Cold. When Wind-Cold invades the body it causes the channels and muscles in the shoulder area to contract, which leads to stagnation of the Qi and Blood, and so causes pain.

When Cold attacks the body in combination with Damp, these may obstruct the channels, collaterals, muscles and tendons, slowing down the circulation of Qi and Blood, and causing pain. Since Damp, a pathogen of the Yin type, is characterised by stagnation and viscosity, it tends to impede the functions of the Qi, particularly the Yang-Qi. Invasion of Wind-Damp causes a long-lasting shoulder pain accompanied by a heavy sensation, or swelling at the shoulder.

Deficiency of Qi

Overstrain, a poor constitution, prolonged sickness and bad diet may cause consumption of the Qi, leading to its deficiency, and then internal Cold forms. When Qi fails to warm the channels and muscles, Cold blocks the channels and muscles, causing shoulder pain.

Stagnation of Qi in the channels

Qi and Blood should circulate freely. If there is stagnation of Qi due to stress, frustration or sadness, or Qi deficiency, the channels will become blocked, which causes pain.

Stagnation of Blood in the channels

Long-standing stagnation of Qi may eventually lead to stagnation of Blood. Traumatic injury or an inappropriate operation on the shoulder may directly damage the muscles, tendons and Blood Vessels, causing the Blood to stagnate. Accumulation of Cold and Damp over a long time in the shoulder area may also cause Blood stagnation. When Blood stasis blocks the channels of the shoulder, shoulder pain occurs.

Accumulation of Damp-Phlegm in the channels

Bad diets and dietary habits, such as eating too much fatty, sweet food, cold, raw or highly flavoured food, or drinking too much alcohol, as well as eating irregularly, may easily damage the physiological function of the Spleen and Stomach. Once the Spleen and Stomach's functions of transportation and transformation are disturbed, then Damp-Phlegm will form. When Damp-Phlegm accumulates it circulates in the body together with the Qi circulation, and may block the channels, thus the free flow of Qi and Blood is impaired and shoulder pain occurs.

Treatment based on differentiation

Differentiation

Differentiation of acute pain and chronic pain

— Acute shoulder pain is often related to invasion of External factors, such as Wind-Cold or Cold-Damp. This kind of shoulder pain is accompanied by External symptoms, for instance, headache, slight fever, an aversion to cold, or muscle pain. Also, this kind of shoulder pain is much related to weather changes. Some acute shoulder pain could also be caused by acute stagnation of Blood resulting from trauma, or some other reasons.
— Chronic pain is often related to stagnation of Qi or Blood in the channels due to emotional disorder, trauma or a history of operations.

Differentiation of character of the pain

— Acute shoulder pain that worsens in cold weather, wandering shoulder pain, an aversion to cold, or slight fever, is often caused by invasion of Wind-Cold.
— Acute shoulder pain with a cold and heavy sensation, which worsens in cold and in rainy weather, alleviation of the shoulder pain by warmth, and sometimes swollen shoulder with difficult movement, is caused by invasion of Cold-Damp.
— Shoulder pain with a distending or numb sensation, aggravation of the pain by stress or emotional upset, with irritability, insomnia or headache, is often due to stagnation of Qi in the channels.
— Long history of shoulder pain with a stabbing sensation and fixed location, history of traumatic injury to the shoulder joint, swelling of the shoulder joint, or aggravation of the pain at night, is usually caused by stagnation of Blood in the channels.
— Chronic shoulder pain with a heavy sensation, limitation of shoulder movement, and soreness or numbness of the muscle, is often caused by accumulation of Damp-Phlegm in the channels.

Treatment

INVASION OF WIND-COLD

Symptoms and signs

Acute shoulder pain, wandering in nature, which is aggravated by exposure to Wind and Cold, accompanied by an aversion to cold, a slight fever, a runny nose, a cough, a pale tongue with a thin coating and a superficial pulse.

Principle of treatment

Dispel Wind and eliminate Cold.

HERBAL TREATMENT

Prescription

FANG FENG TANG
Ledebouriella Decoction
Fang Feng *Radix Ledebouriellae* 10 g
Chuan Xiong *Rhizoma Ligustici Chuanxiong* 10 g
Gan Cao *Radix Glycyrrhizae* 6 g
Fu Ling *Poria* 15 g

Ma Huang *Herba Ephedrae* 6 g
Dang Gui *Radix Angelicae Sinensis* 10 g
Huang Qin *Radix Scutellariae* 6 g
Ge Gen *Radix Puerariae* 12 g
Qin Jiao *Radix Gentianae Macrophyllae* 10 g

Explanations

- Fang Feng, Qin Jiao and Ge Geng dispel Wind-Cold and relieve the pain.
- Ma Huang dispels Wind-Cold, regulates the Qi, and relieves External symptoms and pain.
- Dang Gui and Chuan Xiong promote the circulation of Qi and Blood and also relieve the pain.
- Fu Ling eliminates Damp-Phlegm.
- Huang Qin controls the warming herbs in the prescription.
- Can Cao harmonises the function of the other herbs in the prescription.

Modifications

1. If there is severe pain at night, add Yan Hu Suo *Rhizoma Corydalis* 15 g to relieve the pain.
2. If there is an aversion to cold of the shoulder, add Xi Xin *Herba Asari* 3 g to warm the channels and dispel Cold so as to relieve the pain.
3. If there is a cough with white sputum, add Jie Geng *Radix Platycodi* 10 g to regulate the Lung-Qi and eliminate Phlegm.
4. If there is a fever, add Chai Hu *Radix Bupleuri* 15 g and Sheng Ma *Rhizoma Cimicifugae* 5 g to dispel Wind-Cold and reduce the fever.
5. If there is a runny nose, add Qian Hu *Radix Peucedani* 10 g to promote the circulation of Qi and eliminate Phlegm.

Patent remedy

Feng Shi Pian *Wind-Damp Tablet*

ACUPUNCTURE TREATMENT

LI-4 Hegu, LI-15 Jianyu, Lu-7 Lieque, TE-5 Waiguan, GB-20 Fengchi, SI-9 Jianzhen and SI-11 Tianzong. Reducing method is used on these points. Moxibustion should also be used.

Explanations

- LI–4, the Source point of the Large Intestine channel, dispels Wind-Cold, promotes the circulation of Qi and relieves the pain.

- LU-7, the Connecting point of the Lung channel, dispels Wind-Cold, harmonises the collateral and relieves the pain.
- TE-5, the Connecting point of the Triple Burner channel, dispels Wind-Cold, regulates the circulation of Qi and relieves the pain.
- GB-20 dispels Wind and relieves the pain.
- LI-15, SI-9 and SI-11 are the local points for promoting the circulation of Qi and relieving the shoulder pain.
- Moxibustion warms the channels and dispels Cold.

Modifications

1. If the shoulder pain occurs at the place where the Lung channel passes through, add LU-3, LU-4 and LU-5 to promote the circulation of Qi in the channel and sedate the pain.
2. If the shoulder pain occurs at the place where the Large Intestine channel passes through, add LI-6, LI-7 and LI-14 to regulate the channel and sedate the pain.
3. If the shoulder pain occurs at the place where the Triple Burner channel passes through, add TE-7 and TE-14 to harmonise the collateral and sedate the pain.
4. If the shoulder pain occurs at the place where the Small Intestine channel passes through, add SI-4 and SI-6 to harmonise the collateral and sedate the pain.
5. If there is stiffness and pain in the neck, add GB-21 and SI-14 to promote the circulation of Qi and Blood and relieve the neck stiffness and pain.
6. If there is a headache and feeling of heaviness in the head, add BL-10 and GV-17 to dispel Wind-Cold-Damp, promote the circulation of Qi and relieve the pain.
7. If there is a fever, add LI-11 to clear Heat and reduce the fever.
8. If there is generalised body pain, add ST-40 and BL-63 to harmonise the collateral and sedate the pain.
9. If there is throat pain, add LU-10 and CV-23 to dispel External factors and relieve the throat pain.

INVASION OF COLD-DAMP

Symptoms and signs

Acute shoulder pain with a cold and heavy sensation, which is aggravated by exposure to cold and wind or in rainy weather, and improves with warmth, with occasionally a swollen shoulder with difficult movement, accompanied by a purplish or slight blue colour to the face, a pale tongue with a white and greasy coating and a wiry and tight pulse.

Principle of treatment

Dispel Cold, eliminate Damp, promote circulation of Qi and sedate the pain.

HERBAL TREATMENT

Prescription

JUAN BI TANG
Remove Painful Obstruction Decoction
Qiang Huo *Rhizoma seu Radix Notopterygii* 10 g
Qin Jiao *Radix Gentianae Macrophyllae* 15 g
Dang Gui *Radix Angelicae Sinensis* 12 g
Chuan Xiong *Rhizoma Ligustici Chuangxiong* 10 g
Zhi Gan Cao *Radix Glycyrrhizae Praeparata* 6 g
Sang Zhi *Fructus Gardeniae* 30 g
Cang Zhu *Rhizoma Atractylodis* 10 g
Gui Zhi *Ramulus Cinnamomi* 10 g
Mu Xiang *Radix Aucklandiae* 6 g

Explanations

- Qiang Huo and Qin Jiao dispel Wind, eliminate Damp and relieve the pain.
- Chuan Xiong and Dang Gui promote the circulation of Blood and sedate the pain.
- Mu Xiang promotes the circulation of Qi and relieves the pain.
- Sang Zhi and Gui Zhi together regulate the Qi and Blood, warm the channels and dispel Wind-Cold-Damp.
- Cang Zhu dries Damp and relieves the pain.
- Zhi Gan Cao harmonises the actions of the other herbs in the prescription.

Modifications

1. If there is a heavy sensation of the shoulder, add Jiang Huang *Rhizoma Curcumae Recens* 10 g and Qing Feng Teng *Caulis Sinomenii* 20 g to eliminate Damp and relieve the pain.
2. If there is an aversion to cold, add Fu Zi *Radix Aconiti Lateralis Praeparata* 6 g and Xi Xin *Herba Asari* 3 g to warm the channels and relieve the pain.
3. If the shoulder is swollen, add Tu Fu Ling, *Rhizoma Smilacis Glabrae* 20 g and Ban Xia *Rhizoma Pinelliae* 10 g and eliminate Damp and reduce the swelling.

Patent remedy

Tian Ma Qu Feng Bu Pian *Gastrodia Dispel Wind Formula Tablet*

ACUPUNCTURE TREATMENT

GB-20 Fengchi, LI-15 Jianyu, TE-5 Waiguan, SI-9 Jianzhen, SI-11 Tianzong, ST-36 Zusanli and ST-40 Fenglong. Reducing method is used on all these points.

Explanations

- GB-20 is the meeting point of the Gall Bladder channel and the Yang Linking Vessel. This vessel connects with all the Yang channels and dominates the superficial level of the body. Needling at GB-20 eliminates Wind-Damp to stop the pain.
- LI-15, the meeting point of the Bright Yang channel of the hand and the Yang Heel Vessel, regulates the circulation of Qi in the channels and collateral, eliminates Cold and Damp and relieves the pain.
- SI-9 and SI-11, the local points, relieve the shoulder pain.
- TE-5, the Connecting point of the Triple Burner channel, promotes the circulation of Qi, dispels Cold and Damp and relieves the pain.
- ST-36, the Sea point of the Stomach channel, and ST-40, the Connecting point, promote the circulation of Qi, eliminate Damp and relieve the pain. These two points can be needled whilst moving the shoulder joints to promote the circulation of Qi and relieve the pain.

Modifications

1. If the shoulder pain occurs at the place where the Lung channel passes through, add LU-3, LU-4 and LU-5 to promote the circulation of Qi in the channel and sedate the pain.
2. If the shoulder pain occurs at the place where the Large Intestine channel passes through, add LI-6, LI-7 and LI-14 to regulate the channel and sedate the pain.
3. If the shoulder pain occurs at the place where the Triple Burner channel passes through, add TE-7 and TE-14 to harmonise the collateral and sedate the pain.
4. If the shoulder pain occurs at the place where the Small Intestine channel passes through, add SI-4 and SI-6 to harmonise the collateral and sedate the pain.

5. If there is pain in the scapular region, add SI-10 and SI-11 to harmonise the collateral and sedate the pain.

6. If there is stiffness and pain in the neck, add GB-21 and SI-14 to promote the circulation of Qi and Blood and relieve the neck stiffness and pain.

7. If there is a headache, add Extra Taiyang and Extra Yintang to sedate the headache.

8. If there is an aversion to cold, add moxibustion to dispel Wind-Damp and relieve Cold.

9. If there is nausea and vomiting, add PC-6 and CV-12 to harmonise the Stomach and help the Stomach-Qi to descend.

Case history

A 45-year-old woman had been suffering from left shoulder pain for 6 months. The onset of the pain was gradual and it had worsened recently. She was diagnosed as having periarthritis of the shoulder joint. When she came to the clinic, her shoulder pain was characterised as heaviness, located mainly at the Large Intestine channel and Small Intestine channel, and aggravated by exposure to cold or in rainy weather, improving with warmth. She could not lift her left arm, and also had a pale tongue with a white coating and a wiry pulse.

Diagnosis
Incomplete disappearance of Wind-Cold-Damp.

Principle of treatment
Dispel Wind-Damp, promote Qi circulation and relieve the pain.

Acupuncture treatment
LI-4, LI-15, SI-9, SI-11, GB-21 and ST-39. Reducing method is used on all these points. Treatment was given every other day.

Explanations
- LI-4, the Source point of the Large Intestine channel, promotes the circulation of Qi and relieves the pain.
- GB-21 regulates the circulation of Qi and relieves spasm of the muscles and tendons in the shoulder.
- LI-15, the meeting point of the Bright Yang channel of the hand and the Yang Heel Vessel, regulates the circulation of Qi in the channels and collateral, eliminates Wind-Cold and dispels Damp.
- SI-4, the Source point, is used to promote the circulation of Qi and dispel Wind-Cold and Damp.
- SI-9 and SI-11 are local points for regulating Qi and relieving the pain.
- ST-40, the Connecting point of the Stomach channel, promotes the circulation of Qi, eliminates Damp and relieves the pain.

The patient was required to move her shoulder joint when needled at ST-40. She also received guidance in shoulder exercises every morning.

After 20 days of treatment and exercise, her shoulder pain had disappeared completely. A year later, she was followed up by letter and she stated she had felt no pain after the acupuncture treatment.

STAGNATION OF QI IN THE CHANNELS

Symptoms and signs

Shoulder pain with a distending or numb sensation, no palpable pain spots, which starts or is aggravated by poor mood, accompanied by irritability, insomnia, a migraine headache, irregular menstruation, a poor appetite, hypochondriac pain, lower abdominal pain, a red tongue with a white coating and a wiry pulse.

Principle of treatment

Smooth Liver, regulate the Liver-Qi and relieve the pain.

HERBAL TREATMENT

Prescription

XIAO YAO SAN
Free and Relaxed Powder
Chai Hu *Radix Bupleuri* 10 g
Dang Gui *Radix Angelicae Sinensis* 10 g
Bai Shao *Radix Paeoniae Alba* 20 g
Gan Cao *Radix Glycyrrhizae* 5 g
Bo He *Herba Menthae* 5 g
Sang Zhi *Ramulus Mori* 20 g
Xiang Fu *Rhizoma Cyperi* 6 g

Explanations

- Bai Shao and Dang Gui smooth the Liver, nourish the Blood and strengthen the Liver.
- Chai Hu, Xiang Fu and Bo He regulate and promote the circulation of Liver-Qi so as to remove Qi stagnation in the Liver. These herbs may also serve to relieve pain.
- Sang Zhi regulates the circulation of Qi, harmonises the collateral and relieves shoulder pain.
- Gan Cao harmonises the actions of the other herbs in the prescription.

Modifications

1. If there is a sharp shoulder pain, add Yan Hu Suo *Rhizoma Corydalis* 10 g and Yu Jin *Radix Curcumae* 10 g to promote the circulation of Qi and relieve the pain.

2. If there is a migraine, add Chuan Xiong *Rhizoma Ligustici Chuanxiong* 10 g to regulate the Liver-Qi and sedate the headache.
3. If there is low abdominal pain, add Wu Yao *Radix Linderae* 10 g and Ju He *Semen Citri Reticulatae* 10 g to regulate the circulation of Qi and to relieve the pain.
4. If there is irregular menstruation, add Huai Niu Xi *Radix Achyranthis Bidentatae* 10 g and Yi Mu Cao *Herba Leonuri* 10 g to promote the circulation of Qi and regulate the circulation of Blood.

Patent remedy

Xiao Yao Wan *Free and Relaxed Pill*

ACUPUNCTURE TREATMENT

LI-4 Hegu, TE-5 Waiguan, PC-6 Neiguan, SP-6 Sanyinjiao, LR-3 Taichong and GB-20 Fengchi. Even method is used on these points.

Explanations

- LI-4, the Source point of the Large Intestine channel, promotes the circulation of Qi and relieves the shoulder pain.
- PC-6, the Connecting point of the Pericardium channel, and LR-3, the Source and Stream point of the Liver channel, regulate the circulation of Qi, smooth the Liver and remove the stagnation of Qi.
- TE-5, the Connecting point of the Triple Burner channel, harmonises the collateral and relieves the shoulder pain.
- Long-standing stagnation of Qi may in turn cause stagnation of Blood. SP-6, the crossing point of the three Yin channels of the foot, regulates the Blood and removes Blood stagnation.
- GB-20 calms the Liver, regulates the circulation of Qi and relieves the pain.
- GV-20 calms the Mind and improves the mood.

Modifications

1. If the shoulder pain occurs at the place where the Lung channel passes through, add LU-3, LU-4 and LU-5 to promote the circulation of Qi in the channel and sedate the pain.
2. If the shoulder pain occurs at the place where the Large Intestine channel passes through, add LI-6, LI-7 and LI-14 to regulate the channel and sedate the pain.
3. If the shoulder pain occurs at the place where the Triple Burner channel passes through, add TE-7 and TE-14 to harmonise the collateral and sedate the pain.
4. If the shoulder pain occurs at the place where the Small Intestine channel passes through, add SI-4, SI-6, SI-9 and SI-10 to harmonise the collateral and sedate the pain.
5. If there is pain in the scapular region, add SI-11 and SI-12 to harmonise the collateral and sedate the pain.
6. If there is stiffness and pain of the neck, add GB-21 and SI-14 to promote the circulation of Qi and Blood and relieve the neck stiffness and pain.
7. If there is a headache, add Extra Taiyang and Extra Yintang to sedate the headache.
8. If there is hypochondriac pain, add LR-14 and GB-41 to regulate the circulation of Qi and relieve the pain.
9. If there is lower abdominal pain, add ST-29 and SP-9 to regulate the circulation of Qi and relieve the pain.
10. If there is irregular menstruation, add LR-12 and KI-3 to regulate the menstruation.
11. If there is insomnia, add HT-7 and BL-15 to calm the Heart and tranquillise the Mind.
12. If there is irritability, add LR-2 and GV-20 to regulate the circulation of Qi and calm the Mind.

Case history

A 47-year-old woman had been suffering from shoulder pain on both sides for nearly a year. She complained of shoulder pain with numb limbs when she was angry or during stressful periods. Sometimes she had a headache before her menstrual period. She had a general check-up and was diagnosed as having a climacteric depression. Besides the shoulder pain, she had a headache, irregular menstruation, a dull feeling in her stomach and a sensation of numbness on her tongue. Her tongue was red with a white coating, and her pulse was wiry.

Diagnosis
Stagnation of Liver-Qi.

Principle of treatment
Regulate Liver-Qi, remove Qi stagnation and relieve the pain.

Herbal treatment
XIAO YAO SAN
Free and Relaxed Powder
Chai Hu *Radix Bupleuri* 10 g
Dang Gui *Radix Angelicae Sinensis* 10 g
Bai Shao *Radix Paeoniae Alba* 20 g
Gan Cao *Radix Glycyrrhizae* 5 g
Bo He *Herba Menthae* 3 g
Yu Jin *Radix Curcumae* 10 g

Jiang Huang *Rhizoma Curcumae Longae* 10 g
Huang Qin *Radix Scutellariae* 10 g

Explanations

- Chai Hu promotes the circulation of Qi in the Liver and smoothes the Liver.
- Bai Shao and Dang Gui nourish the Blood and strengthen the physiological function of the Liver.
- Bo He and Huang Qin cool the Liver and promote the circulation of Qi in it.
- Yu Jin helps Chai Hu to regulate the Liver-Qi and relieve the pain.
- Jiang Huang regulates the Qi and relieves shoulder pain.
- Gan Cao harmonises the actions of the other herbs in the prescription.

The patient received daily herbal treatment. Her shoulder pain was relieved after 6 weeks of treatment. A year later, she was followed up by letter and she replied that she had experienced no further shoulder pain since the herbal treatment.

STAGNATION OF BLOOD IN THE CHANNELS

Symptoms and signs

Long-standing shoulder pain with a fixed location, stabbing pain, history of traumatic injury to the shoulder joint, and swelling of the joint, worsening of the pain at night, accompanied by a purplish colour to the face, a purplish tongue with a thin coating and a wiry pulse.

Principle of treatment

Promote circulation of Qi and Blood, remove Blood stasis and sedate the pain.

HERBAL TREATMENT

Prescription

SHEN TONG ZHU YU TANG
Meridian Passage
Qin Jiao *Radix Gentianae Macrophyllae* 10 g
Chuan Xiong *Rhizoma Ligustici Chuanxiong* 12 g
Tao Ren *Semen Persicae* 10 g
Hong Hua *Flos Carthami* 6 g
Qiang Huo *Rhizoma seu Radix Notopterygii* 10 g
Mo Yao *Resina Myrrhae* 6 g
Xiang Fu *Rhizoma Cyperi* 10 g
Di Long *Lumbricus* 10 g
Dang Gui *Radix Angelicae Sinensis* 12 g
Jiang Huang *Rhizoma Curcumae Longae* 10 g
Yan Hu Suo *Rhizoma Corydalis* 15 g
Gan Cao *Radix Glycyrrhizae* 6 g

Explanations

- Dang Gui, Chuang Xiong, Tao Ren and Hong Hua promote the circulation of Blood and eliminate Blood stasis.
- Di Long, Mo Yao and Yan Hu Suo eliminate Blood stasis, promote circulation in the collateral and sedate the pain.
- Xiang Fu promotes the circulation of Qi to reinforce the effect of promoting the circulation of Blood.
- Jiang Huang promotes the circulation of Qi and relieves the shoulder pain.
- Qin Jiao and Qiang Huo eliminate Damp and Wind to stop the pain.
- Gan Cao harmonises the herbs in the formula.

Modifications

1. If the pain is severe, add Xu Chang Qing *Radix Cynanchi Paniculati* 10 g and Wei Ling Xian *Radix Clematidis* 15 g to promote the circulation of Qi and relieve the pain.
2. If there are palpitations, shortness of breath and lassitude, add Dang Shen *Radix Codonopsis Pilosulae* 10 g to reinforce the Qi and regulate the respiration.
3. If there is irritability and insomnia, add Suan Zao Ren *Semen Ziziphi Spinosae* 15 g and Ye Jiao Teng *Caulis Polygoni Multiflori* 15 g to relieve the pain and calm the Mind.

Patent remedy

Xiao Huo Luo Dan *Minor Invigorate the Collaterals Special Pill*

ACUPUNCTURE TREATMENT

SP-6 Sanyinjiao, SP-10 Xuehai, LI-4 Hegu, LR-3 Taichong and Ah Shi points. Reducing method is used on these points.

Explanations

- LI-4, the Source point of the Large Intestine channel, and LR-3, the Stream and Source point of the Liver channel, promote the circulation of Qi and Blood and relieve the pain.
- SP-6, the crossing points of the three Yin channels of the foot, and SP-10 promote the circulation of Blood and remove Blood stasis.
- The Ah Shi points regulate the circulation of Qi and Blood, harmonise the collateral and remove Blood stasis so as to relieve the pain.

Modifications

1. If the shoulder pain occurs at the place where the Lung channel passes through, add LU-3, LU-4 and LU-5 to promote the circulation of Qi in the channel and sedate the pain.
2. If the shoulder pain occurs at the place where the Large Intestine channel passes through, add LI-6, LI-7 and LI-14 to regulate the channel and sedate the pain.
3. If the shoulder pain occurs at the place where the Triple Burner channel passes through, add TE-7 and TE-14 to harmonise the collateral and sedate the pain.
4. If the shoulder pain occurs at the place where the Small Intestine channel passes through, add SI-4, SI-6, SI-9 and SI-10 to harmonise the collateral and sedate the pain.
5. If there is pain at the scapular region, add SI-11 and SI-12 to harmonise the collateral and sedate the pain.
6. If there is stiffness in the shoulder joint, add GB-34 to promote the circulation of Qi, harmonise the collateral and improve joint movement.
7. If there is neck pain, add GB-21 and SI-14 to promote the circulation of Qi and Blood and relieve the neck pain.
8. If there is numbness and heaviness in the shoulder, add ST-40 and SP-9 to promote the circulation of Qi, harmonise the collateral and eliminate Damp.
9. If there is chest pain, add PC-6 and HT-5, the Connecting points, to regulate the circulation of Qi and Blood in the chest and relieve the chest pain.

ACCUMULATION OF DAMP-PHLEGM IN THE CHANNELS

Symptoms and signs

Long-standing shoulder pain, with a heavy sensation, limitation of shoulder movement, and soreness or numbness of the muscle, accompanied by dizziness, lassitude, nausea, painful and swollen joints, a poor appetite, a feeling of fullness on the stomach, a white and sticky tongue coating and a deep and slippery pulse.

Principle of treatment

Promote Qi circulation, dispel Damp-Phlegm and relieve the pain.

HERBAL TREATMENT

Prescription

BAN XIA BAI ZHU TIAN MA TANG
Pinellia–Atractylodes–Gastrodia Decoction
Tian Ma *Rhizoma Gastrodiae* 10 g
Bai Zhu *Rhizoma Atractylodis Macrocephalae* 10 g
Ban Xia *Rhizoma Pinelliae* 10 g
Chen Pi *Pericarpium Citri Reticulatae* 10 g
Fu Ling *Poria* 20 g
Gan Cao *Radix Glycyrrhizae* 5 g
Bai Jie Zi *Semen Sinapis Albae* 10 g
Qing Pi *Pericarpium Citri Reticulatae Viride* 10 g
Sang Zhi *Ramulus Mori* 15 g
Qiang Huo *Rhizoma seu Radix Notopterygii* 10 g

Explanations

- Tian Ma smoothes the Liver and eliminates Wind-Phlegm.
- Ban Xia, Bai Zhu and Fu Ling strengthen the Spleen and Stomach, dry Damp and resolve Phlegm.
- Chen Pi and Qing Pi promote the circulation of Qi and resolve Phlegm.
- Bai Jie Zi eliminates Phlegm in the channels and resolves blockage in them.
- Sang Zhi and Qiang Huo regulate the circulation of Qi in the channels, resolve Damp-Phlegm and relieve the shoulder pain.
- Gan Cao harmonises the actions of the other herbs in the prescription.

Modifications

1. If the shoulder is swollen, add Tong Cao *Medulla Tetrapanacis* 10 g and Gui Zhi *Ramulus Cinnamomi* 6 g to warm the channels and eliminate Phlegm.
2. If the arm is numb or sore, add Chang Pu *Rhizoma Acori Graminei* 10 g and Yuan Zhi *Radix Polygalae* 10 g to eliminate Wind-Phlegm and regulate the circulation of Qi in the channels.
3. If there is fullness of the Stomach, add Guang Mu Xiang *Radix Saussureae Lappae* 10 g and Dan Nan Xing *Rhizoma Arisaematis Praeparatum Cum Felle Bovis* 10 g to resolve Phlegm and calm down the Stomach-Qi.
4. If there is pain at night, add Dang Gui *Radix Angelicae Sinensis* 10 g, Tao Ren *Semen Persicae* 10 g and Shui Zhi *Hirudo* 6 g to remove Blood stagnation.

Patent remedy

Ren Shen Zai Zao Wan *Ginseng Restorative Pills*

ACUPUNCTURE TREATMENT

LI-4 Hegu, LI-15 Jianyu, TE-6 Zhigou, TE-14 Jianliao, SP-6 Sanyinjiao, SP-9 Yinlingquan, ST-40 Fenglong and Ah Shi points. Reducing method is used on these points.

Explanations

- LI-4, the Source point, and LI-15, the local point on the Large Intestine channel, regulate the Qi, eliminate Phlegm and relieve the pain.
- TE-5, the Connecting point of the Triple Burner channel, and TE-14, the local point on the same channel, promote the circulation of Qi, harmonise the collateral and sedate the shoulder pain.
- SP-6, the crossing point of the Spleen, Kidney and Liver channels, SP9, the Sea point, and ST-40, the Connecting point, regulate Qi circulation and eliminate Phlegm in the channels.
- The Ah Shi points promote Qi circulation and relieve the pain.

Modifications

1. If the shoulder pain occurs at the place where the Lung channel passes through, add LU-3, LU-4 and LU-5 to promote the circulation of Qi in the channel and sedate the pain.
2. If the shoulder pain occurs at the place where the Large Intestine channel passes through, add LI-6, LI-7 and LI-14 to regulate the channel and sedate the pain.
3. If the shoulder pain occurs at the place where the Triple Burner channel passes through, add TE-7 and TE-14 to harmonise the collateral and sedate the pain.
4. If the shoulder pain occurs at the place where the Small Intestine channel passes through, add SI-4, SI-6, SI-9 and SI-10 to harmonise the collateral and sedate the pain.
5. If there is pain in the scapular region, add SI-11 and SI-12 to harmonise the collateral and sedate the pain.
6. If the shoulder joint is stiff, add GB-34 to promote the circulation of Qi, harmonise the collateral and improve joint movement.
7. If there is neck pain, add GB-21 and SI-14 to promote the circulation of Qi and Blood and relieve the neck pain.
8. If there is limitation of shoulder movement, add GB-34, the Gathering point for the tendons, to promote the circulation of Qi and increase the range of movement.
9. If the shoulder is swollen, add TE-6 and ST-39 to promote the circulation of Qi, eliminate Phlegm and reduce the swelling.
10. If there is a feeling of dullness or fullness in the stomach, add CV-12, the Front Collecting point of the Stomach and the Gathering point for the Fu organs, and SP-4, the Connecting point, to harmonise the Stomach, help the Stomach-Qi descend and relieve nausea.
11. If the appetite is poor, add SP-3, the Source point, to activate the Spleen and improve the appetite.

Elbow pain 36

肘
痛

Elbow pain may occur in one or both elbows, but is mostly on one side. According to TCM theory, it can be caused either by invasion of External factors or by stagnation of Blood. Elbow pain may be attributed to any of the following disorders in Western medicine: tennis elbow, subluxation of the capitulum radii, rheumatism, rheumatoid arthritis, muscle strain or traumatic injury to the middle of the arm, and deformation or injury to the elbow joint.

Aetiology and pathology

Invasion of External factors

Overexposure to Wind, Cold, Heat or Damp may allow these pathogenic factors to invade the elbow.

Wind has an uprising nature. It usually attacks the body in combination with other pathogenic factors, for instance, Wind-Cold, Wind-Damp or Wind-Cold-Damp. Cold has the characteristics of contraction and stagnation. If Wind-Cold invades, it causes contraction of muscles and tendons around the elbow, leading to stagnation of the Qi and Blood in the channels, which causes elbow pain.

Damp has the characteristics of stagnation and viscosity. When it attacks the body, it tends to obstruct the free flow of Qi and Blood, again leading to stagnation of Qi and Blood, and elbow pain.

Heat has the characteristics of uprising and burning, and a tendency to move upwards. Furthermore, it may consume the Blood and Yin, causing concentration of the Blood and Body Fluids, which again leads to stagnation of Qi and Blood. If Wind-Heat invades the elbow, it manifests as elbow pain with swelling and redness, an aversion to heat, and a preference for cold.

Stagnation of Blood

The Blood should circulate freely in the channels. Overwork, playing too much sport, or overuse of the elbow may impair the tendons and collateral, leading to stagnation of the Blood, and causing elbow pain. Physical trauma, a wound, adhesions after an operation and inappropriate operation may all directly damage the channels and muscles, which leads to stagnation of Blood and causes elbow pain.

Treatment based on differentiation

Differentiation

Differentiation of External invasion or Blood stagnation should be made in order to set up an accurate diagnosis.

— Acute onset of elbow pain with a short duration, accompanied by External symptoms, is usually caused by invasion of External pathogenic factors.
— Acute onset of elbow pain with an obvious history of trauma or operation is usually caused by stagnation of Blood.
— Chronic onset of elbow pain without a history of trauma, but of long duration, and accompanied by symptoms such as stabbing pain, aggravation of the pain at night, or inability to lie on the affected side, is also usually caused by stagnation of Blood

Treatment

INVASION OF EXTERNAL FACTORS

Symptoms and signs

Acute elbow pain, with an aversion to cold or wind, and varying with weather changes, accompanied by limitation of movement, a thin and white tongue coating and a superficial and tight pulse.

Principle of treatment

Dispel Wind and eliminate External factors.

HERBAL TREATMENT

Prescription

FANG FENG TANG
Ledebouriella Decoction
Fang Feng *Radix Ledebouriellae* 10 g
Chuan Xiong *Rhizoma Ligustici Chuanxiong* 10 g
Gan Cao *Radix Glycyrrhizae* 6 g
Fu Ling *Poria* 15 g
Ma Huang *Herba Ephedrae* 6 g
Dang Gui *Radix Angelicae Sinensis* 10 g
Sang Zhi *Ramulus Mori* 12 g
Qin Jiao *Radix Gentianae Macrophyllae* 10 g

Explanations

- Fang Feng, Sang Zhi and Qin Jiao dispel Wind and relieve the pain.
- Ma Huang eliminates Cold, regulates Qi, harmonises the collateral and relieves the pain.
- Dang Gui and Chuan Xiong promote the circulation of Qi and Blood, eliminate Blood stasis and relieve the pain.
- Fu Ling eliminates Damp-Phlegm.
- Can Cao harmonises the function of the other herbs in the prescription.

Modifications

1. If there is severe pain at night, add Xi Xin *Herba Asari* 3 g and Yan Hu Suo *Rhizoma Corydalis* 15 g to promote the circulation of Blood and relieve the pain.
2. If the elbow has an aversion to cold, add Gan Jiang *Rhizoma Zingiberis* 5 g and Gui Zhi *Ramulus Cinnamomi* 10 g to warm the channels and dispel Cold.
3. If there is a fever, add Chai Hu *Radix Bupleuri* 15 g to dispel Wind and reduce the fever.
4. If there is a feeling of heaviness in the elbow, add Qiang Huo *Rhizoma seu Radix Notopterygii* 10 g to eliminate Damp, promote the circulation of Qi and relieve the pain.
5. If the elbow is red and swollen, add Ren Dong Teng *Caulis Lonicerae* 15 g and Xi Xian Cao *Herba Siegesbeckiae* 10 g to dispel Wind and clear Heat.
6. If there is a fever and a burning sensation at the elbow, add Sheng Di Huang *Radix Rehmanniae Recens* 10 g and Chi Shao *Radix Paeoniae Rubra* 10 g to clear Heat, reduce the fever and remove Toxin.
7. If there is neck pain, add Ge Gen *Radix Puerariae* 10 g to harmonise the collateral and relieve the pain in the neck.
8. If there is a headache, add Chuan Xiong *Rhizoma Ligustici Chuanxiong* 10 g and Man Jing Zi *Fructus Viticis* 10 g to dispel Wind and sedate the headache.

Patent remedies

Feng Shi Pian *Wind-Damp Tablet* for invasion of Wind-Cold and Damp
Feng Shi Xiao Tong Pian *Wind-Damp Dispel Pain Pill* for invasion of Wind, Damp and Heat.

ACUPUNCTURE TREATMENT

LI-4 Hegu, LI-10 Shousanli, TE-5 Waiguan, GB-20 Fengchi and Ah Shi points. Reducing method is used on these points.

Explanations

- LI-4, the Source point of the Large Intestine channel, dispels Wind, relieves External symptoms, promotes the circulation of Qi and relieves the pain.
- LI-10 promotes the circulation of Qi in the channel, dispels Wind and relieves the pain.
- TE-5, the Connecting point of the Triple Burner channel, dispels Wind, harmonises the collateral and relieves the pain.
- GB-20 dispels Wind, relieves external symptoms and sedates the pain.
- The Ah Shi points dispel Wind-Cold, promote the circulation of Qi in the locality and relieve the pain.

Modifications

1. If there is pain along the Large Intestine channel, add LI-3, the Stream point, LI-6, the Connecting point, and LI-7, the Accumulation point, to harmonise the Large Intestine collateral, promote circulation in the channel and relieve the pain.
2. If there is pain along the Triple Burner channel, add TE-3, the Stream point, TE-7, the Accumulation point, and TE-10, the Sea point, to harmonise the collateral, promote circulation in the Triple Burner channel and relieve the pain.
3. If there is pain along the Small Intestine channel, add SI-3, the Stream point, and SI-6, the Accumulation point, to harmonise the collateral, promote circulation in the Small Intestine channel and relieve the pain.
4. If there is pain along the Lung channel, add LU-9, the Stream point and Source point from the Lung channel, LU-7, the Connecting point, LU-6, the Accumulation point, and LU-5, the Sea point, to harmonise the collateral, promote circulation in the Lung channel and relieve the pain.
5. If there is pain along the Heart channel, add HT-7, the Stream point, HT-5, the Connecting point, HT-6, the Accumulation point, and HT-3, the Sea point, to harmonise the collateral, promote circulation in the Heart channel and relieve the pain.
6. If the elbow has an aversion to cold, add moxibustion and BI-12 to warm the channels and dispel Cold.
7. If there is a stabbing pain, or an aggravation of pain at night, add SP-6 to promote the circulation of Blood and relieve the pain.
8. If there is a feeling of heaviness in the elbow, add SP-9, the Sea point, and ST-40, the Connecting point, to eliminate Damp, promote the circulation of Qi and relieve the pain.
9. If the elbow is red and swollen, add LI-2 and TE-2, the Spring points, to dispel Wind, clear Heat and reduce the swelling.
10. If there is a constant pain in the elbow, add LI-1 and TE-1, the Well points, to open the collateral and remove obstruction in the channels.
11. If the arm is painful, add LI-15 and TE-14 to promote the circulation of Qi and Blood and relieve the pain.
12. If there is neck pain, add GB-21 and BL-11 to harmonise the collateral, strengthen the bones and relieve the pain.
13. If there is a headache, add Extra Yintang to dispel Wind and sedate the headache.
14. If there is a fever and aversion to cold, add BL-13 to dispel Wind-Cold and relieve External symptoms.
15. If there is generalised body pain, add BL-58, the Connecting point, and BL-63, the Accumulation point, to dispel External factors and relieve the pain.

STAGNATION OF BLOOD

Symptoms and signs

Traumatic history or history of elbow strain, elbow pain of long duration, stabbing pain in the elbow, which is aggravated at night or by immobility, accompanied by a limitation of elbow movement, a dislike of pressure and massage, a purplish tongue and a wiry pulse.

Principle of treatment

Promote the circulation of Blood, eliminate Blood stasis and relieve the pain.

HERBAL TREATMENT

Prescription

SHEN TONG ZHU YU TANG
Meridian Passage
Qin Jiao *Radix Gentianae Macrophyllae* 10 g
Chuan Xiong *Rhizoma Ligustici Chuanxiong* 10 g
Tao Ren *Semen Persicae* 10 g
Hong Hua *Flos Carthami* 6 g
Qiang Huo *Rhizoma seu Radix Notopterygii* 10 g
Xiang Fu *Rhizoma Cyperi* 10 g
Wu Ling Zhi *Faeces Trogopterorum* 6 g
Jiang Huang *Rhizoma Curcumae Longae* 10 g
Di Long *Lumbricus* 10 g
Dang Gui *Radix Angelicae Sinensis* 12 g
Gan Cao *Radix Glycyrrhizae* 6 g

Explanations

- Dang Gui, Chuan Xiong, Tao Ren and Hong Hua promote the circulation of Blood and eliminate Blood stasis.
- Wu Ling Zhi eliminates Blood stasis and sedates the pain.
- Since the circulation of Qi leads to the circulation of Blood, Xiang Fu is used to promote the circulation of Qi so as to reinforce the effect of promoting Blood circulation.
- Jiang Huang promotes the circulation of Qi and Blood in the channels and relieves the elbow pain.
- Di Long promotes circulation in the collateral and removes obstruction in the channels.
- Qiang Huo and Qin Jiao harmonise the collateral and relieve the elbow pain.
- Gan Cao harmonises the function of the other herbs in the prescription.

Modifications

1. If there is severe pain at night, add Yan Hu Suo *Rhizoma Corydalis* 12 g and Mo Yao *Resina Myrrhae* 5 g to remove Blood stasis and relieve the pain.
2. If there is numbness in the elbow, add Mu Xiang *Radix Aucklandiae* 12 g and Gui Zhi *Ramulus Cinnamomi* 6 g to promote the circulation of Qi and Blood.
3. If there is an aversion to cold, add Gan Jiang *Rhizoma Zingiberis* 10 g and Rou Gui *Cortex Cinnamomi* 3 g to warm the channels and dispel Cold.

Patent remedy

Xiao Huo Luo Dan *Minor Invigorate the Collaterals Special Pill*

ACUPUNCTURE TREATMENT

LI-3 Sanjian, LI-4 Hegu, LI-6 Pianli, LI-10 Shousanli, TE-5 Waiguan, TE-10 Tianjing, LR-3 Taichong and SP-6 Sanyinjiao. Reducing method is used on these points.

Explanations

- LI-3, the Stream point, and LI-6, the Connecting point, harmonise the collateral, promote circulation in the channels and relieve the pain.
- LI-4, the Source point of the Large Intestine channel, promotes circulation in the channel and relieves the pain.
- TE-5, the Connecting point, harmonises the collateral and sedates the pain.

- LI-10 and TE-10, two local points, promote the circulation of Qi and Blood in the locality and sedate the pain.
- LR-3, the Source point and the Stream point from the Liver channel, promotes the circulation of Qi and relieves the pain.
- SP-6, the crossing point of three Yin channels, promotes the circulation of Blood and eliminates Blood stasis so as to sedate the pain.

Modifications

1. If there is pain along the Large Intestine channel, add LI-7, the Accumulation point, and LI-8 to harmonise the Large Intestine collateral, promote circulation in the channel and relieve the pain.
2. If the pain is along the Triple Burner channel, add TE-3, the Stream point, and TE-7, the Accumulation point, to harmonise the collateral, promote circulation in the channel and relieve the pain.
3. If the pain is along the Small Intestine channel, add SI-3, the Stream point, and SI-6, the Accumulation point, to harmonise the collateral, promote circulation in the channel and relieve the pain.
4. If the pain is along the Lung channel, add LU-7, the Connecting point, LU-6, the Accumulation point, and LU-5, the Sea point, to harmonise the collateral, promote circulation in the channel and relieve the pain.
5. If the pain is along the Heart channel, add HT-7, the Stream point, HT-5, the Connecting point, HT-6, the Accumulation point and HT-3, the Sea point, to harmonise the collateral, promote circulation in the channel and relieve the pain.
6. If there is limitation of movement in the elbow joint, add one or two points on the knee from the corresponding channel, to regulate the circulation of Qi and improve the joint function.
7. If there is severe pain at night, add BL-17, the Gathering point for the Blood, and HT-7 to promote the circulation of the Blood, calm the Mind and sedate the pain.
8. If the elbow is red and swollen, add LI-2 to clear Heat and reduce the swelling.
9. If there is a stabbing pain in the bones, add LI-1 to promote the circulation of Blood and eliminate Blood stasis in the joint.

Case history

A 27-year-old man had been suffering from right elbow pain at a fixed location for a month. It had started after physical trauma to the elbow. He did not go for treatment immediately. Later on it was diagnosed as tennis elbow. The main manifestations were intermittent stabbing pain in the elbow, with fixed location near to LI-11, which worsened at night, with an inability to lie down on the same side, a slightly purplish tongue with a thin coating and a deep and wiry pulse.

Diagnosis
Elbow pain due to stagnation of Blood.

Principle of treatment
Circulate the Blood, smooth the collateral and sedate the pain.

Herbal treatment
TAO HONG SI WU TANG
Four-Substance Decoction with Safflower and Peach Pit
Dang Gui *Radix Angelicae Sinensis* 10 g
Sheng Di Huang *Radix Rehmanniae Recens* 12 g
Chi Shao *Radix Paeoniae Rubra* 10 g
Chuan Xiong *Rhizoma Ligustici Chuanxiong* 6 g
Jiang Huang *Rhizoma Curcumae* 10 g
Gui Zhi *Ramulus Cinnamomi* 10 g
Tao Ren *Semen Persicae* 10 g
Hong Hua *Flos Carthami* 10 g

Explanations

- Chuan Xiong and Hong Hua promote the circulation of Blood and remove Blood stagnation.
- Dang Gui and Tao Ren regulate the circulation of Blood, remove Blood stagnation and relieve the pain.
- Jiang Huang and Gui Zhi are specific herbs for elbow pain caused by Blood stagnation, and harmonise the collateral and promote circulation in the channels.

- Sheng Di Huang and Chi Shao regulate the circulation of Blood, prevent the formation of Heat in the Blood and relieve the pain.

Acupuncture treatment
LI-4, LI-6, LI-7, LI-11, LR-3 and SP-6. Since the pain was mainly located along the Large Intestine channel, several points from this channel were prescribed. Reducing method was used on these points.

Explanations

- LI-4, the Source point of the Large Intestine channel, and LI-11, the Sea point, promote circulation in the channel and relieve the pain.
- LI-6, the Connecting point, and LI-7, the Accumulation point, harmonise the collateral, promote circulation in the channels and relieve the pain.
- LR-3, the Source point and the Stream point of the Liver channel, promotes the circulation of Qi and relieves the pain.
- SP-6, the crossing point of the three Yin channels of the foot, promotes the circulation of Blood and eliminates Blood stasis so as to sedate the pain.

The patient was given daily treatment. He was advised to warm the painful elbow himself with moxa three times a day, each time for about 10 minutes. He had some elbow movement every day. After a month of treatment his elbow pain was cured. He was followed up a year later and he stated he had experienced no further pain since the herbal treatment.

Wrist pain 37

腕
痛

Wrist pain may occur in one or both wrists, and sometimes the area of pain extends to the palms and arms. According to TCM theory, wrist pain may be caused by invasion of External Wind-Cold, stagnation of Phlegm-Damp in the channels, stagnation of Qi and Blood, or deficiency of Blood.

Wrist pain may be attributed to any of the following disorders in Western medicine: rheumatic pain, rheumatoid arthritis, nerve pain, tenosynovitis, ganglion, sprain of the local muscles or tendons, and tendon injury of the wrist joint.

Aetiology and pathology

Invasion of Wind-Cold

Overexposure to cold, living and working for too long in a cold environment and wearing insufficient clothing can all increase the chance of Wind-Cold invasion. Wind has the characteristic of upward movement; Cold has the characteristic of contraction and stagnation. So if Wind-Cold invades the body it causes the muscles and tendons of the wrist to contract, leading to stagnation of Qi and Blood, and this causes the wrist pain.

Accumulation of Phlegm-Damp in the channels

Living or working for a long time in a damp place, overexertion, and excessive physical labour that places a strain on the wrist may all cause the Qi to stagnate and Phlegm-Damp to accumulate in the channels around the wrist. Also, the circulation of Body Fluids is influenced by the circulation of Qi, so if the Qi stagnates in the locality, then the Body Fluids stagnate as well. If the Body Fluids stagnate this in turn may cause Phlegm-Damp to form. Once Phlegm-Damp blocks the channels, it further disturbs the circulation of Qi and Blood and causes wrist pain and swelling.

Stagnation of Qi and Blood

Qi and Blood should circulate freely in the channels of the wrist. Overstrain, physical trauma, inappropriate movements and inappropriate operations on the wrist may all block the circulation of Qi and Blood in the channels, leading to the stagnation of Qi and Blood, so wrist pain follows.

Deficiency of Blood

Excessive blood loss during the menstrual period, or during an operation, or prolonged chronic disease may lead to consumption of the Qi and Blood, which results in deficiency of Blood. The tendons and joints need to be nourished by Blood if they are to perform their function smoothly. So if there is insufficient Blood circulation in the channels, the wrist is undernourished, and this leads to wrist pain.

Treatment based on differentiation

Differentiation

Differentiation of External or Internal origin

— Acute onset of wrist pain of short duration, accompanied by External symptoms, is usually caused by invasion of External pathogenic factors.
— Chronic onset of wrist pain of long duration, accompanied by symptoms resulting from Internal disorder, is usually caused by disorder of Internal organs.

Differentiation of character of the pain

— Acute wrist pain, swelling with a cold sensation, aggravation of the pain in cold weather, or alleviation of the pain by movement, is usually caused by invasion of Wind-Cold.
— Swelling and pain of the wrist, with limitation of wrist movement, a heavy sensation of wrist and fingers, or formation of soft nodules around the wrist, is usually caused by accumulation of Phlegm-Damp in the channels.
— Chronic wrist pain, or history of traumatic injury at the wrist, or history of operation, or wrist pain with numbness, with worsening of the pain at night, or alleviation of pain by movement, is often due to stagnation of Qi and Blood.
— Slight wrist pain with numbness, weakness of the wrists and hands, a pale complexion and lips, dizziness or palpitations, is often caused by deficiency of Blood.

Treatment

INVASION OF WIND-COLD

Symptoms and signs

Acute wrist pain, swelling and pain of the wrist with a cold sensation, difficulty in relaxing or extending the wrist, worsening of the pain in cold weather, and alleviation with movement, spasm in the fingers or arms, an aversion to cold, a preference for warmth, a purplish tongue with a white coating and a wiry or tight pulse.

Principle of treatment

Dispel Cold, regulate Qi circulation and relieve the pain.

HERBAL TREATMENT

Prescription

DANG GUI SI NI TANG
Angelica Four Rebellious Decoction
Gan Jiang *Rhizoma Zingiberis* 6 g
Gui Zhi *Ramulus Cinnamomi* 10 g
Dang Gui *Radix Angelicae Sinensis* 10 g
Bai Shao *Radix Paeoniae Alba* 20 g
Xi Xin *Herba Asari* 3 g
Qing Feng Teng *Caulis Sinomenii* 20 g
Jiang Huang *Rhizoma Curcumae Longae* 10 g
Gan Cao *Radix Glycyrrhizae* 5 g

Explanations

● Gan Jiang and Gui Zhi dispel Cold, warm the channels and relieve the pain.
● Dang Gui and Bai Shao nourish the tendons, regulate the circulation of Qi and Blood in the channels and relieve the pain.
● Xi Xin is good at dispelling Wind-Cold and relieving the pain.
● Qing Feng Teng and Jiang Huang dispel Wind-Cold, promote the circulation in the channels and relieve the pain.
● Gan Cao harmonises the herbs in the formula.

Modifications

1. If there is an aversion to wind, add Fang Feng *Radix Ledebouriellae* 10 g to dispel Wind and relieve External symptoms.
2. If the wrist is swollen, add Han Fang Ji *Radix Stephaniae Tetrandrae* 10 g and Wu Jia Pi *Cortex Acanthopanacis Radicis* 10 g to eliminate Damp and reduce the swelling.
3. If there is a severe aversion to cold and muscular spasm, add Fu Zi *Radix Aconiti Lateralis Praeparata* 10 g and Rou Gui *Cortex Cinnamomi* 5 g to warm the channels and collateral and relieve the spasm.
4. If the wrist is rigid, add Di Long *Lumbricus* 10 g and Jiang Can *Bombyx Batryticatus* 10 g to relax the tendons and resolve Phlegm-Damp in the channel.
5. If there is generalised body pain, add Qiang Huo *Rhizoma seu Radix Notopterygii* 10 g and Du Huo *Radix Angelicae Pubescentis* 10 g to dispel Wind-Cold and relieve the pain.

Patent remedy

Feng Shi Pian *Wind-Damp Tablet*

ACUPUNCTURE TREATMENT

LI-3 Sanjian, LI-4 Hegu, Lu-7 Lieque, SI-4 Wangu, TE-5 Waiguan, Extra Baxie and Ah Shi points. Reducing method is used on all these points.

Explanations

- LI-3, the Stream point, and LI-4, the Source point, dispel Wind-Cold, promote circulation in the channels and relieve the pain.
- LU-7, the Connecting point of the Lung channels, dispels Wind-Cold and relieves the pain.
- SI-4, the Source point of the Small Intestine channel, and TE-5, the Connecting point of the Triple Burner channel, promote the circulation of Qi and Blood in the wrist and relieve pain.
- The Extra Baxie and Ah Shi points promote the circulation of Qi in the local channels and collateral and stop the pain.

Modifications

1. If there is a severe aversion to cold and muscular spasm, add moxibustion on LI-4, LU-7 and the Ah Shi points to warm the tendons and muscles and relieve the spasm.
2. If the wrist is swollen, add TE-6 to regulate the circulation of Qi, promote the discharge of excessive water and reduce the swelling.
3. If there is generalised body pain, add ST-40 and SP-21 to regulate the circulation of Qi and Blood and relieve the pain.

Case history

A 45-year-old woman had been suffering from wrist and finger pain on both sides for a year. She had a tense pain and in the morning there was rigidity in both wrists. She also had an aversion to cold, fatigue, a pale tongue with a white coating and a wiry pulse. At the hospital her complaint had been diagnosed as rheumatoid arthritis.

Diagnosis
Invasion of Wind-Cold with deficiency of Qi.

Principle of treatment
Dispel Wind-Cold, regulate Qi circulation, tonify Qi and relieve the pain.

Herbal treatment
DANG GUI SI NI TANG
Angelica Four Rebellious Decoction

Gui Zhi *Ramulus Cinnamomi* 10 g
Dang Gui *Radix Angelicae Sinensis* 10 g
Bai Zhu *Rhizoma Atractylodis Macrocephalae* 10 g
Dang Shen *Radix Salviae Miltiorrhizae* 10 g
Qing Feng Teng *Caulis Sinomenii* 30 g
Jiang Huang *Rhizoma Curcumae Longae* 10 g
Xi Xin *Herba Asari* 3 g
Chi Shao *Radix Paeoniae Rubra* 10 g
Huang Qi *Radix Astragali seu Hedysari* 15 g
Fu Zi *Radix Aconiti Praeparata* 10 g
Zhi Gan Cao *Radix Glycyrrhizae Praeparata* 5 g

Explanations

- Gui Zhi, Xi Xin and Fu Zi warm the channels and relieve the pain.
- Dang Gui and Chi Shao promote the circulation of Blood and relieve the wrist pain.
- Dang Shen, Huang Qi and Bai Zhu activate the Spleen and Stomach and tonify the Qi.
- Qing Feng Teng and Jiang Huang are good at dispelling Wind-Cold and relieving the joint pain.
- Zhi Gan Cao tonifies the Qi and harmonises the actions of the other herbs in the formula.

The patient was given daily treatment with this herbal decoction. She was also advised to warm her wrists with the moxa stick three times a day, for 5 to 10 minutes each time. After 1 month of treatment, her wrist and finger pain had disappeared. She was followed up 2 years later, and she stated that she had experienced no more pain since the herbal treatment.

ACCUMULATION OF PHLEGM-DAMP IN THE CHANNELS

Symptoms and signs

Swelling and pain of the wrist, limitation of wrist movement, and a heavy sensation in the wrist and fingers, accompanied by the formation of soft nodules around the wrist, a poor appetite, loose stools, a pale tongue with a white and greasy coating and a deep and slippery pulse.

Principle of treatment

Promote Qi circulation, eliminate Phlegm and relieve the pain.

HERBAL TREATMENT

Prescription

QIANG HUO SHENG SHI TANG
Notopterygium Dispelling Dampness Decoction
Qiang Huo *Rhizoma seu Radix Notopterygii* 10 g
Fu Ling *Poria* 15 g
Chuan Xiong *Rhizoma Ligustici Chuanxiong* 10 g
Gan Cao *Radix Glycyrrhizae* 6 g

Fang Feng *Radix Ledebouriellae* 6 g
Zhi Ban Xia *Rhizoma Pinelliae Praeparata* 10 g
Bai Jie Zi *Semen Sinapis Albae* 10 g

Explanations

- Qiang Huo dispels Wind-Cold-Damp from the upper body and sedates pain.
- Fang Feng dispels Wind-Cold and relieves External symptoms.
- Chuang Xiong promotes the circulation of Blood and expels Wind so as to arrest the pain.
- Zhi Ban Xia and Fu Ling dry Damp and eliminate Phlegm.
- Bai Jie Zi eliminates Phlegm and resolves Damp in the channels.
- Gan Cao coordinates the effects of the other herbs in the prescription.

Modifications

1. If there is swelling and heaviness in the wrist and fingers, add Cang Zhu *Rhizoma Atractylodis* 10 g and Yi Yi Ren *Semen Coicis* 10 g to dry Damp, reduce the swelling and relieve the pain.
2. If there is numbness in the wrist, add Di Long *Lumbricus* 10 g and Si Gua Luo *Retinervous Luffae Fructus* 10 g to resolve Phlegm-Damp in the channels and harmonise the collateral.
3. If there is a stabbing pain, or worsening of the pain at night, add Dan Shen *Radix Salviae Miltiorrhizae* 10 g and Pu Huang *Pollen Typhae* 10 g to promote the circulation of Blood and eliminate Blood stasis.
4. If the appetite is poor, add Ji Nei Jin *Endothelium Corneum Gigeriae Galli* 10 g and Mai Ya *Fructus Hordei Germinatus* 10 g to activate the Spleen and improve the appetite.
5. If there is nausea or vomiting, add Huo Xiang *Herba Agastachis* 10 g and Xuan Fu Hua *Flos Inulae* 10 g to harmonise the Stomach and help the Stomach-Qi to descend.

Patent remedy

Ren Shen Zai Zao Wan *Ginseng Restorative Pill*

ACUPUNCTURE TREATMENT

LI-4 Hegu, LI-5 Yangxi, LU-7 Lieque, TE-4 Yangchi, SI-6 Yanglao, SP-6 Sanyinjiao, SI-40 Fenglong and Ah Shi points. Reducing method was used on these points. Use of a three-edged needle is advised in order to puncture the nodules.

Explanations

- LI-4, the Source point, and LI-5 promote circulation in the channels and relieve the pain.
- LU-7, the Connecting point of the Lung channel, promotes the circulation of Qi, harmonises the collateral and relieves the pain.
- TE-6 regulates the Qi circulation, eliminates Damp and relieves the pain.
- SI-5, the River point of the Small Intestine channel, promotes the circulation of Qi, increases urination and relieves the pain.
- SP-9, the Sea point, and ST-40, the Connecting point, activate the Spleen and Stomach and resolve Damp-Phlegm in the channels.
- The Ah Shi points in the locality regulate the circulation of Qi, reduce swelling and relieve the pain. Three-edged needles are used to eliminate stagnation of Phlegm, reduce swelling and sedate the pain.

Modifications

1. If there is numbness in the wrist, add TE-5 and LI-1 to promote the circulation of Qi, harmonise the collateral and eliminate Phlegm.
2. If there is limitation of movement, add SI-5 and HT-7 to regulate the Qi and remove stagnation of Qi.
3. If the appetite is poor, add CV-12 and SP-3 to regulate the Qi in the Spleen and Stomach, harmonise the Stomach and improve the appetite.

STAGNATION OF QI AND BLOOD

Symptoms and signs

Chronic wrist pain with numbness, or history of traumatic injury to the wrist, or of wrist operation, worsening of the pain at night or with emotional upset, and alleviation with movement, accompanied by cold or purplish hands, a preference for warmth, a purplish tongue and a wiry pulse.

Principle of treatment

Promote Qi and Blood circulation, eliminate Blood stasis and relieve the pain.

HERBAL TREATMENT

Prescription

TAO HONG SI WU TANG
Four-Substance Decoction with Safflower and Peach Pit
Dang Gui *Radix Angelicae Sinensis* 12 g
Chi Shao *Radix Paeoniae Rubra* 10 g

Chuan Xiong *Rhizoma Ligustici Chuanxiong* 12 g
Tao Ren *Semen Persicae* 12 g
Hong Hua *Flos Carthami* 12 g
Mo Yao *Resina Myrrhae* 10 g
Jiang Huang *Rhizoma Curcumae* 10 g
Sang Zhi *Ramulus Mori* 15 g
Ji Xue Teng *Caulis Spatholobi* 20 g
Yu Jin *Radix Curcumae* 10 g

Explanations

- Dang Gui and Chi Shao nourish the Blood and regulate its circulation.
- Chuang Xiong, Tao Ren and Hong Hua promote the circulation of Blood and remove Blood stagnation.
- Mo Yao is also good at removing Blood stasis and relieving the pain.
- Jiang Huang and Yu Jin promote the circulation of Qi and Blood and sedate the pain.
- Sang Zhi promotes the circulation of Qi and Blood in the wrist to relieve the pain.
- Ji Xue Teng and Sang Zhi circulate the Blood, harmonise the collateral and relieve the pain.

Modifications

1. If there is a wandering or heavy pain of the arms due to invasion of Wind-Damp, add Qiang Huo *Rhizoma seu Radix Notopterygii* 10 g and Qin Jiao *Radix Gentianae Macrophyllae* 10 g to dispel the Wind and remove the Damp.
2. If there is a severe pricking pain due to traumatic injury, add Ru Xiang *Resina Olibani* 6 g and Qing Pi *Pericarpium Citri Reticulatae Viride* 10 g to increase the effect of promoting the circulation of Qi and Blood and removing Blood stasis.

Patent remedy

Xiao Huo Luo Dan *Minor Invigorate the Collaterals Special Pill*

ACUPUNCTURE TREATMENT

LI-4 Hegu, PC-7 Daling, LU-9 Taiyuan, HT-7 Shenmen, SI-4 Wangu, SI-5 Yanggu, SP-6 Sanyinjiao, LR-3 Taichong and Extra Baxie. Reducing method is used on these points.

Explanations

- LI-4, the Source point of the Large Intestine channel, and LR-3, the Source point of the Liver channel, smooth the Liver, promote the circulation of Qi and sedate the pain.
- PC-7, the Stream and Source point of the Pericardium channel, SI-4, the Source point of the Small Intestine channel, and SI-5, the River point of the Small Intestine channel, promote the circulation of Qi in the locality and relieve the pain.
- LU-9, the Stream and Source point of the Lung channel and the Gathering point for the Vessels, and SP-6, the crossing point of the three Yin channels of the foot, activate the circulation of Blood, eliminate Blood stasis and relieve the pain.
- HT-7, the Stream and Source point of the Heart channel, promotes the circulation of Blood, removes Blood stasis, calms the Heart and relieves the wrist pain.
- Extra Baxie removes Blood stasis from the locality and relieves the pain.

Modifications

1. If there is wrist pain with a heavy sensation, add TE-6 to promote urination and resolve Damp.
2. If there is numbness of the fingers, add LU-7 and LI-5 to harmonise the collateral and relieve the numbness.
3. If there is emotional upset, add PC-6 and GB-20 to calm the Liver and smooth the emotions.
4. If there is insomnia, add HT-3, the Sea point, to calm the Heart and tranquillise the Mind.

Case history

A 41-year-old man had been suffering from a stabbing pain on the left wrist for a week. He had sprained his left hand after slipping and falling to the ground. The pain was aggravated when he closed or extended his wrist, and the wrist movement was limited. His tongue was purple with a white coating and his pulse was deep and wiry.

Diagnosis
Stagnation of Blood.

Principle of treatment
Promote Qi and Blood circulation, remove Blood stasis and relieve the wrist pain.

Acupuncture treatment
HT-7, PC-6, SI-4, LU-9 and Extra Baxie. Reducing method was used on all the points.

Explanations
- HT-7, the Stream and Source point of the Heart channel, activates the circulation of Qi and relieves the wrist pain.

- SI-4, the Source point of the Small Intestine channel, promotes the circulation of Qi and Blood. PC-6, the Connecting point of the Pericardium channel, promotes the circulation of Blood. The combination of these two points has a strong function in removing Blood stasis and relieving the pain.
- LU-9, the Stream and Source point, promotes the circulation of Qi and Blood and relieves the pain.
- Extra Baxie regulates the circulation of Qi in the locality and relieves the pain.

The patient was cured after 8 days of treatment. He was followed up by letter 2 years later and he reported that he had experienced no more wrist pain since the treatment.

DEFICIENCY OF BLOOD

Symptoms and signs

Slight wrist pain, numbness and slight stiffness of the wrist, and weakness of the wrists and hands, accompanied by a pale complexion, pale lips, dizziness, palpitations, dry stools, a pale tongue with a thin and white coating, and a thready and weak pulse.

Principle of treatment

Tonify Qi, nourish Blood and sedate the pain.

HERBAL TREATMENT

Prescription

BA ZHEN TANG
Eight-Precious Decoction
Dang Gui *Radix Angelicae Sinensis* 12 g
Chuan Xiong *Rhizoma Ligustici Chuanxiong* 10 g
Bai Shao *Radix Paeoniae Alba* 12 g
Shu Di Huang *Radix Rehmanniae Praeparata* 12 g
Ren Shen *Radix Ginseng* 6 g
Bai Zhu *Rhizoma Atractylodis Macrocephalae* 12 g
Fu Ling *Poria* 12 g
Ji Xue Teng *Caulis Spatholobi* 20 g
Qin Jiao *Radix Gentianae Macrophyllae* 10 g
Sang Zhi *Ramulus Mori* 20 g
Gan Cao *Radix Glycyrrhizae* 6 g

Explanations

- Dang Gui, Bai Shao and Shu Di Huang nourish the Blood.
- Ren Shen, Bai Zhu, Fu Ling and Gan Cao strengthen the Spleen and reinforce the Qi.
- Chuan Xiong promotes the circulation of Qi and Blood and relieves obstruction in the channels.

- Sang Zhi is one of the patent herbs to relieve the wrist pain.
- Ji Xue Teng nourishes the Blood, promotes circulation in the channels and relieves the joint pain.
- Qin Jiao eliminates Wind and relieves the joint pain.

Modifications

1. If there is an aversion to cold, or cold limbs, due to deficiency of Yang, add Gui Zhi *Ramulus Cinnamomi* 10 g and San Ji Sheng *Ramulus Loranthi* 10 g to reinforce the Yang-Qi and relieve the pain.
2. If there is dizziness, add Tian Ma *Rhizoma Gastrodiae* 10 g and He Shou Wu *Radix Polygoni Multiflori* 10 g to nourish the Blood and relieve the dizziness.
3. If there is swelling in the fingers due to poor water metabolism resulting from deficiency of Spleen-Qi, add Hai Feng Teng *Caulis Piperis Futokadsure* 15 g and Ze Xie *Rhizoma Alismatis* 15 g to eliminate Damp, reduce swelling and relieve the pain.
4. If the appetite is poor, add Chen Pi *Pericarpium Citri Reticulatae* 10 g to regulate the circulation of Qi and improve the appetite.

Patent remedies

Gui Pi Wan *Tonifying the Spleen Pill*
Shi Quan Da Bu Wan *All-Inclusive Great Tonifying Pill*

ACUPUNCTURE TREATMENT

PC-7 Daling, HT-7 Shenmen, ST-36 Zusanli, SP-6 Sanyinjiao, LU-9 Taiyuan and Ah Shi points. Reinforcing method is used on ST-36 and LU-9. Even method is used on PC-7, HT-7 and the Ah Shi points.

Explanations

- PC-7, the Stream and Source point of the Pericardium channel, nourishes the Blood and relieves the pain.
- ST-36, the Sea point of the Stomach channel, tonifies the Qi, promotes the production of Blood and relieves the pain.
- LU-9, the Stream and Source point of the Lung channel, and the Gathering point of the Vessels, and SP-6, the crossing point of the three Yin channels of the foot, tonify the Qi and Blood, harmonise the collateral and relieve the pain.
- The Ah Shi points regulate the Qi and Blood to relieve the pain.

Modifications

1. If the wrist is swollen, add SP-9 and TE-6 to strengthen the Spleen, eliminate Damp and reduce the swelling.
2. If there is an aversion to cold or coldness of wrist due to deficiency of Yang-Qi, add CV-6 and CV-4 with moxibustion to reinforce the Yang-Qi and dispel Cold.
3. If the appetite is poor, add CV-12 and SP-3 to tonify the Qi in the Middle Burner and improve the digestion.
4. If there are palpitations, add PC-6 and HT-5 to calm the Heart, regulate the circulation of Blood and relieve the pain.

Palmar pain 38

掌
痛

Palmar pain may occur on one or both palms. It may appear as an independent disorder, or exist as one of the symptoms seen in the Bi syndromes (arthritis). It is usually accompanied by a sensation of cold or heat in the palm, painful finger joints, numbness or swelling of the palm, a pale or red skin colour on the palm, and even ulcers. According to TCM theory, palmar pain may be caused by invasion of External Cold-Damp, or of External Damp-Heat, stagnation of Liver-Qi and deficiency of Yang, invasion of Toxic Fire or stagnation of Blood. Palmar pain may be attributed to any of the following disorders in Western medicine: rheumatoid arthritis, rheumatic arthritis, gout, cervical radiculitis, thoracic radiculitis, carpal arthritis, carpal tunnel syndrome, palm infection, fracture of the palm or injury to the soft tissue of the palm.

Aetiology and pathology

Invasion of External Cold-Damp

Damp is a substantial pathogenic factor of the Yin type; it has the characteristics of heaviness and viscosity. Cold is characterised by stagnation and contraction. Therefore, when Cold-Damp invades the palms, it obstructs their physiological function by causing the channels and tendons in the area to contract, which disturbs the circulation of Qi and Blood in the palm. Stagnation of Qi and Blood follows, and pain follows. In addition to causing pain in the palm, Cold-Damp may also invade the finger joints, causing finger pain (see Ch. 39).

Invasion of External Damp-Heat

During a hot and humid summer, External Damp-Heat may easily invade the palm directly. In addition, if Exterior Cold-Damp persists in the body for a long time it may turn into Damp-Heat. Overeating of fatty and sweet food, or drinking too much alcohol, may cause a dysfunction in the Spleen and Stomach, leading to the formation of internal Damp-Heat in the body. When Damp-Heat accumulates it slows down the circulation of Qi and Blood, leading to stagnation of the Qi and Blood in the channels and tendons of the palm, and causing palmar pain.

Stagnation of Liver-Qi with deficiency of Yang

The emotions are closely related to the function of the Liver. Unstable emotional states, or excessive stress or frustration, may cause the circulation of Liver-Qi to slow down, so that it eventually stagnates. In some people with a constitutional Yang deficiency, stagnation of Liver-Qi may lead to stagnation of Cold in the Liver channel; this condition is often seen in women who are exposed to cold environments during their menstrual periods. This occurs because there is a temporary weakness of Blood in the Liver and Yang deficiency during the menstrual period, which attracts the invasion of External Cold. As a result, the circulation of Qi and Blood in the palm becomes blocked and pain occurs.

Invasion of Toxic Fire

A traumatic wound to the palm may leave the person vulnerable to direct invasion of toxic Fire to the muscles and tendons in the area, or even invasion of Toxic Heat into the Blood. When the pathogenic factors spread in the channels of the palm, they may cause stagnation of Qi and Blood in the palm, or even decomposition of the muscle in the locality, leading to palmar pain. Incomplete elimination of Exterior Cold and Damp from the body over a long period of time may also lead to stagnation of Qi and Blood and generate Internal Fire.

Toxic Fire may also form as a result of bad diet and emotional states as well as a poor constitution. For instance, overeating of pungent food or drinking too much alcohol may cause Damp-Heat to form in the body. When this Damp-Heat accumulates in the body over a long period, it may generate Toxic Fire; diabetic patients who suffer with palm pain are usually found to have this condition.

Stagnation of Blood

All the pathological changes mentioned above may eventually influence the circulation of Qi and Blood in the palm. Moreover, physical trauma or inappropriate movement of the hands may directly damage the muscles, tendons and even bones, leading to Qi and Blood stagnation. Inappropriate surgical operations on the palm may also directly cause stagnation of Blood directly. Once the channels of the palm are blocked, pain appears there.

Treatment based on differentiation

Differentiation

Differentiation of External or Internal origin

— Acute onset of palm pain of short duration, accompanied by External symptoms, is usually caused by invasion of External pathogenic factors.

— Chronic onset of palm pain of long duration, accompanied by symptoms resulting from Internal disorder, is usually caused by disorder of Internal organs.

Differentiation of character of the pain

— Palmar pain with a cold and heavy sensation, pale skin on the hands, aggravation of the pain by exposure to cold, or alleviation of pain by warmth, is usually caused by invasion of Cold-Damp.
— Palmar pain with a hot and heavy sensation, redness, swelling and a burning feeling, is often due to invasion of Damp-Heat.
— Formation of ulcers on the palm, and reddish skin of the palm with a hot feeling, aggravation of the pain by pressure, fever, or restlessness, is often due to invasion of Toxin Fire.
— Chronic onset of palmar pain with a cold sensation, and aggravation of the palm pain by emotional upset or exposure to cold, especially during the menstruation, is usually caused by stagnation of Liver-Qi with deficiency of Yang.
— Injury, or history of operation on the palm and fingers, stabbing pain with a fixed location, with aggravation of the pain at night, is usually due to stagnation of Blood.

Treatment

INVASION OF EXTERNAL COLD-DAMP

Symptoms and signs

Palm pain with a cold and heavy sensation, which worsens on exposure to cold and humid weather or by contact with water, and is alleviated by warmth, with swelling of the joints. Other symptoms include pale skin on the hands, a slight fever, an aversion to cold, numb or frigid fingers, cold limbs, a poor appetite, an absence of thirst, clear urine, a pale tongue with a white and moist coating and a floating and tense pulse.

Principle of treatment

Dispel External Cold-Damp and promote Blood circulation.

HERBAL TREATMENT

Prescription

JUAN BI TANG
Remove Painful Obstruction Decoction
Qiang Huo *Rhizoma seu Radix Notopterygii* 10 g

Huang Qi *Radix Astragali seu Hedysari* 10 g
Fang Feng *Radix Ledebouriellae* 10 g
Dang Gui *Radix Angelicae Sinensis* 10 g
Jiang Huang *Rhizoma Curcumae Longae* 15 g
Chi Shao *Radix Paeoniae Rubra* 10 g
Gan Cao *Radix Glycyrrhizae* 6 g
Sheng Jiang *Rhizoma Zingiberis Recens* 10 g

Explanations

- Qiang Huo, Fang Feng and Jiang Huang dispel Wind, Cold and Damp and relieve the pain.
- Dang Gui and Chi Shao promote Blood circulation and relieve the pain.
- Huang Qi strengthens the Antipathogenic Qi and consolidates the skin.
- Sheng Jiang and Gan Cao harmonise the stomach and regulate the herbs in the formula.

Modifications

1. If there is severe coldness in the hands and palms, add Fu Zi *Radix Aconiti Praeparata* 10 g and Rou Gui *Cortex Cinnamomi* 6 g to warm the channels, eliminate Cold-Damp and relieve the pain.
2. If the limbs are pale and cold, add Tao Ren *Semen Persicae* 10 g and Hong Hua *Flos Carthami* 10 g to regulate the circulation of Blood and remove Blood stasis.
3. If there is severe pain, add Xi Xin *Herba Asari* 3 g to warm the channels and relieve the pain.
4. If the joints are swollen, add Han Fang Ji *Radix Stephaniae Tetrandrae* 10 g and Bi Xie *Rhizoma Dioscoreae Septemlobae* 15 g to eliminate Damp and reduce the swelling.

Patent remedy

Feng Shi Pian *Wind-Damp Tablet*

ACUPUNCTURE TREATMENT

LI-4 Hegu, LI-5 Yangxi, TE-5 Waiguan, LU-7 Lieque, SI-3 Houxi and LR-3 Taichong. Reducing method is used on these points.

Explanations

- LI-4, the Source point of the Large Intestine channel, promotes sweating and dispels Wind-Cold and Damp. It can also promote the circulation of Qi and reduce the swelling.
- LI-5, the River point, regulates the circulation of Qi and dispels Wind and Damp to relieve palmar pain.

- TE-5, the Connecting point, dispels Wind-Cold and Damp, promotes the circulation of Qi, harmonises the collateral in the hands and relieves the pain.
- LU-7, the Connecting point, disperses the Lung-Qi, relieves External symptoms, regulates the Qi and relieves the pain.
- SI-3, the Stream point, promotes the circulation of Qi and relieves the pain.
- LR-3, the Source point of the Liver channel, promotes the circulation of Qi and Blood and relieves the palmar pain.

Modifications

1. If there is a cold sensation in the palm, add TE-6 and ST-36 with moxibustion to warm the channels, dispel Cold and relieve the pain.
2. If the palmar joints are swollen, add PC-6 and ST-40 to promote the circulation of Qi, eliminate Damp and reduce the swelling.
3. If the fingers are painful, add Extra Baxie to promote the circulation of Qi and relieve the pain.
4. If there is numbness in the palm, add PC-7 and HT-7 to regulate the circulation of Qi and relieve the numbness.
5. If there is a fever, add GV-14 and LI-11 to promote sweating and reduce the fever.

Case history

A 35-year-old man had been suffering with palmar pain for 6 months. The pain in the palm and finger joints had started when he was caught in a big storm the previous winter. He was diagnosed as having rheumatoid arthritis, and a doctor had given him some painkillers and some Chinese herbal pills. There was some relief of the joint pain, but he still had pain in the palm. Therefore he wanted acupuncture treatment as well as the other therapies. When he arrived at the acupuncture clinic, he had finger and palmar pain in both hands. He also had a slightly rigid and cold sensation in his hands, pale and swollen fingers, an aversion to cold, a poor appetite, an absence of thirst, clear urine, a white tongue and a superficial and wiry pulse.

Diagnosis
Invasion of External Cold.

Principle of treatment
Dispel External Cold, warm the channels and relieve the pain.

Acupuncture treatment
LI-4, TE-5, SI-4, LU-5, SP-3 and LR-3 were needled with reducing method. The patient also used moxa sticks to warm the finger joints twice a day. He was treated with acupuncture every other day. Besides this acupuncture

and moxibustion treatment, he was given a herbal formula Feng Shi Bi Chong Ji to take every day.

Explanations

- LI-4 is the Source point of the Large Intestine channel. TE-5 is the Connecting point of the Triple Burner channel. SI-4 is the Source point of the Small Intestine channel. These three points in combination promote the circulation of Qi, dispel Cold and relieve the pain.
- LU-5 is the Sea point of the Lung channel. SP-3 is the Source point of the Spleen channel. These two points in combination promote the circulation of Qi and dispel Cold in these channels and resolve Damp.
- LR-3 is the Stream and Source point of the Liver channel. The Liver dominates the tendons, so LR-3 regulates the circulation of Qi and relieves the pain in the tendons.
- The moxa treatment strengthens the warming effect, dispels External Cold and relieves the pain.

After 3 weeks, his palm pain was completely under control. He was followed up by telephone a year later and he said he had experienced no more pain in the palm after this treatment.

INVASION OF EXTERNAL DAMP-HEAT

Symptoms and signs

Palmar pain with a hot and heavy sensation, accompanied by redness, swelling and a burning feeling in the finger joints or all the limb joints, a preference for cold, fever, a thirst, yellow urine, restlessness, a red tongue with a yellow coating and a rapid and slippery pulse.

Principle of treatment

Clear Damp-Heat and promote the Blood circulation.

HERBAL TREATMENT

Prescription

BAI HU JIA GUI ZHI TANG
White Tiger Ramulus Cinnamomi Decoction
Shi Gao *Gypsum Fibrosum* 30 g
Zhi Mu *Rhizoma Anemarrhenae* 12 g
Gan Cao *Radix Glycyrrhizae* 6 g
Jing Mi *Semen Oryzae* 30 g
Gui Zhi *Ramulus Cinnamomi* 10 g

Explanations

- Shi Gao and Zhi Mu clear Heat and reduce fever.
- Gan Cao and Jing Mi protect the Stomach-Qi and relieve the pain.

- Gui Zhi eliminates Wind-Damp and promotes the circulation of Blood so as to relieve the palmar pain.

Modifications

1. If there is a fever, add Huang Qin *Radix Scutellariae* 10 g and Da Qing Ye *Folium Isatidis* 10 g to clear Heat and reduce the fever.
2. If the palm and the joints are swollen, add Han Fang Ji *Radix Stephaniae Tetrandrae* 10 g and Jiang Huang *Rhizoma Curcumae Longae* 10 g to eliminate Damp-Heat and reduce the swelling.
3. If the joints are reddish, add Jin Yin Hua *Flos Lonicerae* 10 g, Sang Zhi *Ramulus Mori* 10 g and Luo Shi Teng *Caulis Trachelospermi* 15 g to clear Damp-Heat and cool the Blood.

Patent remedy

Feng Shi Xiao Tong Pian *Wind-Damp Dispel Pain Pill*

ACUPUNCTURE TREATMENT

LI-3 Sanjian, LI-11 Quchi, TE-5 Waiguan, PC-6 Neiguan, SP-6 Sanyinjiao and SP-9 Yinlingquan. Reducing method is used on these points.

Explanations

- LI-3, the Stream point, eliminates Damp-Heat and relieves the pain.
- LI-11, the Sea point, promotes the circulation of Qi and relieves the pain.
- TE-5, the Connecting point of the Triple Burner channel, dispels Wind, eliminates Damp-Heat, regulates the circulation of Qi and relieves the pain.
- PC-6, the Connecting point of the Pericardium channel, regulates the circulation of Qi and relieves the pain.
- SP-6 is the crossing point of the Spleen, Kidney and Liver channels. SP-9 is the Sea point of the Spleen channel. These two points in combination promote urination and eliminate Damp-Heat.

Modifications

1. If there is a fever, add LI-2 and GV-14 to clear Heat and reduce the fever.
2. If the palm and joints are red and swollen, add LI-4 and Extra Baxie to promote the circulation of Qi and reduce the swelling.
3. If there is a heavy sensation in the palm, add TE-6 to promote the circulation of Qi and eliminate Damp.

4. If the appetite is poor, add ST-36 and CV-12 to regulate the circulation of Qi in the Stomach and improve the appetite.
5. If there is restlessness, add HT-7 and LR-3 to regulate the Qi and calm the Mind.
6. If there is a thirst, add LU-8, the Metal point of the Lung channel, to clear Heat and relieve the thirst.

INVASION OF TOXIC FIRE

Symptoms and signs

Formation of ulcers and oedema in the palm, reddish skin on the palm with a hot feeling, aggravation of pain by pressure, itching and a wet palm, thirst with cold drinking, a bitter taste in mouth, fever, an aversion to cold, constipation, scanty and yellow urine, a red tongue with a yellow and dry coating and a rapid pulse.

Principle of treatment

Clear Fire and eliminate Toxin.

HERBAL TREATMENT

Prescription

WU WEI XIAO DU YIN
Five-Ingredient Decoction to Eliminate Toxin
Jin Yin Hua *Flos Lonicerae* 20 g
Ye Ju Hua *Flos Chrysanthemi Indici* 15 g
Pu Gong Ying *Herba Taraxaci* 30 g
Zi Hua Di Ding *Herba Violae* 30 g
Zi Bei Tian Kui *Herba Begonia Fibristipulatae* 15 g

Explanations

- Jin Yin Hua and Pu Gong Ying clear Heat and eliminate Wind to relieve pain and itching of the palm.
- Ye Ju Hua, Zi Hua Di Ding and Zi Bei Tian Kui eliminate Toxin, cool the Blood, reduce swelling and relieve the ulceration.

Modifications

1. If there is a high fever and aversion to cold, add Shi Gao *Gypsum Fibrosum* 15 g to clear Heat and reduce the fever.
2. If there is a severe pain in the palm with a burning feeling, add Huang Lian *Rhizoma Coptidis* 5 g and Da Qing Ye *Folium Isatidis* 10 g to clear Toxic Fire and relieve the pain.

3. If there is a thirst, add Zhi Mu *Rhizoma Anemarrhenae* 10 g and Tian Hua Fen *Radix Trichosanthis* 10 g to clear Heat, promote the secretion of Body Fluids and relieve the thirst.
4. If there is constipation, add Da Huang *Radix et Rhizoma Rhei* 10 g and Mang Xiao *Natrii Sulfas* 10 g to clear Fire and promote defecation.

Patent remedy

Niu Huang Jie Du Pian *Cattle Gallstone Tablet to Resolve Toxin*

ACUPUNCTURE TREATMENT

LI-4 Hegu, LI-11 Quchi, PC-8 Laogong, TE-2 Yemen, SP-6 Sanyinjiao and ST-40 Fenglong. Reducing method is used on these points.

Explanations

- LI-4, the Source point of the Large Intestine channel, regulates the circulation of Qi, clears Fire and relieves the pain.
- LI-11, the Sea point of the Large Intestine channel, clears Fire, reduces fever and relieves the pain.
- PC-8 and TE-2, the Spring points of the Pericardium and the Triple Burner channels respectively, clear Fire and relieve the pain.
- SP-6, the crossing point of the three Yin channels of the foot, clears Fire, reduces fever and promotes urination and defecation.
- ST-40, the Connecting point of the Stomach channel, clears Fire in the muscles and relieves the pain.

Modifications

1. If there is a fever, add GV-14 and LI-2 to clear Fire and reduce the fever.
2. If the palm is swollen, add PC-7 and HT-7 to clear Fire and reduce the swelling.
3. If there is ulceration, add BL-17 and SP-10 to clear Fire and cool the Blood.
4. If there is a bitter taste in the mouth, add GB-40 to eliminate Heat in the Fu organs.
5. If there is a thirst, add LU-5 and LU-8 to clear Fire and relieve the thirst.
6. If there is constipation, add ST-25, the Front Collecting point of the Large Intestine, and ST-37, the Lower Sea point, to clear Fire and remove Qi stagnation.

STAGNATION OF LIVER-QI WITH DEFICIENCY OF YANG

Symptoms and signs

Palmar pain with a distending and cold sensation, which is aggravated by emotional upset or exposure to cold especially during the menstrual period, accompanied by a pale colour to the skin on the hand, hypochondriac pain, fatigue, a poor appetite, a dull feeling in the stomach, irritability, a pale tongue with a white coating and a deep and wiry pulse.

Principle of treatment

Regulate Liver-Qi, warm the Liver channel and dispel Cold.

HERBAL TREATMENT

Prescription

DANG GUI SI NI TANG
Angelica Four Rebellious Decoction
Gui Zhi *Ramulus Cinnamomi* 10 g
Dang Gui *Radix Angelicae Sinensis* 10 g
Bai Shao *Radix Paeoniae Alba* 20 g
Mu Tong *Caulis Akebiae* 6 g
Xi Xin *Herba Asari* 3 g
Gan Cao *Radix Glycyrrhizae* 5 g
Da Zao *Fructus Ziziphi Jujubae* 10 g

Explanations

- Gui Zhi and Dang Gui warm the channels of the hand and promote the circulation of Blood so as to remove Qi stagnation in the Liver channel.
- Bai Shao and Dang Gui harmonise the Liver, nourish the Blood and strengthen the Liver.
- Gui Zhi and Xi Xin warm the interior and dispel Cold from the Liver channels so as to relieve the palmar pain.
- Mu Tong regulates the circulation of Qi in the channels so as to remove Qi stagnation.
- Da Zao tonifies the Qi and Blood.
- Gan Cao harmonises the actions of the other herbs in the formula.

Modifications

1. If there is Liver-Qi stagnation, add Chai Hu *Radix Bupleuri* 10 g and Yu Jin *Radix Curcumae* 10 g to smooth the Liver, regulate the circulation of Liver-Qi and remove Qi stagnation.
2. If there is a sharp pain, add Yan Hu Suo *Rhizoma Corydalis* 10 g and Mo Yao *Resina Myrrhae* 10 g to strengthen the effect of boosting the circulation of Qi so as to relieve the palmar pain.
3. If there is a pain with a cold sensation, add Chuan Xiong *Radix Ligustici Chuanxiong* 10 g and Zhi Fu Zi *Radix Aconiti Praeparata* 10 g to warm the channels, promote the circulation of Blood and relieve the pain.

Patent remedy

Shu Gan Wan *Soothe Liver Pill*

ACUPUNCTURE TREATMENT

LI-4 Hegu, ST-36 Zusanli, PC-6 Neiguan, LR-3 Taichong, GB-20 Fengchi and BL-18 Ganshu. Even method is used on these points.

Explanations

- LI-4, the Source point of the Large Intestine channel, promotes the circulation of Qi and relieves the pain.
- ST-36, the Sea point, tonifies the Yang-Qi and warms the Interior.
- PC-6, the Connecting point of the Pericardium channel, regulates the circulation of Qi and removes its stagnation.
- LR-3, the Source and Stream point of the Liver channel, and BL-18, the Back Transporting point of the Liver, regulate the Liver-Qi and relieve the palmar pain.
- GB-20 calms the Liver, tranquillises the Mind and relieves the palmar pain.

Modifications

1. If there is hypochondriac pain, add LR-14, the Front Collecting point of the Liver, and GB-40 to regulate the circulation of Qi for relieving the pain.
2. If there is emotional instability, add LR-2 and SP-6 to regulate the circulation of Liver-Qi and relieve its stagnation.
3. If there is irregular menstruation, add KI-3, the Source point, and SP-10 to regulate the menstruation.
4. If there is a cold sensation in the palm and fingers, add TE-3 to promote the circulation of Qi and warm the channels.
5. If the skin on the hand has a pale colour, add SI-4 and TE-4 to promote the circulation of Qi and improve the circulation of Blood.

STAGNATION OF BLOOD

Symptoms and signs

Traumatic injury to or operation on the wrist, palm and fingers, long-standing pain in the palm, a stabbing pain with a fixed location, which worsens at night and is alleviated by movement, accompanied by rigidity of the palm or fingers, swelling of the joints and hands, purplish tongue with a thin coating and a wiry and choppy pulse.

Principle of treatment

Promote Qi and Blood circulation and remove Blood stagnation.

HERBAL TREATMENT

Prescription

FU YUAN HUO XUE TANG
Receive Health by Invigorating the Blood Decoction
Chai Hu *Radix Bupleuri* 15 g
Tian Hua Fen *Radix Trichosanthis* 20 g
Hong Hua *Flos Carthami* 10 g
Tao Ren *Semen Persicae* 10 g
Dang Gui *Radix Angelicae Sinensis* 12 g
Da Huang *Radix et Rhizoma Rhei* 6 g
Yan Hu Suo *Rhizoma Corydalis* 20 g
Can Cao *Radix Glycyrrhizae* 6 g

Explanations

- Chai Hu and Tian Hua Fen promote the circulation of Qi and relieve the pain.
- Dang Gui, Tao Ren and Hong Hua promote the circulation of Blood to remove Blood stasis.
- Yan Hu Suo strengthens the function of the prescription in removing Blood stasis. This herb has also a strong effect in relieving the pain.
- Da Huang removes Blood stagnation.
- Gan Cao harmonises the functions of other herbs in the formula.

Modifications

1. If there is fracture, add Du Zhong *Cortex Eucomiae* 10 g and San Qi *Radix Notoginseng* 10 g to strengthen the Kidney, remove Blood stagnation and relieve the pain.
2. If there is a severe pain with a tense sensation, add Qing Pi *Pericardium Citri Reticulatae Viride* 10 g and Mo Yao *Resina Myrrhae* 10 g to regulate the Qi and remove Blood stasis.

3. If the joints are rigid, add San Leng *Rhizoma Sparganii* 10 g and E Zhu *Rhizoma Zedoariae* 10 g to promote the circulation of Blood and remove Blood stagnation in order to relieve the joint rigidity.

Patent remedy

Xiao Huo Luo Dan *Minor Invigorate the Collaterals Special Pill*

ACUPUNCTURE TREATMENT

LI-3 Sanjian, TE-5 Waiguan, Lu-7 Lieque, PC-6 Neiguan, GB-34 Yanglingquan, ST-36 Zusanli and BI-17 Geshu. Reducing method is used on these points.

Explanations

- LI-3, the Stream point of the Large Intestine channel, promotes the circulation of Qi and relieves the pain.
- TE-5, the Connecting point of the Triple Burner channel, promotes the circulation of Qi and removes Blood stagnation.
- LU-7, the Connecting point of the Lung channel, also promotes the circulation of Qi and removes Blood stagnation.
- PC-6, the Connecting point of the Pericardium channel, regulates the circulation of Qi and relieves the pain.
- GB-34, the Gathering point for the tendons, regulates the circulation of Qi and Blood in the tendons so as to relieve the palmar pain.
- ST-36, the Sea point of the Stomach channel, promotes the circulation of Qi and removes Blood stagnation.
- BL-17, the Gathering point for the Blood, regulates the circulation of Blood and removes its stagnation.

Modifications

1. If there is pain due to a fracture, add KI-3 and TE-4 to regulate the Qi and strengthen the Kidney to relieve the pain.
2. If the palmar pain worsens at night, add HT-7 and SP-6 to regulate the circulation of Blood and eliminate its stasis.
3. If the palm is swollen, add PC-7 and Extra Baxie to activate the circulation of Qi and Blood in the locality to reduce the swelling.
4. If the joints are rigid, add LI-3, the Stream point, and SI-4, the Source point, to promote the circulation of Qi to remove Blood stasis.

Case history

A 29-year-old woman had been suffering from palmar pain for 4 months. She had suffered a trauma to her right hand during the previous winter when she slipped and fell in the snow. Her palm was swollen and it was diagnosed as soft tissue injury, for which she received massage therapy. Afterwards, the swelling resolved, but she still felt pain in her palm, especially at night. She had no other symptoms.

Diagnosis
Stagnation of Blood in the channels.

Principle of treatment
Promote Qi and Blood circulation, remove Blood stagnation and relieve the pain.

Herbal treatment
TAO HONG SI WU TANG
Four-Substance Decoction with Safflower and Peach Pit
Dang Gui *Radix Angelicae Sinensis* 10 g
Sheng Di Huang *Radix Rehmanniae Recens* 10 g
Chi Shao *Radix Paeoniae Rubra* 10 g
Chuan Xiong *Rhizoma Ligustici Chuanxiong* 6 g
Tao Ren *Semen Persicae* 10 g

Hong Hua *Flos Carthami* 10 g
Qiang Huo *Rhizoma seu Radix Notopterygii* 10 g
Jiang Huang *Rhizoma Curcumae Longae* 12 g
Yan Hu Suo *Rhizoma Corydalis* 10 g

Explanations
- Chuan Xiong, Chi Shao, Tao Ren and Hong Hua promote the circulation of Blood and remove its stagnation.
- Dang Gui harmonises the Blood, and regulates its circulation and removes its stagnation.
- Qiang Huo and Jiang Huang are good at promoting the circulation of Blood, harmonising the collateral and relieving the upper limb pain.
- Yan Hu Suo regulates the circulation of Blood and relieves the pain.
- As a long-standing stagnation of Blood may generate Heat in the Blood, Sheng Di Huang is used here to cool the Blood and remove Toxin from it.

The patient was given daily treatment with the herbal decoction.

After 2 weeks of treatment, her palmar pain was completely relieved. Nine months later she was followed up by letter; she replied she had experienced no more palmar pain after the treatment.

Finger pain 39

手
指
疼
痛

Finger pain may occur in one or more fingers, and in one or both hands. According to TCM theory, it can often be caused by the accumulation of Cold-Damp, or of Damp-Heat, stagnation of Qi and Blood, deficiency of Blood, or deficiency of the Liver- and Kidney-Essence. Finger pain may be attributed to any of the following disorders in Western medicine: rheumatoid arthritis, rheumatic fever, chilblains, nerve pain, paralysis or injury of the nerves, sprain of the local muscles or tendons, carpal tunnel syndrome and Raynaud's syndrome.

Aetiology and pathology

Accumulation of Cold-Damp in the Channels

Exposure to cold over a long period or living in a cold and damp environment may allow Cold-Damp to invade the body. Overeating of cold food or drinking too many cold beverages may damage the Spleen and Stomach, impeding the Spleen's function of transporting water and damp so that internal Damp forms. Cold has the characteristics of contraction and stagnation; Damp is characteristically heavy, viscous and lingering. Therefore, when Cold-Damp invades or accumulates in the channels, it causes the muscles and tendons of the fingers to contract, leading to stagnation of the Qi and Blood, which triggers the finger pain.

Living or working in a humid and warm place for a long time, or eating of too much fatty, sweet or pungent food, impairs the Spleen and Stomach in their functions of transporting and transforming in the Middle Burner, causing Damp-Heat to form. Once Damp-Heat blocks the channels, it will cause stagnation of the Qi and Blood, so finger pain follows.

Stagnation of Qi and Blood

Qi and Blood should circulate freely in the channels. If there is Qi and Blood stagnation from various causes, such as emotional disturbance, stress, frustration, overstrain, physical trauma, or inappropriate movement of the fingers, the circulation of Qi and Blood slows, leading to blockage in the channels, so finger pain occurs.

Deficiency of Blood

Prolonged chronic disease, excessive bleeding during the menstrual period or during an operation and haemorrhoids may all cause the Qi and Blood to be consumed, resulting in deficiency of Blood. When there is insufficient Blood circulating in the channels, the fingers are not properly nourished and finger pain follows.

Deficiency of Liver and Kidney-Essence

The Kidney dominates the Bones and produces the Marrow; the Liver stores the Blood and dominates the tendons. Overstrain, prolonged sickness or senility and a constitutional weakness may all cause the Kidney-Essence to be consumed, resulting in deficiency of Kidney- and Liver-Essence. In this condition the muscles, tendons and bones are undernourished, causing finger pain to occur.

Treatment based on differentiation

Differentiation

Differentiation of Excess and Deficiency

— Constant finger pain, severe finger pain, aggravation of the finger pain by rest, and alleviation of finger pain by some movement, with swelling on the fingers, is usually caused by Excessive pathogenic factors.
— Intermittent finger pain, slight finger pain, with aggravation of the pain by exertion and movement, or tiredness, is often caused by Deficiency.

Differentiation of the character of the pain

— Finger pain with a cold sensation, swelling, heaviness and numbness, or aggravation of the pain in damp and cold weather, is usually caused by accumulation of Cold-Damp in the channels.
— Swelling, redness and pain of the finger joints, heaviness and numbness of the fingers with a warm or even burning sensation, is usually caused by accumulation of Damp-Heat in the channels.
— Finger pain with a history of trauma or operation, stabbing pain and numbness of the fingers, aggravation of the pain at night, or deformity of the finger joints, is usually caused by stagnation of Qi and Blood.
— Chronic finger pain, numbness of the fingers with stiffness, weakness of the hands, a pale complexion and lips, is often caused by deficiency of Blood.

— Slight finger pain with spasm, shaking, gradual deformity of the fingers, weakness of the fingers, wrists, arms and legs, or lower back pain, is usually caused by deficiency of Essence of Kidney and Liver.

Treatment

ACCUMULATION OF COLD-DAMP IN THE CHANNELS

Symptoms and signs

Swelling and pain in the fingers, heaviness and numbness of the fingers with a cold sensation, which worsens in damp and cold weather, with limitation of joint movement, spasms of the fingers and difficulty in grasping things. Accompanying symptoms include heaviness of the body generally, an aversion to cold, a poor appetite, loose stools, a pale tongue with a white and greasy coating and a deep, slow and slippery pulse or a tight pulse.

Principle of treatment

Dispel Cold, remove Damp, regulate Qi circulation and relieve the pain.

HERBAL TREATMENT

Prescription

DANG GUI SI NI TANG
Angelica Four Rebellious Decoction
Gan Jiang *Rhizoma Zingiberis* 6 g
Fu Ling *Poria* 15 g
Bai Zhu *Rhizoma Atractylodis Macrocephalae* 12 g
Gui Zhi *Ramulus Cinnamomi* 10 g
Dang Gui *Radix Angelicae Sinensis* 10 g
Bai Shao *Radix Paeoniae Alba* 20 g
Xi Xin *Herba Asari* 3 g
Qing Feng Teng *Caulis Sinomenii* 20 g
Gan Cao *Radix Glycyrrhizae* 5 g

Explanations

- Gan Jiang and Gan Cao dispel Cold in the channels and body and warm the Middle Burner.
- Fu Ling and Bai Zhu strengthen the Spleen and remove Damp.
- Gui Zhi and Dang Gui regulate the circulation of Qi and Blood in the channels and also warm the channels.

- Xi Xin and Qing Feng Teng dispel Wind and Damp so as to relieve the pain.
- Bai Shao nourishes the tendons and relieves the pain.

Modifications

1. If there is a severe aversion to cold and muscular spasm, add Fu Zi *Radix Aconiti Lateralis Praeparata* 10 g to warm the channels and collaterals and relieve the spasm.
2. If there is swelling or heaviness in the fingers due to the predominance of the invasion of Damp, add Du Huo *Radix Angelicae Pubescentis* 10 g and Cang Zhu *Rhizoma Atractylodis* 10 g to remove the Damp and sedate the pain.
3. If the appetite is poor, add Ban Xia *Rhizoma Pinelliae* 10 g and Bai Kou Ren *Semen Amomi Rotundus* 5 g to dry Damp and improve the appetite.

Patent remedy

Feng Shi Pian *Wind-Damp Tablet*

ACUPUNCTURE TREATMENT

TE-5 Waiguan, CV-12 Zhongwan, SP-6 Sanyinjiao, SP-9 Yinlingquan, LI-4 Hegu, Extra Baxie and Ah Shi points. Reducing method is used on these points. It is advisable to use moxibustion in all patients who suffer from severe pain.

Explanations

- TE-5, the Connecting point of the Triple Burner channel, promotes the circulation of Qi and relieves the pain.
- CV-12, the Front Collecting point of the Stomach and the Gathering point for all the Fu organs, removes obstructions from the channels, invigorates the circulation of Qi in the collateral and eliminates both Cold and Damp.
- SP-6, the crossing point of the three Yin channels of the foot, promotes urination and eliminates Damp.
- SP-9, the Sea point of the Spleen channel, activates the Spleen and Stomach and eliminates Damp.
- LI-4, the Source point of the Large Intestine channel, promotes the circulation of Qi and Blood in the hands and relieves the finger pain.
- The Extra Baxie and Ah Shi points promote the circulation of Qi in the local channels and collateral and stop the pain.

- Moxibustion warms the needles so as to warm the channels and Middle Burner, dispels Cold and relieves Damp.

Modifications

1. If there is a severe aversion to cold and muscular spasm, add moxibustion on CV-6 to warm the channels and collateral and relieve the spasm.
2. If the fingers are swollen and there is a heavy sensation in the body due to an invasion of Damp, add TE-6 and ST-36 to remove the Damp and reduce the swelling.
3. If the appetite is poor, add LR-13, the Front Collecting point of the Spleen, and SP-3, the Source point, to activate the Spleen and Stomach, regulate the circulation of Qi and improve the appetite.

Case history

A 30-year-old woman had been suffering from finger pain on both sides for 5 months. She had a heavy sensation in both hands, and rigidity of the fingers in the morning, accompanied by a poor appetite, fatigue, abdominal distension, loose stools, a white and watery tongue coating and a soft and slow pulse. At the hospital she was diagnosed as having rheumatoid arthritis.

Diagnosis
Invasion of Cold-Damp in the channels with Spleen and Kidney-Yang deficiency.

Principle of treatment
Dispel Wind, Cold and Damp, tonify the Yang-Qi and sedate the pain.

Herbal treatment
DANG GUI SI NI TANG
Angelica Four Rebellious Decoction
Gui Zhi *Ramulus Cinnamomi* 10 g
Dang Gui *Radix Angelicae Sinensis* 10 g
Qing Feng Teng *Caulis Sinomenii* 30 g
Jiang Huang *Rhizoma Curcumae Longae* 10 g
Xi Xin *Herba Asari* 3 g
Fu Ling *Poria* 15 g
Gan Cao *Radix Glycyrrhizae* 5 g

Explanations

- Gui Zhi and Dang Gui promote the circulation of Blood, tonify the Yang-Qi, warm the channels and relieve the pain.
- Gui Zhi and Xi Xin warm the channels, dispel Cold and relieve the finger pain.
- Fu Ling activates the Spleen and Stomach and eliminates Damp.
- Qing Feng Teng and Jiang Huang are good at dispelling Wind-Damp and relieving the painful joints.
- Gan Cao harmonises the actions of the other herbs in the formula.

The patient had daily treatment with the herbal decoction. She was also advised to wash her painful fingers with the remainder of the hot herbs after decocting them. Every day she kept her fingers warm. After 3 months of treatment, her finger pain had disappeared. She was followed up 2 years later and reported that she had experienced no more finger pain since the herbal treatment.

ACCUMULATION OF DAMP-HEAT IN THE CHANNELS

Symptoms and signs

Swelling, redness and pain in the fingers, which worsens in damp and warm weather, heaviness and numbness in the fingers with a warm or even burning sensation, with difficulty in grasping, limitation of joint movement and spasm of the fingers. Accompanying symptoms include a feeling of heaviness in the body generally, an aversion to cold, a poor appetite, loose stools, a red tongue with a yellow and greasy coating and a deep, slippery and rapid, or tight and rapid, pulse.

Principle of treatment

Dry Damp, clear Heat, regulate the circulation of Qi and relieve the pain.

HERBAL TREATMENT

Prescription

SI MIAO SAN
Four-Marvel Powder
Huang Bai *Cortex Phellodendri* 10 g
Cang Zhu *Rhizoma Atractylodis* 10 g
Yi Yi Ren *Semen Coicis* 10 g
Chuan Niu Xi *Radix Cyathulae* 10 g
Ren Dong Teng *Caulis Lonicerae* 20 g
Dang Gui *Radix Angelicae Sinensis* 10 g
Bai Shao *Radix Paeoniae Alba* 20 g
Qing Feng Teng *Caulis Sinomenii* 20 g
Gan Cao *Radix Glycyrrhizae* 5 g

Explanations

- Huang Bai clears Heat, dries Damp and sedates pain.
- Cang Zhu activates the Spleen and dries Damp.
- Yi Yi Ren and Chuan Niu Xi promote urination, eliminate Damp and reduce the swelling.
- Dang Gui and Bai Shao harmonise the Blood circulation, relax the tendons and muscles and relieve the spasm so as to sedate the finger pain.

- Ren Dong Ten clears Heat in the collateral.
- Qing Feng Teng dispels Damp, circulates the channels and relieves the finger pain.
- Gan Cao harmonises the function of the other herbs in the prescription.

Modifications

1. If there is a fever, add Shi Gao *Gypsum Fibrosum* 20 g and Zhi Mu *Rhizoma Anemarrhenae* 10 g to clear Heat and reduce the fever.
2. If the fingers are swollen and red, add Bi Xie *Rhizoma Dioscoreae Septemlobrae* 10 g and Tu Fu Ling *Rhizoma Smilacis Glabrae* 10 g to clear Heat, eliminate Damp and reduce the swelling.
3. If there is severe spasm in the fingers, add Bai Jiang Cao *Herba Patriniae* 10 g and Bai Hua She *Agkistrodon Acutus* 10 g to promote the circulation in the channels and relax the tendons.
4. If the fingers are deformed, add Wu Jia Pi *Cortex Acanthopanacis Radicis* 10 g and Di Long *Lumbricus* 10 g to strengthen the tendons and bones and relieve obstruction in the channels.
5. If the finger pain worsens at night, add Pu Hung *Pollen Typhae* 10 g and Wu Ling Zhi *Faeces Trogopterorum* 10 g to promote the circulation of Blood and eliminate its stasis.
6. If the appetite is poor, add Shan Zha *Fructus Crataegi* 15 g and Bai Kou Ren *Semen Amomi Rotundus* 5 g to activate the Spleen and Stomach and improve the appetite.

Patent remedy

Feng Shi Xiao Tong Pian *Wind-Damp Dispel Pain Pill*

ACUPUNCTURE TREATMENT

TE-6 Zhigou, CV-12 Zhongwan, LI-2 Erjian, LI-3 Sanjian, LI-4 Hegu, ST-40 Fenglong, ST-44 Neiting, SP-9 Yinlingquan, Extra Baxie and Ah Shi points. Reducing method is used on all these points.

Explanations

- TE-6 eliminates Damp, clears Heat, promotes the circulation of Qi and relieves the pain.
- CV-12, the Front Collecting point of the Stomach and the Gathering point for all the Fu organs, removes Damp from the channels, invigorates the circulation of Qi in the collateral and activates the Stomach.

- LI-3, the Stream point, and LI-4, the Source point, reduce the swelling and promote the circulation of Qi in the channels so as to sedate the finger pain.
- LI-2 and ST-44, the Spring points, clear Heat, reduce the swelling and sedate the finger pain.
- SP-9, the Sea point of the Spleen channel, and ST-40, the Connecting point of the Stomach channel, activate the Spleen and Stomach, eliminate Damp and relieve obstruction in the channels.
- The Extra Baxie and Ah Shi points promote the circulation of Qi in the local channels and collateral and stop the pain.

Modifications

1. If there is severe redness, add TE-2 and SI-2, the Spring points, to clear Heat and reduce the swelling.
2. If there is a fever, add GV-14 and LI-11 to clear Heat and reduce the fever.
3. If there is spasm in the finger, add SI-3 to circulate the channels and collateral and relieve the spasm.
4. If there is swelling of the fingers with a heavy sensation in the body, add ST-36 to remove Damp and reduce the swelling.
5. If the appetite is poor, add LR-13, the Front Collecting point of the Spleen, and SP-3, the Source point, to regulate the circulation of Qi and improve the appetite.

STAGNATION OF QI AND BLOOD

Symptoms and signs

A chronic history of finger pain or a history of trauma or operation, pain and numbness in the fingers, which worsens at night and is better with movement, accompanied by cold or purplish fingers and hands, a preference for warmth, a purplish tongue and a deep and wiry pulse.

Principle of treatment

Promote the Qi and Blood circulation, remove Blood stasis and sedate the pain.

HERBAL TREATMENT

Prescription

TAO HONG SI WU TANG
Four-Substance Decoction with Safflower and Peach Pit
Sheng Di Huang *Radix Rehmanniae Recens* 12 g
Chi Shao *Radix Paeoniae Rubra* 10 g
Dang Gui *Radix Angelicae Sinensis* 12 g

Chuan Xiong *Rhizoma Ligustici Chuanxiong* 12 g
Tao Ren *Semen Persicae* 12 g
Hong Hua *Flos Carthami* 12 g
Mo Yao *Resina Myrrhae* 10 g
Jiang Huang *Rhizoma Curcumae Longae* 10 g

Explanations

- Sheng Di Huang and Chi Shao nourish the Blood and regulate its circulation.
- Chuang Xiong and Hong Hua promote the circulation of Blood and remove its stagnation.
- Dang Gui and Tao Ren regulate the circulation of Blood and remove its stagnation.
- Mo Yao is good at removing Blood stasis and relieving the pain.
- Jiang Huang promotes the circulation of Qi and Blood in the fingers and relieves the pain.

Modifications

1. If there is a wandering finger pain or pain with heavy sensation due to the invasion of Wind-Damp, add Qiang Huo *Rhizoma seu Radix Notopterygii* 10 g and Qin Jiao *Radix Gentianae Macrophyllae* 10 g to dispel the Wind and remove the Damp.
2. If there is a severe stabbing pain due to traumatic injury, add Ru Xiang *Resina Olibani* 6 g and Qing Pi *Pericarpium Citri Reticulatae Viride* 10 g to strengthen the effect of promoting the Qi and Blood circulation and removing the Blood stasis.

Patent remedy

Xiao Huo Luo Dan *Minor Invigorate the Collaterals Special Pill*

ACUPUNCTURE TREATMENT

LI-4 Hegu, LI-11 Quchi, PC-6 Neiguan, LU-7 Lieque, SP-6 Sanyinjiao, Extra Baxie and Ah Shi points. Reducing method is used on these points.

Explanations

- LI-4, the Source point of the Large Intestine channel, promotes the circulation of Qi and relieves the pain.
- LI-11, the Sea point of the Large Intestine channel, activates the circulation of Qi and relieves the pain.
- PC-6, the Connecting point of the Pericardium channel, promotes the circulation of Qi, removes Blood stasis and relieves the finger pain.

- LU-7, the Connecting point of the Lung channel, promotes the circulation of Qi, harmonises the collateral and relieves the pain.
- The Extra Baxie and Ah Shi points remove the obstruction in the channels and collateral.

Modifications

1. If there is severe finger pain, add LI-3 and LR-3 to dispel Wind, circulate the channels and remove Damp.
2. If there is a severe stabbing pain due to traumatic injury, add BL-17 and SI-4 to strengthen the effect of promoting the Qi and Blood circulation and remove Blood stasis.
3. If there is restlessness and insomnia due to pain, add HT-7 to calm the Heart and tranquillise the Mind.

Case history

A 41-year-old man had been suffering from stabbing finger pain in his right hand for 6 months, which occurred after carrying some heavy things. His finger pain had worsened over the preceding 12 days. It also worsened at night and with immobility, when carrying heavy things, and when finger movement was limited. His tongue was purple with a white coating, and his pulse was deep and wiry.

Diagnosis
Stagnation of Blood.

Principle of treatment
Promote Qi and Blood circulation, remove Blood stasis and relieve the finger pain.

Acupuncture treatment
L1-4, PC-6, TE-5, LU-7 and Extra Baxie. Reducing method was used on all these points.

Explanations

- LI-4, the Source point of the Large Intestine channel, activates the circulation of Qi and Blood and relieves the finger pain.
- TE-5, the Connecting point of the Triple Burner channel, promotes the circulation of Qi and Blood and harmonises the collateral.
- PC-6, the Connecting point of the Pericardium channel, promotes the circulation of Qi and Blood and tranquillises the Mind.
- The combination of TE-5 and PC-6 has a strong effect on removing Blood stasis and relieving the pain.
- LU-7 promotes the circulation of Qi, harmonises the collateral and relieves the pain.
- Extra Baxie regulates the circulation of Qi in the locality to relieve the pain.

The patient was cured after 2 months of treatment. He was followed up by letter 2 years later, and he said he had experienced no further finger pain.

DEFICIENCY OF BLOOD

Symptoms and signs

Slight finger pain, numbness of the fingers with stiffness, accompanied by weakness in the hands, a pale complexion, pale lips, dizziness, palpitations, dry stools, a pale tongue with a thin and white coating, and a thready and weak pulse.

Principle of treatment

Tonify the Qi, nourish the Blood and sedate the pain.

HERBAL TREATMENT

Prescription

BA ZHEN TANG
Eight-Precious Decoction
Dang Gui *Radix Angelicae Sinensis* 12 g
Chuan Xiong *Rhizoma Ligustici Chuanxiong* 10 g
Bai Shao *Radix Paeoniae Alba* 12 g
Shu Di Huang *Radix Rehmanniae Praeparata* 12 g
Ren Shen *Radix Ginseng* 6 g
Bai Zhu *Rhizoma Atractylodis Macrocephalae* 12 g
Fu Ling *Poria* 12 g
Sang Zhi *Ramulus Mori* 20 g
Zhi Gan Cao *Radix Glycyrrhizae Praeparata* 6 g

Explanations

- The main function of this prescription is to reinforce the Qi and nourish Blood. When the muscles and collateral are properly nourished, the finger pain disappears spontaneously.
- Dang Gui, Bai Shao and Shu Di Huang nourish the Blood and tonify the Kidney-Essence.
- Ren Shen, Bai Zhu, Fu Ling and Zhi Gan Cao strengthen the Spleen and reinforce the Qi so as to promote the production of Qi and Blood.
- Chuan Xiong activates the circulation of Qi and Blood and relieves the obstruction in the channels.
- Sang Zhi is one of the main herbs for relieving pain in the upper part of the body, especially in the limbs.

Modifications

1. If there is an aversion to cold or cold limbs due to deficiency of Yang-Qi, add Gui Zhi *Ramulus Cinnamomi* 10 g and San Ji Sheng *Ramulus Loranthi* 10 g to reinforce the Yang-Qi and relieve the pain.
2. If the fingers are swollen owing to poor Water metabolism caused by deficiency of Spleen-Qi, add Hai Feng Teng *Caulis Piperis Futokadsurae* 15 g,

Ze Xie *Rhizoma Alismatis* 10 g and Wu Jia Pi *Cortex Acanthopanacis Radicis* 10 g to induce urination, eliminate Damp and relieve the pain.

Patent remedies

Gui Pi Wan *Tonifying the Spleen Decoction*
Shi Quan Da Bu Wan *All-Inclusive Great Tonifying Pill*

ACUPUNCTURE TREATMENT

LI-4 Hegu, PC-6 Neiguan, HT-7 Shenmen, SP-6 Sanyinjiao, ST-36 Zusanli, KI-3 Taixi and Ah Shi points. Even method is used on LI-4, PC-6, CV-6 and HT-7. Reinforcing method is used on ST-36 and SP-6. Reducing method is used on the Ah Shi points. Treatment is given every other day.

Explanations

- LI-4, the Source point of the Large Intestine channel, and PC-6, the Connecting point of the Pericardium channel, promote the circulation of Qi in the channels and relieve the finger pain.
- HT-7, the Stream and Source point, promotes the circulation of Blood and nourishes it.
- ST-36 and SP-6 activate the Spleen and Stomach and promote the production of Qi and Blood.
- KI-3, the Source point, promotes the production of Kidney-Essence so as to promote the production of Blood.
- The Ah Shi points regulate the Qi and Blood and relieve the finger pain.

Modifications

1. If there is an aversion to cold or cold fingers due to deficiency of Yang-Qi, add CV-6 with moxibustion to reinforce the Yang-Qi.
2. If the fingers are swollen, add SP-9 and TE-6 to promote urination and eliminate Damp.
3. If there is generalised tiredness due to deficiency of Qi and Blood, add ST-42 and SP-3, the Source points, to strengthen the Spleen and Stomach and tonify the Qi and Blood.

DEFICIENCY OF ESSENCE OF KIDNEY AND LIVER

Symptoms and signs

Slight finger pain with spasm, gradual deformity of the fingers, weakness of the fingers, wrists, arms and legs, accompanied by tiredness, lower back pain, tinnitus, a poor memory, hair loss, a thin tongue coating and a weak pulse, especially at the Kidney positions.

Principle of treatment

Tonify the Kidney and Liver, nourish the Essence, strengthen the tendons and bones and relieve the finger pain.

HERBAL TREATMENT

Prescription

LIU WEI DI HUANG WAN
Six-Flavour Rehmanniae Pill
Shu Di Huang *Radix Rehmanniae Praeparata* 15 g
Shan Yao *Rhizoma Dioscoreae* 12 g
Shan Zhu Yu *Fructus Corni* 15 g
Tu Si Zi *Semen Cuscutae* 12 g
Dang Gui *Radix Angelicae Sinensis* 12 g
Mu Dan Pi *Cortex Moutan Radicis* 9 g
Sang Zhi *Ramulus Mori* 15 g

Explanations

- Shu Di Huang, Shan Yao and Shan Zhu Yu nourish the Essence of the Liver and Kidney.
- Tu Si Zi nourishes the Kidney-Yin and Kidney-Yang.
- Dang Gui promotes the circulation of Qi and Blood and removes the obstructions in the channels.
- Mu Dan Pi clears Deficient-Heat.
- Sang Zhi promotes the circulation of Qi and Blood and relieves the finger pain.

Modifications

1. If there is lower back pain, add Xu Duan *Radix Dipsaci* 10 g, Sang Ji Sheng *Ramulus Loranthi* 10 g and Bai Shao *Radix Paeoniae Alba* 10 g to strengthen the Kidney and relieve the pain.
2. If there is night sweating and heat in the palms and soles of the feet due to deficiency of Kidney-Yin, add Gui Ban Jiao *Plastrum Testudinis Colla* 10 g and Han Lian Cao *Herba Ecliptae* 10 g to nourish the Kidney-Yin and clear Deficient-Heat.
3. If there is an aversion to cold, impotence and cold hands and feet due to deficiency of Kidney-Yang, add Ba Ji Tian *Radix Morindae Officinalis* 10 g and Gou Ji *Rhizoma Cibotii* 10 g to tonify the Kidney-Yang and dispel Cold.
4. If there is constipation, add Xuan Shen *Radix Scrophulariae* 15 g to nourish the Kidney-Yin and

lubricate the Large Intestine so as to relieve the constipation.

Patent remedies

Liu Wei Di Huang Wan *Six-Flavour Rehmanniae Pill*
Hai Ma Bu Shen Wan *Sea Horse Tonify Kidney Pill*

ACUPUNCTURE TREATMENT

LI-4 Hegu, PC-6 Neiguan, KI-3 Taixi, LR-3 Taichong, SP-6 Sanyinjiao and Ah Shi points. Reinforcing method is used on these points except for the Ah Shi points, on which even method is used.

Explanations

- KI-3, the Source point of the Kidney channel, and LR-3, the Source point of the Liver channel, reinforce the Essence of the Liver and Kidney, and strengthen the tendons and bones.
- SP-6, the crossing point of the three Yin channels of the foot, activates the Spleen and Stomach and promotes the production of Qi and Blood so as to tonify the Essence of the Liver and Kidney.
- LI-4, Source point of the Large Intestine channel, regulates the circulation of Qi and Blood and relieves the finger pain.

- PC-6, the Connecting point of the Pericardium channel, promotes the circulation of Qi, tranquillises the Mind and relieves the pain.
- Even method applied to the Ah Shi points can clear obstructions from the locality and relieve the finger pain.

Modifications

1. If there is lower back pain, add BL-23 and BL-58 to strengthen the lower back and regulate the channels.
2. If there is night sweating, heat in the palms and the soles of the foot and thirst, add KI-7 and HT-6 to nourish Yin and clear Deficient-Heat.
3. If there is a dry throat and thirst, add LU-8 and KI-6 to nourish the Yin, clear Deficient-Fire and promote the secretion of Body Fluids.
4. If there is irritability, add GB-20 to calm the Liver and relieve the irritability.
5. If there is insomnia, add HT-7 and Extra Anmian to calm the Heart and tranquillise the Mind.
6. If there is an aversion to cold, with cold hands and feet, add CV-6 and CV-4 with moxibustion to warm the Interior and dispel Cold.
7. If there is oedema in the legs, add SP-9 and BL-22 to promote urination and relieve the oedema.
8. If the appetite is poor with loose stools due to deficiency of Spleen-Yang, add ST-36 and SP-3 to strengthen the Spleen and improve the appetite.

Part 8

Lower limb pain 下肢疼痛

Hip pain 40

髋
痛

Hip pain may occur on one or both sides of the body, and may refer to the sacrum and coccyx region or to the inguinal regions and thighs. Generally speaking, according to TCM theory it can be caused by invasion of External pathogenic Wind, Cold and Damp, or of Wind, Damp and Heat, stagnation or deficiency of the Qi and Blood, or deficiency of the Liver and Kidney. Hip pain may be attributed to any of the following disorders in Western medicine: rheumatic fever, rheumatic arthritis, arthrosis of the hip joint, hyperosteogeny of the hip joint, gout, fibrositis, nerve pain, piriformis syndrome, synovitis of the hip, snapping hip and coxa plana.

Aetiology and pathology

Invasion of External pathogenic factors

Poor functioning of the Defensive Qi, open skin pores, exposure to wind during sweating after physical exercise or labour, catching cold in the water or dwelling in a damp place for a long time may all cause the hip to be invaded by the External pathogens Wind, Cold and Damp. These impede the circulation of Qi and Blood in the channels, joints, muscles and tendons in the locality of the hip, causing hip pain.

The clinical symptoms and signs vary greatly depending on which pathogenic factors have invaded. Wind is characteristically moving and changing. If Wind invasion is predominant, the hip pain is migrating in nature (e.g. moving from left side to right side, or up and down). Cold is a Yin pathogenic factor, and its characteristics are contraction and stagnation. Pathogenic Cold tends to impair the Yang-Qi of the body and impede the circulation of Qi and Blood. If Cold invasion is predominant, the muscles and tendons around the hip joints contract, leading to stagnation of Qi and Blood, which causes a severe pain with a cold sensation. Damp is characteristically lingering and heavy. So if Damp invasion is predominant, there is obstruction of the channels leading to numbness and a fixed pain in the hip with a feeling of heaviness.

Exposure to Wind-Damp-Heat can also induce hip pain, especially in people with a constitutional excess of Yang or deficiency of Yin. In some other cases, patients who at first suffer invasion of External pathogenic Wind, Cold and Damp may later on suffer from Wind, Damp and Heat, because if Cold remains in the body for a long time it may gradually generate Heat, especially in those with a constitution excess of Yang and Yin deficiency. Heat is characterised by a red colour and a burning nature. Wind, Damp and Heat invasion disturbs the Qi and Blood in the channels, especially the Bright Yang channel of the foot.

When it invades the lower limbs, it causes stagnation of Qi and Blood circulation in the channels and blockage of the channels by Damp-Heat, leading to a hip pain with redness and swelling.

463

Bad diet

Bad diets, such as eating too much sweet and fatty food, or drinking too much alcohol, may impair the Spleen and Stomach, leading to the formation of Damp-Heat in the body. When Damp-Heat flows downward to the lower limbs, it blocks the channels, causing hip pain to occur.

Prolonged persistence of Cold-Damp in the body may also cause gradual generation of Heat, leading to formation of Damp-Heat, so eating foods that tend to encourage Cold (such as raw and cold foods) and Damp (such as dairy products) can also trigger hip pain.

Stagnation of Qi and Blood

Qi and Blood should circulate freely in the channels around the hip. If the Qi and Blood stagnate because of various causes, such as overstrain, physical trauma or inappropriate operations on the hip, they block the channels, leading to a painful and swollen hip joint. In addition, the wrong treatment, such as too forceful manipulation or very vigorous massage of the hip joint, can also be an important cause of Blood stagnation, and should not be ignored.

Deficiency of Qi and Blood

According to TCM theory, there are two major causes of pain, one of which is malnourishment of the channels, collateral, joints, muscles and bones. Excessive strain, prolonged illness and poor diet can all lead to consumption or diminished production of the Qi and Blood, which eventually result in a deficiency of the Qi and Blood, so the hip is not properly nourished, and hip pain occurs.

Deficiency of Liver and Kidney

Overstrain, prolonged sickness or a weak constitution in elderly people may cause consumption of Qi and Blood, and deficiency of the Liver and Kidney. In this condition the tendons, bones, muscles and joints around the hip may not be properly nourished, leading to a painful hip with a feeling of weakness at the joint.

Treatment based on differentiation

Differentiation

Differentiation of External or Internal origin

— Acute onset of hip pain of short duration, accompanied by External symptoms, is usually caused by invasion of External pathogenic factors. Traumatic injury could also cause acute hip pain.
— Chronic onset of hip pain of long duration, accompanied by symptoms resulting from internal disorders, is usually caused by Internal disorder such as deficiency of Qi and Blood, deficiency of Liver and Kidney, or stagnation of Qi and Blood.

Differentiation of character of the pain

— Wandering hip pain, with an aversion to wind, or associated with chills and fever, is usually caused by invasion of Wind-Cold-Damp with predominance of Wind.
— Severe hip pain with a cold sensation, an aversion to cold, alleviation of the hip pain by warmth, aggravation of the pain by cold, or cramp of the muscles, is mainly caused by invasion of Wind-Cold-Damp with predominance of Cold.
— Hip pain with swelling and a fixed localization, heavy sensation of the lower limbs, or sensitivity to humid weather, is usually caused by invasion of Wind-Cold-Damp with predominance of Damp.
— Swollen and painful hip joint with a local burning sensation and redness, is usually caused by invasion of Wind-Heat-Damp.
— Slight and dull pain of the hip joint with rigidity in the morning suggests deficiency of the Liver and Kidney.
— Fixed and pricking pain of the hip joint, with a history of trauma, is mainly caused by stagnation of Qi and Blood.
— Continuous pain in both hips, with numbness and weakness of the lower limbs, is usually caused by deficiency of Qi and Blood.

Differentiation of shape of the hip joint

— A normal-shaped hip joint is usually found in those with hip pain due to invasion of Wind-Cold-Damp.
— Acute onset of swelling and a red hip joint is usually caused by invasion of Wind-Heat-Damp.
— Swelling hip joint with deformity, hyperosteogeny and muscular atrophy, indicates deficiency of Liver and Kidney.
— Swelling hip joint, with red or hard nodules under the skin around the joint, is usually due to stagnation of Qi and Blood.
— Muscular atrophy at the hip or on the legs is usually caused by deficiency of Qi and Blood.

Treatment

INVASION OF WIND-COLD-DAMP WITH PREDOMINANCE OF WIND

Symptoms and signs

Wandering hip pain, with difficult flexion and extension or intorsion and extorsion of the hip joints, which is aggravated in windy conditions, associated with chills and fever, an aversion to wind, a thin white greasy tongue coating and a superficial pulse.

Principle of treatment

Dispel Wind, resolve Damp, eliminate Cold, promote circulation in the channels and stop the pain.

HERBAL TREATMENT

Prescription

FANG FENG TANG
Ledebouriella Decoction
Fang Feng *Radix Ledebouriellae* 10 g
Ma Huang *Herba Ephedrae* 6 g
Dang Gui *Radix Angelicae Sinensis* 12 g
Huai Niu Xi *Radix Achyranthis Bidentatae* 10 g
Qin Jiao *Radix Gentianae Macrophyllae* 10 g
Rou Gui *Cortex Cinnamomi* 6 g
Fu Ling *Poria* 12 g
Sheng Jiang *Rhizoma Zingiberis Recens* 3 g
Da Zao *Fructus Ziziphi Jujubae* 6 g
Gan Cao *Radix Glycyrrhizae* 6 g

Explanations

- Fang Feng and Ma Huang dispel Wind and Cold and relieve External symptoms.
- Qin Jiao and Rou Gui warm the channels and dispel Cold so as to relieve the hip pain.
- Dang Gui promotes the circulation of Blood and removes the obstructions from the collateral.
- Huai Niu Xi promotes the circulation of Blood, strengthens the bone and induces the herbs to reach the hip joints.
- Fu Ling is good at strengthening the Spleen and inducing urination.
- The last three herbs can coordinate all the herbs in the prescription.

Modifications

1. If there is a fever and chills, add Gui Zhi *Ramulus Cinnamomi* 10 g to relieve the Exterior syndrome and reduce the fever.

2. If the hip joints are swollen, add Du Huo *Radix Angelica Pubescentis* 10 g and Han Fang Ji *Radix Stephaniae Tetrandrae* 10 g to dispel Damp, reduce the swelling and sedate the pain.
3. If the hip joint is swollen and red, add Zhi Mu *Rhizoma Anemarrhenae* 10 g and Huang Bai *Cortex Phellodendri* 10 g to clear Heat, eliminate Damp and relieve the swelling and redness.

Patent remedy

Jing Fang Bai Du Pian *Schizonepeta and Ledebouriella Tablet to Overcome Pathogenic Influences*

ACUPUNCTURE TREATMENT

TE-5 Waiguan, LI-4 Hegu, BL-12 Fengmen, GB-30 Huantiao, GB-31 Fengshi, GB-35 Yangjiao, SP-10 Xuehai, SP-6 Sanyinjiao and some local Ah Shi points. Reducing method is used on these points.

Explanations

- TE-5, LI-4 and BL-12 dispel External pathogenic Wind and relieve External symptoms.
- GB-30 is the meeting point of the Gall Bladder channel and the Bladder channel. It eliminates Damp and Wind, invigorates the circulation of Qi in the collateral and removes obstructions in the channels.
- GB-31 dispels External Wind and eliminates Damp in the lower limbs.
- GB-35, the Accumulation point of the Yang Linking Vessel, harmonises the collateral, promotes the circulation of Qi and Blood and relieves hip pain.
- SP-10 activates the circulation of Blood. SP-6 is the crossing point of the Kidney, Spleen, Liver channels, and is good for regulating the Blood and Qi.
- The Ah Shi points around the hip joint are suitable for regulating the circulation of Qi and Blood in the locality.

Modifications

1. If there is a slight fever and chills, add GV-14, the meeting point for all the Yang channels, with moxibustion, to dispel Wind, to relieve Exterior symptoms and reduce the fever.
2. If the hip joint is swollen, add SP-9, the Sea point, to remove Damp and reduce the swelling.
3. If there is redness, swelling and hot sensation of the hip joint, add GB-44, the Spring point of the

Gall Bladder channel, and ST-44, the Spring point of the Stomach channel, to clear Heat and reduce the swelling.

4. If there is hip pain along the Bladder channel, add BL-36, BL-58 and BL-63 to harmonise the collateral and relieve the pain.

5. If there is hip pain along the Gall Bladder channel, add GB-36, GB-34 and GB-41 to promote the circulation of Qi and Blood in the channel and relieve the pain.

6. If there is hip pain along the Stomach channel, add ST-30, ST-31, ST-34, ST-40 and ST-42 to promote the circulation of Qi and Blood in the channel, relieve the blockage and arrest the pain.

7. If there is hip pain along the Liver channel, add LR-3, LR-5, LR-11 and LR-12 to harmonise the collateral, promote the circulation of Qi and Blood in the channel and relieve the pain.

8. Some corresponding points on the shoulder should be applied in order to strengthen the therapeutic effect.

Case history

A 24-year-old man had been suffering from wandering hip pain for more than 2 months. Two months previously, he had caught a cold because of insufficient covering one night during his sleep. To begin with, he had much generalised body pain, a lower back pain, a headache, an aversion to cold and a slight fever. At the same time, he had a slight hip pain on both sides, but worse on the right one. He went to his general practitioner and took some drugs to relieve the cold for a few days. After this medication, his general cold symptoms improved slightly, but his wandering hip pain remained, together with limitation of joint movement. He continued the medications for another 3 weeks. Two weeks previously, he went to the hospital and there he was diagnosed with sciatica.

When he came to the clinic, he had hip pain, especially at the right one. The pain was mainly along the Gall Bladder channel. He also had a lower back pain with a cold feeling, an aggravation of the pain on contact with wind or cold, a thin and white tongue coating and a superficial and wiry pulse.

Diagnosis
Hip pain due to invasion of Wind, Cold and Damp.

Principle of treatment
Dispel Wind, eliminate Cold and Damp, harmonise the collateral and sedate the pain.

Herbal treatment
FANG FENG TANG
Ledebouriella Decoction
Fang Feng *Radix Ledebouriellae* 10 g
Ma Huang *Herba Ephedrae* 6 g
Dang Gui *Radix Angelicae Sinensis* 10 g

Qin Jiao *Radix Gentianae Macrophyllae* 10 g
Du Huo *Radix Angelicae Pubescentis* 10 g
Rou Gui *Cortex Cinnamomi* 6 g
Fu Ling *Poria* 15 g
Gan Cao *Radix Glycyrrhizae* 6 g

Explanations
- Fang Feng and Ma Huang dispel Wind-Cold and relieve External symptoms.
- Qin Jiao and Rou Gui warm the channels and dispel Cold.
- Dang Gui promotes the circulation of Blood and removes obstructions from the collateral.
- Du Huo dispels Wind-Cold-Damp in the lower body and relieves the hip pain.
- Fu Ling eliminates Damp.
- Gan Cao harmonises the actions of the other herbs in the prescription.

Acupuncture treatment
TE-5 Waiguan, GB-30 Huantiao, GB-31 Fengshi, GB-34 Yanglingquan, GB-35 Yangjiao, GB-41 Zulinqi, SP-6 Sanyinjiao, BL-58 Feiyang and two local Ah Shi points. Reducing method was applied on these points. Treatment was given once every day.

Explanations
- TE-5 and GB-41, a special point combination, dispel external pathogenic Wind, Cold and Damp and relieve External symptoms. They can also open the Lesser Yang channels and relieve pain in the sides of the body.
- GB-31 helps the above points to dispel external Wind and eliminate Damp in the lower limbs.
- GB-30, the meeting point of the Gall Bladder channel and the Bladder channel, eliminates Damp and Wind, invigorates the circulation of Qi in the collateral and removes obstructions in the channels.
- GB-34, the Sea point, and GB-35, the Accumulation point of the Yang Linking Vessel, harmonise the collateral, promote the circulation of Qi and Blood in the channel and relieve the hip pain.
- BL-58, the Connecting point, harmonises the collateral, dispels Wind, Cold and Damp and relieves the pain.
- SP-6, the crossing point of the Kidney, Spleen, Liver channels, activates the circulation of Blood and relieves the hip pain.
- The Ah Shi points around hip joint regulate the circulation of Qi and Blood in the locality so as to relieve the hip pain.

The patient was cured after receiving treatment for 3 weeks. He was followed up 6 months later and he stated he had experienced no more hip pain since the herbal and acupuncture treatment.

INVASION OF WIND-COLD-DAMP WITH PREDOMINANCE OF COLD

Symptoms and signs

Severe hip pain with a cold feeling, radiating to legs, which is aggravated by contact with cold and alleviated by warmth, accompanied by an aversion to cold, cold limbs, limited movement in the joint, a white tongue coating and a tight and superficial pulse.

Principle of treatment

Warm the channels, dispel Cold, remove Damp and relieve the hip pain.

HERBAL TREATMENT

Prescription

WU TOU TANG
Aconite Decoction
Zhi Chuan Wu *Radix Aconiti Praeparata* 10 g
Ma Huang *Herba Ephedrae* 6 g
Bai Shao *Radix Paeoniae Alba* 12 g
Gan Cao *Radix Glycyrrhizae* 6 g
Huang Qi *Radix Astragali seu Hedysari* 15 g

Explanations

- Zhi Chuan Wu and Ma Huang, warm in nature, warm the channels and dispel Wind, remove Damp and sedate the pain.
- Bai Shao and Gan Cao relieve muscular spasm and stop the pain.
- Huang Qi reinforces the Qi and consolidates the body surface. It can also promote the circulation of Blood and relieve the pain.

Modifications

1. If there is an aversion to cold, add Xi Xin *Herba Asari* 3 g to eliminate Cold and relieve the Exterior symptoms.
2. If there is hip pain radiating to the legs, add Chuan Niu Xi *Radix Cyathulae* 10 g to sedate the pain.
3. If the hip joints are swollen, add Cang Zhu *Rhizoma Atractylodis* 10 g and Mu Tong *Caulis Akebiae* 6 g to promote urination, eliminate Damp and reduce the swelling.
4. If there is cold in the lower limbs, add Du Huo *Radix Angelicae Pubescentis* 10 g and Rou Gui *Cortex Cinnamomi* 5 g to warm the channels, reinforce Yang and dispel Cold.
5. If there is severe pain, add Jiang Huang *Rhizoma Curcumae Longae* 10 g to regulate the circulation of Blood and relieve the pain.

Patent remedy

Han Shi Bi Chong Ji *Cold-Damp Bi Syndrome Infusion*

ACUPUNCTURE TREATMENT

TE-5 Waiguan, LI-4 Hegu, GB-30 Huantiao, GB-31 Fengshi, GB-41 Zulinqi, ST-36 Zusanli, SP-6 Sanyinjiao, CV-4 Guanyuan and Ah Shi points. Reducing method is used on these points except for ST-36 and CV-4, on which tonifying method is used. Moxibustion is used on TE-5, LI-4, ST-36 and CV-4.

Explanations

- TE-5 and LI-4 dispel External pathogenic Wind, eliminate Cold and relieve External symptoms. Also TE-5 together with GB-41 dispels Wind, Cold and Damp, opens the Lesser Yang channels and relieves pain in the sides of the body.
- The Ah Shi points, GB-30 and GB-31, all the local points, regulate the circulation of Qi and Blood in the local areas so as to relieve the hip pain.
- CV-4 and ST-36, the Sea point, warm the channels and dispel Cold.
- SP-6 activates the circulation of Blood and relieves hip pain.
- Moxibustion is applied to warm the channels, dispel Cold and relieve the pain.

Modifications

1. If there is swelling of the hip joint with a feeling of heaviness, add SP-9 to eliminate Damp and reduce the swelling.
2. If there is a cold sensation in the body and cold limbs, add KI-3 and CV-8 with moxibustion to reinforce the Yang and dispel Cold.
3. If there is a slight fever and chills, add GV-14 with moxibustion to dispel Wind, relieve Exterior symptoms and reduce the fever.
4. If there is a headache, add GB-20 to dispel Wind, Cold and Damp and relieve the headache.
5. If there is a hip pain along the Bladder channel, add BL-36, BL-58 and BL-63 to harmonise the collateral and relieve the pain.
6. If there is a hip pain along the Gall Bladder channel, add GB-36, GB-34 and GB-40 to promote the circulation of Qi and Blood in the channel and relieve the pain.
7. If there is hip pain along the Stomach channel, add ST-30, ST-31, ST-34, ST-40 and ST-42 to promote the circulation of Qi and Blood in the channel, relieve the blockage and arrest the pain.
8. If there is hip pain along the Liver channel, add LR-3, LR-5, LR-11 and LR-12 to harmonise the collateral, promote the circulation of Qi and Blood in the channel and relieve the pain.

9. Some corresponding points on the shoulder should be used in order to strengthen the therapeutic effect.

Case history

A 36-year-old male had been suffering from weakness and pain in the lumbar region for a few years due to herniation between vertebrae L4 and L5. When he arrived at the clinic he had also been suffering from lower back pain and severe pain in the left hip joint with a cold sensation for 5 months. These worsened in cold conditions, when walking, or even when coughing. He also had weakness of the lower limbs, limited intorsion and extorsion of the hip joint, radiation of the lower back pain down the left leg to the toe along the Gall Bladder channel, and a tight, and weak and deep pulse at the Kidney positions.

Diagnosis
Hip pain and lower back pain due to deficiency of Kidney-Yang with invasion of Wind, Cold and Damp.

Principle of treatment
Reinforce Kidney-Yang, dispel Cold, strengthen the back and sedate the pain.

Acupuncture treatment
TE-5, LI-4, GB-30, GB-31, GB-34, GB-36, GB-40, GB-41, SP-6, KI-3 and CV-4. Reducing method was used on these points; tonifying method was used on CV-4 and KI-3. Moxibustion was used on TE-5, LI-4, KI-3 and CV-4.

Explanations
- TE-5 and LI-4 dispel External pathogenic Wind, eliminate Cold and relieve External symptoms. Also, TE-5 together with GB-41 dispels Wind, Cold and Damp, opens the Lesser Yang channels and relieves pain in the sides of the body.
- GB-30 and GB-31, the local points, regulate the circulation of Qi and Blood in the locality so as to relieve the lower back pain and hip pain.
- GB-36, the Accumulation point, GB-34, the Gathering point for the tendons, and GB-40, the Source point, promote the circulation of Qi and Blood in the Gall Bladder channel, harmonise the collateral, eliminate Blood stagnation and relieve the hip pain.
- CV-4 and KI-3 warm the channels, reinforce the Yang and dispel Cold.
- SP-6 activates the circulation of Blood and relieves the lower back pain and hip pain.
- Moxibustion warms the channels, dispels Cold and relieves the pain.

The patient was cured of the hip pain and his lower back pain was greatly improved after 15 treatment sessions, with no relapse at a follow-up a month later.

INVASION OF WIND-COLD-DAMP WITH PREDOMINANCE OF DAMP

Symptoms and signs

Pain and swelling in the hip joints with limited joint movement, which worsen in cloudy and rainy weather conditions, accompanied by numbness of the skin and muscles, a heavy sensation in the buttocks and lower limbs, limping, a white and greasy tongue coating and a soft and slow pulse.

Principle of treatment

Eliminate Damp, dispel Cold and Wind, promote circulation of the collateral and sedate the pain.

HERBAL TREATMENT

Prescription

YI YI REN TANG
Coix Decoction
Yi Yi Ren *Semen Coicis* 15 g
Cang Zhu *Rhizoma Atractylodis* 12 g
Qiang Huo *Rhizoma et Radix Notopterygii* 12 g
Du Huo *Radix Angelicae Pubescentis* 10 g
Fang Feng *Radix Ledebouriellae* 10 g
Zhi Chuan Wu *Radix Aconiti Praeparata* 6 g
Ma Huang *Herba Ephedrae* 10 g
Gui Zhi *Ramulus Cinnamomi* 6 g
Dang Gui *Radix Angelicae Sinensis* 12 g
Chuan Xiong *Radix Ligustici Chuanxiong* 12 g
Sheng Jiang *Rhizoma Zingiberis Recens* 6 g
Gan Cao *Radix Glycyrrhizae* 6 g

Explanations

- Yi Yi Ren and Cang Zhu strengthen the Spleen and remove Damp.
- Qiang Huo, Du Huo and Fang Feng dispel Wind-Cold and eliminate Damp.
- Zhi Chuan Wu, Ma Huang, Gui Zhi warm the channels, dispel Cold and remove Damp.
- Dang Gui and Chuan Xiong nourish the Blood and promote its circulation.
- Sheng Jiang and Gan Cao strengthen the Spleen and regulate the Middle Burner.

Modifications

1. If the joints are swollen, add Bi Xie *Rhizoma Dioscoreae Septemlobae* 15 g and Jiang Huang *Rhizoma Curcumae Longae* 10 g to remove the obstructions from the collateral and reduce the swelling.

2. If there is a feeling of heaviness in the legs, add Fu Ling *Poria* 15 g and Ze Xie *Rhizoma Alismatis* 10 g to promote urination and eliminate Damp.
3. If there is severe hip pain, add Wu Gong *Scolopendra* 3 g to relieve the pain.
4. If there is numbness of the skin, add Hai Tong Pi *Cortex Erythrinae* 10 g and Xi Xian Cao *Herba Siegesbeckiae* 10 g to dispel Wind and clear the collateral.
5. If there is lower back pain, add Du Zhong *Cortex Eucommiae* 10 g and Sang Ji Sheng *Ramulus Loranthi* 10 g to strengthen the lower back and relieve the lower back pain.
6. If there is nausea or vomiting and diarrhoea, add Sha Ren *Fructus Ammomi* 5 g and Bai Zhu *Rhizoma Atractylodis Macrocephalae* 10 g to activate the Spleen and Stomach and relieve Damp in the Middle Burner.

Patent remedies

Feng Shi Pian *Wind-Damp Tablet*
Tian Ma Qu Feng Bu Pian *Gastrodia Dispel Wind Formula Tablet*

ACUPUNCTURE TREATMENT

TE-6 Zhigou, LI-4 Hegu, ST-31 Biguan, ST-40 Fenglong, SP-9 Yinlingquan, GB-29 Juliao, GB-30 Huantiao, BL-12 Fengmen, BL-54 Zhibian, BL-58 Feiyang and Ah Shi points. Reducing method is used on these points.

Explanations

- TE-6, LI-4 and BL-12 dispel External pathogenic Wind, eliminate Cold, resolve Damp and relieve External symptoms.
- BL-58, the Connecting point, dispels Wind, Cold and Damp and harmonises the collateral.
- ST-40, the Connecting point, and SP-9, the Sea point, eliminate Damp in the channels and relieve pain.
- GB-29, GB-30, BL-54, ST-31 and the Ah Shi points promote the circulation of Qi and Blood in the local channels and collateral, remove the obstructions and relieve the pain.

Modifications

1. If there is an aversion to cold and cold in the lower limbs, add moxibustion on CV-4 to warm the body, reinforce the Yang and dispel Cold.

2. If there is numbness in the lower back and hip regions, add moxibustion or Plum Blossom needles on the local areas to promote the circulation of Qi and Blood.
3. If there is hip pain along the Bladder channel, add BL-36, BL-58 and BL-63 to harmonise the collateral and relieve the pain.
4. If there is hip pain along the Gall Bladder channel, add GB-36, GB-34 and GB-40 to promote Qi and Blood circulation in the channel and relieve the pain.
5. If there is hip pain along the Stomach channel, add ST-30, ST-34, ST-40 and ST-42 to promote the circulation of Qi and Blood in the channel, remove the blockage and arrest the pain.
6. If there is hip pain along the Liver channel, add LR-3, LR-5, LR-11 and LR-12 to harmonise the collateral, promote the circulation of Qi and Blood in the channel and relieve the pain.
7. Some corresponding points on the shoulder should be used in order to strengthen the therapeutic effect.

DOWNWARD FLOW OF DAMP-HEAT
Symptoms and signs

Swelling and painful hip joint, which is aggravated by touching, with limited movement, and a burning sensation with redness. Accompanying symptoms include irritability, restlessness, a poor appetite, a bitter taste in the mouth, scanty and yellow urination, occasional fever, a yellow and greasy tongue coating and a slippery and rapid pulse.

In acute pain, beside the swelling, redness and pain of the joint, there are usually some external symptoms, such as an aversion to cold, fever, generalised body pain, a headache, a red tongue with a yellow and greasy coating and a superficial and slippery pulse.

Principle of treatment

Clear Heat, eliminate Damp and sedate the pain. If there is invasion of Wind-Damp-Heat, then add the method for dispelling Wind-Damp-Heat.

HERBAL TREATMENT
Prescription

BAI HU JIA GUI ZHI TANG and **SAN MIAO WAN**
White Tiger plus Ramulus Cinnamon Decoction and *Three-Marvel Pill*
Zhi Mu *Rhizoma Anemarrhenae* 10 g
Shi Gao *Gypsum Fibrosum* 20 g
Gui Zhi *Ramulus Cinnamomi* 8 g

Gan Cao *Radix Glycyrrhizae* 6 g
Jing Mi *Semen Oryzae* 10 g
Huang Bai *Cortex Phellodendri* 10 g
Cang Zhu *Rhizoma Atractylodis* 10 g
Huai Niu Xi *Radix Achyranthis Bidentatae* 10 g
Wei Ling Xian *Radix Clematidis* 10 g
Han Fang Ji *Radix Stephaniae Tetrandrae* 10 g
Sang Zhi *Ramulus Mori* 15 g

Explanations

- Shi Gao and Zhi Mu are the main herbs in Bai Hu Jia Gui Zhi Tang for clearing Heat and reducing fever.
- Gan Cao and Jing Mi benefit the Stomach and reinforce the Body Fluids, moderating the extremely Cold nature of Shi Gao.
- Gui Zhi dispels Wind, harmonises the collateral and promotes the circulation of Blood to relieve hip pain.
- Wei Ling Xian, Fang Ji and Sang Zhi expel pathogenic Wind, eliminate Damp, promote the circulation of Blood and unblock the channels.
- Huang Bai and Cang Zhu dry Damp, clear Heat and reduce the swelling of the hip.
- Huai Niu Xi induces the herbs to the ankle and eliminates Damp in the Lower Burner.

Modifications

1. If there is a fever, add Jin Yin Hua *Flos Lonicerae* 10 g and Lian Qiao *Fructus Forsythiae* 10 g to clear Heat and reduce the fever.
2. If the hip is swollen and red, add Tu Fu Ling *Rhizoma Smilacis* 10 g and Sheng Di Huang *Radix Rehmanniae Recens* 15 g to clear Heat, remove Toxin, reduce swelling and relieve the pain.
3. If there is pus in the hip joint, add Di Fu Zi *Fructus Kochiae* 10 g and Chi Shao *Radix Paeoniae Rubra* 10 g to eliminate Damp-Heat and cool the Blood.
4. If there is severe hip pain, add Jiang Huang *Rhizoma Curcumae Longae* 10 g to clear Heat, promote the circulation of Blood and stop the pain.
5. If the appetite is poor, add Ban Xia *Rhizoma Pinelliae* 10 g and Chen Pi *Pericarpium Citri Reticulatae* 10 g to regulate the Qi and improve the appetite.
6. If there is a thirst, add Xuan Shen *Radix Scrophulariae* 10 g and Ge Gen *Radix Puerariae* 10 g to clear the Heat and relieve the thirst.
7. If there is irritability, add Deng Xin Cao *Medulla Junci* 15 g to clear the Fire and calm the Mind.
8. If there is constipation, add Da Huang *Radix et Rhizoma Rhei* 6 g and Mang Xiao *Natrii Sulfas* 6 g to eliminate Heat, promote defecation and relieve the constipation.

Patent remedies

Feng Shi Xiao Tong Pian *Wind-Damp Dispel Pain Pill*
Shi Re Bi Chong Ji *Damp-Heat Bi Infusion*
San Miao Wan *Three-Marvel Pill*

ACUPUNCTURE TREATMENT

TE-6 Zhigou, LI-4 Hegu, ST-40 Fenglong, SP-6 Sanyinjiao, SP-9 Yinlingquan, BL-64 Jinggu, GB-34 Yanglingquan, GB-40 Qiuxu, GB-43 Xiaxi, ST-44 Neiting and some Ah Shi points. Reducing method is used on these points.

Explanations

- TE-6 and LI-4 dispel External pathogenic factors, promote the circulation of Qi in the channels, eliminate Damp and reduce Heat.
- ST-40, the Connecting point, SP-6, the crossing point of the three Yin channels of the foot, and SP-9 and GB-34, the Sea points, together with GB-40, eliminate Damp in the body and channels and clear the Heat so as to relieve the pain.
- BL-64, the Source point, dispels External pathogenic factors, promotes urination, eliminates Damp and relieves the hip pain.
- ST-44 and GB-43, the Spring points, eliminate Damp-Heat and reduce fever.
- The Ah Shi points eliminate Damp, regulate the circulation of Qi and Blood in the channels and relieve the hip pain.

Modifications

1. If the hip joint is red and painful, add SP-10 to cool the Blood and reduce the swelling.
2. If there is hip pain along the bladder channel, add BL-36, BL-58 and BL-63 to harmonise the collateral and relieve the pain.
3. If there is hip pain along the Gall Bladder channel, add GB-36, GB-35 and GB-41 to promote the circulation of Qi and Blood in the channel and relieve the pain.
4. If there is hip pain along the Stomach channel, add ST-30, ST-31, ST-34 and ST-42 to promote the circulation of Qi and Blood in the channel, remove the blockage and arrest the pain.
5. If there is hip pain along the Liver channel, add LR-3, LR-5, LR-11 and LR-12 to harmonise the collateral, promote the circulation of Qi and Blood in the channel and relieve the pain.
6. Some corresponding points on the shoulder should be added in order to strengthen the therapeutic effects.

7. In case of fever, add GV-14 and LI-11 to clear the Heat and reduce the fever.
8. If there is generalised body pain and headache, add GB-20 to dispel External factors and relieve the body pain.
9. If there is severe nausea and vomiting, add ST-36 and PC-6 to harmonise the Stomach and relieve the vomiting.
10. If there is an inguinal hernia with swelling and a distending pain in the scrotum or testicle, and scanty urine, add CV-2, LR-5 and ST-30 to clear Heat, eliminate Damp, harmonise the collateral and arrest the pain.
11. If there is yellow and scanty urination, add CV-3 to promote urination, clear Heat and eliminate Damp in the body.

STAGNATION OF QI AND BLOOD

Symptoms and signs

Fixed, stabbing or pricking pain of the hip joints, with swelling of the joints, a history of trauma, limited movement of the joint and difficulty in walking, which worsens on rest and at night, and alleviated by movement, associated with red or hard nodules under the skin around the joints, a purplish tongue with purplish spots and a choppy or thready and deep pulse.

Principle of treatment

Promote the Blood circulation, remove the Blood stasis, promote the circulation of the channels and collateral and sedate the pain.

HERBAL TREATMENT

Prescription

SHEN TONG ZHU YU TANG
Meridian Passage
Tao Ren *Semen Persicae* 10 g
Hong Hua *Flos Carthami* 12 g
Chuan Xiong *Rhizoma Chuanxiong* 10 g
Dang Gui *Radix Angelicae Sinensis* 12 g
Qin Jiao *Radix Gentianae Macrophyllae* 10 g
Qiang Huo *Rhizoma et Radix Notopterygii* 12 g
Mo Yao *Resina Myrrhae* 10 g
Wu Ling Zhi *Faeces Trogopterorum* 10 g
Xiang Fu *Rhizoma Cyperi* 12 g
Huai Niu Xi *Radix Achyranthis Bidentatae* 12 g
Di Long *Lumbricus* 10 g
Gan Cao *Radix Glycyrrhizae* 6 g

Explanations

- Tao Ren and Hong Hua promote the Blood circulation and remove Blood stasis, which is the treatment for the root cause.
- Since Qi is the commander of Blood, smoothing the flow of Qi activates the circulation of Blood. Xiang Fu and Chuan Xiong regulate the circulation of Qi and Blood so as to relieve the hip pain.
- Dang Gui nourishes the Blood and promotes its circulation.
- Qin Jiao, Qiang Huo and Di Long eliminate obstructions in the channels and collateral, and sedate the body pain and joint pain.
- Wu Ling Zhi and Mo Yao promote Blood circulation.
- Huai Niu Xi induces the herbs to the lower limbs.
- Gan Cao harmonises the herbs in the formula.

Modifications

1. If there is stagnation of Blood resulting from physical trauma, add Ru Xiang *Resina Olibani* 10 g to promote the circulation of Blood, eliminate Blood stasis, promote healing, reduce swelling and relieve hip pain.
2. If there is a bone fracture, add Xue Jie *Sanguis Draconis* 5 g to promote the circulation of Blood and speed up the bone healing.
3. If there is swelling of the hip joint with formation of pus, add Zao Jiao Ci *Spina Gleditsiae* 10 g and Pu Gong Ying *Herba Taraxaci* 10 g to clear Heat, remove Toxin, subside swelling, eliminate pus and promote healing.
4. If there is restlessness at night due to severe pain, add Long Gu *Os Draconis* 20 g to calm the Mind and improve sleep.
5. If there is a prolonged history of hip pain caused by stagnation of Blood with failure of the routine method to promote Blood circulation, add Xiao Huo Luo Dan *Minor Invigorate the Collaterals Special Pill* (1 pill once a day) to promote the circulation of Blood, eliminate its stasis and remove blockage in the channels.

Patent remedies

Xiao Huo Luo Dan *Minor Invigorate the Collaterals Special Pill*
Jin Gu Die Shang Wan *Muscle and Bone Traumatic Injury Pill*

ACUPUNCTURE TREATMENT

LI-4 Hegu, SP-6 Sanyinjiao, SP-10 Xuehai, BL-17 Geshu, LR-3 Taichong, GB-29 Juliao, GB-30 Huantiao,

ST-31 Biguan and some Ah Shi points. Reducing method is used on these points.

Explanations

- LI-4 and LR-3, the Source points, promote Qi circulation in the channels, eliminate stagnation of Blood and relieve the pain.
- SP-6, the crossing point of the three Yin channels of the foot, BL-17, the Gathering point for the Blood and SP-10 promote the circulation of Blood, eliminate its stasis and relieve the hip pain.
- Ah Shi points, GB-29, GB-30 and ST-31, the local points, are the most important points for removing obstructions in the channels and collateral and relieving the hip pain.

Modifications

1. If there is fracture of the hip bone, add BL-11, the Gathering point for the Bones, and GB-39, the Gathering point for the Marrow, to promote the circulation of Blood and speed up the bone healing.
2. If there is swelling of the hip joint with formation of pus, add SP-9 to clear Heat, remove Toxin, reduce the swelling, eliminate the pus and promote healing.
3. If there is restlessness at night due to severe pain, add HT-3 and HT-7 to calm the Mind and improve the sleep.
4. If there is a sensation of heat in the hip joints, add ST-44 and GB-44, the Spring points, to clear Heat.
5. If the hip pain is of long duration, add ST-40 to harmonise the collateral and relieve the hip pain.
6. If there is hip pain along the Bladder channel, add BL-36, BL-58 and BL-63 to harmonise the collateral and relieve the pain.
7. If there is hip pain along the Gall Bladder channel, add GB-34, GB-35, GV-36 and GB-41 to promote the circulation of Qi and Blood in the channel and relieve the pain.
8. If there is hip pain along the Stomach channel, add ST-30, ST-31, ST-34 and ST-42 to promote the circulation of Qi and Blood in the channel, relieve the blockage and arrest the pain.
9. If there is hip pain along the Liver channel, add LR-3, LR-5, LR-11 and LR-12 to harmonise the collateral, promote the circulation of Qi and Blood in the channel and relieve the pain.
10. Some corresponding points on the shoulder should be added in order to strengthen the therapeutic effect.

Case history

A 38-year-old woman had been suffering from painful swelling of the left hip joint for 3 months. Her hip pain started after she had fallen off her bicycle. To begin with, she did not feel much hip pain, but the following day a big bruise appeared and her left hip became swollen and painful. The movements of the joint were limited. She took some painkillers, which relieved the swelling and pain of the joint a little. At the hospital she was diagnosed with soft tissue injury. In the weeks before arriving at the clinic, the left hip pain had got worse, especially at night; there was also rigidity in the hip joint, aggravation of the pain with pressure or on lying down, a dark purplish tongue and a deep and choppy pulse.

Diagnosis
Hip pain due to obstruction of the channels by stagnation of Qi and Blood.

Principle of treatment
Promote the circulation of Qi and Blood, harmonise the collateral and relieve the pain.

Acupuncture treatment
GB-29, GB-30, GB-31, GB-34, GB-36, GB-41, SP-6, BL-17, SP-10 and TE-5. Reducing method was used on these points. Treatment was given once every 2 days.

Explanations

- SP-6, SP-10 and BL-17 promote the circulation of Blood and remove its stasis so as to relieve the hip pain.
- GB-29, GB-30 and GB-31, the local points, remove the obstructions in the local channel and relieve the pain.
- GB-34, the Sea point, and GB-36, the Accumulation point, eliminate Blood stasis and relieve hip pain.
- TE-5 and GB-41 open the Lesser Yang channels and relieve the pain in the hip joints.

After having treatment for 3 weeks, her hip pain was under control. She was followed up 9 months later and she stated she had experienced no more hip pain since the treatment.

DEFICIENCY OF QI AND BLOOD

Symptoms and signs

Intermittent pain in both hips, which is alleviated by rest or pressure and aggravated by overwork, with numbness and weakness of the lower limbs, and muscular atrophy of hip and on the legs. Accompanying symptoms include tiredness, a pale complexion, a poor appetite, loose stools, shortness of breath, an aversion to cold, a pale tongue with a thin and white coating and a thready and weak pulse.

Principle of treatment

Activate the Spleen, reinforce Qi, tonify Blood and sedate the pain.

HERBAL TREATMENT

Prescription

BA ZHEN TANG
Eight-Precious Decoction
Dang Gui *Radix Angelicae Sinensis* 12 g
Chuan Xiong *Rhizoma Ligustici Chuanxiong* 10 g
Bai Shao *Radix Paeoniae Alba* 12 g
Shu Di Huang *Radix Rehmanniae Praeparata* 12 g
Ren Shen *Radix Ginseng* 6 g
Bai Zhu *Rhizoma Atractylodis Macrocephalae* 12 g
Fu Ling *Poria* 12 g
Gan Cao *Radix Glycyrrhizae* 6 g

Explanations

- Dang Gui, Bai Shao and Shu Di Huang tonify the Kidney-Essence and nourish the Liver-Blood.
- Ren Shen, Bai Zhu, Fu Ling and Gan Cao, the ingredients of Si Jun Zi Tang *Four-Gentlemen Decoction*, strengthen the Spleen and reinforce the Qi.
- Chuan Xiong activates the circulation of Qi and Blood and relieves obstruction in the channels. It can also prevent side-effects due to the use of too many tonics.

Modifications

1. If there is an aversion to cold or cold limbs due to deficiency of Yang, add Gui Zhi *Ramulus Cinnamomi* 6 g and Wu Zhu Yu *Fructus Evodiae* 10 g to reinforce the Yang-Qi and activate the Yang-Qi.
2. If there is swelling of hips or legs due to poor water metabolism caused by deficiency of Spleen-Qi, add Zhu Ling *Polyporus Umbellatus* 15 g and Ze Xie *Rhizoma Alismatis* 12 g to strengthen the Spleen, promote urination and relieve the swelling.

Patent remedies

Shi Quan Da Bu Wan *All-Inclusive Great Tonifying Pill*
Gui Pi Wan *Tonifying the Spleen Pill*

ACUPUNCTURE TREATMENT

GB-30 Huantiao, GB-34 Yanglingquan, GB-39 Xuanzhong, ST-31 Biguan, LR-3 Taichong, KI-3 Taixi, ST-36 Zusanli, SP-6 Sanyinjiao and Ah Shi points. Reinforcing method is used on GB-39, KI-3 and ST-36. Even method is used on the rest of the points.

Explanations

- LR-3 and KI-3, the Source points of the Liver and Kidney channels respectively, tonify the Liver and Kidney and strengthen the tendons and bones. LR-3 can also promote the circulation of Qi and Blood and relieve the hip pain.
- SP-6, the crossing point of the three Yin channels of the foot, strengthens the Spleen, Liver and Kidney and tonifies the Blood.
- GB-39, the Gathering point of Marrow, and GB-34, the Gathering point of the tendons, reinforces the tendons and bones.
- ST-36, the Sea point for the Stomach channel, reinforces the Spleen and Stomach and promotes the production of Qi and Blood.
- GB-30, ST-31 and the Ah Shi points, the local points, harmonise the collateral, promote the circulation of Qi and Blood in the channels and relieve the hip pain.

Modifications

1. If there is hip pain along the Bladder channel, add BL-36, BL-58 and BL-63 to harmonise the collateral and relieve the pain.
2. If there is hip pain along the Gall Bladder channel, add GB-36, GB-35 and GB-40 to promote the circulation of Qi and Blood in the channel and relieve the pain.
3. If there is hip pain along the Stomach channel, add ST-30, ST-34, ST-40 and ST-42 to promote the circulation of Qi and Blood in the channel, relieve the blockage and arrest the pain.
4. If there is hip pain along the Liver channel, add LR-3, LR-5, LR-11 and LR-12 to harmonise the collateral, promote the circulation of Qi and Blood in the channel and relieve the pain.
5. Some corresponding points on the shoulder should be added in order to strengthen the therapeutic effect.
6. If there is an aversion to cold or cold limbs due to deficiency of Yang, add moxibustion on CV-4 and CV-6 to reinforce the Yang-Qi and eliminate Cold.
7. If there is swelling in the hips due to poor water metabolism caused by deficiency of Spleen-Qi, add ST-40 and SP-9 to strengthen the Spleen, promote urination and reduce the swelling.
8. If there is dizziness due to deficiency of Qi and Blood, add GV-20 to activate the Yang-Qi, lift Yang-Qi to the head and relieve the dizziness.

DEFICIENCY OF THE LIVER AND KIDNEY

Symptoms and signs

Chronic hip pain with difficulty in rotation, which is aggravated by overstrain or by standing for too long, with weakness of the lower back and knees, rigidity in the morning, joint deformity and muscular atrophy. Accompanying symptoms include fatigue, lower back pain, an aversion to cold, a thin and white tongue coating and a deep and wiry pulse, and weak pulse on the Kidney position.

Principle of treatment

Strengthen Kidney and Liver, harmonise the collateral and relieve the pain.

HERBAL TREATMENT

Prescription

DU HUO JI SHENG TANG
Angelica Pubescens–Loranthus Decoction
Du Huo *Radix Angelicae Pubescentis* 10 g
Fang Feng *Radix Ledebouriellae* 10 g
Qin Jiao *Radix Gentianae Macrophyllae* 10 g
Xi Xin *Herba Asari* 3 g
Rou Gui *Cortex Cinnamomi* 6 g
Ren Shen *Radix Ginseng* 6 g
Fu Ling *Poria* 12 g
Gan Cao *Radix Glycyrrhizae* 6 g
Dang Gui *Radix Angelicae Sinensis* 12 g
Chuan Xiong *Rhizoma Ligustici Chuanxiong* 10 g
Shu Di Huang *Radix Rehmanniae Praeparata* 15 g
Bai Shao *Radix Paeoniae Alba* 12 g
Du Zhong *Cortex Eucommiae* 12 g
Huai Niu Xi *Radix Achyranthis Bidentatae* 12 g
Sang Ji Sheng *Ramulus Loranthi* 15 g

Explanations

- Du Huo, Fang Feng, Qin Jiao, Xi Xin and Rou Gui disperse Wind, remove Damp, dispel Cold and relieve pain.
- Ren Shen, Fu Ling, Gan Cao, Dang Gui, Chuan Xiong, Sheng Di Huang and Bai Shao reinforce the Qi, nourish the Blood and promote its circulation.
- Du Zhong, Huai Niu Xi, Sang Ji Sheng strengthen the Liver and Kidney and relieve the lower back pain and hip pain.

Modifications

1. If there is an aversion to cold, add Yin Yang Huo *Herba Epimedii* 10 g to warm the Yang, dispel Cold and relieve the pain.

2. If there is lower abdominal pain with a cold sensation, add Wu Zhu Yu *Fructus Evodiae* 5 g to warm the Interior, dispel Cold and relieve the pain.

3. If there is frequent urination at night, add Yi Zhi Ren *Fructus Alpiniae Oxyphyllae* 10 g and San Piao Xiao *Ootheca Mantidis* 10 g to tonify the Kidney-Yang and decrease the urine.

4. If there is deficiency of the Yin of Liver and Kidney, use a modified prescription based on Zhi Bai Di Huang Wan *Ane-phello and Rehmannia Pill* (9 g each time, three times a day) instead of Du Huo Ji Sheng Tang.

5. If there is fatigue, add Huang Qi *Radix Astragali seu Hedysari* 15 g to tonify the Qi and relieve the fatigue.

Patent remedies

Du Huo Ji Sheng Wan *Angelica Pubescens–Loranthus Decoction*
Hai Ma Bu Shen Wan *Sea Horse Tonify Kidney Pill*
Kang Gu Zheng Sheng Pian *Combat Bone Hyperplasia Pill*

ACUPUNCTURE TREATMENT

GB-29 Juliao, GB-30 Huantiao, GB-34 Yanglingquan, ST-31 Biguan, Ah Shi points, KI-3 Taixi, BL-23 Shenshu, BL-18 Ganshu, SP-6 Sanyinjiao, and Extra Huatuojiaji points. Reducing method is used for GB-29, GB-30, GB-34 and the Ah Shi points, and re-inforcing method on the rest of the points. A tapping method with the plum blossom needle is used on the Extra Huatuojiaji points.

Explanations

- This type of hip pain is often seen in old people, caused by decline of the Essence of the Liver and Kidney.
- KI-3, the Source point of the Kidney channel, and BL-23, the Back Transporting point of the Kidney, reinforce both the Liver and Kidney and strengthen the bones.
- BL-18, the Back Transporting point of the Liver, tonifies the Liver-Blood and strengthens the tendons.
- SP-6, the crossing point of the three Yin channels of the foot, tonifies the Spleen, Kidney and Liver.
- GB-29, GB-30, ST-31 and the Ah Shi points are the local points. Reducing on these points can remove obstructions in the local channels. In addition, GB-34 is one of eight Gathering points relating to the tendons.

- The Extra Huatuojiaji points are extremely effective points for tonification. They are the lateral collateral of the Governing Vessel and connect with the first line of the Bladder channel and the Kidney organ. So tapping on the Huatuojiaji points with the Plum Blossom needle is effective for nourishing the Kidney Essence and Marrow, and strengthens the bones and tendons. In addition, this tapping method could activate the Qi and Blood in the channels, and so undernourishment of the muscles and tendons can be relieved.

Modifications

1. If the hip joints are swollen, add SP-9 to dispel Damp and reduce the swelling.
2. If there is a stabbing pain or aggravation of the hip pain at night due to stagnation of Blood, add LI-4 and SP-10 to promote the circulation of Blood and remove the Blood stasis.
3. If there is an extreme aversion to cold and a cold sensation in the joints, moxibustion on the local points and BL-23 could be used.
4. If there is hip pain along the Bladder channel, add BL-36, BL-58 and BL-63 to harmonise the collateral and relieve the pain.
5. If there is hip pain along the Gall Bladder channel, add GB-36, GB-35 and GB-40 to promote the circulation of Qi and Blood in the channel and relieve the pain.
6. If there is hip pain along the Stomach channel, add ST-30, ST-34, ST-40 and ST-42 to promote the circulation of Qi and Blood in the channel, relieve blockage and arrest the pain.
7. If there is hip pain along the Liver channel, add LR-3, LR-5, LR-11 and LR-12 to harmonise the collateral, promote the circulation of Qi and Blood in the channel and relieve the pain.
8. Some corresponding points on the shoulder should be added in order to increase the therapeutic effect.

Knee pain 41

膝
痛

Knee pain may occur in one or both of the knee joints, or the muscles and tendons around the joints. Generally, according to TCM theory it can be caused by invasion of the knee joints by External Wind, Cold, Damp and Heat, deficiency of the Liver and Kidney, or deficiency or stagnation of the Qi and Blood. Knee pain may be attributed to any of the following disorders in Western medicine: rheumatic fever, rheumatic arthritis, rheumatoid gout, hyperosteogeny of the knee joint, fibrositis, nerve pain, injury to the medial and lateral collateral ligaments of the knee joint, synovitis of the knee joint, chondromalacia of the patella, injury to the meniscus and strain of the subpatellar fat pad.

Aetiology and pathology

Invasion of External factors

Weakness of the Defensive Qi may cause failure of the skin pores to open and close properly. In consequence External pathogenic factors can easily invade the body and knees, causing stagnation of the Qi and Blood circulation, so that knee pain occurs. Invasion of Wind-Cold-Damp and Heat usually happens when a person is exposed to strong winds or cold whilst sweating after physical exercise or physical work, has been walking in water or has lived in a damp place for a long time. When External pathogenic factors invade the channels, muscles and joints around the knee, they block the channels, slow down the circulation of Qi and Blood and limit the joint movement, and cause knee pain.

The clinical symptoms and signs vary greatly due to the difference in pathogenic factors: Wind is characteristically moving and changing, so if the Wind invasion is predominant it causes a knee pain that moves from one place to another place and from the left side to the right. Cold has the characteristics of contraction and stagnation. If Cold invasion is predominant, it causes contraction of the muscles and tendons around the knee, leading to stagnation of Qi and Blood, and a severe pain with a cold sensation occurs. Damp is characteristically lingering and heavy, so if Damp invasion is predominant, it obstructs the channels, leading to a knee pain with swelling, numbness and heaviness. Heat is characteristically red in colour and burning. If Wind, Damp and Heat invade the lower body, they disturb the circulation of Qi and Blood in the channels, especially the foot Bright Yang Channel, leading to the accumulation of Damp-Heat and stagnation of Qi and Blood, which block the channels around the knee joint. This causes knee pain with swelling, redness and a burning feeling. If Wind, Cold and Damp remain in the body for a long time they may also generate Damp-Heat, especially in those who have an accumulation of Excessive-Heat or Deficient-Heat in the body.

Bad diet

Bad diets, such as eating too much sweet or fatty food, or drinking too much alcohol, may impair the Spleen and Stomach, leading to the formation of Damp-Heat in the body. When Damp-Heat flows downward to the lower limbs, it blocks the channels, causing knee pain.

Stagnation of Qi and Blood

Qi and Blood should circulate freely in the channels. If the Qi and Blood stagnate because of various causes, such as overstrain, physical trauma or inappropriate operation on the knee, they block the channels, leading to pain and swelling in the knee joint.

In addition, stagnation of Qi and Blood can be caused by bad diet, for instance eating too much greasy or fatty, sweet, cold or raw food, which causes Damp-Phlegm to form in the body and block the channels, leading to knee pain.

Deficiency of Liver and Kidney

Overstrain, prolonged sickness, a weak constitution and old age may all cause consumption of the Qi and Blood and deficiency of the Liver and Kidney. In this condition the tendons are not properly nourished by the Liver and the bone is not properly nourished by the Kidney, causing knee pain with weakness.

Deficiency of Qi and Blood

Overstrain, irregular eating habits, a poor diet and prolonged illness may cause consumption or diminished production of the Qi and Blood, so the knees are not sufficiently nourished, and knee pain follows.

In addition, excessive bleeding during the menstrual period, or chronic bleeding conditions such as haemorrhoids, may result in a gradual and constant blood loss, eventually leading to deficiency of the Qi and Blood, so that knee pain follows.

Treatment based on differentiation

Differentiation

Differentiation of External or Internal origin

— Acute onset of knee pain of a short duration, accompanied by External symptoms, is usually caused by invasion of External pathogenic factors. Traumatic injury could also cause acute knee pain.
— Chronic onset of knee pain of long duration, accompanied by some symptoms resulting from Internal disorders, such as deficiency of Qi and Blood, deficiency of Liver and Kidney, stagnation of Qi and Blood, etc.

Differentiation of character of the pain

— Wandering knee pain, with an aversion to wind, associated with chills and fever, is usually caused by invasion of Wind-Cold-Damp with predominance of Wind.
— Severe knee pain with a cold sensation, an aversion to cold, alleviation of the knee pain by warmth, aggravation of the hip pain by cold, or cramp of the muscles, is mainly caused by invasion of Wind-Cold-Damp with predominance of Cold.
— Knee pain with swelling and a fixed localization, a heavy sensation of lower limbs, or sensitivity to humid weather, is usually caused by invasion of Wind-Cold-Damp with predominance of Damp.
— Swollen and painful knee joint with a local burning sensation and redness, is usually caused by invasion of Wind-Heat-Damp.
— Slight and dull pain of the knee joint, with rigidity in the morning, suggests deficiency of the Liver and Kidney.
— Fixed and pricking pain of the knee joint, with a history of trauma, is mainly caused by stagnation of Qi and Blood.
— Continuous pain in both knees, with numbness and weakness of the lower limbs, is usually caused by deficiency of Qi and Blood.

Differentiation shape of the knee joint

— A normal-shaped knee joint is usually found in those with knee pain due to invasion of Wind-Cold-Damp.
— Acute onset of swelling and a red knee joint is usually caused by invasion of Wind-Heat-Damp.
— A swollen knee joint, with deformity, hyperosteogeny and muscular atrophy, indicates deficiency of Liver and Kidney.
— A swollen knee joint, with red or hard nodules under the skin around the joint, is usually due to stagnation of Qi and Blood.
— Muscular atrophy in the knee or on the legs is usually caused by deficiency of Qi and Blood.

Treatment

INVASION OF WIND-COLD-DAMP AND PREDOMINANCE OF WIND

Symptoms and signs

Wandering knee pain, which is aggravated by wind, with difficulty in flexion and extension, an aversion to wind, accompanied by chills and fever, generalised body pain, headache, a thin white or thin greasy tongue coating and a superficial pulse.

Principle of treatment

Dispel Wind, eliminate Cold and Damp, harmonise the collateral and relieve the pain.

HERBAL TREATMENT

Prescription

FANG FENG TANG
Ledebouriella Decoction
Fang Feng *Radix Ledebouriellae* 10 g
Ma Huang *Herba Ephedrae* 6 g
Dang Gui *Radix Angelicae Sinensis* 12 g
Huai Niu Xi *Radix Achyranthis Bidentatae* 10 g
Qin Jiao *Radix Gentianae Macrophyllae* 10 g
Rou Gui *Cortex Cinnamomi* 6 g
Fu Ling *Poria* 12 g
Sheng Jiang *Rhizoma Zingiberis Recens* 3 g
Da Zao *Fructus Ziziphi Jujubae* 6 g
Gan Cao *Radix Glycyrrhizae* 6 g

Explanations

- Fang Feng and Ma Huang dispel Wind and Cold and relieve External symptoms.
- Qin Jiao and Rou Gui warm the channels and dispel Cold so as to relieve the knee pain.
- Dang Gui promotes the circulation of Blood and removes obstructions from the collateral.
- Huai Niu Xi promotes the circulation of Blood, strengthens the bone and induces the herbs to reach the knee joints.
- Fu Ling is good for strengthening the Spleen and inducing urination.
- The last three herbs can coordinate all the other herbs in the prescription.

Modifications

1. If there is fever and chills, add Gui Zhi *Ramulus Cinnamomi* 10 g to relieve the Exterior symptoms and reduce the fever.

2. If the knee joints are swollen, add Du Huo *Radix Angelica Pubescentis* 10 g and Han Fang Ji *Radix Stephaniae Tetrandrae* 10 g to dispel Damp, reduce the swelling and sedate the pain.
3. If the knee joints are swollen and red, add Zhi Mu *Rhizoma Anemarrhenae* 10 g and Huang Bai *Cortex Phellodendri* 10 g to clear Heat, eliminate Damp and reduce the swelling and redness.
4. If there is a headache, add Man Jing Zi *Fructus Viticis* 10 g to dispel Wind and relieve the headache.

Patent remedy

Jing Fang Bai Du Pian *Schizonepeta and Ledebouriella Tablet to Overcome Pathogenic Influences*

ACUPUNCTURE TREATMENT

TE-5 Waiguan, LI-4 Hegu, GB-31 Fengshi, GB-35 Yangjiao, SP-6 Sanyinjiao and some local Ah Shi points. Reducing method is used on these points.

Explanations

- TE-5 and LI-4 dispel External pathogenic Wind and relieve External symptoms.
- GB-31 dispels External Wind and eliminates Damp in the lower limbs.
- GB-35, the Accumulation point of the Yang Linking Vessel, harmonises the collateral, promotes the circulation of Qi and Blood and relieves the knee pain.
- SP-6, the crossing point of the Kidney, Spleen, Liver channels, activates the circulation of Blood, eliminates its stasis and relieves the knee pain.
- The Ah Shi points around knee joint regulate the circulation of Qi and Blood in the local areas and relieve the knee pain.

Modifications

1. If there is a slight fever and chills, add GV-14, the meeting point for all the Yang channels, with moxibustion to dispel Wind, relieve Exterior symptoms and reduce the fever.
2. If the knee joint is swollen, add SP-9, the Sea point, to remove Damp and reduce the swelling.
3. If there is redness, swelling and a hot sensation in the knee joint, add ST-44 and GB-43, the Spring points of the Stomach and Gall Bladder

channel respectively, to clear Heat and reduce the swelling.

4. If there is knee pain along the Bladder channel, add BL-36, BL-40, BL-58 and BL-63 to harmonise the collateral and relieve the pain.
5. If there is knee pain along the Gall Bladder channel, add GB-34, GB-36, GB-40 and GB-41 to promote the circulation of Qi and Blood in the channel and relieve the pain.
6. If there is knee pain along the Stomach channel, add ST-34, ST-35, ST-36, ST-40 and ST-42 to promote the circulation of Qi and Blood in the channel, relieve the blockage and arrest the pain.
7. If there is knee pain along the Liver channel, add LR-3, LR-5, LR-6 and LR-8 to harmonise the collateral, promote the circulation of Qi and Blood in the channel and relieve the pain.
8. If there is knee pain along the Kidney channel, add KI-3, KI-4, KI-5 and KI-10 to strengthen the Kidney, regulate the circulation of Qi and Blood in the channel and relieve the pain.
9. If there is knee pain along the Spleen channel, add SP-3, SP-4, SP-8 and SP-10 to activate the Spleen, promote the circulation of Qi and Blood in the channel, harmonise the collateral and relieve the pain.
10. Some corresponding points on the elbow should be added in order to increase the therapeutic effect.
11. If there is generalised body pain, add BL-12 to dispel Wind, relieve External symptoms and relieve the body pain.
12. If there is a headache, add GB-20 to dispel Wind and relieve the headache.

INVASION OF WIND-COLD-DAMP WITH PREDOMINANCE OF COLD

Symptoms and signs

Severe knee pain with a cold sensation, which is aggravated by contact with cold and alleviated by warmth, with spasm and a contracting feeling in the knees, and limited movement of the joint. Accompanying symptoms include an aversion to cold and cold limbs, headache, generalised body pain, a thin and white tongue coating and a tight and superficial pulse.

Principle of treatment

Warm the channels and dispel Cold, also dispel Wind and remove Damp.

HERBAL TREATMENT

Prescription

WU TOU TANG
Aconite Decoction
Zhi Chuan Wu *Radix Aconiti Praeparata* 10 g
Ma Huang *Herba Ephedrae* 6 g
Bai Shao *Radix Paeoniae Alba* 12 g
Gan Cao *Radix Glycyrrhizae* 6 g
Huang Qi *Radix Astragali* 15 g

Explanations

- Zhi Chuan Wu and Ma Huang, warm in nature, warm the channels and dispel Wind, remove Damp and sedate the pain.
- Bai Shao and Gan Cao relieve muscle spasm and stop the pain.
- Huang Qi reinforces the Qi and consolidates the body surface. It can also promote the circulation of Blood and relieve the pain.

Modifications

1. If there is an aversion to cold, add Xi Xin *Herba Asari* 3 g to eliminate Cold and relieve the Exterior symptoms.
2. If there is knee pain radiating to the legs, add Chuan Niu Xi *Radix Cyathule* 10 g to strengthen the knee and sedate the pain.
3. If the knee joints are swollen, add Cang Zhu *Rhizoma Atractylodis* 10 g and Mu Tong *Caulis Akebiae* 6 g to promote urination, to eliminate Damp and reduce the swelling.
4. If the lower limbs are cold, add Du Huo *Radix Angelicae Pubescentis* 10 g and Rou Gui *Cortex Cinnamomi* 5 g to warm the channels, reinforce the Yang and dispel Cold.
5. If there is severe pain, add Jiang Huang *Rhizoma Curcumae Longae* 10 g to regulate the circulation of Blood and relieve the pain.

Patent remedy

Han Shi Bi Chong Ji *Cold-Damp Bi Syndrome Infusion*

ACUPUNCTURE TREATMENT

TE-5 Waiguan, LI-4 Hegu, GB-34 Yanglingquan, GB-35 Yangjiao, Extra Xiyan, ST-36 Zusanli, SP-6 Sanyinjiao and Ah Shi points. Reducing method is used on these points, except for ST-36, on which tonifying method is used. Moxibustion is used on TE-5, LI-4 and ST-36.

Explanations

- TE-5 and LI-4 dispel External pathogenic Wind, eliminate Cold and relieve External symptoms.
- ST-36, the Sea point, with moxibustion warms the channels and dispels Cold.
- SP-6 activates the circulation of Blood and relieves the knee pain.
- The Ah Shi points, Extra Xiyan, GB-34 and GB-35 regulate the circulation of Qi and Blood in the locality and relieve the knee pain.
- Moxibustion warms the channels, dispels Cold and relieves pain.

Modifications

1. If there is swelling of the knee with heaviness, add SP-9 to eliminate Damp and reduce the swelling.
2. If there is knee pain along the Bladder channel, add BL-36, BL-40, BL-58 and BL-63 to harmonise the collateral and relieve the pain.
3. If there is knee pain along the Gall Bladder channel, add GB-33, GB-36, GB-40 and GB-41 to promote the circulation of Qi and Blood in the channel and relieve the pain.
4. If there is knee pain along the Stomach channel, add ST-34, ST-35, ST-36, ST-40 and ST-42 to promote the circulation of Qi and Blood in the channel, remove the blockage and arrest the pain.
5. If there is knee pain along the Liver channel, add LR-3, LR-5, LR-6 and LR-8 to harmonise the collateral, promote the circulation of Qi and Blood in the channel and relieve the pain.
6. If there is knee pain along the Kidney channel, add KI-3, KI-4, KI-5 and KI-10 to strengthen the Kidney, regulate the circulation of Qi and Blood in the channel and relieve the pain.
7. If there is knee pain along the Spleen channel, add SP-3, SP-4, SP-8 and SP-10 to activate the Spleen, promote the circulation of Qi and Blood in the channel, harmonise the collateral and relieve the pain.
8. Some corresponding points on the elbow should be added in order to increase the therapeutic effect.
9. If there is a cold sensation in the body and cold limbs, add KI-3 and CV-4 with moxibustion to reinforce the Yang and dispel Cold.
10. If there is a slight fever and chills, add GV-14 with moxibustion to dispel Wind, relieve Exterior symptoms and reduce the fever.
11. If there is a headache, add GB-20 to dispel Wind, Cold and Damp and relieve the headache.

Case history

A 40-year-old male had been suffering from severe pain in both knee joints with a cold sensation for 2 months. To begin with, he had caught a cold, and had generalised body pain, a headache, an aversion to cold and a slight fever. He did not feel too bad so did not visit his doctor. One week later, his general symptoms had improved, but he had started to suffer from knee pain. He also felt a weakness in the lower back region and aggravation of the knee pain in cold weather. He was given no clear diagnosis for his knee pain despite all kinds of investigations. Over the previous 2 months, he often took painkillers when the knee pain was severe.

When he arrived at the clinic, he still had pain in his knees with a cold feeling. The pain was mainly along the Spleen channel, with a slight swelling on the knees, and tenderness at both SP-8 and SP-9. His pulse was superficial and tight, and he had a thin and white tongue coating.

Diagnosis
Knee pain due to incomplete elimination of Wind, Cold and Damp.

Principle of treatment
Dispel Wind, warm Cold, eliminate Damp and relieve the pain.

Acupuncture treatment
TE-5, LI-4, SP-3, SP-4, SP-6, SP-8, SP-9 and SP-10. Reducing method was applied on these points except for SP-3, on which tonifying method was used. Moxibustion was used on TE-5, LI-4 and SP-3. Treatment was given once every 3 days.

Explanations

- TE-5 and LI-4 dispel External pathogenic Wind, and eliminate Cold and Damp.
- SP-3, the Source point, with moxibustion warms the channels and dispels Cold.
- SP-6 and SP-10 activate the circulation of Blood, eliminate its stasis and relieve knee pain.
- SP-4, the Connecting point, SP-8, the Accumulation point, and SP-9, the Sea point, harmonise the collateral, promote circulation in the channels and reduce knee pain.
- Moxibustion was applied to warm the channels, dispel Cold and relieve the pain.

The patient was cured after 6 treatments, and he reported no relapse at the 1 month follow-up.

INVASION OF WIND-COLD-DAMP WITH PREDOMINANCE OF DAMP

Symptoms and signs

Pain and swelling in the knee joints, which worsens on overcast and rainy days, with numbness in the knees and a heavy sensation in the knees and the lower limbs, and limited movement of the knee joints, accompanied by a white and greasy tongue coating and a soft and slow pulse.

Principle of treatment

Eliminate Damp, dispel Cold and Wind, promote circulation in the collateral and sedate the pain.

HERBAL TREATMENT

Prescription

YI YI REN TANG
Coix Decoction
Yi Yi Ren *Semen Coicis* 15 g
Cang Zhu *Rhizoma Atractylodis* 12 g
Qiang Huo *Rhizoma et Radix Notopterygii* 12 g
Du Huo *Radix Angelicae Pubescentis* 10 g
Fang Feng *Radix Ledebouriellae* 10 g
Zhi Chuan Wu *Radix Aconiti Praeparata* 6 g
Ma Huang *Herba Ephedrae* 10 g
Gui Zhi *Ramulus Cinnamomi* 6 g
Dang Gui *Radix Angelicae Sinensis* 12 g
Chuan Xiong *Radix Ligustici Chuanxiong* 12 g
Sheng Jiang *Rhizoma Zingiberis Recens* 6 g
Gan Cao *Radix Glycyrrhizae* 6 g

Explanations

- Yi Yi Ren and Cang Zhu strengthen the Spleen and remove Damp.
- Qiang Huo, Du Huo and Fang Feng dispel Wind-Cold and eliminate Damp.
- Zhi Chuang Wu, Ma Huang, Gui Zhi warm the channels, dispel Cold and remove Damp.
- Dang Gui and Chuan Xiong nourish the Blood and promote its circulation.
- Sheng Jiang and Gan Cao strengthen the Spleen and regulate the Middle Burner.

Modifications

1. If the joints are swollen, add Jiang Huang *Rhizoma Curcumae Longae* 10 g to remove obstructions from the collateral and reduce swelling.
2. If there is a feeling of heaviness in the legs, add Fu Ling *Poria* 15 g and Ze Xie *Rhizoma Alismatis* 10 g to promote urination and eliminate Damp.
3. If there is severe knee pain, add Wu Gong *Scolopendra* 3 g to relieve the pain.
4. If there is numbness of skin, add Hai Tong Pi *Cortex Erythrinae* 10 g and Xi Xian Cao *Herba Siegesbeckiae* 10 g to dispel Wind and clear the collateral.

5. If there is lower back pain, add Du Zhong *Cortex Eucommiae* 10 g and Sang Ji Sheng *Ramus Loranthi* 10 g to strengthen the lower back and relieve the lower back pain.
6. If there is nausea or vomiting and diarrhoea, add Sha Ren *Fructus Ammomi* 5 g and Bai Zhu *Rhizoma Atractylodis Macrocephalae* 10 g to activate the Spleen and Stomach and relieve Damp in the Middle Burner.
7. If there is difficulty in urination, add Bi Xie *Rhizoma Dioscoreae Septemlobae* 15 g to promote urination and relieve painful urination.

Patent remedies

Feng Shi Pian *Wind-Damp Tablet*
Tian Ma Qu Feng Bu Pian *Gastrodia Dispel Wind Formula Tablet*

ACUPUNCTURE TREATMENT

TE-6 Zhigou, LI-4 Hegu, GB-34 Yanglinquan, Extra Xiyan, ST-40 Fenglong, SP-6 Sanyinjiao, SP-9 Yinlingquan and Ah Shi points. Reducing method is used on these points.

Explanations

- TE-5 and LI-4 dispel External pathogenic Wind, eliminate Cold and relieve External symptoms.
- ST-40, the Connecting point, activates the circulation in the channels, harmonises the collateral, eliminates Damp and relieves knee pain.
- SP-6, the crossing point of the three Yin Channels of the foot, and SP-9, the Sea point, activate the Spleen and Stomach, eliminate Damp, promote the circulation of Blood and relieve the knee pain.
- Ah Shi points, Extra Xiyan, GB-34 and GB-35 regulate the circulation of Qi and Blood in the locality and relieve the knee pain.

Modifications

1. If there is numbness in the knees, add moxibustion or Plum Blossom needles in the local area to promote the circulation of Qi and Blood and relieve the numbness.
2. If there is knee pain along the Bladder channel, add BL-36, BL-40, BL-58 and BL-63 to harmonise the collateral and relieve the pain.
3. If there is knee pain along the Gall Bladder Channel, add GB-33, GB-36, GB-40 and GB-41 to promote the circulation of Qi and Blood in the channel and relieve the pain.

4. If there is knee pain along the Stomach channel, add ST-34, ST-35, ST-36, ST-40 and ST-42 to promote the circulation of Qi and Blood in the channel, relieve the blockage and arrest the pain.
5. If there is knee pain along the Liver channel, add LR-3, LR-5, LR-6 and LR-8 to harmonise the collateral, promote the circulation of Qi and Blood in the channel and relieve the pain.
6. If there is knee pain along the Kidney channel, add KI-3, KI-4, KI-5 and KI-10 to strengthen the Kidney, regulate the circulation of Qi and Blood in the channel and relieve the pain.
7. If there is knee pain along the Spleen channel, add SP-3, SP-4, SP-8 and SP-10 to activate the Spleen, promote the circulation of Qi and Blood in the channel, harmonise the collateral and relieve the pain.
8. Some corresponding points on the elbow should be added in order to increase the therapeutic effect.
9. If there is a cold sensation in the body and cold limbs, add KI-3 and CV-4 with moxibustion to reinforce the Yang and dispel Cold.
10. If there is a headache, add GB-20 to dispel Wind, Cold and Damp and relieve the headache.

DOWNWARD FLOW OF DAMP-HEAT

Symptoms and signs

Swelling and painful knee joint, which gets worse on touching, with a burning sensation in the knees, redness and limited joint movement. Accompanying symptoms include irritability, restlessness, a poor appetite, a bitter taste in the mouth, scanty and yellow urination, occasional fever, a yellow and greasy tongue coating and slippery and rapid pulse.

If there is acute pain, as well as swelling, redness and pain in the joint, there are usually some external symptoms such as an aversion to cold, a fever, generalised body pain, a headache, a red tongue with a yellow and greasy coating and a superficial and slippery pulse.

Principle of treatment

Clear Heat, eliminate Damp and sedate the pain. If there is Wind-Damp-Heat invasion then add the method for dispelling Wind-Damp-Heat.

HERBAL TREATMENT

Prescription

BAI HU JIA GUI ZHI TANG and **SAN MIAO WAN**
White Tiger plus Ramulus Cinnamomi Decoction and Three-Marvel Pill

Zhi Mu *Rhizoma Anemarrhenae* 10 g
Shi Gao *Gypsum Fibrosum* 20 g
Gui Zhi *Ramulus Cinnamomi* 8 g
Gan Cao *Radix Glycyrrhizae* 6 g
Jing Mi *Semen Oryzae* 10 g
Huang Bai *Cortex Phellodendri* 10 g
Cang Zhu *Rhizoma Atractylodes* 10 g
Huai Niu Xi *Radix Achyranthis Bidentatae* 10 g
Wei Ling Xian *Radix Clematidis* 10 g
Han Fang Ji *Radix Stephaniae Tetrandrae* 10 g
Sang Zhi *Ramulus Mori* 15 g

Explanations

- Shi Gao and Zhi Mu are the main herbs in Bai Hu Gui Zhi Tang for clearing Heat and reducing fever.
- Gan Cao and Jing Mi benefit the Stomach and reinforce the Body Fluids moderating the extremely Cold nature of Shi Gao.
- Gui Zhi dispels Wind, harmonises the collateral and promotes the circulation of Blood to relieve the knee pain.
- Wei Ling Xian, Han Fang Ji and Sang Zhi expel pathogenic Wind, eliminate Damp, promote the circulation of Blood and unblock the channels.
- Huang Bai and Cang Zhu dry Damp, clear Heat and reduce swelling of the knees.
- Huai Niu Xi leads the herbs to the knee and eliminates Damp in the Lower Burner.

Modifications

1. If there is a fever, add Jin Yin Hua *Flos Lonicerae* 10 g and Lian Qiao *Fructus Forsythiae* 10 g to clear Heat and reduce the fever.
2. If the knees are swollen and red, add Tu Fu Ling *Rhizoma Smilacis* 10 g and Sheng Di Huang *Radix Rehmanniae* 15 g to clear Heat, remove toxin, reduce the swelling and relieve the pain.
3. If there is pus in the knee joint, add Di Fu Zi *Fructus Kochiae* 10 g and Chi Shao *Radix Paeoniae Rubra* 10 g to eliminate Damp-Heat and cool the Blood.
4. If there is severe knee pain, add Jiang Huang *Rhizoma Curcumae Longae* 10 g to clear Heat, promote the circulation of Blood and stop the pain.
5. If the appetite is poor, add Ban Xia *Rhizoma Pinelliae* 10 g and Chen Pi *Pericarpium Citri Reticulatae* 10 g to regulate the Qi and improve the appetite.
6. If there is a thirst, add Xuan Shen *Radix Scrophulariae* 10 g and Ge Gen *Radix Puerariae* 10 g to clear Heat and relieve the thirst.

7. If there is irritability, add Deng Xin Cao *Medulla Junci* 15 g to clear Fire and calm the Mind.

8. If there is constipation, add Da Huang *Radix et Rhizoma Rhei* 6 g and Mang Xiao *Natrii Sulfas* 6 g to eliminate Heat, promote defecation and relieve the constipation.

Patent remedies

Feng Shi Xiao Tong Pian *Wind-Damp Dispel Pain Pill*
Shi Re Bi Chong Ji *Damp-Heat Bi Infusion*
San Miao Wan *Three-Marvel Pill*

ACUPUNCTURE TREATMENT

ST-40 Fenglong, SP-6 Sanyinjiao, SP-9 Yinlingquan, BL-64 Jinggu, GB-34 Yanglingquan, GB-43 Xiaxi, ST-44 Neiting and some Ah Shi points. Reducing method is applied on these points.

Explanations

- ST-40, the Connecting point, and SP-9 and GB-34, the Sea points from the Spleen and Gall Bladder channels respectively, activate the Spleen and Stomach, eliminate Damp-Heat in the body and channels and relieve knee pain.
- SP-6, the crossing point of the three Yin channels of the foot, is used to promote the circulation of Blood, eliminates its stasis and unblocks the channels so as to relieve knee pain.
- BL-64, the Source point, promotes urination, eliminates Damp-Heat and relieves knee pain.
- ST-44 and GB-43, the Spring points, eliminate Damp-Heat and reduce fever.
- The Ah Shi points eliminate Damp, regulate the circulation of Qi and Blood in the channels and relieve knee pain.

Modifications

1. If there is invasion of Wind, Damp and Heat, add TE-6 and LI-4 to dispel External pathogenic factors, promote the circulation of Qi in the channels, eliminate Damp and reduce Heat.

2. If the knee joint is red and painful, add SP-10 to cool the Blood and reduce the swelling.

3. If there is knee pain along the Bladder channel, add BL-36, BL-40, BL-58 and BL-63 to harmonise the collateral and relieve the pain.

4. If there is knee pain along the Gall Bladder channel, add GB-33, GB-36, GB-40 and GB-41 to promote the circulation of Qi and Blood in the channel and relieve the pain.

5. If there is knee pain along the Stomach channel, add ST-34, ST-35, ST-36 and ST-42 to promote the circulation of Qi and Blood in the channel, clear the blockage and arrest the pain.

6. If there is knee pain along the Liver channel, add LR-3, LR-5, LR-6 and LR-8 to harmonise the collateral, promote the circulation of Qi and Blood in the channel and relieve the pain.

7. If there is knee pain along the Kidney channel, add KI-3, KI-4, KI-5 and KI-10 to strengthen the Kidney, regulate the circulation of Qi and Blood in the channel and relieve the pain.

8. If there is knee pain along the Spleen channel, add SP-3, SP-4, SP-8 and SP-10 to activate the Spleen, promote the circulation of Qi and Blood in the channel, harmonise the collateral and relieve the pain.

9. Some corresponding points on the elbow should be added in order to increase the therapeutic effects.

10. If there is a fever, add GV-14 and LI-11 to clear Heat and reduce the fever.

11. If there is generalised body pain and a headache, add GB-20 to dispel External factors and relieve the body pain.

12. If there is nausea and vomiting, add PC-6 to harmonise the Stomach and relieve the vomiting.

13. If there is yellow and scanty urination, add CV-3 to promote urination, clear Heat and eliminate Damp.

STAGNATION OF QI AND BLOOD

Symptoms and signs

Stabbing knee pain with a fixed location and swelling of the joints, which worsens at night or with rest and is alleviated by movement, with a history of trauma, and limited joint movement, accompanied by a purplish tongue or purplish spots on the tongue and a deep and choppy pulse.

Principle of treatment

Promote the Blood circulation and remove the Blood stasis, clear the channels and collateral and sedate pain.

HERBAL TREATMENT

Prescription

SHEN TONG ZHU YU TANG
Meridian Passage
Tao Ren *Semen Persicae* 10 g
Hong Hua *Flos Carthami* 12 g

Chuan Xiong *Rhizoma Ligustici Chuanxiong* 10 g
Dang Gui *Radix Angelicae Sinensis* 12 g
Qin Jiao *Radix Gentianae Macrophyllae* 10 g
Qiang Huo *Rhizoma et Radix Notopterygii* 12 g
Mo Yao *Resina Myrrhae* 10 g
Wu Ling Zhi *Faeces Trogopterorum* 10 g
Xiang Fu *Rhizoma Cyperi* 12 g
Huai Niu Xi *Radix Achyranthis Bidentatae* 12 g
Di Long *Lumbricus* 10 g
Gan Cao *Radix Glycyrrhizae* 6 g

Explanations

- Tao Ren and Hong Hua promote the circulation of Blood and remove its stasis, which is the treatment for the root cause.
- Since the Qi is the commander of the Blood, smoothing the flow of Qi can activate the Blood circulation. Chuan Xiong and Xiang Fu are used to regulate the circulation of Qi and Blood so as to relieve knee pain.
- Dang Gui nourishes the Blood and promotes its circulation.
- Qin Jiao, Qiang Huo and Di Long eliminate obstructions in the channels and collateral, and sedate body and knee pain.
- Mo Yao and Wu Ling Zhi promote Blood circulation.
- Huai Niu Xi induces the herbs to the lower limbs.

Modifications

1. If there is stagnation of Blood resulting from physical trauma, add Ru Xiang *Resina Olibani* 10 g to promote the circulation of Blood, eliminate its Stasis, promote healing, reduce swelling and relieve the knee pain.
2. If there is bone fracture, add Xue Jie *Sanguis Draconis* 5 g to promote the circulation of Blood and speed up the bone healing.
3. If the knee joint is swollen with formation of pus, add Zao Jiao Ci *Spina Gleditsiae* 10 g and Pu Gong Ying *Herba Taraxaci* 10 g to clear Heat, remove Toxin, reduce swelling, eliminate pus and promote healing.
4. If there is restlessness at night due to severe pain, add Long Gu *Os Draconis* 20 g to calm the Mind and improve the sleep.
5. If there is a long history of knee pain caused by stagnation of Blood with failure of the routine method for promoting the circulation of Blood, add Xiao Huo Luo Dan (1 pill once a day) to promote the circulation of Blood, eliminate its stasis and remove blockage in the channels.

Patent remedies

Xiao Huo Luo Dan *Minor Invigorate the Collaterals Special Pill*
Ji Gu Die Shang Wan *Muscle and Bone Traumatic Injury Pill*

ACUPUNCTURE TREATMENT

LI-4 Hegu, SP-6 Sanyinjiao, SP-10 Xuehai, BL-17 Geshu, LR-3 Taichong, GB-35 Yangjiao and some local Ah Shi points. Reducing method is used on these points.

Explanations

- LI-4 and LR-3, the Source points, promote the circulation of Qi in the channels, eliminate stagnation of Blood and relieve the pain.
- SP-6, the crossing point of the three Yin channels of the foot, BL-17, the Gathering point for the Blood, and SP-10 promote the circulation of Blood, eliminate its stasis and relieve knee pain.
- GB-35, the Accumulation point of the Yang Linking Vessel, and some local Ah Shi points, remove obstruction in the channels and collaterals and relieve knee pain.

Modifications

1. If there is knee bone fracture, add BL-11, the Gathering point of the Bones, and GB-39, the Gathering point for the Marrow, to promote the circulation of Blood and speed up bone healing.
2. If the knee joint is swollen with formation of pus, add SP-9 to clear Heat, remove toxin, reduce swelling, eliminate pus and promote healing.
3. If there is knee pain along the Bladder channel, add BL-36, BL-40, BL-58 and BL-63 to harmonise the collateral and relieve the pain.
4. If there is knee pain along the Gall Bladder channel, add GB-33, GB-36, GB-40 and GB-41 to promote the circulation of Qi and Blood in the channel and relieve the pain.
5. If there is knee pain along the Stomach channel, add ST-34, ST-35, ST-36 and ST-42 to promote the circulation of Qi and Blood in the channel, remove the blockage and arrest the pain.
6. If there is knee pain along the Liver channel, add LR-3, LR-5, LR-6 and LR-8 to harmonise the collateral, promote the circulation of Qi and Blood in the channel and relieve the pain.
7. If there is knee pain along the Kidney channel, add KI-3, KI-4, KI-5 and KI-10 to strengthen the Kidney, regulated the circulation of Qi and Blood in the channel and relieve the pain.

8. If there is knee pain along the Spleen channel, add SP-3, SP-4, SP-8 and SP-10 to activate the Spleen, promote the circulation by Qi and Blood in the channel, harmonise the collateral and relieve the pain.

9. Some corresponding points on the elbow should be added in order to increase the therapeutic effect.

10. If there is restlessness at night due to severe pain, add HT-3 and HT-7 to calm the Mind and improve the sleep.

11. If there is a sensation of heat in the knee joints, add ST-44 and GB-43, the Spring points, to clear Heat.

Case history

A 45-year-old woman had been suffering from pain and swelling in the inner right knee for 3 years. It had started after she had fallen from her bicycle and her right knee was injured. To begin with, there was a big bruise on the inner right knee and she could not walk for about 10 days. X-ray examination failed to show any bone fracture, so the general practitioner simply gave her some anti-inflammatory pills. One month after the accident, she still had some pain in her right knee and was given some physiotherapy; however, it did not help the pain much. Since then she has constantly suffered from right knee pain. Usually this worsened when she sat in the same position for too long. Also, she often woke at night because of the pain. In the morning, when she got up, she felt very stiff with pain in her right knee, which improved after moving around. Due to the knee pain, she had to take painkillers from time to time.

When she arrived at the clinic, she had a stabbing pain in her inner right knee, mainly located along the Spleen channel, which was aggravated by touch and pressure, with slight swelling and limitation of the joint movement, accompanied by a slightly purplish tongue with a thin and white coating and a thready and deep pulse.

Diagnosis
Knee pain due to obstruction of channels by stagnated Blood.

Principle of treatment
Promote Blood circulation, harmonise the collateral and relieve the pain.

Acupuncture treatment
LI-4, LR-3, HT-3, SP-3, SP-4, SP-6, SP-8, SP-9 and one local Ah Shi point. Reducing method was used on these points. Treatment was given once every 2 days.

Explanations

- LI-4 and LR-3, the Source point and an Ah Shi point, promote Qi circulation in the channels, eliminate stagnation of Blood and relieve knee pain.
- SP-6, the crossing point of the three Yin channels of the foot, promotes the circulation of Blood, eliminates its stasis and relieves knee pain.

- SP-3, the Source point, and SP-4, the Connecting point, promote circulation in the channel, harmonise the collateral and relieve knee pain.
- SP-8, the Accumulation point, opens the collateral and sedates knee pain.
- SP-9, the local point and the Sea point, removes the obstruction in the Spleen channel, reduces knee swelling and relieves knee pain.
- HT-3 calms the Mind and improves sleep.

After the first treatment, her knee pain was much better for a day, and that night she slept very soundly for the first time in 3 years. After three treatments, her swollen knee had started to improve, and the pain diminished progressively. She stopped taking the painkillers for her knee pain. After ten treatments, her knee pain had gone completely. Six months later, she reported on follow-up that she had not experienced any relapse of the knee pain since the acupuncture treatment.

DEFICIENCY OF LIVER AND KIDNEY

Symptoms and signs

Chronic knee pain with difficulty in rotation, which worsens with excessive strain or standing for too long, with weakness in the lower back and knees, rigidity in the morning, joint deformity and muscular atrophy. Accompanying symptoms include fatigue, lower back pain, an aversion to cold, a thin and white tongue coating, a deep and wiry pulse, and a weak pulse at the Kidney position.

Principle of treatment

Strengthen Kidney and Liver, harmonise the collateral and relieve the pain.

HERBAL TREATMENT

Prescription

DU HUO JI SHENG TANG
Angelica Pubescens and Loranthus Decoction
Du Huo *Radix Angelicae Pubescentis* 10 g
Fang Feng *Radix Ledebouriellae* 10 g
Qin Jiao *Radix Gentianae Macrophyllae* 10 g
Xi Xin *Herba Asari* 3 g
Rou Gui *Cortex Cinnamomi* 6 g
Ren Shen *Radix Ginseng* 6 g
Fu Ling *Poria* 12 g
Gan Cao *Radix Glycyrrhizae* 6 g
Dang Gui *Radix Angelicae Sinensis* 12 g
Chuan Xiong *Rhizoma Chuanxiong* 10 g
Shu Di Huang *Radix Rehmanniae Praeparata* 15 g
Bai Shao *Radix Paeoniae Alba* 12 g
Du Zhong *Cortex Eucommiae* 12 g

Huai Niu Xi *Radix Achyranthis Bidentatae* 12 g
Sang Ji Sheng *Ramulus Loranthi* 15 g

Explanations

- Du Huo, Fang Feng, Qin Jiao, Xi Xin, Rou Gui disperse Wind and remove Damp, dispel Cold and relieve the pain.
- Ren Shen, Fu Ling, Gan Cao, Dang Gui, Chuan Xiong, Shu Di Huang and Bai Shao reinforce the Qi and nourish the Blood and promote its circulation.
- Du Zhong, Huai Niu Xi and Sang Ji Sheng strengthen the Liver and Kidney and relieve the lower back and knee pain.

Modifications

1. If there is an aversion to cold, add Yin Yang Huo *Herba Epimedii* 10 g to warm the Yang, dispel Cold and relieve the pain.
2. If there is lower abdominal pain with a cold sensation, add Wu Zhu Yu *Fructus Evodiae* 5 g to warm the Interior, dispel Cold and relieve the pain.
3. If there is frequent urination at night, add Yi Zhi Ren *Fructus Alpiniae Oxyphyllae* 10 g and Sang Piao Xiao *Ootheca Mantidis* 10 g to tonify the Kidney-Yang and decrease the urine.
4. If there is deficiency of the Yin of Liver and Kidney, use a modified formula based on Zhi Bai Di Huang Wan *Ane-phello and Rehmannia formula* (9 g each time, three times a day) which should be applied instead of Du Huo Ji Sheng Tang.
5. If there is fatigue, add Huang Qi *Radix Astragali seu Hedysari* 15 g to tonify the Qi and relieve the fatigue.

Patent remedies

Du Huo Ji Sheng Wan *Angelica Pubescens and Loranthus Pill*
Hai Ma Bu Shen Wan *Sea Horse Tonify Kidney Pill*
Kang Gu Zheng Sheng Pian *Combat Bone Hyperplasia Pill*

ACUPUNCTURE TREATMENT

GB-34 Yanglingquan, GB-39 Xuanzhong, ST-34 Liangqui, KI-3 Taixi, KI-10 Yingu, SP-6 Sanyinjiao, LR-3 Taichong, LR-8 Ququan and some local Ah Shi points. Reinforcing method is used on these points, except for the local Ah Shi points, on which even method is used.

Explanations

- KI-3, the Source point, and KI-10, the Sea point, reinforce the Kidney and strengthen the bones and knees.
- LR-3, the Source point, and LR-8, the Sea point, tonify the Liver, strengthen the tendons and benefit the knees.
- SP-6, the crossing point of the three Yin channels of the foot, tonifies the Spleen, Kidney and Liver, promotes the circulation of Blood and relieves the pain.
- GB-34, the Gathering point for the tendons, strengthens the tendons and benefits the knees.
- GB-39, the Gathering point for the Marrow, tonifies the Blood and benefits the Kidney-Essence.
- ST-34, the Accumulation point, and the Ah Shi points are local points, which remove obstructions from the local channels and relieve knee pain.

Modifications

1. If there is swelling in the knee joints, add SP-9 to remove Damp and reduce the swelling.
2. If there is a stabbing pain or aggravation of knee pain at night due to stagnation of Blood, add LI-4 and SP-10 to promote the circulation of Blood and remove its stasis.
3. If there is knee pain along the Bladder channel, add BL-36, BL-40, BL-58 and BL-63 to harmonise the collateral and relieve the pain.
4. If there is knee pain along the Gall Bladder channel, add GB-33, GB-36, GB-40 and GB-41 to promote the circulation of Qi and Blood in the channel and relieve the pain.
5. If there is knee pain along the Stomach channel, add ST-34, ST-35, ST-36, ST-40 and ST-42 to promote the circulation of Qi and Blood in the channel, remove the blockage and arrest the pain.
6. If there is knee pain along the Liver channel, add LR-3, LR-5, LR-6 and LR-8 to harmonise the collateral, promote the circulation of Qi and Blood in the channel and relieve the pain.
7. If there is knee pain along the Kidney channel, add KI-3, KI-4, KI-5 and KI-10 to strengthen the Kidney, regulate the circulation of Qi and Blood in the channel and relieve the pain.
8. If there is knee pain along the Spleen channel, add SP-3, SP-4, SP-8 and SP-10 to activate the Spleen, promote the circulation of Qi and Blood in the channel, harmonise the collateral and relieve the pain.
9. Some corresponding points on the elbow should be added in order to increase the therapeutic effect.

10. If there is a severe aversion to cold and a cold sensation in the joints, add moxibustion on the local points and ST-36 to dispel Cold.

DEFICIENCY OF QI AND BLOOD

Symptoms and signs

Intermittent pain of both knees, which is alleviated by rest or massage and aggravated by overwork, with numbness and weakness of the lower limbs, and muscular atrophy in the legs. Accompanying symptoms include tiredness, a pale complexion, lower back pain, shortness of breath after exertion, a poor appetite, a pale tongue with a thin and white coating and a thready and weak pulse.

Principle of treatment

Tonify Qi and Blood, strengthen the knees and sedate the pain.

HERBAL TREATMENT

Prescription

BA ZHEN TANG
Eight-Precious Decoction
Dang Gui *Radix Angelicae Sinensis* 12 g
Chuan Xiong *Rhizoma Ligustici Chuanxiong* 10 g
Bai Shao *Radix Paeoniae Alba* 12 g
Shu Di Huang *Radix Rehmanniae Praeparata* 12 g
Ren Shen *Radix Ginseng* 6 g
Bai Zhu *Rhizoma Atractylodis Macrocephalae* 12 g
Fu Ling *Poria* 12 g
Gan Cao *Radix Glycyrrhizae* 6 g

Explanations

- Dang Gui, Bai Shao and Shu Di Huang tonify the Kidney-Essence and nourish the Liver-Blood.
- Ren Shen, Bai Zhu, Fu Ling and Gan Cao, the ingredients of Si Jun Zi Tang *Four-Gentlemen Decoction*, strengthen the Spleen and reinforce the Qi.
- Chuan Xiong activates the circulation of Qi and Blood and relieves obstruction in the channels. It can also prevent side-effects due to using too many tonics.

Modifications

1. If there is an aversion to cold or cold limbs due to deficiency of Yang, add Gui Zhi *Ramulus*

Cinnamomi 6 g and Wu Zhu Yu *Fructus Evodiae* 10 g to reinforce and activate the Yang-Qi.
2. If there is swelling in the knee or legs due to poor water metabolism caused by deficiency of Spleen-Qi, add Zhu Ling *Polyporus* 15 g and Ze Xie *Rhizoma Alismatis* 12 g to strengthen the Spleen, promote urination and relieve the swelling.
3. If there is fatigue, add Huang Qi *Radix Astragali seu Hedysari* 12 g to tonify the Qi and Blood and relieve the fatigue.

Patent remedies

Shi Quan Da Bu Wan *All-Inclusive Great Tonifying Pill*
Gui Pi Wan *Tonifying the Spleen Pill*

ACUPUNCTURE TREATMENT

GB-34 Yanglingquan, GB-39 Xuanzhong, LR-3 Taichong, KI-3 Taixi, ST-36 Zusanli, SP-6 Sanyinjiao and Ah Shi points. Reinforcing method is used on these points. Reducing method is used on the Ah Shi points.

Explanations

- LR-3 and KI-3, the Source points of the Liver and Kidney channels respectively, tonify the Liver and Kidney, and strengthen the tendons and bones. LR-3 can also promote the circulation of Qi and Blood and relieve knee pain.
- SP-6, the crossing point of the three Yin channels of the foot, strengthens the Spleen, Liver and Kidney and tonifies the Blood.
- GB-39, the Gathering point for the Marrow, and GB-34, the Gathering point for the tendons, reinforce the tendons and bones.
- ST-36, the Sea point of the Stomach channel, reinforces the Spleen and Stomach and promotes the production of Qi and Blood.
- The Ah Shi points harmonise the collateral, promote the circulation of Qi and Blood in the channels and relieve knee pain.

Modifications

1. If there is knee pain along the Bladder channel, add BL-36, BL-40, BL-58 and BL-63 to harmonise the collateral and relieve the pain.
2. If there is knee pain along the Gall Bladder channel, add GB-33, GB-36, GB-40 and GB-41 to promote the circulation of Qi and Blood in the channel and relieve the pain.

3. If there is knee pain along the Stomach channel, add ST-34, ST-35, ST-40 and ST-42 to promote the circulation of Qi and Blood in the channel, relieve the blockage and arrest the pain.

4. If there is knee pain along the Liver channel, add LR-3, LR-5, LR-6 and LR-8 to harmonise the collateral, promote the circulation of Qi and Blood in the channel and relieve the pain.

5. If there is knee pain along the Kidney channel, add KI-4, KI-5 and KI-10 to strengthen the Kidney, regulate the circulation of Qi and Blood in the channel and relieve the pain.

6. If there is knee pain along the Spleen channel, add SP-3, SP-4, SP-8 and SP-10 to activate the Spleen, promote the circulation of Qi and Blood in the channel, harmonise the collateral and relieve the pain.

7. Some corresponding points on the elbow should be used in order to increase the therapeutic effect.

8. If there is an aversion to cold or cold limbs due to deficiency of Yang, add moxibustion on CV-4 and CV-6 to reinforce the Yang-Qi and eliminate Cold.

9. If there is swelling in the knees due to poor water metabolism caused by deficiency of Spleen-Qi, add ST-40 and SP-9 to strengthen the Spleen, promote urination and reduce the swelling.

10. If there is dizziness due to deficiency of Qi and Blood, add GV-20 to activate the Yang-Qi and lift it to the head and relieve the dizziness.

Ankle pain 42

踝
痛

Ankle pain may occur in one or both of the ankle joints. According to TCM theory it is caused mainly by invasion of External factors, deficiency of the Liver and Kidney, or accumulation of Phlegm and stagnation of Blood. Ankle pain may be attributed to any of the following disorders in Western medicine: ankle sprain, dislocation of the long and short peroneal muscles, tarsal tunnel syndrome, dislocation of the ankle joint, traumatic bursal synovitis, rheumatic fever, rheumatic arthritis, rheumatoid arthritis, gout and hyperosteogeny of the ankle joint.

Aetiology and pathology

Invasion of External factors

Exposure to Wind, Cold or Damp over a long period of time, for instance living in damp environment, wandering in cold water, catching a cold, may all lead to invasion of the ankle by these pathogenic factors. When they invade the body they impede the circulation of Qi and Blood in the locality, and cause the pain.

The clinical symptoms and signs vary depending on the pathogenic factor that predominates. Wind is by nature moving and changing, so if it is predominant the ankle pain characteristically moves from one side of the body to the other. Cold has the characteristics of contraction and stagnation, so if it is predominant, it causes the channels and tendons in the ankle to contract, leading to stagnation of Qi and Blood, and causing a severe ankle pain with a cold sensation. Damp is by nature lingering, and its characteristics are heaviness and stagnation. If it predominates, there is obstruction of the channels, leading to numbness and swelling of the ankle and a fixed ankle pain with a heavy sensation.

Exposure to Wind, Damp and Heat can also induce ankle pain, especially in people with an excess of Yang or deficiency of Yin in their body constitution. However, invasion of External pathogenic Wind, Cold and Damp that persists for a long time in the body may also cause Heat to be generated, so that Wind, Damp and Heat accumulates. Heat is characteristically red in colour and burning by nature. Therefore Wind, Damp and Heat invasion or formation disturbs the circulation of Qi and Blood in the channels, so that the Qi and Blood accumulate and stagnate in the joint and the channels are blocked by Damp-Heat. When Cold-Damp persists in the body it may also cause the gradual generation of Heat, leading to formation of Damp-Heat. All of these processes result in pain in the ankle joint, that is accompanied by swelling and redness.

Bad diet

Bad diets, such as eating too much sweet or fatty food, or drinking too much alcohol, may impair the Spleen and Stomach, causing Damp-Heat to form in the body. When Damp-Heat flows downward to the lower limbs, it blocks the channels, and causes ankle pain.

Stagnation of Qi and Blood

When Qi and Blood circulate freely in the ankle region they maintain the normal function of the ankle. If, however, they stagnate because of various causes, such as a sprain, falling over, an inappropriate operation, or overstrain, the channels and collateral become blocked, and the stagnation of Qi and Blood causes ankle pain.

Deficiency of Liver and Kidney

Overstrain, constitutional weakness, standing for too long during work, or prolonged sickness may all cause consumption of the Qi and Blood and deficiency of the Liver and Kidney. Then the tendons are not properly nourished by the Liver-Blood and the bones are not properly nourished by the Kidney, and ankle pain accompanied by weakness or joint deformity follows.

In long-term sickness, a deficiency of Qi and Blood may develop, which leads to a slowing down of the Qi and Blood circulation, and undernourishment of the tendons, causing ankle pain.

Treatment based on differentiation

Differentiation

Differentiation of External or Internal origin

— Acute onset of ankle pain of short duration, accompanied by External symptoms, is usually caused by invasion of External pathogenic factors. Traumatic injury could also cause acute ankle pain.
— Chronic onset of ankle pain of long duration, accompanied by symptoms resulting from Internal disorders, is usually caused by Internal disorders such as deficiency of Liver and Kidney.

Differentiation of character of the pain

— Severe pain, which gets worse with pressure, is usually cause by Excessive pathogenic factors,

such as invasion of Wind-Cold-Damp, or stagnation of Qi and Blood.
— Ankle pain that is dull and lingering often indicates deficiency, such as deficiency of the Liver and Kidney.
— Acute onset of ankle pain with no fixed location is mainly due to pathogenic Wind, such as invasion of external Wind-Cold-Damp with predominance of Wind.
— Severe ankle pain with a cold sensation indicates a Cold syndrome, such as invasion of External Wind-Cold-Damp with predominance of Cold.
— Ankle pain with heavy sensation often indicates pathogenic Dampness, such as invasion of external Wind-Cold-Dampness with predominance of Damp.
— Painful ankle with local redness, swelling and a burring sensation implies pathogenic Heat, such as downward flow of Damp-Heat.

Treatment

INVASION OF WIND-COLD-DAMP WITH PREDOMINANCE OF WIND

Symptoms and signs

Wandering ankle pain, which is aggravated by windy conditions, with difficult movement of the ankle joint, and an aversion to wind, accompanied by a chill and fever, a thin white or thin greasy tongue coating and a superficial pulse.

Principle of treatment

Dispel Wind and unblock the channels, promote Qi and Blood circulation and relieve the pain.

HERBAL TREATMENT

Prescription

FANG FENG TANG
Ledebouriella Decoction
Fang Feng *Radix Ledebouriellae* 10 g
Ma Huang *Herba Ephedrae* 6 g
Dang Gui *Radix Angelicae Sinensis* 10 g
Qin Jiao *Radix Gentianae Macrophyllae* 10 g
Rou Gui *Cortex Cinnamomi* 6 g
Fu Ling *Poria* 15 g
Sheng Jiang *Rhizoma Zingiberis Recens* 6 g
Da Zao *Fructus Ziziphi Jujubae* 10 g
Gan Cao *Radix Glycyrrhizae* 6 g

Explanations

- Fang Feng and Ma Huang dispel Wind and Cold and relieve External symptoms.
- Qin Jiao and Rou Gui warm the channels and dispel Cold so as to relieve the ankle pain.
- Dang Gui promotes the circulation of Blood and removes obstructions from the collaterals. Fu Ling is good at strengthening the Spleen and inducing urination.
- The last three herbs can coordinate all the other herbs in the prescription.

Modifications

1. If there is a fever and chills, add Gui Zhi *Ramulus Cinnamomi* 10 g to relieve the Exterior symptoms and reduce the fever.
2. If the ankle joints are swollen, add Du Huo *Radix Angelica Pubescentis* 10 g and Huai Niu Xi *Radix Achyranthis Bidentatae* 10 g to dispel Damp, reduce the swelling and sedate the pain.
3. If the ankle joint is swollen and red, add Zhi Mu *Rhizoma Anemarrhenae* 10 g and Han Fang Ji *Radix Stephaniae Tetrandrae* 10 g to clear Heat and remove the obstruction from the collateral.

Patent remedy

Jing Fang Bai Du Pian *Schizonepeta and Ledebouriella Tablet to Overcome Pathogenic Influences*

ACUPUNCTURE TREATMENT

TE-5 Waiguan, LI-4 Hegu, BL-12 Fengmen, GB-40 Qiuxu, GB-41 Zulinqi, SP-10 Xuehai, SP-6 Sanyinjiao and some local Ah Shi points. Reducing method is used on these points.

Explanations

- TE-5, LI-4 and BL-12 dispel external pathogenic Wind and relieve External symptoms.
- Ah Shi points and GB-40 and GB-41 around the ankle joint are suitable for regulating the local circulation of Qi and Blood.
- There is a saying 'the Wind will be dispelled automatically when the Blood flows smoothly'. SP-10 activates the circulation of Blood; SP-6 is the crossing point of the Kidney, Spleen, Liver channels, good at regulating the Blood and Qi, so these are useful for eliminating Wind.

Modifications

1. If there is a fever and chills, add GV-14, the meeting point for all the Yang channels, to dispel Wind, relieve Exterior symptoms and reduce the fever.
2. If the ankle joint is swollen, add SP-9, the Sea point, to remove Damp and reduce the swelling.
3. If there is redness, swelling and a sensation of heat in the ankle joint, add LI-11, the Sea point, and ST-44, the Spring point, to clear Heat and reduce the swelling.
4. If there is ankle pain along the Bladder channel, add BL-60, BL-62 and BL-63 to harmonise the collateral and relieve the pain.
5. If there is ankle pain along the Gall Bladder channel, add GB-34 and GB-42 to promote the circulation of Qi and Blood and relieve the pain.
6. If there is ankle pain along the Stomach channel, add ST-41, ST-42 and ST-43 to promote the circulation of Qi and Blood in the channel, relieve blockage and arrest the pain.
7. If there is ankle pain along the Liver channel, add LR-3 and LR-4 to harmonise the collateral and relieve the pain.
8. If there is ankle pain along the Kidney channel, add KI-3, KI-4 and KI-5 to promote the circulation of Qi and Blood and relieve the pain.
9. If there is ankle pain along the Spleen channel, add SP-4 and SP-5 to harmonise the collateral and relieve the pain.
10. Some corresponding points on the wrist should be used in order to increase the therapeutic effect.

Case history

A 30-year-old man had been suffering from wandering ankle pain on both sides for a month. He always wore slippers at home in the winter. A month previously, he started to feel pain in his ankle joint, which got worse when exposed to a wind. The painful areas around the ankle always moved from one ankle to the other, but were mostly around the place where the Bladder channels pass through; he also had a thin white tongue coating and a superficial and tight pulse.

Diagnosis
Ankle pain due to invasion of Wind-Cold.

Principle of treatment
Dispel Wind, expel Cold and relieve the pain.

Herbal treatment
FANG FENG TANG
Ledebouriella Decoction
Fang Feng *Radix Ledebouriellae* 10 g
Ma Huang *Herba Ephedrae* 6 g

Dang Gui *Radix Angelicae Sinensis* 10 g
Qin Jiao *Radix Gentianae Macrophyllae* 10 g
Rou Gui *Cortex Cinnamomi* 6 g
Gan Cao *Radix Glycyrrhizae* 6 g
Qing Feng Teng *Caulis Sinomenii* 20 g

Explanations

- Fang Feng and Ma Huang dispel Wind and Cold and relieve External symptoms.
- Qin Jiao and Rou Gui warm the channels and dispel Cold.
- Dang Gui promotes the circulation of Blood and removes obstructions from the collateral.
- Qing Feng Teng dispels Wind-Cold and relieves the ankle pain.
- Gan Cao harmonises the actions of the other herbs in the prescription.

Acupuncture treatment
TE-5, LI-4, SP-10, SP-6, BL-60, BL-63, wrist point SI-4 and some local Ah Shi points. Reducing method was used on these points. Treatment was given once every day.

Explanations

- TE-5 and LI-4 dispel External pathogenic Wind and relieve External symptoms.
- SP-10, and SP-6, the crossing point of the three Yin channels of the foot, regulate the circulation of the Blood and relieve the pain.
- The Ah Shi points, wrist point SI-4, BL-60 and BL-63 promote the circulation of Qi and Blood around the ankle joint, dispel Wind-Cold and relieve the pain.

After treatment for 2 weeks, the patient's ankle pain disappeared.

INVASION OF WIND-COLD-DAMP WITH PREDOMINANCE OF COLD

Symptoms and signs

Severe pain in the ankle joints with a cold sensation, which is aggravated by contact with cold and alleviated by warmth, accompanied by an aversion to cold, cold limbs, limited movement of the ankle joint in case of pain, a white tongue coating and a tight and slow pulse.

Principle of treatment

Warm the channels, dispel Cold and relieve the pain.

HERBAL TREATMENT

Prescription

WU FU MA XIN GUI JIANG TANG
Decoction of Ephedra, Asari, Cinnamon and Dried Ginger
Chuan Wu Tou *Radix Aconiti Carmichaeli* 10 g, decoct first

Zhi Fu Zi *Radix Lateralis Aconiti Carmichaeli Praeparata* 10 g
Gan Jiang *Rhizoma Zingiberis* 10 g
Ma Huang *Herba Ephedrae* 9 g
Xi Xin *Herba Asari* 3 g
Gui Zhi *Ramulus Cinnamomi* 10 g
Gan Cao *Radix Glycyrrhizae* 6 g

Explanations

- Chuan Wu Tou, Zhi Fu Zi and Gan Jiang, warm in nature, warm the channels, dispel Cold and sedate the pain.
- Ma Huang, Xi Xin and Gui Zhi expel Wind, Cold and Damp.
- Gan Cao moderates all the herbs and minimises the Toxic effects of Chuan Wu Tou and Zhi Fu Zi.

Modifications

1. If there is limitation of the joint movement, add Huai Niu Xi *Radix Achyranthis Bidentatae* 10 g and Bai Shao *Radix Paeoniae Alba* 10 g to strengthen the joints and relieve the pain.
2. If the ankle is swollen, add Mu Tong *Caulis Akebiae* 6 g to promote urination, eliminate Damp and reduce the swelling.
3. If the limbs are cold, add Rou Gui *Cortex Cinnamomi* 5 g to warm the Yang and dispel Cold.
4. If there is severe pain, add Jiang Huang *Rhizoma Curcumae Longae* 10 g to regulate Blood circulation and relieve the pain.

Patent remedy

Han Shi Bi Chong Ji *Cold-Damp Bi Syndrome Infusion*

ACUPUNCTURE TREATMENT

TE-5 Waiguan, LI-4 Hegu, ST-36 Zusanli, SP-6 Sanyinjiao, BL-12 Fengmen, BL-60 Kunlun, BL-63 Jinmen, GB-40 Qiuxu and Ah Shi points. Reducing method is used on these points except for ST-36, on which tonifying method is used. Moxibustion is used on TE-5, LI-4, ST-36, BL-60 and GB-40.

Explanations

- TE-5, LI-4 and BL-12 dispel External pathogenic Wind, eliminate Cold and relieve External symptoms.
- Ah Shi points, GB-40, BL-60 and BL-63, all the local points, regulate circulation of Qi and Blood in the local areas so as to relieve the ankle pain.

- ST-36, the Sea point, tonifies the Qi, warms the channels and dispels Cold.
- SP-6 activates the circulation of Blood and relieves the ankle pain.
- Moxibustion is applied to warm the channels, dispel Cold and relieve the pain.

Modifications

1. If the ankle is swollen, add SP-9 to eliminate Damp and reduce the swelling.
2. If there is a cold sensation in the body and cold limbs, add KI-3 and CV-8 with moxibustion to reinforce the Yang and dispel Cold.
3. If there is ankle pain along the Bladder channel, remove GB-40, and add BL-62 and BL-64 to harmonise the collateral and relieve the pain.
4. If there is ankle pain along the Gall Bladder channel, add GB-34 and GB-41 to promote the circulation of Qi and Blood and relieve the pain.
5. If there is ankle pain along the Stomach channel, add ST-41, ST-42 and ST-43 to promote the circulation of Qi and Blood in the channel, relieve blockage and arrest the pain.
6. If there is ankle pain along the Liver channel, add LR-3 and LR-4 to harmonise the collateral and relieve the pain.
7. If there is ankle pain along the Kidney channel, add KI-3, KI-4 and KI-5 to promote the circulation of Qi and Blood and relieve the pain.
8. If there is ankle pain along the Spleen channel, add SP-4 and SP-5 to harmonise the collateral and relieve the pain.
9. Some corresponding points on the wrist should be used in order to increase the therapeutic effect.
10. If there is a runny nose and coughing, add LU-7 and GB-20 to dispel Wind and eliminate Cold so as to relieve External symptoms.

INVASION OF WIND-COLD-DAMP WITH PREDOMINANCE OF DAMP

Symptoms and signs

Painful and swollen ankle joints with a heavy sensation, and fixed in a certain area, which worsens on overcast or rainy days, with limited movement of the ankle joints, a white and greasy tongue coating and a soft and slow pulse.

Principle of treatment

Eliminate Damp, dispel Wind and Cold, promote circulation of the collateral and sedate the pain.

HERBAL TREATMENT

Prescription

YI YI REN TANG
Coix Decoction
Yi Yi Ren *Semen Coicis* 15 g
Cang Zhu *Rhizoma Atractylodis* 10 g
Qiang Huo *Rhizoma el Radix Notopterygii* 10 g
Du Huo *Radix Angelicae Pubescentis* 10 g
Fang Feng *Radix Ledebouriellae* 10 g
Chuan Wu Tou *Radix Aconiti Carmichaeli* 6 g
Ma Huang *Herba Ephedrae* 6 g
Gui Zhi *Ramulus Cinnamomi* 6 g
Dang Gui *Radix Angelicae Sinensis* 10 g
Chuan Xiong *Radix Ligustici Chuanxiong* 6 g
Sheng Jiang *Rhizoma Zingiberis Recens* 6 g
Gan Cao *Radix Glycyrrhizae* 6 g

Explanations

- Yi Yi Ren and Cang Zhu strengthen the Spleen and remove Damp.
- Qiang Huo, Du Huo and Fang Feng dispel Wind, remove Damp, promote the circulation of Qi and Blood in the channels and relieve the pain.
- Chuang Wu Tou, Ma Huang and Gui Zhi warm the channels, dispel Cold and remove Damp.
- Dang Gui and Chuan Xiong nourish the Blood and promote Blood circulation.
- Sheng Jiang and Gan Cao strengthen the Spleen and regulate the Middle Burner.

Modifications

1. If there is a feeling of heaviness in the ankle joints, add Fu Ling *Poria* 15 g and Ze Xie *Rhizoma Alismatis* 10 g to promote urination and eliminate Damp.
2. If there is severe joint pain, add Wu Gong *Scolopendra* 3 g to relieve the pain.
3. If there is lower back pain, add Du Zhong *Cortex Eucommiae* 10 g and Sang Ji Sheng *Ramus Loranthi* 10 g to strengthen the lower back and relieve the lower back pain.
4. If there is nausea or vomiting and diarrhoea, add Sha Ren *Fructus Ammomi Villosi* 5 g and Bai Zhu *Rhizoma Atractylodis Macrocephalae* 10 g to activate the Spleen and Stomach and relieve Damp in the Middle Burner.

Patent remedies

Feng Shi Pian *Wind-Damp Tablet*
Tian Ma Qu Feng Bu Pian *Gastrodia Dispel Wind Formula Tablet*

ACUPUNCTURE TREATMENT

TE-6 Zhigou, LI-4 Hegu, ST-40 Fenglong, SP-9 Yinlingquan, BL-12 Fengmen, BL-63 Jinmen, BL-64 Jinggu, GB-40 Qiuxu and Ah Shi points. Reducing method is used on these points.

Explanations

- TE-6, LI-4 and BL-12 dispel External pathogenic Wind, eliminate Cold, resolve Damp and relieve External symptoms.
- GB-40, the Source point, BL-63, the Accumulation point, and BL-64, the Source point, which are the local points, eliminate Damp, and regulate the circulation of Qi and Blood in the local areas so as to relieve the ankle pain.
- ST-40, the Connecting point, and SP-9, the Sea point, eliminate Damp in the channels and relieve the pain.
- Ah Shi points promote circulation of Qi and Blood in the local areas so as to relieve the ankle pain.

Modifications

1. If there is swelling of the ankle, add SP-3, the Source point, to eliminate Damp and reduce the swelling.
2. If there is a cold sensation in the body and cold limbs, add CV-8 with moxibustion to reinforce the Yang and dispel Cold.
3. If there is ankle pain along the Bladder channel, remove GB-40, add BL-60 and BL-62 to harmonise the collateral and relieve the pain.
4. If there is ankle pain along the Gall Bladder channel, add GB-34 and GB-41 to promote the circulation of Qi and Blood and relieve the pain.
5. If there is ankle pain along the Stomach channel, add ST-41, ST-42 and ST-43 to promote the circulation of Qi and Blood in the channel, relieve blockage and arrest the pain.
6. If there is ankle pain along the Liver channel, add LR-3 and LR-4 to harmonise the collateral and relieve the pain.
7. If there is ankle pain along the Kidney channel, add KI-3, KI-4 and KI-5 to promote the circulation of Qi and Blood and relieve the pain.
8. If there is ankle pain along the Spleen channel, add SP-4 and SP-5 to harmonise the collateral and relieve the pain.
9. Some corresponding points on the wrist should be used in order to increase the therapeutic effect.
10. If there is nausea, or vomiting and diarrhoea, add CV-12 and ST-25 to regulate the Qi in the Middle Burner and harmonise the Spleen and Stomach.
11. If there is scanty urination, add SP-6 and KI-3 to promote urination and eliminate Damp.
12. If there is a feeling of heaviness in the body generally, add BL-22 and BL-40 to promote urination and eliminate Damp.

Case history

A 46-year-old female had been suffering from rheumatoid arthritis for 4 years. The pain was mainly in the lower limbs, especially in her ankles. In the previous few weeks, her ankle pain had become worse, and caused her difficulty in walking and sleeping. She received some painkillers from her doctor, but they did not help much. There was swelling and a heavy sensation in the ankle joints, the pain worsened on overcast and rainy days, and was located at GB-40. Accompanying symptoms included a poor appetite and occasional loose stools, a white and greasy tongue coating and a soft and slippery pulse.

Diagnosis
Ankle pain due to invasion of Wind-Cold-Damp with predominance of Damp, weakness of Spleen and Stomach.

Principle of treatment
Eliminate Damp, dispel Wind-Cold, activate the Spleen and Stomach and sedate the pain.

Acupuncture treatment
TE-6, ST-40, SP-6, SP-9, BL-12, BL-60, GB-34, GB-40 and corresponding wrist point TE-4. Reducing method is used on these points. Treatment was given once every day.

Explanations
- TE-6 and BL-12 dispel External pathogenic Wind-Cold and eliminate External Damp.
- ST-40, the Connecting point, SP-6, the crossing point of the three Yin channels of the foot, and SP-9, the Sea point, activate the Spleen and Stomach, and eliminate Damp in the body and channels so as to relieve the pain.
- BL-60 dispels External pathogenic factors and relieves the ankle pain.
- GB-34, the Gathering point for the tendons, GB-40, the Source point, and the corresponding wrist point TE-4, the Source point, eliminate Damp, regulate the circulation of Qi and Blood in the Gall Bladder channel and relieve the ankle pain.

Herbal treatment
A prescription based on Yi Yi Ren Tang *Coix Decoction* and Shen Ling Bai Zhu San *Panaxa–Poria–Atractylodis Powder* was given to eliminate Wind-Cold-Damp in the channels and strengthen the Spleen and Stomach. After four treatment sessions, her ankle pain had improved, and the swelling had subsided. After ten treatments, the ankle pain was gone. The herbal treatment was continued for another month in order to regulate her Spleen and Stomach and eliminate Damp from the body.

DOWNWARD FLOW OF DAMP-HEAT

Symptoms and signs

Swelling and painful ankle joints with a local burning sensation and redness, which worsen with touching, and limited movement. Other symptoms include irritability, restlessness, a poor appetite, a bitter taste in the mouth, scanty and yellow urination, occasional fever, a yellow and greasy tongue coating and a slippery and rapid pulse.

In acute ankle pain, as well as swelling, redness and pain in the ankle joint, there are usually some external symptoms, such as an aversion to cold, fever, generalised body pain, headache, a red tongue with a yellow and greasy coating and a superficial and slippery pulse.

Principle of treatment

Clear Heat, eliminate Damp and sedate the pain. If there is invasion of Wind-Damp-Heat, then add the method for dispelling Wind-Damp-Heat.

HERBAL TREATMENT

Prescription

BAI HU JIA GUI ZHI TANG and **SAN MIAO WAN**
White Tiger Ramulus Cinnamon Decoction and *Three-Marvel Pill*
Zhi Mu *Rhizoma Anemarrhenae* 10 g
Shi Gao *Gypsum Fibrosum* 20 g
Gui Zhi *Ramulus Cinnamomi* 8 g
Gan Cao *Radix Glycyrrhizae* 6 g
Jing Mi *Semen Oryzae* 10 g
Huang Bai *Cortex Phellodendri* 10 g
Cang Zhu *Rhizoma Atractylodis* 10 g
Huai Niu Xi *Radix Achyranthis Bidentatae* 10 g
Wei Ling Xian *Radix Clematidis* 10 g
Han Fang Ji *Radix Stephaniae Tetrandrae* 10 g
Sang Zhi *Ramulus Mori* 15 g

Explanations

- Shi Gao and Zhi Mu are the main herbs in Bai Hu Jia Gui Zhi Tang for clearing Heat and reducing fever.
- Gan Cao and Jing Mi benefit the Stomach, reinforce the Body Fluids, and moderate the extremely Cold nature of Shi Gao.
- Gui Zhi dispels Wind, harmonises the collateral and promotes the circulation of Blood to relieve the ankle pain.
- Wei Ling Xian, Han Fang Ji and Sang Zhi expel pathogenic Wind, eliminate Damp, promote the circulation of Blood and unblock the channels.
- Huang Bai and Cang Zhu dry Damp, clear Heat and reduce swelling in the ankle.
- Huai Niu Xi induces the herbs to the ankle and eliminates Damp in the Lower Burner.

Modifications

1. If there is swelling and redness of the ankle, add Tu Fu Ling *Rhizoma Smilacis* 10 g and Sheng Di Huang *Radix Rehmanniae* 15 g to clear Heat, remove Toxin, reduce swelling and relieve the pain.
2. If there is a fever, add Jin Yin Hua *Flos Lonicerae* 10 g and Lian Qiao *Fructus Forsythiae* 10 g to clear Heat and reduce the fever.
3. If the appetite is poor, add Ban Xia *Rhizoma Pinelliae* 10 g and Chen Pi *Pericarpium Citri Reticulatae* 10 g to regulate the Qi and improve the appetite.
4. If there is a thirst, add Xuan Shen *Radix Scrophulariae* 10 g and Ge Gen *Radix Puerariae* 10 g to clear Heat and relieve the thirst.
5. If there is irritability, add Deng Xin Cao *Medulla Junci* 15 g to clear Fire and calm the Mind.
6. If there is constipation, add Da Huang *Radix et Rhizoma Rhei* 6 g and Mang Xiao *Natrii Sulfas* 6 g to eliminate Heat, promote defecation and relieve the constipation.

Patent remedies

San Miao Wan *Three-Marvel Pill*
Feng Shi Xiao Tong Pian *Wind-Damp Dispel Pain Pill*

ACUPUNCTURE TREATMENT

TE-6 Zhigou, LI-4 Hegu, SP-6 Sanyinjiao, BL-60 Kunlun, GB-34 Yanglingquan, GB-40 Qiuxu, GB-41 Zulinqi, ST-44 Neiting and some Ah Shi points. Reducing method is used on these points.

Explanations

- TE-6 and LI-4 dispel External pathogenic factors, promote the circulation of Qi in the channels, eliminate Damp and reduce Heat.
- SP-6, the crossing point of the three Yin channels of the foot, SP-9 and GB-34, the Sea point, together with GB-40, eliminate Damp in the body and channels and clear Heat so as to relieve the pain.
- BL-60 dispels External pathogenic factors, promotes urination, eliminates Damp and relieves the ankle pain.

- ST-44 and GB-41 eliminate Damp-Heat and reduce fever.
- Ah Shi points eliminate Damp, regulate the circulation of Qi and Blood in the channels and relieve the ankle pain.

Modifications

1. If there is redness and pain in the ankle joint, add SP-10 to cool the Blood and reduce the swelling.
2. If there is a fever, add GV-14 and LI-11 to clear Heat and reduce the fever.
3. If there is generalised body pain and headache, add GB-20 to dispel External factors and relieve the body pain.
4. If there is yellow and scanty urination, add CV-3 to promote urination, clear Heat and eliminate Damp in the body.
5. If there is ankle pain along the Bladder channel, remove GB-40, and add BL-59, BL-62 and BL-63 to harmonise the collateral and relieve the pain.
6. If there is ankle pain along the Gall Bladder channel, add GB-42 and GB-43 to promote the circulation of Qi and Blood, clear Heat and relieve the pain.
7. If there is ankle pain along the Stomach channel, add ST-41, ST-42 and ST-43 to promote the circulation of Qi and Blood in the channel, relieve blockage and arrest the pain.
8. If there is ankle pain along the Liver channel, add LR-2, LR-3 and LR-4 to harmonise the collateral and relieve the pain.
9. If there is ankle pain along the Kidney channel, add KI-3, KI-4 and KI-5 to promote the circulation of Qi and Blood and relieve the pain.
10. If there is ankle pain along the Spleen channel, add SP-4 and SP-5 to harmonise the collateral and relieve the pain.
11. Some corresponding points on the wrist should be used in order to increase the therapeutic effect.
12. If there is nausea, or vomiting and diarrhoea, add CV-12 and ST-25 to regulate the Qi in the Middle Burner and harmonise the Spleen and Stomach.
13. If there is a general feeling of heaviness in the body, add BL-22 and BL-40 to promote urination and eliminate Damp.

Case history

A 55-year-old lady had been suffering from ankle pain on both sides for 3 years. Her ankle joints were red and swollen with a hot sensation, and a pain that worsened with touching, with limited movement. The pain didn't change with the weather, but related to her drinking of alcohol and eating fatty food. She liked to eat sweet food. Her doctor forbade her to drink alcohol, but she sometimes still did it. However, each time she drank too much, her ankle started to get swollen and become painful. The pain was mainly located around GB-40. Accompanying symptoms were: a sensation of heat in the head, irritability, nervousness, a poor appetite, a bitter taste in the mouth, deep yellow urine, sometimes painful urination, constipation, a white and greasy coating and a slippery and rapid pulse.

Diagnosis
Ankle pain due to downward flow of Damp-Heat with accumulation of Damp-Heat in the Liver and Gall Bladder.

Principle of treatment
Clear Heat, eliminate Damp, harmonise the Liver and Gall Bladder, promote Blood circulation and relieve the pain.

Herbal treatment
SAN MIAO WAN
Three-Marvel Pill
Huang Bai *Cortex Phellodendri* 10 g
Cang Zhu *Rhizoma Atractylodes* 10 g
Huai Niu Xi *Radix Achyranthis Bidentatae* 10 g
Wei Ling Xian *Radix Clematidis* 10 g
Han Fang Ji *Radix Stephaniae Tetrandrae* 10 g
Sang Zhi *Ramulus Mori* 10 g
Yin Chen Hao *Herba Artemesiae Capillaris* 15 g
Zhi Mu *Rhizoma Anemarrhenae* 10 g
Tu Fu Ling *Rhizoma Smilacis* 10 g
Sheng Di Huang *Radix Rehmanniae Recens* 10 g
Da Huang *Radix et Rhizoma Rhei* 6 g

Explanations
- Huang Bai and Cang Zhu dry Damp, clear Heat and reduce swelling of the ankle.
- Huai Niu Xi leads the herbs to the ankle and eliminates Damp in the Lower Burner.
- Wei Ling Xian, Han Fang Ji and Sang Zhi eliminate Damp-Heat in the channels and promote the circulation of Blood and unblock the channels.
- Yin Chen Hao and Zhi Mu eliminate Damp-Heat in the Liver and Gall Bladder and harmonise the Liver and Gall Bladder.
- Tu Fu Ling and Sheng Di Huang clear Heat, remove toxin and eliminate Damp-Heat in the body.
- Da Huang clears Heat, promotes defecation and relieves constipation.

Acupuncture treatment
TE-6 Zhigou, SP-6 Sanyinjiao, SP-9 Yinlingquan, GB-34 Yanglingquan, GB-40 Qiuxu, GB-41 Zulinqi, LR-2 Xingjian and corresponding wrist point TE-4. Reducing method was used on these points. Treatment was given once every day.

Explanations
- TE-6 promotes the physiological function of the Triple Burner and the circulation of Qi in the channels, eliminates Damp and reduces Heat.

- SP-9 and GB-34, the Sea point, activate the Spleen, eliminate Damp-Heat and harmonise the tendons.
- GB-40 and GB-41 eliminate Damp-Heat in the channel so as to relieve the pain.
- SP-6, the crossing point of the three Yin channels of the foot, and LR-2, the Spring point, harmonise the Liver and Gall Bladder, and clear Damp-Heat in the body and channels.
- The corresponding wrist point TE-4 eliminates Damp-Heat, regulates the circulation of Qi and Blood in the Lesser Yang channel and relieves the ankle pain.

After treatment for 2 weeks, her ankle pain was much better, and the redness and swelling had diminished. Meanwhile, she was asked to stop drinking alcohol completely, and eat less sweet food. After treatment for a month, her ankle pain was under control. Then the acupuncture was stopped and she was asked to continue with the herbal treatment only for another 2 months. One year later she was followed up by letter and she said she had experienced no more pain in her ankle.

STAGNATION OF QI AND BLOOD

Symptoms and signs

Ankle pain with a fixed location, which worsens at night, with pressure or on movement, with swelling and bruising laterally or medially, a history of trauma, limited movement of the joint, and lameness due to the pain. During the acute stage, there may be no changes on the tongue and the pulse might be tight or wiry, but during the chronic stage there may be a light purple tongue and a choppy pulse.

Principle of treatment

Promote Qi and Blood circulation, remove Blood stasis, smooth the collateral and relieve the pain.

HERBAL TREATMENT

Prescription

Acute stage

QI LI SAN (patent pill) 0.5 g each time twice a day for oral intake
Seven-Thousandths of a Tael Powder
Xue Jie *Sanguis Draconis*
She Xiang *Secretio Mischus*
Bing Pian *Borneolum Syntheticum*
Ru Xiang *Resina Olibani*
Mo Yao *Resina Myrrhae*
Hong Hua *Flos Carthami*
Er Cha *Catechu*

Take 0.2 g of Qi Li San twice daily, orally with Chinese rice wine each time. Apply the proper amount of Qi Li San (2 g) mixed with Chinese rice wine topically to the affected area.

Explanations

- Xue Jie is the main herb for stopping bleeding.
- Hong Hua, Ru Xiang and Mo Yao are good at promoting the circulation of Qi and Blood, reducing swelling and relieving pain.
- She Xiang and Bing Pian are pungent, and promote Blood circulation and clear away the obstruction in the collateral.
- Er Cha, astringent in taste and Cool in nature, arrests bleeding and promotes the growth of new tissue.

Middle and restoration stage

XIAO HUO LUO DAN (patent pill)
Minor Invigorate the Collaterals Special Pill
Zhi Nan Xing *Rhizoma Arisaematis Praeparata*
Zhi Chuan Wu *Radix Aconiti Praeparata*
Zhi Cao Wu *Radix Aconiti Kusnezoffii Praeparata*
Di Long *Lumbricus*
Ru Xiang *Resina Olibani*
Mo Yao *Resina Myrrhae*

Take one bolus once daily, with Chinese rice wine each time.

Explanations

- Zhi Chuan Wu and Zhi Cao Wu, pungent in flavour and Hot in nature, have a strong effect in warming the channels and eliminating pain.
- Zhi Nan Xing eliminates Phlegm-Damp in the channels and stops pain.
- Ru Xiang, Mo Yao and Chinese rice wine promote the circulation of Qi and Blood.
- Di Long smoothes the collateral and conducts all the herbs to the collateral.

Patent remedies

Xiao Huo Luo Dan *Minor Invigorate the Collaterals Special Pill*
Jin Gu Die Shang Wan *Muscle and Bone Traumatic Injury Pill*

ACUPUNCTURE TREATMENT

LI-4 Hegu, SP-6 Sanyinjiao, SP-10 Xuehai, BL-17 Geshu, LR-3 Taichong, GB-34 Yanglingquan and some Ah Shi points. Reducing method is used on these points.

Explanations

- LI-4 and LR-3, the Source points, promote the circulation of Qi in the channels, eliminate stagnation of Blood and relieve the pain.
- SP-6, the crossing point of the three Yin channels of the foot, BL-17, the Gathering point of the Blood, and SP-10 eliminate Blood stasis and relieve pain.
- GB-34, the Sea point, strengthens the tendons and harmonises the movement of the joints.
- Ah Shi points regulate the circulation of Qi and Blood in the channels and relieve the ankle pain.

Modifications

1. If there is ankle pain along the Bladder channel, add BL-59, BL-62 and BL-63 to harmonise the collateral and relieve the pain.
2. If there is ankle pain along the Gall Bladder channel, add GB-40, GB-42 and GB-43 to promote the circulation of Qi and Blood and relieve the pain.
3. If there is ankle pain along the Stomach channel, add ST-41, ST-42 and ST-43 to promote the circulation of Qi and Blood in the channel, relieve blockage and arrest the pain.
4. If there is ankle pain along the Liver channel, add LR-2, LR-3 and LR-4 to harmonise the collateral and relieve the pain.
5. If there is ankle pain along the Kidney channel, add KI-3, KI-4 and KI-5 to promote the circulation of Qi and Blood and relieve the pain.
6. If there is ankle pain along the Spleen channel, add SP-4 and SP-5 to harmonise the collateral and relieve the pain.
7. Some corresponding points on the wrist should be used in order to increase the therapeutic effects.
8. If there is restlessness and insomnia, add HT-3 and PC-6 to calm the Mind and improve the sleep.
9. If the ankle is swollen, add Extra Bafeng to promote the circulation of Qi and Blood and reduce the swelling.
10. If the ankle is a purplish colour, add GB-44 and BL-67, the Well points, to promote the circulation of Blood and relieve the pain.

Case history

A 19-year-old man had fallen from his bicycle a month previously, and the outside of his left ankle had been injured. He went to his doctor but the doctor found nothing wrong except a slight soft tissue sprain. The man was asked to rest at home for 2 days. After this, because the pain was not much improved, he was sent for X-ray 2 days before he came to the acupuncture clinic, but nothing abnormal was found.

When he arrived at the clinic, his ankle pain was still present, especially during the night. It was mainly located around BL-62, and the ankle was still swollen and painful, and aggravated by pressure. There was limitation of the ankle joint movement on the left side. The patient also had a light red tongue with a thin white coating and a tight pulse.

Diagnosis
Ankle pain due to obstruction of channels by stagnated Blood.

Treatment principle
Promote Blood circulation, smooth the collateral and relieve the pain.

Acupuncture treatment
LI-4, SP-6, SP-10, LR-3, GB-34, BL-60, BL-62, two Ah Shi points and corresponding wrist point SI-5. Reducing method was used on these points. Treatment was given once every 2 days.

Explanations

- LI-4 and LR-3, the Source points, promote the circulation of Qi in the channels, eliminate stagnation of Blood and relieve the pain.
- SP-6, the crossing point of the three Yin channels of the foot, and SP-10 eliminate Blood stasis and relieve the pain.
- GB-34, the Sea point, strengthens the tendons and harmonises the movement of the joints.
- BL-60 and BL-62, together with Ah Shi points and the corresponding wrist point SI-5 regulate the circulation of Qi and Blood in the channels and relieve ankle pain.

After the first treatment, he felt no pain for about 5 hours. After the second treatment, he had no ankle pain at night for 3 days. After four treatments, his ankle pain was almost gone. In total, he received ten treatments, after which he had no more ankle pain.

DEFICIENCY OF ESSENCE OF LIVER AND KIDNEY

Symptoms and signs

Chronic ankle pain with difficulty in rotation, flexion and extension, which is aggravated by overstrain or standing for too long, with weakness of the knees and ankle, rigidity in the morning, joint deformity and muscular atrophy. Accompanying symptoms include fatigue, lower back pain, an aversion to cold, a thin and white tongue coating, and a deep and wiry pulse, with a weak pulse at the Kidney position.

Principle of treatment

Tonify the Kidney and Liver, strengthen the tendons and bones, smooth the channels and relieve the pain.

HERBAL TREATMENT

Prescription

DU HUO JI SHENG TANG
Angelica Pubescens–Loranthus Decoction
Du Huo *Radix Angelicae Pubescentis* 9 g
Fang Feng *Radix Ledebouriellae* 6 g
Qin Jiao *Radix Gentianae Macrophyllae* 6 g
Xi Xin *Herba Asari* 6 g
Rou Gui *Cortex Cinnamomi* 6 g
Ren Shen *Radix Ginseng* 6 g
Dang Gui *Radix Angelicae Sinensis* 6 g
Chuan Xiong *Radix Ligustici Chuanxiong* 6 g
Shu Di Huang *Radix Rehmanniae Praeparata* 10 g
Du Zhong *Cortex Eucommiae* 10 g
Huai Niu Xi *Radix Achyranthis Bidentatae* 10 g
Sang Ji Sheng *Ramulus Loranthi* 10 g
Gan Cao *Radix Glycyrrhizae* 6 g

Explanations

- Du Huo, Fang Feng and Qin Jiao dispel external factors, smooth the channels and relieve pain.
- Xi Xin and Rou Gui warm the channels, tonify the Kidney-Yang, dispel Cold and relieve the pain.
- Ren Shen and Dang Gui tonify the Qi and Blood so as to nourish the Liver and Kidney.
- Chuan Xiong and Huai Niu Xi promote the circulation of Blood and eliminate its stasis so as to relieve the ankle pain.
- Shu Di Huang tonifies the Liver and Kidney and strengthens the tendons and bones.
- Du Zhong and Sang Ji Sheng benefit the Liver and Kidney, and strengthen the lower back, tendons and bones.
- Gan Cao harmonises the herbs in the formula.

Modifications

1. If the ankles are swollen, add Fu Ling *Poria* 10 g to promote urination and eliminate the swelling.
2. If there is weakness in the knees, legs and ankles, add Xu Duan *Radix Dipsaci* 10 g to tonify the Kidney and strengthen the lower back.
3. If there is lower back pain with a cold feeling, add Yin Yang Huo *Herba Epimedii* 10 g to warm the Kidney-Yang and promote the circulation of Blood.
4. If there is lower abdominal pain with a cold sensation, add Wu Zhu Yu *Fructus Evodiae* 5 g to warm the Interior, dispel Cold and relieve the pain.
5. If there is frequent urination at night, add Yi Zhi Ren *Fructus Alpiniae Oxyphyllae* 10 g and Sang Piao Xiao *Ootheca Mantidis* 10 g to tonify the Kidney-Yang and reduce the urine.

6. If there is deficiency of Yin of Liver and Kidney, use a modification based on Zhi Bai Di Huang Wan *Ane-phello and Rehmannia Formula* (9 g each time, three times a day) instead of Du Huo Ji Sheng Tang.

Patent remedies

Hai Ma Bu Shen Pian *Sea Horse Tonify Kidney Tablet*
Du Huo Ji Sheng Wan *Angelica Pubescens–Loranthus Pill*
Kang Gu Zheng Sheng Pian *Combat Bone Hyperplasia Tablet*

ACUPUNCTURE TREATMENT

GB-39 Xuanzhong, GB-34 Yanglingquan, LR-3 Taichong, KI-3 Taixi, ST-36 Zusanli and SP-6 Sanyinjiao. Even method is used on GB-34, LR-3 and SP-6. Reinforcing method is used on the rest of the points.

Explanations

- This type of ankle pain is often seen in old people as the functioning of the Liver and Kidney tends to decline with age, so the Blood and Kidney-Essence become unable to nourish the tendons and bones sufficiently. Therefore the Kidney and Liver should be strengthened first.
- LR-3 and KI-3, the Source points of Liver and Kidney channels respectively, tonify the Liver and Kidney, and strengthen the tendons and bones.
- SP-6, the crossing point of the three Yin channels of the foot, strengthens the Spleen, Liver and Kidney and tonifies the Blood.
- GB-39, the Gathering point for the Marrow, and GB-34, the Gathering point for the tendons, reinforce the tendons and bones.
- ST-36, the Sea point of the Stomach channel, reinforces the Spleen and Stomach and promotes the production of Blood.

Modifications

1. If there is ankle pain along the Bladder channel, add BL-59, BL-62 and BL-63 to harmonise the collateral and relieve the pain.
2. If there is ankle pain along the Gall Bladder channel, add GB-40, GB-42 and GB-43 to promote the circulation of Qi and Blood and relieve the pain.
3. If there is ankle pain along the Stomach channel, add ST-41, ST-42 and ST-43 to promote the circulation of Qi and Blood in the channel, relieve blockage and arrest the pain.

4. If there is ankle pain along the Liver channel, add LR-2, LR-3 and LR-4 to harmonise the collateral and relieve the pain.

5. If there is ankle pain along the Kidney channel, add KI-3, KI-4 and KI-5 to promote the circulation of Qi and Blood and relieve the pain.

6. If there is ankle pain along the Spleen channel, add SP-4 and SP-5 to harmonise the collateral and relieve the pain.

7. Some corresponding points on the wrist should be added in order to increase the therapeutic effect.

8. If there is swelling of ankle joints due to water retention, add SP-9 to eliminate Damp and reduce the swelling.

9. If there is swelling and even deformity of the ankle joints due to stagnation of Blood, add SP-10 to promote the circulation of Blood and remove the Blood stasis.

10. If there is an aversion to cold and a cold sensation in the joints, add moxibustion on the local points.

11. If there is restlessness and insomnia, add HT-3 and PC-6 to calm the Mind and improve sleep.

Heel pain 43

足
跟
疼
痛

Heel pain may occur in one or both heels, and may appear as an isolated disorder, or may be one of a group of symptoms classified in TCM as a Bi syndrome (arthritis). It can be accompanied by a cold or heat sensation on the heel, ankle pain, numbness or swelling of heels. According to TCM theory, heel pain can be caused by invasion of External Wind-Damp, invasion of Toxic Fire, downward flow of Damp-Heat, stagnation of Qi and Blood in the channels, deficiency of Qi and Blood, and deficiency of Yin of Liver and Kidney. Heel pain may be attributed to any of the following disorders in Western medicine: rheumatoid arthritis, rheumatic arthritis, gout, heel infection, fracture or soft tissue injury of the heels and formation of a heel spur.

Aetiology and pathology

Invasion of External Wind, Cold and Damp

Wind is a pathological factor existing in all four seasons; Cold is characterised by stagnation and contraction; Damp is characterised by heaviness, downward flowing and viscosity. When these three pathogenic factors invade the heels, they may obstruct the local channels, leading to stagnation of the Qi and Blood circulation, and causing heel pain.

This situation happens most often when the heels are exposed for too long to the cold air, after walking or working in cold water, or living in a cold and humid place.

Invasion of Toxic Fire

Local wounds or skin ulcers on the heel, with lack of personal hygiene of the foot, wearing of inappropriate footware, and insect bites may all cause invasion of Toxic Fire to the heels, leading to injury of the muscles, channels and tendons in the heels; the heel pain occurs because of the stagnation of the Qi and Blood that follows.

In addition, if Excessive-Heat accumulates in the body, or there is a deficiency of Yin, then toxic Heat may gradually form as a result. If this toxic Heat remains in the body for some time then it may generate toxic Fire, which burns the skin, muscles and tendons in the heels, causing heel pain.

Downward flow of Damp-Heat

Bad diets, such as eating too much sweet or fatty food, or drinking too much alcohol, may impair the Spleen and Stomach, causing Damp-Heat to form in the body. When Damp-Heat flows downward to the lower limbs, it blocks the channels around the heels. Furthermore, if Wind-Damp-Heat invades the lower limbs, it may cause the circulation of Qi and Blood in the channels to stagnate and once again the channels become blocked by Damp-Heat. Both of these circumstances result in heel pain.

Finally, if Cold-Damp remains in the body then over time it may cause the gradual generation of Heat, leading to the formation of Damp-Heat, and again resulting in heel pain.

Stagnation of Qi and Blood in the channels

Inappropriate exercise and movement may injure and cause trauma to the channels and tendons of the heel, which in turn results in stagnation of the Qi and Blood in the area, and causes heel pain. Standing, walking or running for too long, or remaining for too long in the same sitting position, may also lead to Qi and Blood stagnation so that heel pain follows.

Exposure to excessive heat or cold, and excessive strain on the heel, are other possible causes of stagnation of Qi and Blood that may lead to heel pain.

Deficiency of Qi and Blood

Excessive physical work, or stress, a poor diet and chronic disease may all result in the consumption of or poor production of the Qi and Blood. This leads to the heel not being properly nourished, and causes heel pain to occur.

Deficiency of Yin of Liver and Kidney

The Kidney dominates the Bones and lower back, and also produces the Marrow. The Liver dominates the tendons and regulates the Blood in the body. Excessive strain, excessive sexual activity, giving birth to several children, prolonged sickness, excessive bleeding in menstruation, chronic bleeding conditions such as haemorrhoids, or old age may all cause consumption of the Kidney-Essence and deficiency of Liver-Blood. As a result, the tendons, bones and channels are not well nourished, and heel pain occurs.

Treatment based on differentiation

Differentiation

Differentiation of acute and chronic pain

— Usually acute heel pain is often caused by Excessive pathogenic factors, such as invasion of External Cold or Toxic Fire.

— Chronic cases are often caused by Deficiency, such as deficiency of Qi and Blood or deficiency of Kidney-Essence. Downward flow of Damp-Heat could also be a chronic case, or a chronic case with acute aggravation.

Differentiation of the character of the pain

— Heel pain with a cold and heavy sensation, swelling of the heel, aggravation of the heel pain by exposure to cold weather or humid weather, or alleviation of pain by warmth, is often caused by invasion of Wind, Cold and Damp.
— Acute heel pain with a hot and burning sensation, redness and swelling on the heel, aggravation of the heel pain by warmth and alleviation by cold, fever, thirst, a red tongue with a dry and yellow coating and a rapid pulse, is often caused by invasion of Toxic Fire.
— Heel pain with a hot and heavy sensation, red and swollen heel, aggravation of the pain by warmth, heaviness of the body, nausea, diarrhoea, and a red tongue with a yellow and greasy coating, is usually caused by downward flow of Damp-Heat.
— Heel pain with a dull sensation or numbness, aggravation of the heel pain by walking, tiredness and exertion, alleviation by rest, lassitude, shortness of breath, palpitations, a pale complexion, a pale tongue and weak pulse, is often caused by deficiency of Qi and Blood.
— Chronic heel pain on rotation, flexion and extension, with aggravation of the heel pain by overstrain or standing for too long, alleviation by rest, weakness of the knees and ankle, muscular atrophy, lower back pain, and a weak pulse on the Kidney position, is usually deficiency of Essence of the Liver and Kidney.

Treatment

INVASION OF WIND, COLD AND DAMP

Symptoms and signs

Heel pain with a cold and heavy sensation, which worsens on exposure to cold or in cold weather or water and is alleviated by warmth, with swelling of the joints. Accompanying symptoms include a slight fever, an aversion to cold, numb or frigid toes, cold limbs, a poor appetite, an absence of thirst, clear urine, a pale tongue with a white and moist coating and a superficial and tense pulse.

Principle of treatment

Dispel Wind, Cold and Damp, promote Qi and Blood circulation and relieve the pain.

HERBAL TREATMENT

Prescription

JUAN BI TANG
Remove Painful Obstruction Decoction
Qiang Huo *Rhizoma seu Radix Notopterygii* 10 g
Fang Feng *Radix Ledebouriellae* 10 g
Sang Zhi *Ramulus Mori* 10 g
Ji Xue Teng *Caulis et Radix Milletiae* 10 g
Hai Feng Teng *Caulis Piperis Futokadsurae* 10 g
Chuan Niu Xi *Radix Cyathulae* 10 g
Dang Gui *Radix Angelicae Sinensis* 10 g
Jiang Huang *Rhizoma Curcumae* 15 g
Chi Shao *Radix Paeoniae Rubra* 10 g
Chuan Xiong *Rhizoma Ligustici Chuanxiong* 10 g
Gan Cao *Radix Glycyrrhizae* 6 g
Sheng Jiang *Rhizoma Zingiberis Recens* 10 g

Explanations

- Qiang Huo, Fang Feng and Jiang Huang dispel Wind, Cold and Damp and relieve heel pain.
- Sang Zhi, Ji Xue Teng and Hai Feng Teng harmonise the collateral, eliminate Wind, Cold and Damp in the channels, promote Blood circulation and relieve heel pain.
- Dang Gui, Chi Shao and Chuan Xiong promote Blood circulation, remove Blood stasis and relieve heel pain.
- Chuan Niu Xi eliminates Damp and removes the blockage of the channels by the Damp. Also, it is a good herb for promoting the circulation of Blood and inducing the action of this formula to reach the heel.
- Gan Cao and Sheng Jiang harmonise the Stomach and the actions of all the other herbs in the prescription.

Modifications

1. If there is swelling of the joints on the foot, add Bi Xie *Rhizoma Dioscoreae Septemlobae* 15 g to eliminate Damp and reduce the swelling of the joints.
2. If there is a stabbing pain, add Tao Ren *Semen Persicae* 10 g and Hong Hua *Flos Carthami* 10 g to regulate the circulation of Blood and remove Blood stasis.
3. If there is severe cold in the foot, add Zhi Fu Zi *Radix Aconiti Praeparata* 10 g and Rou Gui *Cortex*

Cinnamomi 5 g to warm the channels, eliminate Cold-Damp and relieve the pain.
4. If there is generalised tiredness, shortness of breath and frequent sweating due to deficiency of Qi, add Huang Qi *Radix Astragali seu Hedysari* 10 g to tonify the Qi and relieve the tiredness.
5. If the appetite is poor, add Ban Xia *Rhizoma Pinelliae* 10 g and Fu Ling *Poria* 10 g to harmonise the Stomach and improve the appetite.

Patent remedies

Feng Shi Pian *Wind-Damp Tablet*
Jing Fang Bai Du Pian *Schizonepeta and Ledebouriella Tablet to Overcome Pathogenic Toxin*
Tian Ma Qu Feng Bu Pian *Gastrodia Dispel Wind Formula Tablet*

ACUPUNCTURE TREATMENT

TE-5 Waiguan, LI-4 Hegu, SI-4 Wangu, BL-58 Feiyang, BL-60 Kunlun, BL-63 Jinmen, BL-64 Jinggu, KI-3 Taixi and SP-6 Sanyinjiao. Reducing method is used on these points.

Explanations

- TE-5 and LI-4 dispel Wind, Cold and Damp and relieve External symptoms.
- BL-58, the Connecting point, dispels External Wind-Damp, harmonises the collateral, promotes the circulation of Qi and relieves the heel pain.
- BL-60, the River point, BL-63, the Accumulation point, BL-64 and SI-4, the Source points, dispel Wind-Damp, promote the circulation of Qi and Blood in the channels and relieve the heel pain.
- SP-6, the crossing point of the three Yin channels of the foot, promotes the circulation of Blood, eliminates Blood stasis and Damp and relieves the heel pain.
- KI-3, the Stream and Source point, warms the channels, dispels Cold and relieves the heel pain.

Modifications

1. If there is a cold sensation in the heel, add moxibustion on BL-60 and KI-3 to warm the channels, promote the circulation of Qi, dispel Cold and relieve the pain.
2. If there is swelling of the heel, add SP-9 to promote the circulation of Qi, eliminate Damp and relieve the swelling.
3. If there is a numb heel, add Plum-Blossom needle on the heel to regulate the circulation of Qi and relieve the numbness.

4. If there is heel pain along the Kidney channel, add KI-4 and KI-5 to harmonise the collateral, promote the Qi and Blood circulation and relieve the pain.
5. If there is heel pain along the Bladder channel, add BL-59 and BL-62 to promote the Qi and Blood circulation, dispel Wind, Cold and Damp and relieve the heel pain.
6. If there are painful toes, add Extra Bafeng to promote the circulation of Qi in the locality and relieve the pain.
7. If there is a fever, add GV-14 to dispel Wind, promote sweating and reduce the fever.
8. If there is a headache, add GB-20 to dispel Wind-Cold and relieve the headache.
9. If there is generalised body pain, add GB-35 to dispel Wind, Cold and Damp, harmonise the collateral and relieve the body pain.

Case history

A 35-year-old man had been suffering from painful heels on both sides for a month. His heel pain had started soon after being caught in a big snowstorm on a mountain during a trip. Besides the heel pain, he was also suffering from generalised body pain, neck pain, headache, an aversion to cold, a slight fever and a poor appetite. Because of the severe heel pain, he went to the doctor and was given some aspirin. Two days later, his cold was generally a lot better, but he still had the heel pain.

When he arrived at the acupuncture clinic, he had heel pain on both sides, obvious tenderness at the place where the Bladder channel passes through, difficulty in walking, aversion to exposing the heel to wind and cold, and a preference for keeping it warm, and no colour change on the heels. He also had a poor appetite, no thirst, clear urine, a thin and white tongue coating and a tight pulse.

Diagnosis
Heel pain due to invasion of Wind, Cold and Damp.

Principle of treatment
Dispel external Wind, Cold and Damp, warm the channels and relieve the pain.

Acupuncture treatment
TE-5, SI-3, SI-4, BL-58, BL-59, BL-60, BL-63, BL-64 and SP-6. Reducing method was used on these points. Moxibustion was applied on BL-58, BL-59, BL-60, BL-63 and BL-64. Treatment was given once every 2 days.

Explanations
- TE-5 and SI-3 dispel Wind, Cold and Damp and relieve External symptoms.
- BL-58, the Connecting point, dispels External Wind-Damp, harmonises the collateral, promotes the circulation of Qi and relieves the heel pain.
- BL-59, the Accumulation point of the Yang Heel Vessel, BL-60, the River point, BL-62, the Confluence point of the Yang Heel Vessel, BL-63, the Accumulation point,

BL-64 and SI-4, the Source points, dispel Wind-Damp, promote the Qi and Blood circulation in the channels and relieve the heel pain.
- SP-6, the crossing point of the three Yin channels of the foot, promotes the circulation of Blood, eliminates its stasis and Damp and relieves the heel pain.
- Moxibustion dispels Cold, warms the channels, promotes the Qi and Blood circulation and relieves the heel pain.

Immediately after the first treatment, he felt that his heel pain had improved, and he could walk better. The pain came back after half a day. After the second session, his heel pain improved greatly, and stayed better for 2 days. After six treatments his heel pain had completely cleared and he did not need to take any more painkillers.

INVASION OF TOXIC FIRE

Symptoms and signs

Acute occurrence of heel pain, which worsens in warmth and is better with cold, together with heat and burning, redness and swelling on the heel, formation of ulcers or even pus on the heel. Other symptoms include fever, an aversion to cold, thirst, restlessness, insomnia, yellow urine, constipation, a red tongue with a yellow and dry coating and a rapid and forceful pulse.

Principle of treatment

Clear Fire, eliminate Toxin, promote Blood circulation and relieve the pain.

HERBAL TREATMENT

Prescription

PU JI XIAO DU YIN
Universal Benefit Decoction to Eliminate Toxin
Huang Qin *Radix Scutellariae* 10 g
Huang Lian *Rhizoma Coptidis* 10 g
Xuan Shen *Radix Scrophulariae* 6 g
Zhi Zi *Fructus Gardeniae* 10 g
Ban Lan Gen *Radix Isatidis* 6 g
Lian Qiao *Fructus Forsythiae* 3 g
Jiang Can *Bombyx Batryticatus* 3 g
Sheng Ma *Rhizoma Cimicifugae* 3 g
Da Qing Ye *Folium Isatidis* 10 g
Zhe Bei Mu *Bulbus Fritillariae Thunbergii* 10 g
Gan Cao *Radix Glycyrrhizae* 6 g

Explanations

- Huang Qin, Huang Lian and Zhi Zi clear Heat, reduce the swelling and eliminate Toxin.
- Sheng Ma and Xuan Shen eliminate Toxin.

- Ban Lan Gen, Lian Qiao and Da Qing Ye dispel Heat, reduce fever and eliminate Toxin.
- Jiang Can and Zhe Bei Mu resolve Phlegm, harmonise the collateral and reduce swelling.
- Gan Cao harmonises the actions of the other herbs in the prescription and eliminates Toxin.

Modifications

1. If there is redness and swelling of the feet, add Sheng Di Huang *Radix Rehmanniae Recens* 10 g and Long Dan Cao *Radix Gentianae* 5 g to clear Damp-Heat and reduce the swelling.
2. If there is itching on the feet, add Bai Xian Pi *Cortex Dictamni* 10 g and Ku Shen *Radix Sophorae Flavescentis* 10 g to clear Damp-Heat and relieve the itching.
3. If there is a stabbing pain at the heel, add Pu Huang *Pollen Typhae* 10 g and Dan Shen *Radix Salvia Miltiorrhizae* 10 g to promote the circulation of Blood and eliminate its stasis.
4. If there is a wound on the heel, add San Qi *Radix Notoginseng* 10 g to eliminate toxin and promote healing of the wound.
5. If there is a fever, add Shi Gao *Gypsum Fibrosum* 20 g and Zhi Mu *Rhizoma Anemarrhenae* 10 g to clear Heat and reduce fever.
6. If there is nervousness, add Xia Ku Cao *Spica Prunellae* 10 g to clear Heat in the Liver and calm Liver-Fire.
7. If there is a throat pain with swelling, add Ma Bo *Lasiosphaera seu Calvatia* 5 g to benefit the throat and reduce swelling in it.
8. If there is coughing with expectoration of yellow phlegm, add Niu Bang Zi *Fructus Arctii* 5 g to eliminate Phlegm and relieve the cough.
9. If there is restlessness and insomnia, add Dan Zhu Ye *Herba Lophatgeri* 10 g to clear Heat from the Heart.
10. If there is constipation due to blockage of the Large Intestine by Heat, add Da Huang *Radix et Rhizoma Rhei* 10 g to clear Heat and promote defection so as to relieve the constipation.

Patent remedies

Feng Shi Xiao Tong Wan *Wind-Damp Dispel Pain Pill*
Niu Huang Jie Du Pian *Cattle Gallstone Tablet to Resolve Toxin*

ACUPUNCTURE TREATMENT

TE-6 Zhigou, LI-4 Hegu, LI-11 Quchi, ST-44 Neiting, SP-6 Sanyinjiao, SP-10 Xuehai, BL-60 Kunlun, BL-63 Jinmen, SI-4 Wangu and KI-2 Rangu. Reducing method is used on these points.

Explanations

- TE-6 promotes the function of the Triple Burner and eliminates Heat and toxin from the body.
- ST-44, the Spring point, clears Heat and reduces Fire so as to eliminate redness and swelling. It is also a Water point according to the Five Element theory, and Water controls Fire, so it is a suitable point.
- LI-4, the Source point, and LI-11, the Sea point, have a function in relieving Heat and circulating the channel so as to sedate the pain. In most cases with invasion of toxic Heat, there could be fever. When these two points are applied together, the fever reduction will be greater.
- SP-6, the crossing point of the three Yin channels of the foot, and SP-10 cool the Blood, eliminate toxin, reduce swelling and relieve the heel pain.
- KI-2, the Spring point, clears Heat, reduces fever and reduces the swelling of the heels.
- BL-60, the River point, BL-63, the Accumulation point, BL-64 and SI-4, the Source points, dispel Wind-Damp, promote the Qi and Blood circulation in the channels and relieve the heel pain.

Modifications

1. If there is redness and swelling of the foot, add GB-43 to clear Damp-Heat and reduce the swelling.
2. If there is heel pain along the Kidney channel, add KI-4 and KI-5 to harmonise the collateral, promote the Qi and Blood circulation and relieve the pain.
3. If there is itching on the feet, add LR-2 to clear Damp-Heat and relieve the itching.
4. If there is a stabbing pain at the heel, add KI-1 to sedate the heel pain.
5. If there is a wound on the heel, add Extra Bafeng to eliminate Toxin and promote healing of the wound.
6. If there is a fever, add GV-14 to clear Heat and reduce the fever.
7. If there is nervousness, add GB-20 to clear Heat in the Liver and calm Liver-Fire.
8. If there is throat pain with swelling, add LU-10 to benefit the throat and reduce the swelling there.
9. If there is coughing with expectoration of yellow phlegm, add LU-5 to eliminate Phlegm and relieve the cough.
10. If there is restlessness and insomnia, add HT-8 to clear Heat from the Heart.

11. If there is constipation due to blockage of the Large Intestine by Heat, add ST-25 to clear Heat and promote defecation so as to relieve the constipation.

STAGNATION OF QI AND BLOOD

Symptoms and signs

Trauma to the heel with swollen muscles or tendons, long duration of pain on the heel, or history of operation or injury on the heel, stabbing pain with a fixed location, which worsens at night, with rigidity of the ankle joints and a purplish colour to the skin on the heel. There is usually also a purplish tongue with a thin coating and a wiry and choppy pulse.

Principle of treatment

Promote Qi and Blood circulation, eliminate Blood stasis and relieve the pain.

HERBAL TREATMENT

Prescription

FU YUAN HUO XUE TANG
Revive Health by Invigorating the Blood Decoction
Chai Hu *Radix Bupleuri* 5 g
Tian Hua Fen *Radix Trichosanthis* 10 g
Hong Hua *Flos Carthami* 10 g
Tao Ren *Semen Persicae* 10 g
Dang Gui *Radix Angelicae Sinensis* 12 g
Da Huang *Radix et Rhizoma Rhei* 6 g
Yan Hu Suo *Rhizoma Corydalis* 20 g
Gan Cao *Radix Glycyrrhizae* 6 g

Explanations

- Chai Hu promotes the circulation of Qi and relieves pain.
- Tian Hua Fen reduces swelling and relieves pain.
- Dang Gui, Tao Ren and Hong Hua promote the circulation of Blood, eliminate its stasis and relieve the heel pain.
- Yan Hu Suo promotes the circulation of Blood. This herb has also a strong pain-relieving effect.
- Da Huang removes Blood stagnation and promotes healing.
- Gan Cao harmonises the functions of the other herbs in the formula.

Modifications

1. If there is bone fracture, add Xu Duan *Radix Dipsaci* 10 g and Du Zhong *Cortex Eucommiae* 10 g to strengthen the Kidney, promote bone healing and relieve the heel pain.
2. If there is a severe sharp pain in the heel, add Xu Chang Qing *Radix Cynanchi Paniculati* 10 g and Qing Pi *Pericardium Citri Reticulatae Viride* 5 g to promote the circulation of Qi and relieve the pain.
3. If there is a severe stabbing pain, add San Qi *Radix Notoginseng* 10 g and Mo Yao *Resina Myrrhae* 5 g to regulate the Qi and Blood circulation, remove Blood stasis and relieve the heel pain.
4. If there is rigidity of the ankle joints, add Wei Ling Xian *Radix Clematidis* 10 g, San Leng *Rhizoma Sparganii* 10 g and E Zhu *Rhizoma Zedoariae* 10 g to promote the circulation of Blood, harmonise the collateral and relieve joint rigidity.

Patent remedies

Jin Gu Die Shang Wan *Muscle and Bone Traumatic Injury Pill*
Xiao Huo Luo Dan *Minor Invigorate the Collaterals Special Pill*

ACUPUNCTURE TREATMENT

LI-4 Hegu, SP-6 Sanyinjiao, LR-3 Taichong, SI-3 Houxi, GB-34 Yanglingquan, SI-4 Wangu and BL-60 Kunlun. Reducing method is used on these points.

Explanations

- LI-4 and LR-3, the Source points, promote the circulation of Qi in the channels, eliminate stagnation of Blood and relieve the pain.
- SP-6, the crossing point of the three Yin channels of the foot, promotes the circulation of Blood, eliminates Blood stasis and relieves the pain.
- GB-34, the Sea point, strengthens the tendons and relieves heel pain.
- SI-3, the Stream point, SI-4, the Source point, and BL-60 promote the Qi and Blood circulation, eliminate Blood stasis in the greater Yang channels and relieve the heel pain.

Modifications

1. If there is heel pain along the Kidney channel, add KI-3, KI-4 and KI-5 to harmonise the collateral, promote the Qi and Blood circulation and relieve the pain.
2. If there is heel pain along the Bladder channel, add BL-59, BL-60, BL-62, BL-63 and BL-64 to

promote the Qi and Blood circulation, dispel Wind, Cold and Damp and relieve the heel pain.

3. If there is swelling on the feet, add Extra Bafeng to promote the Qi and Blood circulation and reduce the swelling.

4. If there is a purplish colour to the feet, add BL-67, the Well point, to promote the circulation of Blood and relieve the pain.

5. If there is a bone fracture in the foot, add GB-39 and KI-3 to tonify the Kidney and benefit the bones.

6. If there are red spots on the foot due to formation of Heat in the Blood, add SP-10 to cool the Heat in the Blood and promote the circulation of Blood.

7. If there is depression, add LR-14 and CV-17 to smooth the Liver, promote the circulation of Qi and relieve the depression.

8. If there is an aversion to cold, or the foot is cold, add ST-36 and KI-3 with moxibustion to warm the channels and dispel Cold.

9. If there is restlessness and insomnia, add HT-3 and PC-6 to calm the Mind and improve the sleep.

DOWNWARD FLOW OF DAMP-HEAT

Symptoms and signs

Heel pain with a feverish and heavy sensation, redness and swelling, which is aggravated by contact with warmth and alleviated by cold. Other symptoms include a bitter taste in the mouth, a poor appetite, fever, a feeling of heaviness in the legs, painful urination, loose stools, abdominal pain and distension, deep yellow urine, a red tongue, with a yellow and greasy coating at the back and a slippery and rapid pulse.

Principle of treatment

Eliminate Damp, clear Heat, harmonise the collateral and relieve pain.

HERBAL TREATMENT

Prescription

SI MIAO WAN
Four-Marvel Pill
Huang Bai *Cortex Phellodendri* 12 g
Cang Zhu *Rhizoma Atractylodis* 10 g
Yi Yi Ren *Semen Coicis* 15 g
Fu Ling *Poria* 10 g
Chuan Xiong *Rhizoma Ligustici Chuanxiong* 10 g
Huai Niu Xi *Radix Achyranthis Bidentatae* 10 g
Gan Cao *Radix Glycyrrhizae* 6 g

Explanations

- Huang Bai clears Heat, dries Damp in the Lower Burner, reduces swelling and sedates heel pain.
- Cang Zhu helps Huang Bai eliminate Damp-Heat in the Lower Burner and relieve heel pain.
- Yi Yi Ren and Fu Ling activate the Spleen and Stomach and eliminate Damp in the body. Fu Ling also tonifies the Kidney and promotes urination.
- Huai Niu Xi promotes the circulation of Blood in the body and in the channels and eliminates Damp and Blood stasis. Moreover, this herb induces all the herbs to descend to the heel so as to relieve heel pain.
- Chuan Xiong promotes the Qi and Blood circulation and relieves heel pain.
- Gan Cao harmonises the actions of the other herbs in the prescription.

Modifications

1. If there is redness and swelling of the heel, add Sheng Di Huang *Radix Rehmanniae* 15 g, Chi Shao *Radix Paeoniae Rubra* 10 g and Pu Gong Ying *Herba Taraxaci* 15 g to clear Heat in the Blood, remove toxin and reduce the swelling.

2. If there is a burning feeling in the heel, add Zhi Mu *Rhizoma Anemarrhenae* 10 g to clear Heat and relieve the burning feeling.

3. If there is itching on the heel and feet, add Bai Xian Pi *Cortex Dicatamni* 10 g and Ku Shen *Radix Sophorae Flavescentis* 10 g to clear Damp-Heat and relieve the itching.

4. If there is a stabbing pain in the heel, add Pu Huang *Pollen Typhae* 10 g and Dan Shen *Radix Salvia Miltiorrhizae* 10 g to promote the circulation of Blood, eliminate its stasis and relieve the heel pain.

5. If there is a wound in the heel, add San Qi *Radix Notoginseng* 10 g to eliminate toxin and promote the healing of the wound.

6. If there is a fever, add Zhi Zi *Fructus Gardeniae* 10 g to clear Heat and reduce the fever.

7. If there is a bitter taste in the mouth, add Long Dan Cao *Radix Gentianae* 5 g and Yin Chen Hao *Herba Artemesiae Capillaris* 10 g to eliminate Damp-Heat, harmonise the Gall Bladder and relieve the bitter taste in the mouth.

8. If there is insomnia and restlessness, add Huang Lian *Rhizoma Coptidis* 10 g to clear Heat in the Heart, calm the Mind and improve the sleep.

9. If the appetite is poor, add Ji Nei Jin *Endothelium Corneum Gigeriae Galli* 15 g and Mai Ya *Fructus Hordei Germinatus* 30 g to activate the Spleen and Stomach and improve appetite.

10. If there is constipation due to predominance of Heat in the Large Intestine, add Da Huang *Radix et Rhizoma Rhei* 10 g to clear Heat, promote defecation and relieve the constipation.

Patent remedy

San Miao Wan *Three-Marvel Pill*

ACUPUNCTURE TREATMENT

TE-6 Zhigou, SI-3 Houxi, SI-4 Wangu, BL-63 Jinmen, BL-64 Jinggu, KI-2 Rangu, SP-6 Sanyinjiao, SP-9 Yinlingquan and GB-34 Yanglingquan. Reducing method is applied on these points.

Explanations

- TE-6 eliminates Damp-Heat and relieves heel pain.
- SI-4 and BL-64, the Source points, promote defecation and urination and eliminate Damp.
- SI-3, the Stream point, and BL-63, the Accumulation point, harmonise the collateral, promote the Qi and Blood circulation in the channels and relieve the heel pain.
- KI-2, the Spring point, clears Heat, promotes urination and eliminates Damp-Heat in the Lower Burner.
- SP-6, the crossing point of the three Yin channels of the foot, promotes the Qi and Blood circulation in the body and channels and eliminates Blood stasis so as to relieve the heel pain.
- SP-9 and GB-34, the Sea points, eliminate Damp-Heat in the Lower Burner and relieve heel pain.

Modifications

1. If there is a sharp pain, add LI-4 and LR-3 to promote the circulation of Qi and relieve the pain.
2. If there is a heavy sensation on the feet, add KI-6 to promote urination and eliminate Damp.
3. If there is heel pain along the Kidney channel, add KI-3, KI-4 and KI-5 to harmonise the collateral, promote the circulation of Qi and Blood and relieve the pain.
4. If there is heel pain along the Bladder channel, add BL-59, BL-60, BL-62 and BL-65 to promote the circulation of Qi and Blood, dispel Wind, Cold and Damp and relieve the heel pain.
5. If there is redness on the feet, add SP-10 to cool the Blood and reduce the redness.
6. If there are ulcers on the feet, add ST-44, the Spring point, to clear Heat, remove Toxin and promote healing.

7. If there is itching at the heel, add Extra Bafeng to dispel Wind and eliminate Damp-Heat.
8. If there is a fever, add GV-14 and LI-11 to clear Heat and reduce the fever.
9. If there is a poor appetite and nausea, add CV-12 and SP-4 to harmonise the Stomach and promote the appetite.
10. If there is leucorrhoea with itching in the genital region, add GB-41 and LR-5 to eliminate Damp-Heat in the body and relieve the itching.

DEFICIENCY OF QI AND BLOOD

Symptoms and signs

Heel pain with a dull sensation, which is aggravated by tiredness and exertion and alleviated by rest, with a slight diffused tenderness at the heel, lassitude, shortness of breath, a low voice, spontaneous sweating, a poor appetite, lower back pain, nycturia, a pale tongue and a weak pulse.

Principle of treatment

Tonify Qi and Blood, nourish muscles and tendons and relieve the pain.

HERBAL TREATMENT

Prescription

BA ZHEN TANG
Eight-Precious Decoction
Dang Gui *Radix Angelicae Sinensis* 12 g
Chuan Xiong *Rhizoma Chuanxiong* 10 g
Bai Shao *Radix Paeoniae Alba* 12 g
Shu Di Huang *Radix Rehmanniae Praeparata* 12 g
Ren Shen *Radix Ginseng* 6 g
Bai Zhu *Rhizoma Atractylodis Macrocephalae* 12 g
Fu Ling *Poria* 12 g
Huai Niu Xi *Radix Achyranthis Bidentatae* 10 g
Gan Cao *Radix Glycyrrhizae* 6 g

Explanations

- Dang Gui, Bai Shao and Shu Di Huang tonify the Kidney-Essence and nourish the Liver-Blood.
- Ren Shen, Bai Zhu, Fu Ling and Gan Cao, the ingredients of Si Jun Zi Tang *Four-Gentlemen Decoction*, strengthen the Spleen and reinforce the Qi.
- Chuan Xiong activates the Qi and Blood circulation and relieves obstruction in the channels. It can also prevent side-effects from the use of too many tonics.

- Huai Niu Xi promotes the circulation of Blood in the body and the channels and eliminates Damp and Blood stasis. Moreover, it induces all the herbs to descend to the heel so as to relieve the heel pain.

Modifications

1. If there is an aversion to cold or cold limbs due to deficiency of Yang, add Gui Zhi *Ramulus Cinnamomi* 6 g and Wu Zhu Yu *Fructus Evodiae* 10 g to reinforce and activate the Yang-Qi.
2. If there is swelling in the legs due to poor water metabolism caused by deficiency of Spleen-Qi, add Zhu Ling *Polyporus* 15 g and Ze Xie *Rhizoma Alismatis* 12 g to strengthen the Spleen, promote urination and reduce the swelling.
3. If there is dizziness, add Tian Ma *Rhizoma Gastrodiae* 10 g and Gou Qi Zi *Fructus Lycii* 10 g to nourish the Liver-Blood and calm Liver-Wind.
4. If there are palpitations add Suan Zao Ren *Semen Ziziphi Spinosae* 10 g and Bai Zi Ren *Semen Biotae* 10 g to nourish the Heart-Blood and calm the Mind.
5. If the appetite is poor, add Sha Ren *Fructus Amomi* 5 g, Mu Xiang *Radix Aucklandiae* 10 g and Pei Lan *Herba Eupatorii* 10 g to activate the Stomach, promote the Spleen-Qi circulation and improve the appetite.

Patent remedy

Shi Quan Da Bu Wan *All-Inclusive Great Tonifying Pill*

ACUPUNCTURE TREATMENT

SI-3 Houxi, SI-4 Wangu, BL-63 Jinmen, BL-64 Jinggu, SP-6 Sanyinjiao, ST-36 Zusanli, GB-39 Xuanzhong and GB-34 Yanglingquan. Reducing method is used on these points.

Explanations

- SI-4 and BL-64, the Source points, promote defecation and urination and eliminate Damp.
- SI-3, the Stream point, and BL-63, the Accumulation point, harmonise the collateral, promote the Qi and Blood circulation in the channels and relieve the heel pain.
- SP-6, the crossing point of the three Yin channels of the foot, ST-36, the Sea point, and GB-39, the Gathering point for the Marrow, promote the production of Qi and Blood, benefit the marrow and strengthen the bones.

- GB-34, the Sea point, tonifies the tendons, benefits the heel and relieves the heel pain.

Modifications

1. If there is heel pain along the Kidney channel, add KI-3, KI-4 and KI-5 to promote Qi and Blood circulation in the channel, harmonise the collateral and relieve the pain.
2. If the appetite is poor, add SP-3 and CV-12 to activate the Spleen and Stomach, tonify the Spleen-Qi and improve the appetite.
3. If there is dizziness, add GV-20 and GB-20 to lift up the Yang-Qi to the head, dispel Wind and relieve the dizziness.
4. If there is diarrhoea, add SP-9 to activate the Spleen, eliminate Damp and relieve the diarrhoea.

DEFICIENCY OF ESSENCE OF LIVER AND KIDNEY

Symptoms and signs

Chronic heel pain with difficulty in rotation, flexion and extension, which is aggravated by overstrain or standing for too long and alleviated by rest, with weakness of the knees and ankles, rigidity in the morning, joint deformity and muscular atrophy. Other symptoms include fatigue, lower back pain, an aversion to cold, a thin and white tongue coating, and a deep and wiry pulse, and weak pulse on the Kidney regions.

Principle of treatment

Tonify the Kidney and Liver, strengthen the tendons and bones, smooth the channels and relieve the pain.

HERBAL TREATMENT

Prescription

LIU WEI DI HUANG WEN
Six-Flavour Rehmanniae Pill
Shu Di Huang *Radix Rehmanniae Praeparata* 12 g
Shan Zhu Yu *Fructus Corni* 10 g
Shan Yao *Rhizoma Dioscoreae* 10 g
Fu Ling *Poria* 10 g
Ze Xie *Rhizoma Alismatis* 10 g
Dang Gui *Radix Angelicae Sinensis* 6 g
Chuan Xiong *Radix Ligustici Chuanxiong* 6 g
Du Zhong *Cortex Eucommiae* 10 g
Huai Niu Xi *Radix Achyranthis Bidentatae* 10 g
Sang Ji Sheng *Ramulus Loranthi* 10 g
Gan Cao *Radix Glycyrrhizae* 6 g

Explanations

- Shu Di Huang, Shan Zhu Yu and Shan Yao tonify the Blood and the Essence of the Liver and Kidney.
- Ze Xie promotes urination and clears Heat.
- Fu Ling strengthens the Spleen, eliminates Damp and tonifies the Qi.
- Dang Gui tonifies the Qi and Blood so as to nourish the Liver and Kidney.
- Huai Niu Xi, Du Zhong and Sang Ji Sheng tonify the Liver and Kidney, and strengthen the tendons and bones.
- Chuan Xiong promotes the circulation of Qi and Blood and eliminates Blood stasis so as to stop the heel pain.
- Gan Cao harmonises the actions of the other herbs in the prescription.

Modifications

1. If there is heel pain that is sometimes influenced by the weather changes, add Du Huo *Radix Angelicae Pubescentis* 9 g and Qin Jiao *Radix Gentianae Macrophyllae* 6 g to harmonise the collateral, dispel Wind, Cold and Damp and relieve the heel pain.
2. If there is an aversion to exposing the heel to cold and cold limbs, add Xi Xin *Herba Asari* 6 g and Rou Gui *Cortex Cinnamomi* 6 g to warm the channels, dispel Cold and relieve the heel pain.
3. If there is weakness in the knees, legs and lower back, add Xu Duan *Radix Dipsaci* 10 g to tonify the Kidney and strengthen the lower back.
4. If there is impotence, add Yin Yang Huo *Herba Epimedii* 10 g to warm the Kidney-Yang and promote potency.
5. If there is lower abdominal pain with a cold sensation, add Wu Zhu Yu *Fructus Evodiae* 5 g to warm the Interior, dispel Cold and relieve the pain.
6. If there is frequent urination at night, add Yi Zhi Ren *Fructus Alpiniae Oxyphyllae* 10 g and Sang Piao Xiao *Ootheca Mantidis* 10 g to tonify the Kidney-Yang and decrease urination.
7. If there is tiredness and shortness of breath due to deficiency of Qi, add Ren Shen *Radix Ginseng* 6 g to tonify the Qi and activate the Spleen and Stomach.
8. If there is deficiency of the Yin of Liver and Kidney, use a modification based on Zhi Bai Di Huang Wan *Ane-phello and Rehmannia Pill* (9 g each time, three times a day) instead of Liu Wei Di Huang Wan.

Patent remedies

Liu Wei Di Huang Wan *Six-Flavour Rehmanniae Pill*
Hai Ma Bu Shen Wan *Sea Horse Tonify Kidney Pill*
Kang Gu Zheng Sheng Pian *Combat Bone Hyperplasia Pill*

ACUPUNCTURE TREATMENT

GB-39 Xuanzhong, GB-34 Yanglingquan, LR-3 Taichong, KI-3 Taixi, SI-3 Houxi, BL-63 Jinmen, ST-36 Zusanli and SP-6 Sanyinjiao. Even method is used on GB-34, LR-3 and SP-6. Reinforcing method is used on the rest of the points.

Explanations

- This type of heel pain is often seen in old people because of the decline in function of the Liver and Kidney. The heel pain occurs because of insufficiency of the Blood and Kidney-Essence and failure of the tendons and bones to be properly nourished.
- LR-3 and KI-3, the Source points of the Liver and Kidney channels respectively, tonify the Liver and Kidney, and strengthen the tendons and bones.
- SP-6, the crossing point of the three Yin channels of the foot, strengthens the Spleen, Liver and Kidney and tonifies the Blood.
- GB-39, the Gathering point for the Marrow, and GB-34, the Gathering point for the tendons, reinforce the tendons and bones.
- SI-3, the Stream point, and BL-63, the Accumulation point, harmonise the collateral, promote the Qi and Blood circulation in the channels and relieve the heel pain.
- ST-36, the Sea point of the Stomach channel, reinforces the Spleen and Stomach and promotes the production of Blood.

Modifications

1. If there is heel pain along the Kidney channel, add KI-4 and KI-5 to promote the circulation of Qi and Blood in the channel, harmonise the collateral and relieve the heel pain.
2. If there is heel pain that is sometimes influenced by the weather changes, add TE-5, the Connecting point, to harmonise the collateral, dispel Wind, Cold and Damp and relieve the heel pain.
3. If there is an aversion to exposing the heel to cold and cold limbs, add moxibustion on KI-3 and CV-6 to warm the channels, dispel Cold and relieve the heel pain.

4. If there is weakness in the knees, legs and lower back, add BL-23 to tonify the Kidney and strengthen the lower back.

5. If there is impotence, add CV-4 to warm the Kidney-Yang and increase potency.

6. If there is lower abdominal pain with a cold sensation, add ST-25 to warm the Interior, dispel Cold and relieve the pain.

7. If there is frequent urination at night, add KI-10 to tonify the Kidney-Yang and decrease urination.

8. If there is tiredness and shortness of breath due to deficiency of Qi, add GV-20 to tonify the Qi and relieve the tiredness.

9. If there is deficiency of the Yin of Liver and Kidney, add KI-6 and KI-7 to nourish the Yin, tonify the Kidney and clear Deficient-Heat.

Case history

A 65-year-old woman had been suffering from painful heels for 5 months. She had a slight pain in both knees and heels, which was mainly located along the Kidney channels. The pain usually got worse when she walked too much, and was alleviated by rest. After massage treatment, there was some improvement in her knee pain. However, she still had the heel pain. As well as the heel pain, she had a lower back pain, weakness in her knees and ankles, dizziness, tinnitus, lassitude, a dry mouth, thirst, night sweating, a red tongue with a scanty coating, and a thin and rapid pulse.

Diagnosis
Heel pain due to deficiency of Yin of Liver and Kidney.

Principle of treatment
Nourish Yin, tonify the Liver and Kidney and relieve the heel pain.

Herbal treatment
LIU WEI DI HUANG WAN
Six-Flavour Rehmanniae Pill
Shu Di Huang *Radix Rehmanniae Praeparata* 12 g
Shan Zhu Yu *Fructus Corni* 10 g
Shan Yao *Rhizoma Dioscoreae* 10 g
Fu Ling *Poria* 10 g
Ze Xie *Rhizoma Alismatis* 10 g
Dang Gui *Radix Angelicae Sinensis* 6 g
Chuan Xiong *Radix Ligustici Chuanxiong* 6 g
Du Zhong *Cortex Eucommiae* 10 g

Huai Niu Xi *Radix Achyranthis Bidentatae* 10 g
Sang Ji Sheng *Ramulus Loranthi* 10 g
Gui Ban Jiao *Testudinis Plastri Colla* 15 g
Han Lian Cao *Herba Ecliptae* 10 g
Gan Cao *Radix Glycyrrhizae* 6 g
Herbal decoction from this formula was given once every day.

Explanations
- Shu Di Huang, Shan Zhu Yu and Shan Yao tonify the Blood and the Essence of the Liver and Kidney.
- Ze Xie promotes urination and clears Heat.
- Fu Ling strengthens the Spleen, eliminates Damp and Tonifies the Qi.
- Dang Gui tonifies the Qi and Blood so as to nourish the Liver and Kidney.
- Huai Niu Xi, Du Zhong and Sang Ji Sheng tonify the Liver and Kidney, and strengthen the tendons and bones.
- Chuan Xiong promotes the circulation of Qi and Blood and eliminates Blood stasis so as to stop the heel pain.
- Gui Ban Jiao and Han Lian Cao nourish the Kidney-Yin and clear Deficient-Heat.
- Gan Cao harmonises the actions of the other herbs in the prescription.

Acupuncture treatment
GB-39, GB-34, LR-3, KI-3, KI-4, KI-5, SI-3 and SP-6. Even method was used on GB-34, LR-3 and SP-6. Reinforcing method was used on the rest of the points. Treatment was given once every 3 days.

Explanations
- LR-3 and KI-3, the Source points of the Liver and Kidney channels respectively, tonify the Liver and Kidney, and strengthen the tendons and bones.
- KI-3, KI-4 and KI-5 promote the circulation of Qi and Blood in the channel, harmonise the collateral and relieve the heel pain.
- SP-6, the crossing point of the three Yin channels of the foot, strengthens the Spleen, Liver and Kidney and tonifies the Blood.
- GB-39, the Gathering point for the Marrow, and GB-34, the Gathering point for the tendons, reinforce the tendons and bones.
- SI-3, the Stream point, harmonises the collateral, promotes the circulation of Qi and Blood in the channels and relieves the heel pain.

After treatment for 3 months, the heel pain had disappeared.

Sole pain 44

足
心
疼
痛

Sole pain may occur in one or both soles, but is mostly found in only one sole. It is often accompanied by difficulty in walking, restlessness and insomnia. According to TCM theory, sole pain may be caused by the invasion of External pathogenic factors, or of Toxic Heat, downward flow of Damp-Heat, stagnation of Qi and Blood or deficiency of the Essence of Liver and Kidney. Sole pain may be attributed to any of the following disorders in Western medicine: injury to the soft tissue of the sole, metatarsalgia, plantar fibrositis, plantar aponeurositis, fracture of metatarsal bone, bunion and hallux valgus.

Aetiology and pathology

Invasion of External pathogenic factors

Invasion of External pathogenic factors, such as Wind, Cold, Heat and Damp, is a common cause of sole pain. When these factors invade the foot they block the channels there, the Qi and Blood stagnate, and pain follows. Wind is characterised by constant movement, so if there is invasion of External pathogenic factors with a predominance of Wind, there is a sole pain that changes its location. Cold is characterised by contraction and stagnation, so if there is invasion of external pathogenic factors with a predominance of Cold, there is severe sole pain with a cold sensation. Damp is characterised by heaviness and viscosity, so if there is invasion of External pathogenic factors with a predominance of Damp, there is sole pain with a heavy sensation and swelling in the ankle and feet. Heat is characterised by burning, so if there is invasion of Heat in combination with the other pathogenic factors, the Heat will burn the muscles, tendons and channels, leading to the consumption of Body Fluids and Blood and to stagnation of Qi and Blood, so sole pain with a burning sensation, redness and swelling occurs.

Bad diet

Overconsumption of cold drinks and food, such as salad and fruit, may cause Cold to invade the Spleen and Stomach and impair the Yang of the Middle Burner; this impairs the Spleen's function of transportation and transformation, so Damp-Phlegm forms in the body. When Damp-Phlegm blocks the channels around the sole, the Qi and Blood stagnate, causing sole pain.

In contrast, consumption of too much spicy food, coffee, alcohol, fatty food, sweet food or milk products may generate Heat and Damp in the Middle Burner, which leads to the formation of Damp-Heat in the body. Since Damp is characterised by heaviness, when Damp-Heat accumulates in the Middle Burner it can cause the Damp-Heat to Flow downward to the sole. This slows down the Qi and Blood circulation and blocks the channels, causing a sole pain with a burning feeling and swelling.

Furthermore, bad eating habits, such as not eating enough, or not eating sufficient nutritious food, or eating irregularly, may weaken the Spleen and Stomach, leading to a deficiency of Qi and Blood, so that the sole is not properly nourished, and sole pain occurs.

Traumatic injury

Trauma, wounding, adhesions after an operation or after an acute or chronic infection in the sole, may all cause stagnation of the Qi and Blood, blockage in the channels and impairment of the muscles and tendons in the sole, so that sole pain follows.

Deficiency of Essence of Liver and Kidney

A weak constitution, prolonged chronic disease, old age, bad diets, overstrain, excessive sexual activity, and giving birth to several children, may all cause weakness of the Essence of the Liver and Kidney. As a consequence, the tendons, bones and muscles are not properly nourished, causing sole pain.

Deficiency of Qi and Blood

A weak constitution, prolonged chronic diseases, bad diets, overstrain and excessive bleeding, may all cause weakness of the Qi and Blood, leading to their deficiency, so that the tendons, bones, muscles and channels are not properly nourished, and sole pain follows.

Treatment based on differentiation

Differentiation

Differentiation of the pain due to Excess or Deficiency

— Sole pain due to Excess pathogenic factors includes the following types: invasion of Cold-Damp, or invasion of Damp-Heat, or stagnation of Qi and Blood.
— Sole pain due to Deficient factors includes the following types: deficiency of Qi and Blood, or deficiency of Kidney Essence.

Differentiation of character of the pain

— Sole pain with a heavy sensation, an aversion to cold, preference for warmth, aggravation of the sole pain in cold and humid weather, or heavy and cold limbs, is often caused by invasion of Cold-Damp.
— Sole pain with a hot and heavy sensation, or swelling of the sole with a heavy sensation, is usually due to invasion of Damp-Heat.
— Sole pain with a fixed location, history of trauma such as muscle strain, falling down, bone fracture, or operation, a purplish colour to the sole, stabbing pain, or aggravation of the pain at night, is usually caused by the stagnation of Qi and Blood.
— Sole pain, with aggravation of the sole pain by tiredness and exertion, lassitude, shortness of breath, a pale complexion, lips and tongue, is often caused by deficiency of Qi.
— Slight sole pain, with numbness at the soles, aggravation of the sole pain around the time of menstruation, accompanied by fatigue, dizziness, blurred vision, palpitations, insomnia, or numbness of limbs, is usually caused by deficiency of Blood.
— Sole pain that gets worse when tired and better with rest, with lassitude in the loins and knees, dizziness and tinnitus or deafness, or loose teeth, is usually caused by deficiency of Kidney-Essence.

Treatment

INVASION OF WIND, COLD AND DAMP

Symptoms and signs

Acute sole pain, which is aggravated in wind, cold and damp weather, with a heavy sensation in the leg and feet, an absence of any colour change on the foot, and difficulty in walking. Other external symptoms include generalised body pain, an aversion to wind and cold, headache, a thin and white or slightly greasy tongue coating and a superficial and tight pulse.

Principle of treatment

Dispel Wind-Cold, dry Damp, promote Qi and Blood circulation and sedate the pain.

HERBAL TREATMENT

Prescription

QIANG HUO SHENG SHI TANG
Notopterygium Dispelling Dampness Decoction
Qiang Huo *Rhizoma seu Radix Notopterygii* 10 g

Du Huo *Radix Angelicae Pubescentis* 10 g
Chuan Xiong *Rhizoma Ligustici Chuanxiong* 10 g
Man Jing Zi *Fructus Viticis* 10 g
Fang Feng *Radix Ledebouriellae* 6 g
Gao Ben *Rhizoma et Radix Ligustici* 10 g
Cang Zhu *Rhizoma Atractylodis* 10 g
Chuan Niu Xi *Radix Cyathulae* 10 g
Gan Cao *Radix Glycyrrhizae* 6 g

Explanations

- Qiang Huo dispels Wind, Cold and Damp from the upper body and relieves pain. Du Huo dispels Wind, Cold and Damp from the lower body. The combination can also eliminate Wind, Cold and Damp in the joints, muscles and channels of the whole body and relieve the pain.
- Fang Feng dispels Wind-Cold and relieves External symptoms.
- Chuang Xiong promotes the circulation of Blood, expels Wind and relieves the sole pain.
- Man Jing Zi and Gao Ben dispel Wind-Cold and relieve generalised body pain and headache.
- Cang Zhu and Chuan Niu Xi eliminate Damp and unblock the channels. Chuan Niu Xi is also a good herb for promoting the circulation of Blood and inducing the herbs in this formula to reach the sole.
- Gan Cao coordinates the effects of the other herbs in the prescription.

Modifications

1. If there is a cold sensation on the feet, add Gui Zhi *Ramulus Cinnamomi* 10 g to dispel Cold, warm the channels and relieve the pain.
2. If there is swelling in the feet, add Ze Xie *Rhizoma Alismatis* 10 g and Fu Ling *Poria* 10 g to promote urination and relieve the swelling.
3. If the appetite is poor, add Ji Nei Jin *Endothelium Corneum Gigeriae Galli* 15 g and Mai Ya *Fructus Hordei Germinatus* 10 g to activate the Stomach and improve the appetite.
4. If there is a nasal discharge and sneezing, add Huo Xiang *Herba Agastachis* 12 g to dispel External symptoms and stop the sneezing.
5. If there is diarrhoea, add Fu Ling *Poria* 10 g to activate the Spleen, eliminate Damp and relieve the diarrhoea.

Patent remedies

Feng Shi Pian *Wind-Damp Tablet*
Han Shi Bi Chong Ji *Cold-Damp Bi Syndrome Infusion*
Tian Ma Qu Feng Bu Pian *Gastrodia Dispel Wind Formula Tablet*

ACUPUNCTURE TREATMENT

TE-5 Waiguan, LI-4 Hegu, SI-3 Houxi, SI-4 Wangu, BL-63 Jinmen, BL-64 Jinggu, LR-3 Taichong and SP-6 Sanyinjiao. Reducing method is used on these points. Moxibustion is used on the first six points.

Explanations

- TE-5, the Connecting point of the Triple Burner channel, and LI-4, the Source point, dispel External pathogenic factors and relieve External symptoms.
- SI-4 and BL-64, the Source points, dispel Wind, Cold and Damp, promote urination and eliminate Damp.
- SI-3, the Stream point, and BL-63, the Accumulation point, harmonise the collateral, promote the Qi and Blood circulation in the channels and relieve the sole pain.
- LR-3, the Stream and Source point of the Liver channel, and SP-6, the crossing point of the three Yin channels of the foot, promote the Qi and Blood circulation in the body and channels and eliminate Blood stasis so as to relieve the sole pain.
- Moxibustion warms the channels, dispels Cold and relieves the pain.

Modifications

1. If there is a sharp pain with cold sensation, add BL 60 and ST-44 to promote the circulation of Qi and relieve the pain.
2. If there is a heavy sensation of the feet, add SP-9 to promote urination and eliminate Damp.
3. If there is an obvious aversion to exposing the feet to cold, add ST-36 with moxibustion to promote the circulation of Qi and dispel External Cold.
4. If there is generalised body pain and headache, add GB-20 to dispel Wind and Cold and relieve External symptoms.
5. If the appetite is poor, add SP-3, the Source point, and CV-12, the Front Collecting point of the Stomach, to activate the Spleen, regulate the Stomach-Qi and improve the appetite.

Case history

A 40-year-old woman had been suffering from pain in both soles for 3 days. One week before attending the clinic, she had caught a cold after walking in the rain. She suffered from generalised body pain and heaviness in her legs. To begin with, she did not pay enough attention to it. Four days later, she woke up during the night with pain in the both soles. This pain had got worse and worse over the last 2 days.

When she arrived at the clinic, her main complaints were sole pain, extreme tenderness around KI-1, aggravation of the pain with pressure and alleviation with warmth, and difficulty in walking. In addition, she had an absence of colour changes in the feet, a slight headache, an aversion to cold, a slight fever (37.7 °C), generalised body pain, neck pain, restlessness, insomnia for 3 nights, a thin and white tongue coating and a superficial and tight pulse.

Diagnosis
Sole pain due to invasion of Wind, Cold and Damp.

Principle of treatment
Dispel External Cold-Damp, promote Qi circulation and relieve the pain.

Herbal treatment
QIANG HUO SHENG SHI TANG
Notopterygium Dispelling Dampness Decoction
Qiang Huo *Rhizoma seu Radix Notopterygii* 10 g
Du Huo *Radix Angelicae Pubescentis* 10 g
Fang Feng *Radix Ledebouriellae* 6 g
Chuan Xiong *Rhizoma Ligustici Chuanxiong* 10 g
Fu Ling *Poria* 10 g
Cang Zhu *Rhizoma Atractylodis* 10 g
Huai Niu Xi *Radix Achyranthis Bidentatae* 10 g
Gan Cao *Radix Glycyrrhizae* 6 g

Explanations
- Qiang Huo and Du Huo dispel Wind, Cold and Damp in the superficial levels of the body and relieve External symptoms.
- Fang Feng dispels Wind-Cold and relieves headache.
- Chuang Xiong promotes the circulation of Blood, expels Wind and relieves the sole pain.
- Huai Niu Xi dispels Wind-Damp, promotes the circulation of Blood and relieves the sole pain. It can also help other herbs to reach the sole so as to relieve the sole pain.
- Fu Ling and Cang Zhu promote urination and eliminate Damp.
- Gan Cao coordinates the effects of the other herbs in the prescription.

The patient took this herbal decoction every day. After 2 days, her sole pain was much better, and her general external symptoms were also much improved. After taking the herbs for a week, her sole pain was almost under control and the external symptoms were gone. After treatment for 2 weeks, the sole pain had disappeared completely.

INVASION OF TOXIC HEAT

Symptoms and signs

Acute occurrence of sole pain, swelling, redness, heat and severe pain of the soles, and an inability of the sole to touch the ground. Other symptoms include high fever, restlessness, insomnia, thirst, constipation, red tongue with a yellow and dry coating, and a rapid and forceful pulse.

Principle of treatment

Clear Heat, remove Toxin, subside swelling and relieve the pain.

HERBAL TREATMENT
Prescription

PU JI XIAO DU YIN
Universal Benefit Decoction to Eliminate Toxin
Huang Qin *Radix Scutellariae* 10 g
Huang Lian *Rhizoma Coptidis* 10 g
Xuan Shen *Radix Scrophulariae* 6 g
Zhi Zi *Fructus Gardeniae* 10 g
Ban Lan Gen *Radix Isatidis* 6 g
Lian Qiao *Fructus Forsythiae* 3 g
Jiang Can *Bombyx Batryticatus* 3 g
Sheng Ma *Rhizoma Cimicifugae* 3 g
Da Qing Ye *Folium Isatidis* 10 g
Zhe Bei Mu *Bulbus Fritillariae Thunbergii* 10 g
Gan Cao *Radix Glycyrrhizae* 6 g

Explanations
- Huang Qin, Huang Lian and Zhi Zi clear Heat, reduce swelling and remove Toxin.
- Sheng Ma and Xuan Shen eliminate Toxin.
- Ban Lan Gen, Lian Qiao and Da Qing Ye dispel Heat, reduce fever and clear Toxin.
- Jiang Can and Zhe Bei Mu resolve Phlegm and harmonise the collateral and reduce the swelling.
- Gan Cao harmonises the herbs in the prescription and removes Toxin.

Modifications
1. If there is redness and swelling of the feet, add and Sheng Di Huang *Radix Rehmanniae Recens* 10 g and Long Dan Cao *Radix Gentianae* 5 g to clear Damp-Heat and reduce the swelling.
2. If there is itching on the feet, add Bai Xian Pi *Cortex Dictamni Radicis* 10 g and Ku Shen *Radix Sophorae Flavescentis* 10 g to clear Damp-Heat and relieve the itching.
3. If there is a stabbing pain in the sole, add Pu Huang *Pollen Typhae* 10 g and Dan Shen *Radix Salvia Miltiorrhizae* 10 g to promote the circulation of Blood and eliminate its stasis.
4. If there is a wound on the sole, add San Qi *Radix Notoginseng* 10 g to eliminate Toxin and promote healing of the wound.
5. If there is a fever, add Shi Gao *Gypsum Fibrosum* 20 g and Zhi Mu *Rhizoma Anemarrhenae* 10 g to clear Heat and reduce the fever.

6. If there is nervousness, add Xia Ku Cao *Spica Prunellae* 10 g to clear Heat in the Liver and calm Liver-Fire.
7. If there is throat pain and swelling, add Ma Bo *Lasiosphaera seu Calvatia* 5 g to benefit the throat and reduce the swelling.
8. If there is coughing with expectoration of yellow phlegm, add Niu Bang Zi *Fructus Arctii* 5 g to eliminate Phlegm and relieve the cough.
9. If there is restlessness and insomnia, add Dan Zhu Ye *Herba Lophatheri* 10 g to clear Heat from the Heart.
10. If there is constipation due to blockage of the Large Intestine by Heat, add Da Huang *Radix et Rhizoma Rhei* 10 g to clear Heat and promote defecation so as to relieve the constipation.

Patent remedy

Niu Huang Jie Du Pian *Cattle Gallstone Tablet to Resolve Toxin*

ACUPUNCTURE TREATMENT

TE-6 Zhigou, LI-4 Hegu, LI-11 Quchi, ST-44 Neiting, SP-6 Sanyinjiao, SP-10 Xuehai and KI-2 Rangu. Reducing method is used on these points.

Explanations

- TE-6 promotes the function of the Triple Burner and eliminates Heat and Toxin from the body.
- ST-44, the Spring point, clears Heat and reduces Fire, so as to eliminate redness and swelling. It is also a Water point according to the Five Element theory, and Water controls Fire, so it is a suitable point.
- LI-4, the Source point, and LI-11, the Sea point, relieve Heat and circulate the channel so as to sedate the pain. In most cases of invasion of Toxic Heat, there is fever. When these two points are applied together, the reduction of fever will be greater.
- SP-6, the crossing point of the three Yin channels of the foot, and SP-10 cool the Blood, eliminate toxin, reduce the swelling and relieve sole pain.
- KI-2, the Spring point, clears Heat, reduces fever and reduces the swelling in the soles.

Modifications

1. If there is redness and swelling of the feet, add GB-43 to clear Damp-Heat and reduce the swelling.
2. If there is itching on the feet, add LR-2 to clear Damp-Heat and relieve the itching.
3. If there is a stabbing pain in the sole, add KI-1 to sedate the pain.
4. If there is a wound in the sole, add Extra Bafeng to eliminate Toxin and promote healing of the wound.
5. If there is a fever, add GV-14 to clear Heat and reduce the fever.
6. If there is nervousness, add GB-20 to clear Heat in the Liver and calm Liver-Fire.
7. If there is throat pain and swelling, add LU-10 to benefit the throat and reduce the swelling.
8. If there is coughing with expectoration of yellow phlegm, add LU-5 to eliminate Phlegm and relieve the cough.
9. If there is restlessness and insomnia, add HT-8 to clear Heat from the Heart.
10. If there is constipation due to blockage of the Large Intestine by Heat, add ST-25 to clear Heat and promote defecation so as to relieve the constipation.

DOWNWARD FLOW OF DAMP-HEAT

Symptoms and signs

Sole pain with a feverish and heavy sensation, redness and swelling, which is aggravated by contact with warmth and alleviated by cold. Other symptoms include a bitter taste in the mouth, a poor appetite, fever, heaviness in the legs, painful urination, loose stools, abdominal pain and distension, deep yellow urine, a red tongue with a yellow and greasy coating at the back and a slippery and rapid pulse.

Principle of treatment

Eliminate Damp, clear Heat, harmonise the collateral and relieve the pain.

HERBAL TREATMENT

Prescription

SI MIAO WAN
Four-Marvel Pill
Huang Bai *Cortex Phellodendri* 12 g
Cang Zhu *Rhizoma Atractylodis* 10 g
Yi Yi Ren *Semen Coicis* 15 g
Fu Ling *Poria* 10 g
Chuan Xiong *Rhizoma Ligustici Chuanxiong* 10 g
Huai Niu Xi *Radix Achyranthis Bidentatae* 10 g
Gan Cao *Radix Glycyrrhizae* 6 g

Explanations

- Huang Bai clears Heat, dries Damp in the Lower Burner, reduces swelling and sedates the sole pain.
- Cang Zhu helps Huang Bai to eliminate Damp-Heat in the Lower Burner and relieve the sole pain.
- Yi Yi Ren and Fu Ling activate the Spleen and Stomach and eliminate Damp in the body. Fu Ling also tonifies the Kidney and promotes urination.
- Huai Niu Xi promotes the circulation of Blood in the body and channels and eliminates Damp and Blood stasis. Moreover, this herb induces all the herbs to descend to the sole so as to relieve the sole pain.
- Chuan Xiong promotes the circulation of Qi and Blood and relieves the sole pain.
- Gan Cao harmonises the actions of the other herbs in the prescription.

Modifications

1. If there is redness and swelling of the feet, add Sheng Di Huang *Radix Rehmanniae Recens* 15 g, Chi Shao *Radix Paeoniae Rubra* 10 g and Pu Gong Ying *Herba Taraxaci* 15 g to clear Heat in the Blood, remove toxin and reduce the swelling.
2. If there is a burning feeling in the sole, add Zhi Mu *Rhizoma Anemarrhenae* 10 g and Ren Dong Teng *Caulis Lonicerae* 20 g to clear Heat and relieve the burning feeling.
3. If there is itching of the feet, add Bai Xian Pi *Cortex Dictamni* 10 g and Ku Shen *Radix Sophorae Flavescentis* 10 g to clear Damp-Heat and relieve the itching.
4. If there is a stabbing pain in the sole, add Pu Huang *Pollen Typhae* 10 g and Dan Shen *Radix Salvia Miltiorrhizae* 10 g to promote the circulation of Blood and eliminate its stasis.
5. If there is a wound on the sole, add San Qi *Radix Notoginseng* 10 g to eliminate Toxin and promote healing of the wound.
6. If there is a fever, add Zhi Zi *Fructus Gardeniae* 10 g to clear Heat and reduce the fever.
7. If there is a bitter taste in the mouth, add Long Dan Cao *Radix Gentianae* 5 g and Yin Chen Hao *Herba Artemesiae Capillaris* 10 g to eliminate Damp-Heat, harmonise the Gall Bladder and relieve the bitter taste.
8. If there is insomnia and restlessness, add Huang Lian *Rhizoma Coptidis* 10 g to clear Heat in the Heart, calm the Mind and improve the sleep.
9. If the appetite is poor, add Ji Nei Jin *Endothelium Corneum Gigeriae Galli* 15 g and Mai Ya *Fructus Hordei Germinatus* 30 g to activate the Spleen and Stomach and improve the appetite.
10. If there is constipation due to predominance of Heat in the Large Intestine, add Da Huang *Radix et Rhizoma Rhei* 10 g to clear Heat, promote defecation and relieve the constipation.
11. If there is diarrhoea with a foul smell, or bloody stools, add Bai Tou Weng *Radix Pulsatillae* 10 g to eliminate Damp-Heat in the Large Intestine, cool the Blood and stop the diarrhoea.
12. If there is a thirst, add Mai Dong *Radix Opiopogonis* 12 g to promote secretion of the Body Fluids and relieve the thirst.

Patent remedy

San Miao Wan *Three-Marvel Pill*
Feng Shi Xiao Tong Wan *Wind-Damp Dispel Pain Pill*

ACUPUNCTURE TREATMENT

TE-6 Zhigou, SI-3 Houxi, SI-4 Wangu, BL-63 Jinmen, BL-64 Jinggu, KI-2 Rangu, SP-6 Sanyinjiao, SP-9 Yinlingquan and GB-34 Yanglingquan. Reducing method is used on these points.

Explanations

- TE-6 eliminates Damp-Heat and relieves sole pain.
- SI-4 and BL-64, the Source points, promote urination and eliminate Damp.
- SI-3, the Stream point, and BL-63, the Accumulation point, harmonise the collateral, promote the circulation of Qi and Blood in the channels and relieve the sole pain.
- KI-2, the Spring point, clears Heat, promotes urination and eliminates Damp-Heat in the Lower Burner.
- SP-6, the crossing point of the three Yin channels of the foot, promotes the circulation of Qi and Blood in the body and channels and eliminates Blood stasis so as to relieve the sole pain.
- SP-9 and GB-34, the Sea points, eliminate Damp-Heat in the Lower Burner and relieve the sole pain.

Modifications

1. If there is a sharp pain, add LI-4 and LR-3 to promote the circulation of Qi and relieve the pain.
2. If there is a heavy sensation on the foot, add KI-6 to promote urination and eliminate Damp.
3. If there is redness of the feet, add SP-10 to cool the Blood and reduce the redness.
4. If there are ulcers on the foot, add ST-44, the Spring point, to clear Heat, remove Toxin and promote healing.

5. If there is itching of the sole, add Extra Bafeng to dispel Wind and eliminate Damp-Heat.
6. If there is a fever, add GV-14 and LI-11 to clear Heat and reduce the fever.
7. If there is a headache, add GB-20 to clear Heat and relieve the headache.
8. If there is a poor appetite and nausea, add CV-12 and SP-4 to harmonise the Stomach and restore the appetite.
9. If there is leucorrhoea with itching in the genital regions, add GB-41 and LR-5 to eliminate Damp-Heat in the body and relieve the itching.
10. If there is difficult and painful urination, add KI-4 and KI-5 to promote urination and relieve the pain.
11. If there is diarrhoea, add ST-37 to regulate the Large Intestine and relieve the diarrhoea.

STAGNATION OF QI AND BLOOD

Symptoms and signs

Long-lasting sole pain with a fixed location, and a stabbing nature, which is aggravated at night or by rest and alleviated by movement, usually with a history of bone fracture, strain, operation or trauma to the sole or the foot, accompanied by a purplish colour to the feet, a purplish tongue with a thin coating and a wiry and choppy pulse.

Principle of treatment

Promote Qi and Blood circulation, smooth the collateral and relieve the pain.

HERBAL TREATMENT

Prescription

TAO HONG SI WU TANG
Four-Substance Decoction with Safflower and Peach Pit
Chuan Xiong *Rhizoma Ligustici Chuanxiong* 12 g
Tao Ren *Semen Persicae* 10 g
Hong Hua *Flos Carthami* 6 g
Dang Gui *Radix Angelicae Sinensis* 12 g
Chi Shao *Radix Paeoniae Rubra* 10 g
Huai Niu Xi *Radix Achyranthis Bidentatae* 10 g
Sheng Di Huang *Radix Rehmanniae Recens* 12 g

Explanations

- Chuan Xiong, Tao Ren and Hong Hua promote the circulation of Blood and remove its stasis to sedate the sole pain.

- Dang Gui tonifies the Blood and moistens Dryness so as to remove Blood stasis without impairing the Yin.
- Huai Niu Xi promotes the circulation of Blood in the body and the channels. Moreover, this herb induces all the other herbs to descend to the sole so as to relieve the sole pain.
- Long-lasting Blood stagnation may cause Heat to form in the Blood. Chi Shao and Sheng Di Huang clear Heat in Blood.

Modifications

1. If there is a severe sharp pain due to the predominance of Qi stagnation, add Mu Xiang *Radix Aucklandiae* 12 g and Xiang Fu *Rhizoma Cyperi* 10 g to promote the circulation of Qi and relieve the pain.
2. If there is bone fracture in the foot, or a wound on the sole, add San Qi *Radix Notoginseng* 10 g to eliminate toxin and promote healing of the bones or wound.
3. If there is spasm in the foot, add Mu Gua *Fructus Chaenomelis* 10 g to strengthen the tendons and relieve the spasm.

Patent remedies

Xiao Huo Luo Dan *Minor Invigorate the Collaterals Special Pill*
Jin Gu Die Da Wan *Muscle and Bone Traumatic Injury Pill*

ACUPUNCTURE TREATMENT

LI-4 Hegu, SP-6 Sanyinjiao, LR-3 Taichong, GB-34 Yanglingquan, SI-3 Houxi, SI-4 Wangu and BL-60 Kunlun. Reducing method is used on these points.

Explanations

- LI-4 and LR-3, the Source points, promote the circulation of Qi in the channels, eliminate stagnation of Blood and relieve the pain.
- SP-6, the crossing point of the three Yin channels of the foot, promotes the circulation of Blood, eliminates its stasis and relieves the pain.
- GB-34, the Sea point, strengthens the tendons and relieves the sole pain.
- ST-3, the Stream point, SI-4, the Source point, and BL-60 promote Qi and Blood circulation, eliminate Blood stasis in the Greater Yang channels and relieve the sole pain.

Modifications

1. If there is swelling of the feet, add Extra Bafeng to promote the Qi and Blood circulation and reduce the swelling.
2. If there is a purplish colour to the feet, add GB-44 and BL-67, the Well points, to promote the circulation of Blood and relieve the pain.
3. If there is bone fracture in the foot, add GB-39 and KI-3 to tonify the Kidney and benefit the bones.
4. If there are red spots on the feet due to the formation of Heat in the Blood, add SP-10 to cool the Blood and promote its circulation.
5. If there is depression, add LR-14 and CV-17 to smooth the Liver, promote the circulation of Qi and relieve the depression.
6. If there is an aversion to cold, or coldness of the feet, add ST-36 and KI-3 with moxibustion to warm the channels and dispel Cold.
7. If there is restlessness and insomnia, add HT-3 and PC-6 to calm the Mind and improve the sleep.

DEFICIENCY OF QI

Symptoms and signs

Sole pain that worsens with tiredness and is better for rest, with a lack of obvious tenderness at the sole, lassitude, shortness of breath, a low voice, spontaneous sweating, a poor appetite, lower back pain, nycturia, a pale tongue and a weak pulse.

PRINCIPLE OF TREATMENT

Tonify the Qi and relieve the pain.

HERBAL TREATMENT

Prescription

SI JUN ZI TANG
Four-Gentlemen Decoction
Ren Shen *Radix Ginseng* 6 g
Bai Zhu *Rhizoma Atractylodis Macrocephalae* 10 g
Fu Ling *Poria* 10 g
Qing Jiao *Radix Gentianae Macrophyllae* 10 g
Chuan Xiong *Rhizoma Ligustici Chuanxiong* 12 g
Huai Niu Xi *Radix Achyranthis Bidentatae* 10 g
Gan Cao *Radix Glycyrrhizae* 6 g

Explanations

- Ren Shen strengthens the Spleen and Stomach and greatly tonifies the Qi.

- Bai Zhu and Fu Ling strengthen the Spleen and Stomach and eliminate Damp.
- Qing Jiao harmonises the collateral and relieves the sole pain.
- Chuan Xiong promotes the Qi and Blood circulation and relieves the sole pain.
- Huai Niu Xi promotes the circulation of Blood in the body and the channels. Moreover, this herb induces all the herbs to descend to the sole so as to relieve the sole pain.
- Gan Cao tonifies the Qi and harmonises the actions of the other herbs in the prescription.

Modifications

1. If there is spasm in the feet, add Mu Gua *Fructus Chaenomelis* 10 g to strengthen the tendons and relieve the spasm.
2. If there is an aversion to exposing the foot to cold, add Gui Zhi *Ramulus Cinnamomi* 6 g to warm the channels, dispel Cold and promote the circulation of Blood.
3. If there is generalised tiredness, add Huang Qi *Radix Astragali Seu Hedysari* 15 g to tonify the Qi and relieve the tiredness.
4. If there is spontaneous sweating, add Mu Li *Concha Ostreae* 20 g to stop the sweating.
5. If there is shortness of breath, add Wu Wei Zi *Fructus Schisandrae* 10 g to tonify the Lung and relieve the shortness of breath.
6. If the appetite is poor, add Ji Nei Jin *Endothelium Corneum Gigeriae Galli* 15 g and Mai Ya *Fructus Hordei Germinatus* 20 g to activate the Spleen and Stomach and improve the appetite.
7. If there is diarrhoea, add Bu Gu Zhi *Fructus Psoraleae* 10 g to stop this.
8. If there is a sensation of fullness in the abdomen, add Mu Xiang *Radix Aucklandiae* 10 g to promote the circulation of Qi and relieve the fullness in the abdomen.

Patent remedy

Bu Zhong Yi Qi Wan *Tonifying the Middle and Benefiting Qi Pill*

ACUPUNCTURE TREATMENT

SI-3 Houxi, SI-4 Wangu, SP-6 Sanyinjiao, ST-36 Zusanli, KI-3 Taixi, GB-34 Yanglingquan, BL-60 Kunlun, BL-64 Jinggu and LR-3 Taichong. Reducing method is used on these points.

Explanations

- SI-3, the Stream point, SI-4, the Source point, and BL-60 promote the Qi and Blood circulation in the Greater Yang channels and relieve the sole pain.
- SP-6, the crossing point of the three Yin channels of the foot, and ST-36, the Sea point, activate the Spleen and Stomach and promote the production of Qi.
- BL-64, KI-3 and LR-3, the Source points, tonify the Liver and Kidney and strengthen the bones and tendons.

Modifications

1. If there is spasm in the feet, add GB-34 to strengthen the tendons and relieve the spasm.
2. If there is an aversion to exposing the foot to cold, add ST-42, the Source point, with moxibustion to warm the channels, dispel Cold and promote the circulation of Blood.
3. If there is generalised tiredness, add CV-4 to tonify the Qi and relieve the tiredness.
4. If there is spontaneous sweating, add LU-9 to tonify the Lung-Qi and stop the sweating.
5. If there is shortness of breath, add LU-1 and BL-13 to tonify the Lung and relieve the shortness of breath.
6. If the appetite is poor, add SP-3 to activate the Spleen and Stomach and improve the appetite.
7. If there is diarrhoea, add ST-25 to relieve this.
8. If there is a sensation of fullness in the abdomen, add ST-40 to promote the circulation of Qi and relieve the feeling of fullness.

DEFICIENCY OF BLOOD

Symptoms and signs

Slight sole pain, which in women worsens around the time of menstruation, with numbness in the soles, accompanied by weakness in the knees and feet, a pale complexion, pale lips, easily broken nails, fatigue, dizziness, blurred vision, palpitations, insomnia, limbs numbness, scanty or delayed menstruation or amenorrhoea, a thin and white tongue coating and a thready and weak pulse.

PRINCIPLE OF TREATMENT

Nourish Blood, tonify the Kidney-Essence and relieve the pain.

HERBAL TREATMENT

Prescription

BA ZHEN TANG
Eight-Precious Decoction
Dang Gui *Radix Angelicae Sinensis* 12 g
Chuan Xiong *Rhizoma Ligustici Chuanxiong* 10 g
Bai Shao *Radix Paeoniae Alba* 12 g
Shu Di Huang *Radix Rehmanniae Praeparata* 12 g
Ren Shen *Radix Ginseng* 6 g
Bai Zhu *Rhizoma Atractylodis Macrocephalae* 12 g
Fu Ling *Poria* 12 g
Huai Niu Xi *Radix Achyranthis Bidentatae* 10 g
Gan Cao *Radix Glycyrrhizae* 6 g

Explanations

- Dang Gui, Bai Shao and Shu Di Huang tonify the Kidney-Essence and nourish the Liver-Blood.
- Ren Shen, Bai Zhu, Fu Ling and Gan Cao, the ingredients of Si Jun Zi Tang *Four-Gentlemen Decoction* strengthen the Spleen and reinforce the Qi.
- Chuan Xiong activates the Qi and Blood circulation and relieves obstruction in the channels. It can also prevent side-effects from using too many tonics.
- Huai Niu Xi promotes the circulation of Blood in the body and the channels. Moreover, it also induces all the herbs to descend to the sole so as to relieve the sole pain.

Modifications

1. If there is an aversion to cold or cold limbs due to deficiency of Yang, add Gui Zhi *Ramulus Cinnamomi* 6 g and Wu Zhu Yu *Fructus Evodiae* 6 g to reinforce and activate the Yang-Qi.
2. If the feet are swollen, add Zhu Ling *Polyporus Umbellatus* 15 g and Ze Xie *Rhizoma Alismatis* 12 g to strengthen the Spleen, promote urination and reduce the swelling.
3. If there is fatigue, add Huang Qi *Radix Astragali seu Hedysari* 12 g to tonify the Qi and Blood and relieve the fatigue.
4. If there is insomnia, add Yuan Zhi *Radix Polygalae* 5 g and Dan Shen *Radix Salviae Miltiorrhizae* 10 g to calm the Mind and improve the sleep.
5. If there is bleeding, add E Jiao *Colla Corii Asini* 10 g to tonify the Blood and stop the bleeding.

Patent remedies

Ba Zhen Pian *Eight-Precious Tablet*
Shi Quan Da Bu Wan *All-Inclusive Great Tonifying Pill*

ACUPUNCTURE TREATMENT

SI-3 Houxi, SI-4 Wangu, SP-6 Sanyinjiao, ST-36 Zusanli, KI-3 Taixi, GB-34 Yanglingquan, GB-39 Xuanzhong, CV-6 Qihai and LR-3 Taichong. Reducing method is used on these points.

Explanations

- SI-3, the Stream point, and SI-4, the Source point, promote the Qi and Blood circulation in the Greater Yang channels and relieve the sole pain.
- SP-6, the crossing point of the three Yin channels of the foot, and ST-36, the Sea point, activate the Spleen and Stomach and promote the production of Qi and Blood.
- KI-3 and LR-3, the Source points, and GB-39, the Gathering point for the Marrow, tonify the Liver and Kidney and strengthen the bones and tendons.
- CV-16 tonifies the Qi and Essence and relieves the tiredness.
- GB-34, the Gathering point for the tendons, strengthens the tendons and relieves the sole pain.

Modifications

1. If the feet are swollen, add ST-40 and SP-9 to strengthen the Spleen, promote urination and reduce the swelling.
2. If there is an aversion to cold or cold limbs due to deficiency of Yang, add CV-4 and moxibustion on CV-4 and CV-6 to reinforce the Yang-Qi and eliminate Cold.
3. If there is dizziness, add GV-20 to activate the Yang-Qi and lift it to the head and relieve the dizziness.
4. If there is insomnia, add HT-3 to calm the Mind and improve the sleep.

DEFICIENCY OF KIDNEY-ESSENCE

Symptoms and signs

Sole pain, which gets worse with tiredness and is better from rest, with difficulty in walking, flaccidity in the feet, weakness in the lower back and knees, dizziness, tinnitus or deafness, loose teeth, infertility, irregular menstruation, a thin tongue coating and a thready pulse.

If the deficiency is of Kidney-Yin, there will also be hot flushes, night sweating, thirst, a dry throat, dry stools, a red tongue with a thin and scanty coating and a thready and rapid pulse. If the deficiency is of Kidney-

Yang, there will be an aversion to cold, cold limbs, oedema, profuse clear urine, a pale tongue with a thin and white coating and a slow, deep and thready pulse.

Principle of treatment

Tonify the Kidney, benefit the Essence, strengthen the bones and relieve the sole pain.

HERBAL TREATMENT

Prescription

ZUO GUI WAN
Restoring the Left Pill
Shu Di Huang *Rhizoma Rehmanniae Praeparata* 12 g
Shan Yao *Rhizoma Dioscoreae* 12 g
Gou Qi Zi *Fructus Lycii* 12 g
Shan Zhu Yu *Fructus Corni* 12 g
Chuan Niu Xi *Radix Cyathulae* 9 g
Tu Si Zi *Semen Cuscutae* 12 g
Lu Jiao *Colla Cornus Cervi* 8 g
Gui Jiao *Colla Plastri Testudinis* 8 g

Explanations

- Shu Di Huang, Tu Si Zi and Shan Zhu Yu tonify the Kidney and benefit the Kidney-Essence so as to strengthen the bones and tendons.
- Shan Yao activates the Spleen and tonifies the Kidney.
- Gou Qi Zi tonifies the Kidney-Essence and improves the vision.
- Lu Jiao and Gui Jiao tonify the Kidney, benefit the Kidney-Essence and strengthen the bones and tendons.
- Chuan Niu Xi tonifies the Liver and Kidney, and promotes the circulation of Blood in the body and the channels. Moreover, it induces all the herbs to descend to the sole so as to relieve the sole pain.

Modifications

1. If there are cold limbs and an aversion to cold, add Rou Gui *Cortex Cinnamomi* 10 g to warm the body and Kidney and dispel Cold.
2. If there is shortness of breath, add Wu Wei Zi *Fructus Schisandrae* 10 g to tonify the Lung and Kidney and relieve the shortness of breath.
3. If there is oedema, add Fu Ling *Poria* 12 g and Ze Xie *Rhizoma Alismatis* 10 g to promote urination and reduce the oedema.
4. If there is diarrhoea, add Bu Gu Zhi *Fructus Psoraleae* 10 g to stop this.

5. If there is profuse urination, add Yi Zhi Ren *Fructus Alpiniae Oxyphyllae* 12 g to tonify the Kidney and reduce urination.
6. If there is amenorrhoea, add Yi Mu Cao *Herba Leonuri* 15 g to promote and regulate the menstruation.
7. If there is a tidal fever, and heat in the palms and soles, add Di Gu Pi *Cortex Lycii Radicis* 12 g to clear Deficient-Heat and relieve the tidal fever.
8. If there is profuse night sweating, add Mu Li *Concha Ostreae* 20 g to stop the sweating.

Patent remedies

Du Huo Ji Sheng Wan *Angelica Pubescens–Loranthus Pill*

Kang Gu Zheng Sheng Pian *Combat Bone Hyperplasia Pill*

ACUPUNCTURE TREATMENT

LR-3 Taichong, LR-8 Ququan, SP-6 Sanyinjiao, KI-3 Taixi, KI-4 Dazhong, KI-5 Shuiquan, KI-10 Yingu and BL-64 Jinggu. Reinforcing method is used on these points.

Explanations

- LR-3 and KI-3, the Source points, together with LR-8 and KI-10, the Sea points, tonify the Liver and Kidney, benefit the Kidney-Essence and strengthen the bones and tendons so as to relieve the sole pain.
- KI-4, the Connecting point, and KI-5, the Accumulation point, harmonise the collateral, promote the Qi and Blood circulation in the Kidney channel and relieve the sole pain.
- SP-6, the crossing point of the three Yin channels of the foot, tonifies the Liver, Spleen and Kidney, promotes Qi and Blood production and benefits the Kidney-Essence.
- BL-64, the Source point, promotes the Qi and Blood circulation in the Bladder channel and relieves the sole pain.

Modifications

1. If there is dizziness, add GV-20 to lift the Kidney-Essence to the head and benefit the brain.
2. If there are cold limbs and an aversion to cold, add GV-4 with moxibustion to warm the body and Kidney and dispel Cold.
3. If there is shortness of breath, add LU-9 to tonify the Lung and Kidney and relieve the shortness of breath.
4. If there is weakness in the knees, add GB-34 to benefit the tendons and strengthen the knees.
5. If there is oedema, add SP-9 to promote urination and reduce the oedema.
6. If there is diarrhoea, add SP-3 to activate the Spleen and stop the diarrhoea.
7. If there is profuse urination, add CV-6 to tonify the Kidney and reduce urination.
8. If there is amenorrhoea, add SP-4 to promote and regulate the menstruation.
9. If there is a tidal fever, and heat in the palms and soles, add KI-7 and KI-2 to clear Deficient-Heat and relieve the fever.
10. If there is profuse night sweating, add HT-6 to stop the sweating.

Toe pain

足
趾
疼
痛

Toe pain may occur in one toe, or several toes, and in one or both feet. According to TCM theory, it can be caused by invasion of External factors, the downward flow of Damp-Heat, a deficiency of Liver and Kidney, or stagnation or deficiency of Qi and Blood. Toe pain may be attributed to any of the following disorders in Western medicine: rheumatoid arthritis, hallux bunion, tenosynovitis, gout, osteoarthritis of the tarsometatarsal joint and stenosing tenovaginitis of the long flexor muscle of great toe.

Aetiology and pathology

Invasion of External factors

Long-term exposure to Wind, Cold and Damp, for instance living in a damp environment, walking in cold water and catching cold, may cause the toes to be invaded by these pathogenic factors. The pathogenic factors block the circulation of Qi and Blood in the channels of the feet, slowing down the circulation of Qi and Blood so that stagnation of Qi and Blood occurs, and toe pain follows.

The clinical symptoms and signs will vary depending on which factor is predominant. Wind is characteristically moving and changing, so if this factor predominates in the invasion, there will be a toe pain that tends to move around from place to place. Cold is characterised by contraction and stagnation, so if this factor predominates in the invasion there is contraction of the channels and tendons in the feet, leading to stagnation of Qi and Blood, and causing a severe cold pain in the toe. Damp is characterised by heaviness and stagnation, so if it is predominant there will be obstruction of the foot channels, leading to a toe pain accompanied by feelings of numbness and heaviness.

If the body fails to eliminate the External pathogenic factors so that they accumulate over time, they may gradually generate Heat, leading to the formation of Wind, Damp and Heat. This condition often occurs in those who have an accumulation of Heat in the body or a deficiency of Yin with formation of Deficient-Heat. Direct invasion of the toe by Wind, Damp and Heat may also occur. Heat is characterised by redness and a burning sensation, so if Wind, Damp and Heat invade the body they disturb the Qi and Blood in the channels, leading to stagnation of Qi and Blood circulation and blockage of the channels by Damp-Heat. Qi and Blood accumulate in the toes, so that a toe pain with swelling, redness and hotness occurs.

Prolonged persistence of Cold-Damp in the body may cause a gradual generation of Heat, also leading to formation of Damp-Heat, and resulting in toe pain.

Bad diet

Bad diets, such as habitual eating of sweet or fatty food, or drinking too much alcohol, may impair the Spleen and Stomach, leading to the formation of Damp-Heat in the body. When Damp-Heat flows downward to the lower limbs, it blocks the channels, causing toe pain.

Deficiency of Qi and Blood

Overstrain, eating too little, a constitutional weakness and prolonged sickness may all cause the consumption of Qi and Blood, and deficiency of the Liver and Kidney. In this condition the tendons are not properly nourished by the Liver-Blood and the bones fail to be nourished by Kidney-Essence, so that toe pain with weakness in the feet and joint occurs.

In long-term sickness, the external pathogens may not be completely expelled, leading to stagnation of Qi and Blood in the channels, and causing toe pain.

Stagnation of Qi and Blood

Stagnation of Qi and Blood in the channels of the feet can be caused by various factors, including emotional disturbance, sprain, overstrain and inappropriate operations. When the circulation of Qi and Blood through the feet is blocked in the channels, it leads to toe pain.

Treatment based on differentiation

Differentiation

Differentiation of External or Internal origin

— Acute onset of toe pain of a short duration, accompanied by External symptoms, is usually caused by invasion of External pathogenic factors. Traumatic injury could also cause acute toe pain.
— Chronic onset of toe pain of long duration, accompanied by some symptoms resulting from Internal disorders, such as deficiency of Liver and Kidney, is usually caused by disorder of the Internal organs.

Differentiation of character of the pain

— Severe pain, which gets worse with pressure, is usually cause by Excessive pathogenic factors, such as invasion of Wind-Cold-Damp, or

stagnation of Qi and Blood. Toe pain that is dull and lingering often indicates Deficiency, such as deficiency of Liver and Kidney.
— Acute onset of toe pain with no fixed location is mainly due to pathogenic Wind, such as invasion of External Wind-Cold-Damp with predominance of Wind.
— Severe toe pain with a cold sensation indicates Cold syndrome, such as invasion of External Wind-Cold-Damp with predominance of Cold.
— Toe pain with a heavy sensation often indicates pathogenic Dampness, such as invasion of External Wind-Cold-Dampness with predominance of Damp.
— Painful toe with local redness, swelling and a burring sensation implies pathogenic Heat, such as downward flow of Damp-Heat.
— Constant pain but not severe in a toe or toes, with rigidity of the toe in the morning, hyperosteogeny, muscular atrophy, aggravation of the toe pain by walking, or fatigue, is usually caused by deficiency of the Liver and Kidney.
— Stabbing toe pain with a fixed location, purplish and swollen toe or toes, history of trauma, aggravation of the toe pain by pressure or by movement and at night, is usually caused by stagnation of Blood.

Treatment

INVASION OF WIND-COLD-DAMP WITH PREDOMINANCE OF WIND

Symptoms and signs

Wandering toe pain, which is aggravated by exposure to wind, with difficult movement of the toes, and an aversion to wind, accompanied by chills and fever, a thin white or thin greasy tongue coating and a superficial pulse.

Principle of treatment

Dispel Wind, Cold and Damp, unblock the channels, promote Qi and Blood circulation and calm the pain.

HERBAL TREATMENT

Prescription

FANG FENG TANG
Ledebouriella Decoction
Fang Feng *Radix Ledebouriellae* 10 g
Ma Huang *Herba Ephedrae* 5 g

Dang Gui *Radix Angelicae Sinensis* 10 g
Qin Jiao *Radix Gentianae Macrophyllae* 10 g
Rou Gui *Cortex Cinnamomi* 5 g
Ge Gen *Radix Puerariae* 10 g
Fu Ling *Poria* 10 g
Qiang Huo *Rhizoma et Radix Notopterygii* 10 g
Gui Zhi *Ramulus Cinnamomi* 10 g
Sheng Jiang *Rhizoma Zingiberis Recens* 10 g
Da Zao *Fructus Ziziphi Jujubae* 5 g
Gan Cao *Radix Glycyrrhizae* 3 g

Explanations

- Fang Feng, Ge Gen and Ma Huang dispel Wind, Cold and Damp.
- Dang Gui and Qin Jiao promote the Blood circulation and remove obstructions from the collateral.
- Fu Ling strengthens the Spleen and induces urination so as to eliminate Damp.
- Qiang Huo disperses Wind, Cold and Damp and stops the pain.
- Gui Zhi and Rou Gui activate Yang and warm the channels so as to sedate the pain.
- The last three herbs coordinate all the herbs in this prescription.

Modifications

1. If there is spasm of the toe due to predominance of Cold invasion, add Bai Zhi *Radix Angelicae Dahuricae* 10 g to eliminate Cold and relieve the spasm.
2. If there is stiffness of the toes due to invasion of Wind-Cold, add Ge Gen *Radix Puerariae* 15 g to eliminate Damp and relieve the stiffness.
3. If there is swelling of the toes, add Du Huo *Radix Angelica Pubescentis* 10 g and Huai Niu Xi *Radix Achyranthis Bidentatae* 10 g to dispel Damp, reduce swelling and sedate the pain.
4. If there is swelling and redness of the toes, add Zhi Mu *Rhizoma Anemarrhenae* 10 g and Fang Ji *Radix Stephaniae Tetrandrae* 10 g to clear Heat and remove obstructions from the collateral.
5. If there is fever and chills, add Gui Zhi *Ramulus Cinnamomi* 10 g to relieve the Exterior syndrome and reduce the fever.
6. If there is a headache due to Wind-Cold invasion, add Chuan Xiong *Rhizoma Ligustici Chuanxiong* 6 g to dispel the Wind-Cold and relieve the headache.
7. If there is a poor appetite due to invasion of Wind-Cold, add Ban Xia *Rhizoma Pinelliae* 10 g and Chen Pi *Pericarpium Citri Reticulatae* 10 g to improve the appetite.

Patent remedies

Feng Shi Pian *Wind-Damp Tablet*
Tian Ma Qu Feng Bu Pian *Gastrodia Dispel Wind Formula Tablet*
Han Shi Bi Chong Ji *Cold-Damp Bi Syndrome Infusion*

ACUPUNCTURE TREATMENT

TE-5 Waiguan, LI-4 Hegu, BL-12 Fengmen, BL-60 Kunlun, GB-40 Qiuxu, SP-6 Sanyinjiao and Extra Bafeng. Reducing method is used on these points.

Explanations

- TE-5, LI-4 and BL-12 dispel External pathogenic Wind and relieve External symptoms.
- BL-60 and GB-40 are suitable for regulating the local circulation of Qi and Blood.
- SP-6 is the crossing point of Kidney, Spleen, Liver channels, and is good at regulating the Blood and Qi.
- Extra Bafeng dispels Wind, Cold and Damp and promotes Qi and Blood circulation on the feet so as to relieve the toe pain.

Modifications

1. If there is fever and chills, add GV-14, the meeting point for all the Yang channels, to dispel Wind, relieve Exterior symptoms and reduce the fever.
2. If there is swelling of the foot and toes, add SP-9, the Sea point, to remove Damp and reduce the swelling.
3. If there is redness, swelling and a hot sensation in the toe, add LI-11, the Sea point, and ST-44, the Spring point, to clear Heat and reduce the swelling.
4. Some corresponding points on the finger should be added in order to increase the therapeutic effect.
5. If there is a headache, add GB-20 to dispel Wind and relieve the headache.
6. If the appetite is poor, add SP-4 and ST-36 to activate the Spleen and improve the appetite.

Case history

A 50-year-old woman had been suffering from toe pain for 3 years. She was diagnosed as having 'rheumatoid arthritis', and often took painkillers and anti-inflammatory drugs to relieve the toe pain.

During the previous 2 weeks, she had been suffering a lot of toe pain after an infection, and was unable to sleep because of the pain. Besides the toe pain, she also had generalised body pain, a slight fever (37.5°C) during the day, an aversion to cold, a headache, a thin and white tongue coating, and a superficial and wiry pulse.

Diagnosis
Toe pain due to invasion of Wind-Cold-Damp.

Principle of treatment
Dispel Wind, expel Cold, eliminate Damp, smooth the channels and collateral and relieve the pain.

Herbal treatment
FANG FENG TANG
Ledebouriella Decoction
Fang Feng *Radix Ledebouriellae* 10 g
Ge Gen *Radix Puerariae* 15 g
Ma Huang *Herba Ephedrae* 6 g
Dang Gui *Radix Angelicae Sinensis* 10 g
Rou Gui *Cortex Cinnamomi* 6 g
Xi Xin *Herba Asari* 3 g
Sheng Jiang *Rhizoma Zingiberis Recens* 10 g
Gan Cao *Radix Glycyrrhizae* 6 g
The prescription was taken once a day.

Explanations

- Fang Feng, Ge Gen and Ma Huang dispel Wind, Cold and Damp.
- Dang Gui promotes the circulation of Blood and removes obstructions from the channels; promoting the Blood circulation also can quench Wind.
- Rou Gui and Xi Xin dispel Wind-Cold and relieve pain.
- Sheng Jiang and Gan Cao strengthen the Spleen and coordinate the actions of all the other herbs in the prescription.

After 20 days of treatment, the pain had disappeared. A year later she was followed up and she reported that she had experienced no more pain since the treatment.

INVASION OF WIND-COLD-DAMP WITH PREDOMINANCE OF COLD

Symptoms and signs

Cold and severe pain in the toes, which is aggravated by contact with cold and alleviated by warmth, with an aversion to cold and cold limbs, limited movement of the toes in cases of severe pain, a white tongue coating and a tense or deep and slow pulse.

Principle of treatment

Warm the channels, dispel Cold, Wind and Damp.

HERBAL TREATMENT

Prescription

WU FU MA XIN GUI JIANG TANG
Decoction of Ephedra, Asari, Cinnamon and Dried Ginger
Chuan Wu *Radix Aconiti Carmichaeli* 10 g
Fu Zi *Radix Aconiti Carmichaeli Praeparata* 10 g

Gan Jiang *Rhizoma Zingiberis* 10 g
Ma Huang *Herba Ephedrae* 6 g
Xi Xin *Herba Asari* 3 g
Gui Zhi *Ramulus Cinnamomi* 6 g
Gan Cao *Radix Glycyrrhizae* 6 g

Explanations

- Wu Tou, Fu Zi and Gan Jiang are Warm in nature, so they can warm the channels, dispel Cold and sedate the pain.
- Ma Huang, Xi Xin and Gui Zhi expel Wind, Cold and Damp.
- Gan Cao can moderate all the herbs and minimise the Toxic effects of the other herbs.

Modifications

1. If there is limitation of movement in the toe joints, add Dang Gui *Radix Angelicae Sinensis* 10 g to regulate the Qi and Blood circulation to improve the joint function.
2. If the limbs are cold, add Rou Gui *Cortex Cinnamomi* 6 g and Gan Jiang *Rhizoma Zingiberis* 10 g to warm the channels and dispel Cold.
3. If there is a heavy sensation in the joints, add Qin Jiao *Radix Gentianae Macrophyllae* 10 g and Fu Ling *Poria* 15 g to eliminate Damp.
4. If there is a chill and fever, add Ge Gen *Radix Puerariae* 15 g and Fang Feng *Radix Ledebouriellae* 10 g to dispel External factors and reduce the fever.

Patent remedy

Han Shi Bi Chong Ji *Cold-Damp Bi Syndrome Infusion*

ACUPUNCTURE TREATMENT

TE-5 Waiguan, LI-4 Hegu, SP-6 Sanyinjiao, BL-12 Fengmen, BL-60 Kunlun, BL-63 Jinmen, GB-40 Qiuxu and Extra Bafeng. Reducing method is applied on these points, with moxibustion on TE-5, LI-4, BL-60, GB-40 and Extra Bafeng.

Explanations

- TE-5, LI-4 and BL-12 dispel External pathogenic Wind, eliminate Cold and relieve External symptoms.
- GB-40, BL-60, BL-63 and Extra Bafeng, all the local points, regulate the circulation of Qi and Blood in the locality so as to relieve the toe pain.
- SP-6 activates the circulation of Blood and relieves the toe pain.

- Moxibustion warms the channels, dispels Cold and relieves the pain.

Modifications

1. If the feet are swollen, add SP-9 to eliminate Damp and reduce swelling.
2. If there is a cold sensation in the body and cold limbs, add CV-8 with moxibustion to reinforce the Yang and dispel Cold.
3. The corresponding points on the fingers should be added in order to increase the therapeutic effect.
4. If there is a runny nose and coughing, add LU-7 to dispel Wind and eliminate Cold so as to relieve External symptoms.
5. If there is a headache, add GB-20 to dispel Wind and Cold and relieve the headache.

INVASION OF WIND-COLD-DAMP WITH PREDOMINANCE OF DAMP

Symptoms and signs

Pain and swelling in the toes with a heavy sensation, which worsens on overcast or rainy days, with limited movement of the toes, a poor appetite, loose stools, a white and greasy tongue coating and a soft and slow pulse.

Principle of treatment

Eliminate Damp, dispel Cold and Wind, and circulate the collateral and sedate the pain.

HERBAL TREATMENT

Prescription

YI YI REN TANG
Coix Decoction
Yi Yi Ren *Semen Coicis* 10 g
Cang Zhu *Rhizoma Atractylodis* 10 g
Qiang Huo *Rhizoma et Radix Notopterygii* 10 g
Du Huo *Radix Angelicae Pubescentis* 10 g
Fang Feng *Radix Ledebouriellae* 10 g
Chuan Wu *Radix Aconiti Carmichaeli* 5 g
Ma Huang *Herba Ephedrae* 5 g
Dang Gui *Radix Angelicae Sinensis* 6 g
Chuan Xiong *Radix Ligustici Chuanxiong* 6 g
Gan Cao *Radix Glycyrrhizae* 5 g

Explanations

- Yi Yi Ren and Cang Zhu strengthen the Spleen and remove Damp.

- Qiang Huo, Du Huo and Fang Feng are good at dispelling Wind and removing Damp.
- Chuan Wu and Ma Huang dispel Cold, warm the channels and remove Damp.
- Dang Gui and Chuan Xiong nourish the Blood and promote its circulation.
- Gan Cao strengthens the Spleen and regulates the Middle Burner.

Modifications

1. If there is a heavy sensation in the joints, add Fu Ling *Poria* 15 g to dry Damp and improve the joint function.
2. If there is limitation of joint movement, add Qin Jiao *Radix Gentianae Macrophyllae* 10 g and Ge Gen *Radix Puerariae* 15 g to eliminate Wind and Damp, and improve joint movement.
3. If the appetite is poor, add Sheng Jiang *Rhizoma Zingiberis Recens* 10 g to promote the circulation of Qi in the Middle Burner and improve the appetite.
4. If there are loose stools, add Chen Pi *Pericarpium Citri Reticulatae* 10 g and Bai Zhu *Rhizoma Atractylodis* 10 g to dry Damp and dry the stool.
5. If there is nausea or vomiting and diarrhoea, add Sha Ren *Fructus Amomi* 5 g and Bai Zhu *Rhizoma Atractylodis Macrocephalae* 10 g to activate the Spleen and Stomach and relieve Damp in the Middle Burner.

Patent remedies

Feng Shi Pian *Wind-Damp Tablet*
Tian Ma Qu Feng Bu Pian *Gastrodia Dispel Wind Formula Tablet*

ACUPUNCTURE TREATMENT

TE-6 Zhigou, LI-4 Hegu, ST-40 Fenglong, SP-9 Yinlingquan, BL-12 Fengmen, BL-63 Jinmen, BL-64 Jinggu, GB-40 Qiuxu and Extra Bafeng. Reducing method is applied on these points.

Explanations

- TE-6, LI-4 and BL-12 dispel External pathogenic Wind, eliminate Cold, resolve Damp and relieve External symptoms.
- GB-40, the Source point, BL-63, the Accumulation point, and BL-64, the Source point, which are the local points, eliminate Damp and regulate the circulation of Qi and Blood in the locality so as to relieve the toe pain.

- ST-40, the Connecting point, Extra Bafeng and SP-9, the Sea point, eliminate Damp in the channels and relieve the pain.

Modifications

1. If the feet are swollen, add SP-3, the Source point, to eliminate Damp and reduce the swelling.
2. If there is a cold sensation in the body and cold limbs, add CV-8 with moxibustion to reinforce the Yang and dispel Cold.
3. If there is nausea, or vomiting and diarrhoea, add CV-12 and ST-25 to regulate the Qi in the Middle Burner and harmonise the Spleen and Stomach.
4. If there is scanty urination, add SP-6 and KI-3 to promote urination and eliminate Damp.
5. If there is a general feeling of heaviness in the body, add BL-22 and BL-40 to promote urination and eliminate Damp from the body generally.

DOWNWARD FLOW OF DAMP-HEAT

Symptoms and signs

Pain and swelling in the toes which is aggravated by touching, with a burning sensation and redness, and limited movement, accompanied by irritability, restlessness, a slight fever, a poor appetite, scanty and yellow urination, constipation, or loose stools, a desire for cold drinks, a yellow and greasy tongue coating, and a slippery and rapid pulse.

Principle of treatment

Clear Heat, remove Wind and Damp and sedate the pain.

HERBAL TREATMENT

Prescription

BAI HU JIA GUI ZHI TANG
White Tiger Ramulus Cinnamomi Decoction
Zhi Mu *Rhizoma Anemarrhenae* 10 g
Shi Gao *Gypsum Fibrosum* 25 g
Gui Zhi *Ramulus Cinnamomi* 10 g
Gan Cao *Radix Glycyrrhizae* 6 g
Jing Mi *Semen Oryzae* 10 g
Huang Bai *Cortex Phellodendri* 10 g
Wei Ling Xian *Radix Clematidis* 10 g
Fang Ji *Radix Stephaniae Tetrandrae* 10 g
Sang Zhi *Ramulus Mori* 10 g

Explanations

- Shi Gao and Zhi Mu are the main herbs in Bai Hu Jia Gui Zhi Tang to clear Heat and relive irritability, nourish the Stomach and promote the production of Body Fluids.
- Gan Cao and Jing Mi benefit the Stomach, reinforce the Body Fluids and moderate the extremely Cold nature of Shi Gao and Zhi Mu.
- Gui Zhi dispels Wind and promotes the function of the collateral.
- Huang Bai clears Heat and dries Damp.
- Wei Ling Xian, Han Fang Ji and Sang Zhi expel pathogenic Wind and Damp in the channels, promote the circulation of Blood and unblock the channels.

Modifications

1. If there is a sensation of heat in the joints, add Ye Ju Hua *Flos Chrysanthemi* 15 g to clear Fire and relieve the pain.
2. If there is irritability, add Xia Ku Cao *Spica Prunellae* 10 g to reduce Liver-Fire.
3. If there is constipation, add Da Huang *Radix et Rhizoma Rhei* 6 g and Mang Xiao *Natrii Sulfas* 10 g to clear Fire and promote defecation.
4. If there is a bitter taste in the mouth, add Huang Qin *Radix Scutellariae* 10 g to clear Heat in the Gall Bladder and improve the taste.
5. If there is a fever, add Zhi Zi *Fructus Gardeniae* 10 g to clear Heat and reduce the fever.

Patent remedies

San Miao Wan *Three-Marvel Pill*
Feng Shi Xiao Tong Pian *Wind-Damp Dispel Pain Pill*

ACUPUNCTURE TREATMENT

TE-6 Zhigou, LI-4 Hegu, SP-6 Sanyinjiao, SP-9 Yinlingquan, BL-60 Kunlun, GB-34 Yanglingquan, GB-40 Qiuxu, GB-41 Zulinqi, ST-44 Neiting and Extra Bafeng. Reducing method is used on these points.

Explanations

- TE-6 and LI-4 dispel External pathogenic factors, promote the circulation of Qi in the channels, eliminate Damp and reduce Heat.
- SP-6, the crossing point of the three Yin channels of the foot, SP-9 and GB-34, the Sea points, together with GB-40 eliminate Damp in the body and channels and clear Heat so as to relieve the pain.

- BL-60 dispels External pathogenic factors, promotes urination, eliminates Damp and relieves toe pain.
- ST-44 and GB-41 eliminate Damp-Heat and reduce fever.
- Extra Bafeng eliminates Damp, regulates the circulation of Qi and Blood in the channels and relieves the toe pain.

Modifications

1. If there is redness and pain in the toes, add SP-10 to cool the Blood and reduce swelling.
2. If there is fever, add GV-14 and LI-11 to clear Heat and reduce fever.
3. If there is generalised body pain and headache, add GB-20 to dispel External factors and relieve the body pain.
4. If there is yellow and scanty urination, add CV-3 to promote urination, clear Heat and eliminate Damp from the body.
5. The corresponding points on the fingers should be added in order to increase the therapeutic effect.
6. If there is nausea, or vomiting and diarrhoea, add CV-12 and ST-25 to regulate the Qi in the Middle Burner and harmonise the Spleen and Stomach.
7. If there is a general feeling of heaviness in the body, add BL-22 and BL-40 to promote urination and eliminate Damp from the body generally.

Case history

A 40-year-old-lady had been suffering from toe pain for a year. The pain was mainly in the two big toes, was aggravated by touch, warmth and walking, as well as by eating fatty, sweet foods and drinking alcohol, and was accompanied by redness and swelling, limited movement of the toes, restlessness and irritability. At the hospital she was diagnosed with gout. Accompanying symptoms included a bitter taste in the mouth, yellow urine, constipation, a poor appetite, a white and greasy tongue coating and a slippery and rapid pulse.

Diagnosis
Toe pain due to downward flow of Damp-Heat.

Principle of treatment
Clear Heat, remove Damp and relieve the pain.

Herbal treatment
BAI HU JIA GUI ZHI TANG
White Tiger Ramulus Cinnamomi Decoction
Shi Gao *Gypsum Fibrosum* 20 g
Zhi Mu *Rhizoma Anemarrhenae* 10 g
Gui Zhi *Ramulus Cinnamomi* 10 g
Gan Cao *Radix Glycyrrhizae* 6 g
Jing Mi *Semen Oryzae* 10 g
Du Huo *Radix Angelicae Pubescentis* 10 g

Han Fang Ji *Radix Stephaniae Tetrandrae* 10 g
Sang Zhi *Ramulus Mori* 10 g
Tu Fu Ling *Rhizoma Smilacis* 10 g
Sheng Di Huang *Radix Rehmanniae Recens* 15 g

The patient took the decoction twice a day.

Explanations
- Shi Gao and Zhi Mu clear Heat and relive irritability, nourish the Stomach and increase production of Body Fluids.
- Gan Cao and Jing Mi benefit the Stomach, reinforce the Body Fluids, and moderate the extremely Cold nature of Shi Gao and Zhi Mu.
- Gui Zhi dispels Wind and promotes the function of the collateral.
- Du Huo, Han Fang Ji and Sang Zhi eliminate Damp, promote the circulation of Blood and unblock the channels.
- Tu Fu Ling and Sheng Di Huang clear Heat, remove toxin, reduce the swelling and relieve the pain.

Acupuncture treatment
The same points as mentioned above were used. Acupuncture treatment was given once every 2 days.
  After treatment for a month, the toes were no longer painful. Two years later, she was followed up and she stated she had experienced no more pain since the treatment.

DEFICIENCY OF LIVER AND KIDNEY

Symptoms and signs

A constant but not severe pain in one or more toes, which is aggravated by walking, with rigidity of the toe in the morning, hyperosteogeny, muscular atrophy, soreness and weakness in the loin and knees, fatigue, a pale tongue with a thin and white coating, and a thready and weak pulse.

Principle of treatment

Replenish the Qi and Blood, strengthen the Kidney and Liver, dispel Wind-Cold-Damp, and smooth the channels and collateral.

HERBAL TREATMENT

Prescription

DU HUO JI SHENG TANG
Angelica Pubescens–Loranthus Decoction
Du Huo *Radix Angelicae Pubescentis* 9 g
Fang Feng *Radix Ledebouriellae* 6 g
Qin Jiao *Radix Gentianae Macrophyllae* 10 g
Xi Xin *Herba Asari* 3 g
Rou Gui *Cortex Cinnamomi* 5 g
Ren Shen *Radix Ginseng* 10 g

Fu Ling *Poria* 10 g
Dang Gui *Radix Angelicae Sinensis* 10 g
Chuan Xiong *Radix Ligustici Chuanxiong* 6 g
Shu Di Huang *Radix Rehmanniae Praeparata* 10 g
Bai Shao *Radix Paeonia Alba* 10 g
Du Zhong *Cortex Eucommiae* 10 g
Huai Niu Xi *Radix Achyranthis Bidentatae* 10 g
Sang Ji Sheng *Ramulus Loranthi* 10 g
Gan Cao *Radix Glycyrrhizae* 6 g

Explanations

- Du Huo, Fang Feng, Qin Jiao, Xi Xin and Rou Gui dispel Wind, remove Damp, dispel Cold and relieve the pain.
- Ren Shen, Fu Ling and Gan Cao tonify the Qi.
- Dang Gui, Chuan Xiong, Shu Di Huang and Bai Shao nourish the Blood and promote its circulation.
- Du Zhong, Huai Niu Xi and Sang Ji Sheng tonify the Liver and Kidney and strengthen the tendons and bones.

Modifications

1. If there is morning rigidity, add Wu Zhu Yu *Fructus Evodiae* 10 g to warm the channels and regulate the circulation of Blood.
2. If there is muscular atrophy, add Yin Yang Huo *Herba Epimedii* 10 g to warm the Kidney-Yang and promote the circulation of Blood.
3. If there is lower back pain with soreness, add Yi Zhi Ren *Fructus Alpiniae Oxyphyllae* 10 g and Gui Ban *Plastrum Testudinis* 10 g to tonify the Kidney-Essence.
4. If there is fatigue, add Huang Qi *Radix Astragali seu Hedysari* 15 g to activate the Spleen and tonify the Qi.

Patent remedies

Hai Ma Bu Shen Pian *Sea Horse Tonify Kidney Pill*
Du Huo Ji Sheng Wan *Angelica Pubescens–Loranthus Decoction*
Kang Gu Zheng Sheng Pian *Combat Bone Hyperplasia Pill*

ACUPUNCTURE TREATMENT

GB-39 Xuanzhong, GB-34 Yanglingquan, LR-3 Taichong, KI-3 Taixi, ST-36 Zusanli, SP-6 Sanyinjiao and Extra Bafeng. Even method is used on GB-34, LI-3, SP-6 and Extra Bafeng. Reinforcing method is used on the rest of the points.

Explanations

- This type of toe pain is often seen in old people due to the decline in the functions of the Liver and Kidney, so the Blood and Kidney-Essence become insufficient to nourish the tendons and bones. Therefore the Kidney and Liver should be strengthened first.
- LR-3 and KI-3, the Source points of the Liver and Kidney channels respectively, tonify the Liver and Kidney, and strengthen the tendons and bones.
- SP-6, the crossing point of the three Yin channels of the foot, strengthens the Spleen, Liver and Kidney and tonifies the Blood.
- GB-39, the Gathering point for the Marrow, and GB-34, the Gathering point for the tendons, reinforce the tendons and bones.
- ST-36, the Sea point of the Stomach channel, reinforces the Spleen and Stomach and promotes the production of the Blood.
- Extra Bafeng promotes the Qi and Blood circulation and relieves the toe pain.

Modifications

1. If there is swelling on the toes and feet, add SP-9 to eliminate Damp and reduce the swelling.
2. If there is swelling and even deformity in the toes due to stagnation of Blood, add SP-10 to promote the circulation of Blood and remove its stasis.
3. If there is a severe aversion to cold and a cold sensation in the joints, add moxibustion on the local points to dispel Cold.
4. If there is restlessness and insomnia, add HT-3 and PC-6 to calm the Mind and improve the sleep.
5. The corresponding points on the fingers should be added in order to increase the therapeutic effect.

STAGNATION OF QI AND BLOOD

Symptoms and signs

A fixed pain and purplish and swollen toe or toes, which is aggravated by pressure or movement and at night, with a history of trauma, no changes on the tongue, and a tight or wiry pulse.

Principle of treatment

Promote the Qi and Blood circulation, eliminate Blood stasis, smooth the channels and collateral and calm the pain.

HERBAL TREATMENT

Prescription

Acute stage

QI LI SAN (patent pill) 0.5 g each time, twice a day for oral intake
Seven-Thousandths of a Tael Powder
Xue Jie *Sanguis Draconis*
She Xiang *Secretio Mischus*
Bing Pian *Bomeolum Syntheticum*
Ru Xiang *Resina Olibani*
Mo Yao *Resina Myrrhae*
Hong Hua *Flos Carthami*
Er Cha *Catechu*
Apply the proper amount of Qi Li San (2 g) mixed with wine to the affected area.

Explanations

- Xue Jie is the main herb for arresting bleeding.
- Hong Hua, Ru Xiang and Mo Yao are good at promoting the circulation of Qi and Blood to eliminate the swelling and pain.
- She Xiang and Bing Pian promote the circulation of Blood to clear away obstruction in the channels.
- Er Cha, astringent in taste and Cool in nature, arrests bleeding and promotes the growth of new tissues.

Middle and restoration stage

BA XIAN XIAO YAO TANG
Ease of Decoction of Eight Ingredients
Fang Feng *Radix Ledebouriellae* 3 g
Jing Jie *Herba Schizonepetae* 3 g
Chuan Xiong *Radix Ligustici Chuanxiong* 3 g
Gan Cao *Radix Glycyrrhizae* 3 g
Dang Gui *Radix Angelicae Sinensis* 6 g
Cang Zhu *Rhizoma Atractylodis* 10 g
Chuan Jiao *Pericarpium Zanthoxyli Bungeani* 10 g
Ku Shen *Radix Sophorae Flavescentis* 15 g
Huang Bai *Cortex Phellodendri* 6 g
Soak the toes in a decoction of the above herbs once daily.

Explanations

- Fang Feng and Jing Jie disperse Wind.
- Chuan Xiong and Dang Gui remove Blood stagnation in the channels. Also, Chuan Xiong warms the channels, eliminates Cold and relieves the pain.
- Ku Shen and Huang Bai clear Heat and eliminate Damp.

- Gan Cao harmonises the actions of all the other herbs in the prescription.
- Chuan Jiao promotes circulation in the collaterals and stops the pain.
- This prescription disperses Wind, promotes the circulation of Blood and unblocks the channels.

Modifications

1. If there is dizziness, add Tian Ma *Rhizoma Gastrodiae* 10 g to regulate the circulation of Qi.
2. If there is insomnia, add Suan Zao Ren *Semen Ziziphi Spinosae* 10 g and Bai Zi Ren *Semen Biotae* 10 g to nourish the Heart-Blood and calm the Mind.
3. If there are dry stools, add Xuan Shen *Radix Scrophulariae* 10 g and Lu Hui Pasta *Aloes* 4 g to nourish the Yin and soften the stools.

Patent remedies

Xiao Huo Luo Dan *Minor Invigorating the Collaterals Special Pill*
Jin Gu Die Shang Wan *Muscle and Bone Traumatic Injury Pill*

ACUPUNCTURE TREATMENT

LI-4 Hegu, SP-6 Sanyinjiao, SP-10 Xuehai, BL-17 Geshu, LR-3 Taichong, GB-34 Yanglingquan and Extra Bafeng. Reducing method is used on these points.

Explanations

- LI-4 and LR-3, the Source points, promote the circulation of Qi in the channels, eliminate stagnation of Blood and relieve the pain.
- SP-6, the crossing point of the three Yin channels of the foot, BL-17, the Gathering point for the Blood, and SP-10 eliminate Blood stasis and relieve the pain.
- GB-34, the Sea point, strengthens the tendons and harmonises the movement of the joints.
- Extra Bafeng regulates the circulation of Qi and Blood in the channels and relieves the toe pain.

Modifications

1. The corresponding points on the fingers should be added in order to increase the therapeutic effect.
2. If there is restlessness and insomnia, add HT-3 and PC-6 to calm the Mind and improve the sleep.
3. If the feet and toes are swollen, add SP-3 to reduce the swelling.
4. If the toe has a purplish colour, add GB-44 and BL-67, the Well points, to promote the circulation of Blood and relieve the pain.

Leg pain 46

腿
痛

Leg pain may occur in the thighs or the lower legs, and in one or both legs.

All the three Yang channels of the foot and the three Yin channels of the foot pass through the leg. Any disturbance of these channels, whether due to external invasion or to internal disorders, may cause leg pain. According to TCM theory, leg pain can be caused by invasion of Wind-Cold-Damp in the channels, stagnation or deficiency of Qi and Blood, the downward flow of Damp-Heat in the channels, accumulation of Phlegm-Damp in the channels and collateral, or deficiency of Kidney-Essence.

Leg pain may be attributed to any of the following disorders in Western medicine: sciatica, rheumatic fever, nerve pain, paralysis or injury of the common peroneal nerve, a protrusion of the intervertebra disc, sprain of local muscles and thromboangiitis obliterans.

Aetiology and pathology

Invasion of Wind, Cold and Damp

Overexposure to windy, cold and damp weather, or living in a cold and damp environment may allow the pathogenic factors Wind, Cold and Damp to invade the lower limbs. Cold is characterised by contraction and stagnation; Damp is marked by heaviness and lingering. If Cold-Damp invades the lower limbs, therefore, there is contraction of the collateral and muscles in the leg, leading to stagnation of Qi and Blood, and causing leg pain. This kind of leg pain usually has the characteristic that it is aggravated by cold and humid weather.

When there is invasion of Wind, Damp-Heat to the body and lower limbs, it may cause stagnation of Qi and Blood circulation in the channels and blockage of the channels by Damp-Heat, which results in leg pain. Prolonged persistence of Cold-Damp in the body may also cause a gradual generation of Heat, leading to formation of Damp-Heat, and again resulting in leg pain.

Bad diet

Bad diets, such as eating too much sweet, pungent or fatty food, or milk products, or drinking too much alcohol, may impair the Spleen and Stomach, leading to the formation of Damp-Heat in the body. When Damp-Heat flows downward to the lower limbs, it blocks the channels, and causes leg pain.

Stagnation of Qi and Blood

Qi and Blood should circulate freely in the channels and collateral. If there is stagnation of Qi and Blood due to various causes, such as overstrain, physical trauma, or inappropriate operation on the leg, the channels will become blocked by the impeded Qi and Blood circulation, leading to leg pain with a stabbing nature.

Deficiency of Qi and Blood

In TCM one of the two causes for pain is undernourishment of the channels and collaterals. This may happen as a result of excessive strain or prolonged illness, which may consume the Qi and Blood, resulting in a deficiency of Qi and Blood. When there is insufficient Qi and Blood to nourish the leg properly, the leg pain occurs.

Downward flow of Damp-Heat

Since Damp has the characteristics of heaviness and lingering, if external Damp-Heat invasion is not eliminated in time, it may cause a flow of Damp-Heat down the leg. When Damp-Heat blocks the leg channels it triggers leg pain.

Bad diets or bad eating habits impair the Spleen and Stomach; this causes Damp-Heat to form in the Middle Burner. When Damp-Heat remains in the Middle Burner over a long period, it may flow downward into the leg, and leg pain then occurs because the channels become blocked by Damp-Heat, which leads to stagnation of Qi and Blood.

Accumulation of Phlegm-Damp in the channels and collaterals

Overeating of fatty or sweet food, or milk products as well as raw and cold food, may cause internal Damp to form. These kinds of food are rich of energy and nutrition, but are more difficult to digest than other kinds of food and drinks. Too much raw and cold food can also impair the Yang of the Spleen. All these foods therefore will place a burden on the Spleen and Stomach, and their physiological functions will be damaged. When the Spleen fails to transport and transform food properly, then internal Damp forms.

Internal Phlegm-Damp also tends to be produced by some people who have poor water metabolism, whether resulting from a constitutional weakness in the Spleen and Stomach, or from overstrain or an irregular diet.

When Phlegm-Damp forms, like Damp-Heat it may flow downward to the leg and disturb the Qi and Blood circulation in the channels, causing leg pain.

Deficiency of Kidney-Essence

The Kidney dominates the Bones, and the lower back is the house of the Kidney. Because of excessive strain, a prolonged sickness, a poor constitution, or old age the Kidney-Essence may be consumed, which results in deficiency of the Kidney-Essence and weakness of the Qi and Blood; in this condition the lower back and leg are not properly nourished, so that weakness of the legs with pain occurs. This kind of leg pain is often characterised by weakness in the lower back, knees and legs, an aggravation of the pain by standing for too long and alleviation with rest.

Treatment based on differentiation

Differentiation

Differentiation of External or Internal origin

— Acute onset of leg pain of short duration, accompanied by External symptoms, is usually caused by invasion of External pathogenic factors. Traumatic injury could also cause acute leg pain.
— Chronic onset of leg pain of long duration, accompanied by some symptoms resulting from internal disorders, is usually caused by disorders of the internal organs such as deficiency of Qi and Blood, deficiency of Liver and Kidney, downward flow of Damp-Heat, or stagnation of Qi and Blood.

Differentiation of the pain due to Excess or Deficiency

— Severe or constant leg pain is usually caused by an Excess syndrome, such as invasion of Wind, Cold and Damp, accumulation of Phlegm-Damp in the channels and collaterals, downward flow of Damp-Heat, or stagnation of Qi and Blood.
— Intermittent or slight leg pain is usually caused by Deficiency, such as deficiency of Qi and Blood, or deficiency of Kidney-Essence.

Differentiation of the character of the pain

— Acute onset of leg pain with a cold sensation and heaviness, accompanied by an aversion to cold, slight fever, or cold limbs, is usually caused by invasion of Wind, Cold and Damp.

— Gradual onset of a dull leg pain with heaviness and swelling, accompanied by nausea, poor appetite, or loose stools, is usually caused by accumulation of Phlegm-Damp in the channels and collaterals.

— Stabbing leg pain with a fixed location, swelling and hardening of the muscles, aggravation of the pain at night, or a purplish tongue, is usually caused by stagnation of Qi and Blood.

— Gradual onset of leg pain with numbness and weakness of the lower limbs, aggravation of the leg pain by exertion, tiredness, or a pale complexion, is due to deficiency of Qi and Blood.

— Leg pain with burning, heaviness and redness, is usually caused by downward flow of Damp-Heat.

— Chronic leg pain, with lower back pain, weakness of the legs and knees, muscular atrophy, hair loss, or poor memory, is usually caused by deficiency of Kidney-Essence.

Treatment

INVASION OF WIND, COLD AND DAMP

Symptoms and signs

Leg pain with cold and heavy sensation, which worsens in cold and damp weather, with difficult movements of the lower limbs, an aversion to cold, slight generalised body pain, a slight fever, neck pain, a headache, a slight cough, a thin, white and greasy tongue coating and a deep and tight pulse.

Principle of treatment

Dispel Wind, eliminate Cold, remove Damp, promote circulation in the channels and relieve the pain.

HERBAL TREATMENT

Prescription

GAN JIANG LING ZHU TANG

Licorice, Ginger, Poria and Atractylodis Decoction
Gan Jiang *Rhizoma Zingiberis* 6 g
Gan Cao *Radix Glycyrrhizae* 6 g
Fu Ling *Poria* 15 g
Bai Zhu *Rhizoma Atractylodis Macrocephalae* 12 g
Gui Zhi *Ramulus Cinnamomi* 6 g
Huai Niu Xi *Radix Achyranthis Bidentatae* 15 g

Explanations

● Fu Ling and Bai Zhu strengthen the Spleen and remove the Damp. The Spleen dominates the muscles and transports Damp. If the Spleen-Yang is deficient, there may be invasion of Wind, Cold and Damp to the muscles, leading to leg pain.

● Gan Jiang and Gan Cao dispel Wind-Cold and warm the Middle Burner.

● Gui Zhi dispels Wind, Cold and Damp and relieves External symptoms. It can also promote circulation in the collateral and relieve the leg pain.

● Huai Niu Xi promotes Qi and Blood circulation in the channels, and eliminates Damp and Blood stagnation in the muscles. Moreover, this herb can also induce the other herbs in the prescription to reach the lower leg.

Modifications

1. If there is a severe aversion to cold and muscular spasm, add Fu Zi *Radix Aconiti Lateralis Praeparata* 10 g to warm the channels and collateral and relieve the spasm.

2. If there is swelling in the legs or a heavy sensation in the lower limbs, add Du Huo *Radix Angelicae Pubescentis* 10 g and Cang Zhu *Rhizoma Atractylodis* 10 g to remove Damp and sedate the pain.

3. If there are cold limbs and lower back pain due to deficiency of Kidney-Yang, add Tu Si Zi *Semen Cuscutae* 10 g and Du Zhong *Cortex Eucommiae* 10 g to reinforce the Kidney-Yang.

4. If there is a headache, add Man Jing Zi *Fructus Viticis* 10 g to dispel Wind and sedate the headache.

5. If there is scanty urination, add Che Qian Zi *Semen Plantaginis* 10 g to promote urination and eliminate Damp.

Patent remedies

Han Shi Bi Chong Ji *Cold-Damp Bi Syndrome Infusion*
Jing Fang Bai Du Pian *Schizonepeta and Ledebouriella Tablet to Overcome Pathogenic Influences*
Tian Ma Qu Feng Bu Pian *Gastrodia Dispel Wind Formula Tablet*
Feng Shi Pian *Wind-Damp Tablet*

ACUPUNCTURE TREATMENT

TE-5 Waiguan, LI-4 Hegu, BL-12 Fengmen, GB-30 Huantiao, GB-31 Fengshi, GB-35 Yangjiao, SP-6 Sanyinjiao and some local Ah Shi points. Reducing method is used on these points. Moxibustion is used on all the points except SP-6.

Explanations

- TE-5, LI-4 and BL-12 dispel External pathogenic Wind, Cold and Damp and relieve External symptoms.
- GB-30, the meeting point of the Gall Bladder and the Bladder channels, eliminates Damp and Wind, invigorates the circulation of Qi in the collateral, and removes obstructions in the channels so as to relieve the leg pain.
- GB-31 dispels External Wind and eliminates Damp in the lower limbs.
- GB-35, the Accumulation point of the Yang Linking Vessel, harmonises the collateral, promotes the Qi and Blood circulation and relieves the leg pain.
- The local Ah Shi points are suitable for regulating the circulation of Qi and Blood in the locality.
- SP-6, the crossing point of the Kidney, Spleen and Liver channels, regulates the Blood and Qi and relieves the leg pain.
- Moxibustion warms the channels and dispels Cold.

Modifications

1. If there is a severe aversion to cold and muscular spasm, add moxibustion on CV-4 to warm the channels and collateral and relieve the spasm.
2. If there is swelling or a heavy sensation in the lower limbs, add SP-9 to remove the Damp and sedate the pain.
3. If there is leg pain along the Bladder channel, add BL-36, BL-58, BL-63 and BL-64 to harmonise the collateral and relieve the pain.
4. If there is leg pain along the Gall Bladder channel, add GB-36, GB-34, GB-40 and GB-41 to promote the Qi and Blood circulation in the channel and relieve the pain.
5. If there is leg pain along the Stomach channel, add ST-30, ST-31, ST-34, ST-40 and ST-42 to promote the Qi and Blood circulation in the channel, relieve the blockage and arrest the pain.
6. If there is leg pain along the Liver channel, add LR-3, LR-5, LR-11 and LR-12 to harmonise the collateral, promote the Qi and Blood circulation in the channel and relieve the pain.
7. If there is leg pain along the Spleen channel, add SP-3, SP-4, SP-8 and SP-11 to promote the Qi and Blood circulation in the channel, harmonise the collateral and relieve the leg pain.
8. If there is leg pain along the Kidney channel, add KI-4, KI-5, KI-8 and KI-10 to regulate the Qi and Blood circulation in the channel and relieve the leg pain.
9. If there are cold limbs and lower back pain due to deficiency of Kidney-Yang, add KI-3 and BL-23 to reinforce the Kidney-Yang, dispel Cold and strengthen the lower back.
10. If there is a headache, add GB-20 to dispel Wind and sedate the headache.
11. If there is scanty urination, add BL-64, the Source point, to promote urination and eliminate Damp.

STAGNATION OF QI AND BLOOD

Symptoms and signs

Pricking pain or stabbing pain on the leg with long history, which is aggravated at night or with rest and is alleviated during the day or by movement, accompanied by limited movement of legs, a dark and purple tongue with a thin and white tongue coating and a wiry and hesitant pulse.

Principle of treatment

Promote Qi and Blood circulation, remove Blood stasis, clear the channels and collateral and sedate the pain.

HERBAL TREATMENT

Prescription

SHEN TONG ZHU YU TANG
Meridian Passage
Dang Gui *Radix Angelicae Sinensis* 12 g
Chuan Xiong *Rhizoma Ligustici Chuanxiong* 12 g
Tao Ren *Semen Persicae* 12 g
Hong Hua *Flos Carthami* 12 g
Mo Yao *Resina Myrrhae* 10 g
Wu Ling Zhi *Faeces Trogopterorum* 10 g
Xiang Fu *Rhizoma Cyperi* 12 g
Huai Niu Xi *Radix Achyranthis Bidentatae* 15 g

Explanations

- Dang Gui, Chuan Xiong, Tao Ren and Hong Hua promote the circulation of Blood and remove its stasis.
- Mo Yao and Wu Ling Zhi relieve the swelling and sedate the pain. These two herbs can also promote the circulation of Blood and remove its stasis.
- Xiang Fu promotes the circulation of Qi so as to promote the circulation of Blood.

- Huai Niu Xi removes Blood stasis in the lower limbs and strengthens the lumbar area and lower limbs.

Modifications

1. If there is severe leg pain due to traumatic injury, add Ru Xiang *Resina Olibani* 6 g and San Qi *Radix Notoginseng* 10 g to strengthen the function of promoting the Qi and Blood circulation, remove Blood stasis, promote healing and relieve the leg pain.
2. If there is leg pain due to invasion of Wind, Cold and Damp, add Du Huo *Radix Angelicae Pubescentis* 10 g and Qin Jiao *Radix Gentianae Macrophyllae* 10 g to dispel the Wind-Cold and remove the Damp.
3. If there is aggravation of the leg pain by emotional disturbance, add Qing Pi *Pericarpium Citri Reticulatae Viride* 10 g and Zhi Ke *Fructus Aurantii* 10 g to smooth the Liver, promote the circulation of Liver-Qi and regulate the emotions.
4. If there is insomnia due to leg pain, add Long Gu *Os Draconis* 20 g and Fu Shen *Sclerotium Poriae Pararadicis* 10 g to calm the Mind and improve the sleep.

Patent remedies

Jin Gu Die Shang Wan *Muscle and Bone Traumatic Injury Pill*
Xiao Huo Luo Dan *Minor Invigorate the Collaterals Pill*

ACUPUNCTURE TREATMENT

LI-4 Hegu, SP-6 Sanyinjiao, BL-17 Geshu, LR-3 Taichong, GB-30 Huantiao and some Ah Shi points. Reducing method is used on these points.

Explanations

- LI-4 and LR-3, the Source points, promote the circulation of Qi in the channels, eliminate stagnation of Blood and relieve the pain.
- SP-6, the crossing point of the three Yin channels of the foot, and BL-17, the Gathering point for the Blood, promote the circulation of Blood, eliminate its stasis and relieve the leg pain.
- GB-30, the meeting point of the Gall Bladder and the Bladder channels, eliminates Damp and Wind, invigorates the circulation of Qi in the collateral and removes obstructions in the channels so as to relieve the leg pain.

- The Ah Shi points remove obstructions in the channels and collateral and relieve the leg pain.

Modifications

1. If there is leg pain due to bone fracture, add BL-11, the Gathering point for the Bones, and GB-39, the Gathering point for the Marrow, to promote the circulation of Blood and speed up the bone healing.
2. If the leg is swollen, add SP-9 to promote circulation in the channels and reduce swelling.
3. If there is restlessness at night or insomnia due to severe pain, add HT-3 and HT-7 to calm the Mind and improve the sleep.
4. If there is a sensation of heat in the leg due to formation of Heat in the Blood resulting from prolonged duration of Blood stagnation, add SP-10 to clear Heat in the Blood and promote Blood circulation.
5. If there is leg pain along the Bladder channel, add BL-36, BL-58, BL-63 and BL-64 to harmonise the collateral and relieve the pain.
6. If there is leg pain along the Gall Bladder channel, add GB-36, GB-34, GB-40 and GB-41 to promote the circulation of Qi and Blood in the channel and relieve the pain.
7. If there is leg pain along the Stomach channel, add ST-30, ST-31, ST-34, ST-40 and ST-42 to promote the circulation of Qi and Blood in the channel, relieve the blockage and arrest the pain.
8. If there is leg pain along the Liver channel, add LR-3, LR-5, LR-11 and LR-12 to harmonise the collateral, promote the circulation of Qi and Blood in the channel and relieve the pain.
9. If there is leg pain along the Spleen channel, add SP-3, SP-4, SP-8 and SP-11 to promote the circulation of Qi and Blood in the channel, harmonise the collateral and relieve the leg pain.
10. If there is leg pain along the Kidney channel, add KI-4, KI-5, KI-8 and KI-10 to regulate the circulation of Qi and Blood in the channel and relieve the leg pain.

Case history

A 51-year-old male had been suffering from a pricking pain in his left leg for 3 years, and this had worsened during the previous 30 days. Three years previously, he had suffered lumbago on his left side caused by lifting some heavy items. He was diagnosed as having a hernia between vertebrae L4 and L5. He received two epidural injections of corticosteroids, but this did not help very much.

When he arrived at the clinic, he stated that he had a pricking pain in the leg, which was mainly located along the Gall Bladder channel down to the fourth toe. His pain was aggravated when he had a cough, and worsened especially at night. It usually improved if he walked around a bit. He had limited movement in his left leg, a purplish tongue with a thin and white coating, and a wiry pulse.

Diagnosis
Leg pain due to stagnation of Qi and Blood.

Principle of treatment
Promote Qi and Blood circulation, remove Blood stasis, harmonise the collateral and sedate the pain.

Acupuncture treatment
LI-4, SP-6, BL-11, BL-17, BL-15, GB-30, GB-34, GB-36, GB-40 and GB-44. Reducing method was used on these points. Treatment was given once every 3 days.

Explanations

- LI-4, the Source point, promotes the circulation of Qi in the channels, eliminates stagnation of Blood and relieves the pain.
- SP-6, the crossing point of the three Yin channels of the foot, and BL-17, the Gathering point for the Blood, promote the circulation of Blood, eliminate its stasis and relieve the leg pain.
- GB-30, the meeting point of the Gall Bladder and the Bladder channels, GB-34, the Gathering point for the tendons, GB-36, the Accumulation point of the Gall Bladder channel, and GB-40, the Source point, harmonise the collateral, invigorate the Qi and Blood circulation in the collateral and remove Blood stasis so as to relieve the leg pain.
- BL-11, the Gathering point for the Bones, strengthens the bones in the lower back regions.
- BL-15, the Back Transporting point of the Heart, calms the Mind and improves the sleep.

The pain was much better after five treatment sessions. Meanwhile, he was required to avoid putting strain on his back and take care of how he moved his back.

DEFICIENCY OF QI AND BLOOD

Symptoms and signs

Intermittent slight leg pain, which is alleviated by pressure and rest and aggravated by standing for too long and on exertion, with numbness and weakness of the lower limbs, tiredness, a pale complexion, shortness of breath, lower back pain, nycturia, a pale tongue with a thin and white coating and a deep and weak pulse.

Principle of treatment

Reinforce Qi and nourish Blood, tonify the Kidney-Essence and sedate the pain.

HERBAL TREATMENT

Prescription

BA ZHEN TANG
Eight-Precious Decoction
Dang Gui *Radix Angelicae Sinensis* 12 g
Chuan Xiong *Rhizoma Ligustici Chuanxiong* 10 g
Bai Shao *Radix Paeoniae Alba* 12 g
Shu Di Huang *Radix Rehmanniae Praeparata* 12 g
Ren Shen *Radix Ginseng* 6 g
Bai Zhu *Rhizoma Atractylodis Macrocephalae* 12 g
Fu Ling *Poria* 12 g
Zhi Gan Cao *Radix Glycyrrhizae* 6 g

Explanations

- Dang Gui, Bai Shao and Shu Di Huang nourish the Blood and tonify the Kidney-Essence.
- Ren Shen, Bai Zhu, Fu Ling and Zhi Gan Cao strengthen the Spleen and Stomach and reinforce the Qi.
- Chuan Xiong activates the circulation of Qi and Blood and relieves obstruction in the channels.
- When the Qi and Blood are tonified and the muscles and collateral are properly nourished, the leg pain will disappear.

Modifications

1. If there is an aversion to cold or cold limbs due to deficiency of Qi, add Gui Zhi *Ramulus Cinnamomi* 10 g and Wu Zhu Yu *Fructus Evodiae* 6 g to reinforce the Yang-Qi and dispel Cold.
2. If there is swelling in the legs due to water retention, add Zhu Ling *Polyporus Umbellatus* 15 g and Ze Xie *Rhizoma Alismatis* 15 g to strengthen the Spleen, promote urination and relieve the leg swelling.
3. If there is shortness of breath and a pale complexion, add Huang Qi *Radix Astragali seu Hedysari* 12 g and Shan Yao *Rhizoma Dioscoreae* 10 g to activate the Spleen, tonify the Qi and relieve the shortness of breath.
4. If there are loose stools or diarrhoea, add Ge Gen *Radix Puerariae* 10 g and Yi Yi Ren *Semen Coicis* 15 g to lift the Spleen-Qi and relieve the diarrhoea.

Patent remedy

Shi Quan Da Bu Wan *All-Inclusive Great Tonifying Pill*

ACUPUNCTURE TREATMENT

GB-34 Yanglingquan, GB-39 Xuanzhong, LR-3 Taichong, KI-3 Taixi, ST-36 Zusanli, SP-6 Sanyinjiao and Ah Shi points. Reinforcing method is used on these points except for the Ah Shi points, on which even method is used.

Explanations

- LR-3 and KI-3, the Source points of the Liver and Kidney channels respectively, tonify the Liver and Kidney, and strengthen the tendons and bones. LR-3 can also promote the circulation of Qi and Blood and relieve the leg pain.
- SP-6, the crossing point of the three Yin channels of the foot, strengthens the Spleen, Liver and Kidney and tonifies the Blood.
- GB-39, the Gathering point for the Marrow, and GB-34, the Gathering point for the tendons, reinforce the tendons and bones.
- ST-36, the Sea point of the Stomach channel, reinforces the Spleen and Stomach and promotes the production of Qi and Blood.
- The Ah Shi points, the local points, harmonise the collateral, promote the circulation of Qi and Blood in the channels and relieve the leg pain.

Modifications

1. If there is an aversion to cold or cold limbs due to deficiency of Qi, add moxibustion on CV-4 to reinforce the Yang-Qi and dispel Cold.
2. If there is swelling in the legs due to water retention, add SP-9 to strengthen the Spleen and promote urination and reduce the swelling.
3. If there is leg pain along the Bladder channel, add BL-36, BL-58, BL-63 and BL-64 to harmonise the collateral and relieve the pain.
4. If there is leg pain along the Gall Bladder channel, add GB-36, GB-34, GB-40 and GB-41 to promote the circulation of Qi and Blood in the channel and relieve the pain.
5. If there is leg pain along the Stomach channel, add ST-30, ST-31, ST-34, ST-40 and ST-42 to promote the circulation of Qi and Blood in the channel, relieve the blockage and arrest the pain.
6. If there is leg pain along the Liver channel, add LR-3, LR-5, LR-11 and LR-12 to harmonise the collateral, promote the circulation of Qi and Blood in the channel and relieve the pain.
7. If there is leg pain along the Spleen channel, add SP-3, SP-4, SP-8 and SP-11 to promote the circulation of Qi and Blood in the channel, harmonise the collateral and relieve the leg pain.
8. If there is leg pain along the Kidney channel, add KI-4, KI-5, KI-8 and KI-10 to regulate the circulation of Qi and Blood in the channel and relieve the leg pain.
9. If there is shortness of breath and pale complexion, add CV-6 and CV-17 to tonify the Qi, relax the chest and relieve the shortness of breath.
10. If there are loose stools or diarrhoea, add ST-25, the Front Collecting point of the Large Intestine, and SP-3, the Source point, to lift the Spleen-Qi and relieve the diarrhoea.

Case history

A 50-year-old man had been suffering from dull leg pain in both legs for more than 6 months, which worsened after exertion. He also had numbness and swelling in his legs, dizziness, scanty urination, shortness of breath, palpitations, a thin and white tongue coating and a deep and weak pulse.

Diagnosis
Leg pain due to deficiency of Qi and Blood.

Acupuncture treatment
GB-34, GB-39, KI-3, SP-6, SP-9, BL-18, BL-20 and Ah Shi points. Reinforcing method was used on these points, except for the Ah Shi points, on which even method was used. Treatment was given once every 3 days.

Explanations

- KI-3, the Source point, BL-18, the Back Transporting point of the Liver, and BL-20, the Back Transporting point of the Spleen, tonify the Spleen, Liver and Kidney, and strengthen the tendons and bones.
- SP-6, the crossing point of the three Yin channels of the foot, strengthens the Spleen, Liver and Kidney and tonifies the Blood.
- SP-9, the Sea point, activates the Spleen, eliminates Damp and reduces the swelling.
- GB-39, the Gathering point for the Marrow, and GB-34, the Gathering point for the tendons, reinforce the tendons and bones and tonify the Blood.
- The Ah Shi points, the local points, harmonise the collateral, promote the circulation of Qi and Blood in the channels and relieve the leg pain.

After treatment for 2 months, his leg pain was much improved and his legs were no longer swollen. Six months later, he was followed up by telephone and he stated that he had experienced no more leg pain since the treatment.

DOWNWARD FLOW OF DAMP-HEAT

Symptoms and signs

Leg pain with a burning and heavy sensation, which is aggravated by touching or worsens on hot or rainy days and is alleviated by movement, with redness, ulceration and swelling in the leg, accompanied by scanty and yellow urination, a yellow and greasy tongue coating, and a slippery and rapid pulse.

Principle of treatment

Clear Heat, eliminate Damp, harmonise the collateral and sedate the pain.

HERBAL TREATMENT

Prescription

SI MIAO WAN
Four-Marvel Pill
Cang Zhu *Rhizoma Atractylodis* 10 g
Huang Bai *Cortex Phellodendri* 12 g
Yi Yi Ren *Semen Coicis* 15 g
Huai Niu Xi *Radix Achyranthis Bidentatae* 15 g
Hua Shi *Talcum* 15 g

Explanations

- Cang Zhu, Warm in nature and bitter in flavour, activates the Spleen and dries Damp.
- Huang Bai clears Heat in the Lower Burner and dries Damp.
- Hua Shi and Yi Yi Ren promote urination and eliminate Damp-Heat in the Lower Burner.
- Huai Niu Xi strengthens the lower limbs and promotes the circulation of Blood so as to relieve the leg pain. This herb also induces the other herbs to reach the legs.

Modifications

1. If there is a red tongue, thirst, and restlessness, add Zhi Zi *Rhizoma Gardeniae* 10 g and Huang Lian *Rhizoma Coptidis* 5 g to clear Heat and remove Toxin.
2. If there is a fever, add Zhi Mu *Rhizoma Anemarrhenae* 10 g and Shi Gao *Gypsum Fibrosum* 20 g to clear Heat and reduce the fever.
3. If there is scanty urination, add Ze Xie *Rhizoma Alismatis* 12 g and Mu Tong *Caulis Akebiae* 6 g to promote urination and eliminate Damp.
4. If there is redness of the legs and ulceration, add Pu Gong Ying *Herba Taraxaci* 15 g and Zi Hua Di Ding *Herba Violae* 15 g to clear Toxin, remove Heat and promote healing.
5. If there is weakness of the legs, dry throat and a sensation of heat in the palms and soles of the feet due to damage to the Kidney-Yin caused by prolonged duration of Damp-Heat, add Nu Zhen Zi *Fructus Ligustri Lucidi* 10 g and Han Lian Cao

Herba Ecliptae 10 g to nourish the Kidney-Yin and clear Deficient-Heat.
6. If there is itching of the legs with oozing, add Di Fu Zi *Fructus Kochiae* 10 g and Chi Shao *Radix Paeoniae Rubra* 10 g to eliminate Damp-Heat and cool the Blood.
7. If there is severe leg pain, add Jiang Huang *Rhizoma Curcumae Longae* 10 g to clear Heat, promote the circulation of Blood and stop the pain.
8. If the appetite is poor, add Ban Xia *Rhizoma Pinelliae* 10 g and Chen Pi *Pericarpium Citri Reticulatae* 10 g to regulate the Qi in the Middle Burner and improve the appetite.
9. If there is a thirst, add Xuan Shen *Radix Scrophulariae* 10 g and Ge Gen *Radix Puerariae* 10 g to clear Heat and relieve the thirst.
10. If there is irritability, add Deng Xin Cao *Medulla Junci* 15 g to clear Fire and calm down the Mind.
11. If there is constipation, add Da Huang *Radix et Rhizoma Rhei* 6 g and Mang Xiao *Natrii Sulfas* 6 g to eliminate Heat, promote defecation and relieve the constipation.

Patent remedies

San Miao Wan *Three-Marvel Pill*
Feng Shi Xiao Tong Wan *Wind-Damp Dispel Pain Tablet*

ACUPUNCTURE TREATMENT

TE-6 Zhigou, LI-4 Hegu, ST-40 Fenglong, SP-6 Sanyinjiao, SP-9 Yinlingquan, GB-34 Yanglingquan, ST-44 Neiting and some Ah Shi points. Reducing method is used on these points.

Explanations

- TE-6 and LI-4 promote the circulation of Qi in the channels, eliminate Damp and reduce Heat.
- ST-40, the Connecting point, SP-6, the crossing point of the three Yin channels of the foot, and SP-9 and GB-34, the Sea points, eliminate Damp in the body and channels and clear Heat so as to relieve the pain.
- BL-64, the Source point, dispels External pathogenic factors, promotes urination, eliminates Damp and relieves the leg pain.
- ST-44, the Spring point, eliminates Damp-Heat and reduces fever.
- The Ah Shi points eliminate Damp, regulate circulation of Qi and Blood in the channels and relieve the leg pain.

Modifications

1. If there is leg pain along the Bladder channel, add BL-36, BL-58, BL-63 and BL-64 to harmonise the collateral and relieve the pain.
2. If there is leg pain along the Gall Bladder channel, add GB-36, GB-34 and GB-40 to promote Qi and Blood circulation in the channel and relieve the pain.
3. If there is leg pain along the Stomach channel, add ST-30, ST-31, ST-34, ST-40 and ST-42 to promote Qi and Blood circulation in the channel, relieve the blockage and arrest the pain.
4. If there is leg pain along the Liver channel, add LR-3, LR-5, LR-11 and LR-12 to harmonise the collateral, promote Qi and Blood circulation in the channel and relieve the pain.
5. If there is leg pain along the Spleen channel, add SP-3, SP-4, SP-8 and SP-11 to promote Qi and Blood circulation in the channel, harmonise the collateral and relieve the pain.
6. If there is leg pain along the Kidney channel, add KI-4, KI-5, KI-8 and KI-10 to regulate Qi and Blood circulation in the channel and relieve the pain.
7. If there is a red tongue, thirst and restlessness, add SP-10 and HT-3 to clear Heat and remove Toxin.
8. If there is a fever, add GV-14 to clear Heat and reduce the fever.
9. If there is scanty urination, add CV-2 to promote urination and eliminate Damp.
10. If there is redness on the legs and ulceration, add BL-66 and GB-43, the Spring points, to clear toxin, remove Heat and promote healing.
11. If there is weakness in the legs, dry throat and a sensation of heat in the palms and soles of the foot due to damage to the Kidney-Yin caused by prolonged duration of Damp-Heat, add KI-6 and KI-7 to nourish the Kidney-Yin and clear Deficient-Heat.
12. If there is itching in the legs with oozing, add GB-41 to eliminate Damp-Heat and cool the Blood.
13. If there is severe leg pain, add LR-3 to promote Qi and Blood circulation and stop the pain.
14. If the appetite is poor, add SP-3 to activate the Spleen, regulate the Qi in the Middle Burner and improve the appetite.
15. If there is a thirst, add CV-12 to clear Heat and relieve the thirst.
16. If there is irritability, add GB-20 to clear Fire and calm the Mind.
17. If there is constipation, add ST-25, the Front Collecting point of the Large Intestine, to eliminate Heat, promote defecation and relieve the constipation.

Case history

A 35-year-old man had been suffering from leg pain in his right side with a heavy sensation for 6 months. He also had a slight sensation of heat in his right leg. The pain was aggravated by touching and worsened on rainy days and with limited movement. The pain was mainly along the Bladder Channel. His doctor told him that he had inflammation of the muscles in the leg and gave him some painkillers, but these did not much improve the leg pain.

Accompanying symptoms were: nausea, a bitter taste in the mouth, a thirst but no desire to drink, scanty yellow urine, constipation, a poor appetite, a yellow and greasy tongue coating and a slippery and rapid pulse.

Diagnosis
Leg pain due to downward flow of Damp-Heat.

Principle of treatment
Clear Heat, remove Damp, harmonise the collateral and sedate the pain.

Acupuncture treatment
ST-40, SP-6, SP-9, GB-34, BL-36, BL-40, BL-58, BL-63 and BL-64. Reducing method was applied on these points. The treatment was given once every 3 days.

Explanations

- ST-40, the Connecting point, SP-6, the crossing point of the three Yin channels of the foot, and SP-9 and GB-34, the Sea points, eliminate Damp in the body and channels and clear Heat so as to relieve the pain.
- BL-36, the local point, BL-40, the Sea point, BL-58, the Connecting point, BL-63, the Accumulation point and BL-64, the Source point, promote urination, eliminate Damp, harmonise the collateral, promote circulation in the channel and relieve the leg pain.

After treatment for 2 weeks, his leg pain had started to improve, his urination was much easier. His appetite and defecation had also improved. After treatment for 2 months, the leg pain had disappeared.

ACCUMULATION OF PHLEGM-DAMP IN THE CHANNELS AND COLLATERAL

Symptoms and signs

Chronic onset of leg pain with a heavy sensation, which worsens on rainy days and is alleviated by movement, accompanied by oedema in the legs, formation of nodules on the legs, a lower back pain with a heavy feeling, nausea, dizziness, a poor appetite, loose stools, or diarrhoea, a swollen tongue with tooth marks and a white and greasy coating, and a slippery and deep pulse.

Principle of treatment

Remove Phlegm, eliminate Damp, promote circulation in the channels and collateral, and sedate the pain.

HERBAL TREATMENT

Prescription

ER CHEN TANG
Two-Cured Decoction
Ban Xia *Rhizoma Pinelliae* 12 g
Chen Pi *Pericarpium Citri Reticulatae* 12 g
Fu Ling *Poria* 15 g
Gan Cao *Radix Glycyrrhizae* 6 g
Qiang Huo *Rhizoma et Radix Notopterygii* 12 g
Bai Zhu *Rhizoma Atractylodis Macrocephalae* 12 g
Sheng Jiang *Rhizoma Zingiberis Recens* 3 g
Huai Niu Xi *Radix Achyranthis Bidentatae* 15 g

Explanations

- Ban Xia, Warm in nature and pungent in flavour, dries Damp and removes Phlegm. It can also regulate the Stomach-Qi and relieve the nausea.
- Chen Pi smoothes the circulation of Qi in the Middle Burner and resolves Phlegm.
- Fu Ling and Bai Zhu activate the Spleen and Stomach and promote transportation of Phlegm.
- Qiang Huo removes Phlegm-Damp in the channels and collaterals as well as in the muscles. It can also relieve the leg pain.
- Huai Niu Xi promotes circulation in the channels and collaterals, eliminates Blood stasis and relieves the leg pain.
- Sheng Jiang harmonises the Stomach and resolves Phlegm-Damp.
- Gan Cao coordinates the actions of the other herbs in the formula and regulates the Middle Burner.

Modifications

1. If there are nodules on the legs, add Zhi Shi *Fructus Aurantii Immaturus* 10 g and Kun Bu *Thallus Laminariae* 10 g to soften and eliminate the nodules and promote the circulation of Qi.
2. If there is swelling of the legs due to water retention, add Zhu Ling *Polyporus Umbellatus* 15 g and Ze Xie *Rhizoma Alismatis* 15 g to strengthen the Spleen, promote urination and reduce the swelling.
3. If there is an aversion to cold or cold limbs due to deficiency of Qi, add Gui Zhi *Ramulus Cinnamomi* 10 g and Wu Zhu Yu *Fructus Evodiae* 6 g to reinforce the Yang-Qi and dispel Cold.

4. If there is itching of the legs with oozing, add Di Fu Zi *Fructus Kochiae* 10 g to eliminate Damp and stop the itching.
5. If there is a cough with profuse sputum due to accumulation of Phlegm in the Lung, add Dan Nan Xing *Arisaema cum Bile* 10 g and Zhu Ru *Caulis Bambusae in Taeniam* 10 g to resolve Phlegm, help the Lung-Qi descend and relieve the cough.
6. If the appetite is poor, add Sha Ren *Fructus Amomi* 10 g and Mai Ya *Fructus Hordei Germinatus* 15 g to regulate the Qi in the Middle Burner, activate the Stomach and improve the appetite.
7. If there are loose stools or diarrhoea, add Ge Gen *Radix Puerariae* 10 g and Yi Yi Ren *Semen Coicis* 15 g to lift the Spleen-Qi and relieve the diarrhoea.

Patent remedy

Ren Shen Zai Zao Wan *Ginseng Restorative Pill*

ACUPUNCTURE TREATMENT

TE-6 Zhigou, LI-4 Hegu, SP-3 Taibai, SP-6 Sanyinjiao, SP-9 Yinlingquan, ST-36 Zusanli, ST-40 Fenglong, GB-30 Huantiao, BL-40 Weizhong and Ah Shi points. Reducing method is used on the rest of the points.

Explanations

- TE-6 and LI-4 promote the circulation of Qi in the channels, eliminate Damp and reduce the leg pain.
- ST-40, the Connecting point, SP-9, the Sea point, and GB-30, the meeting point of the Gall Bladder and the Bladder channels, eliminate Phlegm-Damp in the body and channels, promote the circulation of Qi and Blood and relieve the leg pain.
- SP-6, the crossing point of the three Yin channels of the foot, promotes the circulation of Blood, eliminates Blood stasis and relieves the leg pain.
- ST-36, the Sea point, and SP-3, the Source point, activate the Spleen and Stomach, tonify the Qi and eliminate Phlegm-Damp.
- BL-40, the Sea point, promotes urination, reduces swelling in the legs and relieves the leg pain.
- The Ah Shi points eliminate Damp, regulate the circulation of Qi and Blood in the channels and relieve the leg pain.

Modifications

1. If there is leg pain along the Bladder channel, add BL-36, BL-58, BL-63 and BL-64 to harmonise the collateral and relieve the pain.

2. If there is leg pain along the Gall Bladder channel, add GB-36, GB-34 and GB-40 to promote the Qi and Blood circulation in the channel and relieve the pain.
3. If there is leg pain along the Stomach channel, add ST-30, ST-31, ST-34 and ST-42 to promote the Qi and Blood circulation in the channel, remove blockage and arrest the pain.
4. If there is leg pain along the Liver channel, add LR-3, LR-5, LR-11 and LR-12 to harmonise the collateral, promote the Qi and Blood circulation in the channel and relieve the pain.
5. If there is leg pain along the Spleen channel, add SP-4, SP-8 and SP-11 to promote the Qi and Blood circulation in the channel, harmonise the collateral and relieve the pain.
6. If there is leg pain along the Kidney channel, add KI-4, KI-5, KI-8 and KI-10 to regulate the Qi and Blood circulation in the channel and relieve the pain.
7. If there is scanty urination and swelling of the legs, add BL-39 to promote urination and eliminate Damp.
8. If there is an aversion to cold or cold limbs due to deficiency of Qi, add CV-4 with moxibustion to reinforce the Yang-Qi and relieve Cold in the body.
9. If there is coughing with profuse sputum due to Phlegm attacking the Lung, add LU-5 to cause the Lung-Qi to descend and resolve Phlegm in the Lung.
10. If the appetite is poor, add CV-12 to activate the Stomach, regulate the Qi in the Middle Burner and improve the appetite.
11. If there are loose stools or diarrhoea, add ST-37 to relieve the diarrhoea.

DEFICIENCY OF KIDNEY-ESSENCE

Symptoms and signs

Intermittent leg pain, which is aggravated by exertion and alleviated by rest, with a lower back pain and weakness, weakness of the knees and legs, difficulty in walking and standing for long, tiredness, a poor memory and concentration, a thin and white tongue coating and a thready and deep pulse.

Principle of treatment

Reinforce Kidney-Essence, strengthen the bones and tendons and sedate the pain.

HERBAL TREATMENT

Prescription

YOU GUI YIN
Restoring the Right Decoction
Shu Di Huang *Radix Rehmanniae Praeparata* 15 g
Shan Yao *Rhizoma Dioscoreae* 12 g
Shan Zhu Yu *Fructus Corni* 15 g
Gou Qi Zi *Fructus Lycii* 15 g
Du Zhong *Cortex Eucommiae* 12 g
Tu Si Zi *Semen Cuscutae* 12 g
Dang Gui *Radix Angelicae Sinensis* 12 g

Explanations

- Shu Di Huang, Shan Yao, Shan Zhu Yu and Gou Qi Zi reinforce the Kidney-Essence and strengthen the bones and tendons.
- Du Zhong strengthens the lower back and lower limbs and relieves the leg pain.
- Blood is stored in the Liver, and Essence is stored in the Kidney. The Liver-Blood and Kidney-Essence nourish each other. Tu Si Zi is used to nourish the Essence in the Kidney, and Dang Gui is used to tonify the Liver-Blood. Dang Gui can also promote the circulation of Blood in the channels and remove obstruction so as to relieve the leg pain.

Modifications

1. If there is irritability, insomnia, a dry throat, flushed cheeks, a red tongue and a thready and rapid pulse due to deficiency of Kidney-Yin, add Gui Ban Jiao *Colla Plastrium Testudinis* 15 g and Han Lian Cao *Herba Ecliptae* 10 g to nourish the Kidney-Yin and clear Deficient-Heat.
2. If there is an aversion to cold and cold limbs due to deficiency of Kidney-Yang, add Fu Zi *Radix Aconiti Praeparata* 10 g to tonify the Kidney-Yang and dispel Interior Cold.
3. If there is a feeble voice, poor appetite and loose stools due to deficiency of Spleen-Qi and Spleen-Yang, add Dang Shen *Radix Codonopsis Pilosulae* 10 g and Bai Zhu *Rhizoma Atractylodis Macrocephalae* 10 g to tonify the Spleen-Qi, strengthen the Spleen and relieve the diarrhoea.

Patent remedies

Liu Wei Di Huang Wan *Six-Flavour Rehmanniae Pill*
Hai Ma Bu Shen Wan *Sea Horse Tonify Kidney Pill*
Kang Gu Zhengsheng Pian *Combat Bone Hyperplasia Pill*

ACUPUNCTURE TREATMENT

GB-34 Yanglingquan, GB-39 Xuanzhong, KI-3 Taixi, BL-23 Shenshu, BL-18 Ganshu, SP-6 Sanyinjiao and some local Ah Shi points. Reinforcing method is used on these points.

Explanations

- This type of leg pain is often seen in old people due to decline of the Essence of the Liver and Kidney.
- KI-3, the Source point of the Kidney channel, and BL-23, the Back Transporting point of the Kidney, reinforce both the Liver and Kidney and strengthen the bones.
- GB-34, the Gathering point for the tendons, and BL-18, the Back Transporting point of the Liver, tonify the Liver-Blood and strengthen the tendons.
- SP-6, the crossing point of the three Yin channels of the foot, tonifies the Spleen, Kidney and Liver.
- The local Ah Shi points promote the circulation of Qi and Blood, eliminate stasis in the channels and relieve the leg pain.

Modifications

1. If there is leg pain along the Bladder channel, add BL-36, BL-58, BL-63 and BL-64 to harmonise the collateral and relieve the pain.
2. If there is leg pain along the Gall Bladder channel, add GB-36, GB-34 and GB-40 to promote the Qi and Blood circulation in the channel and relieve the pain.
3. If there is leg pain along the Stomach channel, add ST-30, ST-31, ST-34 and ST-42 to promote the Qi and Blood circulation in the channel, relieve blockage and arrest the pain.
4. If there is leg pain along the Liver channel, add LR-3, LR-5, LR-11 and LR-12 to harmonise the collateral, promote the Qi and Blood circulation in the channel and relieve the pain.
5. If there is leg pain along the Spleen channel, add SP-4, SP-8 and SP-11 to promote the Qi and Blood circulation in the channel, harmonise the collateral and relieve the pain.
6. If there is leg pain along the Kidney channel, add KI-4, KI-5, KI-8 and KI-10 to regulate the Qi and Blood circulation in the channel and relieve the pain.
7. If there is scanty urination, add BL-39 to promote urination and eliminate Damp.
8. If there is swelling in the legs, add SP-9 to remove Damp and reduce the swelling.
9. If there is a stabbing pain, or aggravation of the leg pain at night due to stagnation of Blood, add LI-4 and SP-10 to promote the Blood circulation and remove the Blood stasis.
10. If there is a severe aversion to cold and a cold sensation in the joints, add moxibustion on the local points and BL-23 to warm the channels and dispel Cold.
11. If there is night sweating, a sensation of heat in the palms and soles of the foot and a thirst, add KI-7 to nourish the Yin and clear Deficient-Heat.
12. If there is insomnia, add HT-3 and PC-6 to calm the Mind and improve sleep.
13. If there is generalised tiredness, add GV-20 to lift the Yang-Qi and relieve the tiredness.

Pain in all four limbs 47

四
肢
疼
痛

In the TCM it is not unusual to see pain occurring in all four limbs, including the joints, tendons and muscles, and sometimes accompanied by generalised body pain and other Internal symptoms. Many pathogenic factors may cause pain in the limbs, such as invasion of External Wind-Cold-Damp, accumulation of Damp-Phlegm in the channels, stagnation of Qi and Blood in the channels, deficiency of Qi and Blood, or deficiency of Spleen-Yang. Pain in all the limbs may be attributed to any of the following disorders in Western medicine: cold infection, influenza, rheumatic fever, rheumatoid arthritis, nerve pain, cervical spondylosis, sprain of the local muscles, depression, peripheral nerve injury or multiple neuritis.

Aetiology and pathology

Invasion of External Wind-Cold-Damp

Carelessness in daily habits, such as wearing too few clothes, standing in a windy or cold environment after sweating profusely from work or exercise, or working and living in a windy and cold place, may cause opening of the skin pores, leaving the person vulnerable to the invasion of Wind-Cold. Wind has the characteristics of upward movement and constant change; Cold has the characteristics of stagnation and viscosity. Therefore, when Wind-Cold invades the channels, it blocks the circulation of Qi and Blood in the body, leading to stagnation of the Qi and Blood, and causing pain in all the limbs.

Overexposure to cold and damp weather, or working and living in a cold and damp environment, may allow Cold-Damp to invade the limbs. Damp has the characteristics of heaviness, lingering and stagnation. If there is invasion of Wind-Cold-Damp, then the channels and muscles in all the limbs contract, leading to stagnation of the Qi and Blood, and causing generalised limb pain.

Accumulation of Damp-Phlegm in the Channels

If external Cold-Damp, Damp-Phlegm and Damp-Heat are not eliminated after an invasion, they may block the channels, leading to stagnation of the Qi and Blood. Bad diets, such as overeating of pungent, fatty or greasy food, may impair the Spleen and Stomach's function of transportation and transformation, so that Damp-Phlegm forms in the Middle Burner. Once Damp-Phlegm forms, it may circulate with the Qi and reach the limbs. Since Damp has the characteristics of stagnation and lingering, it may block the channels and cause the Qi and Blood to stagnate, and pain in the limbs follows.

If Damp-Phlegm remains in the body it may cause Heat to be generated, so that Damp-Heat forms. This may further slow the circulation of Qi and Blood and causes pain in all four limbs.

Emotional disturbance

Emotional disorders impair the physiological functioning of the channels and the Internal Zang-Fu organs, especially the Liver, Lung, Heart and Spleen.

The Liver function is closely related to the emotional state, and also it regulates the circulation of Qi and stores the Blood. Therefore, emotional disturbance, such as habitual anger, or excessive stress or frustration, may disturb the Liver's function of regulating the Qi and Blood circulation, so that the Liver-Qi stagnates. The Lung is in charge of dispersing the Qi and regulating water. Excessive grief may slow down the circulation of Qi in the Lung, causing the Lung-Qi to stagnate and Damp-Phlegm to form in the body. The Heart is in charge of housing the Mind and circulating the Blood. Excessive meditation may cause the Qi circulation in the Heart to slow down, which leads to the stagnation of Qi and Blood in the Heart. Habitual worrying may cause the Spleen-Qi to stagnate, so that Damp-Phlegm can form in the body.

Once there the Qi and Blood stagnate or Damp-Phlegm forms, the channels become blocked, so that pain in all the limbs follows.

Stagnation of Qi and Blood

Prolonged chronic sickness, physical trauma to the limbs, inappropriate limb movements, inappropriate operations, incomplete elimination of External pathogenic factors after invasion, deficiency of Qi and the formation of Damp-Phlegm, may all cause the Qi and Blood to stagnate, leading to damage to the channels, tendons and muscles, and causing pain in the four limbs.

Deficiency of Qi and Blood

The limbs function smoothly provided they are nourished properly by the Qi and Blood. However, if the Qi and Blood become deficient as a result of overstrain or prolonged sickness, the limbs will not be properly nourished, and pain in the four limbs will follow.

The Qi is part of the Yang; therefore prolonged Qi deficiency may in turn lead to Yang deficiency, and allow Interior Cold to form. Cold has the characteristic of contraction, so when interior Cold forms the tendons, muscles and channels contract and are not properly warmed, and pain in the four limbs occurs.

Treatment based on differentiation

Differentiation

Differentiation of External and Internal origin

Pain in all the limbs can be caused by External pathological factors as well as Internal disorders or trauma.

— If the pain is caused by invasion of External factors, it is usually acute, and accompanied by External symptoms, such as fever, an aversion to cold, or joint pain.
— If the pain is caused by Internal disorders, then it is usually chronic and has no External symptoms, but symptoms of Internal origin.

Differentiation of character of the pain

— Pain in all the limbs with a heavy and cold sensation, stiffness of the limbs, aggravation of the pain by cold and damp weather, an aversion to cold, or slight fever, is often caused by invasion of External Wind-Cold or Wind-Cold-Damp.
— Pain in all the limbs with a hot and heavy sensation, red and swelling joints, aggravation of pain by hot weather, or alleviation by cold, is often caused by accumulation of Damp-Heat.
— Pain in all the limbs with a distending feeling, wandering in nature, aggravation of the pain by stress or emotional upset, is often caused by stagnation of Liver-Qi. Some women patients with this kind of pain have worsening of the pain before or at the beginning of the menstrual period.
— Fixed pain in all the limbs with recent or historical physical trauma or operation, stabbing pain, limitation of the movement, or aggravation of the pain at night, is usually caused by stagnation of the Blood.
— Chronic pain in all the limbs with soreness of the muscles, prolonged sickness, a pale complexion, fatigue, or shortness of breath, is usually caused by deficiency of Qi and Blood.
— Pain in all the limbs with a cold sensation, cold hands and cold feet, soreness or numbness of limbs, oedema of the limbs, lassitude, an aversion to cold, constitutional weakness or chronic disease history, or a pale complexion, is often caused by deficiency of Spleen-Yang.

Treatment

INVASION OF EXTERNAL WIND-COLD-DAMP

Symptoms and signs

Pain in all four limbs, which worsens in cold or damp weather or with a cold infection, with a heavy and cold sensation in the limbs, difficult movement of the limbs, an aversion to cold, a slight fever, a poor appetite, a slight red tongue with a white and greasy coating and a deep and slow pulse.

Principle of treatment

Dispel Cold, eliminate Wind, remove Damp and relieve the pain.

HERBAL TREATMENT

Prescription

QIANG HUO SHENG SHI TANG
Notopterygium Dispelling Dampness Decoction
Qiang Huo *Rhizoma seu Radix Notopterygii* 10 g
Du Huo *Radix Angelicae Pubescentis* 10 g
Gao Ben *Rhizoma et Radix Ligustici* 10 g
Fang Feng *Radix Ledebouriellae* 10 g
Chuan Xiong *Rhizoma Ligustici Chuanxiong* 10 g
Zhi Gan Cao *Radix Glycyrrhizae* 6 g
Ma Huang *Herba Ephedrae* 6 g
Gui Zhi *Ramulus Cinnamomi* 10 g
Fu Ling *Poria* 15 g

Explanations

- Qiang Huo, Du Huo, Fang Feng and Gao Ben dispel Wind-Damp and relieve the pain.
- Ma Huang and Gui Zhi dispel Wind-Cold, promote the circulation of Qi and relieve the pain.
- Chuan Xiong invigorates the circulation of Blood and promotes the circulation of Qi in the channels.
- Fu Ling promotes urination in order to eliminate Damp.
- Gan Cao harmonises the actions of the other herbs in the formula.

Modifications

1. If there is an aversion to cold, add Gan Jiang *Rhizoma Zingiberis* 5 g and Rou Gui *Cortex Cinnamomi* 5 g to warm the Interior and dispel Cold.
2. If the joints are swollen, add Fang Ji *Radix Stephaniae Tetrandrae* 10 g and Tu Fu Ling *Rhizoma Smilacis Glabrae* 15 g to eliminate Damp.
3. If the muscles are sore, add Mu Gua *Fructus Chaenomelis* 10 g and Yi Yi Ren *Semen Coicis* 10 g to eliminate Damp and regulate the circulation of Qi.
4. If there is a feeling of heaviness in the limbs, add Can Sha *Excrementum Bombycis Mori* 10 g and Ze Xie *Rhizoma Alismatis* 15 g to promote urination and eliminate Damp.
5. If there is severe muscle pain with a contracting feeling, add Xi Xin *Herba Asari* 3 g and Bai Shao *Radix Paeoniae Alba* 10 g to warm the channels, relax the muscles and relieve the pain.
6. If the appetite is poor, add Ban Xia *Rhizoma Pinelliae* 10 g and Sha Ren *Fructus Amomi* 6 g to dry Damp and improve the appetite.

Patent remedy

Feng Shi Pian *Wind-Damp Tablet*

ACUPUNCTURE TREATMENT

LU-7 Lieque, LI-4 Hegu, LI-11 Quchi, SP-6 Sanyinjiao, GB-34 Yanglingquan, BL-58 Feiyang and BL-60 Kunlun. Reducing method is used on these points. Moxibustion is used if there is severe pain.

Explanations

- LU-7, the Connecting point, and LI-4, the Source point, regulate the skin pores, dispel Wind-Cold-Damp, promote the circulation of Qi and relieve the pain.
- LI-11, the Sea point of the Large Intestine channel, helps LI-4 regulate the circulation of Qi and relieves the pain.
- SP-6, the crossing point of the Spleen, Kidney and Liver channels, eliminates Damp and promotes urination.
- GB-34, the Sea point of the Gall Bladder channel and the Gathering point for the tendons, regulates the circulation of Qi and relieves the pain in the tendons.
- BL-58, the Connecting point of the Bladder channel, and BL-60, the River point, promote the circulation of Qi, eliminate Wind-Damp and relieve the pain.
- Moxibustion, a warming method, warms the channels, eliminates Wind-Damp-Cold and relieves the pain.

Modifications

1. If there is pain along the Large Intestine channel, add LI-3, the Stream point, LI-6, the Connecting point, LI-7, the Accumulation point, and LI-15 to harmonise the Large Intestine collateral, promote circulation in the channel and relieve the pain.
2. If there is pain along the Triple Burner channel, add TE-3, the Stream point, TE-7, the Accumulation point, TE-10, the Sea point, and TE-14 to harmonise the collateral, promote circulation in the channel and relieve the pain.
3. If there is pain along the Small Intestine channel, add SI-3, the Stream point, LI-6, the Connecting point, SI-6, the Accumulation point, SI-9 and SI-10 to harmonise the collateral, promote circulation in the channel and relieve the pain.
4. If there is pain in the scapular region, add SI-11, SI-12 and SI-14 to harmonise the collateral and sedate the pain.
5. If there is pain along the Lung channel, add LU-9, the Stream point and Source point, LU-6, the Accumulation point, LU-5, the Sea point, LU-3 and LU-1, the Front Collecting point of the Lung, to harmonise the collateral, promote circulation in the channel and relieve the pain.
6. If there is muscular numbness, add SP-9, the Sea point and ST-40, the Connecting point, to promote the circulation of Qi, resolve Damp, eliminate Phlegm and relieve the numbness.
7. If there is a low fever, add GV-14 to promote sweat, eliminate Wind-Damp and reduce the fever.
8. If there is a severe pain, add BL-11, the Gathering point for the Bones, and Ah Shi points to regulate the circulation of Qi and relieve the pain.
9. If there is a headache, add GB-20 to promote sweating and relieve the headache.
10. If the appetite is poor, add CV-12, the Front Collecting point of the Stomach, and ST-36, the Sea point, to promote the circulation of Qi and improve the appetite.

Case history

A 20-year-old woman had been suffering from a wandering pain in all her limbs with a cold sensation for 3 months. The pain was mainly located along the Large Intestine channel. At the hospital she was diagnosed as having rheumatic arthritis. As well as painful limbs, she also had a low fever, an aversion to cold, aggravation of the pain by exposure to cold and in humid weather, a poor appetite, loose stools, a pale tongue with a white coating and a superficial and rapid pulse.

Diagnosis
Invasion of Wind-Cold.

Principle of treatment
Dispel Wind-Cold, promote Qi circulation and sedate the pain.

Herbal treatment
FANG FENG TANG
Ledebouriella Decoction
Fang Feng *Radix Ledebouriellae* 10 g
Chuan Xiong *Rhizoma Ligustici Chuanxiong* 10 g
Gan Cao *Radix Glycyrrhizae* 6 g
Fu Ling *Poria* 15 g
Chai Hu *Radix Bupleuri* 15 g
Dang Gui *Radix Angelicae Sinensis* 10 g
Qin Jiao *Radix Gentianae Macrophyllae* 10 g
Qing Feng Teng *Caulis Sinonenii* 30 g
Gui Zhi *Ramulus Cinnamomi* 10 g

Explanations

- Fang Feng, Qin Jiao and Qing Feng Teng dispel Wind and relieve the pain.
- Gui Zhi eliminates Cold, regulates the circulation of Qi and Blood and relieves the pain.
- Dang Gui and Chuan Xiong promote the circulation of Qi and Blood and relieve the pain.
- Fu Ling eliminates Wind-Damp and strengthens the Spleen.
- Chai Hu dispels Wind, promotes the circulation of Qi and reduces fever.
- Gan Cao harmonises the functions of other herbs in the prescription.

Acupuncture treatment
LI-3, LI-4, LI-6, LI-14, LI-15, TE-5, BL-58 and BL-60. Reducing method is used on these points. Moxibustion is used where there is severe pain.

Explanations

- LI-3, the Stream point, and LI-4, the Source point, regulate the skin pores, dispel Wind-Cold-Damp, promote the circulation of Qi and relieve the pain.
- LI-6, the Connecting point, and LI-7, the Accumulation point, harmonise the collateral, promote the circulation of Qi in the channels and sedate the pain.
- LI-14 and LI-15, the local points, regulate the circulation of Qi and relieve the pain.
- TE-5, the Connecting point from the Triple Burner channel, BL-58, the Connecting point of the the Bladder channel, and BL-60, the River point, dispel external pathogenic factors, promote the circulation of Qi, harmonise the collateral and relieve the pain.

The patient was treated with a daily herbal decoction, and acupuncture was given once every other day. The pain in her limbs was under control after a month. She was followed up a year later and she stated she had experienced no more pain after the herbal treatment.

ACCUMULATION OF DAMP-HEAT

Symptoms and signs

Pain in the four limbs with a hot and heavy sensation, which is aggravated by warmth and alleviated by cold, with swollen joints, lower back pain, scanty and yellow urine, constipation, or loose stools, fever and an aversion to cold, a headache, a bitter taste in the mouth, thirst, a red tongue with a thick and yellow coating and a slippery and rapid pulse.

Principle of treatment

Clear Heat, eliminate Damp and relieve the pain.

HERBAL TREATMENT

Prescription

BAI HU JIA GUI ZHI TANG
White Tiger Ramulus Cinnamomi Decoction
Shi Gao *Gypsum Fibrosum* 30 g
Zhi Mu *Rhizoma Anemarrhenae* 10 g
Jing Mi *Semen Oryzae* 15 g
Gui Zhi *Ramulus Cinnamomi* 10 g
Qiang Huo *Rhizoma seu Radix Notopterygii* 10 g
Du Huo *Radix Angelicae Pubescentis* 10 g
Qing Feng Teng *Caulis Sinomenii* 30 g
Tu Fu Ling *Rhizoma Smilacis Glabrae* 30 g
Zhi Gan Cao *Radix Glycyrrhizae Praeparata* 6 g

Explanations

- Shi Gao and Zhi Mu clear Heat and reduce fever.
- Gui Zhi dispels Wind, harmonises the collateral and eliminates Damp.
- Jing Mi and Gan Cao tonify the Qi and harmonise the Stomach-Qi.
- Qiang Huo and Du Huo help Gui Zhi to eliminate Wind and relieve painful limbs.
- Qing Feng Teng dispels Wind-Damp and relieves the pain.
- Tu Fu Ling eliminates Damp and clears Heat.
- Gan Cao harmonises the actions of the other herbs in the formula.

Modifications

1. If there is severe pain, add Luo Shi Teng *Caulis Trachelospermi* 20 g and Hu Zhang *Rhizoma Polygoni Cuspidati* 15 g to dispel Wind, eliminate Damp-Heat and relieve the pain.
2. If there is a fever, add Sheng Ma *Rhizoma Cimicifugae* 10 g and Chai Hu *Radix Bupleuri* 12 g to clear Heat, reduce the fever and relieve the pain.

3. If there is swelling in the limbs, add Ku Shen *Radix Sophorae Flavescentis* 10 g and Jin Yin Hua *Flos Lonicerae* 10 g to eliminate Damp-Heat, reduce the swelling and relieve the pain.
4. If there is constipation, add Da Huang *Radix et Rhizoma Rhei* 6 g and Mang Xiao *Natrii Sulfas* 10 g to clear Heat, promote defecation and relieve the constipation.
5. If there is diarrhoea, add Cang Zhu *Rhizoma Atractylodis* 10 g and Ge Gen *Radix Puerariae* 10 g to activate the Spleen and relieve the diarrhoea.

Patent remedy

Feng Shi Xiao Tong Pian *Wind-Damp Dispel Pain Tablet*

ACUPUNCTURE TREATMENT

LI-4 Hegu, LI-11 Quchi, TE-6 Zhigou, SP-6 Sanyinjiao, SP-9 Yinlingquan and GB-34 Yanglingquan. Reducing method is used on these points.

Explanations

- LI-4, the Source point of the Large Intestine channel, promotes sweating, regulates the circulation of Qi and relieves the pain.
- LI-11, the Sea point of the Large Intestine channel, regulates the circulation of Qi, reduces fever and eliminates Damp-Heat.
- TE-6 promotes the circulation of Qi, eliminates Damp-Heat and relieves the pain.
- SP-6, the crossing point of the three Yin channels of the foot, SP-9, the Sea point of the Spleen channel, GB-34, the Sea point and the Gathering point for the tendons, eliminate Damp, clear Heat and relieve the pain.

Modifications

1. If there is pain along the Large Intestine channel, add LI-3, the Stream point, LI-6, the Connecting point, LI-7, the Accumulation point, and LI-15 to harmonise the collateral, promote circulation in the channel and relieve the pain.
2. If there is pain along the Triple Burner channel, add TE-3, the Stream point, TE-7, the Accumulation point, TE-10, the Sea point, and TE-14 to harmonise the collateral, promote circulation in the channel and relieve the pain.
3. If there is pain along the Small Intestine channel, add SI-3, the Stream point, SI-6, the Accumulation point, SI-9 and SI-10 to harmonise

the collateral, promote circulation in the channel and relieve the pain.

4. If there is pain in the scapular region, add SI-11, SI-12 and SI-14 to harmonise the collateral and sedate the pain.

5. If there is pain along the Lung channel, add LU-9, the Stream point and the Source point, LU-6, the Accumulation point, LU-5, the Sea point, LU-3, and LU-1, the Front Collecting point of the Lung, to harmonise the collateral, promote circulation in the channel and relieve the pain.

6. If there is muscle numbness, add SP-9, the Sea point, and ST-40, the Connecting point, to promote the circulation of Qi, resolve Damp, eliminate Phlegm and relieve the numbness.

7. If there is a fever, add LI-2, the Spring point, and GV-14, the meeting point of all the Yang channels, to clear Heat and reduce the fever.

8. If there is a headache, add GB-20 to promote sweating and relieve the headache.

9. If the appetite is poor, add CV-12, the Front Collecting point of the Stomach, and ST-36, the Sea point, to promote the circulation of Qi and improve the appetite.

10. If there is diarrhoea, add ST-25, the Front Collecting point of the Large Intestine, and ST-36, the Sea point, to activate the Spleen and eliminate Damp.

STAGNATION OF QI

Symptoms and signs

Pain in the four limbs which is aggravated by stress, anger, excessive thinking, excessive grief and meditation, with a distending feeling, headache, dizziness, insomnia, irritability, palpitations, irregular menstruation, a poor appetite, a feeling of dullness in the stomach, lower abdominal pain, a red tongue with a white coating and a wiry pulse.

Principle of treatment

Regulate Qi, remove Qi stagnation and sedate the pain.

HERBAL TREATMENT

Prescription

XIAO YAO SAN
Free and Relaxed Powder
Chai Hu *Radix Bupleuri* 10 g
Dang Gui *Radix Angelicae Sinensis* 10 g

Bai Shao *Radix Paeoniae Alba* 20 g
Bai Zhu *Rhizoma Atractylodis Macrocephalae* 10 g
Fu Ling *Poria* 15 g
Gan Cao *Radix Glycyrrhizae* 5 g
Bo He *Herba Menthae* 3 g
Jiang Huang *Rhizoma Curcumae* 10 g
Sang Zhi *Ramulus Mori* 15 g

Explanations

- Chai Hu and Bo He regulate and promote circulation of the Liver-Qi so as to remove Qi stagnation from the Liver.
- Bai Shao and Dang Gui nourish the Blood, strengthen the Liver and relieve the pain.
- Bai Zhu and Fu Ling strengthen the Spleen and Stomach.
- Jiang Huang and Sang Zhi regulate the circulation of Qi and relieve the pain.
- Gan Cao harmonises the actions of the other herbs in the formula.

Modifications

1. If there is a headache, add Chuan Xiong *Radix Ligustici Chuanxiong* 10 g and Qiang Huo *Rhizoma seu Radix Notopterygii* 10 g to regulate the circulation of Qi and relieve the headache.

2. If there is depression and sadness, add Xiang Fu *Rhizoma Cyperi* 10 g and Yu Jin *Radix Curcumae* 10 g promote the circulation of Liver-Qi and remove Qi stagnation.

3. If there is mental disturbance, add Bai Zi Ren *Semen Biotae* 10 g and Long Gu *Os Draconis* 15 g to calm the Heart and tranquillise the Mind.

4. If there is irritability, add Xia Ku Cao *Spica Prunellae* 10 g to clear Heat and smooth the Liver.

5. If there is irregular menstruation, add Huai Niu Xi *Radix Achyranthis Bidentatae* 10 g and Yi Mu Cao *Herba Leonuri* 10 g to regulate the menstruation.

ACUPUNCTURE TREATMENT

LI-4 Hegu, LR-3 Taichong, PC-6 Neiguan, GB-20 Fengchi, SP-6 Sanyinjiao and Ah Shi points. Even methods are used on these points.

Explanations

- LI-4, the Source point of Large Intestine channel, promotes the circulation of Qi and relieves the pain.

- LR-3, the Source and Stream point of the Liver channel, and PC-6, the Connecting point, regulate the circulation of Qi, calm the Mind and relieve the limb pain.
- GB-20 calms the Mind and regulates the circulation of Qi.
- SP-6, the crossing point of the three Yin channels of the foot, promotes the circulation of Blood, regulates the Liver and relieves the pain.
- Ah Shi points promote the circulation of Qi in the locality and relieve the pain.

Modifications

1. If there is pain along the Large Intestine channel, add LI-3, the Stream point, LI-6, the Connecting point, LI-7, the Accumulation point, and LI-15 to harmonise the collateral, promote circulation in the channel and relieve the pain.
2. If there is pain along the Triple Burner channel, add TE-3, the Stream point, TE-7, the Accumulation point, TE-10, the Sea point, and TE-14 to harmonise the collateral, promote circulation in the channel and relieve the pain.
3. If there is pain along the Small Intestine channel, add SI-3, the Stream point, SI-6, the Accumulation point, SI-9 and SI-10 to harmonise the collateral, promote the circulation in the channel and relieve the pain.
4. If there is pain in the scapular region, add SI-11, SI-12 and SI-14 to harmonise the collateral and sedate the pain.
5. If there is pain along the Lung channel, add LU-9, the Stream point and Source point, LU-6, the Accumulation point, LU-5, the Sea point, LU-3 and LU-1, the Front Collecting point of the Lung, to harmonise the collateral, promote circulation in the channel and relieve the pain.
6. If there is headache, add GV-20 to suppress the Liver and sedate the headache.
7. If there is depression, add CV-17, the Gathering point for the Qi, and LR-14, the Front Collecting point of the Liver, to smooth the Liver and promote the circulation of Qi.
8. If there is nervousness and irritability, add LR-2, the Spring point, to clear Heat and calm the Liver.
9. If there are palpitations, add HT-7, the Source point, to calm the Heart and tranquillise the Mind.
10. If the appetite is poor, add ST-36 and SP-4 to regulate the circulation of Qi and improve the appetite.
11. If there is irregular menstruation, add SP-10 and KI-3 to regulate the menstruation.

Case history

A 45-year-old woman had been suffering from pain in all four limbs for a year. The pain moved up and down, and was aggravated when she was stressed or nervous. In the hospital she was diagnosed as having menopausal syndrome. In addition to Western medical treatment, she asked for acupuncture treatment. Beside the painful limbs, she had irregular menstruation, lumbago, hot flushes, tiredness, dizziness, palpitations, irritability, a poor appetite, a pale tongue with a white coating and a deep wiry pulse.

Diagnosis
Stagnation of Liver-Qi.

Principle of treatment
Regulate Liver-Qi, remove Qi stagnation and relieve the pain.

Acupuncture treatment
LI-4, HT-7, PC-6, GB-20, LR-3, SP-6 and ST-36. Even method was used on these points.

Explanations

- LI-4, the Source point of the Large Intestine channel, promotes the circulation of Qi.
- HT-7, the Source point of the Heart channel, regulates the circulation of Qi, calms the Heart and tranquillises the Mind.
- PC-6, Connecting point of the Pericardium channel, regulates the circulation of Qi and calms the Mind.
- GB-20, and LR-3, the Stream and Source point of the Liver channel, calm the Mind, regulate the circulation of Qi and remove its stagnation.
- SP-6, the crossing point of the three Yin channels of the foot, regulates the Qi and calms the Mind.
- ST-36, the Sea point of the Stomach channel, strengthens the Spleen and the Stomach and improves the appetite.

Acupuncture treatment was given daily. Besides this, the patent herbal pill Xiao Yao Wan *Free and Relaxed Pill* was prescribed, eight pills each time, three times a day. After 6 weeks of treatment, her limb pain was under control. Two years later she was followed up by letters, and stated she had experienced no more pain since the acupuncture treatment.

STAGNATION OF BLOOD IN THE CHANNELS

Symptoms and signs

History of physical trauma or operation, long duration of limb pain with a fixed location, occasional stabbing pain, and joint pain, which is aggravated by certain postures or movement, and worsens at night, accompanied by thirst without much desire to drink, a purplish tongue with a white coating and a deep pulse.

Principle of treatment

Promote Blood circulation, remove Blood stagnation and sedate the pain.

HERBAL TREATMENT

Prescription

TAO HONG SI WU TANG
Four-Substance Decoction with Safflower and Peach Pit
Dang Gui *Radix Angelicae Sinensis* 10 g
Sheng Di Huang *Radix Rehmanniae Recens* 12 g
Chi Shao *Radix Paeoniae Rubra* 10 g
Chuan Xiong *Rhizoma Ligustici Chuanxiong* 6 g
Tao Ren *Semen Persicae* 10 g
Qin Jiao *Radix Gentianae Macrophyllae* 10 g
Huai Niu Xi *Radix Achyranthis Bidentatae* 10 g
Qiang Huo *Rhizoma seu Radix Notopterygii* 10 g
Hong Hua *Flos Carthami* 10 g

Explanations

- Sheng Di Huang and Chi Shao regulate the circulation of Blood and relieve pain. Since long-term stagnation of Blood may produce Heat in the Blood, these two herbs are included to clear Heat in the Blood.
- Chuan Xiong, Dang Gui, Tao Ren and Hong Hua promote the circulation of Blood and remove its stagnation.
- Qin Jiao, Qiang Huo and Huai Niu Xi promote the circulation of Blood and relieve the limb pain.

Modifications

1. If there is a severe stabbing pain, add Yan Hu Suo *Rhizoma Corydalis* 10 g and Pu Huang *Pollen Typhae* 10 g to strengthen the circulation of Blood and relieve the pain.
2. If there is joint pain, add Chuan Shan Long *Rhizoma Dioscoreae Nipponicae* 10 g and Jiang Huang *Rhizoma Curcumae Longae* 10 g to regulate the circulation of Qi in the channels and relieve the joint pain.
3. If there is limitation of joint movement, add Ji Xue Teng *Caulis Spatholobi* 10 g and Yu Jin *Radix Curcumae* 10 g to regulate the circulation of Blood and improve the joint movement.

Patent remedy

Xiao Huo Luo Dan *Minor Invigorate the Collaterals Special Pill*

ACUPUNCTURE TREATMENT

LI-4 Hegu, LI-11 Quchi, TE-5 Waiguan, PC-6 Neiguan, LR-3 Taichong, SP-6 Sanyinjiao, BL-17 Geshu and GB-34 Yanglingquan. Reducing method is used on these points.

Explanations

- LI-4, the Source point, and LI-11, the Sea point, promote the circulation of Qi and Blood and relieve the pain.
- TE-5, the Connecting point, harmonises the collateral and relieves the pain.
- SP-6, the crossing point of the three Yin channels of the foot, and BL-17, the Gathering point for the Blood, promote the circulation of Blood, eliminate its stasis and sedate the pain.
- Since the circulation of Qi leads to the circulation of Blood, PC-6, the Connecting point of the Pericardium channel, and LR-3, the Stream and Source point of the Liver channel, are useful for regulating the circulation of Qi and removing Blood stasis.
- GB-34, the Gathering point for the tendons, strengthens the tendons and relieves the pain.

Modifications

1. If there is pain along the Large Intestine channel, add LI-3, the Stream point, LI-6, the Connecting point, LI-7, the Accumulation point, and LI-15 to harmonise the collateral, promote circulation in the channel and relieve the pain.
2. If there is pain along the Triple Burner channel, add TE-3, the Stream point, TE-7, the Accumulation point, TE-10, the Sea point, and TE-14 to harmonise the collateral, promote circulation in the channel and relieve the pain.
3. If there is pain along the Small Intestine channel, add SI-3, the Stream point, SI-6, the Accumulation point, SI-9 and SI-10 to harmonise the collateral, promote the circulation in the channel and relieve the pain.
4. If there is pain in the scapular region, add SI-11, SI-12 and SI-14 to harmonise the collateral and sedate the pain.
5. If there is pain along the Lung channel, add LU-9, the Stream point and Source point, LU-6, the Accumulation point, LU-5, the Sea point, LU-3 and LU-1, the Front Collecting point of the Lung, to harmonise the collateral, promote the circulation in the channel and relieve the pain.
6. If there is a headache, add GV-20 to suppress the Liver and sedate the headache.

7. If the pain worsens at night, add HT-7 and KI-6 to promote the circulation of Blood, remove its stasis and calm the Mind.
8. If there is limitation of joint movement, add ST-40, the Connecting point of the Stomach channel, to harmonise the collateral, resolve Phlegm, promote the Qi and Blood circulation and relieve the pain.

DEFICIENCY OF QI AND BLOOD

Symptoms and signs

Slight pain in the four limbs over a long period, with soreness in the muscles, fatigue, shortness of breath, dizziness, excessive sweating after slight exertion, an aversion to wind, dizziness, palpitations, a poor appetite, diarrhoea with loose stools, a pale tongue with a white coating and a weak and threadly pulse.

Principle of treatment

Tonify Qi and Blood and relieve the pain.

HERBAL TREATMENT

Prescription

BU ZHONG YI QI TANG
Tonifying the Middle and Benefiting Qi Decoction
Huang Qi *Radix Astragali seu Hedysari* 20 g
Gan Cao *Radix Glycyrrhizae* 5 g
Ren Shen *Radix Ginseng* 10 g
Dang Gui *Radix Angelicae Sinensis* 10 g
Ju Pi *Pericarpium Citri Reticulatae* 6 g
Sheng Ma *Rhizoma Cimicifugae* 3 g
Chai Hu *Radix Bupleuri* 3 g
Qin Jiao *Radix Gentianae Macrophyllae* 10 g
Ge Gen *Radix Puerariae* 15 g
Fang Feng *Radix Ledebouriellae* 10 g
Bai Zhu *Rhizoma Atractylodis Macrocephalae* 10 g

Explanations

- Ren Shen, Huang Qi, Bai Zhu and Gan Cao strengthen the Spleen and tonify the Qi of the Spleen and Stomach.
- Sheng Ma and Chai Hu lift up the Yang-Qi, which is deficient.
- Dang Gui, a companion of Chai Hu, tonifies the Blood and smoothes the Liver.
- Ju Pi promotes the circulation of Qi and strengthens the Spleen and Stomach.
- Ge Gen, Qin Jiao and Fang Feng dispel Wind and relieve the limb pain.

Modifications

1. If there is muscular pain, add Qiang Huo *Rhizoma seu Radix Notopterygii* 10 g and Du Huo *Radix Angelicae Pubescentis* 10 g to regulate the circulation of Qi and relieve the pain.
2. If there is dizziness, add Tian Ma *Rhizoma Gastrodiae* 10 g and Man Jing Zi *Fructus Viticis* 10 g to regulate the circulation of Qi and relieve the dizziness.
3. If the appetite is poor, add Sha Ren *Fructus Amomi* 6 g and Mu Xiang *Radix Aucklandiae* 10 g to activate the Spleen and improve the appetite.
4. If there are palpitations, add Dan Shen *Radix Salviae Miltiorrhizae* 10 g and Ji Xue Teng *Caulis Spatholobi* 15 g to nourish the Blood and calm the Mind.

Patent remedy

Shi Quan Da Bu Wan *All-Inclusive Great Tonifying Pill*

ACUPUNCTURE TREATMENT

LI-4 Hegu, TE-5 Waiguan, PC-6 Neiguan, GV-20 Baihui, SP-6 Sanyinjiao and ST-36 Zusanli. Reinforcing method is used on these points. Moxibustion is recommended on GV-20 and ST-36.

Explanations

- LI-4, the Source point of the Large Intestine channel, regulates the Qi and relieves the pain.
- PC-6, the Connecting point of the Pericardium channel, regulates the circulation of Qi and calms the Mind.
- GV-20, the crossing point of the Governing Vessel and the Bladder channel, can promote the physiological function of the Yang-Qi and reinforce the Internal organs.
- ST-36, the Stream point of the Stomach, activates the Spleen and Stomach and tonifies the Qi so as to promote the production of Qi and Blood.
- SP-6, the crossing point of the three Yin channels of the foot, promotes the production of Blood, regulates the Blood and calms the Mind.

Modifications

1. If there is pain along the Large Intestine channel, add LI-3, the Stream point, LI-6, the Connecting point, LI-7, the Accumulation point, and LI-15 to

harmonise the collateral, promote circulation in the channel and relieve the pain.

2. If there is pain along the Triple Burner channel, add TE-3, the Stream point, TE-7, the Accumulation point, TE-10, the Sea point, and TE-14, to harmonise the collateral, promote circulation in the channel and relieve the pain.

3. If there is pain along the Small Intestine channel, add SI-3, the Stream point, SI-6, the Accumulation point, SI-9 and SI-10, to harmonise the collateral, promote circulation in the channel and relieve the pain.

4. If there is pain in the scapular region, add SI-11, SI-12 and SI-14 to harmonise the collateral and sedate the pain.

5. If there is pain along the Lung channel, add LU-9, the Stream point and Source point, LU-6, the Accumulation point, LU-5, the Sea point, LU-3 and LU-1, the Front Collecting point of the Lung, to harmonise the collateral, promote circulation in the channel and relieve the pain.

6. If there is a headache, add Extra Yintang to harmonise the collateral and sedate the headache.

7. If the appetite is poor, add CV-12 and SP-3 to regulate the Spleen and Stomach and improve the appetite.

8. If there is fatigue, add CV-8 with moxibustion to tonify the Yang and relieve the tiredness.

DEFICIENCY OF SPLEEN-YANG

Symptoms and signs

Pain in the four limbs with a cold sensation, with constitutional weakness or chronic disease, soreness or numbness of the limbs, lassitude, an aversion to cold, a pale complexion, dizziness, diarrhoea, a poor appetite, a pale tongue with a white coating and a deep, slow and thready pulse.

Principle of treatment

Reinforce the Spleen, warm the channels and relieve the pain.

HERBAL TREATMENT

Prescription

GUI ZHI JIA FU ZI TANG
Cinnamon Twig Plus Prepared Aconite Decoction
Gui Zhi *Ramulus Cinnamomi* 10 g
Fu Zi *Radix Aconiti Carmichaeli Praeparata* 10 g
Bai Shao *Radix Paeoniae Alba* 30 g
Bai Zhu *Rhizoma Atractylodis Macrocephalae* 10 g
Wu Zhu Yu *Fructus Evodiae* 10 g
Ren Shen *Radix Ginseng* 10 g

Explanations

- Fu Zi and Gui Zhi reinforce the Spleen-Yang, warm the channels and relieve the pain.
- Wu Zhu Yu warms the Middle Burner and relieves the pain.
- Bai Shao nourishes the Blood and relieves the pain.
- Bai Zhu and Ren Shen tonify the Qi, improve its circulation and relieve the pain.

Modifications

1. If the pain has a cold sensation, add Xi Xin *Herba Asari* 3 g and Gan Jiang *Rhizoma Zingiberis* 10 g to warm the channels and relieve the pain.

2. If there is tiredness, add Huang Qi *Radix Astragali seu Hedysari* 10 g to tonify the Spleen-Yang and relieve the tiredness.

3. If there is an aversion of the abdomen to cold, add Rou Gui *Cortex Cinnamomi* 5 g to warm the Interior and dispel Cold.

4. If there is dizziness, add Tian Ma *Rhizoma Gastrodiae* 10 g to suppress interior Wind and relieve the dizziness.

5. If there is diarrhoea, add Shan Yao *Rhizoma Dioscoreae* 10 g and Bu Gu Zhi *Fructus Psoraleae* 10 g to reinforce the Yang of the Spleen and Kidney and stop the diarrhoea.

ACUPUNCTURE TREATMENT AND MODIFICATIONS

(See Deficiency of Qi and Blood, p. 557.)

Part 9

Genital pain 外阴疼痛

Genital pain 48

外
阴
疼
痛

Genital pain may occur in the penis, testicles, female pudendum or vagina, and is often accompanied by painful urination, lower abdominal pain or lower back pain. According to TCM theory, it may be caused by invasion of External Cold, Excessive-Fire in the Terminal Yin channel of the Liver, accumulation of Damp-Heat in the Terminal Yin channel, stagnation of Liver-Qi, stagnation of Blood in the Liver channel or deficiency of the Yin of Liver and Kidney. Genital pain may be attributed to any of the following disorders in Western medicine: acute bartholinitis, vaginitis, urethritis, testitis, prostatitis, seminal vesiculitis, inguinal hernia and external injury to the genitals.

Aetiology and pathology

Invasion of External Cold

Invasion of Exogenous Cold and Damp-Cold are two common factors that cause genital pain. Cold has a contracting nature, and may obstruct the channels, collateral, muscles and tendons, slowing down the circulation of Qi. In this way stagnation of Qi occurs and genital pain follows.

Damp is a substantial Yin pathogenic factor. It is characterised by heaviness and viscosity, so, combined with Cold, it may easily obstruct the circulation of Qi and Blood. These two pathogenic factors may directly invade the body through the Lower Burner. If there is an invasion of Cold or of Cold-Damp, it causes contraction of the Terminal Yin channel and the tendons around the genitals, leading to a local stagnation of Qi and Blood, which causes pain.

Excessive Fire in the Terminal Yin channel

Excessive stress or anger may cause disharmony of the Liver in its function of promoting the circulation of Qi. This leads to stagnation of Qi in the Liver, and prolonged Liver-Qi stagnation may generate Liver-Fire. Also, if External Cold or Cold and Damp persist in the body over a long time they may cause the Qi to stagnate and these pathogenic factors may also turn into Internal Fire. Eating of too much pungent, fat, greasy or sweet food, or drinking too much alcohol, may also gradually produce Internal Fire. When Internal Fire spreads in the channels, it may disturb the circulation of Qi and damage the Yin in the body, leading to genital pain. Moreover, an invasion of Exterior Toxic Fire to the genital region may also cause disharmony in the Terminal Yin channel, damage the local tendons and muscles and result in genital pain.

Accumulation of Damp-Heat in the Terminal Yin channel of the Liver

Bad diets, such as eating too much fat or sweet food, or dairy products, or drinking too much alcohol, may also damage the Spleen and Stomach, leading to the generation of Damp-Heat in the body. Damp flows downward by nature, so the Lower Burner will eventually be affected as well, resulting in genital pain.

Lack of personal hygiene, a prolonged stay in a humid place, or walking and working in the rain, may lead to a direct invasion of External Damp-Heat to the genitals, resulting in stagnation of the Qi and Blood there, and causing genital pain.

Stagnation of Liver-Qi

Emotional disturbance, such as excessive stress, frustration or anger, may cause the Liver-Qi to stagnate. The Liver's function is to store the Blood and to regulate its circulation, therefore stagnation of Liver-Qi may lead in turn to stagnation of Blood. Eventually this may block the circulation of Qi and Blood in the Liver and its channel and cause genital pain.

Excessive leg movements (as in overstrenuous exercise) may also injure the tendons around the genital region, resulting in local stagnation of the Liver-Qi and causing genital pain.

Stagnation of Blood

Incomplete elimination of Exterior Cold after an invasion may cause contraction of the muscles and tendons; if Damp invades or accumulates it may block the channels and tendons; stagnation of Liver-Qi may influence the Blood circulation. All of these circumstances may eventually influence the circulation of Qi and Blood, leading to Blood stagnation and causing genital pain.

In addition, physical trauma, inappropriate operation or excessive leg movement may all directly damage the channels and muscles, leading to a stagnation of Qi and Blood and causing genital pain.

Deficiency of Yin of Liver and Kidney

A poor constitution, prolonged febrile disease or eating too much spicy food may all cause Internal Heat to form and result in the consumption of Yin of the Liver and Kidney. Also, old age, chronic disease and excessive sexual activity may all cause consumption of the Qi and Yin of the Kidney. The Liver and Kidney share the same origin; therefore, deficiency of Yin of the Kidney may cause deficiency of Liver-Yin. If there is Yin deficiency, the tendons and channels in the genital region will not be properly nourished, and genital pain will occur.

Treatment based on differentiation

Differentiation

Differentiation of acute and chronic pain

Since genital pain is not only a local complaint, but also related to general body conditions, differentiation should be made based on the local pain in the genitals and whole body complaints.

— Acute genital pain with a cold sensation is often due to invasion of External Cold.
— Chronic genital pain, or chronic genital pain with acute aggravation, is usually caused by disorder of the Internal organs.

Differentiation of character of the pain

— Acute genital pain with a cold sensation, contraction of the scrotum with occasional pain, aggravation of the genital pain by exposure to cold, is often caused by invasion of External Cold.
— Acute sharp pain in the genitals with a burning sensation, redness and swelling of the genitals, or dark yellow urine, is usually caused by Excessive-Fire in the Terminal Yin channel.
— Genital pain with a hot and itching sensation, yellow and sticky discharge from the genitals with a foul smell, leucorrhoea, itching of the vulvae, or itching, red and wet scrotum, and a yellow and greasy tongue coating, is usually caused by accumulation of Damp-Heat in the Terminal Yin channel.
— Genital pain with a distending sensation, aggravation of the pain by emotional upset or stress, or hypochondriac pain, is often caused by stagnation of Liver-Qi.
— Sharp genital pain, or stabbing pubic pain, with a history of trauma or operation in the genital region, is often related to stagnation of the Blood in the Terminal Yin channel.
— Chronic genital pain with a dry and itchy feeling, lower back pain with soreness, tidal fever, or night sweating, are usually caused by deficiency of the Yin of Liver and Kidney.

Treatment

INVASION OF EXTERNAL COLD

Symptoms and signs

Acute onset of genital pain with a cold sensation, and pain radiating to the lower abdomen, which is aggravated by exposure to cold and alleviated by warmth, with contraction of the scrotum with a cold sensation, or swelling of the scrotum, cold limbs, a poor appetite, an absence of thirst, clear urine, clear leucorrhoea, loose stools, a pale tongue with a white and moist coating and a wiry and tense pulse.

Principle of treatment

Dispel External Cold, warm the Liver channel and relieve the pain.

HERBAL TREATMENT

Prescription

TIAN TAI WU YAO SAN
Top-Quality Lindera Powder
Wu Yao *Radix Linderae* 12 g
Mu Xiang *Radix Aucklandiae* 6 g
Xiao Hui Xiang *Fructus Foeniculi* 6 g
Qing Pi *Pericarpium Citri Reticulatae Viride* 6 g
Gao Liang Jiang *Rhizoma Alpiniae Officinarum* 9 g
Bing Lang *Semen Arecae* 9 g
Chuan Lian Zi *Fructus Meliae Toosendan* 12 g

Explanations

- Wu Yao, Qing Pi, Mu Xiang, Bing Lang and Chuan Lian Zi promote the circulation of Liver-Qi and stop the pain.
- Xiao Hui Xiang and Gao Liang Jiang warm the channels, dispel Cold and relieve the pain.

Modifications

1. If there is severe cold, add Rou Gui *Cortex Cinnamomi* 6 g and Wu Zhu Yu *Fructus Evodiae* 5 g to warm the Liver channel and to relieve the pain.
2. If there is dysmenorrhoea, add Chuan Xiong *Radix Ligustici Chuanxiong* 10 g, Hong Hua *Flos Carthami* 10 g and Dang Gui *Radix Angelicae Sinensis* 10 g to remove Blood stasis and to regulate the menstruation.
3. If there is severe pain in the testicles, add Ju He *Semen Citri Peticulatae* 10 g and Li Zhi He *Semen Litchi* 10 g to regulate the circulation of Qi in the Liver channel and to relieve the pain.
4. If there is lower abdominal pain, add Gan Jiang *Rhizoma Zingiberis* 6 g and Yan Hu Suo *Rhizoma Corydalis* 10 g to warm the Lower Burner in order to relieve the pain.
5. If there is a swollen scrotum, add Fu Ling *Poria* 15 g, Ze Xie *Rhizoma Alismatis* 10 g and Che Qian Zi *Semen Plantaginis* 10 g to promote urination in order to eliminate Damp.

Patent remedy

Tian Tai Wu Yao Wan *Top-Quality Lindera Pill*

ACUPUNCTURE TREATMENT

LI-4 Hegu, TE-5 Waiguan, LR-3 Taichong, LR-5 Ligou and SP-6 Sanyinjiao. Reducing method is used on these points. Moxibustion is also recommended.

Explanations

- LI-4 and TE-5 dispel External Cold and relieve External symptoms.
- LR-3, the Stream and Source point of the Liver channel, warms the channel and regulates the circulation of Qi. LR-5, the Connecting point, eliminates External Cold, harmonises the collateral and relieves pain. These two points are both treated with moxibustion to warm the Liver channel and to dispel External Cold.
- SP-6, the crossing point of the three Yin channels of the leg, regulates the circulation of Qi and Blood and relieves the pain.

Modifications

1. If there are painful testicles, add LR-8 and LR-12 to regulate the circulation of Qi in the Liver channel and to relieve the pain.
2. If there is a painful vagina, add ST-29 and CV-2 to warm the channel and to relieve the pain.
3. If there are swollen genitals, add ST-30 and SP-9 to eliminate Damp and to relieve the swelling.
4. If there is lower abdomen pain, add CV-3 and ST-28 to warm the channels and to relieve the pain. At the same time, moxibustion treatment on CV-4 is recommended.
5. If there is perineal pain, add KI-10 to regulate the circulation of Qi and to relieve the pain.

Case history

A 43-year-old man came to the acupuncture department with pain at the right side of his lower abdomen, which he had had for the past 20 days. The pain had an acute onset: it was there one morning when he woke up in an air-conditioned room. The pain radiated from the genitals to the interior aspect of the right thigh and there was a slight feeling of stiffness and pain with a cold sensation in the scrotum. He had already visited a doctor who gave him some painkillers and advised bed rest. He was known to have an inguinal hernia on his right side, but it was never operated on. His tongue was white and moist, and his pulse was superficial and wiry.

Diagnosis
Invasion of External Cold to the Liver channel.

Principle of treatment
Warm the Liver channel, eliminate the External Cold and relieve the genital pain.

Acupuncture treatment
LR-3, LR-8, LR-12, ST-29 and CV-4 were needled with reducing method. Treatment was given once every other day.

Explanations

- LR-3, the Source point of the Liver channel, and LR-8, the Sea point, regulate the Liver-Qi and dispel External Cold in the channel.
- LR-12, the local point, harmonises the collateral and stops the pain.
- CV-4 warms the channels and regulates the circulation of Qi in the local area, especially for genital disorders.
- ST-29 circulates the Qi in the genital region and relieves the pain.

After 2 weeks, the genital pain was completely relieved. Upon follow-up a year later, the man said that since the treatment he had experienced no more genital pain.

EXCESSIVE-FIRE IN THE TERMINAL YIN CHANNEL

Symptoms and signs

A sharp pain with a hot sensation in the genitals, redness, swelling and a burning feeling in the pudendum, fever, thirst, constipation, yellow leucorrhoea, dark yellow urine, restlessness, a red tongue with a yellow and dry coating and a rapid and slippery pulse.

Principle of treatment

Clear Heat, reduce Fire and stop the pain.

HERBAL TREATMENT

Prescription

PU JI XIAO DU YIN
Universal Benefit Decoction to Eliminate Toxin
Huang Qin *Radix Scutellariae* 15 g
Huang Lian *Rhizoma Coptidis* 9 g
Xuan Shen *Radix Scrophulariae* 6 g
Chai Hu *Radix Bupleuri* 6 g
Ban Lan Gen *Radix Isatidis* 6 g
Jie Geng *Radix Platycodi* 6 g
Lian Qiao *Fructus Forsythiae* 3 g
Ma Bo *Lasiosphaerae seu Calvatia* 3 g
Niu Bang Zi *Fructus Arctii* 3 g
Bo He *Herba Menthae* 3 g
Jiang Can *Bombyx Batryticatus* 3 g
Sheng Ma *Rhizoma Cimicifugae* 3 g
Gan Cao *Radix Glycyrrhizae* 6 g
Chen Pi *Pericarpium Citri Reticulatae* 6 g

Explanations

- Huang Qin, Huang Lian, Ma Bo and Ban Lan Gen clear Heat and remove Fire.
- Chai Hu, Sheng Ma and Bo He regulate the circulation of Liver-Qi and relieve the pain.
- Xuan Shen, Jie Geng and Gan Cao nourish the Yin and reduce the swelling.
- Lian Qiao, Niu Bang Zi and Jiang Can dispel Wind and reduce Liver-Fire.
- Chen Pi promotes the circulation of Qi and reduces the swelling.

Modifications

1. If there is a high fever, add Shi Gao *Gypsum Fibrosum* 15 g, Da Qing Ye *Folium Isatidis* 10 g and Zhi Mu *Rhizoma Anemarrhenae* 10 g to clear Fire and to reduce the fever.
2. If there is severe swelling and pain, add Pu Gong Ying *Herba Taraxaci* 10 g and Ye Ju Hua *Flos Chrysanthemi* 10 g to remove Toxin, reduce the swelling and to relieve the pain.
3. If there is itching of the genitals, use Tu Fu Ling *Rhizoma Smilacis Glabrae* 10 g, Bai Xian Pi *Cortex Dictamni Radicis* 10 g, Ku Shen *Radix Sophorae Flavescentis* 10 g and She Chuang Zi *Fructus Cnidii* 10 g as a lotion to wash the genitals twice a day in order to relieve the itching, reduce swelling and stop the pain.
4. If there is constipation, add Mang Xiao *Natrii Sulfas* 10 g and Da Huang *Radix et Rhizoma Rhei* 6 g to clear Excessive-Fire and to eliminate Toxin by means of defecation.

Patent remedy

Niu Huang Jie Du Pian *Cattle Gallstone Tablet to Resolve Toxin*

ACUPUNCTURE TREATMENT

LR-3 Taichong, LR-8 Ququan, SP-6 Sanyinjiao, SP-9 Yinlingquan, KI-10 Yingu, CV-2 Qugu and PC-6 Neiguan. Reducing method is used on these points.

Explanations

- LR-3, the Stream and Source point of the Liver channel, promotes the circulation of Liver-Qi and reduces Liver-Fire.
- LR-8, the Sea point and the Water point of the Liver channel, clears Fire in the channel.
- SP-6, the crossing point of the Spleen, Kidney and Liver channels, and SP-9, the Sea point of the Spleen channel, reduce Fire and regulate the circulation of Qi in the Lower Burner.
- KI-10, the Sea point of the Kidney channel, nourishes the Kidney-Yin in order to clear Liver-Fire.
- CV-2, the point where the Liver channel and the Directing Vessel cross, reduces Liver-Fire and relieves the redness and swelling in the genitals.
- PC-6, the Connecting point of the Pericardium channel and Confluence point of the Yin Linking Vessel, tranquillises the Mind and clears Liver-Fire.

Modifications

1. If there is fever due to the flaming up of Liver-Fire, add LR-2, the Spring point, LI-4, the Source point, and LI-11, the Sea point of the Large Intestine channel, to reduce Liver-Fire and clear the fever.
2. If there is redness and swelling of the genitals, add ST-29 to reduce Fire in order to relieve the redness and swelling.
3. If there is painful urination, add KI-2, the Spring point, to clear Heat, promote urination and relieve the pain.
4. If there is restlessness, add HT-3, the Source point, and HT-8, the Spring point of the Heart channel, to reduce Fire and tranquillise the Mind.
5. If there is constipation, add ST-25, the Front Collecting point, and ST-37, the Lower Sea point of the Large Intestine, to promote the circulation of Qi and to relieve the constipation.

Case history

A 4-year-old boy had been suffering from painful genitals for 5 days. He had had an acute parotitis 14 days before, when he was treated with Ban Lan Gen *Radix Isatidis* herbal powder and painkillers. The local pain and swelling had improved. When he came to the clinic he had a slight swelling of the parotid glands on the right side of his face, and his scrotum was a little swollen and painful. Also, he was thirsty and had constipation, his tongue was red with a dry and yellow coating and his pulse was rapid.

Diagnosis
Invasion of toxic Fire to the Liver channel.

Principle of treatment
Clear Fire and eliminate Toxin.

Herbal treatment
PU JI XIAO DU YIN
Universal Benefit Decoction to Eliminate Toxin
Huang Qin *Radix Scutellariae* 5 g
Huang Lian *Rhizoma Coptidis* 5 g
Xuan Shen *Radix Scrophulariae* 6 g
Chai Hu *Radix Bupleuri* 6 g
Ban Lan Gen *Radix Isatidis* 6 g
Long Dan Cao *Radix Gentianae* 5 g
Bo He *Herba Menthae* 3 g
Jiang Can *Bombyx Batryticatus* 3 g
Sheng Ma *Rhizoma Cimicifugae* 3 g
Gan Cao *Radix Glycyrrhizae* 6 g
Chen Pi *Pericarpium Citri Reticulatae* 6 g

Explanations

- Huang Qin, Long Dan Cao, Huang Lian and Ban Lan Gen clear Heat and remove Toxin.
- Chai Hu, Sheng Ma and Bo He regulate the circulation of Liver-Qi and relieve the pain.
- Xuan Shen and Gan Cao nourish the Yin and reduce the swelling.
- Jiang Can dispels Wind and clears Fire.
- Chen Pi promotes the circulation of Qi and relieves the swelling.

The boy received herbal treatment every day. After 15 days of treatment, the genital pain was completely gone. Upon follow-up 6 months later, his mother said her son had experienced no more pain since the last treatment.

ACCUMULATION OF DAMP-HEAT IN THE TERMINAL YIN CHANNEL

Symptoms and signs

Redness and swelling of the genitals with a hot sensation, aggravation of pain during urination, scanty and yellow urine, yellow and smelling leucorrhoea, itching vulvae, itching and wet scrotum, urethral mucus, constipation, low abdominal pain, lower back pain, a fever, a bitter taste in the mouth, a thick and yellow tongue coating and a wiry and rapid pulse.

Principle of treatment

Clear Heat and eliminate Damp.

HERBAL TREATMENT

Prescription

LONG DAN XIE GAN TANG
Gentiana Draining the Liver Decoction
Long Dan Cao *Radix Gentianae* 6 g
Huang Qin *Radix Scutellariae* 9 g
Zhi Zi *Fructus Gardeniae* 9 g
Ze Xie *Rhizoma Alismatis* 12 g
Mu Tong *Caulis Akebiae* 9 g
Che Qian Zi *Semen Plantaginis* 9 g
Dang Gui *Radix Angelicae Sinensis* 3 g
Sheng Di Huang *Radix Rehmanniae Recens* 9 g
Chai Hu *Radix Bupleuri* 6 g
Gan Cao *Radix Glycyrrhizae* 6 g

Explanations

- Long Dan Cao and Huang Qin clear Heat and dry Damp.
- Zhi Zi, Mu Tong, Ze Xie and Che Qian Zi clear Heat, promote urination and eliminate Damp.
- Dang Gui and Sheng Di Huang nourish the Yin and Blood and protect them from being damaged by Fire.
- Chai Hu regulates the Liver-Qi and relieves Qi stagnation.
- Gan Cao harmonises the actions of the other herbs in the formula.

Modifications

1. If the genitals are swollen and painful, add Huang Bai *Cortex Phellodendri* 6 g, Ku Shen *Radix Sophorae Flavescentis* 10 g and Tu Fu Ling *Rhizoma Smilacis Glabrae* 10 g to eliminate Damp-Heat and relieve the pain.
2. If the testicles are painful, add Ju He *Semen Citri Reticulatae* 10 g and Li Zhi He *Semen Litchi* 10 g to regulate Liver-Qi and to relieve the pain.
3. If there is yellow leucorrhoea, add Ku Shen *Radix Sophorae Flavescentis* 10 g and Bai Xian Pi *Cortex Dictamni Radicis* 10 g to eliminate Damp-Heat in the Lower Burner.
4. If there is constipation, add Da Huang *Radix et Rhizoma Rhei* 6 g and Mang Xiao *Natrii Sulfas* 10 g to clear Fire and to promote defecation.

Patent remedy

Long Dan Xie Gan Wan *Gentiana Draining the Liver Pill*

ACUPUNCTURE TREATMENT

LR-2 Xingjian, LR-4 Zhongfeng, SP-3 Taibai, SP-9 Yinlingquan, KI-3 Taixi, BL-18 Ganshu and CV-2 Qugu. Reducing method is used on these points.

Explanations

- LR-2, the Spring point, and LR-4, the River point of the Liver channel, eliminate Damp-Heat in this channel.
- SP-3, the Source point, and SP-9, the Sea point of the Spleen channel, activate the Spleen and remove Damp-Heat.
- KI-3, the Source point of the Kidney channel, eliminates Damp-Heat and nourishes the Yin.
- BL-18, the Back Transporting point of the Liver, reduces Liver-Fire.
- CV-2, the crossing point of the Directing Vessel and the Liver channel, regulates the circulation of Qi in these two channels and relieves the pain.

Modifications

1. If there is fever caused by Damp-Heat, add LI-4 and GV-14 to clear Heat and reduce the fever.
2. If there is swelling of the genitals, add SP-6 and LR-12 to eliminate Damp-Heat and reduce the swelling.
3. If the testicles are painful, add ST-29 and ST-30 to regulate the Qi and to remove its stagnation in order to relieve the pain.
4. If there is a painful vagina with leucorrhoea, add SP-8, the Accumulation point of the Spleen channel and ST-29 to eliminate Damp-Heat and relieve the pain.
5. If there is painful urination, add ST-30 and KI-2 to promote urination and to relieve the pain.
6. If there is lower back pain, add BL-23, the Back Transporting point of the Kidney, and BL-58, the Connecting point of the Bladder, to strengthen the lower back and relieve the pain.

STAGNATION OF LIVER-QI

Symptoms and signs

Genital pain which is aggravated by emotional upset or stress, with a distending sensation, depression, hypochondriac pain, irregular menstruation, a poor appetite, distension in the stomach, insomnia, irritability, lower abdominal pain, a red tongue with a white coating and a wiry pulse.

Principle of treatment

Regulate the Liver, remove Qi stagnation and relieve the pain.

HERBAL TREATMENT

Prescription

DAN ZHI XIAO YAO SAN
Free and Relaxed Powder with Moutan and Gardenia
Chai Hu *Radix Bupleuri* 10 g
Dang Gui *Radix Angelicae Sinensis* 10 g
Bai Shao *Radix Paeoniae Alba* 20 g
Bai Zhu *Rhizoma Atractylodis Macrocephalae* 10 g
Fu Ling *Poria* 15 g
Gan Cao *Radix Glycyrrhizae* 5 g
Bo He *Herba Menthae* 3 g
Mu Dan Pi *Cortex Moutan Radicis* 10 g
Zhi Zi *Fructus Gardeniae* 10 g
Sheng Jiang *Rhizoma Zingiberis Recens* 5 g

Explanations

- Chai Hu and Bo He regulate and promote the circulation of Liver-Qi in order to remove Qi stagnation in the Liver.
- Bai Shao and Dang Gui nourish the Blood and strengthen the Liver. These two herbs can also directly relieve the genital pain.
- Dan Pi and Zhi Zi clear internal Heat produced by Qi stagnation.
- Bai Zhu, Fu Ling and Sheng Jiang tonify the Spleen and Stomach.
- Gan Cao harmonises the actions of the other herbs in the prescription.

Modifications

1. If there is a pain in the lower abdomen, add Wu Yao *Radix Linderae* 5 g and Ju He *Semen Citri Reticulatae* 10 g to regulate the circulation of Qi and relieve the pain.
2. If there is a sharp pain, add Yan Hu Suo *Rhizoma Corydalis* 10 g and Mo Yao *Resina Myrrhae* 10 g to promote the circulation of Qi and Blood and relieve the pain.
3. If there is irregular menstruation, add Chuan Xiong *Radix Ligustici Chuanxiong* 10 g and Yi Mu Cao *Herba Leonuri* 10 g to regulate the menstruation.

Patent remedies

Xiao Yao Wan *Free and Relaxed Pill*
Shu Gan Wan *Soothe Liver Pill*

ACUPUNCTURE TREATMENT

LR-3 Taichong, LR-8 Ququan, PC-6 Neiguan, CV-2 Qugu, GV-20 Baihui and BL-18 Ganshu. Even method is used for these points.

Explanations

- LR-3, the Source and Stream point of the Liver channel, and LR-8, the Sea point, regulate the Liver-Qi and relieve the genital pain.
- BL-18, the Back Transporting point of the Liver, regulates the Liver-Qi and removes Qi stagnation in the Liver.
- CV-2 relieves the genital pain.
- PC-6, the Connecting point of the Pericardium channel and Confluence point of the Yin Linking Vessel, regulates the circulation of Qi and removes its stagnation.
- GV-20 is the patent point for calming the Mind and regulating the circulation of Qi.

Modifications

1. If there is pain in the hypochondrium, add TE-5 and GB-34 to regulate the circulation of Qi and relieve the pain.
2. If there is pain in the lower abdomen, add ST-29 and BL-25 to regulate the local circulation of Qi and relieve the pain.
3. If there is irregular menstruation, add SP-6 and KI-3 to regulate the menstruation.
4. If there is insomnia, add HT-7 and Extra Anmian to calm the Mind and improve sleep.
5. If there is irritability, add LR-2 and GB-20 to calm the Liver, clear Heat in the Liver and calm the Mind.

Case history

A 41-year-old woman had been suffering from genital pain for 3 months, which worsened when she got angry. She had been diagnosed with mild depression, for which she was given tranquillisers. However, she preferred to have acupuncture treatment. She also mentioned she had irregular menstruation, a poor appetite and low abdominal pain. Her tongue was red at the sides and had a white coating, and her pulse was wiry.

Diagnosis
Stagnation of Liver-Qi.

Principle of treatment
Regulate the Liver and relieve Qi stagnation.

Acupuncture treatment
LR-3, SP-6, ST-29, BL-25 and PC-6 were selected. Even method was used on these points. In the first week

treatment was given daily; in the second week treatments were given every other day.

Explanations

- LR-3 is the Stream and Source point of the Liver channel. PC-6 is the Connecting point of the Pericardium channel and Confluence point of the Yin Linking Vessel. These two points together regulate the circulation of Liver-Qi and calm the Mind.
- SP-6 is the crossing point of the three Yin channels of the foot. It regulates the circulation of Qi and relieves the genital pain.
- ST-29 and BL-25 regulate the circulation of Qi in the lower abdomen and relieve the genital pain.

After 2 months of treatment, her genital pain was under control. Six months later she came back to the clinic with a headache. She stated that she had experienced no more genital pain since the treatment.

STAGNATION OF BLOOD

Symptoms and signs

A prolonged, sharp pain with a fixed location, or a stabbing pubic pain radiating to the lower abdomen or lower back when moving, which worsens at night, with a a rigid scrotum, a purplish tongue with a thin coating and a wiry and choppy pulse.

Principle of treatment

Circulate Qi and Blood, regulate the collateral and sedate the pain.

HERBAL TREATMENT

Prescription

SHAO FU ZHU YU TANG
Drive Out Blood Stasis in the Lower Abdomen Decoction
Xiao Hui Xiang *Fructus Foeniculi* 6 g
Gan Jiang *Rhizoma Zingiberis* 6 g
Yan Hu Suo *Rhizoma Corydalis* 9 g
Mo Yao *Resina Myrrhae* 6 g
Dang Gui *Radix Angelicae Sinensis* 12 g
Rou Gui *Cortex Cinnamomi* 6 g
Chuan Xiong *Radix Ligustici Chuanxiong* 6 g
Chi Shao *Radix Paeoniae Rubra* 9 g
Pu Huang *Pollen Typhae* 12 g
Wu Ling Zhi *Faeces Trogopterorum* 9 g

Explanations

- Xiao Hui Xiang and Chuan Xiong regulate the circulation of Liver-Qi and relieve the pain.

- Gan Jiang and Rou Gui warm the channels and collateral in order to promote the circulation of Blood.
- Dang Gui, Pu Huang, Wu Ling Zhi, Mo Yao, Chi Shao and Yan Hu Suo remove Blood stagnation and relieve the pain.

Modifications

1. If there is lower back pain, add Du Zhong *Cortex Eucommiae* 10 g and Gou Ji *Rhizoma Cibotii* 10 g to strengthen the Kidney and relieve the pain.
2. If there is lower abdominal pain, add Qing Pi *Pericarpium Citri Reticulatae Viride* 10 g and Wu Yao *Radix Linderae* 5 g to regulate the Qi and relieve the pain.
3. If there is pain around the testicles, add Ju He *Semen Citri Peticulatae* 10 g and Li Zhi He *Semen Litchi* 10 g to regulate the Liver-Qi and relieve the pain.

Patent remedies

Yan Hu Suo Zhi Tong Pian *Corydalis Stop Pain Tablet*
Jie Ji Wan *Dispel Prostate Swelling Pill*

ACUPUNCTURE TREATMENT

LR-3 Taichong, SP-10 Xuehai, BL-17 Geshu, BL-18 Ganshu and CV-2 Qugu. Reducing method is used on these points.

Explanations

- BL-18 is the Back Transporting point of the Liver, and can regulate the Liver-Qi. LR-3 is the Stream and Source point of the Liver channel. Since the Qi guides the Blood, BL-18 and LR-3 together can regulate the circulation of Qi in order to promote the circulation of Blood.
- SP-10 is the patent point for treating Blood stagnation and lower abdominal pain. BL-17 is the Gathering point for the Blood and promotes its circulation. These two points together promote the circulation of Blood, eliminate its stasis and relieve the pain.
- CV-2 is the crossing point of the Directing Vessel and the Liver channel. It may be used to regulate the circulation of Qi and relieve pain in this area.

Modifications

1. If there is pain around the testicles, add LR-12 and ST-30 to regulate the local circulation of Qi.

2. If there is lower back pain, add BL-58, the Connecting point, and BL-63, the Accumulation point of the Bladder channel, to regulate the circulation of Qi and Blood and relieve the pain.
3. If there is pain in the lower abdomen, add ST-29 and KI-12 to activate the local circulation of Qi and Blood and relieve the pain.
4. If the pain worsens at night, add HT-3 and SP-6 to promote the circulation of Qi and remove Blood stasis.

Case history

A 36-year-old man had been suffering from testicle pain for 6 months since a bicycle accident. The pain was mainly on the right side and got worse at night. He could no longer ride a bicycle. He had a normal tongue and a wiry pulse.

Diagnosis
Stagnation of Blood in the Liver channel.

Principle of treatment
Regulate Liver-Qi, remove Blood stagnation and relieve the pain.

Acupuncture treatment
LR-2, SP-10, BL-17, ST-30 and CV-2 were selected for treatment every other day. Even method was used for these points.

Explanations

- LR-2 is the Spring point of the Liver channel. ST-10 is the patent point for promoting the circulation of Blood. These two points together regulate the Liver-Qi and promote the Blood circulation in order to remove Blood stagnation in the Liver Channel.
- BL-17 is one of the eight Gathering points. It is good for removing Blood stasis. In this treatment it was used to relieve the genital pain.
- CV-12 and ST-30 regulate the local circulation of Qi and Blood, harmonise the collateral and relieve the pain.

After 3 weeks of treatment, the testicle pain had disappeared.

DEFICIENCY OF YIN OF LIVER AND KIDNEY

Symptoms and signs

Chronic genital pain, with a dry and itchy feeling and perineal pain, accompanied by lumbago with soreness, scanty and frequent urination, a tidal fever, night sweating, a dry mouth, a poor appetite, restlessness, insomnia, lassitude, tinnitus, sensations of heat in the palms and soles of the feet, constipation and diminished menstruation with a pale colour, a red tongue with little coating and a thready and rapid pulse.

Principle of treatment

Tonify the Yin of the Liver and Kidney.

HERBAL TREATMENT

Prescription

LIU WEI DI HUANG WAN
Six-Flavour Rehmanniae Pill
Shu Di Huang *Radix Rehmanniae Praeparata* 24 g
Shan Zhu Yu *Fructus Corni* 12 g
Shan Yao *Rhizoma Dioscoreae* 12 g
Fu Ling *Poria* 9 g
Mu Dan Pi *Cortex Moutan Radicis* 9 g
Ze Xie *Rhizoma Alismatis* 9 g

Explanations

- Shu Di Huang, Shan Zhu Yu and Shan Yao tonify the Blood and Essence of the Liver and Kidney.
- Ze Xie promotes urination and clears Deficient-Heat.
- Mu Dan Pi cools the Blood and activates the circulation of Blood.
- Fu Ling strengthens the Spleen and drains Damp.

Modifications

1. If there is insomnia, add Suan Zao Ren *Semen Ziziphi Spinosae* 10 g and Wu Wei Zi *Fructus Schisandrae* 10 g to calm the Mind.
2. If there is lower back pain, add Xu Duan *Radix Dipsaci* 10 g, Sang Ji Sheng *Ramulus Loranthi* 10 g and Bai Shao *Radix Paeoniae Alba* 15 g to strengthen the Kidney and relieve the pain.
3. If there is constipation, add Sheng Di Huang *Radix Rehmanniae Recens* 15 g and Xuan Shen *Radix Scrophulariae* 10 g to tonify the Kidney-Yin, to lubricate the Large Intestine and to relieve the constipation.

Patent remedy

Zhi Bai Di Huang Wan *Anemarrhena, Phellodendron and Rehmannia Pill*

ACUPUNCTURE TREATMENT

LR-3 Taichong, KI-3 Taixi, KI-7 Fuliu, SP-6 Sanyinjiao, CV-3 Zhongji and BL-23 Shenshu. Reinforcing method is used on these points.

Explanations

- LR-3 is the Stream and Source point of the Liver channel. It nourishes the Liver-Yin.

- KI-3, the Stream and Source point of the Kidney channel, and KI-7, the Metal point, nourish the Kidney-Yin as well as the Liver-Yin, because the Liver and Kidney share the same origin.
- CV-3 is the Front Collecting point of the Bladder, the crossing point of the Directing Vessel and the three Yin channels of the leg. It is often used to tonify the Liver and Kidney.
- SP-6 is the crossing point of the Spleen, Kidney and Liver channels. It can nourish the Yin and clear Deficient-Fire.
- BL-23 is the Back Transporting point of the Kidney. It may be used to tonify the Kidney-Yin and nourish the Liver-Yin indirectly.

Modifications

1. If there is lower back pain with soreness, add BL-25 and BL-58 to relieve the pain.
2. If there is scanty and frequent urination, add CV-4 to tonify the Kidney-Qi and diminish the frequency of urination.
3. If there is restlessness and insomnia, add PC-6 and HT-3 to tranquillise the Mind.
4. If there is a poor appetite and lassitude, add ST-36 and CV-12 to promote the circulation of Qi and nourish the Stomach-Yin.
5. If there is constipation, add ST-25 to nourish the Yin in the Large Intestine and relieve the constipation.

Pain associated with 49
urination 小便疼痛

Pain associated with urination may be a stabbing, burning or colicky pain that may occur either during or after urination. This pain, according to TCM theory, may be caused by invasion of Damp-Heat, stagnation of Liver-Qi, deficiency of Spleen-Qi or deficiency of Kidney-Yin. Pain on urination may be attributed to any of the following disorders in Western medicine: infection of the urinary tract, urinary tract lithiasis, tuberculous urinary tract or prostatitis.

Aetiology and pathology

Accumulation of Damp-Heat in the Lower Burner

Invasion of external Damp-Heat is a major cause of accumulation of Damp-Heat in the Lower Burner. Bad diets, such as eating too much pungent or greasy food, or drinking too much alcohol, may damage the Spleen and Stomach in their function of transportation and transformation; this causes Damp-Heat to form in the Middle Burner. Since Damp has the characteristics of heaviness and downward flow, when Damp-Heat forms in the Middle Burner it eventually causes Damp-Heat to accumulate in the Lower Burner, leading to blockage or damage of the collateral and Blood vessels in the bladder and urinary tract. This impedes its function of transforming Qi, causing urination pain.

Stagnation of Liver-Qi

The Liver has a relationship to the emotional balance and the free flow of Qi. If there is excessive stress, anger, frustration or depression, the flow of Qi becomes impaired and the circulation of Qi in the Liver slows down, leading to stagnation of the Liver-Qi. Stagnation of Liver-Qi may in turn influence the circulation of Qi in the bladder, so urination pain occurs.

Deficiency of Spleen-Qi

Irregular eating habits, an unbalanced diet, prolonged sickness and excessive physical work may all damage the Spleen-Qi in its function of transporting and transforming, so that Damp accumulates in the body and the Spleen-Qi becomes deficient. Since the proper circulation of Qi and Blood depends on the amount of Qi being sufficient, when there is insufficient Spleen-Qi the circulation of Qi and Blood slows and stagnates. Stagnation of Qi and Blood in the Lower Burner causes urination pain.

Deficiency of Kidney-Yin

Prolonged febrile disease, prolonged presence of Damp-Heat in the Lower Burner or excessive sexual activity may all gradually damage and consume the Kidney-Yin, and lead to the generation of Deficient-Fire. When this Deficient-Fire burns the collateral and the Blood vessels in the Lower Burner, then urination pain occurs.

Treatment based on differentiation

Differentiation

Before giving a treatment, special attention should be paid to differentiating clearly the symptoms and signs. The factors to be taken into consideration include the quality and the duration of the pain, the accompanying symptoms, and the conditions that trigger the pain, aggravate it or alleviate it.

The quality of the pain

— Urination pain with a distending sensation in the lower abdomen is usually caused by stagnation of Liver-Qi.
— Urination pain with a stabbing nature is usually caused by stagnation of Blood.
— Urination pain with a burning sensation is usually caused by accumulation of Damp-Heat.
— Urination pain of an indistinct nature combined with lower back pain is usually caused by deficiency of Kidney-Yin.

Duration of the pain

— Acute urination pain is usually caused by Excessive factors.
— Chronic urination pain accompanied by other weakness is usually caused by Deficiency.

Accompanying symptoms

— Fever, an aversion to cold and urination pain with a hot sensation is usually caused by invasion of Damp-Heat.
— Urination pain with irritability, hypochondriac pain and abdominal distension is usually caused by stagnation of Liver-Qi.
— Chronic urination pain with a poor appetite, lassitude and tiredness is usually caused by deficiency of Spleen-Qi.

— Chronic urination pain with lower back pain or soreness and fatigue is usually caused by deficiency of Kidney-Yin.

Conditions that trigger, aggravate or alleviate the pain

— When urination pain is triggered or aggravated after eating spicy or pungent food, it is usually due to Damp-Heat.
— When urination pain is triggered or aggravated by emotional disturbance, it is usually caused by stagnation of Liver-Qi.
— Urination pain that begins after prolonged persistence of Damp-Heat is usually caused by deficiency of Kidney-Yin.
— Urination pain that begins after chronic diarrhoea or an abdominal operation is usually due to deficiency of Spleen-Qi.
— Urination pain that is worsened by pressure on the abdomen is caused by an Excess syndrome.
— Urination pain that is relieved by pressure on the abdomen is caused by Deficient syndrome.

Treatment

INVASION OF DAMP-HEAT IN THE BLADDER

Symptoms and signs

Scanty and frequent urination with a stabbing and burning pain, and with pain and fullness of the lower abdomen and lower back pain, accompanied by an aversion to cold, fever, a bitter taste in the mouth, nausea or constipation, a red tongue with a yellow greasy coating and a soft and rapid pulse.

Principle of treatment

Promote urination and eliminate Damp-Heat.

HERBAL TREATMENT

Prescription

BA ZHENG SAN
Eight-Herb Powder for Rectification
Che Qian Zi *Semen Plantaginis* 10 g
Qu Mai *Herba Dianthi* 15 g
Bian Xu *Herba Polygoni Avicularis* 12 g
Hua Shi *Talcum* 20 g
Zhi Zi *Fructus Gardeniae* 12 g
Gan Cao *Radix Glycyrrhizae* 6 g

Tong Cao *Medulla Tetrapanacis* 10 g
Da Huang *Radix et Rhizoma Rhei* 6 g

Explanations

- Bian Xu, Qu Mai, Tong Cao, Che Qian Zi and Hua Shi promote urination, clear Heat and eliminate Damp.
- Zhi Zi clears Heat and eliminates Damp.
- Da Huang clears Internal Fire and reduces fever.
- Gan Cao harmonises the actions of the other herbs in the prescription.
- All the herbs are used to stop urination pain caused by Damp-Heat.

Modifications

1. If there is a fever and an aversion to cold, add Chai Hu *Radix Bupleuri* 10 g to dispel Heat and to relieve the External symptoms.
2. If there is blood in the urine, add Hu Po *Succinum* 2 g and San Qi *Radix Notoginseng* 10 g to stop the bleeding.
3. If there is constipation and a feeling of fullness in the abdomen, add Mang Xiao *Natrii Sulfas* 10 g to assist Da Huang in promoting defecation.
4. If there is deficiency of Yin caused by Damp-Heat, manifesting as night sweating, heat in the palms and soles of the feet, thirst and a dry mouth and throat, add Zhi Mu *Rhizoma Anemarrhenae* 10 g to nourish the Yin and clear Deficient-Heat.
5. If there is a feeling of fullness in the chest and abdomen, add Qing Pi *Pericarpium Citri Reticulatae Viride* 10 g to regulate the circulation of Qi and remove its stagnation.
6. If there is a stabbing pain due to stagnation of Blood, add Hong Hua *Flos Carthami* 10 g to regulate the circulation of Blood and remove its stasis.
7. If there is urinary lithiasis, add Jin Qian Cao *Herba Lysimachiae* 15 g to eliminate the stones and promote urination.

Patent remedies

Ba Zheng Wan *Eight-Herb Pill for Rectification*
Qian Lie Xian Wan *Prostate Gland Pill*

ACUPUNCTURE TREATMENT

TE-5 Waiguan, SP-6 Sanyinjiao, SP-9 Yinlingquan, CV-3 Zhongji, LR-5 Ligou and ST-28 Shuidao. Reducing method is used on these points.

Explanations

- TE-5, the Connecting point of the Triple Burner channel, dispels Damp-Heat and relieves External symptoms.
- SP-6, the crossing point of the three Yin channels of the foot, and SP-9, the Sea point of the Spleen channel, promote urination and clear Damp-Heat in the Bladder.
- CV-3, the crossing point of the Directing Vessel and the three Yin channels of the foot, and the Front Collecting point of the Bladder, clears Damp-Heat and relieves the pain.
- LR-5, the Connecting point of the Liver channel, harmonises the collateral, regulates the circulation of Qi in the channel and relieves the pain.
- ST-28, the local point, promotes urination, eliminates Damp-Heat and relieves urinary pain.

Modifications

1. If there is fever and aversion to cold, add LU-7, the Connecting point, and LI-4, the Source point, to eliminate Damp-Heat and relieve the external symptoms.
2. If there is blood in the urine, add SP-10 to clear Heat and to stop the bleeding.
3. If there is lithiasis, add KI-4 and SP-29 to promote urination, eliminate the stones and to relieve the pain.
4. If there is severe urination pain, add BL-32 and BL-66 to clear Heat, eliminate Damp and relieve the pain.
5. If there is lower abdominal pain, add SP-8 and ST-40 to regulate the circulation of Qi and relieve the pain.
6. If there is constipation, add TE-6 and BL-25 to clear Heat in the Large Intestine and promote defecation.
7. If there is lower back pain, add BL-23 and BL-58 to regulate the circulation of Qi and to relieve the pain.

Case history

A 44-year-old woman had been suffering from urination pain for about 15 days. She was diagnosed as having acute urethritis and received antibiotics for 13 days, but this did not help her much. So she came to the acupuncture clinic. As well as the urination pain, she had a fever (38.6°C), frequent urination with a sensation of heat, a bitter taste in her mouth, thirst, low back pain and constipation. Her tongue was red with a yellow and greasy coating and her pulse was slippery and rapid.

Diagnosis
Invasion of External Damp-Heat to the Lower Burner.

Principle of treatment
Clear Damp-Heat and relieve the pain.

Acupuncture treatment
TE-5, LR-2, LR-5, BL-64, SP-6, SP-9 and ST-29 were needled daily with reducing method.

Explanations

- TE-5, the Connecting point of the Triple Burner channel, dispels Damp-Heat and relieves External symptoms.
- LR-2, the Spring point, and LR-5, the Connecting point of the Liver channel, clear Damp-Heat in the Lower Burner and relieve the pain.
- SP-6, the crossing point of the three Yin channels of the foot, and SP-9, the Sea point of the Spleen channel, promote urination and eliminate Damp Heat.
- BL-64, the Source point of the Bladder channel, promotes urination and clears Damp-Heat.
- ST-29 regulates the circulation of Qi in the locality in order to relieve the pain.

After 10 days of treatment, the patient had no more urinary pain.

STAGNATION OF LIVER-QI

Symptoms and signs

Urination pain, which may worsen with emotional upset, scanty and frequent urination, or dribbling urination, emotional instability, depression, stress, a feeling of fullness and pain in the chest, lower abdominal pain, palpitations, insomnia, a thin and white tongue coating and a wiry pulse.

Principle of treatment

Smooth the Liver, regulate the circulation of Liver-Qi and sedate the urinary pain.

HERBAL TREATMENT

Prescription

CHEN XIANG SAN
Aquilaria Powder
Chen Xiang *Lignum Aquilariae Resinatum* 10 g
Shi Wei *Folium Pyrrosiae* 10 g
Hua Shi *Talcum* 20 g
Dang Gui *Radix Angelicae Sinensis* 12 g
Chen Pi *Pericarpium Citri Reticulatae* 6 g
Bai Shao *Radix Paeoniae Alba* 6 g
Dong Kui Zi *Fructus Malvae Verticillatae* 10 g
Gan Cao *Radix Glycyrrhizae* 6 g
Wang Bu Liu Xing *Semen Vaccariae* 6 g

Explanations

- Chen Xiang and Chen Pi promote the circulation of Qi in the Liver and the Lower Burner.
- Dang Gui and Bai Shao soothe the Liver and harmonise the circulation of Qi.
- Shi Wei, Hua Shi, Dong Kui Zi and Wang Bu Liu Xing promote urination and relieve the pain.
- Gan Cao clears Heat in the Lower Burner and harmonises the actions of the other herbs in the prescription.

Modifications

1. If there is a stabbing pain due to stagnation of Blood, add Hong Hua *Flos Carthami* 10 g to regulate the circulation of Blood and remove Blood stasis.
2. If there is a sensation of fullness in the chest and abdomen, add Qing Pi *Pericarpium Citri Reticulatae Viride* 5 g to regulate the Liver-Qi and remove the Qi stagnation.
3. If there are palpitations, add Yuan Zhi *Radix Polygalae* 10 g and Yu Jin *Radix Curcumae* 10 g to regulate the circulation of Liver-Qi and calm the Mind.
4. If there is insomnia, add Ci Shi *Magnetitum* 15 g and Suan Zhao Ren *Semen Ziziphi Spinosae* 15 g to calm the Mind and improve sleep.

Patent remedies

Shu Gan Wan *Soothe Liver Pill*
Xiao Yao Wan *Free and Relaxed Pill*

ACUPUNCTURE TREATMENT

LR-3 Taichong, LR-5 Ligou, LR-12 Jimai, PC-6 Neiguan, SP-6 Sanyinjiao and GV-20 Baihui. Even method is used on these points.

Explanations

- LR-3, the Stream and Source point, and LR-5, the Connecting point of the Liver channel, together with LR-12, smooth the Liver, regulate the circulation of Liver-Qi and relieve the pain.
- PC-6 is the Connecting point of the Pericardium channel; SP-6 is the crossing point of the three Yin channels of the foot. These two points, together with GV-20, regulate the circulation of Qi and calm the Mind in order to relieve the pain.

Modifications

1. If there is lower abdominal pain, add ST-28 and BL-25 to remove Qi stagnation and relieve the pain.
2. If there is a feeling of fullness and pain in the chest, add CV-17 and BL-15 to regulate the circulation of Qi and relieve the fullness.
3. If there are palpitations, add HT-7 and KI-3 to regulate the circulation of Qi and Blood and relieve the palpitations.
4. If there is insomnia, add HT-3 and Extra Anmian to regulate the circulation of Qi and calm the Mind.
5. If there is emotional instability, add LR-14 and BI-18 to smooth the Liver and harmonise the emotions.

DEFICIENCY OF SPLEEN-QI

Symptoms and signs

Prolonged duration of urination pain, low abdominal pain with a heavy and bearing-down sensation, accompanied by a pale complexion, a poor appetite, fatigue, palpitations, dizziness, diarrhoea with loose stools, a pale tongue and a weak pulse.

Principle of treatment

Tonify the Spleen-Qi, raise the Spleen-Yang and relieve the pain.

HERBAL TREATMENT

Prescription

BU ZHONG YI QI TANG
Tonifying the Middle and Benefiting Qi Decoction
Ren Shen *Radix Ginseng* 10 g
Huang Qi *Radix Astragali seu Hedysari* 15 g
Bai Zhu *Rhizoma Atractylodis Macrocephalae* 10 g
Gan Cao *Radix Glycyrrhizae* 6 g
Dang Gui *Radix Angelicae Sinensis* 12 g
Chen Pi *Pericarpium Citri Reticulatae* 6 g
Sheng Ma *Rhizoma Cimicifugae* 3 g
Chai Hu *Radix Bupleuri* 3 g

Explanations

- Huang Qi replenishes Qi and elevates the Yang.
- Ren Shen, Bai Zhu and Gan Cao invigorate the Spleen and replenish the Spleen-Qi.
- Chen Pi promotes the circulation of Qi while Dang Gui tonifies the Blood.

- Sheng Ma and Chai Hu together raise the Spleen-Yang.

Modifications

1. If there is a sensation of fullness in the chest and abdomen, add Zhi Qiao *Fructus Aurantii* 10 g to regulate and raise the Spleen-Qi.
2. If there is stagnation of Blood due to deficiency of Qi, add Hong Hua *Flos Carthami* 10 g to regulate the circulation of Blood and eliminate its stasis.
3. If there is blood in the urine, add San Qi *Radix Notoginseng* 10 g to regulate the circulation of Blood and stop the bleeding.
4. If there is diarrhoea, add Shan Yao *Rhizoma Dioscoreae* 10 g to tonify the Spleen-Qi, activate the Spleen and stop the diarrhoea.
5. If the appetite is poor, add Sha Ren *Fructus Amomi* 15 g to improve the appetite.

Patent remedy

Bu Zhong Yi Qi Wan *Tonifying the Middle and Benefiting Qi Pill*

ACUPUNCTURE TREATMENT

CV-4 Guanyuan, CV-12 Zhongwan, ST-36 Zusanli, SP-6 Sanyinjiao and BL-20 Pishu. Reinforcing method is used on these points. Moxibustion is recommended on CV-4, CV-12 and ST-36.

Explanations

- CV-4, the crossing point of the Directing Vessel and the three Yin channels of the foot, and the Front Collecting point of the Small Intestine, is a key point for tonifying the Qi and Yang of the body, dispelling Cold and relieving the weakness.
- CV-12, the Gathering point for the Fu organs and the Front Collecting point of the Stomach, ST-36, the Sea point of the Stomach channel, and BL-20, the Back Transporting point for the Spleen, tonify the Spleen-Qi and activate the Spleen and Stomach.
- SP-6, the crossing point of the three Yin channels of the foot, regulates the circulation of Qi and Blood in the Lower Burner and relieves the pain.

Modifications

1. If the appetite is poor, add SP-3, the Source point of the Spleen channel, and BL-21, the Back Transporting point of the Stomach, to regulate the Stomach-Qi and improve the appetite.

2. If there is dizziness, add GV-20 and BL-18 to raise the Yang-Qi and relieve the dizziness.
3. If there is fatigue, add CV-6 with moxibustion to tonify the Yang-Qi and increase the energy.
4. If there is diarrhoea, add SP-9 and ST-25 to regulate Stomach-Qi and stop the diarrhoea.
5. If there is blood in the urine, add ST-10 and KI-3 to tonify the Qi and regulate Blood circulation in order to stop the bleeding.

DEFICIENCY OF KIDNEY-YIN

Symptoms and signs

Long-term urinary tract infection or other urinary disease, urinary pain with a sensation of heat, scanty urination, dark yellow urine or blood in the urine, irritability, palpitation, soreness in the lower back and knees, fatigue, a low fever, night sweating, a red tongue with no coating and a thready pulse.

Principle of treatment

Nourish the Kidney-Yin and relieve the pain.

HERBAL TREATMENT

Prescription

ZUO GUI WAN
Left Metal Pill
Shu Di Huang *Radix Rehmanniae Praeparatae* 12 g
Shan Yao *Rhizoma Dioscoreae* 15 g
Shan Zhu Yu *Fructus Corni* 10 g
Tu Si Zi *Semen Cuscutae* 12 g
Gou Qi Zi *Fructus Lycii* 12 g
Chuan Niu Xi *Radix Cyathulae* 10 g
Lu Jiao Jiao *Colla Cervi Cornus* 6 g
Gui Ban Jiao *Colla Plastri Testudinis* 6 g

Explanations

- Shu Di Huang and Shan Zhu Yu tonify the Kidney-Yin.
- Gou Qi Zi, Lu Jiao Jiao, Tu Si Zi and Gui Ban Jiao tonify the Kidney-Essence, strengthen the Kidney and relieve the weakness.
- Shan Yao tonifies the Spleen-Qi.
- Chuan Niu Xi strengthens the Kidney, promotes urination and relieves the pain.

Modifications

1. If there is low back pain, add Xu Duan *Radix Dipsaci* 10 g to tonify the Kidney and to relieve the pain.

2. If there is night sweating, add Mu Li *Concha Ostreae* 10 g and Dan Pi *Cortex Moutan Radicis* 10 g to clear Deficient-Heat and stop the sweating.
3. If there is blood in the urine, add Han Lian Cao *Herba Ecliptae* 10 g and Xiao Ji *Herba Cephalanoploris* 10 g to cool the Blood and stop the bleeding.
4. If there is dizziness, add Ju Hua *Flos Chrysanthemi* 10 g to nourish the Yin and subdue Liver-Yang hyperactivity.
5. If there is irritability, add Suan Zhao Ren *Semen Ziziphi Spinosae* 10 g and Bai Zi Ren *Semen Biotae* 10 g to calm the Mind.

Patent remedies

Qi Ju Di Huang Wan *Lycium Fruit, Chrysanthemum and Rehmannia Pill*
Zhi Bai Di Huang Wan *Anemarrhena, Phellodendron and Rehmannia Pill*

ACUPUNCTURE TREATMENT

KI-3 Taixi, LR-3 Taichong, LR-12 Jimai, SP-6 Sanyinjiao, CV-3 Qugu, BL-23 Shenshu and BL-18 Ganshu. Reinforcing method is used on these points.

Explanations

- KI-3 is the Stream and Source point of the Kidney channel. It tonifies the Kidney-Yin and clears Deficient-Fire.
- LR-3 is the Stream point and Source point of the Liver channel. Together with LR-12 it harmonises the collateral, promotes the circulation of Qi and relieves the pain.
- SP-6, the crossing point of the three Yin channels of the foot, regulates the circulation of Qi and Blood and relieves the pain.
- CV-3, the crossing point of the Directing Vessel and the three Yin channels of the foot, and the Front Collecting point of the Bladder, relieves the urination pain.
- BL-23, the Back Transporting point of the Kidney, and BL-18, the Back Transporting point of the Liver, nourish the Kidney-Yin and Liver-Yin and relieve the urination pain.

Modifications

1. If there is scanty urination with pain, add SP-9 and KI-10, the Sea points of the Spleen and Kidney channels respectively, to promote urination, nourish the Yin and relieve the pain.

2. If there is a low fever, add KI-6 and HT-6 to nourish Yin and clear Deficient-Fire.
3. If there is night sweating, add HT-7 and LU-8 to clear Deficient-Fire and stop the sweating.
4. If there is soreness and pain in the lower back, add BL-25 and BL-58 to strengthen the Kidney and Liver and relieve the pain.
5. If there is haematuria, add SP-10 to cool the Blood and stop the bleeding.
6. If there is irritability, add GV-20 and LR-2 to clear Liver-Fire and calm the Mind.

Case history

A 65-year-old woman had been suffering from urination pain during the previous 3 months. A year before she had been diagnosed as suffering from chronic urethritis, and was treated with antibiotics and herbal tablets. Her present complaint was pain on urination and a dry and itching sensation in the vagina. She also mentioned lumbago with soreness, frequent and scanty urination, lassitude, a dry mouth and night sweating. Her tongue was red with no coating, and her pulse was thready and rapid.

Diagnosis
Deficiency of Kidney-Yin.

Principle of treatment
Nourish the Kidney-Yin and relieve the pain.

Acupuncture treatment
LR-3, KI-3, KI-10, SP-6, CV-3 and BL-23. LR-3 was needled with reducing method. The rest of the points were needled with reinforcing method. She was treated every other day.

Explanations

- LR-3 is the Stream and Source point of the Liver channel. It regulates the Liver-Qi, nourishes the Liver-Yin and relieves the pain.
- KI-3 is the Stream and Source point of the Kidney channel. BL-23 is the Back Transporting point of the Kidney. These two points together tonify the Kidney-Yin and clear Deficient-Fire.
- CV-4 is the crossing point of the Directing Vessel and the three Yin channels of the foot. SP-6 is the crossing point of the three Yin channels of the foot. These two points in combination nourish the Yin, regulate the circulation of Qi in the Lower Burner, promote urination and relieve the pain.

After 4 weeks of treatment the urination pain was completely gone.

Pain during ejaculation 50

射
精
疼
痛

Pain that occurs in the penis during ejaculation may in some cases be accompanied by perineal pain, pain in the lower abdomen or in the lower back. According to TCM theory, ejaculation pain may be caused by invasion of External Cold, downward flow of Damp-Heat in the Terminal Yin channel, stagnation of Liver-Qi, stagnation of Blood in the Lower Burner, deficiency of Yin of the Liver and Kidney or deficiency of Kidney-Yang. Ejaculation pain may be attributed to any of the following disorders in Western medicine: acute or chronic urethritis, testitis, prostatitis, seminal vesiculitis, inguinal herniation.

Aetiology and pathology

Invasion of External Cold

Exposure to a cold environment may allow External Cold to invade the genitals. Cold has the characteristics of contraction and stagnation, so when Cold invades the genitals, it may cause the channels and the tendons of the penis to contract and the circulation of Qi in the Terminal Yin Channel to stagnate, and ejaculation pain follows.

Downward flow of Damp-Heat in the Terminal Yin channel

External Damp-Heat may invade the penis directly, causing an invasion of Damp-Heat in the Lower Burner. In addition, eating too much hot, pungent, sweet or fat food, or drinking too much alcohol, may impair the Spleen's functions of transportation and transformation, allowing Damp-Heat to form in the Stomach and Spleen. This Damp-Heat may then flow down the channels to the genitals, blocking the circulation of Qi and Blood in the penis and causing ejaculation pain.

Stagnation of Liver-Qi

The Liver plays an important role in the relationship between emotions and the body. For example, stress, depression and fear may all lead to a slowing down in the circulation of Qi in the Liver, so that the Liver-Qi stagnates. This stagnant Liver-Qi may block the penis during sexual intercourse and ejaculation, so that ejaculation pain occurs.

Stagnation of Blood

Prolonged disease, stagnation of Liver-Qi or persistence of Damp-Heat in the Lower Burner, as well as deficiency of Qi, may all cause the circulation of Blood to slow down, gradually leading to Blood stagnation. When Blood stasis blocks the free circulation of Qi and Blood in the channels around the genitals, ejaculation pain appears.

As well as these causes, physical trauma to the genitals or an inappropriate operation on the penis may directly damage the channels and collaterals, leading to stagnation of Qi and Blood and therefore once again to ejaculation pain.

Deficiency of Yin of Liver and Kidney

Long febrile and chronic diseases and excessive sexual activity may both consume the Yin of the Liver and Kidney. This causes a deterioration of the tendons and muscles around the genitals because they do not receive proper nourishment, so ejaculation pain follows. This syndrome can often be seen in elderly men.

Deficiency of Kidney-Yang

Ageing, a weak constitution, too many operations and prolonged Cold diseases may all gradually damage the Kidney-Yang, so that interior Cold forms and the genitals fail to be properly warmed. Since Cold has characteristics of contraction and stagnation, naturally there is ejaculation pain. Also, sexual activity expends a lot of energy in patients with Kidney-Yang deficiency, so ejaculation pain occurs.

Treatment based on differentiation

Differentiation

Differentiation of External or Internal origin

— Acute ejaculation pain with a cold sensation in the genital regions, accompanied by some External symptoms, such as an aversion to cold, slight fever, or generalised muscle pain, is due to invasion of External Cold.
— Chronic ejaculation pain, or chronic ejaculation pain with acute aggravation, is usually caused by disorder of the Internal organs.

Differentiation of the character of pain

— Ejaculation pain with a cold and cramping sensation in the genitals and lower abdomen, aggravation of the pain by exposure to cold, or alleviation by warmth, is usually caused by invasion of External Cold.

— Ejaculation pain with a hot sensation, itching of the urethral orifice, red and swollen genitals, and aggravation of the pain by urination, fever, or a bitter taste in the mouth, is often caused by downward flow of Damp-Heat.
— Severe pain on ejaculation, sometimes a stabbing pain in the lower abdomen, with aggravation of the pain by emotional stress or irritability, nervousness, or a purplish tongue, is often caused by stagnation of Liver-Qi with formation of Liver-Fire.

Treatment

INVASION OF EXTERNAL COLD

Symptoms and signs

Ejaculation pain, which is aggravated by exposure to cold and alleviated by warmth, with a cold and dull sensation in the genital region radiating to the lower abdomen, or a contracting sensation in the perineum, frequent urination of clear urine, cold limbs, a poor appetite, a pale tongue with a white coating and a wiry pulse.

Principle of treatment

Eliminate External Cold and warm the Liver channel.

HERBAL TREATMENT

Prescription

DANG GUI SI NI TANG
Angelica Four Rebellious Decoction
Dang Gui *Radix Angelicae Sinensis* 12 g
Gui Zhi *Ramulus Cinnamomi* 9 g
Bai Shao *Radix Paeoniae Alba* 9 g
Xi Xin *Herba Asari* 1.5 g
Gan Cao *Radix Glycyrrhizae* 5 g
Tong Cao *Medulla Tetrapanacis* 3 g
Da Zao *Fructus Ziziphi Jujubae* 8 pieces

Explanations

- Gui Zhi and Xi Xin warm the channels and dispel External Cold.
- Tong Cao and Gui Zhi invigorate the circulation of Blood and remove Blood stagnation.
- Dang Gui and Bai Shao nourish the Blood and the tendons in order to relieve the spasm.

- Gan Cao and Da Zao tonify the Qi and protect against External Cold.

Modifications

1. If there is a severe cold feeling in the genital region, add Wu Zhu Yu *Fructus Evodiae* 5 g and Gao Liang Jiang *Rhizoma Alpiniae Officinarum* 10 g to warm the Liver channel and relieve the pain.
2. If there is perineal pain, add Wu Yao *Radix Linderae* 5 g and Li Zhi He *Semen Litchi* 10 g to regulate the circulation of Qi in the Liver channel and relieve the perineal pain.
3. If there is pain in the lower abdomen, add Gan Jiang *Rhizoma Zingiberis* 10 g, Yan Hu Suo *Rhizoma Corydalis* 10 g and Xiao Hui Xiang *Fructus Foeniculi* 6 g to warm the Lower Burner and relieve the abdominal pain.
4. If there is severe testicle pain, add Ju He *Semen Citri Peticulatae* 10 g and Chuan Lian Zi *Fructus Meliae Toosendan* 10 g to regulate the circulation of Qi in the Liver channel and relieve the pain.
5. If there is swelling of the scrotum, add Fu Ling *Poria* 10 g and Che Qian Zi *Semen Plantaginis* 10 g to eliminate Damp and reduce the swelling.

Patent remedy

Tian Tai Wu Yao Wan *Top-Quality Lindera Powder*

ACUPUNCTURE TREATMENT

LR-3 Taichong, KI-10 Yingu, SP-9 Yinlingquan, BL-23 Shenshu and CV-3 Zhongji. Reducing method is used for LR-3, KI-10 and SP-9. BL-23 and CV-3 are needled with reinforcing method. These two points can be treated with moxibustion as well.

Explanations

- LR-3, the Stream and Source point of the Liver channel, warms the channels and regulates the circulation of Qi.
- KI-10 is the Sea point of the Kidney channel. It may eliminate Cold, regulate the circulation of Qi in the Channel and relieve the pain.
- SP-9 is the Sea point of the Spleen channel. It may regulate the circulation of Qi and dispel Cold so as to stop the pain.
- CV-3 is the crossing point of the Directing Vessel and the three Yin channels of the foot. It is also the Front Collecting point of the Bladder. It can increase the activity of the Yang-Qi, warm the genitals and eliminate External Cold in the Lower Burner.
- BL-23 is the Back Transporting point of the Kidney. It can eliminate external Cold from the Kidney and warm the genitals.

Modifications

1. If there is perineal pain, add CV-2 and KI-12 to warm the channels and relieve the pain.
2. If the testicles are painful, add LR-5 and SP-9 to regulate the circulation of Liver-Qi, harmonise the collateral and relieve the pain.
3. If there is lower abdominal pain, add CV-4 and BL-25 to warm the channels and relieve the pain. CV-4 can be warmed by moxibustion.
4. If there is a sharp pain with a contracting sensation, add CV-1 to remove External Cold and relieve the pain.

Case history

A 30-year-old man had been suffering with ejaculation pain for 4 days. He had suffered with acute urethritis the previous week, which was controlled by antibiotics. A week previously, after playing sport, he had taken a cold shower. The same night, the ejaculation pain had started. His family doctor gave him some painkillers. Two days later, however, the ejaculation pain returned. When he arrived at the acupuncture clinic, he had only a slight rigid sensation on his scrotum with a cold feeling. His tongue was pale with a white coating, and his pulse was superficial and tight.

Diagnosis
Invasion of External Cold to the Liver channel. The key symptom of this case was the ejaculation pain. It was caused by a sudden cold shower after sweating, leading to the invasion of External Cold in the Liver channel through the opened skin pores. The white coating and the superficial and tight pulse were symptoms of the invasion of External Cold.

Principle of treatment
Warm the Liver channel, eliminate the External Cold and relieve the pain.

Herbal treatment
DANG GUI SI NI TANG (modified)
Angelica Four Rebellious Decoction (modified)
Gui Zhi *Ramulus Cinnamomi* 10 g
Dang Gui *Radix Angelicae Sinensis* 10 g
Bai Shao *Radix Paeoniae Alba* 20 g
Wu Zhu Yu *Fructus Evodiae* 10 g
Xi Xin *Herba Asari* 3 g
Gan Cao *Radix Glycyrrhizae* 5 g
Chuan Lian Zi *Fructus Meliae Toosendan* 10 g
Xiao Hui Xiang *Fructus Foeniculi* 6 g

Explanations

- Gui Zhi and Dang Gui promote the circulation of Blood and remove the stagnation of Qi from the Liver channel.
- Bai Shao and Dang Gui nourish Blood and strengthen the Liver.
- Gui Zhi and Xi Xin warm the Liver channel, dispel external Cold and relieve External symptoms.
- Wu Zhu Yu and Xiao Hui Xiang warm the Liver channel and regulate the circulation of Qi in the channels, as well as relieving the pain.
- Chuan Lian Zi regulates the circulation of Qi in the Liver channel and relieves the pain.
- Gan Cao harmonises the actions of the other herbs in the prescription.

The patient used this herbal decoction daily. One week later the ejaculation pain was almost completely relieved. Then one more herb, Yan Hu Suo *Rhizoma Corydalis* 10 g was added to the prescription in order to increase the therapeutic effect. Two weeks later the ejaculation pain was definitely gone. Upon follow-up 2 years later he reported that after the treatment the pain did not return.

DOWNWARD FLOW OF DAMP-HEAT IN THE TERMINAL YIN CHANNEL

Symptoms and signs

Red and swollen External urethral orifice of the penis, and ejaculation pain with a sensation of heat, which is aggravated by urination, with itching of the urethral orifice, and dark yellow urine with viscous secretion. Other symptoms included restlessness, constipation, lower abdominal pain, lower back pain, a bitter taste in the mouth, a yellow and sticky tongue coating and a wiry and slippery pulse.

Principle of treatment

Clear Heat, eliminate Damp and relieve the pain.

HERBAL TREATMENT

Prescription

LONG DAN XIE GAN TANG
Gentiana Draining the Liver Decoction
Long Dan Cao *Radix Gentianae* 6 g
Huang Qin *Radix Scutellariae* 9 g
Zhi Zi *Fructus Gardeniae* 9 g
Ze Xie *Rhizoma Alismatis* 12 g
Mu Tong *Caulis Akebiae* 9 g
Che Qian Zi *Semen Plantaginis* 9 g
Dang Gui *Radix Angelicae Sinensis* 3 g
Sheng Di Huang *Radix Rehmanniae Recens* 9 g
Chai Hu *Radix Bupleuri* 6 g
Gan Cao *Radix Glycyrrhizae* 6 g

Explanations

- Long Dan Cao and Huang Qin clear Heat and dry Damp.
- Zhi Zi, Mu Tong, Ze Xie and Che Qian Zi clear Heat and promote urination in order to eliminate Damp.
- Dang Gui and Sheng Di Huang nourish the Yin and Blood and prevent damage to the Yin by the other herbs in the prescription.
- Chai Hu regulates the Liver-Qi and removes Qi stagnation.
- Gan Cao harmonises the actions of the other herbs used in the prescription.

Modifications

1. If there is swelling of the penis, add Huang Bai *Cortex Phellodendri* 10 g and Tu Fu Ling *Rhizoma Smilacis Glabrae* 10 g to eliminate Damp-Heat and reduce the swelling.
2. If the testicles are painful, add Ju He *Semen Citri Reticulatae* 10 g and Li Zhi He *Semen Litchi* 10 g to regulate the Liver-Qi and to relieve the testicle pain.
3. If there is secretion of yellow viscous liquid from the urethral orifice, add Ku Shen *Radix Sophorae Flavescentis* 10 g and Che Qian Zi *Semen Plantaginis* 10 g to eliminate Damp-Heat in the Lower Burner and remove Toxin.
4. If there is constipation, add Da Huang *Radix et Rhizoma Rhei* 6 g and Mang Xiao *Natrii Sulfas* 10 g to clear Fire, promote defecation and relieve the constipation.

Patent remedies

Long Dan Xie Gan Wan *Gentiania Draining the Liver Pill*
Qian Lie Xian Wan *Prostate Gland Pill*

ACUPUNCTURE TREATMENT

LR-4 Zhongfeng, SP-6 Sanyinjiao, SP-9 Yinlingquan, KI-3 Taixi, BL-23 Shenshu and CV-2 Qugu. Reducing method is used on these points.

Explanations

- LR-4 is the River point of the Liver channel. It may regulate the Liver-Qi and relieve the pain.

- SP-6 is the crossing point of the three Yin channels of the foot. SP-9 is the Sea point of the Spleen channel. These two points in combination eliminate Damp-Heat in the Lower Burner.
- KI-3, a Stream and Source point, nourishes the Yin and eliminates Damp-Heat.
- BL-23 is the Back Transporting point of the Kidney, which regulates the circulation of Qi in the Lower Burner and relieves the ejaculation pain.
- CV-2 is the crossing point of the Directing Vessel and the Liver channel. It regulates the circulation of Qi in these two channels, eliminates Damp-Heat and relieves the pain.

Modifications

1. If there is swelling and redness of the external urethral orifice, add KI-2, the Spring point of the Kidney channel, and LR-5, the Connecting point of the Liver channel, to eliminate Damp-Heat and to reduce the swelling.
2. If the testicles are painful, add ST-29 and KI-8 to regulate the circulation of Qi, remove Qi stagnation and relieve the testicle pain.
3. If there is painful urination, add KI-4 and SP-9 to eliminate Damp and relieve the pain.
4. If there is lower back pain, add BL-23 and BL-58 to strengthen the back, harmonise the collateral and relieve the pain.
5. If there is perineal pain, add CV-1 to regulate the circulation of Qi, harmonise the collateral and relieve the pain.

Case history

A 35-year-old man had been diagnosed with a chronic prostatitis for the last 5 years. He was suffering from ejaculation pain. Long-term use of antibiotics brought him no relief. Therefore he asked for acupuncture treatment for this complaint. As well as the ejaculation pain he mentioned itching of the penis, dark yellow urine, a thirst and a bitter taste in his mouth. His tongue was red with a yellow and greasy coating and his pulse was rapid and slippery.

Diagnosis
Accumulation of Damp-Heat in the Lower Burner.

Principle of treatment
Clear Damp-Heat, regulate the circulation of Qi and relieve the pain.

Acupuncture treatment
LR-2, LR-4, SP-9, CV-2 and ST-28 were selected with reducing method. Treatment was given once every other day. He also used Long Dan Xie Gan Wan *Gentiana Draining the Liver Pill* 6 pills, 2 a day every day.

Explanations

- LR-2 is the Spring and LR-4 is the River point of the Liver channel. These two points eliminate Damp-Heat from this channel.
- SP-9, the Sea point of the Spleen channel, eliminates Damp-Heat and promotes urination.
- CV-2 and ST-28 regulate the circulation of Qi, eliminate Damp-Heat and relieve the pain.

After 20 days of treatment, the ejaculation pain was under control. Upon follow-up 2 years later he declared that he was completely cured by the treatment.

STAGNATION OF LIVER-QI WITH FORMATION OF LIVER-FIRE

Symptoms and signs

Ejaculation pain, which is aggravated by emotional strain or stress, with impotence, headache, a poor appetite, a dull feeling in the stomach, hypochondriac pain, irritability, insomnia, lower abdominal pain, a red tongue with a white or yellow coating and a wiry pulse.

Principle of treatment

Regulate the Liver-Qi, reduce Liver-Fire and relieve the pain.

HERBAL TREATMENT

Prescription

XIAO YAO SAN
Free and Relaxed Powder
Chai Hu *Radix Bupleuri* 30 g
Dang Gui *Radix Angelicae Sinensis* 30 g
Bai Shao *Radix Paeoniae Alba* 30 g
Bai Zhu *Rhizoma Atractylodis Macrocephalae* 30 g
Fu Ling *Poria* 30 g
Gan Cao *Radix Glycyrrhizae* 15 g
Bo He *Herba Menthae* 3 g
Sheng Jiang *Rhizoma Zingiberis Recens* 3 g

Explanations

- Chai Hu and Bo He regulate and promote the circulation of Liver-Qi in order to remove Qi stagnation in the Liver channel.
- Bai Shao and Dang Gui nourish the Liver-Blood and strengthen the physiological function of the Liver. These two herbs can also directly relieve the pain.
- Bai Zhu, Fu Ling and Sheng Jiang tonify the Spleen and Stomach.
- Gan Cao harmonises the actions of the other herbs in the prescription.

Modifications

1. If there is lower abdominal pain, add Wu Yao
   Radix Linderae 5 g and Ju He *Semen Citri Reticulatae*
   10 g to regulate the circulation of Qi and relieve
   the abdominal pain.
2. If there is impotence, add Yu Jin *Radix Curcumae*
   10 g and Wu Gong *Scolopendra* 1 g to regulate the
   circulation of Qi and Blood and improve the
   potency.
3. If there is insomnia, add Suan Zao Ren *Semen
   Ziziphi Spinosae* 10 g and Mu Li *Concha Ostreae* 15 g
   to calm the Mind and to improve the sleep.
4. If the appetite is poor, add Shan Zha *Fructus
   Crataegi* 10 g and Sha Ren *Fructus Amomi* 6 g to
   improve the appetite.

Patent remedy

Xiao Yao Wan plus Zhi Bai Di Huang Wan
Anemarrhena, Phellodendron and Rehmannia Pill

ACUPUNCTURE TREATMENT

LR-3 Taichong, SP-6 Sanyinjiao, PC-6 Neiguan, CV-3
Zhongji, LI-4 Hegu and GV-20 Baihui. Reducing
method is used on these points.

Explanations

- LR-3 is the Source and Stream point of the Liver
  channel. It may soothe the Liver, regulate the
  circulation of Liver-Qi and relieve blockage in the
  channel in order to treat ejaculation pain.
- SP-6 is the crossing point of the three Yin channels
  of the foot. PC-6 is the Connecting point of the
  Pericardium channel. These two points in
  combination regulate the circulation of Liver-Qi
  and calm the Mind.
- CV-3 is the crossing point of the Directing Vessel
  with the three Yin channels of the foot and the
  Front Collecting point of the Bladder. It promotes
  the local circulation of Qi and relieves ejaculation
  pain.
- GV-20, the crossing point of the Directing Vessel
  with the Bladder channel, and LI-4, the Source
  point, calm the Mind and reduce Liver-Fire.

Modifications

1. If there is a headache, add LR-2 and GB-20 to
   regulate the circulation of Liver-Qi, to reduce
   Liver-Fire and relieve the headache.
2. If there is hypochondriac pain, add LR-14, LR-5
   and GB-41 to regulate the circulation of Liver-Qi,
   harmonise the collateral and relieve the pain.

Pain during copulation 51

房

事

疼

痛

Pain during copulation may occur in men in the penis or testes, or in women in the pudendum or vagina. Sometimes this is accompanied by lower abdominal pain or lower back pain. According to TCM theory, it may be caused by invasion of External Cold, accumulation of Damp-Heat in the Liver channel, stagnation of Liver-Qi, deficiency of Spleen-Qi or deficiency of Kidney-Yin with flaring-up of Liver-Fire. Painful copulation may be attributed to any of the following disorders in Western medicine: testitis, prostatitis, prostatomegaly, seminal vesiculitis, hernia, vaginismus, bartholinitis, vaginitis and urethritis.

Aetiology and pathology

Invasion of External Cold

Exposure to cold surroundings after heavy physical work, giving birth, or a major operation may cause External Cold to invade the vulva or penis. Cold has the characteristic of contraction, so when it invades Cold may block the free flow of Qi circulation, leading to stagnation of Qi in the Lower Burner. It may also directly cause the tendons in the genitals to contract, leading to copulation pain.

Accumulation of Damp-Heat in the Liver Channels

Lack of personal hygiene may allow Damp-Heat to invade the penis or vagina, damaging the local channels and collateral, and causing copulation pain.

Bad diets, such as habitual eating of pungent, sweet, or fatty food, or drinking too much alcohol, may cause Damp-Heat to accumulate in the Stomach and Spleen. Since Damp characteristically moves downward, this Damp-Heat flows down to the genitals, disturbing the channels and collaterals there, causing copulation pain. In addition, accumulation of Damp-Heat in the Lower Burner may disturb the circulation of Qi and Blood, again leading to copulation pain.

Stagnation of Liver-Qi

The circulation of Qi in the body is directly related to the emotional state, which is dominated not only by the Heart, but also especially by the Liver. Mental disturbances, such as excessive stress or depression, may impede the Liver's physiological function of promoting the free flow of Qi around the body, which could result in stagnation of Liver-Qi. Since the genital region is very closely related to the Liver channel and stagnation of Liver-Qi tends to cause dysfunction in the Liver channel, copulation pain will probably occur as a consequence of Liver-Qi stagnation.

Deficiency of Spleen-Qi

Long-term chronic disease, a weak constitution, malnutrition, excessive physical work, menorrhagia, giving birth to several children and having operations may all cause consumption of the Spleen-Qi. This may lead to deficiency or even sinking of the Spleen-Qi. Although the genital region is most related to the Liver and Kidney channels, the Spleen is the resource of Qi and Blood after birth. This means that the genitals need to be nourished by Qi and Blood produced by the physiological function of the Spleen in transportation and transformation. In the case of deficiency of Spleen-Qi, there would be deficiency of Qi and Blood, so the genitals would fail to be nourished properly and become dry or painful, which may result in copulation pain.

Deficiency of Kidney-Yin and flaring up of Liver-Fire

The Kidney stores the Original Essence and the Liver stores the Blood; these all belong to the Yin of the human body. Ageing, chronic febrile disease, excessive sexual activity or prolonged sickness may all cause consumption of the Blood and Yin of the body. Also, the Liver and Kidney have the same origin, so Kidney-Yin deficiency may in turn produce Liver-Yin deficiency. The physiological function of the genitals depends on the proper nourishment of Kidney-Yin and Liver-Yin. When there is insufficient Yin in the Liver channels to nourish the tendons and muscles, then painful copulation occurs.

Treatment based on differentiation

Differentiation

Differentiation of External or Internal origin

— Acute onset of copulation pain with a cold sensation in the genital regions, accompanied by External symptoms, such as an aversion to cold, slight fever, or generalised muscle pain, is due to invasion of External Cold.
— Chronic onset of copulation pain, or chronic copulation pain with acute aggravation, is usually caused by disorder of the Internal organs.

Differentiation of character of the pain

— Painful copulation with a spastic and cold sensation around the penis or vagina, radiation of the pain to the lower abdomen, aggravation of the pain by exposure to cold, or alleviation by warmth, is usually caused by invasion of external Cold.
— Painful copulation, reddish and swelling genitals with a hot or even burning sensation, aggravation of the genital pain on discharge of urine, or scanty and yellow urine, is often due to accumulation of Damp-Heat in the Liver channel.
— Painful copulation with a distending sensation in the lower abdomen, irritability, or aggravation of the pain by emotional stress and insomnia, is usually caused by stagnation of Liver-Qi.
— Gradual onset of painful copulation, with a low sexual drive, lassitude, a pale complexion, or history of chronic disease, is often due to deficiency of Spleen-Qi.
— Painful copulation, with itching of the penis or vagina, dryness of the vagina, irregular menstruation, weakness of the knees and legs, hot flushes, or night sweating, is usually caused by deficiency of Kidney-Yin with flaring up of Liver-Fire.

Treatment

INVASION OF EXTERNAL COLD

Symptoms and signs

Pain on copulation with spastic penis or vagina, which is aggravated by exposure to cold and alleviated by warmth, with a cold sensation in the lower abdomen, or a contracted scrotum with a cold sensation, a slight fever, an aversion to cold, muscle pain, dysmenorrhoea, excessive clear leucorrhoea, cold limbs, a pale tongue with a white and thin coating and a wiry pulse.

Principle of treatment

Dispel External Cold and warm the Liver channel.

HERBAL TREATMENT

Prescription

QU FENG DING TONG TANG
Dispel Wind Relieve Pain Decoction
Chuan Xiong *Rhizoma Ligustici Chuanxiong* 6 g
Dang Gui *Radix Angelicae Sinensis* 10 g
Du Huo *Radix Angelicae Pubescentis* 10 g

Fang Feng *Radix Ledebouriellae* 10 g
Jing Jie *Herba Schizonepetae* 10 g
Rou Gui *Cortex Cinnamomi* 6 g
Fu Ling *Poria* 12 g
Da Zao *Fructus Ziziphi Jujubae* 5 pieces

Explanations

- Du Huo, Fang Feng and Jing Jie dispel External Cold and relieve the pain.
- Chuan Xiong and Dang Gui regulate the circulation of Blood and relieve the pain.
- Rou Gui warms the Liver channel and promotes the circulation of Blood.
- Fu Ling activates the spleen and tonifies Spleen-Qi.
- Da Zao moderates the actions of the other herbs in the formula.

Modifications

1. If there is severe Cold, add Xi Xin *Herba Asari* 5 g and Wu Zhu Yu *Fructus Evodiae* 6 g to warm the Liver channel and relieve the pain.
2. If there is dysmenorrhoea, add Tao Ren *Semen Persicae* 10 g, Hong Hua *Flos Carthami* 10 g and Yi Mu Cao *Herba Leonuri* 10 g to remove Blood stasis and relieve the pain.
3. If there is severe pain in the testes, add Ju He *Semen Citri Peticulatae* 10 g and Li Zhi He *Semen Litchi* 10 g to regulate the circulation of Qi in Liver channel and relieve the pain.
4. If there is pain in the lower abdomen, add Gan Jiang *Rhizoma Zingiberis* 10 g and Yan Hu Suo *Rhizoma Corydalis* 10 g to warm the Lower Burner and relieve the pain.

Patent remedy

Tian Tai Wu Yao Wan *Top-Quality Lindera Pill*

ACUPUNCTURE TREATMENT

LI-4 Hegu, TE-5 Waiguan, LR-3 Taichong, SP-8 Diji, CV-3 Zhongji, KI-10 Yingu and BL-18 Ganshu. Reducing method is applied for these points, with moxibustion on LI-4 and TE-5. Reinforcing method is used on CV-3.

Explanations

- LI-4, the Source point, and TE-5, the Connecting point, dispel External Cold and relieve External symptoms.
- LR-3, the Stream and Source point of the Liver channel, warms the channel and regulates the circulation of Qi.
- SP-8, the Accumulation point of the Spleen channel, regulates the circulation of Qi, harmonises the collateral and relieves the pain.
- KI-10, the Sea point of the Kidney channel, regulates the circulation of Qi, dispels Cold from the channel and relieves the pain.
- CV-3, the crossing point of the Directing Vessel and the three Yin channels of the foot, and the Front Collecting point of the Bladder, can improve the Yang-Qi, warm the channels and relieve pain.
- BL-18, the Back Transporting point of the Liver, removes Qi stagnation and relieves painful copulation.

Modifications

1. If the testicles are painful, add LR-5 and LR-8 to regulate the circulation of Qi in the Liver channel and relieve the pain.
2. If the vagina is painful, add ST-29 and CV-2 to warm the channel and relieve the pain.
3. If there is spastic penis, add ST-40 and SP-9 to regulate the circulation of Qi, harmonise the collateral and relieve the pain.
4. If there is lower abdomen pain, add ST-25 to warm the channels and relieve the pain. At the same time, moxibustion treatment on CV-8 is recommended.
5. If there is perineal pain, add KI-10 to regulate the circulation of Qi and relieve the pain.

Case history

A 32-year-old man had been suffering from painful copulation for 2 days. He had caught a cold infection the previous week, with an aversion to cold, abdominal pain and a low fever. He had been given antibiotics and painkillers. The previous night he had a sudden pain in the penis with a spastic sensation when he and his wife had sexual intercourse. When he arrived at the clinic, he had the following symptoms: lower abdominal pain with a cold sensation, lower back pain, aversion to cold, cold limbs and a pale complexion. He also had a white and wet tongue coating and a wiry pulse.

Diagnosis
Invasion of External Cold to the Liver channel.

Principle of treatment
Warm the Liver channel, eliminate External Cold and relieve the pain.

Acupuncture treatment
LR-3, KI-10, ST-29, BL-23 and CV-4 were needled with reducing method. One treatment was given every day. Moxibustion was carried out on CV-8.

Explanations

- LR-3 is the Source point of the Liver channel. KI-10 is Sea point of the Kidney channel. These two points in combination regulate the circulation of Qi and dispel External Cold.
- ST-29 promotes the circulation of Qi in the locality and relieves the pain.
- BL-23 is the Back Transporting point of the Kidney. CV-4 is the crossing point of the Directing Vessel and the three Yin channels of the foot, and the Front Collecting point of the Small Intestine. These two points in combination warm the channels, dispel external Cold and relieve painful copulation.
- Moxibustion on CV-8 warms the body and channels and dispels Cold.

After 10 days of treatment, the pain of copulation had disappeared. He was followed up 9 months later and he stated he had experienced no more painful copulation since the acupuncture treatment.

ACCUMULATION OF DAMP-HEAT IN THE LIVER CHANNEL

Symptoms and signs

Painful copulation, reddish and swelling genitals with a sensation of heat, scanty and yellow urine, yellow and smelling leucorrhoea, urethral mucus, constipation, or diarrhoea, lower abdominal pain, lower back pain, a bitter taste in the mouth, a thick and yellow tongue coating and a wiry and rapid pulse.

It is often seen in the following diseases, testitis, vaginitis and urethritis.

Principle of treatment

Clear Heat and eliminate Damp.

HERBAL TREATMENT

Prescription

LONG DAN XIE GAN TANG
Gentiana Draining the Liver Decoction
Long Dan Cao *Radix Gentianae* 6 g
Huang Qin *Radix Scutellariae* 9 g
Zhi Zi *Fructus Gardeniae* 9 g
Ze Xie *Rhizoma Alismatis* 12 g
Mu Tong *Caulis Akebiae* 9 g
Che Qian Zi *Semen Plantaginis* 9 g
Dang Gui *Radix Angelicae Sinensis* 3 g
Sheng Di Huang *Radix Rehmanniae Recens* 9 g
Chai Hu *Radix Bupleuri* 6 g
Gan Cao *Radix Glycyrrhizae* 6 g

Explanations

- Long Dan Cao and Huang Qin clear Heat and dry Damp.
- Zhi Zi, Mu Tong, Ze Xie and Che Qian Zi clear Heat, promote urination and eliminate Damp.
- Dang Gui and Sheng Di Huang nourish the Yin and Blood and prevent the other herbs from injuring the Yin.
- Chai Hu regulates the Liver-Qi and removes Qi stagnation.
- Gan Cao harmonises the actions of the other herbs in the formula.

Modifications

1. If the genitals are swollen and painful, use the following herbs to make a body lotion to wash the genitals: Huang Bai *Cortex Phellodendri* 10 g, Ku Shen *Radix Sophorae Flavescentis* 10 g and Tu Fu Ling *Rhizoma Smilacis Glabrae* 10 g, to eliminate Damp-Heat and relieve the pain.
2. If the testicles are painful, add Ju He *Semen Citri Reticulatae* 10 g and Li Zhi He *Semen Litchi* 10 g to regulate the Liver-Qi and relieve the pain.
3. If there is yellow leucorrhoea, add Ku Shen *Radix Sophorae Flavescentis* 10 g and Bai Xian Pi *Cortex Dictamni Radicis* 10 g to eliminate Damp-Heat in the Lower Burner.
4. If there is constipation, add Da Huang *Radix et Rhizoma Rhei* 6 g and Mang Xiao *Natrii Sulfas* 10 g to clear Fire, promote defecation and relieve the constipation.
5. If there is a painful perineum, add Yin Hua *Flos Lonicerae* 10 g and Yu Jin *Radix Curcumae* 10 g to clear Heat and relieve the pain.

Patent remedy

Long Dan Xie Gan Wan *Gentiaria Draining the Liver Pill*

ACUPUNCTURE TREATMENT

LR-2 Xingjian, SP-9 Yinlingquan, KI-2 Rangu, KI-10 Yingu, BL-18 Ganshu and CV-2 Qugu. Reducing method is used on these points.

Explanations

- LR-2, the Spring point of the Liver channel, eliminates Damp-Heat in the channel.
- SP-9, the Sea point of the Spleen channel, removes Damp-Heat and activates the Spleen.

- KI-2, the Spring point of the Kidney channel, and KI-10, the Sea point, promote urination and eliminate Damp-Heat.
- BL-18, the Back Transporting point of the Liver, reduces Liver-Fire.
- CV-2, the crossing point of the Directing Vessel and the Liver channel, regulates the circulation of Qi in these two channels, eliminates Damp-Heat and relieves the pain.

Modifications

1. If there is a painful perineum, add CV-1 and KI-6 to clear Damp-Heat and relieve the pain in the perineum.
2. If there are swollen genitals, add SP-6 to eliminate Damp-Heat and reduce the swelling.
3. If the testicles are painful, add ST-29 and LR-12 to regulate the Qi, remove its stagnation and relieve the pain.
4. If there is a painful vagina with leucorrhoea, add ST-30 and HT-8 to eliminate Damp-Heat and relieve the pain.
5. If there is painful urination, add KI-4 and LR-5 to clear Damp-Heat, promote urination and relieve the pain.
6. If there is lower back pain, add BL-23 and BL-58 to strengthen the lower back and relieve the pain.

STAGNATION OF LIVER-QI

Symptoms and signs

Painful copulation, lower abdominal pain with distension, hypochondriac pain, headache, dizziness, palpitations, irregular menstruation, a poor appetite, a feeling of fullness in the stomach, irritability, insomnia, a white and thin tongue coating and a wiry pulse.

Principle of treatment

Regulate the Liver-Qi, remove Qi stagnation and relieve the pain.

HERBAL TREATMENT

Prescription

XIAO YAO SAN
Free and Relaxed Powder
Chai Hu *Radix Bupleuri* 10 g
Dang Gui *Radix Angelicae Sinensis* 10 g
Bai Shao *Radix Paeoniae Alba* 20 g
Bai Zhu *Rhizoma Atractylodis Macrocephalae* 10 g

Fu Ling *Poria* 15 g
Gan Cao *Radix Glycyrrhizae* 5 g
Bo He *Herba Menthae* 3 g
Sheng Jiang *Rhizoma Zingiberis Recens* 5 g

Explanations

- Chai Hu and Bo He regulate and promote the circulation of Liver-Qi so as to remove Qi stagnation in the Liver channel.
- Bai Shao and Dang Gui nourish the Blood and strengthen the Liver. These two herbs can also relieve the pain directly.
- Bai Zhu, Fu Ling and Sheng Jiang tonify the Spleen and Stomach.
- Gan Cao harmonises the actions of the other herbs in the formula.

Modifications

1. If there is lower abdominal pain, add Wu Yao *Radix Linderae* 5 g and Ju He *Semen Citri Reticulatae* 10 g to regulate the circulation of Qi and relieve the pain.
2. If there is a sharp pain, add Yan Hu Suo *Rhizoma Corydalis* 10 g and Mo Yao *Resina Myrrhae* 10 g to promote the circulation of Qi and relieve the pain.
3. If there is low potency, add Yu Jin *Radix Curcumae* 10 g and Wu Gong *Scolopendra* 3 g to regulate the Qi and Blood circulation in the Liver channel and improve the potency.
4. If there is irregular menstruation, add Chuan Xiong *Radix Ligustici Chuanxiong* 10 g and Yi Mu Cao *Herba Leonuri* 10 g to regulate the menstruation.

Patent remedies

Xiao Yao Wan *Free and Relaxed Pill*
Yan Hu Suo Zhi Tong Pian *Corydalis Stop Pain Tablet*

ACUPUNCTURE TREATMENT

LR-3 Taichong, LR-8 Ququan, PC-6 Neiguan, CV-3 Zhongji, GB-20 Fengchi and BL-18 Ganshu. Even method is used on these points.

Explanations

- LR-3, the Source and Stream point of the Liver channel, and LR-8, the Sea point, regulate the Liver-Qi in order to relieve the pain.
- BL-18, the Back Transporting point of the Liver channel, smoothes the Liver, regulates the Liver-Qi and removes Qi stagnation in the channel.

- CV-3, the crossing point of the Liver channel and the three Yin channels of the foot, relieves the pain.
- PC-6, the Connecting point of the Pericardium channel and the Confluence point of the Yin Linking Vessel, regulates the circulation of Qi and removes its stagnation.
- GB-20 calms the Mind and regulates the circulation of Qi.

Modifications

1. If there is hypochondriac pain, add TE-5 and GB-41 to regulate the circulation of Qi and relieve the pain.
2. If there is lower abdominal pain, add ST-29 and BL-25 to regulate the circulation of Qi in the locality and relieve the pain.
3. If there is low potency, add KI-10, the Sea point, and SP-6, the crossing point of the three Yin channels of the foot, to tonify the Kidney and regulate the Liver in order to improve the potency.
4. If there is irregular menstruation, add SP-10 and KI-3 to regulate the menstruation.
5. If there is insomnia, add HT-7 to calm the Mind and improve the sleep.
6. If there is irritability, add LR-3 and HT-8, the Spring points, to clear Heat from the Liver and Heart and calm the Mind.

Case history

A 52-year-old woman had been suffering from painful copulation for 2 months. She complained she had a dry and painful feeling during sexual intercourse. She also stated that she got this complaint soon after she was terrified by a group of thugs at home. She was very upset about this situation. She went to the hospital and was given some tranquillisers. Besides painful copulation, she also had a headache, nervousness, a dry sensation in her eyes, palpitations, a poor appetite and lower abdominal pain. Her tongue was red with a thin coating, and her pulse was wiry.

Diagnosis
Stagnation of Liver-Qi with formation of Liver-Fire.

Principle of treatment
Smooth the Liver, remove Qi stagnation and clear Liver-Fire.

Herbal treatment
XIAO YAO SAN (modified)
Free and Relaxed Powder (modified)
Chai Hu *Radix Bupleuri* 10 g
Dang Gui *Radix Angelicae Sinensis* 10 g
Bai Shao *Radix Paeoniae Alba* 20 g
Long Dan Cao *Radix Gentianae* 6 g
Huang Qin *Radix Scutellariae* 9 g
Zhi Zi *Fructus Gardeniae* 9 g

Fu Ling *Poria* 15 g
Bo He *Herba Menthae* 3 g
Gan Cao *Radix Glycyrrhizae* 5 g

Explanations
- Chai Hu and Bo He regulate and promote the circulation of Liver-Qi so as to remove Qi stagnation in the Liver channel.
- Bai Shao and Dang Gui harmonise the Liver and nourish the Blood in the Liver in order to strengthen it. These two herbs can also relieve pain directly.
- Fu Ling tonifies the Spleen and Stomach.
- Long Dan Cao, Zhi Zi and Huang Qin clear Liver-Fire.
- Gan Cao harmonises the actions of the other herbs in the formula.

Acupuncture treatment
LR-2, LR-3, LR-12, CV-1, SP-6, GB-20, BL-18 and PC-6 were selected. Reducing method was used on these points. Treatment was given every other day.

Explanations
- LR-2, the Spring point of the Liver channel, and LR-3, the Stream and Source point, promote Liver-Qi circulation and clear Liver-Fire.
- CV-1, the crossing point of the Directing, Governing and Penetrating Vessels, and LR-12, the local point, remove Qi stagnation in the genital region and relieve the pain.
- PC-6, the Connecting point of the Pericardium channel and Confluence point of the Yin Linking Vessel, and GB-20 regulate the circulation of Liver-Qi and calm the Mind.
- SP-6, the crossing point of the three Yin channels of the foot, regulates the circulation of Qi and relieves the copulation pain.
- BL-18, the Back Transporting point of the Liver, smoothes the Liver and regulates the Liver-Qi circulation.

After 2 months of treatment, her painful copulation was relieved completely. She was followed up 2 years later and she stated that she had experienced no further painful copulation since the treatment.

DEFICIENCY OF SPLEEN-QI

Symptoms and signs

Gradual occurrence of painful copulation, a low sexual drive, lassitude, a pale complexion, a poor appetite, diarrhoea, palpitations, prolapse of the uterus or anus, irregular menstruation, menorrhagia, a pale tongue with a white coating and a feeble pulse. Usually these patients have some chronic disease, weak constitution, malnutrition or a history of multiple births.

Principle of treatment

Activate the Spleen and Stomach and tonify the Spleen-Qi.

HERBAL TREATMENT

Prescription

BU ZHONG YI QI TANG
Tonifying the Middle and Benefiting Qi Decoction
Huang Qi *Radix Astragali seu Hedysari* 20 g
Gan Cao *Radix Glycyrrhizae* 5 g
Ren Shen *Radix Ginseng* 10 g
Dang Gui *Radix Angelicae Sinensis* 10 g
Ju Pi *Pericarpium Citri Reticulatae* 6 g
Sheng Ma *Rhizoma Cimicifugae* 3 g
Chai Hu *Radix Bupleuri* 3 g
Bai Zhu *Rhizoma Atractylodis Macrocephalae* 10 g

Explanations

- Ren Shen, Huang Qi, Bai Zhu and Gan Cao strengthen the Spleen and tonify the Qi of the Spleen and Stomach.
- Sheng Ma and Chai Hu lift the Yang-Qi.
- Dang Gui tonifies the Blood in the Liver. It is also a companion of Chai Hu in the treatment of Liver disorder.
- Ju Pi promotes the circulation of Qi in the Middle Burner and strengthens the Spleen and Stomach.

Modifications

1. If there is low potency, add Yin Yang Huo *Herba Epimedii* 10 g and Wu Gong *Scolopendra* 1 g to regulate the circulation of Blood and improve the potency.
2. If there is menorrhagia, add Bai Ji *Rhizoma Bletillae* 10 g, San Qi *Radix Notoginseng* 10 g and Xue Yu Tan *Crinis Carbonisatus* 10 g to stop the bleeding.
3. If there is prolapse of the uterus or anus, add Qing Pi *Pericarpium Citri Reticulatae Viride* 10 g and Zhi Qiao *Fructus Aurantii* 10 g to regulate the circulation of Qi and lift up the uterus and anus.
4. If there are palpitations, add Suan Zhao Ren *Semen Ziziphi Spinosae* 10 g and Bai Zi Ren *Semen Biotae* 10 g to tonify the Blood and calm the Mind.
5. If the appetite is poor, add Sha Ren *Fructus Amomi* 6 g and Mu Xiang *Radix Aucklandiae* 10 g to regulate the Spleen-Qi and improve the appetite.

Patent remedy

Bu Zhong Yi Qi Wan *Tonifying the Middle and Benefiting Qi Pill*

ACUPUNCTURE TREATMENT

LR-3 Taichong, KI-3 Taixi, CV-4 Guanyuan, CV-12 Zhongwan, BL-20 Pishu and ST-36 Zusanli. Reinforcing method is used on these points. Moxibustion treatment is recommended on CV-4, KI-3 and ST-36.

Explanations

- LR-3 is the Stream and Source point of the Liver channel. KI-3 is the Stream and Source point of the Kidney channel. These two points in combination can tonify the Liver and Kidney.
- BL-20 is the Back Transporting point of the Spleen. ST-36 is the Sea point of the Stomach channel. CV-12 is the Front Collecting point of the Stomach, the Gathering point for the Fu organs, and the crossing point of the Directing Vessel with the three Yang channels of the hand. These three points in combination tonify the Spleen and Stomach-Qi.
- CV-4 tonifies the Original Qi and improves the constitution.
- Moxibustion tonifies the Qi and warms the interior organs.

Modifications

1. If the appetite is poor, add SP-3, the Source point, to tonify the Spleen-Qi and improve the appetite.
2. If there is low potency, add CV-6 and LR-5 to tonify the Kidney and regulate the circulation of Qi.
3. If there are palpitations, add PC-6 and HT-3 to calm the Mind and stop the palpitations.
4. If there is prolapse of the anus or uterus, add GV-20 and moxibustion on CV-8 to tonify and lift the Yang-Qi.
5. If there is chronic diarrhoea, add ST-25 and SP-4 to tonify the Spleen and stop the diarrhoea.
6. If there is irregular menstruation, add SP-6 and BI-23 to tonify the Qi and Blood and regulate the menstruation.

DEFICIENCY OF KIDNEY-YIN AND FLARING UP OF LIVER-FIRE

Symptoms and signs

Painful copulation, dry and itching on the penis or vagina, irregular menstruation, menopausal syndrome, lower back pain with soreness, scanty and frequent urination, dry mouth, restlessness, insomnia, lassitude, tinnitus, hot sensation in the hands and soles, constipation, red tongue with less coating, thready and rapid pulse.

Principle of treatment

Nourish Kidney-Yin and reduce Liver-Fire.

HERBAL TREATMENT

Prescription

ZHI BAI DI HUANG WAN

Anemarrhena, Phellodendron and Rehmannia Pill
Shu Di Huang *Radix Rehmanniae Praeparata* 24 g
Shan Zhu Yu *Fructus Corni* 12 g
Shan Yao *Rhizoma Dioscoreae* 12 g
Fu Ling *Poria* 9 g
Mu Dan Pi *Cortex Moutan Radicis* 9 g
Ze Xie *Rhizoma Alismatis* 9 g
Zhi Mu *Rhizoma Anemarrhenae* 10 g
Huang Bai *Cortex Phellodendri* 10 g

Explanations

- Shu Di Huang, Shan Zhu Yu and Shan Yao tonify the Essence of the Liver and Kidney.
- Ze Xie promotes urination and clears Deficient-Heat.
- Mu Dan Pi cools Heat and activates the circulation of Blood.
- Fu Ling strengthens the Spleen and promotes the production of Qi and Blood.
- Zhi Mu and Huang Bai reduce Liver-Fire.

Modifications

1. If there is low potency, add Dang Gui *Radix Angelicae Sinensis* 10 g and Wu Gong *Scolopendra* 1 g to improve the potency.
2. If there is insomnia, add Suan Zao Ren *Semen Ziziphi Spinosae* 10 g and Wu Wei Zi *Fructus Schisandrae* 10 g to calm the Mind.
3. If there is irregular menstruation, add Chuan Xiong *Rhizoma Ligustici Chuanxiong* 10 g and Chuan Niu Xi *Radix Cyathulae* 10 g to regulate the menstruation.
4. If there is lower back pain, add Xu Duan *Radix Dipsaci* 10 g, Sang Ji Sheng *Ramulus Loranthi* 10 g and Bai Shao *Radix Paeoniae Alba* 10 g to strengthen the lower back and relieve the pain.
5. If there is constipation, add Sheng Di Huang *Radix Rehmanniae* 15 g and Xuan Shen *Radix Scrophulariae* 12 g to tonify the Kidney-Yin and lubricate the Large Intestine.

Patent remedy

Zhi Bai Di Huang Wan *Six-Flavour Rehmannia Pill with Anemarrhena and Phellodendri*

ACUPUNCTURE TREATMENT

LR-3 Taichong, LR-8 Ququan, KI-3 Taixi, KI-10 Yingu, SP-6 Sanyinjiao, CV-4 Guanyuan and BL-23 Shenshu. Reinforcing method is used on these points.

Explanations

- LR-3 is the Stream and Source point of the Liver channel; LR-8 is the Sea point. These two points in combination smooth the Liver and clear Liver-Fire.
- KI-3 is the Stream and Source point of the Kidney channel, and KI-10 is the Sea point. BL-23 is the Back Transporting point of the Kidney. These three points together tonify the Kidney-Yin and clear Deficient-Heat.
- CV-4 is the Front Collecting point of the Small Intestine and the crossing point of the Directing Vessel and the three Yin channels of the foot. It tonifies the Yin of the Liver and Kidney.
- SP-6 is the crossing point of the Spleen, Kidney and Liver channels. It nourishes the Yin and clears Deficient-Fire.

Modifications

1. If there is irregular menstruation, add BL-18 and SP-9 to regulate the menstruation.
2. If there is low potency, add CV-6 and LR-12 to improve the potency.
3. If there is lower back pain, add BL-58 and GB-36 to harmonise the collateral and relieve the pain.
4. If there is scanty and frequent urination, add CV-3 to relieve the urination problems.
5. If there is restlessness and insomnia, add PC-6 and GV-20 to tranquillise the Mind.
6. If there is a poor appetite and lassitude, add ST-36 and CV-12 to activate the Spleen and improve the appetite.
7. If there is constipation, add ST-25 and ST-37 to regulate the Large Intestine and promote defecation.

Case history

A 55-year-old man had been suffering from pain on copulation for 5 months. He had been suffering with chronic prostitis for about 2 years, and lately often had pain on copulation with itching of his penis. Sometimes he also suffered from impotence. Meanwhile, he had lower back pain with soreness, frequent and scanty urination, lassitude, a dry mouth with a bitter taste in his mouth, night sweating, restlessness, occasional headache, a red tongue with a scanty coating and a wiry and rapid pulse.

Diagnosis
Deficiency of Kidney-Yin and flaring-up of Liver-Fire.

Principle of treatment
Nourish Kidney-Yin and reduce Liver-Fire.

Acupuncture treatment
LR-3, LR-8, KI-3, CV-3, SP-6 and BL-23. LR-3 and LR-8 were needled with reducing method. KI-3, CV-3, SP-6 and BL-23 were needled with reinforcing method. Treatment was carried out once every other day.

Explanations

- LR-3 is the Stream and Source point of the Liver channel. LR-8 is the Sea point. These two points in combination reduce Liver-Fire resulting from deficiency of Kidney-Yin.
- KI-3 is the Stream and Source point of the Kidney channel. BL-23 is the Back Transporting point of the Kidney. These two points in combination tonify the Kidney-Yin.

- CV-3 is the crossing point of the Directing Vessel and the three Yin channels of the foot. SP-6 is the crossing point of the three Yin channels of the foot. These two points in combination nourish the Yin and regulate the circulation of Qi in the Lower Burner to relieve the painful copulation.

After 6 weeks of treatment, his painful copulation was under control.

Anal pain 52

肛
门
疼
痛

Anal pain may occur in the anus or rectum during defecation, sitting or walking. In severe cases it may be accompanied by local swelling with a feeling of heat, bleeding, or even difficulty in defecation, difficulty in sitting and lying down or an uncomfortable feeling when walking. According to TCM theory, the anus is the place where the Directing and Governing Vessels meet, and it is the exit of the Large Intestine. Therefore a painful anus can be caused by disorders in one of these Vessels or by disorders of the Large Intestine, including accumulation of Toxic Heat or of Damp-Heat in the Large Intestine, as well as deficiency or stagnation of Qi and Blood. Anal pain may be attributed to any of the following disorders in Western medicine: haemorrhoids, anusitis, fissure in ano, anal fistula, perianal abscess, anal prolapse and rectum carcinoma.

Aetiology and pathology

Accumulation of Toxic Heat in the Large Intestine

Overconsumption of spicy, pungent or sweet foods or alcohol may cause internal Heat to form in the Large Intestine and may gradually damage it. Furthermore, overeating may cause accumulation and stagnation of food in the Middle Burner, which obstructs the circulation of Qi in the Large Intestine. In the long run this causes anal pain.

Accumulation of Damp-Heat in the Large Intestine

Drinking too much alcohol or eating too many pungent, sweet, fat or greasy foods may damage the Stomach and Spleen's function of transportation and transformation, and result in the formation of Damp-Heat. Damp has the characteristic of downward flow, so when Damp combines with Heat, it may flow downwards to the Lower Burner, damaging the Large Intestine so that anal pain occurs. Accumulation of Damp-Heat in the Lower Burner can also cause stagnation of Qi, so that its movement in the Large Intestine slows or even stops, and anal pain follows.

Constitutional Qi deficiency of Spleen may also cause internal Damp to accumulate so that the Qi stagnates, and this causes the generation of internal Heat.

Stagnation and deficiency of Qi and Blood

Prolonged sitting or walking, a disharmony of Cold and Warmth, accumulation of Damp in the Lower Burner, excessive stress, anger and frustration and lack of sufficient movement may all cause a slowing down or a stagnation of Qi in the Large Intestine, resulting in anal pain.

Since the Qi guides the Blood, if Qi stagnation persists it may in turn influence the circulation of the Blood, leading to stagnation of Blood in the Large Intestine and causing anal pain. Furthermore, physical trauma or an inappropriate operation on the anus may directly damage the channels and muscles in this area, bringing about a local stagnation of Qi and Blood, and causing anal pain.

A deficiency of Qi and Blood can also cause anal pain. Excessive physical work or walking for long distances with a heavy pack consumes the Spleen-Qi. When the Qi is not sufficient to produce the Blood, this results in a deficiency of the Blood. Sexual hyperactivity, giving birth to several children and prolonged sickness may all cause consumption of Kidney-Essence, which indirectly leads to deficiency of Qi and Blood. Sinking of the Spleen-Qi may also cause a prolapse of the anus and pain in the anal region.

Treatment based on differentiation

Differentiation

Differentiation of acute and chronic anal pain

Generally speaking, anal pain is classified into acute type and chronic type.

— The acute cases are often related to invasion of Toxic Heat or Damp-Heat.
— The chronic cases are often due to stagnation of Qi and Blood, or deficiency of Qi and Blood resulting from chronic sickness.

Differentiation of character of the pain

— Acute anal pain with a burning or pricking sensation, constipation, blood in the stool, pyogenic anus, fever, or aversion to cold, is often caused by invasion of Toxic Heat to the Large Intestine.
— Acute or chronic anal pain with a burning and itching sensation, swelling and redness of the anus, tenesmus, or loose stools with a foul smell, is usually caused by accumulation of Damp-Heat in the Large Intestine.
— Chronic anal pain with a stabbing feeling, aggravation of the anal pain by pressure, stools with purplish blood, a history of operation or trauma in the anus, is usually caused by stagnation of Blood in the anus.

— Chronic anal pain with a bearing-down sensation in the anus, anal prolapse, lassitude, a pale complexion, cold hands and feet, or shortness of breath, is often caused by deficiency of Qi and Blood.

Treatment

ACCUMULATION OF TOXIC HEAT IN THE LARGE INTESTINE

Symptoms and signs

Pain in the anus with a burning or pricking sensation, which worsens during defecation, with blood in the stools, pyogenic anus, fever, an aversion to cold, a thirst, dark yellow urine, constipation, a red tongue with a sticky and yellow coating and a slippery and rapid pulse.

Principle of treatment

Clear Heat, eliminate Toxin and relieve the pain.

HERBAL TREATMENT

Prescription

XIAN FANG HUO MING YIN
Sublime Formula for Sustaining Life
Bai Zhi *Radix Angelicae Dahuricae* 3 g
Bei Mu *Bulbus Fritillariae Thungergii* 3 g
Fang Feng *Radix Ledebouriellae* 3 g
Chi Shao *Radix Paeoniae Rubra* 3 g
Tian Hua Fen *Radix Trichosanthis* 3 g
Ru Xiang *Resina Olibani* 3 g
Dang Gui *Radix Angelicae Sinensis* 3 g
Jin Yin Hua *Flos Lonicerae* 9 g
Gan Cao *Radix Glycyrrhizae* 3 g
Zao Jiao Ci *Spina Gleditsiae* 3 g
Chuan Shan Jia *Squama Manitis* 3 g
Ju Pi *Pericarpium Citri Reticulatae* 9 g
Mo Yao *Resina Myrrhae* 3 g

Explanations

- Jin Yin Hua and Gan Cao clear Heat and remove Toxin.
- Dang Gui, Mo Yao, Ru Xiang and Chi Shao invigorate the circulation of Blood and resolve stagnation in order to reduce swelling and to stop pain.
- Chuan Shan Jia and Zao Jiao Ci promote the circulation of Blood and eliminate pus.

- Fang Feng and Bai Zhi remove Qi stagnation and expel Intestinal Wind.
- Bei Mu and Tian Hua Fen clear Heat and resolve swelling caused by Toxin.
- Ju Pi regulates the circulation of Qi.

Modifications

1. If there is a fever, add Lian Qiao *Fructus Forsythiae* 10 g, Pu Gong Ying *Herba Taraxaci* 10 g and Jing Jie *Herba Schizonepetae* 10 g to clear Heat and to reduce the fever.
2. If there is constipation, add Da Huang *Radix et Rhizoma Rhei* 6 g and Mang Xiao *Natrii Sulfas* 10 g to eliminate Heat and to promote defecation.
3. If there is blood in the stools, add Bai Tou Weng *Radix Pulsatillae* 10 g, Sheng Di Huang *Radix Rehmanniae Recens* 10 g to cool the Blood and to stop the bleeding.

Patent remedy

Huang Lian Su Pian *Coptis Extract Tablet*

ACUPUNCTURE TREATMENT

GV-1 Changqiang, BL-25 Tianzhu, BL-30 Baihuanshu, SP-9 Sanyinjiao, LI-2 Erjian and LI-4 Hegu. Reducing method is used on these points.

Explanations

- GV-1, the Connecting point of the Governing Vessel, harmonises the collateral and relieves the anal pain.
- BL-25, the Back Transporting point of the Large Intestine, clears Toxic Heat in the Large Intestine and promotes defecation.
- BL-30 regulates the circulation of Qi in the Lower Burner and relieves the anal pain.
- SP-9, the Sea point of the Spleen channel, clears Heat and relieves the anal pain.
- LI-2, the Spring point of the Large Intestine channel, and LI-4, the Source point, remove toxic Heat in the Large Intestine, promote defecation and relieve the anal pain.

Modifications

1. If there is a fever, add GV-14, the meeting point for all the Yang channels, and LI-11, the Sea point of the Large Intestine channel, to clear Heat and reduce the fever.

2. If there is anal soreness and swelling, add SP-6 and LI-6 to relieve the soreness and reduce the swelling.
3. If there is constipation, add ST-37, the Lower Sea point of the Large Intestine, to clear Heat in the Large Intestine and promote defecation.
4. If there is blood in the stools, add BL-40 and BL-57 to clear Heat in the Large Intestine and stop the bleeding.

Case history

A 45-year-old man had been suffering from anal pain for 5 days. He complained that he always had a painful anus after eating hot foods such as peppers. Sometimes there was fresh blood in his stools when he strained during defecation. A previous diagnosis of 'fissure in ano' had been made. Besides anal pain, he had a bitter taste in the mouth, constipation, irritability and yellow urine, a red tongue with a dry yellow coating and a rapid pulse.

Diagnosis
Accumulation of toxic Heat in the Large Intestine and hyperactivity of Liver-Fire.

Principle of treatment
Clear Toxic Heat and relieve the pain.

Herbal treatment
XIAN FANG HUO MING YIN (modified)
Subime Formula for Sustaining Life (modified)
Bai Zhi *Radix Angelicae Dahuricae* 3 g
Fang Feng *Radix Ledebouriellae* 3 g
Chi Shao *Radix Paeoniae Rubra* 3 g
Tian Hua Fen *Radix Trichosanthis* 3 g
Dang Gui *Radix Angelicae Sinensis* 3 g
Jin Yin Hua *Flos Lonicerae* 9 g
Gan Cao *Radix Glycyrrhizae* 6 g
Zao Jiao Ci *Spina Gleditsiae* 3 g
Ju Pi *Pericarpium Citri Reticulatae* 9 g
Zhi Zi *Fructus Gardeniae* 10 g

Explanations

- Jin Yin Hua, Zhi Zi and Gan Cao clear Heat in the Large Intestine, reduce Liver-Fire and remove Toxin.
- Dang Gui and Chi Shao invigorate the circulation of Blood and resolve stagnation in order to reduce the swelling and stop the pain.
- Zao Jiao Ci promotes the circulation of Blood.
- Fang Feng and Bai Zhi remove Qi stagnation and relieve Intestinal Wind.
- Tian Hua Fen clears Heat and reduces swelling.
- Ju Pi regulates the circulation of Qi.

The patient took this herbal prescription daily. After 6 days his anal pain was under control. Upon follow-up 6 months later, he reported being free of the pain since the treatment.

ACCUMULATION OF DAMP-HEAT IN THE LARGE INTESTINE

Symptoms and signs

Biting pain in the anus with a burning sensation, which worsens during defecation, with oozing, swelling and redness of the anus, dark yellow urine, yellow leucorrhoea, constipation with tenesmus, itching in the anus, a sticky and yellow tongue coating and a slippery and rapid pulse.

Principle of treatment

Eliminate Damp and clear Heat.

HERBAL TREATMENT

Prescription

QIN JIAO FANG FENG TANG
Chin-Chia and Siler Decoction
Qin Jiao *Radix Gentianae Macrophyllae* 12 g
Fang Feng *Radix Ledebouriellae* 12 g
Dang Gui *Radix Angelicae Sinensis* 12 g
Chuang Xiong *Radix Ligustici Chuangxiong* 9 g
Sheng Di Huang *Radix Rehmanniae Recens* 12 g
Bai Shao *Radix Paeoniae Alba* 10 g
Fu Ling *Poria* 12 g
Lian Qiao *Fructus Forsythiae* 10 g
Di Yu *Radix Sanguisorbae* 12 g
Zhi Qiao *Fructus Aurantii* 12 g
Huai Jiao *Fructus Sophorae* 10 g
Bai Zhi *Radix Angelicae Dahuricae* 9 g
Cang Zhu *Rhizoma Atractylodis* 12 g
Gan Cao *Radix Glycyrrhizae* 6 g

Explanations

- Qin Jiao, Fang Feng and Bai Zhi expel intestinal Wind and eliminate Damp in the Large Intestine.
- Dang Gui and Chuan Xiong remove Blood stagnation and relieve the pain.
- Sheng Di Huang, Lian Qiao, Huai Jiao and Di Yu clear Heat and cool the Blood.
- Fu Ling and Cang Zhu strengthen the Spleen and eliminate Damp.
- Zhi Qiao regulates the circulation of Qi and removes the Qi stagnation.
- Bai Shao and Gan Cao relieve spasm in the Large Intestine and stop the anal pain.

Modifications

1. If there is constipation, add Da Huang *Radix et Rhizoma Rhei* 6 g and Mang Xiao *Natrii Sulfas* 10 g to eliminate Heat and promote defecation.

2. If there is itching in the anus, use a warm lotion obtained from Huang Bai *Cortex Phellodendri* 10 g, Ku Shen *Radix Sophorae Flavescentis* 10 g and She Chuang Zi *Fructus Cnidii* 10 g to wash the anus in order to clear Heat, remove Damp and relieve the itching.
3. If there is swelling and redness of anus, add Jin Yin Hua *Flos Lonicerae* 10 g, Lian Qiao *Fructus Forsythiae* 10 g and Xuan Shen *Radix Scrophulariae* 10 g to clear Heat and remove Toxin as well as relieve the swelling.

Patent remedies

Huang Lian Su Pian *Coptis Extract Tablet*
San Miao Wan *Three-Marvel Pill*

ACUPUNCTURE TREATMENT

GV-1 Changqiang, BL-25 Dachangshu, BL-57 Chengshan, BL-58 Feiyang, SP-9 Yinlingquan, ST-40 Fenglong and LI-4 Hegu. Reducing method is used on these points.

Explanations

- GV-1, the Connecting point of the Governing Vessel, specially harmonises the collateral and relieves the anal pain.
- BL-25, the Back Transporting point of the Large Intestine, and LI-4, the Source point of the Large Intestine channel, clear Toxic Heat in the Large Intestine and promote defecation.
- SP-9, the Sea point of the Spleen channel, and ST-40, the Connecting point of the Stomach channel, clear Heat and relieve the anal pain.
- BL-57 and BL-58, the Connecting point of the Bladder channel, harmonise the collateral, eliminate Damp-Heat and relieve the anal pain.

Modifications

1. If there is anal bleeding, add SP-6 and LI-11 to clear Heat, cool the Blood and stop the bleeding.
2. If there is redness and swelling of the anus, add BL-25 and BL-35 to clear Damp-Heat in the Large Intestine and reduce the swelling.
3. If there is constipation, add ST-25 and ST-37 to promote defecation and relieve the constipation.

DEFICIENCY OF QI AND BLOOD

Symptoms and signs

Prolonged persistence of a slight pain in the anus, with a bearing-down sensation in the anus, anal prolapse, lassitude, a pale complexion, dizziness, a poor appetite, palpitations, loose stools, a pale tongue with tooth marks and a white coating and a weak and deep pulse.

Principle of treatment

Activate the Spleen, tonify the Spleen-Qi and relieve the pain.

HERBAL TREATMENT
Prescription
BU ZHONG YI QI TANG
Tonifying the Middle and Benefiting Qi Decoction
Huang Qi *Radix Astragali seu Hedysari* 20 g
Gan Cao *Radix Glycyrrhizae* 5 g
Ren Shen *Radix Ginseng* 10 g
Dang Gui *Radix Angelicae Sinensis* 10 g
Ju Pi *Pericarpium Citri Reticulatae* 6 g
Sheng Ma *Rhizoma Cimicifugae* 3 g
Chai Hu *Radix Bupleuri* 3 g
Bai Zhu *Rhizoma Atractylodis Macrocephalae* 10 g

Explanations
- Ren Shen, Huang Qi, Bai Zhu and Gan Cao strengthen the Spleen and tonify the Qi of the Spleen and Stomach.
- Sheng Ma and Chai Hu raise the Yang-Qi.
- Dang Gui aids Chai Hu to regulate the Liver-Qi and Liver-Blood.
- Ju Pi promotes the Qi and strengthens the Spleen and Stomach.

Modifications
1. If there is blood in the stools, add Bai Ji *Rhizoma Bletillae* 10 g, San Qi *Radix Notoginseng* 10 g and Xue Yu Tan *Crinis Carbonisatus* 10 g to stop the bleeding.
2. If there is prolapse of the anus, add Qing Pi *Pericarpium Citri Reticulatae Viride* 10 g and Zhi Qiao *Fructus Aurantii* 10 g to regulate the circulation of Qi and to lift the anus.
3. If the appetite is poor, add Sha Ren *Fructus Amomi* 6 g, Mu Xiang *Radix Aucklandiae* 10 g and Pei Lan *Herba Eupatorii* 10 g to promote the Spleen-Qi in order to improve the appetite.

Patent remedy
Bu Zhong Yi Qi Wan *Tonifying the Middle and Benefiting Qi Pill*

ACUPUNCTURE TREATMENT

GV-1 Changqiang, GV-4 Mingmen, GV-20 Baihui, BL-25 Dachangshu and BL-23 Shenshu. Reinforcing method is used on these points. Moxibustion treatment is recommended.

Explanations
- GV-1, the Connecting point of the Governing Vessel, harmonises the collateral and relieves the anal pain.
- BL-25, the Back Transporting point of the Large Intestine, regulates the Large Intestine and relieves the anal pain.
- GV-20, the crossing point of the Governing Vessel and the Bladder channel, promotes the function of Yang-Qi to lift the Internal organs.
- GV-4 tonifies the Yang-Qi.
- BL-23, the Back Transporting point of the Kidney, tonifies the Kidney and warms the Yang-Qi in order to dispel Internal Cold.

Modifications
1. If the appetite is poor, add ST-36 and CV-12 to tonify the Spleen-Qi and improve the appetite.
2. If there is anal prolapse, add CV-4 to tonify and raise the Yang-Qi and to relieve the prolapse.
3. If there is constipation, add ST-25 and ST-37 to promote defecation and relieve the constipation.

Case history

A 56-year-old woman had been suffering from haemorrhoids for 24 years. She complained about anal pain, which had worsened 6 months before after a haemorrhoid operation, and about a prolapse of the anus. She looked pale, had a poor appetite, dizziness, fatigue, palpitations, constipation, a pale tongue and a weak pulse.

Diagnosis
Deficiency of Qi and Blood.

Principle of treatment
Tonify Qi and Blood to lift the Internal organs.

Acupuncture treatment
GV-1, GV-4, BL-20, BL-23 and BL-25 were selected. Reinforcing method was used. Treatment was given once every other day. Besides this, the patient was asked to warm CV-12 and CV-14 with moxa daily for 15 minutes.

Explanations
- GV-1 is the Connecting point of the Governing Vessel and the patent point for treating anal disorders.

- GV-4 tonifies the Qi and Blood to treat haemorrhoids with anal prolapse.
- BL-20 is the Back Transporting point of the Spleen, and BL-23 is the Back Transporting point of the Kidney. These two points in combination tonify the Qi and Blood.
- BL-25, the Back Transporting point of the Large Intestine, relieves the anal pain.
- Moxibustion promotes the Yang-Qi and supports the internal organs in order to relieve the prolapse.

After 2 months the pain and prolapse were under control. Then Bu Zhong Yi Qi Wan *Tonifying the Middle and Benefiting Qi Pill* was prescribed to stabilise the treatment effect. Upon follow-up 2 years later she reported being free of the prolapse and pain since the treatment.

STAGNATION OF QI AND BLOOD WITH FORMATION OF HEAT IN THE BLOOD

Symptoms and signs

Prolonged anal pain with a fixed location, or stabbing pain with a hot sensation, which is aggravated by pressure, defecation and when walking, thirst, swelling and redness of the anus, constipation, restlessness, a purplish tongue and a wiry or choppy pulse.

Principle of treatment

Circulate Qi and Blood, clear Heat, remove Blood stasis and sedate the pain.

HERBAL TREATMENT

Prescription

LIANG XUE DI HUANG TANG
Rehmannia Decoction to Cool Blood
Dang Gui *Radix Angelicae Sinensis* 12 g
Sheng Di Huang *Radix Rehmanniae Recens* 12 g
Di Yu *Radix Sanguisorbae* 12 g
Huai Jiao *Fructus Sophorae* 12 g
Huang Lian *Rhizoma Coptidis* 9 g
Tian Hua Fen *Radix Trichosanthis* 12 g
Chi Shao *Radix Paeoniae Rubra* 12 g
Sheng Ma *Rhizoma Cimicifugae* 10 g
Zhi Qiao *Fructus Aurantii* 12 g
Huang Qin *Radix Astragali seu Hedysari* 10 g
Jing Jie *Herba Schizonepetae* 10 g
Wu Ling Zhi *Faeces Trogopterorum* 10 g
Dan Shen *Radix Salviae Miltiorrhizae* 12 g

Explanations

- Zhi Qiao and Jing Jie regulate the circulation of Qi.

- Tian Hua Fen, Sheng Ma, Sheng Di Huang, Huang Lian and Huang Qin clear Heat in the Blood.
- Dan Shen, Dang Gui and Chi Shao cool the Blood and remove Blood stagnation.
- Di Yu, Huai Jiao and Wu Ling Zhi remove Blood stagnation and stop the bleeding.

Modifications

1. If there is swelling and redness of the anus, wash the anus with a lotion obtained from Ku Shen *Radix Sophorae Flavescentis* 10 g, and Mang Xiao *Natrii Sulfas* 10 g to reduce the swelling and relieve the redness.
2. If there is constipation, add Da Huang *Radix et Rhizoma Rhei* 10 g, Mang Xiao *Natrii Sulfas* 10 g to promote defecation and relieve the anal pain.
3. If there is restlessness, add Long Dan Cao *Radix Gentianae* 10 g and Xuan Shen *Radix Scrophulariae* 10 g to clear Heat and relieve the restlessness.

Patent remedies

Qiang Li Hua Zhi Ling *Better Strength Dissolve-Haemorrhoids Efficacious Cure*

ACUPUNCTURE TREATMENT

GV-1 Changquang, BL-17 Geshu, BL-18 Ganshu, BL-57 Chengshan, BL-58 Feiyang and LI-4 Hegu. Even method is used on these points.

Explanations

- GV-1, the Connecting point of the Governing Vessel, regulates the circulation of Qi and harmonises the collateral in order to relieve the anal pain.
- BL-17, the Gathering point for the Blood, promotes the circulation of Blood and removes its stasis.
- BL-18, the Back Transporting point of the Liver, regulates the circulation of Qi and Blood and removes Blood stagnation.
- LI-4, the Source point of the Large Intestine channel, clears Intestinal Heat and promotes defecation, as well as relieving the anal pain.
- BL-57 and BL-58, the Connecting point of the Bladder channel, harmonise the collateral, regulate the circulation of Qi in the Large Intestine and relieve the anal pain.

Modifications

1. If there is a sharp or stabbing pain around the anus, add LU-6 and LI-7, both Accumulation

points, to promote the circulation of Blood in the Large Intestine and relieve the pain around the anus.

2. If the pain worsens at night owing to severe stagnation of Blood, add BL-30 and BL-36 to regulate the circulation of Blood and relieve the anal pain.

3. If there is pain caused by constipation, add SP-6 and KI-6 to promote the production of Body Fluids and relieve the constipation.

Case history

A 36-year-old man had been diagnosed as suffering from haemorrhoids and anal fistula 3 years previously. During the last 2 years he also complained about a painful anus. Chinese herbal treatment had given some relief, but for 2 weeks the pain had been unbearable. Prolonged sitting or riding his bicycle caused a sharp pain, and as well as the painful anus he also had a hot sensation in his anus and constipation. His tongue was purplish and his pulse was wiry.

Diagnosis
Blood stagnation with accumulation of Heat in the Large Intestine.

Principle of treatment
Clear Heat, regulate the circulation of Qi and Blood and remove Blood stagnation.

Acupuncture treatment
The points GV-1, BL-17, BL-40 and SP-10 were needled with even method every other day. The blood-letting method was used on BL-40.

Explanations

- GV-1, the Connecting point of the Governing Vessel and the patent point for anal disorders, harmonises the Collateral and relieves the anal pain.
- BL-17, the Gathering point for the Blood, regulates the circulation of Blood and removes its stasis.
- SP-10 clears Heat and eliminates Blood stasis.
- BL-40, the Sea point of the Bladder channel, relieves anal pain. Bleeding at this point can also clear Heat in the Large Intestine.

After 20 days of treatment, the anal pain was under control. Upon follow-up a year later he reported being free of the pain since the treatment.

Pain during defecation 53

大
便
疼
痛

Pain occurring during defecation may be accompanied by a sensation of heat, swelling and congestion. In severe cases, there might be blood in the stools, constipation and problems in defecating as well. According to TCM theory, defecation pain can be caused by bad dietary habits, Dryness-Heat in the Large Intestine, downward flow of Damp-Heat in the Large Intestine, deficiency of Spleen-Qi and stagnation of Blood, etc. Defecation pain may be attributed to the following disorders in Western medicine: rectitis, dysentery, chronic constipation, rectalgia, rectostenosis, haemorrhoids, anusitis, anal fissures, prolapse of the rectum or rectum carcinoma.

Aetiology and pathology

Invasion of Wind-Heat

Lifestyle and dietary habits, such as exposure to Dryness or too-strong wind and eating seafood, may cause Wind-Heat to invade the Stomach and Spleen, which disturbs the circulation of Qi in the Middle Burner. This may impair the Spleen's function of transportation and transformation of food, so food stagnates in the Large Intestine, and defecation pain will follow.

An invasion of Wind-Heat in the Large Intestine can also directly injure the collateral, and might cause bleeding. As a result there will be diarrhoea, blood in the stools and defecation pain.

Accumulation of Dry-Heat in the Large Intestine

Eating too much pungent, hot, sweet, greasy or deep-fried food, may cause Dry-Heat to form in the Large Intestine; that may consume the Body Fluids in the Intestines so that the transportation in the Large Intestine slows down. If Dryness-Heat persists over a longer period it will cause stagnation in the Large Intestine, leading to constipation, dry stools and defecation pain.

Downward flow of Damp-Heat in the Large Intestine

Consuming unhygienic or unhealthy food (too much sweet, pungent or greasy food), as well as drinking too much alcohol, may impair the Spleen and Stomach, so that Damp-Heat forms in the Middle Burner. Damp has the characteristics of viscosity, stagnation and downward flow, so when Damp-Heat forms in the Middle Burner it may flow downward to the Large Intestine causing the Qi and Blood there to stagnate, and defecation pain occurs. Also if Damp-Heat persists in the Large Intestine it may injure the collateral, resulting in blood in the stools and defecation pain.

Lack of personal hygiene in the genital and anal area can be another route for Damp-Heat to attack the Large Intestine. Moreover, anal sex may also damage the rectum, resulting in defecation pain.

Deficiency of Spleen-Qi

Spleen-Qi is a key energy in the body, as it keeps the Internal organs in their proper position. A weak constitution, malnutrition, physical exhaustion, irregular eating patterns and prolonged sickness may all weaken the Spleen-Qi, which may result in prolapse of the anus, so that defecation pain follows. Moreover, when the Spleen is weak, its function or transportation will also be weak, so that food stagnates in the Large Intestine, again causing defecation pain.

Stagnation of Blood

Stagnation of Qi, accumulation of Damp-Heat, stagnation of food in the Large Intestine and deficiency of Qi will all impair the circulation of Blood in the Large Intestine. This will lead to Blood stagnation and thus to defecation pain. Prolonged disease, as anusitis, perianal abscess and anal fissures, may also influence the circulation of Blood in the Large Intestine, resulting in its stagnation.

Physical trauma to the anus, or inappropriate operation, may directly damage the channels and the muscles, causing defecation pain due to stagnation of Blood.

Treatment based on differentiation

Differentiation

Differentiation of acute and chronic defecation pain

Occurrence of defecation pain is often related to heat in the Large Intestine or disorder of Qi and Blood.

— Acute cases of defecation pain are often caused by invasion of Wind-Heat or Dryness-Heat, frequently induced or aggravated by consumption of spicy food.
— Chronic defecation pain could be caused by deficiency of Spleen-Qi or stagnation of Blood. Usually these cases are caused by a chronic disease or an inappropriate operation.

Differentiation of character of the pain

— Acute defecation pain with fresh blood in the stool, accompanied by other symptoms such as headache, fever, aversion to cold, or muscle pain, is usually caused by invasion of Wind-Heat. Invasion of Wind-Heat sometimes takes place after eating food such as fish, shrimps, pepper or onions.
— Defecation pain with a burning or pricking sensation, constipation, dry stools, or dry mouth with desire for cold drinks, is often caused by formation of Dryness-Heat in the Large Intestine. This type of defecation pain could be either the acute or chronic type of defecation pain.
— Slight defecation pain with intermittent occurrence, prolapse of the anus, fatigue, a pale complexion, poor appetite, or history of chronic diarrhoea or dysentery, is often caused by deficiency of Spleen-Qi.
— Long-term defecation pain with a stabbing feeling, history of trauma or operation to the large intestine or anus, purplish blood mixed with the stool, diarrhoea or constipation, is usually caused by stagnation of Blood.

Treatment

INVASION OF WIND-HEAT

Symptoms and signs

Acute onset of the pain, which is aggravated by foods such as fish, shrimps, pepper or onions, with fresh blood in the stools, a sore throat, a dry mouth, coughing, abdominal pain with the urge to defecate, dry stools or diarrhoea and an itching sensation in the anus. External symptoms include headache, fever, an aversion to cold and pain in the entire body, a red tongue with a dry yellow coating and a rapid pulse.

Principle of treatment

Dispel Wind-Heat and relieve the pain.

HERBAL TREATMENT

Prescription

DI YU SAN
Sanguisorba Powder
Di Yu *Radix Sanguisorbae* 12 g
Qian Cao *Radix Rubiae* 12 g
Huang Qin *Radix Scutellariae* 9 g
Huang Lian *Rhizoma Coptidis* 9 g
Zhi Zi *Fructus Gardeniae* 9 g
Fu Ling *Poria* 15 g

Explanations

- Di Yu and Qian Cao clear Wind-Heat and stop the bleeding.
- Huang Qin, Huang Lian and Zhi Zi clear Heat and eliminate Toxin from the Large Intestine.
- Fu Ling activates the Spleen and eliminates Damp.

Modifications

1. If there are external symptoms, add Jing Jie *Herba Schizonepetae* 10 g, Fang Feng *Radix Ledebouriellae* 10 g and Su Ye *Folium Perillae* 6 g to dispel Wind, stop the itching and relieve the External symptoms.
2. If there is diarrhoea, add Ge Geng *Radix Puerariae* 10 g and Hua Shi *Talcum* 10 g to eliminate Damp and to relieve the diarrhoea.
3. If there is constipation, add Da Huang *Radix et Rhizoma Rhei* 6 g and Lu Hui *Pasta Aloes* 10 g to eliminate Heat in the Large Intestine and relieve the constipation.
4. If there is a sore throat, add Yin Hua *Flos Lonicerae* 10 g and Pu Gong Ying *Herba Taraxaci* 10 g to clear Wind-Heat in the Upper Burner and relieve the sore throat.

Patent remedy

Ge Gen Qin Lian Pian *Kudzu, Coptis and Scutellaria Tablet*

ACUPUNCTURE TREATMENT

GV-1 Changqiang, BL-25 Dachangshu, BL-36 Chengfu, SP-3 Taibai and ST-37 Shangjuxu. Reducing method is used on these points.

Explanations

- GV-1, the Connecting point of the Governing Vessel and a patent point for anal disorders, harmonises the collateral and relieves defecation pain.
- BL-25, the Back Transporting point of the Large Intestine, clears Wind-Heat in the Large Intestine, promotes its physiological function and relieves defecation pain.
- BL-36 is the patent point for treating disorders of the anus.
- SP-3, the Stream and Source point of the Spleen channel, eliminates Wind-Heat in the Middle Burner and relieves the defecation pain.
- ST-37, the Lower Sea point of the Large Intestine, clears Wind Heat and relieves defecation pain.

Modifications

1. If there is constipation, add ST-25, the Front Collecting point of the Large Intestine, to promote defecation and relieve the constipation.
2. If there is diarrhoea, add SP-9, the Sea point of the Spleen channel, and ST-40, the Connecting point of the Stomach channel, to regulate the Spleen and Stomach and stop the diarrhoea.
3. If there is loss of bright red blood, add SP-10 and BL-57 to stop the bleeding.
4. If there is abdominal pain, add ST-34, the Accumulation point, and ST-36, the Sea point of the Stomach channel, to regulate the circulation of Qi and relieve the pain.

Case history

A 31-year-old woman had been suffering from defecation pain during the past month, which had started with diarrhoea after eating some sea fish. She was diagnosed by the doctor as having acute colitis, for which she was treated with antibiotics. There had been some improvement in her diarrhoea, but the defecation pain persisted. As well as pain when defecating, she had pain in her left lower abdomen, a sore throat, a burning sensation in her anus, thirst, sometimes a fever, dark yellow urine, a red tongue with a thin yellow coating and a rapid pulse.

Diagnosis
Invasion of Wind-Heat in the Large Intestine.

Principle of treatment
Dispel Wind, clear Heat and relieve the pain.

Acupuncture treatment
BL-58, BL-36, LI-4, TE-5, ST-25 and ST-37 were selected. Reducing method was used on these points. She was treated daily.

Explanations

- BL-36 is the patent point for anal disorders.
- BL-58, the Connecting point of the Bladder channel, harmonises the collateral, dispels Wind-Heat and relieves defecation pain.
- LI-4 and TE-5 dispel Wind-Heat and relieve External symptoms.
- ST-25, the Front Collecting point, and ST-37, the Lower Sea point of the Large Intestine, clear Wind-Heat and regulate the Large Intestine in order to relieve defecation pain.

After a week of treatment the pain had stopped. Upon follow-up a year later she reported she had been free of the defecation pain since the last acupuncture treatment.

ACCUMULATION OF DRYNESS-HEAT IN THE LARGE INTESTINE

Symptoms and signs

Defecation pain with a burning or pricking sensation, swelling and redness of the anus, constipation, dry and hard stools, blood in the stools, thirst, a preference for cold drinks, a bitter taste in the mouth, deep yellow urine, a red tongue with a dry and yellow coating and a rapid pulse.

Principle of treatment

Moisten the Large Intestine, clear Heat and relieve the pain.

HERBAL TREATMENT

Prescription

ZENG YE CHENG QI TANG
Increase the Fluids and Order the Qi Decoction
Xuan Shen *Radix Scrophulariae* 15 g
Sheng Di Huang *Radix Rehmanniae Recens* 15 g
Mai Dong *Radix Ophiopogonis* 15 g
Da Huang *Radix et Rhizoma Rhei* 6 g
Mang Xiao *Natrii Sulfas* 10 g

Explanations

- Sheng Di Huang nourishes Yin and clears Dryness-Heat in the Lower Burner.
- Xuan Shen and Mai Dong moisten the Large Intestine and clear Heat.
- Da Huang and Mang Xiao clear Dryness-Heat and promote defecation.

Modifications

1. If there is blood in the stools, add Bai Tou Weng *Radix Pulsatillae* 10 g and Chi Shao *Radix Paeoniae Rubra* 10 g to cool the Blood and to stop the bleeding.
2. If there is a thirst, add Tian Hua Fen *Radix Trichosanthis* 10 g and Lu Gen *Rhizoma Phragmitis* 10 g to promote the formation of Body Fluids and relieve the thirst.
3. If there is a bitter taste in the mouth, add Huang Lian *Rhizoma Coptidis* 5 g and Huang Qin *Radix Scutellariae* 10 g to clear the Heat and relieve the bitter taste.

Patent remedies

Fang Feng Tong Sheng Wan *Ledebouriella Powder that Sagely Unblocks*
Er Zhi Wan *Two-Ultimate Pill*

ACUPUNCTURE TREATMENT

GV-1 Changqiang, BL-25 Dachangshu, BL-58 Feiyang, KI-10 Yingu and SP-6 Sanyinjiao. GV-1, BL-25 and BL-58 are needled with reducing method; KI-10 and SP-6 are needled with reinforcing method.

Explanations

- GV-1 is the Connecting point of the Governing Vessel and the patent point for disorders of the anus. It harmonises the collateral and relieves defecation pain.
- BL-25, the Back Transporting point of the Large Intestine, clears Dry-Heat in the Large Intestine, promotes its physiological function and relieves defecation pain.
- BL-58, the Connecting point of the Bladder channel, harmonises the collateral and relieves defecation pain.
- KI-10, the Sea point of the Kidney channel, and SP-6, the crossing point of the three Yin channels of the foot, nourish the Yin, moisten the Large Intestine and clear Dryness-Heat.

Modifications

1. If there is a thirst, add LU-9 to clear Dryness-Heat and relieve the thirst.
2. If there is anal soreness, add BL-56 and BL-57 to relieve this.
3. If there is constipation, add ST-25 and ST-37 to clear Dryness-Heat in the Large Intestine and promote defecation.
4. If there is blood in the stools, add SP-10 and SP-1 to clear Heat in the Blood and stop the bleeding.

DOWNWARD FLOW OF DAMP-HEAT IN THE LARGE INTESTINE

Symptoms and signs

Defecation pain, a burning sensation in the anus, oozing from the anus with local swelling and redness, an itching and pyogenic anus, constipation, tenesmus, blood in the stools, a red tongue with a sticky and yellow coating and a slippery and rapid pulse.

Principle of treatment

Eliminate Damp, clear Heat and relieve the pain.

HERBAL TREATMENT

Prescription

LONG DAN XIE GAN TANG
Gentiana Draining the Liver Decoction
Long Dan Cao *Radix Gentianae* 6 g
Huang Qin *Radix Scutellariae* 9 g
Zhi Zi *Fructus Gardeniae* 9 g
Ze Xie *Rhizoma Alismatis* 12 g
Mu Tong *Caulis Akebiae* 6 g
Che Qian Zi *Semen Plantaginis* 9 g
Dang Gui *Radix Angelicae Sinensis* 3 g
Sheng Di Huang *Radix Rehmanniae Recens* 9 g
Chai Hu *Radix Bupleuri* 6 g
Gan Cao *Radix Glycyrrhizae* 6 g

Explanations

- Long Dan Cao and Huang Qin clear Heat and dry Damp.
- Zhi Zi, Mu Tong, Ze Xie and Che Qian Zi clear Heat and promote urination in order to eliminate Damp.
- Dang Gui and Sheng Di Huang nourish the Yin and Blood.
- Chai Hu regulates the Liver-Qi and removes Qi stagnation.
- Gan Cao harmonises the actions of the other herbs in the formula.

Modifications

1. If there is swelling and redness of the anus, add Huang Bai *Cortex Phellodendri* 6 g, Ku Shen *Radix Sophorae Flavescentis* 10 g and Tu Fu Ling *Rhizoma Smilacis Glabrae* 15 g to eliminate Damp-Heat and relieve the local symptoms.
2. If there is constipation, add Da Huang *Radix et Rhizoma Rhei* 6 g and Mang Xiao *Natrii Sulfas* 10 g to eliminate Heat, promote defecation and relieve the constipation.
3. If there is itching in the anus, add Ku Shen *Radix Sophorae Flavescentis* 10 g and She Chuang Zi *Fructus Cnidii* 10 g to clear Heat, remove Damp and relieve the itching.

Patent remedies

Long Dan Xie Gan Wan *Gentiana Draining the Liver Pill*
Huang Lian Su Pian *Coptis Extract Tablet*

ACUPUNCTURE TREATMENT

GV-1 Changqiang, BL-25 Dachangshu, BL-58 Feiyang, SP-9 Yinlingquan, ST-37 Shangjuxu and ST-40 Fenglong. Reducing method is used on these points.

Explanations

- GV-1, the Connecting point of the Governing Vessel and the patent point for disorders of the anus, harmonises the collateral and relieves defecation pain.
- BL-25, the Back Transporting point of the Large Intestine, clears Dryness-Heat in the Large Intestine, promotes its physiological function and relieves defecation pain.
- BL-58, the Connecting point of the Bladder channel, harmonises the collateral and relieves defecation pain.
- SP-9, the Sea point of the Spleen channel, ST-37, the Lower Sea point of the Large Intestine, and ST-40, the Connecting point of the Stomach channel, activate the Spleen and Stomach, eliminate Damp, promote defecation and relieve the pain.

Modifications

1. If there is itching of the anus, add BL-57 and KI-2 to clear Damp-Heat in the Large Intestine and relieve the itching.
2. If there is redness and swelling of the anus, add SP-6 and BL-32 to clear Damp-Heat in the Large Intestine and reduce the swelling.
3. If there is constipation, add ST-25 to promote defecation and to clear Damp-Heat.
4. If there is anal blood loss, add LI-11 and SP-10 to clear Damp-Heat and to stop the bleeding.

Case history

A 47-year-old man had been suffering from defecation pain for about 10 days. Two years previously he had been diagnosed with haemorrhoids and anal fissure, and in the interim he had been working in an office, sitting down all day. Eating pungent food resulted in blood in his stools and defecation pain. He also had constipation, an oozing and itching anus, dark yellow urine, a red tongue with a sticky, yellow and greasy coating and a wiry, slippery and rapid pulse.

Diagnosis
Accumulation of Damp-Heat in the Large Intestine.

Principle of treatment
Eliminate Damp-Heat and relieve the pain.

Herbal treatment
LONG DAN XIE GAN TANG
Gentiana Draining the Liver Decoction
Long Dan Cao *Radix Gentianae* 6 g
Huang Qin *Radix Scutellariae* 9 g
Zhi Zi *Fructus Gardeniae* 9 g
Ze Xie *Rhizoma Alismatis* 12 g

Mu Tong *Caulis Akebiae* 6 g
Che Qian Zi *Semen Plantaginis* 9 g
Dang Gui *Radix Angelicae Sinensis* 3 g
Sheng Di Huang *Radix Rehmanniae Recens* 20 g
Ku Shen *Radix Sophorae Flavescentis* 10 g
Huang Bai *Cortex Phellodendri* 10 g
Tu Fu Ling *Rhizoma Smilacis Glabrae* 15 g
Gan Cao *Radix Glycyrrhizae* 6 g

Explanations

- Long Dan Cao and Huang Qin clear Heat and dry Damp.
- Zhi Zi, Mu Tong, Ze Xie and Che Qian Zi clear Heat and promote urination in order to eliminate Damp.
- Dang Gui and Sheng Di Huang nourish the Yin and Blood.
- Chai Hu regulates the Liver-Qi and removes Qi stagnation.
- Ku Shen, Tu Fu Ling and Huang Bai eliminate Damp-Heat and relieve the pain.
- Gan Cao harmonises the actions of the other herbs in the formula.

After using the herbs for 2 weeks, his defecation pain was relieved. Upon follow-up 2 years later he reported being free of the pain since then.

DEFICIENCY OF SPLEEN-QI

Symptoms and signs

A history of chronic diarrhoea or dysentery, slight defecation pain, sometimes blood in the stools, prolapse of the anus, a bearing-down sensation in the abdomen and anus, lassitude, a pale complexion, a poor appetite, palpitations, a pale tongue with a white coating and a feeble pulse.

Principle of treatment

Tonify Spleen-Qi and relieve the pain.

HERBAL TREATMENT

Prescription

BU ZHONG YI QI TANG
Tonifying the Middle and Benefiting Qi Decoction
Huang Qi *Radix Astragali seu Hedysari* 20 g
Gan Cao *Radix Glycyrrhizae* 5 g
Ren Shen *Radix Ginseng* 10 g
Dang Gui *Radix Angelicae Sinensis* 10 g
Ju Pi *Pericarpium Citri Reticulatae* 6 g
Sheng Ma *Rhizoma Cimicifugae* 3 g
Chai Hu *Radix Bupleuri* 3 g
Bai Zhu *Rhizoma Atractylodis Macrocephalae* 10 g

Explanations

- Ren Shen, Huang Qi, Bai Zhu and Gan Cao strengthen the Spleen and tonify the Qi of the Spleen and Stomach.
- Sheng Ma and Chai Hu raise the Yang-Qi.
- Dang Gui aids Chai Hu to regulate the Qi and Blood of the Liver.
- Ju Pi promotes the Qi and strengthens the Spleen and Stomach.

Modifications

1. If there is blood in the stools, add Bai Ji *Rhizoma Bletillae* 10 g and San Qi *Radix Notoginseng* 10 g to stop the bleeding.
2. If there is prolapse of the anus, add Qing Pi *Pericarpium Citri Reticulatae Viride* 10 g and Zhi Qiao *Fructus Aurantii* 10 g to regulate the circulation of Qi and lift up the anus.
3. If there are palpitations, add Suan Zao Ren *Semen Ziziphi Spinosae* 10 g and Bai Zhi Ren *Semen Biotae* 10 g to tonify the Blood and to calm the Mind.
4. If the appetite is poor, add Sha Ren *Fructus Amomi* 6 g and Mu Xiang *Radix Aucklandiae* 10 g to promote the Spleen-Qi in order to improve the appetite.

Patent remedy

Bu Zhong Yi Qi Wan *Tonifying the Middle and Benefiting Qi Pill*

ACUPUNCTURE TREATMENT

GV-20 Baihui, CV-12 Zhongwan, CV-4 Guanyuan, BL-20 Pishu and BL-23 Shenshu. Reinforcing method is used on these points. Moxibustion treatment is recommended.

Explanations

- GV-20 is the crossing point of the Governing Vessel and the Bladder channel. It can promote the function of the Yang-Qi and lift the Internal organs.
- BL-20 is the Back Transporting point of the Spleen and Bl-23 is the Back Transporting point of the Kidney. These two points in combination tonify the Qi of the Spleen and Kidney.
- CV-12 is the Front Collecting point of the Stomach, the Gathering point for the Fu organs, and the crossing point of the Directing Vessel with the three Yang channels of the hand. CV-4 is the

crossing point of the Directing Vessel with the three Yin channels of the foot. These two points in combination tonify the Spleen-Qi, regulate the Fu organs and strengthen the body.

Modifications

1. If the appetite is poor, add ST-36 and SP-3 to tonify the Spleen-Qi and improve the appetite.
2. If there are palpitations, add PC-6 and SP-6 to tonify the Yin and Blood and calm the Mind.
3. If there is anal prolapse, add CV-8 (moxibustion treatment) and ST-25 to tonify and raise the Yang-Qi.
4. If there is chronic diarrhoea, warm GV-4 with moxa to warm the Spleen and the Kidney in order to stop the diarrhoea.

Case history

A 62-year-old man had been suffering from chronic colitis for 30 years. He said that eating greasy foods or getting cold would result in defecation pain and loose stools. In combination with this, severe diarrhoea with anal prolapse occasionally occurred. He often felt cold and had a pale complexion, cold limbs, a poor appetite, lassitude, palpitations, lower back pain and low sexual potency. His tongue looked pale and his pulse was deep and weak.

Diagnosis
Deficiency of Yang of Spleen and Kidney.

Principle of treatment
Tonify the Spleen-Qi and warm the Yang of the Spleen and Kidney.

Acupuncture treatment
GV-4, BL-20, BL-23, BL-25, ST-25 and CV-12 were needled with reinforcing method. Moxibustion was applied on CV-8. Treatment was given every other day. Besides the patent medicine Bu Zhong Yi Qi Wan *Tonifying the Middle and Benefiting Qi Pill* was prescribed 6 g 3 times per day.

Explanations
- GV-4 is used to tonify the Qi and Blood in order to treat the diarrhoea combined with the prolapse of the anus. BL-20 is the Back Transporting point of the Spleen and BL-23 is the Back Transporting point of the Kidney. These two points in combination tonify the Qi and Blood and activate the Spleen and Kidney.
- BL-25, the Back Transporting point of the Large Intestine, and ST-25, the Front Collecting point of the Large Intestine, regulate the Large Intestine and relieve defecation pain.
- CV-12, the Front Collecting point of the Stomach, tonifies the Stomach-Qi.
- CV-8 with moxa the warms and tonifies the Spleen-Qi.

- Moxibustion can promote the function of the Yang-Qi, dispel Cold and support the Internal organs.

After 3 months of treatment, his anal prolapse and defecation pain were under control. Upon follow-up 2 years later he reported complete recovery after the treatment.

STAGNATION OF BLOOD

Symptoms and signs

A long history of anal inflammation, trauma or operation in the area of the anus, defecation pain with a fixed location, stabbing pain, swelling and redness of the anus, bleeding during defecation, constipation, restlessness, thirst, a purplish tongue with thin coating and a wiry pulse.

Principle of treatment

Circulate Qi and Blood, clear Heat and remove Blood stasis to sedate the pain.

HERBAL TREATMENT

Prescription

TAO HONG SI WU TANG
Four-Substance Decoction with Safflower and Peach Pit
Dang Gui *Radix Angelicae Sinensis* 10 g
Sheng Di Huang *Radix Rehmanniae Recens* 12 g
Chi Shao *Radix Paeoniae Rubra* 10 g
Chuan Xiong *Rhizoma Ligustici Chuanxiong* 6 g
Tao Ren *Semen Persicae* 10 g
Hong Hua *Flos Carthami* 10 g

Explanations

- Sheng Di Huang and and Chi Shao nourish the Yin and clear Heat in the Large Intestine.
- Chuan Xiong and Hong Hua promote the circulation of Blood and remove its stagnation.
- Dang Gui and Tao Ren regulate the circulation of Blood and remove its stasis. These two herbs can also lubricate the Large Intestine in order to promote defecation.

Modifications

1. If there is bleeding on defecation, add Di Yu *Radix Sanguisorbae* 10 g and Huai Hua *Flos Sophorae* 10 g to cool the Blood and stop the bleeding.
2. If there is swelling and redness of the anus, use a lotion made from Ku Shen *Radix Sophorae*

Flavescentis 10 g and Dang Gui *Radix Angelicae Sinensis* 10 g to wash the anus in order to relieve the swelling and redness.

3. If there is constipation, add Da Huang *Radix et Rhizoma Rhei* 6 g and Mang Xiao *Natrii Sulfas* 10 g to relieve the constipation

4. If there is restlessness, add Long Dan Cao *Radix Gentianae* 5 g and Dan Shen *Radix Salviae Miltiorrhizae* 10 g to clear Heat and to calm the Mind.

Patent remedy

Qiang Li Hua Zhi Ling *Better Strength Dissolve-Haemorrhoids Efficacious Cure*

ACUPUNCTURE TREATMENT

GV-1 Changqiang, BL-17 Geshu, BL-36 Chengfu, ST-37 Shangjuxu and SP-4 Gongsun. Even method is used on these points.

Explanations

- GV-1, the Connecting point of the Governing Vessel, harmonises the collateral, regulates the circulation of Qi and relieves defecation pain.

- BL-17, the Gathering point for the Blood, promotes the circulation of Blood, removes its stagnation and relieves defecation pain.

- SP-4, the Connecting point of the Spleen channel and the point that connects with the Penetrating Vessel, promotes the circulation of Qi in the Large Intestine and relieves defecation pain.

- BL-36 is the patent point for treating anal disease.

- ST-37, the Lower Sea point of the Large Intestine, promotes defecation, regulates the circulation of Qi in the Large Intestine and relieves defecation pain.

Modifications

1. If there is bleeding on defecation, add BL-57 and SP-10 to relieve the pain and stop the bleeding.

2. If there is a sharp pain around the anus, add LU-6, the Accumulation point of the Lung channel, and LI-4, the Source point of the Large Intestine channel, to promote the circulation of Blood, remove its stagnation and relieve the pain.

3. If there is swelling of the anus, add BL-32 and BL-36 to regulate the circulation of Blood and reduce the swelling.

4. If there is constipation, add ST-25, the Front Collecting point of the Large Intestine, and ST-40, the Connecting point of the Stomach channel, to regulate the Qi circulating in the Large Intestine, promote defecation and relieve the constipation.

References and bibliography 参考书目

References

参
考
书
目

Antkiewicz-Michaluk L, Romanska I, Michaluk J 1991 Role of calcium channels in effects of antidepressant drugs on responsiveness to pain. Psychopharmacology (Berlin) 105(2):269–274

Ardid D, Guilbaud G 1992 Antinociceptive effects of acute and 'chronic' injections of tricyclic antidepressant drugs in a new model of mononeuropathy in rats. Pain 49(2):279–287

Ardid D, Marty H, Fialip J, Privat A M, Eschalier A, Lavarenne J 1992 Comparative effects of different uptake inhibitor antidepressants in two pain tests in mice. Fundamentals of Clinical Pharmacology 6(2):75–82

Bank J 1994 A comparative study of amitriptyline and fluvoxamine in migraine prophylaxis. Headache 34(8):476–478

Becker R O, Selden G 1985 The body electric: electromagnetism and the foundation of life. William Morrow, New York

Chao Yuanfang 1955 (first published in AD 611) General treatise on the causes and symptoms of diseases (Zhu Bing Yuan Hou Lun). People's Health Publishing, Beijing, p. 105

Chen Shigong 1997 Orthodox manual of external diseases (Wai Ke Zheng Zong). Collection of Famous Books on TCM Surgery and Traumatology. Huaxia Press, Beijing, p. 435

Chinese Academy of Traditional Chinese Medicine 1976 Reference of Research on Traditional Chinese Medicine 2:25

Chinese Academy of Traditional Chinese Medicine 1977 Journal of New Medicine 2(3):27

Chinese Academy of Traditional Chinese Medicine 1978 Acupuncture Anaesthesia 1:65

Danysz W, Minor B G, Post C, Archer T 1986 Chronic treatment with antidepressant drugs and the analgesia induced by 5-methoxy-N, N-dimethyltryptamine: attenuation by desipramine. Acta Pharmacologica Toxicologia (Copenhagen) 59(2):103–112

Fujian Provincial Research Institute for Traditional Chinese Medicine 1979 Abstracts of Proceedings of National Conference on Acupuncture and Acupuncture Anaesthesia 1:221

Ge Zi et al 1983 Chinese Acupuncture 3(3):20–22

Han Jisheng 1978 Chinese Science (5):579

Han Jisheng et al 1979 Abstracts of Proceedings of National Conference on Acupuncture and Acupuncture Anaesthesia 2:115

Huo Tuo 1985 (first published c. AD 180) The classic of the secret transmission (Zhong Cang Jing). Jiansu Scientific Publishing, Jiansu

Jin Guozhang et al 1979 Abstracts of Proceedings of National Conference on Acupuncture and Acupuncture Anaesthesia 2:90

Lei Yongzhong 1982 Clinical analysis of 184 cases with oesophagus carcinoma treated by traditional Chinese herbs. Liaoning Journal of Traditional Chinese Medicine (5):25

Li Baojiao 1981 Fujian Journal of Traditional Chinese Medicine 1(1):24

Lin Guochu et al 1984 Acupuncture anaesthesia for stomatological and facial surgery. In: Weng Enqi et al (eds) Acupuncture anaesthesia (Zhen Jiu Ma Zhui). Shanghai Science and Technology Publishing, Shanghai, p. 126

Ling Shu 1963 Discussion on nine needles (Ling Shu Jing). People's Health Publishing, Beijing, p. 145

Ling Shu 1963 Five changes (Ling Shu Jing). People's Health Publishing, Beijing, p. 89

Ling Shu 1963 Five changes (Ling Shu Jing). People's Health Publishing, Beijing pp. 23, 27, 69

Liu Hengrui 1998 Discussion on pain. Three medical book, volume 2. Experience on various kinds of diseases. China Press of Traditional Chinese Medicine, p. 141

Liu Jiaxiang 1981 Observation of therapeutic results on large intestinal carcinoma treated by TCM. Journal Of Traditional Chinese Medicine 12:33

Lu Guowe et al 1979 Abstracts of Proceedings of National Conference on Acupuncture and Acupuncture Anaesthesia 1:160

Nanjing College of Traditional Chinese Medicine 1979 (first published c. AD 198) An explanation of the classic of difficulties (Nan Jing Jiao Shi). People's Health Publishing, Beijing, p. 151

Qi Kun 1997 (first published in 1965) A complete book of external diseases (Wai Ke Da Cheng). Collection of Famous Books on TCM Surgery and Traumatology. Huaxia Press, Beijing, p. 565

Qiu Maoliang et al 1989 Science of acupuncture (Zhen Jiu Xue). Shanghai Science and Technology Publishing, Shanghai, pp. 321–322

Ren Zhai Zhi Zhi 1982 Discussion on attached formulas. (Ren Zhai Zhi Zhi Fu Yi Fang Lun), volume 22. Xin Wen Feng Press, Taiwan, p. 883

Shanghai No 1 People's Hospital 1977 Chinese Journal of Surgery 1:19

Wang Qingren 1991 (first published in 1830) Correction on the errors of medical works (Yi Lin Gai Cuo). People's Health Publishing, Beijing

Wu Jianping et al 1979 Abstracts of Proceedings from National Conference on Acupuncture and Acupuncture Anaesthesia 2:43

Ye Qiang et al 1984 Acupuncture anaesthesia for gastrectomy. In: Weng Enqi et al (eds) Acupuncture anaesthesia. (Zhen Jiu Ma Zhui). Shanghai Science and Technology Publishing, Shanghai, p. 159

Yellow Emperor's classic of internal medicine: simple questions (Huang Di Nei Jing Su Wen) 1956 (first published c. 100 BC). People's Health Publishing, Beijing, pp.17, 62, 80–81, 190

Yi Qingchen et al 1978 Chinese Science 29(1):83

Yu Chang 1999 Principle of Prohibition of Medical Profession (Yi Men Fa Lu). Collection of Chinese Medical Books, volume 27. China Press of Ancient Books, p. 34

Zhang Jingyue 1991 (first published in 1624) Complete Works (Jing Yue Quan Shu). People's Health Publishing, Beijing, p. 479

Zhu Dinger 1980 Chinese Journal of Medicine 60(8):460–463

Zhuang Xinliang 1984 Acupuncture anaesthesia for neck surgery. In: Weng Enqi et al (eds) Acupuncture anaesthesia (Zhen Jiu Ma Zhui). Shanghai Science and Technology Publishing, Shanghai, p. 135

Bibliography

参考书目

Ancient classics

Chen Shou 1959 (written in the Jin Dynasty) Monograph on three states (San Guo Zhi), China Publishing, Beijing.

Guo Aichun 1989 An explanation of revision for canon of medicine (Huang Di Nei Jing Ling Shu Jiao Zhu Yu Yi). Tianjin Science and Technology Publishing, Tianjin

Li Dongyuan 1976 (first published in the 13th century) Discussion on stomach and spleen (Pi Wei Lun). People's Health Publishing, Beijing

Nanjing College of Traditional Chinese Medicine 1960 (first published c. AD 198) An explanation of the Classic of difficulties (Nan Jing Yi Shi). Shanghai Science and Technology Publishing, Shanghai

Shangdong College of TCM 1979 An explanation of the ABC of acupuncture (Zhen Jiu Jia Yi Jing Jiao Yi). People's Health Publishing, Beijing

Shi Maqian 1959 (written in the Han Dynasty) Monograph on history—biography on Bian Que (Shi Ji Bian Que Cang Gong Lie Zhuan). China Publishing, Beijing

Wang Qingren 1991 (first published in 1830) Correction on the errors of medical works (Yi Lin Gai Cuo). People's Health Publishing, Beijing

Yang Jizhou 1960 (first published in 1624) 1980 Compendium of acupuncture (Zhen Jiu Da Chen). People's Health Publishing, Beijing

Yellow Emperor's classic of internal medicine: Simple questions (Huang Di Nei Jing Su Wen). People's Health Publishing, Beijing 1963 (written in BC 475–221, first published c. 100 BC)

Yu Chang 1983 (first published in 1658) Principle and prohibition for medical profession (Yi Men Fa Lu). Shanghai Science and Technology Publishing, Shanghai

Zhang Jingyue 1984 (first published in 1624) The complete book of Jing Yue (Jing Yue Quan Shu) Shanghai Science and Technology Publishing, Shanghai

Zhu Danxi 1986 (first published in 1481) Essential methods of Dan Xi (Dan Xi Xin Fa). China Beijing Bookstore Publishing, Beijing

---

English language texts

Bensky D, Gamble A, Kaptchuck T 1986 Chinese herbal medicine: materia medica. Eastland, Seattle

Bensky D, Barolet R 1990 Formulas and strategies. Eastland, Seattle

Chen Song Yu, Li Fei 1993 A clinical guide to Chinese herbs and formulae. Churchill Livingstone, New York

Ellis A et al 1988 Fundamentals of Chinese acupuncture. Paradigm, USA

Frakin J 1986 Chinese herbal patent formulas. Institute for Traditional Medicine, Portland, Oregon; Shya Publications, Boulder, CO

Frank D 1995 Low back pain. Blue Poppy Press, USA

Geng Junying et al 1991 Herbal formulas. New World Press, Beijing

Geng Junying et al 1995 Selecting the right acupoints—a handbook on acupuncture therapy. New World Press, Beijing

Li Zhulan, Xuan Jiasheng et al 1990 Gynecology—the English Chinese encyclopedia of practical traditional Chinese medicine—Fu Ke Xue—Ying Han Shi Yong Zhong Yi Yao Da Quan. Higher Education Press, Beijing

Maciocia G 1994 The practice of Chinese medicine. Churchill Livingstone, New York

Vangemeersch L, Sun Peilin 1994 Bi-syndrome or rheumatic disorders. Satas, Belgium

Wiseman N, Bass K 1990 Glossary of Chinese medical terms and acupuncture points. Paradigm, Brookline, MA

Modern texts

Beijing College of TCM 1975 Science of normal human being (Zheng Chang Ren Ti Xue). People's Publishing, Beijing

Chen Kezheng 1993 Essential experiences of ancient and modern acupuncture (Gu Jin Zhen Jiu Zhi Yan Jing Hua). China Press of Traditional Chinese Medicine, Beijing

Guangdong College of TCM 1975 Surgery and traumatology (Wai Shang Ke Xue). Shanghai People's Publishing, Shanghai

Guo Guangwen et al 1986 Color pictures of human anatomy (Ren Ti Jie Pou Cai Se Tu Pu). People's Publishing, Beijing

Han Jisheng 1987 Neurochemical mechanism of pain control by acupuncture analgesia (Zhen Jiu Zheng Tong De Sheng Jing Hua Xue Yuan Li). China Medicine, Science and Technology Publishing, Beijing

He Puren 1990 Treatment of pain with acupuncture and moxibustion (Zhen Jiu Zhi Tong). Science and Technology Literature Publishing, Beijing

Hu Ximing et al 1991 Clinical guide of acupuncture and moxibustion (Zhen Jiu Ling Chuan Zhi Na). People's Publishing, Beijing

Li Jingwei et al 1995 Dictionary of traditional Chinese medicine (Zhong Yi Da Ci Dian). People's Health Publishing, Beijing

Li Qingye 1989 Chinese herbal formulas (Fang Ji Xue). Chinese Medical Science and Technology Publishing, Beijing

Ling Yikui et al 1984 Chinese materia medica (Zhong Yao Xue). Science and Technology Publishing, Shanghai

Peng Rongchen 1994 Dictionary of acupuncture formulas (Zhen Jiu Chu Fang Da Ci Dian). Beijing Publishing, Beijing

Qiu Maoliang et al 1989 Science of acupuncture (Zhen Jiu Xue). Shanghai Science and Technology Publishing, Shanghai

Selection of old TCM doctor's experience (Beijing Shi Lao Zhong Yi Jing Yan Xuan Bian). 1982 Beijing Publishing, Beijing

Shangdong Medical College 1980 Science of diagnosis (Zhen Duan Xue). People's Health Publishing, Beijing

Shanghai University of Medicine 1993 (first publication 1952) Practical internal medicine (Shi Yong Nei Ke Xue). People's Health Publishing, Beijing

Shi Xuemin et al 1998 Therapeutics of acupuncture and moxibustion (Zhen Jiu Zhi Liao Xue). Shanghai Science and Technology Publishing, Shanghai

Su Chenglian et al 1993 Pain syndrome treated by traditional Chinese medicine (Zhong Yi Tong Zheng Da Cheng). Fujian Science and Technology Publishing, Fuzhou

Wang Dai et al 1990 Prescriptions of acupuncture and moxibustion (Zhen Jiu Chu Fang Xue). Beijing Publishing, Beijing

Wang Yongyan et al 1997 Internal medicine of traditional Chinese medicine (Zhong Yi Nei Ke Xue). Shanghai Science and Technology Publishing, Shanghai

Wang Yuyi 1992 Traumatic disease treated with acupuncture (Shang Ke Zhen Jiu Zhi Liao Xue). Sichuan Science and Technology Publishing, Sichuan

Xu Jiqun et al 1985 Chinese herbal formulas (Fang Ji Xue). Shanghai Science and Technology Publishing, Shanghai

Yang Changshen 1988 The therapy of acupuncture and moxibustion (Zhen Jiu Zhi Liao Xue). Science and Technology Publishing, Shanghai

Yang Jiasan et al 1884 Acupuncture points (Shu Xue Xue). Shanghai Science and Technology Publishing, Shanghai

Zhang Boyu et al 1985 Internal medicine of traditional Chinese medicine (Zhong Yi Nei Ke Xue). Shanghai Science and Technology Publishing, Shanghai

Zhang Xiaoping 1983 Study on mechanism of acupuncture function (Zhen Jiu Zuo Yong Ji Li Yan Jiu). Anhui Science and Technology Publishing, Anhui

Zhongshan Medical College 1978 Pathology (Bing Li Xue). People's Health Publishing, Beijing

Appendix

List of the main channels and acupuncture points

Lung channel of the hand

LU-1   Zhongfu
LU-2   Yunmen
LU-3   Tianfu
LU-4   Xiabai
LU-5   Chize
LU-6   Kongzui
LU-7   Lieque
LU-8   Jingqu
LU-9   Taiyuan
LU-10   Yuji
LU-11   Shaoshang

Large Intestine channel

LI-1   Shangyang
LI-2   Erjian
LI-3   Sanjian
LI-4   Hegu
LI-5   Yangxi
LI-6   Pianli
LI-7   Wenliu
LI-8   Xialian
LI-9   Shanglian
LI-10   Shousanli
LI-11   Quchi
LI-12   Zhouliao
LI-13   Shouwuli
LI-14   Binao
LI-15   Jianyu
LI-16   Jugu
LI-17   Tianding
LI-18   Futu
LI-19   Kouheliao
LI-20   Yingxiang

Stomach channel of the foot

ST-1   Chengqi
ST-2   Sibai
ST-3   Juliao
ST-4   Dicang
ST-5   Daying
ST-6   Jiache
ST-7   Xiaguan
ST-8   Touwei
ST-9   Renying
ST-10 Shuitu
ST-11 Qishe
ST-12 Quepen
ST-13 Qihu
ST-14 Kufang
ST-15 Wuyi
ST-16 Yingchuang
ST-17 Ruzhong
ST-18 Rugen
ST-19 Burong
ST-20 Chengman
ST-21 Liangmen
ST-22 Guanmen
ST-23 Taiyi
ST-24 Huaroumen
ST-25 Tianshu
ST-26 Wailing
ST-27 Daju
ST-28 Shuidao
ST-29 Guilai
ST-30 Qichong

ST-31   Biguan
ST-32   Futu
ST-33   Yinshi
ST-34   Liangqiu
ST-35   Dubi
ST-36   Zusanli
ST-37   Shangjuxu
ST-38   Tiaokou
ST-39   Xiajuxu
ST-40   Fenglong
ST-41   Jiexi
ST-42   Chongyang
ST-43   Xiangu
ST-44   Neiting
ST-45   Lidui

Spleen channel of the foot

SP-1   Yinbai
SP-2   Dadu
SP-3   Taibai
SP-4   Gongsun
SP-5   Shangqiu
SP-6   Sanyinjiao
SP-7   Lougu
SP-8   Diji
SP-9   Yinlingquan
SP-10   Xuehai
SP-11   Jimen
SP-12   Chongmen
SP-13   Fushe
SP-14   Fujie
SP-15   Daheng
SP-16   Fuai
SP-17   Shidou
SP-18   Tianxi
SP-19   Xiongxiang
SP-20   Zhourong
SP-21   Dabao

Heart channel of the hand

HT-1   Jiquan
HT-2   Qingling
HT-3   Shaohai
HT-4   Lingdao
HT-5   Tongli
HT-6   Yinxi
HT-7   Shenmen
HT-8   Shaofu
HT-9   Shaochong

Small Intestine channel of the hand

SI-1   Shaoze
SI-2   Qiangu
SI-3   Houxi
SI-4   Wangu
SI-5   Yanggu
SI-6   Yanglao
SI-7   Zhizheng
SI-8   Xiaohai
SI-9   Jianzhen
SI-10   Naoshu
SI-11   Tianzong
SI-12   Bingfeng
SI-13   Quyuan
SI-14   Jianwaishu
SI-15   Jianzhongshu
SI-16   Tianchuang
SI-17   Tianrong
SI-18   Quanliao
SI-19   Tinggong

Bladder channel of the foot

BL-1   Jingming
BL-2   Zanzhu
BL-3   Meichong
BL-4   Quchai
BL-5   Wuchu
BL-6   Chengguang
BL-7   Tongtian
BL-8   Luoque
BL-9   Yuzhen
BL-10   Tianzhu
BL-11   Dashu
BL-12   Fengmen
BL-13   Feishu
BL-14   Jueyinshu
BL-15   Xinshu
BL-16   Dushu
BL-17   Geshu
BL-18   Ganshu
BL-19   Danshu
BL-20   Pishu
BL-21   Weishu
BL-22   Sanjiaoshu
BL-23   Shenshu
BL-24   Qihaishu
BL-25   Dachangshu
BL-26   Guanyuanshu
BL-27   Xiaochangshu
BL-28   Pangguangshu

BL-29	Zhonglushu
BL-30	Baihuanshu
BL-31	Shangliao
BL-32	Ciliao
BL-33	Zhongliao
BL-34	Xialiao
BL-35	Huiyang
BL-36	Chengfu
BL-37	Yinmen
BL-38	Fuxi
BL-39	Weiyang
BL-40	Weizhong
BL-41	Fufen
BL-42	Pohu
BL-43	Gaohuang
BL-44	Shentang
BL-45	Yixi
BL-46	Geguan
BL-47	Hunmen
BL-48	Yanggang
BL-49	Yishe
BL-50	Weicang
BL-51	Huangmen
BL-52	Zhishi
BL-53	Baohuang
BL-54	Zhibian
BL-55	Heyang
BL-56	Chengjin
BL-57	Chengshan
BL-58	Feiyang
BL-59	Fuyang
BL-60	Kunlun
BL-61	Pushen (*Pucan*)
BL-62	Shenmai
BL-63	Jinmen
BL-64	Jinggu
BL-65	Shugu
BL-66	Zutonggu
BL-67	Zhiyin

Kidney channel of the foot

KI-1	Yongquan
KI-2	Rangu
KI-3	Taixi
KI-4	Dazhong
KI-5	Shuiquan
KI-6	Zhaohai
KI-7	Fuliu
KI-8	Jiaoxin
KI-9	Zhubin
KI-10	Yingu
KI-11	Henggu
KI-12	Dahe
KI-13	Qixue
KI-14	Siman
KI-15	Zhongzhu
KI-16	Huangshu
KI-17	Shangqu
KI-18	Shiguan
KI-19	Yindu
KI-20	Futonggu
KI-21	Youmen
KI-22	Bulang
KI-23	Shenfeng
KI-24	Lingxu
KI-25	Shencang
KI-26	Yuzhong
KI-27	Shufu

Pericardium channel of the hand

PC-1	Tianchi
PC-2	Tianquan
PC-3	Quze
PC-4	Ximen
PC-5	Jianshi
PC-6	Neiguan
PC-7	Daling
PC-8	Laogong
PC-9	Zhongchong

Triple Burner (Energiser) channel of the hand

TE-1	Guanchong
TE-2	Yemen
TE-3	Zhongzhu
TE-4	Yangchi
TE-5	Waiguan
TE-6	Zhigou
TE-7	Huizong
TE-8	Sanyangluo
TE-9	Sidu
TE-10	Tianjing
TE-11	Qinglengyuan
TE-12	Xiaoluo
TE-13	Naohui
TE-14	Jianliao
TE-15	Tianliao
TE-16	Tianyou
TE-17	Yifeng
TE-18	Chimai (*Qimai*)
TE-19	Luxi

TE-20 Jiaosun
TE-21 Ermen
TE-22 Heliao
TE-23 Sizhukong

Gall Bladder channel of the foot

GB-1 Tongziliao
GB-2 Tinghui
GB-3 Shangguan
GB-4 Hanyan
GB-5 Xuanlu
GB-6 Xuanli
GB-7 Qubin
GB-8 Shuaigu
GB-9 Tianchong
GB-10 Fubai
GB-11 Qiaoyin
GB-12 Wangu
GB-13 Benshen
GB-14 Yangbai
GB-15 Toulinqi
GB-16 Muchuang
GB-17 Zhengying
GB-18 Chengling
GB-19 Naokong
GB-20 Fengchi
GB-21 Jianjing
GB-22 Yuanye
GB-23 Zhejin
GB-24 Riyue
GB-25 Jingmen
GB-26 Daimai
GB-27 Wushu
GB-28 Weidao
GB-29 Juliao
GB-30 Huantiao
GB-31 Fengshi
GB-32 Zhongdu
GB-33 Xiyangguan
GB-34 Yanglingquan
GB-35 Yangjiao
GB-36 Waiqiu
GB-37 Guangming
GB-38 Yangfu
GB-39 Xuanzhong
GB-40 Qiuxu
GB-41 Zulinqi
GB-42 Diwuhui
GB-43 Xiaxi
GB-44 Zuqiaoyin

Liver channel of the foot

LR-1 Dadun
LR-2 Xingjian
LR-3 Taichong
LR-4 Zhongfeng
LR-5 Ligou
LR-6 Zhongdu
LR-7 Xiguan
LR-8 Ququan
LR-9 Yinbao
LR-10 Zuwuli
LR-11 Yinlian
LR-12 Jimai
LR-13 Zhangmen
LR-14 Qimen

Governing Vessel

GV-1 Changqiang
GV-2 Yaoshu
GV-3 Yaoyangguan
GV-4 Mingmen
GV-5 Xuanshu
GV-6 Jizhong
GV-7 Zhongshu
GV-8 Jinsuo
GV-9 Zhiyang
GV-10 Lingtai
GV-11 Shendao
GV-12 Shenzhu
GV-13 Taodao
GV-14 Dazhui
GV-15 Yamen
GV-16 Fengfu
GV-17 Naohu
GV-18 Qiangjian
GV-19 Houding
GV-20 Baihui
GV-21 Qianding
GV-22 Xinhui
GV-23 Shangxing
GV-24 Shenting
GV-25 Suliao
GV-29 Renzhong (*Shuigou*)
GV-27 Duiduan
GV-28 Yinjiao

Directing (Conception) Vessel

CV-1	Huiyin
CV-2	Qugu
CV-3	Zhongji
CV-4	Guanyuan
CV-5	Shimen
CV-6	Qihai
CV-7	Yinjiao
CV-8	Shenque
CV-9	Shuifen
CV-10	Xiawan
CV-11	Jianli
CV-12	Zhongwan
CV-13	Shangwan
CV-14	Juque
CV-15	Jiuwei
CV-16	Zhongting
CV-17	Tanzhong
CV-18	Yutang
CV-19	Zigong
CV-20	Huagai
CV-21	Xuanji
CV-22	Tiantu
CV-23	Lianquan
CV-24	Chengjiang

Index